Pediatric Surgery

Prem Puri · Michael Höllwarth

Editors

Pediatric Surgery

Diagnosis and Management

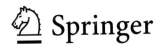 Springer

Editors

Prof. Prem Puri, MS FRCS FRCS (Ed)
  FACS FAAP (Hon)
Children's Research Centre
Our Lady's Children's Hospital
Dublin 12
Ireland
prem.puri@ucd.ie

Prof. Michael Höllwarth, MD
Department of Paediatric Surgery
Medical University
Auenbruggerplatz 34
A-8036 Graz
Austria
Michael.hoellwarth@meduni-graz.at

ISBN: 978-3-540-69559-2   e-ISBN: 978-3-540-69560-8
DOI: 10.1007/978-3-540-69560-8
Springer Dordrecht Heidelberg London New York

Library of Congress Control Number: 2008939393

Cover design: Frido Steinen–Broo, e-Studio Calamar, Spain

Printed on acid-free paper

Springer is part of Springer-Science + Business Media (www.springer.com)

To Veena and Susan for their love and patience.

Preface

During the last two decades there has been a dramatic improvements and expansion in the field of paediatric surgery. Major advances in perinatal diagnosis, imaging, resuscitation, intensive care, minimally invasive surgery, transplantation and improved operative techniques have radically altered the management of infants and children with surgical conditions. Surgical procedures are now routinely performed in neonates and children with serious and complex disorders. Monitoring techniques for the sick child pre and post operatively have become more sophisticated and there is now greater emphasis on physiological aspects of the child undergoing surgery.

This book, which is primarily aimed at paediatric surgical trainees and young paediatric surgeons, provides a comprehensive description of various surgical conditions in infants and children with major emphasis on diagnosis and management. The book contains contributions from outstanding and well known paediatric surgeons and paediatric urologists. Each contributor was selected to provide an authoritative, comprehensive and complete account of their respective topic. Most chapters are well illustrated with the use of tables, radiographic images, clinical photographs and operative techniques.

This book comprises of 97 chapters from 119 contributors from all five continents of the world. We wish to thank all the contributors most sincerely for their outstanding work in producing this innovative text book. We wish to express our gratitude to Vanessa Woods and Silvia Harding (Dublin) and Gudrun Raber (Graz) for their skilful secretarial help. Finally, we wish to thank the editorial staff of Springer, particularly Ms Gabriele Schroeder and Ms Stephanie Benko, who have been behind each step of this book from its original concept to its delivery.

Prem Puri
Michael Höllwarth

Contents

Part X   Spina Bifida and Hydrocephalus

Part XI   Genitourinary

Contributors

Yves Aigrain, MD, PhD Service de Chirurgie Pédiatrique et Urologie Pédiatrique, Hôpital Robert Debré, AP-HP Université Paris VII, 48 bd Serurier, 75019 Paris, France

Atif Awan Consultant Paediatric Nephrologist, Department of Nephro-urology & Transplantation, The Children's University Hospital, Temple Street, Dublin 1, Ireland, e-mail: kidney.unit@cuh.ie

Richard G. Azizkhan, MD Cincinnati Children's Hospital Medical Center, ML3018, 3333 Burnet Avenue, Cincinnati, OH 45229, USA, e-mail: Richard.Azizkhan@cchmc.org

Maria Marcela Bailez Pediatric Surgery, J.P. Garrahan Children's Hospital, Pichincha 1850, Buenos Aires, Argentina, e-mail: mbailez@speedy.com.ar

Bruce S. Bauer, MD, FACS, FAAP Chief, Division of Plastic Surgery, The Children's Memorial Hospital, Professor of Surgery, The Feinberg School of Medicine at Northwestern University, Chicago, IL, USA, e-mail: bbauer@northwestern.edu

Klaas(N) M.A. Bax, MD, PhD, FRCS(Ed) Professor of Pediatric Surgery and Head of the Department of Pediatric Surgery, Sophia Children's Hospital, Erasmus Medical Center, P.O. 2060, 3000 CB Rotterdam, The Netherlands, e-mail: n.bax@erasmusmc.nl

László Bognár Department of Paediatrics/Surgical Unit, Pécs University, József A. str. 7, 7623 Pécs, Hungary

Desmond Bohn Hospital for Sick Children, Toronto, ON, Canada

Paolo Caione Division of Paediatric Urology, "Bambino Gesù" Children's Hospital, Piazza S. Onofrio, 5, 00165 Rome, Italy, e-mail: caione@opbg.net

Victoria Camerini Children's Hospital Los Angeles, 4650 W Sunset Blvd, Los Angeles, CA 90027, USA, e-mail: vcamerini@chla.usc.edu

Donna A. Caniano, MD Professor of Surgery and Pediatrics, H. William Clatworthy Professor of Pediatric Surgery, Ohio State University College of Medicine and Public Health, Columbus, OH, USA
Surgeon-in-Chief, Columbus Children's Hospital, Columbus, OH 43205, USA

Robert Carachi, FRCS Division of Developmental Medicine, Section of Surgical Paediatrics, University of Glasgow, The Royal Hospital for Sick Children, Yorkhill, Glasgow G3 8SJ, Scotland, UK, e-mail: R.Carachi@clinmed.gla.ac.uk

Boris Chertin, MD Department of Urology, Shaare Zedek Medical Center, P.O. Box 3235, Jerusalem 91031, Israel, e-mail: bchertin@yahoo.com

Emily Christison-Lagay, MD Department of Surgery, Children's Hospital Boston, 300 Longwood Ave., Fegan 3, Boston, MA 02115, USA, e-mail: Steven.fishman@childrens.harvard.edu

Melanie C. Clark Murdoch Children's Research Institute, Royal Children's Hospital, Melbourne, VIC, Australia, e-mail: hutsonj@crytic.rch.unimelb.edu.au

Paul M. Colombani, MD Children's Surgeon in Charge, The John Hopkins Hospital, The John Hopkins University School of Medicine, Baltimore, MD, USA

Martin T. Corbally, MCh, FRCSI, FRCS (Paed), FRCSEd Consultant Paediatric Surgeon, Our Lady's Children's Hospital, Crumlin, Dublin 12, Ireland
Associate Professor of Paediatric Surgery, Royal College of Surgeons in Ireland, Dublin, Ireland

Julia Corcoran, MD, FACS, FAAP Assistant Professor of Surgery (Plastic), Northwestern University Feinberg School of Medicine, Attending Surgeon, Children's Memorial Hospital, Chicago, IL 60614, USA

Sarah M. Creighton, MD, FRCOG Consultant Gynaecologist, University College Hospital, Great Ormond Street Hospital, London, UK, e-mail: sarah.creighton@uclh.nhs.uk

Mark Davenport, ChM, FRCS (Paeds), FRCPS (Glas), FRCS (Eng) Department of Paediatric Surgery, King's College Hospital, Denmark Hill, London SE5 9RS, UK, e-mail: Markdav2@ntlworld.com, Mark.Davenport@kingsch.nhs.uk

Duane S. Duke, MD Pediatric Surgery Fellow, Department of Surgery, Drexel College of Medicine, St. Christopher's Hospital for Children, Erie Avenue at Front Street, Philadelphia, PA 19134, USA, e-mail: mzschwartz@msn.com

Simon Eaton, BSc (Hons), PhD Department of Paediatric Surgery, The Institute of Child Health and Great Ormond Street Hospital for Children NHS Trust, University College London, London, UK

Hans G. Eder, MD Professor for Neurosurgery, Head of Pediatric Neurosurgery, Department of Neurosurgery, Medical University, Graz, Austria

Jack S. Elder, MD Department of Urology, Henry Ford Hospital, K-9, 2799 West Grand Blvd, Detroit, MI 48202, USA

Alaa El Ghoneimi, MD, PhD Service de Chirurgie Pédiatrique et Urologie Pédiatrique, Hôpital Robert Debré, AP-HP Université Paris VII, 48 bd Serurier, 75019 Paris, France

Mary E. Fallat, MD Division of Pediatric Surgery, Department of Surgery, University of Louisville School of Medicine, 315 E. Broadway Street, Suite 565, Louisville, KY 40202, USA, e-mail: mefall01@gwise.louisville.edu

Eva E. Fischerauer, MD Department of Paediatric Surgery, Medical University, Auenbruggerplatz 36, 8034 Graz

Steven J. Fishman, MD Department of Surgery, Children's Hospital Boston, 300 Longwood Ave., Fegan 3, Boston, MA 02115, USA, e-mail: Steven.fishman@childrens.harvard.edu

Henri R. Ford, MD Children's Hospital Los Angeles, 4650 W Sunset Blvd, MS 72, Los Angeles, CA 90027, USA, e-mail: hford@chla.usc.edu

Heidi Friedrich Department of Paediatric and Adolescent Surgery, Medical University of Graz, Auenbruggerplatz 34, 8036 Graz, Austria

Takao Fujimoto, MD, PhD Director, Department of Pediatric Surgery, Aiiku Maternal Children's Medical Center, 5-6-8, Minami Azabu, Minato-ku, Tokyo 106-8580, Japan, e-mail: tfujimoto@aiiku.net

Michael W.L. Gauderer, MD, FACS, FAAP Professor of Pediatric Surgery and Pediatrics, University of South Carolina, School of Medicine, Columbia, SC, USA Chief, Division of Pediatric Surgery, Greenville Hospital System University Medical Center, 890 W. Faris Road, MMOB, Suite 440, Greenville, SC 29605-4253, USA, e-mail: mgauderer@ghs.org

John P. Gearhart Brady Urological Institute, Johns Hopkins Hospital, Baltimore, MD, USA, e-mail: jgearhart@jhmi.edu

Keith Georgeson, MD University of Alabama Health Services, Children's Hospital, 1600 7th Ave. S, Ste 300, Birmingham, AL 35233-1785, USA, e-mail: Keith.georgeson@ccc.uab.edu

John Gillick Our Lady's Children's Hospital, Crumlin, Dublin 12, Ireland, e-mail: johngillick@excite.com

David M. Gourlay, MD Assistant Professor of Surgery, Division of Pediatric Surgery, Medical College of Wisconsin, 999 N. 92nd Ave., Suite 320, Milwaukee, WI 53226, USA, e-mail: dgourlay@chw.org

Andrew Green, MB, PhD, FRCPI, FFPath (RCPI) Director, National Centre for Medical Genetics, Our Lady's Children's Hospital, Dublin, Ireland

D.K. Gupta Professor and Head, Department of Pediatric Surgery, All India Institute of Medical Sciences, New Delhi 110029, India, e-mail: devendra6@hotmail.com, profdkgupta@gmail.com

G. Gupte Department of Paediatric Surgery, Birmingham Children's Hospital, Steelhouse Lane, Birmingham B4 6NH, UK, e-mail: ksharif@hotmail.com

Alaa F. Hamza, MD, FRCS, FAAP (Hon.) Department of Pediatric Surgery, Ain-Shams University, 45 Remiss Street, Heliopolis, 11341 Cairo, Egypt, e-mail: shamza@idsc.net.eg

Michael S. Harney, FRCSI (ORL) Specialist Registrar in Otolaryngology, Our Lady's Hospital for Sick Children, Dublin, Ireland, e-mail: michaelsharney@eircom.net

Barry A. Hicks, MD Children's Medical Center, Dallas, 3rd Floor, West Tower, 1935 Motor St, Dallas, TX 75235, USA, e-mail: Barry.hicks@childrens.com

George W. Holcomb, III, MD, MBA Surgeon-in-Chief, Children's Mercy Hospital, 2401 Gillham Rd, Kansas City, MO 64108, USA, e-mail: gholcomb@cmh.edu

Michael Höllwarth, MD Department of Paediatric Surgery, Medical University, Auenbruggerplatz 36, 8034 Graz, Austria, e-mail: Michael.hoellwarth@meduni-graz.at

Catherine J. Hunter Children's Hospital Los Angeles, 4650 W Sunset Blvd, MS 72, Los Angeles, CA 90027, USA, e-mail: hford@chla.usc.edu

John M. Hutson General Surgery/Urology Departments, Royal Children's Hospital, Flemington Road, Parkville, Melbourne, VIC 3052, Australia, e-mail: john.hutson@rch.org.au

Romeo C. Ignacio, Jr Fellow, Pediatric Surgery, Department of Surgery, University of Louisville, Louisville, KY, USA

Edwin C. Jesudason, MA, FRCS(Paed), MD Senior Clinical Lecturer/Consultant Paediatric Surgeon, Division of Child Health, University of Liverpool, Alder Hey Children's Hospital, Liverpool L12 2AP, UK, e-mail: e.jesudason@liv.ac.uk

Paul R.V. Johnson Academic Paediatric Surgery Unit, Nuffield Department of Surgery, Level 6, John Radcliffe Hospital, Headley Way, Oxford OX3 9DU, UK, e-mail: paul.johnson@nds.ox.ac.uk

Martin Kaefer Riley Children's Hospital, Indiana University Medical School, Indianapolis, IN 46202, USA, e-mail: mkaefer@iupui.edu

Jonathan Saul Karpelowsky Department of Paediatric Surgery, Red Cross War Memorial, Children's Hospital, Cape Town, South Africa, e-mail: Jonathan.karpelowsky@uct.ac.za

Yoshifumi Kato Department of Paediatric and Urogenital Surgery, Juntendo University School of Medicine, 2-1-1 Hongo, Bunkyo-ku, Tokyo 113-8421, Japan, e-mail: yama@med.juntendo.ac.jp

Robert E. Kelly, Jr, MD, FACS, FAAP Children's Surgical Specialty Group, 601 Children's Ln, Ste 5b, Norfolk, VA 23507, USA, e-mail: dnuss@chkd.org

Martin A. Koyle, MD Pediatric Urology, The Children's Hospital, 1056 E. 19th Avenue, B463, Denver, CO 80218, USA, e-mail: koyle.martin@tchden.org

Göran Läckgren Section of Urology, University Children's Hospital, Uppsala, Sweden

Kokila Lakhoo Consultant Paediatric Surgeon, Children's Hospital, Oxford OX3 9DU, UK, e-mail: Kokila.lakhoo@paediatrics.ox.ac.uk

Jacob C. Langer, MD Rm 1526, Hospital for Sick Children, 555 University Ave., Toronto, ON, Canada M5G 1X8, e-mail: jacob.langer@sickkids.on.ca

Michael La Quaglia, MD, FACS, FRCS (Edin) Department of Surgery (Ped. Surg.), Memorial Sloan-Kettering Cancer Center, 1275 York Ave., New York, NY 10021, USA, e-mail: laquaglm@mskcc.org

Marc A. Levitt, MD Colorectal Center for Children, Cincinnati Children's Hospital Medical Center, Pediatric Surgery, 3333 Burnet Avenue, ML 2023, Cincinnati, OH 45229, USA, e-mail: marc.levitt@cchmc.org

Thom E. Lobe, MD Professor of Pediatrics, University of Tennessee Health Science Center, Memphis, TN, USA
Clinical Professor of Surgery, University of Iowa, Iowa City, IA, USA
Pediatric Surgeon, Blank Children's Hospital, 1200 Pleasant Street, Des Moines, IA 50309, USA, e-mail: Lobet2@ihs.org

Paul D. Losty, MD, FRCS(Paed) Professor of Paediatric Surgery, Division of Child Health, The Royal Liverpool Children's Hospital (Alder Hey), University of Liverpool, Liverpool, UK

Conor Mallucci Royal Liverpool Children's Hospital, Alder Hey, Eaton Road, Liverpool L12 2AP, UK

Alexander Margulis, MD Senior Lecturer, Hebrew University School of Medicine, Jerusalem, Israel
Attending Surgeon, Department of Plastic Surgery, Hadassah Medical Center, Jerusalem, Israel, e-mail: margul3@yahoo.com

Martin L. Metzelder Department of Pediatric Surgery, Hannover Medical School, Hannover, German

Lina Michala, MRCOG Specialist Registrar, Department of Obstetrics and Gynaecology, King's College Hospital, London, UK

A.J.W. Millar Red Cross Children's Hospital, Cape Town, South Africa

Alan Mortell Children's Research Centre, Our Lady's Children's Hospital, Crumlin, Dublin 12, Ireland, e-mail: Alan.mortell@ucd.ie

Dhanya Mullassery, MRCS(Eng) Paediatric Surgical Research Fellow, Division of Child Health, The Royal Liverpool Children's Hospital (Alder Hey), University of Liverpool, Liverpool, UK

Jeremy B. Myers, MD Department of Surgery, Division of Urology, University of Colorado Health Sciences Center, Denver, CO, USA

Nana Nakazawa, MD Pediatric General and Urogenital Surgery, Juntendo University School of Medicine, Tokyo, Japan, e-mail: nana.nakazawa@gmail.com

Simona Nappo Division of Paediatric Urology, "Bambino Gesù" Children's Hospital, Research Institute, Rome, Italy

L.T. Nguyen, MD Montreal Children's Hospital, 2300 Tupper St., Rm C-1132, Montreal, QC, Canada QCH3H 1P3, e-mail: Luong.nguyen@muhc.mcgill.ca

Agneta Nordenskjöld, MD, PhD Professor of Pediatric Surgery, Department of Women and Child Health, Karolinska University Hospital, Stockholm, Sweden

Amanda C. North Brady Urological Institute, Johns Hopkins Hospital, Baltimore, MD, USA, e-mail: Jgearhart@jhmi.edu

A. Numanoglu Department of Paediatric Surgery, Red Cross War Memorial Children's Hospital, University of Cape Town, Cape Town, South Africa

Donald Nuss, MB, CHB, FRCS (C), FACS Children's Surgical Specialty Group, 601 Children's Ln, Ste 5b, Norfolk, VA 23507, USA, e-mail: dnuss@chkd.org

Benedict C. Nwomeh, MD Department of Pediatric Surgery, ED 379, Columbus Children's Hospital, 700 Children's Drive, Columbus, OH 43205, USA, e-mail: nwomehbe@chi.osu.edu

Christian J. Ochoa Children's Hospital Los Angeles, 4650 W Sunset Blvd, MS 72, Los Angeles, CA 90027, USA

Keith T. Oldham, MD Professor and Chief, Division of Pediatric Surgery, Medical College of Wisconsin, Marie Z. Uihlein Chair and Surgeon-in-Chief, Children's Hospital of Wisconsin, Milwaukee, WI, USA, e-mail: koldham@chw.org

Mikko Pakarinen Children's Hospital, University of Helsinki, Stenbackinkatu 11, P.O. Box 281, 00029 HUS, Finland, e-mail: mikko.pakarinen@hus.fi

Joey C. Papa, MD Stanley Morgan Children's Hospital, New York, NY, USA

Richard H. Pearl, MD University of IL Peoria, Children's Hospital of IL, 420 NE Glen Oak, Ste 201, Peoria, IL 61603, USA, e-mail: rhpearl@uic.edu

Alberto Peña, MD Director, Colorectal Center for Children, Professor of Pediatric Surgery, Department of Pediatric Surgery, Cincinnati Children's Hospital, University of Cincinnati, 3333 Burnet Avenue, ML 2023, Cincinnati, OH 45229, USA, e-mail: alberto.pena@cchmc.org

Agostino Pierro, MD, FRCS (Eng), FRCS (Ed), FAAP Professor of Paediatric Surgery, Department of Paediatric Surgery, Institute of Child Health, 30, Guilford Street, London WC1N 1EH, UK, e-mail: pierro.sec@ich.ucl.ac.uk

Andrew B. Pinter Department of Paediatrics/Surgical Unit, Pécs University, József A. str. 7, 7623 Pécs, Hungary, e-mail: andras.pinter@aok.pte.hu

Prem Puri, MS, FRCS, FRCS (Ed), FACS Children's Research Centre, Our Lady's Children's Hospital, Dublin 12, Ireland, e-mail: prem.puri@ucd.ie

Priya Ramachandran, FRCS, PhD 25 Nageswava Road, Nungambakkam, Chennai, India, e-mail: kidsurg@hotmail.com

Michael Riccabona Department of Radiology, Division of Pediatric Radiology, University Hospital Graz, Auenbruggerplatz, 8036 Graz, Austria, e-mail: michael.riccabona@klinikum-graz.at

Risto J. Rintala Professor of Paediatric Surgery, Hospital for Children and Adolescents, University of Helsinki, P.O. Box 281, 00029 HUS, Finland, e-mail: risto.rintala@hus.fi, risto.rintala@saunalahti.fi

Massimo Rivosecchi Chief, Department of Pediatric Surgery, "Bambino Gesù" Children's Hospital, Palidoro, Rome, Italy

Heinz Rode Department of Paediatric Surgery, Red Cross War Memorial Children's Hospital, University of Cape Town, Cape Town, South Africa

Udo Rolle Department of Paediatric Surgery, University of Leipzig, Leipzig, Germany

Jerard Ross Royal Liverpool Children's Hospital, Alder Hey, Eaton Road, Liverpool L12 2AP, UK, e-mail: rossjerad@jross101.freeserve.co.uk, mallucci@ntlworld.com

Jonathan H. Ross, MD Head, Section of Pediatric Urology, Glickman Urological Institute, Cleveland Clinic Childrens Hospital, 9500 Euclid Avenue/Desk A100, Cleveland, OH 44195, USA, e-mail: rossj@ccf.org

John Russell, FRCSI (ORL) Consultant Otolaryngologist/Paediatric Airway Surgeon, Our Lady's Hospital for Sick Children, Dublin, Ireland

David E. Sawaya, Jr, MD Chief, Division of Pediatric Surgery, The John Hopkins University School of Medicine, Children's Surgeon in Charge, The John Hopkins Hospital, Baltimore, MD, USA

Amulya K. Saxena, MD Associate Professor, Department of Pediatric and Adolescent Surgery, Medical University of Graz, Auenbruggerplatz 34, 8036 Graz, Austria

Marshall Z. Schwartz, MD Professor of Surgery and Pediatrics, Drexel University College of Medicine, Philadelphia, PA, USA
Surgeon-in-Chief, Pediatric Surgery, St. Christopher's Hospital for Children, Erie Avenue at Front Street, Philadelphia, PA 19134, USA, e-mail: mzschwartz@msn.com

K. Sharif Department of Paediatric Surgery, Birmingham Children's Hospital, Steelhouse Lane, Birmingham B4 6NH, UK, e-mail: ksharif@hotmail.com

Shilpa Sharma Assistant Professor of Pediatric Surgery, Post Graduate Institute of Medical Sciences, Dr RML Hospital, New Delhi, India

S.J. Shochat Department of Surgery, St Jude Children's Research Hospital, 332 N Lauderdake, Memphis, TN 38105, USA, e-mail: Stephen.shochat@stjude.org

Owen Patrick Smith, MA, MB, BA Mod.(Biochem.), FRCPCH, FRCPI, FRCPEdin, FRCPLon, FRCPGlasg, FRCPath Consultant Paediatric Haematologist, National Paediatric Haematology/Oncology and Bone Marrow Transplant Centre, Haematology Division, Our Lady's Children's Hospital, Crumlin, Dublin 12, Ireland, e-mail: owen.smith@olhsc.ie
Professor of Haematology, Trinity College Dublin, Dublin, Ireland

Bridget R. Southwell, PhD Murdoch Children's Research Institute, Royal Children's Hospital, Melbourne, VIC, Australia, e-mail: hutsonj@crytic.rch.unimelb.edu.au

Thambipillai Sri Paran, FRCS(I) Children's Research Centre, Our Lady's Children's Hospital, Dublin, Ireland

Charles J.H. Stolar, MD Stanley Morgan Children's Hospital, New York, NY, USA

Shawn D. St. Peter, MD Director, Center for Prospective Clinical Trials, Department of Surgery, Children's Mercy Hospital, 2401 Gillham Rd, Kansas City, MO 64108, USA, e-mail: sspeter@cmh.edu

Mark D. Stringer, BSc, MS, MRCP, FRCS, FRCS (Paed.), FRCSEd Professor of Paediatric Surgery, St. James's University Hospital, Leeds, UK
Department of Anatomy and Structural Biology, Otago School of Medical Sciences, University of Otago, P.O. Box 913, Dunedin, New Zealand, e-mail: mark.stringer@anatomy.otago.ac.nz

Steven Stylianos, MD Children's Hospital of New York Presbyterian, 3959 Broadway, New York, NY 10032, USA, e-mail: Steven.Stylianos@mch.com

Yechiel Sweed, MD Head, Department of Pediatric Surgery, Western Galilee Hospital, Nahariya 22100, Israel, e-mail: yechiel.sweed@naharia.health.gov.il

Paul K.H. Tam Division of Paediatric Surgery, Department of Surgery, University of Hong Kong, Queen Mary Hospital, Hong Kong SAR, China

Juan A. Tovar, MD, PhD Departamento de Cirugía Pediátrica, Hospital Universitario "La Paz", P. de la Castellana, 261, 28046 Madrid, Spain, e-mail: jatovar.hulp@salud.madrid.org

Jeffrey S. Upperman Children's Hospital Los Angeles, 4650 W Sunset Blvd, MS 72, Los Angeles, CA 90027, USA

Christian Urban, MD Division of Pediatric Hematology/Oncology, Department of Pediatrics and Adolescent Medicine, Medical University Graz, 8036 Graz, Austria, e-mail: christian.urban@meduni-graz.at

Benno M. Ure, MD Director/Chairman, Professor of Pediatric Surgery, Hannover Medical School, Carl-Neuberg-Str. 1, 30625 Hannover, Germany, e-mail: ure.benno@mh-hannover.de

Declan Warde Department of Anaesthesia, Children's University Hospital, Temple Street, Dublin 1, Ireland, e-mail: dwarde@indigo.ie

Tomas Wester Department of Paediatric Surgery, University Hospital, 751 85 Uppsala, Sweden, e-mail: tomas.wester@surgsci.uu.se

Kenneth Kak Yuen Wong, MBChb (Ed), FRCS (Ed) Division of Paediatric Surgery, Department of Surgery, University of Hong Kong Medical Centre, Queen Mary Hospital, Pokfulam Road, Hong Kong, e-mail: kkywong@hkucc.hku.hk

Atsuyuki Yamataka, MD Department of Pediatric and Urogenital Surgery, Juntendo University School of Medicine, 2-1-1 Hongo, Bunkyo-ku, Tokyo 113-8421, Japan, e-mail: yama@med.juntendo.ac.jp

Mohammed Zamakhshary, MD, MEd Fellow, Pediatric General Surgery, University of Toronto, Hospital for Sick Children, Toronto, ON, Canada

Moritz M. Ziegler, MD The Children's Hospital, 13123 East 16th Avenue, B323, Aurora, Cal. 80045, USA, e-mail: Ziegler.moritz@tchden.org

The Epidemiology of Birth Defects

1

Edwin C. Jesudason

Contents

1.1 Introduction

The surgical correction of birth defects helped create the speciality of paediatric surgery during the middle of the last century. Around this time, pioneering neonatal operations were successfully performed to allow survival of babies with conditions like oesophageal atresia or congenital diaphragmatic hernia (CDH). Indeed, along with innovations such as parenteral nutrition, the concentration of surgical, anaesthetic, nursing and critical care expertise now allows high survival rates to be achieved for many previously fatal anomalies. For certain conditions that have high mortality and morbidity, fetal surgery aims to further reduce the harm of birth defects.

1.2 Birth Defects Are Leading Causes of Global Infant Mortality

Given the huge progress made in the treatment of infectious diseases in particular, birth defects are now emerging as the leading cause of infant mortality. Moreover, this state of affairs pertains not only to places with expensive healthcare systems but in fact anywhere that infant mortality rates have significantly fallen. Hence, as progress against other infant killer diseases continues it is likely that birth defects will gradually become one of the most significant global causes of infant mortality. In addition, birth defects are a leading contributor to both premature birth (itself a major cause of infant mortality) and chronic disability (with its substantial personal and societal costs). Tragically, many such problems are already preventable; for example, the birth defects associated with congenital rubella syn-

P. Puri and M. Höllwarth (eds.), *Pediatric Surgery: Diagnosis and Management*,
DOI: 10.1007/978-3-540-69560-8_1, © Springer-Verlag Berlin Heidelberg 2009

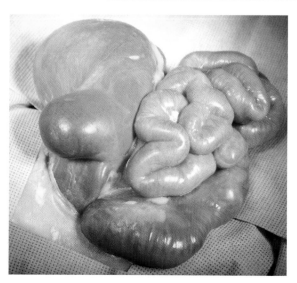

Fig. 1.1 Gastroschisis – a birth defect on the move? Data from birth defect registries indicate a real and unexplained increase in gastroschisis prevalence. It remains to be seen if the severity of gastroschisis is also increasing: in this example, in addition to the gut, most of the liver lies outside the neonatal abdomen (image used with permission, courtesy of the author)

drome may be virtually eradicated by an effective programme of maternal immunisation. Furthermore, a subset of neural tube defects continues to occur due to inadequate implementation of pre-conceptual folate prophylaxis. However, the epidemiological challenges for clinicians extend beyond the known, preventable defects to unsolved conditions and their changing circumstances (for instance, the increasing prevalence of gastroschisis Fig. 1.1).

1.3   Birth Defects Epidemiology and Teratology

Although birth defects have been described with horror and fascination since antiquity, teratology and scientific birth defects epidemiology date, like paediatric surgery, from the mid-twentieth century. Key historical developments include the recognition of congenital rubella syndrome (noted by clinical ophthalmological examination) and the thalidomide disaster (phocomelia and other defects associated with maternal thalidomide administration for morning sickness). These episodes vividly illustrated the devastating consequences of prenatal infection and drug exposure. In addition, these chastening experiences highlighted the urgent need to formalise birth defects surveillance. Such monitoring

of birth defects can now be said to serve a range of important purposes including early warning of an outbreak, identification of possible environmental or genetic causes, rational planning for neonatal surgical provision, facilitation of prenatal counselling based on accurate data, establishment of associations between birth defects and comparison of outcomes.

1.4   Causation of Birth Defects Remains Often Complex and Uncertain

Before considering the methods of birth defects surveillance, it is worth sketching the developmental biology that underpins birth defects from a surgeon's perspective. Causes of birth defects can be classified as parental, fetal and environmental. Examples of the former include the impact of maternal and paternal age on the prevalence of Downs and Aperts Syndromes, respectively. Alternatively, maternal diseases such as diabetes are well-described risk factors for the formation of birth defects. Fetal causes include genetically determined inborn errors of metabolism such as those causing intersex anomalies in congenital adrenal hyperplasia, chromosomal lesions such as Downs Syndrome, Edwards Syndrome etc. and twinning with its increased risk of birth anomalies. Environmental causes include those related to prenatal addiction and drug exposure, such as alcohol, smoking, thalidomide, valproate, phenytoin, warfarin etc., as well as the impact of intrauterine infections, such as toxoplasmosis, rubella and cytomegalovirus. The impact of assisted reproductive technologies such as in vitro fertilisation and intracytoplasmic sperm injection on the prevalence of birth defects are actually quite difficult to assess. The suggestion that anomaly rates are higher in such assisted pregnancies needs to contend with the confounding increased rates of multiple pregnancy. Also, given the parents' need to use assisted reproductive technology, it may be that they are importantly different to parents conceiving naturally; increased anomaly risk could therefore be due to parental abnormality and predisposition rather than a result of the techniques themselves.

Other environmental contributors to birth defects include "endocrine disrupters"; these oestrogenic compounds are conjectured to contribute to anomalies of sexual development in fetal males (e.g. hypospadias) as well as putative impairment of adult male sperm quality. In light of such difficulties in attributing causes, it is important to recognise that only a minority of birth defects are known to arise from a simple genetic or environmental cause. At present, the majority of birth defects appear to have multi-factorial origins. Therefore, it is helpful to consider birth defect causation as the result of complex interactions between genes and environment. Hence some cases of spina bifida may result from micronutrient deficiency in the context of predisposing enzyme polymorphisms. Similarly, teratogenic drugs may interact with pharmacogenomic predispositions to help explain why certain pregnancies are affected. Beyond considerations of even complex causation, it remains likely that simple chance has a major role to play (similar to stochastic effects seen in radiation biology).

1.5 Birth Defects Appear to Arise Typically (But Not Exclusively) in the First Trimester

Developmental biologists refer to "competence windows" to describe periods in development when particular cells and tissues are capable of responding appropriately to certain growth and transcription factors. In a similar manner, developing organs are contended to have particular temporal windows when an otherwise non-specific teratogenic stimulus will impact disproportionately on the formation of that organ system.

During the first trimester, organ morphogenesis predominates while later trimesters are devoted to organ growth and maturation. Unsurprisingly, therefore, sensitivity to teratogens is held to peak during the first trimester. Hence, pregnant women are advised to avoid medications during this part of gestation in particular. Teleologically, "morning sickness" that peaks during the first trimester is postulated to help reduce ingestion of potential teratogens during this period of maximum vulnerability. While the model of first trimester teratogenesis appears appropriate for many birth defects, it is now clear that certain anomalies may arise during later development as a result of fetal events, such as amniotic band formation or vascular accident. Gastroschisis and intestinal atresia may be considered in this latter category. Indeed, the contrast between exomphalos and gastroschisis in terms of associated anomalies (and hence prognosis) can be considered due to the different times they are held to originate during development. Exomphalos is considered an embryonic lesion that is accompanied by contemporaneous lesions of organogenesis in other systems such as the heart. In contrast, intestinal atresia in gastroschisis is thought to result from a discrete fetal vascular accident and hence lacks extra-intestinal manifestations. A similar contrast between duodenal atresia and small bowel atresia may be likewise understood as the result of their differing onsets and aetiologies. Duodenal atresia is commonly explained as an embryonic failure of luminal recanalisation; as expected, therefore it is strongly associated with other dysorganogenesis, such as cardiac, Downs and oesophageal atresia. In contrast, small bowel atresiae are thought to follow mesenteric vascular occlusion usually in fetal life. Hence, aside from gastroschisis, associated structural lesions are unlikely. Between these two "extremes" are birth defects where an embryonic lesion has deleterious "knock-on" effects later in fetal development; based on experimental models, the neurological sequelae of spina bifida are postulated to result from not only the primary failure of neural tube closure but also from consequent exposure of the neural placode to amniotic fluid. Similarly, lung hypoplasia in CDH may emerge as an embryonic lesion prior to CDH only for compression by the visceral hernia to exacerbate the pulmonary lesion. In circumstances such as these, where the pathology is thought to progress during fetal life, prenatal surgical correction has been a logical proposal to meet the challenge of refractory mortality and morbidity.

1.6 Classification of Birth Defects for Epidemiological Purposes

Birth defect epidemiology involves the registration of anomalies by type. At present, birth defects registries such as EUROCAT (European Surveillance of Congenital Anomalies) use a classification scheme based around organ systems (see Table 1.1), specific diagnoses and ICD codes (see Table 1.2; both tables are derived from data published by EUROCAT—http://www.eurocat.ulster.ac.uk/pubdata/tables.html).

Cooperation between registries helps by pooling data and also by building consensus on issues such as the exclusion of minor anomalies without major and long-term sequelae (e.g. cryptorchidism or congenital hydrocoele) or on how abnormalities of gut fixation in CDH might be recorded. Although anomalies are

Table 1.1 Birth prevalence of malformations 1980–2004 grouped by EUROCAT category. Note, rates for each category are inclusive of cases with chromosomal lesions and derived from registries with full EUROCAT membership

Organ system	Live birth + fetal death + termination/10,000 births
All	210
Cardiac	62
Limb	40
Chromosomal	31
Urinary	27
Nervous system	23
Digestive system	19
Genital	15
Musculo-skeletal	11
Other malformations	10
Abdominal wall defects	4.7
Eye	4.7
Genetic syndromes + microdeletions	4.6
Ear, face, neck	4.4
Teratogenic syndromes (inc. infection)	0.9

Table 1.2 Birth prevalence of malformations of relevance to paediatric surgery (1980–2004) grouped by diagnosis from registries with full EUROCAT membership

Anomaly	Live birth + fetal death + termination/10,000 births
Down's	18
Hypospadias	11
Congenital hydronephrosis	8.5
Spina bifida	5.4
Cystic kidney disease	5.3
Edward's	3.7
Anorectal malformations	3.0
Diaphragmatic hernia	2.8
Exomphalos	2.8
OA/TOF	2.3
Gastroschisis	1.8
Bilateral renal agenesis	1.7
Duodenal atresia/stenosis	1.2
Hirschsprung disease	0.87
Posterior urethral valves/ prune belly	0.8
Indeterminate sex	0.8
Intestinal atresia/stenosis	0.74
Bladder extrophy/epispadias	0.58
Situs inversus	0.54
Amniotic band	0.35
CCAM	0.33
Biliary atresia	0.28
Conjoined twins	0.18

Note (a) rates for each category are inclusive of cases with chromosomal lesions; (b) the time frame examined (1980–2004) may obscure recent rising incidence of gastroschisis and, for example, the impact of modern prenatal diagnosis of CCAM; (c) these are birth prevalences (including fetal death/terminations) and not necessarily the prevalences at paediatric surgical units.

currently classified by structural anomaly (e.g. CDH, oesophageal atresia) or defined diagnosis (e.g. Downs), it is likely that, in the future, anomalies may be classified or at least subgrouped by genotypic differences rather than anatomic details alone. Such distinctions may be prognostically and therapeutically important, e.g. in contrast to isolated omphalocoeles, exomphalos in Beckwith-Wiedemann syndrome is associated with hypoglycaemia, macrosomia and increased tumour risk due to disordered gene imprinting. Hence, the anatomic defect (exomphalos) becomes less important than the genetics and its multi-system sequelae. Similarly, it is postulated that subgroups of spina bifida may be folate resistant due to underlying genetic or enzymatic variation. Designing pre-conceptual prophylaxis for birth defects may need to acknowledge pharmacogenomically distinct subgroups to avoid benefits within one subgroup being overlooked due to a larger surrounding non-responder cohort.

Having a system of classification is however only part of the task. Notification and classification in practice are subject to local variations. When resources exist for expert-mediated classification of birth defects by diagnosis, this approach to birth defects epidemiology appears the best currently available. However, even some North American registries lack clinician input in the classification and assignment of observed birth defects. The consequence(s) of this omission for data quality remain to

be determined. In the contrasting circumstances of rural China, expert-led assignment of cases has been substituted by simple photographic recording of malformations; this system not only allows the registry to function but also allows difficult cases to be assigned later after remote assessment of images by experts. In addition, the photographs potentially allow the classifiers to calibrate their judgments against those from other registries.

1.7 Counting of Birth Defects Is Affected by the Definition of Stillbirth

The epidemiology of birth defects becomes difficult whenever the classification of defects is not uniform or straightforward. This task is complicated by practical barriers to case ascertainment (e.g. inadequate resources), the definition of stillbirth and the effects of prenatal diagnosis and terminations.

Recording of anomaly prevalence lies at the core of birth defects epidemiology. To account for the unknown incidence of a defect among vast numbers of naturally miscarried pregnancies, epidemiologists measure the prevalences of defects within a defined birth cohort, i.e. the number of live and stillborn cases of the defect, as a proportion of all births (live and stillborn). This definition depends on the artificial distinction between miscarriage and stillbirth; EUROCAT's recommendation is that spontaneous pregnancy losses prior to 20 weeks of gestation are counted as miscarriages (and do not contribute to anomaly prevalence), while similar losses at 20 weeks of gestation and beyond are counted as stillbirths (and included in prevalence statistics).

Despite these guidelines, several countries have established different demarcations (e.g. 24 or 28 weeks or even 500 g weight). Clearly, some estimate of prenatal birth defects is required to avoid seriously underestimating overall prevalences. However, the demarcation of stillbirths begins to complicate matters. Countries where later gestational cut-off points are used may underestimate the prevalence of birth defects compared to registries where 20 weeks is used. Hence, minor changes in convention can lead to large but artificial differences in anomaly prevalence. While a definition of stillbirths is needed for data collection, the sharp demarcation (whether 20 weeks or later) also appears arbitrary from a biological perspective. Consider a hypothetical prenatal medical therapy that reduces the prevalence of a specific birth defect. When the anomaly is rare (as most are), it may be difficult to determine whether an observed reduction in prevalence is truly due to fewer malformations or instead due to the promotion of earlier loss of affected pregnancies (i.e. prior to the 20 weeks or other agreed margin). This latter phenomenon, termed "terathanasia", has even been invoked to explain how folate supplementation reduces neural tube defect prevalence.

1.8 Prenatal Diagnosis: The Greatest Challenge to Birth Defect Epidemiology?

While classification of birth defects and the definition of stillbirth make anomaly surveillance complex, the impact of prenatal diagnosis is arguably still more important. Prenatal diagnosis (in particular non-specific ultrasound screening) confounds birth defects surveillance in a number of ways: (i) it increases identification of birth defects within the cohort of assessment (still and liveborn) by diagnosing those who may otherwise have perished prenatally (and uncounted), or those who may have presented beyond the neonatal period (if at all). For example, in prenatal identification of cystic lung lesions, some would never have been diagnosed (either regressing spontaneously or persisting asymptomatically), while even symptomatic lesions would often have presented later (beyond the scope of the birth defects registry); (ii) prenatal diagnosis alters antenatal management and results in terminations (or fetal intervention) that affect the numbers of birth defects being counted; most registries therefore attempt to keep separate data on terminations for birth defects. However, where prohibitions on termination exist, such data becomes still harder to find; (iii) prenatal diagnosis may be inaccurate but unchecked; pathological verification after termination may be incomplete or absent, yet the diagnosis is included in the birth defect tally; (iv) resources and expertise to perform prenatal sonography vary with location thereby hampering national and international comparison of the prevalence of birth defects. In summary, the apparently simple task of counting live and stillborn cases for birth defects surveillance is fraught with difficulty once (a) the arbitrary definition of stillbirth is imposed and (b) ubiquitous prenatal imaging prompts both terminations and identification of previously occult "cases".

Given these challenges in data collection, epidemiologists are aided by being able to compare a variety of surveillance databases. Many European registries are incorporated into the EUROCAT initiative. Similarly, several other registries feed into birth defects' surveillance data furnished by the World Health Organisation (WHO). Their Birth Defects Atlas is an interesting publication available in the public domain (http://www.who.int/genomics/publications/en/). Most importantly it is instructive to read and consider the caveats that EUROCAT and WHO place on their data. The interpretational issues raised highlight not only the problems discussed in the previous sections but also allude to the ongoing challenge of inadequate resources and expertise for reporting birth defects. This in turn impairs the data accuracy and may help explain insufficient action upon findings.

1.9   Paediatric Surgeons Often Report Institutional Series of Birth Defects

Given the difficulties in collecting and interpreting data from population-based registries, it should come as no surprise that similar issues afflict institutional series that are the staple of paediatric surgeons' reporting. Again, ascertainment is the most significant problem; prenatal diagnosis, terminations, or deaths prior to transfer, of high-risk cases can give the misleading impression that changed institutional practice is impacting on outcome (when in fact it is pre-institutional interventions that are changing the results). Moreover, paediatric surgeons like to estimate disease severity in their cohort to show that their (good) results are not simply the product of low-risk caseload. However, in such circumstances it can be highly misleading to use the frequency of interventions (e.g. decision to patch and use ECMO or nitric oxide in CDH) to estimate severity in a birth defect cohort; use of these techniques may in fact owe more to institutional protocols rather than any pathophysiological differences between cases. Ultimately, institutional series are subject to often substantial biases (with apparently poorer results perhaps not even being submitted for publication).

1.10   The Challenge for Modern Paediatric Surgery

Despite its confounding influence on modern birth defects surveillance, the impact of prenatal diagnosis will not disappear. On the contrary, advances in prenatal imaging may only serve to identify more "defects" of unknown significance. Moreover, functional fetal imaging and genotyping may evolve to allow better prenatal prognostication and hence case selection for future fetal therapies. In the midst of all these potentially exciting developments, paediatric surgeons retain a key role; using the best available birth defects epidemiology, we may gradually learn to match the defects with the required type and time of intervention appropriately. To achieve this, paediatric surgeons need to keep abreast of birth defects epidemiology and work collaboratively with other surgeons, perinatologists, obstetricians and public health physicians. As a model for such cooperative endeavours, the organisation, previously termed the UK Children's Cancer Study Group (UKCCSG), was led by collaborating paediatric oncologists and surgeons; they achieved remarkably high recruitment rates of paediatric cancer cases into multicentre trials that helped transform clinical management. A similar consortium approach to birth defects and their surgical correction may allow paediatric surgeons to retain a central role in this evolving field. Conversely, overlong adherence to single institution reporting may see the speciality sidelined as governments are advised by public health specialists and others on the pre- and post-natal management of birth defects. Given the opportunities generated by "Web 2.0", the tools for such networked initiatives are within our grasp. As a beginning, the British Association of Paediatric Surgeons Congenital Anomalies Surveillance System (BAPS-CASS) has undertaken a year's census of gastroschisis in the UK (that is, in part, a response to the UK Chief Medical Officer's concerns about rising gastroschisis prevalence). Hence, as birth defects emerge as the leading cause of infant mortality, this project will help us establish how paediatric surgeons can work together to understand these human healthcare problems.

Further Reading

Carmona RH (2005) The global challenges of birth defects and disabilities. Lancet 366(9492):1142–1144

Cragan JD, Khoury MJ (2000) Effect of prenatal diagnosis on epidemiologic studies of birth defects. Epidemiology 11(6):695–699

Davidson N, Halliday J, Riley M, King J (2005) Influence of prenatal diagnosis and pregnancy termination of fetuses with birth defects on the perinatal mortality rate in Victoria, Australia. Paediatr Perinat Epidemiol 19(1):50–55

Howse JL, Howson CP, Katz M (2005) Reducing the global toll of birth defects. Lancet 365(9474):1846–1847

Khoury MJ (1989) Epidemiology of birth defects. Epidemiol Rev 11:244–248

Khoury MJ, Millikan R, Little J, Gwinn M (2004) The emergence of epidemiology in the genomics age. Int J Epidemiol 33(5):936–944

Li S, Moore CA, Li Z et al (2003) A population-based birth defects surveillance system in the People's Republic of China. Paediatr Perinat Epidemiol 17(3):287–293

Lin AE, Forrester MB, Cunniff C, Higgins CA, Anderka M (2006) Clinician reviewers in birth defects surveillance programs: Survey of the National Birth Defects Prevention Network. Birth Defects Res A Clin Mol Teratol 76(11): 781–786

Puri P, Höllwarth ME (eds) (2006) Pediatric Surgery. Springer, Berlin, Heidelberg

Shiota K, Yamada S (2005) Assisted reproductive technologies and birth defects. Congenit Anom (Kyoto) 45(2): 39–43

Fetal Counselling for Surgical Congenital Malformations

2

Kokila Lakhoo

Contents

2.1 Introduction

Paediatric surgeons are often called to counsel parents once a surgical abnormality is diagnosed on a prenatal scan. The referral base for a paediatric surgeon now includes the perinatal period. Expertise in surgical correction of congenital malformations may favourably influence the perinatal management of prenatally diagnosed anomalies by changing the site of delivery for immediate postnatal treatment; altering the mode of delivery to prevent obstructed labour or haemorrhage; early delivery to prevent ongoing fetal organ damage; or treatment in utero to prevent, minimise or reverse fetal organ injury as a result of a structural defect. Favourable impact of prenatal counselling has been confirmed to influence the site of delivery in 37% of cases, change the mode of delivery in 6.8%, reverse the decision to terminate a pregnancy in 3.6% and influence the early delivery of babies in 4.5%.

Counselling parents about prenatally suspected surgically correctable anomalies should not be solely performed by obstetricians or paediatricians. Similarly the paediatric surgeon performing these prenatal consultations must be aware of differences between the prenatal and postnatal natural history of the anomaly. There is often a lack of understanding of the natural history and prognosis of a condition presenting in the newborn and the same condition diagnosed prenatally.

The diagnosis and management of complex fetal anomalies require a team effort by obstetricians, neonatologists, geneticists, paediatricians and paediatric surgeons to deal with all the maternal and fetal complexities of a diagnosis of a structural defect. This team should be able to provide information to prospective parents on fetal outcomes, possible interventions, appropriate setting, time and route of delivery and expected postnatal outcomes. The role of the surgical consultant in this team is to present information regarding the prenatal and postnatal natural history of an anomaly, its surgical management and the long-term outcome.

2.2 Congenital Malformation

Congenital malformations account for one of the major causes of perinatal mortality and morbidity. Single major birth defects affect 3% of newborns and multiple defects affect 0.7% of babies. The prenatal hidden mortality is higher since the majority abort spontaneously. Despite improvements in perinatal care, serious birth defects still account for 20% of all deaths in the newborn period and an even greater percentage of serious morbidity later in infancy and childhood. The major causes of congenital malformation are chromosomal abnormalities, mutant genes, multifactorial disorders and teratogenic agents.

2.3 Prenatal Diagnosis

Prenatal diagnosis has remarkably improved our understanding of surgically correctable congenital malformations. It has allowed us to influence the delivery of the baby, offer prenatal surgical management and discuss the options of termination of pregnancy for seriously handicapping or lethal conditions. Antenatal diagnosis has also defined an in utero mortality for some lesions such as diaphragmatic hernia and sacrococcygeal teratoma so that true outcomes can be measured. Prenatal ultrasound scanning has improved since its first use 30 years ago, thus providing better screening programmes and more accurate assessment of fetal anomaly. Screening for Down's syndrome may now be offered in the first trimester (e.g. nuchal scan combined test) or second trimester (e.g. Triple blood test). Better resolution and increased experience with ultrasound scans has led to the recognition of ultrasound soft markers that have increased the detection rate of fetal anomalies but at the expense of higher false positive rates.

Routine ultrasound screening identifies anomalies and places these pregnancies in the high-risk categories with maternal diabetes, hypertension, genetic disorders, raised alpha fetoprotein, etc. High-risk pregnancies may be offered further invasive diagnostic investigations such as amniocentesis or chorionic villous sampling. Structural abnormalities difficult to define on ultrasound such as hindbrain lesions or in the presence of oligohydramnios are better imaged on ultra fast magnetic resonance imaging. With the increasing range of options and sophistication of diagnostic methods, parents today are faced with more information, choice and decisions than ever before, which can create as well as help to solve dilemmas. The different tests and screening procedures commonly in use are outlined below.

2.3.1 Ultrasound Examination

Ultrasound scan is routinely performed at 18–20 weeks gestation as part of the prenatal screening for all pregnancies in England and Wales. Older mothers are routinely screened and in addition are offered invasive testing. Pregnancies with maternal risk factors such as raised alpha fetoprotein levels, genetic disorders and family history of chromosomal abnormalities or monochorionic twins that carry a high risk for chromosomal anomalies are offered scans in the first trimester. Abnormalities such as diaphragmatic hernia may be detected as early as 11 weeks of gestation. First trimester scans are also useful for accurately dating pregnancies and defining chorionicity in multiple pregnancies.

More recently, nuchal translucency (NT) measurements have emerged as an independent marker of chromosomal abnormalities with a sensitivity of 60%, structural anomalies (particularly cardiac defects) and for some rare genetic syndromes. It involves measuring the area at the back of the fetal neck at 11–14 weeks of gestation (Fig. 2.1). The mechanisms by which some abnormalities give rise to this transient anatomical change of nuchal translucency are poorly understood. Although some abnormalities can be seen at the time of the nuchal scan (11–14 weeks), most are detected at the 18–20 week anomaly scan. Some abnormalities such as gastroschisis have a higher detection rate on a scan than others, for example, cardiac abnormalities.

If the nuchal translucency measurement is increased and the karyotype is normal, there is a higher risk for a cardiac anomaly and these high-risk fetuses may be

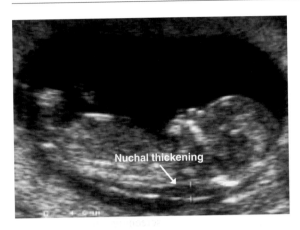

Fig. 2.1 Nuchal translucency scan

obtained is dependent on the expertise and experience of the person performing the scan. In a recent study, congenital anomalies noted at birth were diagnosed on prenatal scan in 64% of cases with 0.5% opting for termination.

2.4 Invasive Diagnostic Tests

Amniocentesis and chorionic villous sampling (CVS) are the two most commonly performed invasive diagnostic tests.

2.4.1 Amniocentesis

Amniocentesis is commonly used for detecting chromosomal abnormalities and less often for molecular studies, metabolic studies and fetal infection. It is performed after 15 weeks of gestation and carries a low risk of fetal injury or loss (0.5–1%). Full karyotype analysis takes approximately 2 weeks but newer RAPID techniques using FISH (fluorescent *in situ* hybridisation) or PCR (polymerase chain reaction) can give limited (usually for trisomies 21,18,13) results within 2–3 days.

2.4.2 Chorionic Villous Sampling (CVS)

CVS is the most reliable method for first trimester diagnosis and may be performed at 10–14 weeks of gestation. The test involves ultrasound-guided biopsy of the chorionic villi. The added risk for fetal loss is approximately 1–2%. The samples obtained may be subjected to a variety of tests including full karyotype, rapid karyotyping (FISH—PCR), enzyme analysis or molecular studies. Approximate timing of chromosomal results is 1–2 weeks for karyotyping and 2–3 days for FISH and PCR.

2.4.3 Prenatal Maternal Serum Screening

Interest in detecting circulating fetal cells in maternal blood for diagnostic purposes has grown since the

referred for fetal echocardiography, which provides better prenatal cardiac assessment than the routine screening scan. Ultrasound surveillance is essential during the performance of invasive techniques such as amniocentesis, CVS and shunting procedures. It is also useful for assessing fetal viability before and after such procedures. Some abnormalities such as tracheo-oesophageal fistula, bowel atresia, diaphragmatic hernia and hydrocephaly may present later in pregnancy and thereby may not be detected during the routine 18-weeks scan.

Overall, around 60% of structural birth defects are detected prenatally but the detection rate varies from 0% (isolated cleft palate) to close to 100% (gastroschisis) depending on the defect. True wrong diagnoses are rare but false positive diagnoses do occur; some are due to natural prenatal regression, but most are due to ultrasound "soft markers".

Ultrasound "soft markers" are changes noted on prenatal scan that are difficult to define. Examples are echogenic bowel, hydronephrosis and nuchal thickening. Their presence creates anxiety among sonographers because the finding may be transient with no pathological relevance or may be an indicator of significant anomalies such as chromosomal abnormalities, cystic fibrosis (echogenic bowel), Down's syndrome (nuchal thickening) or renal abnormalities (hydronephrosis). Once soft markers are detected, the dilemma faced by obstetricians is whether they should be reported or further invasive tests offered. Reporting these markers has increased detection rates at the expense of high false positive rates.

Ultrasound is routinely performed as a prenatal screening test. The reliability of the information

advent of fluorescence-activated cell sorting (FACS). The observation of high levels of AFP (alpha fetoprotein) in the amniotic fluid of pregnancies complicated by open neural tube defects (NTDs) popularised this test. However, with increasing accuracy of ultrasound diagnosis, maternal serum screening of AFP solely for identification of NTDs cannot be justified. The more popular maternal serum screening test is the triple test (HCG, AFP, oestrogen) used in combination with the nuchal scan.

2.4.4 Fetal Blood Sampling (FBS)

Rapid karyotyping of CVS and amniotic fluid samples FISH and PCR has replaced fetal blood sampling for many conditions. However, FBS is still required for the diagnosis and treatment of haematological conditions and some viral infections. When required it is best performed by ultrasound guided needle sampling after 18 weeks of gestation rather than the more invasive fetoscopic technique. Mortality from this procedure is reported to be 1–2%.

2.4.5 Fetal Surgery

There is a spectrum of interventions ranging from simple aspiration of cysts to open fetal surgery. Minimally invasive techniques such as ablation of vessels in sacrococcygeal teratoma, fetoscopic ablation of posterior urethal valves, tracheal occlusion for congenital diaphragmatic hernia, etc. are currently under trial. However, laser ablation in twin-to-twin transfusion is now well established.

2.4.6 Genetic Diagnoses

Antenatal detection of genetic abnormalities is increasing especially in high-risk pregnancies. Previously undiagnosed conditions such as cystic fibrosis, Beckwith-Wiedemann syndrome, Hirshsprung's disease, sickle cell disease, etc. may be detected prenatally following invasive testing and genetic counselling and assessment offered early in pregnancy.

2.4.7 Future Developments

The aim of prenatal diagnosis and testing is to ensure 100% accuracy without fetal loss or injury and no maternal risk. National plans to improve Down's screening using ultrasound and biochemical combination tests are now in place in the UK. Research into new markers for chromosomal abnormalities is ongoing. The fetal nasal bone is one such example, which may assist, in detecting babies with chromosomal abnormalities.

Management of Rhesus disease is showing promise whereby fetal blood groups may be determined from maternal blood samples through detection of free fetal DNA. The search for fetal components in maternal blood is an exciting and expanding field of research since past and present efforts to isolate and use them for diagnosis have met with little success. Rapid detection techniques versus traditional cultures for karyotyping are currently under debate.

Three-dimensional images from new ultrasound machines may have a useful role in diagnosis and assessment of facial deformities such as cleft lip and palate. Magnetic resonance imaging (MRI) may assist in better defining some lesions difficult to view on conventional prenatal scanning such as the presacral teratoma, posterior urethral valves in the presence of oligohydramnios and hindbrain lesions. At present, MRI is unlikely to replace conventional ultrasound scans.

2.5 Specific Surgical Conditions

2.5.1 Congenital Diaphragmatic Hernia (CDH)

CDH accounts for 1 in 3,000 live birth and challenges the neonatologist and paediatric surgeons in the management of this high-risk condition. Mortality remains high (more than 60%) when the "hidden" mortality of in utero death and termination of pregnancy are considered. Lung hypoplasia and pulmonary hypertension account for most deaths in isolated CDH newborns. Associated anomalies (30–40%) signify a grave prognosis with a survival rate of less than 10%.

In the UK, most CDHs are diagnosed at the 20-week anomaly scan with a detection rate approaching 60%, although as early as 11 weeks gestation has been reported. Magnetic resonance imaging (MRI) has a useful role in accurately differentiating CDH from cystic lung lesions and may be useful in measuring fetal lung volumes as a predictor of outcome. Cardiac anomalies (20%), chromosomal anomalies of trisomy 13 and 18 (20%) and urinary, gastrointestinal and neurological (33%) anomalies can co-exist with CDH and should be ruled out by offering the patient fetal echocardiogram, amniocentesis and detailed anomaly scans. In these CDH patients, early detection, liver in the chest, polyhydramnios and fetal lung head ratio (LHR) of less than 1 are implicated as poor predictors of outcome. In these patients with poor prognostic signs, fetal surgery for CDH over the last 2 decades has been disappointing; however, benefit from fetal intervention with tracheal occlusion (FETO) awaits randomised studies. A favourable outcome in CDH with the use of antenatal steroids has not been resolved in the clinical settings. Elective delivery at a specialised centre is recommended with no benefit from caesarean section.

Post-natal management is aimed at reducing barotrauma to the hypoplastic lung by introducing high frequency oscillatory ventilation (HFOV) or permissive hypercapnea, and treating severe pulmonary hypertension with nitric oxide. No clear benefits for CDH with ECMO (extra corporeal membrane oxygenation) have been concluded in a 2002 Cochrane ECMO study.

Surgery for CDH is no longer an emergency procedure. Delayed repair following stabilisation is employed in most paediatric surgical centres. Primary repair using the trans-abdominal route is achieved in 60–70% of patients with the rest requiring a prosthetic patch. Complications of sepsis or reherniation with prosthetic patch requiring revision are recorded in 50% of survivors. Minimally invasive techniques have been successful in repairing diaphragmatic defects in "stable" infants.

Long-term survivors of CDH are reported to develop chronic respiratory insufficiency (48%), gastro-oesophageal reflux (89%) and neurodevelopment delay (30%).

2.5.2 Cystic Lung Lesions

Congenital cystic adenomatoid malformations (CCAMs), bronchopulmonary sequestrations (BPS) or "hybrid" lesions containing features of both are common cystic lung lesions noted on prenatal scan. Less common lung anomalies include bronchogenic cysts, congenital lobar emphysema and bronchial atresia. Congenital cystic lung lesions are rare anomalies with an incidence of 1 in 10,000 to 1 in 35,000.

Prenatal detection rate of lung cysts at the routine 18–20 week scan is almost 100% and may be the commonest mode of actual presentation. Most of these lesions are easily distinguished from congenital diaphragmatic hernia; however, sonographic features of CCAM or BPS are not sufficiently accurate and correlate poorly with histology. Magnetic resonance imaging (MRI), though not routinely used, may provide better definition for this condition; however, inaccuracies were reported in 11% of cases.

Bilateral disease and hydrops fetalis are indicators of poor outcome, whereas mediastinal shift, polyhydramnios and early detection are not poor prognostic signs. In the absence of termination, the natural fetal demise of antenatally diagnosed cystic lung disease is 28%. It is well documented that spontaneous involution of cystic lung lesions can occur but complete post-natal resolution is rare, and apparent spontaneous "disappearance" of antenatally diagnosed lesions should be interpreted with care, as nearly half of these cases subsequently require surgery.

In only 10% of cases the need for fetal intervention arises. The spectrum of intervention includes simple centesis of amniotic fluid, thoracoamniotic shunt placement, percutaneous laser ablation and open fetal surgical resection. Maternal steroid administration has also been reported to have a beneficial effect on some CCAMs although the mechanism is unclear. A large cystic mass and hydrops in isolated cystic lung lesions are the only real indication for fetal intervention.

Normal vaginal delivery is recommended unless maternal conditions indicate otherwise. Large lesions are predicted to become symptomatic shortly after birth (as high as 45% in some series); thus, delivery at a specialised centre would be appropriate. However, smaller lesions are less likely to be symptomatic at birth and could be delivered at the referring institution with follow up in a paediatric surgery clinic.

Post-natal management is dictated by clinical status at birth. Symptomatic lesions require urgent radiological evaluation with chest radiograph and ideally CT scan (Fig. 2.2) followed by surgical excision. In asymptomatic cases, post-natal investigation consists of chest

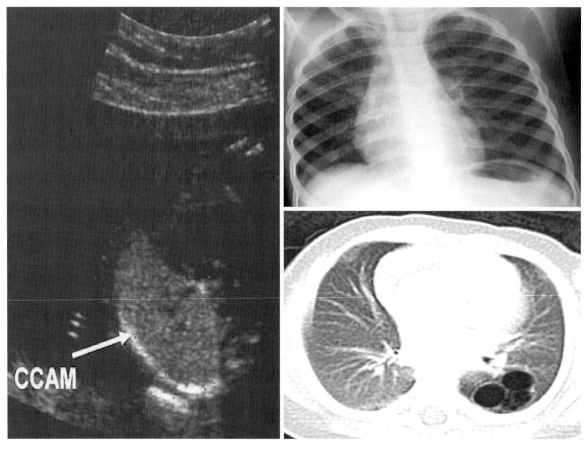

Fig. 2.2 Prenatal scan and post-natal radiological features of CCAM

CT scan within 1 month of birth, even if regression or resolution is noted on prenatal scanning. Plain radiography should not be relied on, because it will miss and underestimate many lesions.

Surgical excision of post-natal asymptomatic lesions remains controversial, with some centres opting for conservative management. The approach to treating this asymptomatic group has evolved in some centres, whereby a CT scan is performed within 1 month post birth, followed by surgery before 6 months of age due to the inherent risk of infection and malignant transformation. Small lesions less than 3 cm may be managed expectantly with annual CT scan, bearing in mind that the true resolution of these lesions is exceptional. Successful outcome of greater than 90% have been reported for these surgically managed asymptomatic lung lesions.

2.6 Abdominal Wall Defects

Exomphalos and gastroschisis are both common but distinct abdominal wall defects with an unclear aetiology and a controversial prognosis. Attention may be drawn to their presence during the second trimester because of raised maternal serum alpha-fetoprotein level or abnormal ultrasound scans.

2.6.1 Exomphalos

Exomphalos is characteristically a midline defect, at the insertion point of the umbilical cord, with a viable sac composed of amnion and peritoneum containing herniated abdominal contents. Incidence is known to be 1 in 4,000 live births. Associated major abnormalities that include trisomy 13, 18 and 21, Beckwith-Wiedemann syndrome (macroglossia, gigantism, exomphalos), Pentology of Cantrell (sternal, pericardial, cardiac, abdominal wall and diaphragmatic defect), cardiac, gastrointestinal and renal abnormalities are noted in 60–70% of cases; thus, karyotyping, in addition to detailed sonographic review and fetal echocardiogram, is essential for complete prenatal screening. Fetal intervention is unlikely in this condition. If termination is not considered, normal vaginal delivery at a centre with neonatal surgical expertise is recommended and delivery by caesarean section only is reserved for large exomphalos with exteriorised liver to prevent damage.

Surgical repair includes primary closure or a staged repair with a silo for giant defects. Occasionally in vulnerable infants with severe pulmonary hypoplasia or complex cardiac abnormalities the exomphalos may be left intact and allowed to slowly granulate and epithelialise by application of antiseptic solution. Post-natal morbidity occurs in 5–10% of cases. Malrotation and adhesive bowel obstruction does contribute to mortality in isolated exomphalos; however, the majority of these children survive to live normal lives.

2.6.2 Gastroschisis

Gastroschisis is an isolated lesion that usually occurs on the right side of the umbilical defect with evisceration of the abdominal contents directly into the amniotic cavity. The incidence is increasing from 1.66 per 10,000 births to 4.6 per 10,000 births affecting mainly young mothers typically less than 20 years old. Associated anomalies are noted in only 5–24% of cases with bowel atresia the most common co-existing abnormality. On prenatal scan with a detection rate of 100%, the bowel appears to be free floating, and the loops may appear to be thickened due to damage by amniotic fluid exposure causing a "peel" formation. Dilated loops of bowel (Fig. 2.3) may be seen from obstruction secondary to protrusion from a defect or atresia due to intestinal ischaemia.

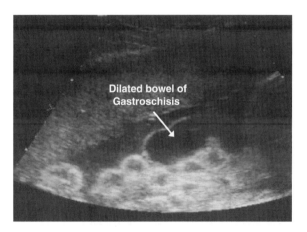

Fig. 2.3 Dilated bowel in gastroschisis

Predicting outcome in fetuses with gastroschisis based on prenatal ultrasound finding remains a challenge. There is some evidence that maximum small bowel diameter may be predictive; however, thickened matted bowel and Doppler measurements of the superior mesenteric artery are not accurate predictors of outcome. To reduce the rate of third trimester fetal loss, serial ultrasounds are performed to monitor the development of bowel obstruction and delivery around 37 weeks recommended at a centre with neonatal surgical expertise.

Recently a randomised control trial has challenged elective preterm delivery. Delivery by caesarean section has no advantage to normal vaginal route. Despite efforts to plan elective delivery, 50% of cases will require emergency caesarean section due to development of fetal distress.

Various methods of post-natal surgical repair include the traditional primary closure, reduction of bowel without anaesthesia, reduction by preformed silo, or by means of a traditional silo. Co-existing intestinal atresia could be repaired by primary anastamosis or staged with stoma formation. Variation in achieving full enteral feeding due to prolonged gut dysmotility is expected in all cases.

The long-term outcome in gastroschisis is dependent on the condition of the bowel. In uncomplicated cases the outcome is excellent in more than 90% of cases. The mortality of live born infants is 5% with further 5% suffering short bowel syndrome and 10% requiring surgery for adhesive bowel obstruction. Late third trimester fetal loss should always be mentioned during fetal counselling.

2.7 Tracheo-Oesophageal Fistula (TOF) and Oesophageal Atresia (OA)

Repair of TOF/OA is a condition that measures the skill of paediatric surgeons from trainees to independent surgeons. The incidence is estimated at 1 in 3,000 births. Prenatally, the condition may be suspected from maternal polyhydramnios and absence of a fetal stomach bubble at the 20-week anomaly scan. Prenatal scan diagnosis of TOF/OA is estimated to be less than 42% sensitive with a positive predicted value of 56%. Additional diagnostic clues are provided by associated anomalies such as trisomy (13,18,21), VACTERL sequence (vertebral, anorectal, cardiac, tracheo-oesophageal, renal, limbs) and CHARGE association (coloboma, heart defects, atresia choanae, retarded development, genital hypoplasia, ear abnormality). Associated anomalies are present in more than 50% of cases and worsen the prognosis; hence, prenatal karyotyping is essential. Duodenal atresia may co-exist with TOF/OA. The risk of recurrence in subsequent pregnancies for isolated TOF/OA is less than 1%. Delivery is advised at a specialised centre with neonatal surgical input.

Postnatal surgical management is dependent on the size and condition of the baby, length of the oesophageal gap and associated anomalies. Primary repair of the oesophagus is the treatment of choice; however, if not achieved, staged repair with upper oesophageal pouch care and gastrostomy or organ replacement with stomach or large bowel are other options. Associated anomalies require evaluation and treatment. Advanced paediatric endosurgical centres may offer minimally invasive thoracoscopic approach to the repair of TOF. Early outcome of a high leak rate and oesophageal stricture requiring dilatation in 50% of cases are expected where the anastamosis of the oesophagus is created under tension.

Improved perinatal management and inherent structural and functional defects in the trachea and oesophagus indicate long-term outcome. In early life, growth of the child is reported to be below the 25th centile in 50% of cases, respiratory symptoms in two-thirds of TOF/OA and gastro-oesophageal reflux recorded in 50% of patients. Quality of life is better in the isolated group with successful primary repair as compared to those with associated anomalies and delayed repair.

2.8 Gastrointestinal Lesions

The presence of dilated loops of bowel (>15 mm in length and 7 mm in diameter) on prenatal ultrasound scan is indicative of bowel obstruction.

Duodenal atresia has a characteristic "double bubble" appearance on prenatal scan, resulting from the simultaneous dilatation of the stomach and proximal duodenum. Detection rate on second trimester anomaly scan is almost 100% in the presence of polyhydramnios and the "double bubble" sign. Associated anomalies are present in approximately 50% of cases with most notably trisomy 21 in 30% of cases, cardiac anomalies in 20% and the presence of VACTERL association (vertebral, anorectal, cardiac, tracheo-oesophageal, renal and limbs).

The incidence of duodenal atresia is 1 in 5,000 live births. The postnatal survival rate is >95% with associated anomalies, low birth weight and prematurity contributing to the <5% mortality. Temporary delay in enteral feeding occurs due to the dysmotility in the dilated stomach and duodenum.

Many bowel abnormalities may be noted on prenatal scanning (dilated bowel, ascites, cystic masses, hyperparistalsis, poyhydramnios and echogenic bowel); however, none is absolutely predictive of postnatal outcome. Patients with obstruction frequently have findings (especially in the third trimester) of bowel dilatation, polyhydramnios and hyperparistalsis, but ultrasound is much less sensitive in diagnosing anomalies in the large bowel than those in the small bowel. Since the large bowel is mostly a reservoir, with no physiologic function in utero, defects in this region such as anorectal malformations or Hirschsprung's disease are very difficult to detect. Bowel dilatation and echogenic bowel may be associated with cystic fibrosis; therefore, all such fetuses should undergo postnatal evaluation for this disease. Prenatally diagnosed small bowel atresia does not select for a group with a worse prognosis and survival rates are 95–100%.

2.9 Sacrococcygeal Teratoma

Sacrococcygeal teratoma (SCT) is the commonest neonatal tumour accounting for 1 in 35,000 to 40,000 births. Four types have been defined:

Type 1 external tumour with a small presacral component

Type 2 external tumours with a large presacral component

Type 3 predominantly presacral with a small external component

Type 4 entirely presacral

The latter carry the worst prognosis due to delay in diagnosis and malignant presentation. Doppler ultrasound is the diagnostic tool; however, fetal MRI provides better definition of the intrapelvic component. SCT is a highly vascular tumour and the fetus may develop high cardiac output failure, anaemia and ultimately hydrops with a mortality of almost 100%. Fetal treatment of tumour resection or ablation of the feeding vessel has been attempted in hydropic patients. Caesarean section may be offered to patients with large tumours to avoid the risk of bleeding during delivery. Post-natal outcomes following surgery in type 1 and 2 lesions are favourable; however, type 3 and 4 tumours may present with urological problems and less favourable outcomes. Long-term follow up with alpha fetoprotein and serial pelvic ultrasounds are mandatory to exclude recurrence of the disease.

2.10 Renal Anomalies

Urogenital abnormalities are among the commonest disorders seen in the perinatal period and account for almost 20% of all prenatally diagnosed anomalies. The routine use of antenatal ultrasound scans has resulted in the early detection of these conditions and in selected cases has led to the development of management strategies including fetal intervention aimed at preservation of renal function. Two major issues are the indications for intervention in bladder outlet obstruction and early pyeloplasty in infancy in cases with hydronephrosis.

Prenatal evaluation of a dilated urinary tract is based on serial ultrasound scans as well as measurement of urinary electrolytes. Ultrasonography provides measurements of the renal pelvis, assessment of the renal parenchyma as well as the detection of cysts

in the cortex. In severe disease, lack of amniotic fluid may make ultrasound assessment of the renal tract difficult and MRI may be helpful. Oligohydramnios is indicative of poor renal function and poor prognosis owing to the associated pulmonary hypoplasia. Urogenital anomalies co-exist with many other congenital abnormalities and amniocentesis should be offered in appropriate cases. It is estimated that 3% of infants will have an abnormality of the urogenital system and half of these will require some form of surgical intervention.

2.10.1 Upper Urinary Tract Obstruction

Antenatal hydronephrosis accounts for 0.6–0.65% pregnancies. The most common cause of prenatal hydronephrosis is pelvi-ureteric junction obstruction (PUJ), others being transient hydronephrosis, physiological hydronephrosis, multicystic kidney, posterior urethral valves, ureterocele, ectopic ureter, etc. The prognosis of antenatally diagnosed hydronephrosis in unilateral disease and in renal pelvic diameter of <10mm is excellent. Spontaneous resolution is noted in 20% of patients at birth and 80% at 3 years of age. Only 17% of prenatally diagnosed hydronephrosis need surgical intervention. Post-natal management of hydronephrosis requires ultrasound at birth and at 1 month of age, and further evaluation with radiology and scintigraphy if an abnormality is suspected. The non-operative treatment of antenatally detected hydronephrosis has been carefully monitored over a 17-year period, and from an analysis of six patient series the conclusion is that this approach is safe.

2.10.2 Lower Urinary Tract Obstruction

Posterior urethral valves (PUV) are the most common cause for lower urinary tract obstruction in boys with an incidence of 1 in 2,000 to 4,000 live male births. The diagnosis of PUV is suspected on the prenatal ultrasound finding of bilateral hydronephrosis associated with a thickened bladder and decreased amniotic fluid volume. Serial fetal urine analysis may provide prognostic information on renal function.

Prenatal diagnosis for patients with PUV is a poor prognostic sign with 64% incidence of renal failure and transient pulmonary failure, compared to 33% in the postnatally diagnosed patients. Pulmonary hypoplasia secondary to oligohydramnios largely contributes to the morbidity and mortality from fetal urethral obstruction. Outcomes of fetal intervention with vesicoamniotic shunting or fetal cystoscopic ablation of urethal valve are still under review and await a multi-center trial.

Postnatal management includes ultrasound confirmation of the diagnosis, bladder drainage via a suprapubic or urethral route and contrast imaging of the urethra. Primary PUV ablation, vesicostomy or ureterostomy are postnatal surgical options. The overall outcome from this disease is unfavourable.

2.11 Conclusion

The boundaries of paediatric surgical practice have been extended by prenatal diagnosis. The care of patients with surgically correctable defects can now be planned prenatally with the collaborative effort of obstetricians, geneticists, neonatologists and paediatric surgeons. The understanding of the specific surgical condition's prenatal natural history, the limitations of prenatal diagnosis, the detection of associated anomalies, the risks and indications of fetal intervention programmes and postnatal outcomes are essential to prenatal counselling. Prenatal counselling is an essential component of paediatric surgical practice and should be ensured in the training programme for future paediatric surgeons.

Further Reading

Black R, Boyd P (2004) What's new in prenatal diagnosis? Trends Urol Gynaecol Sex Health 9:9–11

Boyd PA, Keeling JW (2007) Congenital abnormalities, prenatal diagnosis and screening. In JW Keeling (ed) Fetal and Neonatal Pathology, 4th edn. Springer-Verlag, New York

Harrison MR (2006) The fetus as a patient. In JL Grosfeld, JA O'Neill, EW Fonkalsrud, AG Coran (eds) Pediatric Surgery. Mosby, Philadelphia, pp 77–88

Lakhoo K (2007) Fetal counselling for congenital malformations. PSI 23:509–519

Lakhoo K et al (2006) Best clinical practice: surgical conditions of the fetus and newborn. Early Hum Dev 82(5):281–324

Puri P, Höllwarth ME (eds) (2006) Pediatric Surgery. Springer, Berlin, Heidelberg

Sylvester K, Albanese CT (2005) The fetus as a patient. In KT Oldham, PM Colombani, RP Foglia, MA Skinner, (eds) Principles and Practice of Pediatric Surgery. Lippincott Williams & Wilkins, Philadelphia, PA, pp 27–47

Transport of the Surgical Neonate

3

Prem Puri and Udo Rolle

Contents

3.1 Introduction

The successful outcome of an operation performed on a newborn with congenital anomalies depends not only on the skill of the paediatric surgeon but also on that of a large team consisting of a paediatrician, anaesthetist, radiologist, pathologist, biochemist, nurses, and others necessary for dealing satisfactorily with the newborn infant subjected to surgery. Advances in neonatal intensive care dictate that effective and efficient treatment of the sickest neonates can only be available by concentrating resources such as equipment and skilled staff in a few specialist paediatric centres that have responsibilities to a particular region. It is well established that the outcome of critically ill neonates is better if they are cared for in specialised tertiary centres. In addition, it has been shown that the prognosis for ill neonates is better if postnatal care is given in the same hospital in which they were born. However, not every critically ill neonate can and must be antenatally transferred. Neonates with congenital malformations will therefore have to be transported safely to the specialised centres, sometimes over considerable distances.

3.2 Prenatal Transfer

The prenatal transport of term foetuses with antenatally diagnosed surgical abnormalities does not improve the outcome if the quality of care before and during transport is good. However, many studies support the in-utero transportation of the high-risk foetus, particularly the very low birth weight (VLBW) babies and those with life-threatening neonatal surgical problems.

P. Puri and M. Höllwarth (eds.), *Pediatric Surgery: Diagnosis and Management,*
DOI: 10.1007/978-3-540-69560-8_3, © Springer-Verlag Berlin Heidelberg 2009

Hypothermia remains a main problem in these babies and it adversely affects neonatal outcome. Poor post-transfer temperature seems to be an independent predictor of death. Therefore, whenever possible, threatening preterm delivery before 28 weeks of gestation should be converted to in-utero transport.

3.3 Pre-transfer Management

Transferring a newborn without proper stabilisation is associated with increased morbidity and mortality. The golden rule still is that no neonate should be transported unless his or her condition has been sufficiently stabilised to survive the expected duration of the journey.

Prior to the transportation the newborn needs to be resuscitated and stabilised. This period has to be managed by the local team. The key issues in stabilising neonates for the transfers are airways and breathing; circulation; temperature; blood glucose; infection; parent's information and transfer team information (Table 4.1).

Careful attention to the pre-transfer management will provide a higher margin of safety during the journey, when access to the patient is restricted and it may be difficult to provide adequate treatment should problems arise. Therefore, a standard protocol for the pre-transfer management is recommended.

All babies must be properly resuscitated before the journey is undertaken. Thermoregulation requires critical attention. Hypothermia causes an increase in the neonate's metabolic rate with a subsequent increase in glucose and oxygen use resulting in acidosis and, if not reversed, persistent pulmonary hypertension develops. This can be avoided by warming the baby to a core temperature of at least 35°C and using a pre-warmed transport incubator in a pre-warmed ambulance, with the thermal environment adjusted so as to maintain correct rectal temperature. It should be ensured that the airway is clear and that the baby is well oxygenated and that ventilation can be maintained during transport. If any risk of deterioration in spontaneous breathing is present, the child should be intubated before departure. Every neonate requiring transport must have a functioning nasogastric tube of adequate size to prevent vomiting and aspiration. It should be taped securely in position and kept on open drainage or attached to a low pressure suction pump

Table 4.1 Standard protocol for neonatal transportation (Modified from Fenton et al. 2004)

Airway/breathing
Intubation must be considered before transfer if:
Oxygen requirement > 50%
Rising $PaCO_2$
Recurrent apnoea
<30 weeks of gestation
Control of the correct tube position
Respiratory support
Circulation
Arterial access
Repeated blood gases
Measurement of blood pressure
Intravenous access
Fluids
Inotropes
Coagulation
Vitamin K
Gastrointestinal
Nasogastric tube
Temperature
Support for transport
Blood glucose
Measurement and stabilization
Secure intravenous access
Infection
Screening if indicated
Start of treatment
Parents information
Transfer team/receiving centre information

that should be aspirated every 10–20 min to prevent aspiration. Two reliable and secure routes of venous access should be in place. Many surgical newborn infants have abnormal losses of water, electrolytes and proteins, which must be replaced to prevent hypovolaemia and shock. Intravenous fluids must be initiated immediately and sometimes initiation of inotropic vasopressors such as dopamine or dobutamine may be warranted. Also, glucose homeostasis must be maintained and close monitoring of glucose blood levels should be performed regularly and corrected if necessary. Furthermore, a number of essential data should be transferred with the infant, which are the clinical history, X-ray films and laboratory reports. It should be clearly documented whether vitamin K was administered. Prophylactic broad-spectrum antibiotics should be started if there is a risk of infection. A sample of maternal blood should be sent to facilitate cross-matching. Signed parental consent for operation, signed by the mother if the parents are not married, should be sent together with a contactable phone number in order to explain the surgical condition of the child and the operation procedure to the parents.

Special attention needs to be focussed on the interaction between the referring and the transfer team. The main issue is to ensure a high quality communication between the teams with special emphasis on the appreciation of each other to provide a safe transportation for the child.

3.3.1 Transport Team

Local and individual circumstances will determine whether the referring or specialist centre will send a transport team. Also, the composition of the team may vary from institution to institution. It has been clearly shown that the presence of a highly skilled transport team at a high-risk preterm delivery improves the quality of neonatal resuscitation by increasing intubation success rates and achieving early vascular access. Neonates resuscitated by dedicated neonatal retrieval teams were less likely to become significantly hypothermic. The team should ideally consist of a paediatrician and a trained neonatal nurse familiar with and able to anticipate potential problems associated with specific lesions.

A very interesting study published recently compared neonatal transport teams with and without a physician and showed that non-physician teams (advanced practice nurse) responded more quickly and spent less time at the referring facility. This is an important factor because there is evidence of an association between duration of transport and increased neonatal mortality.

3.3.2 Transport Vehicles

Selection of a transport vehicle is dependent on the distance travelled, geography, weather conditions, the nature of the infant's problem and the need for speed. A variety of conveyances are in popular use, including ground ambulances, helicopters and fixed-wing aircraft. Ambulance transport is generally preferable

to helicopter but is rather slow. Air transport has several disadvantages. A major disadvantage is that separate ground transport must be arranged at both ends to move the baby between the airport and the hospital. The noise, vibrations and poor lighting make in-flight monitoring of the infant difficult in a rotary-wing aircraft (helicopter). This problem is much less in a fixed-wing aircraft. The transport incubator should be securely strapped in case of turbulence of the plane. The infant in the incubator should be fixed well with a lockable piece of cloth. Moreover, the space in a plane is limited and can cause difficulties in manipulating the airway. Negative effects of altitude on the neonate's body can be detrimental. With increasing altitude, the partial pressure of oxygen decreases, therefore diffusion of oxygen across the alveolar membranes becomes more difficult. To maintain the same level of oxygenation, a higher percentage of oxygen may be required. Moreover, the barometric pressure will also decrease with increasing altitude, the volume of gas will increase and any air trapped in a body cavity will expand. This could have a dramatic effect on pulmonary function. It is very important to have medical and nursing equipment functioning well. Monitoring is essential during transfer because clinical assessment can be limited due to suboptimal lighting, noise, vibration and lack of space. Invasive and non-invasive measures of arterial pressure, pulse oxymetry, electrocardiograph (ECG), core temperature measurement and pressure transducers for central venous and intracranial pressure readouts must be present. All monitors and syringe pumps should be battery operated. A range of airway and ventilatory equipment including self-inflating resuscitation bags, masks, airways, laryngoscope handles and blades, uncuffed neonatal endotracheal tubes of various size, humidifiers, portable suction apparatus and oxygen supplies must be available in case airway problems should occur. Additionally, an appropriately stocked box including intravenous (IV) supplies with intraosseous needles, chest tubes and umbilical catheter kits with sterile equipment and emergency drugs should be present. After each transport, record documenting equipment used should be filled in and the equipment unit checked and restocked. The equipment kit should be controlled weekly by the neonatal transport nurse on duty and servicing of the transport incubator and the monitoring equipment should be carried out.

3.3.3 Transport Incubators

Portable incubator is the central piece of equipment for neonatal transfer to provide warmth, visibility and access. It should be equipped with a cardiorespiratory monitor, pulse oxymeter, infusion pump, oxygen analyser, oxygen and air cylinders, double Plexiglas walls and shock-absorbing wheels. The incubator must be able to run on batteries and be capable of providing heat for an extended period of time in various ambient temperature extremes.

3.3.4 Transport Procedure

A save and effective transport procedure involves early and effective communication between the referring centre and the receiving centre, stabilisation of the baby pre-transfer and provision of special care during transport. All too often, transport is hastily arranged and conducted in a vacuum of communication, resulting in preventable catastrophes such as vomiting and aspiration, hypothermia, hypovolaemia and airway obstruction. Once a surgical neonate is identified as potentially needing transfer, this should be arranged by personnel with appropriate expertise, i.e. on senior level. We introduced a standardised transfer-form booklet in our institution. A form is filled in during the initial conversation with the referring centre. It contains all the necessary medical and practical details regarding actual transfer and specific management of the surgical problem of the newborn. By increasing awareness of potential problems, referring hospitals will be less inclined to neglect precise instructions concerning specific surgical conditions.

3.3.5 The Receiving Centre

Continuation of care is essential to improve neonatal outcome. On arrival at the tertiary centre, a brief report of prenatal, labour, and delivery history should be given by the transport nurse to the newborn intensive care nurse, together with details of the newborn's resuscitation and any problems experienced during transfer. The accompanying paediatrician should review the baby and all documents together with the accepting surgeon and anaesthetist if necessary. The parents should be introduced to all staff who will be involved in the care of their baby. Every procedure should be explained in a clear and comprehensive language to avoid confusion and parental fear. The consent form should be updated if need be. Blood tests and radiological examinations can be ordered subsequently.

3.4 Special Considerations

3.4.1 Gastroschisis

There is clear evidence that antenatal transfer of a child with abdominal wall defects is preferable but not essential. Appropriate post-natal transfer has no negative influence on the outcome.

The baby with gastroschisis is at higher risk of hypothermia, excessive fluid loss and shock, infection, intestinal strangulation, necrosis and obstruction due to the small size of the paraumbilical defect and to the lack of a covering peritoneal or amniotic membrane. Treatment starts immediately after delivery in order to prevent water and heat loss. Heat loss is a frequent problem and hypothermia can result. Therefore, radiant heating should be available in the room and the baby should be kept in a warmed incubator with temperature monitored frequently. Intubation and ventilation is done if required. A nasogastric tube is passed for intestinal decompression and prevention of pulmonary aspiration. The exposed bowel and the nasogastric aspirates might result in a fluid and protein loss of up to 30 ml/kg/day. Therefore, immediate resuscitation with adequate IV-fluids (120 ml/kg/24 h) to overcome substantial water, electrolyte and protein losses is started. Pulse rate and mean arterial pressure is observed and blood and glucose are taken. At the same time, vitamin K is administered and broad-spectrum antibiotics (ampicillin, gentamycine and metronidazole) are commenced to reduce contamination of the exposed intestinal loops. A urinary catheter is passed to decompress the bladder and to monitor urinary output. The bowel is localised in the centre of the abdomen and cling film is used to encircle the exposed intestine and is wrapped around the baby. Dry sterile gauze dressing is draped around the cling film to support and protect the highly mobile bowel additionally and to prevent mesenteric injury or venous congestion.

3.4.2 Omphalocele

The initial objectives for the neonatologist are to assess and treat respiratory distress, to protect the sac from rupture and infection and to minimise heat loss. A nasogastric tube is passed immediately to decompress the stomach and bowel. The sac should be stabilised in the middle of the abdomen to prevent kinking of the vessels and covered with a sterile, dry, non-adherent dressing to prevent trauma and heat loss. Intravenous fluids, broad-spectrum antibiotics and vitamin K should be started.

3.4.3 Pierre Robin Syndrome

Babies with Pierre Robin syndrome carry a high risk of tongue swallowing and asphyxiation. The baby should be nursed prone and should have an appropriate assessment of the anatomically site of the airway obstruction. A secure oropharyngeal airway needs to be established for the transport.

3.4.4 Choanal Atresia

Neonates with choanal atresia suffer from intermittent hypoxia. The baby should be nursed with an oral airway of appropriate size to keep the mouth open (i.e. laryngeal mask airway) or teeth with the end cut off.

3.4.5 Myelomeningocele

The infant with myelomeningocele should be nursed prone in order to prevent trauma and pressure on the spinal area. A warm sterile, saline-soaked dressing is placed over the lesion and cling film wrapped around the baby to prevent drying and dehiscence. If the sac ruptures and cerebrospinal fluid (CSF) leaks or if the myelomeningocele is open, it should be covered with Betadine-soaked gauze and broad-spectrum antibiotics started. Care must be taken to prevent faecal contamination in sacral lesions. Careful observation and documentation of neurological function is essential before, during and after transport including evaluation of the sensorimotor level and assessment of the degree of hydrocephalus. Furthermore, it is important to provide a latex-free care for these neonates since children with spina bifida have a high index of latex allergy.

3.4.6 Bladder Exstrophy

At birth, the umbilical cord should be ligated close to the abdominal wall and the umbilical clamp removed to prevent mechanical damage to the bladder mucosa and excoriation of the bladder surface. Trauma and damage to the exposed bladder mucosa and plate should be avoided by covering the defect with cling film wrapped around the baby to prevent the mucosa from sticking to clothing or diapers; this will allow urine to escape while establishing a barrier between the environment and the fragile bladder mucosa. Old urine, mucus and any detritus should be washed from the surface of the bladder with body temperature sterile saline at each nappy change and a clean layer of cling film applied, also during transfer. Prophylactic antibiotics should be started immediately.

3.4.7 Oesophageal Atresia with Tracheo-Oesophageal Fistula

Once the diagnosis of oesophageal atresia is suspected, the baby should be transferred to a tertiary referral centre for further investigation and surgery. Some babies will require endotracheal intubation and ventilation (Table 4.1). These infants are particularly at risk because mechanical ventilation is relatively ineffective due to presence of a fistula. Therefore, the tip of the endotracheal tube should be placed proximal to the carina but distal to the fistula. Urgent transfer and ligation of the fistula are essential. Generally, the infant should be handled with care and crying avoided to reduce the risk of aspiration and abdominal distension and thereby, respiratory distress. Moreover, the baby should be well oxygenated at all times and kept in a warm environment. Regurgitation of gastric contents through the fistula during transport can be prevented by keeping the head of the baby in a slightly elevated position or nurse the baby prone or in a right lateral position and thereby decrease the work of breathing and improve oxygenation. The blind upper oesophageal pouch should be kept empty. A Replogle sump catheter should be placed in the pouch and connected to low-intermittent or low-continuous suction in order to prevent accumulation of saliva. The perforations along the side of the catheter are located only near the tip and therefore the possibility of suctioning oxygenated air away from the larynx is minimised. However, these double lumen oesophageal tubes have a tendency to become blocked with mucus and therefore should be irrigated at frequent intervals during transport. Intravenous fluids should be started to provide maintenance and supplemental fluids and electrolytes to compensate oesophageal secretion losses. Infection should be prevented and any existing pneumonitis treated by broad-spectrum antibiotics. Vitamin K should be administered prior to transfer.

3.4.8 Congenital Diaphragmatic Hernia

The initial objective for the neonatologist and anaesthetist is to stabilise the critically ill neonate before transport to the referral centre. A large calibre nasogastric tube should be passed immediately on diagnosis to decompress the gastrointestinal tract and to prevent further compression of the lung. Endotracheal intubation should be performed promptly in a baby with respiratory difficulty or poor gas exchange. Full sedation and paralysis will reduce the risk of barotrauma. Mask ventilation should be avoided because it will distend the stomach and further compromise the respiratory status. Hyperventilation, using low pressures and high oxygen content, correction of acidosis and prevention of thermal and metabolic stress are recommended to prevent pulmonary hypertension. IV-fluids, fresh frozen plasma and dopamine, if necessary, should be started to maintain adequate peripheral perfusion. Prophylactic antibiotics should be started and vitamin K administered. Venous access through the umbilicus is useful for obtaining mixed venous blood gas specimens.

Arterial access with an umbilical artery catheter will allow monitoring of systemic blood pressure and blood gas measurements at the post-ductal level. The baby will also need a right radial arterial line to measure preductal blood gases. This can be inserted on arrival at the referral centre. Acute deterioration of the infant's condition can occur during transfer due to a pneumothorax. Equipment for intercostal drainage must be available since it can be a life-saving manoeuvre. There has been a tremendous growth in the use of extra-corporeal life support for neonatal cardiopulmonary failure in the last two decades. Extra-corporeal membrane oxygenation (ECMO) has been used as a salvage procedure with 50–80% survival in high-risk neonates with congenital diaphragmatic hernia who fail to respond to mechanical ventilation and meet entry criteria. The number of centres providing ECMO is still limited, so special services are needed to transport critically ill neonates to these centres. These special transport teams should be familiar with the pathophysiology of cardiac and respiratory failure and be equipped to continue the monitoring and treatment started at the referring centre, to maintain that level of care during transport and to treat complications of the disease or therapy itself. Now, transportable ECMO systems exist that can effectively stabilise and transport high-risk neonates to an ECMO-competent centre. ECMO transportation has demonstrated acceptable survival but is a high-risk modality and should not replace early referral to an ECMO center.

3.4.9 Intestinal Obstruction

Intestinal obstruction can occur as a result of a number of conditions, e.g. malrotation, duplications of the alimentary tract, intestinal atresias, necrotising enterocolitis, Hirschsprung's disease, meconium ileus and anorectal anomalies. The principles of care are the same irrespective of the level or cause of the obstruction. The main objectives are to decompress the bowel and prevent aspiration, accurately estimate and correct fluid losses and minimise heat loss. A nasogastric tube should be passed and suction carried out every 15–30 min and left on free drainage between aspirations prior to and during transport. Intravenous fluids should be started to correct acid–base and volume deficits and reviewed and adjusted on a 6–8 hourly basis according to the needs of the infant. Broad-spectrum antibiotics are started prophylactically.

3.4.10 Necrotising Enterocolitis

Neonates with necrotising enterocolitis usually are transferred only if surgery is required in case of perforation of the gangrenous bowel resulting in pneumoperitoneum or progressive clinical deterioration with evidence of peritonitis. Usually they are critically ill with sepsis and shock. Preferably the transfer is done while the infant's condition is as stable as possible. Resuscitation with crystalloids, colloids or blood to correct acidosis is started prior to departure. Ventilation with intermittent positive pressure and inotropic support is often required. A sump nasogastric tube on continuous suction is passed and suctioned regularly prior and during transport. Broad-spectrum antibiotics are started.

3.5 Conclusion

The approach to the care of the high-risk newborn has changed dramatically in the past 30 years. The newborn infant with a serious congenital malformation requires assessment and stabilisation by experienced staff prior to and during transport to the receiving centre. Standard protocols need to be established for appropriate stabilisation of the high-risk newborn before transport, which will result in a reduction in perinatal morbidity and mortality.

Further Reading

De la Hunt MN (2006) The acute abdomen in the newborn. Sem Fetal Neonatal Med 11:191–197

Drewett M, Michailidis GD, Burge D (2006) The perinatal management of gastroschisis. Early Hum Dev 82:305–312

Jaimovich DG, Vidyasagr D (2002) Handbook of Pediatric and Neonatal Transport Medicine, 2nd edn. Hanley & Belfus, Philadelphia

King BR, King TM, Foster RL, McCans KM (2007) Pediatric and neonatal transport teams with and without a physician: A comparison of outcomes and interventions. Pediatr Emerg Care 23(2):77–82

Lloyd DA (1996) Transfer of the surgical newborn infant. Semin Neonatol 1:241–248

McNair C, Hawes J, Urguhart H (2006) Caring for the newborn with an omphalocele. Neonatal Netw 25(5):319–327

Mori R, Fujimura M, Shiraishi J, et al (2007) Duration of interfacility neonatal transport and neonatal mortality: Systematic review and cohort study. Pediatr Int 49(4):452–458

Phibbs CS, Baker LC, Caughey AB, Danielsen B, Schmitt SK, Phibbs RH (2007) Level and volume of neonatal intensive care and mortality in very-low-birth-weight infants. N Engl J Med 356(21):2165–2175

Puri P, De Caluwe D (2003) Transport of the surgical neonate. In Puri P (ed) Newborn Surgery. Arnold, London, pp 39–44

Puri P, Höllwarth M (2006) Pediatric Surgery. Springer, Berlin, Heidelberg

Shah PS, Shah V, Qui Z, Ohlsson A, Lee SK (2005) Canadian neonatal network. Improved outcomes of outborn preterm infants if admitted to perinatal centers versus freestanding pediatric hospitals. J Pediatr 146(5):626–631

Pre-operative Management and Vascular Access

4

John Gillick and Prem Puri

Contents

4.1 Introduction

The surgical procedure performed by the paediatric surgeon forms only a part of the continuum of care provided by paediatric surgeons to their patients. The operation is preceded by pre-operative management involving the assessment and optimisation of each individual patient for the surgical procedure. The operation itself is then followed by a post-operative course where the patient's recovery is followed and managed appropriately. This chapter deals with pre-operative management in the paediatric patient with specific reference to vascular access.

4.2 Prenatal Diagnosis

Many of the congenital defects that are of interest to the paediatric surgeon can now be detected before birth; thus, the pre-operative assessment of the newborn with congenital anomaly starts in utero. When serious malformations incompatible with post-natal life are diagnosed early enough, the family may have the option of terminating the pregnancy. Therefore, it is important for every paediatric surgeon who is familiar with the management of congenital anomalies after birth to be involved in the management decisions and family counselling before birth. The main goal of prenatal diagnosis is to improve prenatal care by maternal transport to an appropriate centre and deliver the baby in the time and mode that are appropriate for the specific fetal malformation.

During the past two decades there have been significant advances in modes and techniques for prenatal diagnosis. These include amniocentesis, amniography,

P. Puri and M. Höllwarth (eds.), *Pediatric Surgery: Diagnosis and Management,*
DOI: 10.1007/978-3-540-69560-8_4, © Springer-Verlag Berlin Heidelberg 2009

fetoscopy, fetal sampling and ultrasonography. The latter enables direct imaging of the fetal anatomy and is a non-invasive technique that is safe for both the fetus and the mother. However, it is important to remember that sonography is operator-dependent and the reliability of the information obtained is directly proportional to the skill and experience of the sonographer. With further advances in screening techniques and with the combination of various antenatal screening modalities, such as the Serum, Urine and Ultrasound Screening Study (SURUSS) for Downs syndrome, the efficacy and safety of antenatal screening have improved.

Serial sonographic evaluations are particularly useful for following the progression or regression of any fetal disease. All this important information is an integral part of the pre-operative assessment of a newborn with any kind of congenital malformation.

Neonates born with congenital malformations are usually in urgent need of surgery and, in addition to their surgical problem, may suffer from a multitude of medical problems. Furthermore, they are at a period when significant physiological and maturational changes of transition from fetal to extrauterine life occur. Surgical and anaesthetic intervention at this time may affect this transition by interfering with normal homeostatic controls of circulation, ventilation, temperature, fluid and metabolic balance. To facilitate a smooth pre-operative course, close coordination among the obstetrician, neonatologist, paediatric surgeon and paediatric anaesthesiologist is necessary. An ideally planned delivery should take place in a centre of paediatric surgical excellence.

All neonates undergoing surgery must be carefully assessed pre-operatively, particularly paying attention to the following:

- History and physical examination
- Maintenance of body temperature
- Respiratory function
- Cardiovascular status
- Metabolic status
- Coagulation abnormalities
- Laboratory investigations
- Vascular access
- Fluid and electrolytes, and metabolic responses

4.3 History and Physical Examination

The history of the newborn starts months before delivery, as many of the congenital malformations (e.g. Bochdalek hernia, omphalocele, gastrochisis, sacrococcygeal teratoma and others) nowadays are known to the paediatric surgeon, prenatally. Not only are the anatomical and structural anomalies important but metabolic abnormalities or chromosomal aberrations are even more important, which must be diagnosed prenatally or immediately after birth.

Anticipation of a problem in the delivery room is often based on prenatal diagnosis. For example, identification of a trisomy 21 in the fetus will increase the neonatologist's awareness in evaluating the infant for those abnormalities closely associated with this chromosomal defect, e.g. evaluation for duodenal atresia and congenital heart disease. Conversely, prenatal identification of specific fetal anomalies should signal the paediatrician to evaluate the infant for a chromosomal abnormality.

The most recent advance in prenatal detection of anatomical problems has been the development of fetal ultrasonography, and, in experienced hands, this mode of imaging can be used to detect a wide range of fetal problems, ranging from relatively minor abnormalities to major structural defects. However, this anatomical prenatal diagnosis is only one of the tools that aids in planning care management. An accurate and well documented family history may increase the suspicion that an infant is at risk for an anatomical defect linked to an inherited disorder. In other cases, only the evidence of polyhydramnios should significantly increase suspicion of congenital anomalies.

Most problems are best managed expectantly by natural labour and vaginal delivery at term. Certain malformations, however, such as conjoined twins, giant omphalocele, sacrococcygeal teratoma or large cystic hygroma, often require caesarean section for delivery. Opinion remains divided on the benefits of elective caesarean section for abdominal wall defects, with some authorities finding only limited usefulness, and others suggesting that elective preterm delivery for gastroschisis results in an improved surgical outcome. A recent development is the EX utero Intrapartum Treatment (EXIT) procedure in which the infant is delivered by elective caesarean section, while maintaining feto-placental circulation. This technique has been utilised in a number of congenital malformations in order to establish the child's airway in a controlled manner.

After birth, the assessment of the degree of prematurity, which is an integral part of the physical examination, and the specific type of congenital anomaly must be identified and recorded because of the profound anaesthetic and post-operative implications that are involved. The normal full-term infant has a gestational age of 37 weeks or more and a body weight greater than 2,500 g. Infants born with a birth weight of less than 2,500 g are defined as being of low birth weight (LBW). Babies may be of LBW because they have been born too early (preterm—earlier than 37 weeks' gestational age), or because of intrauterine abnormalities affecting growth (growth retardation). "Small-for-gestational-age" (SGA) infants are those whose birth weight is less than the 10th percentile for their age. Infants may, of course, be both growth retarded and born preterm.

The principle features of prematurity are as follows:

- A head circumference below the 50th percentile
- A thin, semi-transparent skin
- Soft, malleable ears
- Absence of breast tissue
- Absence of plantar creases
- Undescended testicles with flat scrotum and, in females, relatively enlarged labia minora

The physiological and clinical characteristics of these babies are as follows:

- Apnoeic spells
- Bradycardia
- Hypothermia
- Sepsis
- Hyaline membrane disease
- Blindness and lung injury due to use of high levels of oxygen
- Patent ductus arteriosus

In the SGA infant, although the body weight is low, the body length and head circumference approach that of an infant of normal weight for age. These babies are older and more mature. Their clinical and physiological characteristics are given below:

- Higher metabolic rate
- Hypoglycaemia
- Thermal instability
- Polycythemia
- Increased risk of meconium aspiration syndrome

In relation to these differences, three important observations have been reported:

1. LBW infants have a mortality rate that is ten times that of full-sized infants.
2. More than 75% of overall perinatal mortality is related to clinical problems of LBW infants.
3. The rate of anatomical malformation in LBW infants is higher than for infants at term.

4.4 Maintenance of Body Temperature

The mean and range of temperature for newborns are lower than previously described and most temperatures $\leq 36.3°C$ are, in fact, within normal range. Newborn infants, particularly premature infants, have poor thermal stability because of a higher surface area to weight ratio, a thin layer of insulating subcutaneous fat and a high thermoneutral temperature zone. The newborn readily loses heat by conduction, convection, radiation and evaporation, with the major mechanism being radiation. Shivering thermogenesis is absent in the neonate, and the heat producing mechanism is limited to non-shivering thermogenesis through the metabolising of brown fat. Cold stress in these neonates leads to an increased metabolic rate and oxygen consumption, and calories are consumed to maintain body temperature. If prolonged, this leads to depletion of the limited energy reserve and predisposes to hypothermia and increased mortality. Hypothermia can also suggest infection and should trigger diagnostic evaluation and antibiotic treatment if required.

Body temperature in the premature neonate has been found to be an independent risk factor for mortality. Illness in the newborn, particularly when associated with prematurity, further compounds the problems in the maintenance of body temperature. The classic example for such an illness is the newborn with omphalocele or gastroschisis. In a group of 23 neonates with gastroschisis, Muraji et al. found that hypothermia (31–35.4°C), which was found in seven patients on arrival at the hospital, was the most serious pre-operative problem. To minimise heat losses, it is desirable that most sick neonates be nursed in incubators within controlled temperatures. These incubators are efficient for maintaining the baby's temperature, but do not allow adequate access to the sick baby for active resuscitation and observation. Overhead radiant heaters, servocontrolled by a temperature probe on the baby's skin, are preferred and effective in maintaining the baby's temperatures; they also provide visual and electronic monitoring and access for nursing and medical procedures. Hyperthermia should be avoided, because it is associated with perinatal respiratory depression and hypoxic brain injury.

The environmental temperature must be maintained near the appropriate thermoneutral zone for each individual patient because the increase in oxygen consumption is proportional to the gradient between the skin and the environmental temperature. This is 34–35°C for LBW infants up to 12 days of age and 31–32°C at 6 weeks of age. Infants weighing 2,000–3,000 g have a thermoneutral zone of 31–34°C at birth and 29–31°C at 12 days. In an incubator, either the ambient temperature of the incubator can be monitored and maintained at thermoneutrality, or a servo-system can be used. The latter regulates the incubator temperature according to the patient's skin temperature, which is monitored by means of a skin probe on the infant. The normal skin temperature for a full-term infant is 36.2°C, but because of many reasons, benign factors such as excessive bundling and ambient temperature may affect body temperature. Diurnal and seasonal variations in body temperature have also been described. Thus, the control of the thermal environment of the newborn and especially the ill baby with congenital malformations is of utmost importance to the outcome.

4.5 Respiratory Function

Assessment of respiratory function is essential in all neonates undergoing surgery. The main clinical features of respiratory distress are restlessness, tachypnoea, grunting, nasal flaring, sternal recession, retractions and cyanosis. These symptoms are occasionally present in the delivery room due to the anatomical abnormalities involving the airway and lungs and require the most urgent therapy. Conditions that can present with respiratory distress include diaphragmatic hernia (Bochalek), lobar emphysema, pneumothorax, oesophageal atresia with or without tracheo-esophageal fistula, congenital airway obstruction, congenital cystic adenomatoid malformation of the lung, meconium aspiration syndrome

and aspiration pneumonia. It is important to recognise that more than one condition may be present in the same patient. If there is any clinical suspicion or sign of respiratory insufficiency, a chest X-ray should be obtained immediately after the resuscitation to determine the cause of the respiratory distress. All babies with respiratory distress should have a radio-opaque nasogastric tube passed and a radiograph taken that includes the chest and abdomen in order to localise the oesophagus, stomach and bowel gas, and to avoid misdiagnosis of, for example, a diaphragmatic hernia that can be mistaken for a cystic adenomatoid malformation of the lung.

Blood gas studies are essential in the diagnosis and management of respiratory distress. Arterial PO_2 and PCO_2 indicate the state of oxygenation and ventilation, respectively. In the newborn, repeated arterial blood samples may be obtained either by catheterisation of an umbilical artery or by cannulation of radial, brachial or posterior tibial arteries. An important alternative is non-invasive monitoring technique with transcutaneous PO_2 monitors or pulse oximeters. More recently, combined transcutaneous measurement of both SaO_2 and $PaCO_2$ has proved possible. Monitoring of arterial pH is also essential in patients with respiratory distress. Acidosis in the neonate produces pulmonary arterial vasoconstriction and myocardial depression. Respiratory alkalosis causes decreased cardiac output, decreased cerebral blood flow, diminished oxyhemoglobin dissociation and increased airway resistance with diminished pulmonary compliance.

Respiratory failure is the leading cause of death in the neonate. High-frequency ventilation, use of surfactant, use of inhaled nitric oxide (iNO) and extracorporeal membrane oxygenation (ECMO) have been shown to improve survival dramatically in selected neonates. ECMO provides long-term cardiopulmonary support for patients with reversible pulmonary and cardiac insufficiency. It is well accepted as a standard of treatment for neonatal respiratory failure refractory to conventional techniques of pulmonary support. Typically, patients considered for ECMO are 34 gestational weeks or older or weigh more than 2,000 g, have no major cardiac lesions, intracranial haemorrhages less than grade 2, no significant coagulopathies and have had mechanical ventilation for fewer than 10–14 days. It is limited to those infants who have a 20% or less chance of survival if treated with only conventional therapies.

The Extracorporeal Life Support Registry (ELSO) database now contains outcome data on over 20,000 patients with survival rates of more than 80% in neonates. The National ECMO Registry in Ann Arbour, MI, USA, collected reports from all 46 ECMO centres, summarising their collective experience with 1,489 newborns with an overall survival rate of 81.8%. Of this group of neonates, two-thirds of the 139 newborns with congenital diaphragmatic hernia and who underwent ECMO survived. Failure of ventilatory treatment to reverse hypoxemia, acute clinical deterioration after a "honeymoon period" and an alveolar-arterial oxygen gradient >600 mmHg for 12 h were the principle criteria that justified ECMO in these babies. Premature infants were at the highest risk and intracranial bleeding was the most common cause of death in these anticoagulated newborns. The role of ECMO in congenital diaphragmatic hernia is still being studied. Survivors have significant long-term mortality and morbidity. It is important to emphasise that emergency surgery for congenital diaphragmatic hernia is not necessary and that repair should be done only when the patient has been stabilised using conventional ventilation, high frequency ventilation or ECMO if necessary. Neonatal survival rates with an antenatal diagnosis now exceed 80% in some centers. ECMO is an accepted form of therapy in the treatment of neonates with otherwise lethal persistent pulmonary hypertension related to meconium aspiration and sepsis. This mode of therapy has been tried successfully in neonates with congenital cystic lesions of the lung who developed severe pulmonary hypertension following lobectomy and other life-threatening respiratory problems. However, the long-term effects on its survivors are unknown. At present, the reported morbidity still ranges between 13% and 33%. The developmental outcome is normal in most patients. Severe developmental delay has been found in only 2–8% of neonatal patients who undergo ECMO therapy.

Only one randomised trial of conventional therapy versus ECMO in 185 full-term infants has been published recently. Of the infants included in the trial, 68% who were randomised to ECMO therapy survived compared to 41% in the conventionally treated group. Because of the institution of new therapies and differing management styles for treatment of respiratory failure, there has been a marked decrease in neonatal patients treated with ECMO over time.

Surfactant replacement is commonly used in the clinical management of neonates with respiratory distress syndrome (RDS). It may also be effective in other forms of lung disease, such as meconium aspiration syndrome (MAS), neonatal pneumonia, the "adult" form of acute respiratory distress syndrome (ARDS) and congenital diaphragmatic hernia (CDH). It ensues that alveolar stability is promoted, atelectasis is reduced, oedema formation is decreased and the overall work of respiration is minimised.

iNO is available for treatment of persistent pulmonary hypertension of the neonate (PPHNP). It decreases pulmonary vascular resistance leading to diminished extrapulmonary shunt and has a microselective effect that improves ventilation and perfusion matching. It appears to have a role in decreasing the incidence of chronic lung disease in preterm infants. Clinical trials indicate that the need for ECMO in term newborns with PPHN is diminished by iNO. Unfortunately, its beneficial role in the treatment of congenital diaphragmatic hernia has become more uncertain.

In newborns with severe lung disease, HFOV is frequently used to optimise lung inflation and minimise lung injury. The combination of HFOV and iNO is reported to cause the greatest improvement in oxygenation in some newborns with severe PPHN complicated by diffuse parenchymal lung disease and under inflation.

In summary, the type of respiratory care in particular neonates will always depend on clinical and radiological findings supported by blood gas estimations.

4.6 Cardiovascular Status

At birth, the circulation undergoes rapid transition from fetal to neonatal pattern. The ductus arteriosus normally closes functionally within a few hours after birth, while anatomical closure occurs 2–3 weeks later. Prior to birth, the pulmonary arterioles are relatively muscular and constricted. With the first breath, total pulmonary resistance falls rapidly because of the unkinking of vessels with the expansion of the lungs and also because of the vasodilatory effect of inspired oxygen. However, during the first few weeks of life, the muscular pulmonary arterioles retain a significant capacity for constriction, and any constricting influences such as hypoxia may result in rapid return of pulmonary hypertension.

The management of neonates with congenital malformation is frequently complicated by the presence of congenital heart disease. At this time of life, recognition of heart disease is particularly difficult. There may be no murmur audible on first examination, but a loud murmur can be audible a few hours, days or a week later. A newborn undergoing surgery should have a full cardiovascular examination and a chest X-ray. The presence of cyanosis, respiratory distress, cardiac murmurs, abnormal peripheral pulses or congestive heart failure should be recorded. If there is suspicion of a cardiac anomaly, the baby should be examined by a paediatric cardiologist. In recent years the use of the non-invasive technique of echocardiography allows accurate anatomical diagnosis of cardiac anomalies in many cases prenatally.

4.7 Metabolic Status

4.7.1 Acid–Base Balance

The buffer system, renal function and respiratory function are the three major mechanisms responsible for the maintenance of normal acid–base balance in body fluids. Most newborn infants can adapt competently to the physiological stresses of extrauterine life and have a normal acid–base balance. However, clinical conditions such as RDS, sepsis, congenital renal disorders and gastrointestinal disorders may result in gross acid–base disturbances in the newborn. Four basic disturbances of acid–base physiology are metabolic acidosis, metabolic alkalosis, respiratory acidosis and respiratory alkalosis. In a newborn undergoing surgery, identification of the type of disorder, whether metabolic or respiratory, simple or mixed, is of great practical importance to permit the most suitable choice of therapy, and for it to be initiated in a timely fashion. The acid–base state should be determined by arterial blood gases and pH estimation, and must be corrected by appropriate metabolic or respiratory measures prior to operation

4.7.2 Hypoglycaemia

The mechanisms of glucose homeostasis are not well developed in the early post-natal period; this predisposes the neonate, especially the premature neonate, to the risk of both hypoglycaemia and hyperglycaemia.

Prenatally, the glucose requirements of the fetus are obtained almost entirely from the mother, with very little derived from fetal gluconeogenesis. Following delivery, the limited liver glycogen stores are rapidly depleted and the blood glucose level depends on the infant's capacity for gluconeogenesis, the adequacy of substitute stores and energy requirements. Three mechanisms may lead to infantile hypoglycaemia: (1) those with limited glycogen stores, (2) hyperinsulinism and (3) diminished glucose production. Infants at high risk of developing hypoglycaemia include LBW infants (especially SGA infants), infants of toxemic or diabetic mothers and infants requiring surgery who are unable to take oral nutrition and who have the additional metabolic stresses of their disease. Blood glucose level should be maintained above 2.5 mmol/L (45 mg%) at all times. The symptomatic infant should be treated urgently with 50% dextrose, 1–2 ml/kg intravenously, and maintenance i.v. dextrose 10–15% at 80–100 ml/kg/24 h.

Neonates are susceptible to electrolyte imbalances such as hypocalcaemia and hypomagnesemia, particularly in association with prematurity and SGA. Correction of these deficiencies may be required in the pre-operative period.

4.7.3 Hyperbilirubinaemia

Jaundice in the newborn is a common physiological problem observed in 25–50% of all normal newborn infants and in a considerably higher percentage of premature and SGA infants.

It is the result of a combination of shortened red cell survival, with a consequent increase in bilirubin load, and an immature glucuronyl transferase enzyme system with a limited capacity for conjugating bilirubin. This results in transient physiological jaundice that reaches a maximum at the age of 3–4 days, but returns to normal levels at the end of the first week and the bilirubin level does not exceed 170 mmol/L.

Hyperbilirubinaemia in the newborn may have a pathological basis such as sever sepsis, Rh and ABO incompatibilities and congenital haemolytic anaemias. Neonatal haemolytic jaundice usually appears during the first 24 h of life, whereas physiological jaundice, as mentioned before, reaches a peak between 2 and 5 days of life. Other causes for prolonged hyperbilirubinaemia, including those often associated with surgical conditions are biliary obstruction, hepatocellular dysfunction and upper intestinal tract obstruction. Extra-hepatic biliary obstruction should be diagnosed as early as possible, because early operation for biliary atresia is essential to obtain good short-term as well as long-term results. The major concern in neonatal hyperbilirubinaemia (high levels of unconjugated bilirubin) is the risk of kernicterus that can result in brain damage.

Predisposing factors include hypoalbuminaemia (circulating bilirubin is bound to albumin), hypothermia, acidosis, hypoglycaemia, hypoxia, caloric deprivation and the use of drugs (e.g. gentamicin, digoxin and furosemide). When the serum bilirubin concentration approaches a level at which kernicterus is likely to occur, hyperbilirubinaemia must be treated. In most patients, other than those with severe haemolysis, phototherapy is a safe and effective method of treating hyperbilirubinaemia. When the serum indirect bilirubin level rises early and rapidly and exceeds 340 mmol/L, haemolysis is usually the reason, and exchange transfusion is indicated.

4.7.4 Coagulation Abnormalities

Coagulation abnormalities in the neonate should be sought pre-operatively and treated. The newborn is deficient in vitamin K and 1 mg of the same should be administered prior to the operation in order to prevent hypoprothrombinaemia and haemorrhagic disease in the newborn. Although given routinely in most developed countries immediately after birth, its administration should be confirmed with the labour suite. Neonates with severe sepsis, such as those with necrotizing enterocolitis, may develop disseminated intravascular coagulopathy with a secondary platelet deficiency. Such patients should be given fresh-frozen plasma, fresh blood or platelet concentrate, pre-operatively.

Bleeding is one of the major risks associated with neonatal ECMO—a risk that has a particularly devastating outcome. In their group of 45 patients, Weiss and colleagues reported on 12 (27%) patients who sustained haemorrhagic complications. Most of these haemorrhages were intracranial and were the most serious complication. Other less frequent sites of bleeding included the cannulation site, the gastrointestinal tract and chest tube sites. Although the haemorrhage was related to systematic heparinisation, no correlation was found between the activated clotting time or the amount of heparin used and the haemorrhagic complications. An increased risk of haemorrhage was associated with lower platelet counts; hence, aggressive platelet transfusion remains important in preventing haemorrhagic complications using ECMO, although platelet dysfunction may still persist. Attempts at correcting any coagulopathy should be undertaken before the initiation of ECMO. Future directions include the development of heparin-bonded circuits and non-thrombogenic plastic tubing that would allow ECMO circuits without systemic anti-coagulation.

The potential of an increased rate of intraventricular haemorrhage (IVH) has also been reported in term and preterm neonates following iNO therapy. INO leads to a prolonged bleeding time and inhibits platelet aggregation.

4.7.5 Laboratory Investigations

A newborn undergoing surgery should have blood drawn on admission for various investigations, including full blood count, serum sodium, potassium and chloride, urea, calcium, magnesium, glucose, bilirubin and group and cross-match. Blood gases and pH estimation should also be obtained to assess acid–base state and the status of gas exchange. The availability of micro methods in the laboratory has minimised the amount of blood required to do the above blood test. The coagulation status of infants who have been asphyxiated may be abnormal and should be evaluated. Neonatal sepsis can result in disseminated intravascular clotting and sever thrombocytopenia. A platelet count <50 000/mm^3 in the neonate is an indication for pre-operative platelet transfusion. Blood cultures should be obtained wherever there is any suspicion of sepsis.

4.7.6 Fluid and Electrolytes, and Metabolic Responses

Estimation of the parental fluid and electrolyte requirements is an essential part of management of newborn infants with surgical conditions. Inaccurate assessment of fluid requirements, especially in premature babies and LBW infants, may result in a number of serious complications. Inadequate fluid intake may lead to dehydration, hypotension, poor perfusion with acidosis, hypernatremia and cardiovascular collapse. Administration of excessive fluid may result in pulmonary oedema, congestive heart failure, opening of ductal shunts, bronchopulmonary dysphasia and cerebral intraventricular haemorrhage.

In order to plan accurate fluid and electrolyte therapy for the newborn, it is essential to understand the normal body "water" consumption and the routes through which water and solute are lost from the baby. In fetal life around 16 weeks' gestation, total body water (TBW) represents approximately 90% of total body weight, and the proportions of extracellular and intracellular water components are 65% and 25%, respectively. At term, these two compartments constitute about 45% and 30%, respectively, of total body weight, indicating that (1) a shift from extracellular water to intracellular water occurs during development from fetal to neonatal life and (2) relative total body and extracellular fluid volume both decrease with increasing gestational age.

In very small premature infants, water constitutes as much as 85% of total body weight and in the term infants it represents 75% of body weight. The total body water decreases progressively during the first few months of life, falling to 65% of body weight at the age of 12 months, after which it remains fairly constant. The extracellular and intracellular fluid volumes also change with growth.

The objectives of parenteral fluid therapy are to provide the following:

- Maintenance fluid requirements needed by the body to maintain vital functions
- Replacement of pre-existing deficits and abnormal losses
- Basic maintenance requirement of water for growth

Maintenance fluid requirement consists of water and electrolytes that are normally lost through insensible loss, sweat, urine and stools. The amount lost through various sources must be calculated to determine the volume of fluid to be administered. Insensible loss is the loss of water from the pulmonary system and evaporative loss from the skin. Approximately 30% of the insensible water loss occurs through the pulmonary system as moisture in the expired gas; the remainder (about 70%) is lost through the skin. Numerous factors are known to influence the magnitude of insensible water loss. These include the infant's environment (ambient humidity and ambient temperature), metabolic rate, respiratory rate, gestational maturity, body size, surface area, fever and the use of radiant warmers and phototherapy. In babies weighing less than 1,500 g at birth, insensible loss may be up to three times greater than that estimated for term infants. Faranhoff and colleagues found insensible water loss in infants weighing less than 1,250 g to be 60–120 ml/kg/day. Chief among the factors that affect insensible water loss are the gestational age of the infant and the relative humidity of the environment. The respiratory water loss is approximately 5 ml/kg/24 h and is negligible when infants are intubated and on a ventilator. Water loss through sweat is generally negligible in the newborn except in patients with cystic fibrosis, severe congestive heart failure or high environmental temperature. Fectal water losses are 5–20 ml/kg/day

4.7.7 Renal Function, Urine Volume and Concentration in the Newborn

The kidneys are the final pathway regulating fluid and electrolyte balance of the body. The urine volume is dependent on water intake, the quantity of solute for excretion and the maximal concentrating and diluting abilities of the kidneys. Renal function in the newborn infant varies with gestational age and should be evaluated in this context. Very preterm infants younger than 34 weeks gestational age have reduced glomerular filtration rate (GFR) and tubular immaturity in the handling of the filtered solutes when compared to term infants. Premature infants between 34 and 37 weeks gestational age undergo rapid maturation of renal function similar to term infants with rapid establishment of glomerulotubular balance early in the post-natal period. The full-term newborn infant can dilute urine to osmolarities of 30–50 mmol/L and can concentrate it to 550 mmol/L by approximately 1 month of age. The solute for urinary excretion in infants varies from 10 to

20 mmol/100 cal metabolised, which is derived from endogenous tissue catabolism and exogenous protein and electrolyte intake. In this range of renal solute load, a urine volume of 50–80 ml/100 cal would provide a urine concentration between 125 and 400 mmol/L.

If the volume of fluid administered is inadequate, urine volume falls and concentration increases. With excess fluid administration, the opposite occurs. We aim to achieve a urine output of 2 ml/kg/h, which will maintain a urine osmolarity of 250–290 mmol/kg (specific gravity 1,009–1,012) in newborn infants. For older infants and children, hydration is adequate if the urine output is 1–2 ml/kg/h, with an osmolarity between 280 and 300 mmol/kg.

Accurate measurements of urine flow and concentration are fundamental to the management of critically ill infants and children, especially those with surgical conditions and extensive tissue destruction or with infusion of high osmolar solution. In these situations, it is recommended that urine volume be collected and measured accurately.

4.7.8 Pre-operative Management in the Older Child

Many of the pre-operative management strategies used in the neonate are equally applicable to the older child. Pre-operative management needs to be tailored according to a number of factors, including the urgency of the surgery, the age of the child and any associated medical conditions affecting the patient. In the setting of a sick patient requiring an urgent operation, aggressive resuscitation according to Advanced Paediatric Life Support protocols may be required. In the elective setting there is usually more time for a through and meticulous pre-operative course.

Pre-operative evaluation in older children should involve the children themselves understanding and consenting to the planned procedure. The patient may demonstrate sufficient knowledge of the proposed surgery to give or withhold consent and the issue of "Gillick competence" will require evaluation when obtaining informed consent. The level of maturity possessed by the patient may well dictate the provision of in-depth explanation of the planned surgery, including play therapy, modelling, operating room tour and coping skills for the parents. Authors have stressed the importance of the availability of these facilities in order to optimise the psychological pre-operative preparation of the child. The unfortunate alternative that is still commonplace involves the physical restraint of an extremely anxious, non-compliant child in the operating theatre.

Associated medical conditions in paediatric surgical practice may have significant bearing on pre-operative management of these patients. There has been a significant shift in favour of day case paediatric surgery in recent years. The incidence of unplanned admission following day case surgery remains low at approximately 2%. Close liaison between paediatric surgeons and their anaesthetic colleagues pre-operatively should minimise post-operative complications such as unplanned admission following day surgery. In an ideal situation the anaesthetist would review the child in the outpatient setting in partnership with the surgical team.

Although the majority of children undergoing anaesthesia are healthy, it is crucial to detect any underlying risk factor that may lead to an unexpected adverse event in the peri-operative period. However, pre-operative assessment should not involve unnecessary tests that create a stressful environment for the child and the family prior to surgery. Especially for ambulatory patients, a focussed pre-operative clinic that could be nurse-led may be of benefit.

Unfortunately, accurate pre-operative assessment of paediatric patients for peri-operative surgical and anaesthetic risk remains difficult. One of the most utilised tools for risk assessment, the American Society of Anaesthesiologists (ASA) grade, has been shown to have a significant degree of intraoperator variability. There is a need for a more refined tool for pre-operative physical status grading.

As in the neonatal population, adequate pre-operative preparation may involve investigations such as routine bloodwork, radiological studies and identification and correction of underlying medical conditions that might be supposed to contribute to peri-operative morbidity. If blood loss is anticipated, the availability of cross-matched blood should be ensured. Also, it is imperative that all relevant radiological investigations should be present in the operating room at the time of surgery. This is particularly crucial if unexpected operative findings arise and especially when operating on paired organs.

4.8 Vascular Access

In the neonatal period, most infants with surgical conditions cannot be fed in the operative and early postoperative period. It is essential, therefore, to administer fluids in these patients by the i.v. route. With the availability of 22–24 gauge plastic cannulas, percutaneous cannulation of veins has become possible even in small premature infants. Scalp veins and veins of the dorsum of the hand and palmar surface of the wrist are the most common sites used for starting i.v. infusions. With the improvements of techniques and equipment, it is now rarely necessary to perform a "cut-down" in order to administer i.v. fluids. The availability of a dedicated nurse-provided i.v. access team in our institute has greatly enhanced the success rate of obtaining intravenous access in neonates and the older child with "difficult veins". In older children, larger bore canulas, such as 20–18 gauge, are frequently more appropriate. In the resuscitation scenario, where large volumes of fluid may need to be given quickly, it is important to remember Poiseuille's equation, in that the flow rate through a canula is proportional to the 4th power of the canula's radius, thus emphasising the importance of wide-bore canulas in the trauma setting in the older child.

Longer term venous access can be obtained with fine percutaneous intravascular central catheters inserted at bedside without general anaesthesia—the so-called PICC lines (percutaneously inserted central venous catheters). These catheters can be successfully inserted by dedicated nursing personnel to provide long-term venous access with a reduced incidence of thromboembolic complications. A variety of peripheral veins lend themselves to the placement of PICC lines, particularly the scalp veins in most neonates (Fig. 4.1).To minimise thrombotic complications, it is important to ensure that the catheter tip resides in a central vein.

Adequacy of the intravascular volume and the function of the heart can be assessed by a central venous catheter (CVC), which can be inserted through the internal jugular vein and subclavian vein. Usually catheters are placed using the Seldinger technique. This central line is often mandatory and is a basic monitoring aid for the anaesthetist at the time of operation, and sometimes can be performed at the theatre immediately before starting the operation. It is a useful instrument for fluid resuscitation, administration of medication and central venous pressure monitoring.

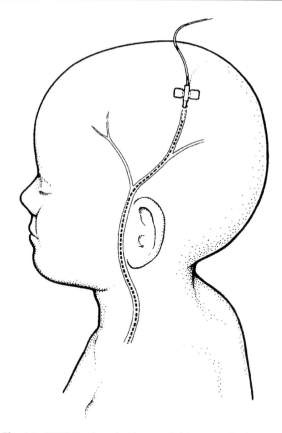

Fig. 4.1 PICC line insertion in superficial temporal vein
Source: (Spitz and Coran 2006)

The next step in the venous access hierarchy is the tunnelled central line (commonly Hickman or Broviac). These are commonly placed in either the neck or groin vein in neonates, and in older children the jugular and subclavian veins are the preferred sites, either approached via an open technique or percutaneously, respectively (Figs. 4.2, 4.3). An alternative site for a tunnelled line in neonates and older children is the saphenous vein, which is easily approached through a groin skin crease incision. (Fig. 4.4) Catheters inserted in the groin site in NICU babies seem to have higher incidence of complications. An advantage of central lines in the paediatric population is that the number of skin punctures required to maintain i.v. access is reduced. Also, in neonates, central lines do not seem to have a higher incidence of sepsis or death, when compared to peripheral lines.

PICC and tunnelled central lines are relatively comparable in terms of efficacy and complications; however if access is required for longer than 15 days a

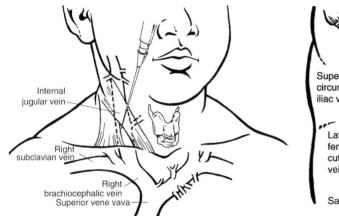

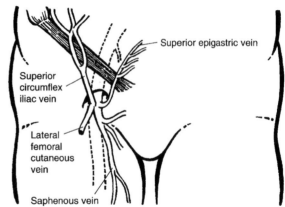

Fig. 4.2 Central venous access sites on the right side of the neck. *Source*: (O'Neill et al. 2004)

Fig. 4.4 Venous access sites in the right groin. *Source*: (O'Neill et al. 2004)

tunnelled central line is more suitable. However, CVC lines are not free from risks. Incidence of sepsis in neonates with central lines has been reported at 24%, and in these patients the presence of a stoma is strongly linked with sepsis. Most catheter-related bloodstream infections respond to appropriate antibiotic treatment and catheter removal.

A final option for obtaining long-term venous access is to insert a totally implantable venous device or "port" (Fig. 4.5). These are particularly suited when i.v. access is only required intermittently and to enable the patient

to carry out many day-to-day activities such as swimming. The tip of the canula should reside in the right atrial and superior vena caval junction parallel to the vein wall. It is our practice to insert the reservoir subcutaneously in the axilla, where it is readily accessible but cosmetically inconspicuous. It is important that a noncoring "Huber" needle is used to access the silicone membrane of the port in order to avoid damage.

Critically ill patients will require an arterial line especially at the time of operation, either because of the surgery, when it is expected to result in significant fluid

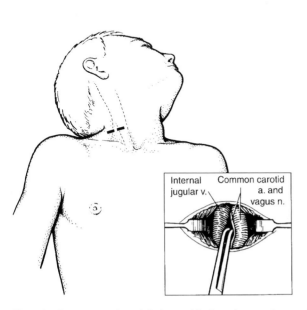

Fig. 4.3 Open approach to right internal juglar vein cannulation. *Source*: (Spitz and Coran 2006)

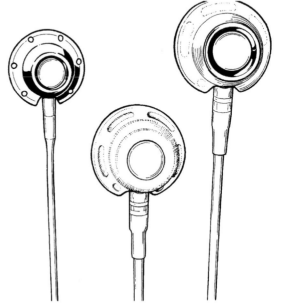

Fig. 4.5 Implantable devices for longterm vascular access. *Source*: (Spitz and Coran 2006)

shift and haemodynamic instability, or in a neonate, because of a significant underlying cardiopulmonary disease of the newborn. This arterial line is for monitoring the haemodynamic and biochemical status, especially throughout the operative procedure. In the neonate, right radial artery percutaneous catheterisation is preferred because it allows sampling of preductal blood for measurement of oxygen tension. If the baby has already had an umbilical artery catheter, it is safer to use it strictly for the purpose of blood pressure monitoring and blood sampling and not for the administration of drugs. In older children, the radial arteries are the preferred sites, generally followed by the posterior tibial and femoral arteries. Access to the relevant artery is generally obtained by a percutaneous technique but also may be approached via a formal cut-down.

Occasionally obtaining vascular access can be anticipated to be particularly difficult. This frequently occurs in the setting of a child who has had multiple previous central venous lines. Screening modalities such as Doppler ultrasound or magnetic resonance venograms may give information on the patency of the remaining veins. Unfortunately, sites that are more difficult to access may have to be considered in order to obtain adequate vascular access. These can include trans-hepatic broviac insertion via a percutaneous approach, formal thoracotomy with canulation of the azygos vein or in extreme circumstances insertion of a central line through the auricle of the right atrium.

In an emergency, temporary vascular access can also be obtained by the intraosseous route. The most common site for intraosseous infusion is the proximal tibia, with secondary sites including the distal tibia and femur. It is important to remember that positive pressure is required to infuse intravenous fluids via the intraosseous route.

Good fixation of all venous and arterial lines is essential to avoid dislodgement, and re-insertion of these vascular lines can be very difficult.

Further Reading

Aplin S, Baines D, De Lime J (2007) Use of the ASA Physical Status Grading System in pediatric practice. Paediatr Anaesth 17(3):216–222

Harting MT, Lally KP (2007) Surgical management of neonates with congenital diaphragmatic hernia. Semin Pediatr Surg 16(2):109–114

MacFaul R, Werneke U (2001) Recent trends in hospital use by children in England. Arch Dis Child 85(3):203–207

Mackway-Jones K (2005) Advanced Paediatric Life Support: The Practical Approach, 1st vol, 4th edn. BMJ Blackwell London/Malden, MA

O'Neil JA Jr, Grosfeld JL, Fonkalsrud EW, Coran AG, Caldamone A (2004) Principles of Pediatric Surgery. Mosby New York

Puri P, De Caluwe (2003) Preoperative assessment. In P Puri (ed) Newborn Surgery. Arnold, London, pp 45–58

Spitz L, and Coran AG (2006) Operative Pediatric Surgery, vol xiv, 6th edn. Hodder Arnold, London, 1060 p

Wheeler R (2006) Gillick or Fraser? A plea for consistency over competence in children. BMJ 332(7545):807

Wilson D, Verklan MT, Kennedy KA (2007) Randomized trial of percutaneous central venous lines versus peripheral intravenous lines. J Perinatol 27(2):92–96

Anaesthesia and Analgesia

5

Declan Warde

Contents

P. Puri and M. Höllwarth (eds.), *Pediatric Surgery: Diagnosis and Management*,
DOI: 10.1007/978-3-540-69560-8_5, © Springer-Verlag Berlin Heidelberg 2009

5.1 Introduction

Over the past 70 years or so, provision of anaesthesia for the child requiring surgery has developed from being a relatively haphazard affair to achieving the status of a recognized subspecialty. The improved outcomes seen following surgery, where even very young and ill infants and children are concerned, have been due in no small part to advances in anaesthetic management. Equally important has been an increased appreciation of the need for an efficient smooth-working team. The success of major paediatric surgery depends on the maximum cooperation between surgeon, anaesthetist, paediatrician, and nursing and paramedical personnel. It is appropriate therefore that everyone involved in the care of the hospitalized child, whether working inside or outside the operating theatre, should be familiar with the basic techniques used in maintaining a favourable physiologic milieu in the face of surgical intrusion, while at the same time ensuring adequate anaesthesia.

5.2 Pre-operative Evaluation and Preparation

The cornerstones of pre-operative anaesthetic management are a detailed knowledge of the child's personal and family history combined with a physical examination. Consideration must also be given to the specific surgical procedure to be undertaken and its implications in terms of potential blood loss, monitoring requirements and post-operative care.

5.2.1 History

Particular attention should be paid to a history of prematurity, respiratory disease, e.g. bronchopulmonary dysplasia or asthma, congenital heart disease, any suggestion of neuromuscular disease (patients with conditions like Duchenne's muscular dystrophy may exhibit severe adverse reactions following exposure to certain anaesthetic agents), recent upper respiratory tract infection or vaccination (see below), and any family history of anaesthesia-related problems. Allergies and current or recent drug therapy should be recorded.

5.2.2 Physical Examination

The anaesthetist should make a brief appraisal of the child's overall condition and follow this with a careful physical examination, paying particular attention to the respiratory and cardiovascular systems. Airway anatomy should be carefully assessed in order that potential difficulties with endotracheal intubation can be anticipated.

5.2.3 Laboratory Investigations

Most older children presenting for minor surgery do not require any pre-operative laboratory workup. Minimum laboratory data required for infants and children undergoing major surgery include full blood count, blood urea and serum electrolytes, blood glucose and calcium, coagulation profile and urine specific gravity. Additional investigations may be required in specific circumstances.

5.2.4 Premedication

Sedative premedication is not used in neonates or in other situations where it may cause increased risk, e.g. children with airway compromise. Its use in other children appears to have declined in recent years—this may be due in part to the fact that increased parental involvement in perioperative care serves to reduce the incidence of separation anxiety. Midazolam and diazepam (for older children) are the most commonly used premedicant drugs.

5.3 Operating Theatre and Anaesthetic Equipment

The primary objectives of anaesthesia are the provision of sleep, analgesia, life support, intensive surveillance and appropriate operating conditions for the patient, irrespective of age, requiring surgery. In order for these to be achieved it is imperative that both operating theatre environmental conditions and anaesthetic equipment be appropriate for infants and children. Appropriate measures should be taken to minimize the risk of heat loss, especially where surgery on infants is concerned.

5.3.1 Breathing Systems

An appropriate anaesthetic circuit for use in infants and children needs to be light, have minimal resistance and dead space, allow for warming and humidifying of inspired gases and be adaptable to spontaneous, assisted or controlled ventilation. The most widely used system continues to be the T-piece designed by Philip Ayre and later modified by Rees. Connectors and tubes should also offer minimal flow resistance and dead space. Knowledge of the probable diameter and length of the endotracheal tube appropriate for any given child is essential. Use of an endotracheal tube (ET) of too large a diameter may result in tracheal wall damage, while excess length leads to endobronchial intubation. The presence of a cuff limits the diameter of the tube that can be used, with consequent increased resistance to airflow. Face-masks are generally used for only brief periods in infants and children, but should provide a good fit and have a low dead space. Use of the laryngeal mask airway (LMA) is increasing in paediatric anaesthesia practice.

5.3.2 Laryngoscopes

Because of the anatomical peculiarities of the infant's airway, most anaesthetists prefer to use a laryngoscope with a straight blade in this age group, lifting the epiglottis forwards from behind to facilitate endotracheal

intubation. Standard curved blades, available in various sizes, are appropriate for older children.

5.3.3 Ventilators

Most infants and children can be ventilated using standard adult ventilators provided the ventilator is of low internal compliance and equipped with paediatric breathing tubes. The ventilator should be capable of delivering small tidal volumes and rapid respiratory rates, and have an adjustable inspiratory flow rate and inspiratory to expiratory ratio so that peak airway pressure is kept as low as possible. Pressure-controlled ventilation is widely used in order to minimize the risk of pulmonary barotrauma. A suitable temperature-controlled humidifier should be incorporated in the inspiratory side of the ventilator circuit. The ability to deliver air and oxygen mixtures through the ventilator or the anaesthetic circuit should be available.

5.3.4 Monitoring Equipment

A complete range of monitoring equipment suitable for paediatric use is required.

5.4 Induction of Anaesthesia

The anaesthetic agents employed in infants and children are identical to those used in adults. The choice of induction technique depends on (a) the age, size and physical status of the child, (b) the relative hazard of regurgitation, and (c) the personal preference of the anaesthetist. Where the older child is concerned, his or her preference may also be taken into consideration. The introduction of local anaesthetic creams has helped reduce the "fear factor" for those children needing intravenous (i.v.) cannulation prior to induction of anaesthesia, especially those requiring multiple anaesthetics. Many are also helped by having a parent remain with them until they are asleep—this was almost unknown 30 years ago but is now commonplace. Inhalational induction is still preferred, especially in younger children, by many paediatric anaesthetists, and is particularly appropriate when difficulty with venous access is anticipated, where a slower induction is desired because of concern regarding loss of airway control, or when the child specifically requests it.

5.5 Intravenous Agents

Sodium thiopentone was for many years the drug of choice for i.v. induction of anaesthesia in patients of all ages. It has now been replaced in most centres by propofol, which provides an equally rapid and smooth induction combined with more rapid and complete recovery, and also has an anti-emetic effect. Pain on injection can be prevented in most instances by the prior addition of lignocaine to the propofol solution. Ketamine is associated with greater cardiovascular stability than many other anaesthetic drugs and is a potent analgesic. It may be used with beneficial effect on the rare occasions when it is necessary to induce anaesthesia in the shocked child.

5.6 Inhalational Agents

5.6.1 Halothane

For decades, halothane was the most popular volatile anaesthetic for inhalational induction in infants and young children. This is largely because it is usually associated with a smooth induction without irritant effects on the airway. Its use has been superseded to such an extent in adult practice by newer agents that it has become difficult to obtain, much to the chagrin of many paediatric anaesthetists who still consider that it has a useful role.

5.6.2 Isoflurane

Inhalational induction of anaesthesia with isoflurane is not as rapid or as smooth as with halothane. Indeed, this agent has been shown to be associated with a significant incidence of hypoxic episodes during induction of anaesthesia in older children. It has considerable potentiating effects on non-depolarizing muscle relaxants, so that lower doses of the latter can be used. It is an excellent agent for maintenance of anaesthesia.

5.6.3 Enflurane

This agent is not widely used in paediatric anaesthesia because its irritant effects render it relatively unsatisfactory for inhalational induction while it offers few particular advantages during the maintenance period.

5.6.4 Desflurane

Airway irritant effects also render desflurane unsuitable for inhalational induction. However, recovery times in infants are shorter than those following other volatile anaesthetics. The agent has been recommended for maintenance of anaesthesia in the ex-premature infant prone to apnoea and ventilatory depression.

5.6.5 Sevoflurane

Induction time with sevoflurane is shorter than with halothane in older children. However, this does not appear to be the case where infants are concerned. The agent has been reported to cause more respiratory depression than halothane in infants and young children, but perhaps not to a degree that is clinically significant. It has become the most widely used volatile agent for inhalational induction and is also popular for maintenance of anaesthesia.

5.6.6 Nitrous Oxide

This gas does not provide adequate anaesthesia when used alone with oxygen. It is most often employed as a carrier that supplements potent volatile anaesthetics, thereby reducing the concentration required and minimizing cardiovascular depressant effects. One limitation to its use is the fact that it is many times more soluble in blood than is nitrogen. As a result, the inhalation and subsequent diffusion of the gas causes an increase in the volume of compliant spaces. It follows that the agent should not be used in patients with congenital diaphragmatic hernia, lobar emphysema or bowel obstruction.

5.7 Neuromuscular Blocking Agents

5.7.1 Succinylcholine

Because of the number of side-effects, including brady-cardia, hyperkalaemia and triggering of malignant hyper-pyrexia reactions associated with this agent, its use has declined dramatically in recent years. However, it remains pre-eminent in rapidly providing optimum conditions for endotracheal intubation, and therefore retains a limited place in emergency paediatric anaesthetic practice. For elective surgery, intubation is now more frequently facilitated by either deep inhalational anaesthesia or use of a non-depolarizing muscle relaxant.

5.7.2 Atracurium and Vecuronium

These two drugs are the most widely used muscle relaxants in paediatrics. They were originally introduced because their duration of action was intermediate between that of succinylcholine and older agents such as pancuronium and because they offered increased cardiovascular stability. In addition, atracurium is attractive in that its metabolism is independent of hepatic and renal function. Because of their pharmacokinetic profiles, both drugs are suitable for use by continuous intravenous infusion, although atracurium infusion requirements show marked individual variation.

5.7.3 Mivacurium

Mivacurium is a short-acting non-depolarizing neuro-muscular agent that is rapidly hydrolysed by plasma pseudocholinesterase. The time course of block produced by the drug is more rapid in younger paediatric patients. Satisfactory intubating conditions are not achieved as quickly as with succinylcholine but serious side-effects occur less frequently.

5.7.4 Rocuronium

This agent has a relatively rapid onset and intermediate duration of action in most children, although neuromuscular blockade may be prolonged in young infants.

5.8 Maintenance of Anaesthesia

Because of the vulnerability of the infant's respiratory system, spontaneous respiration is not used for long periods in the anaesthetized neonate. Mechanical ventilation helps ensure adequate gas exchange and also leaves the hands of the anaesthetist free to perform other tasks. Manual ventilation allows rapid detection of airway obstruction or disconnection, and is particularly useful during thoracic surgery.

The most widely used agents for maintenance of anaesthesia in the paediatric population are isoflurane, sevoflurane and desflurane, usually combined with 50% oxygen in nitrous oxide, along with a small dose of relaxant. Consideration should be given to the use of air and oxygen mixtures in preterm neonates. Older children may be allowed to breathe spontaneously for longer periods; the use of mechanical ventilation often being dictated by the nature of the surgical procedure.

5.9 Reversal and Extubation

If a volatile agent has been used for the maintenance of anaesthesia, it should be discontinued shortly prior to the end of surgery. When muscle relaxants have been used in intubated patients any residual relaxation is reversed by either neostigmine (0.06 mg/kg) or edrophonium (1 mg/kg) combined with either atropine (0.02–0.03 mg/kg) or glycopyrrolate (0.01 mg/kg) once surgery has been completed. Controlled ventilation is continued with 100% oxygen or with oxygen in air until spontaneous respiration has returned. Infants should not be extubated until fully awake and breathing adequately. In most cases, reversal of neuromuscular blockade and resumption of spontaneous respiration occurs rapidly. If difficulty is encountered this may be due to hypothermia, acidosis or hypocalcaemia, or the fact that an incremental dose of relaxant has been given too close to the end of surgery.

5.10 Recovery from Anaesthesia

Immediate recovery from anaesthesia and surgery should be in a fully equipped recovery area with a one-to-one ratio of personnel trained in paediatric nursing. Monitoring of vital signs, adequacy of protective airway reflexes, and correct positioning to prevent airway obstruction, regurgitation and aspiration are the priorities. The recovery room nurse also monitors the wound site for bleeding, checks the security of dressings, and the adequacy of pain relief. The main factors influencing the rate of recovery in children include the use of premedicant drugs, the induction and maintenance techniques, the age of the child, and the duration of surgery. Parental involvement in the early recovery phase is now encouraged in many units.

5.11 Post-operative Care

Most children may be offered a drink or light snack as soon as they have recovered consciousness. Exceptions should be made following endotracheal intubation, some dental or oral procedures, and when local anaesthetic drugs have been used on the upper or lower airway. In addition to post-discharge guidance provided by the surgical team, parents or guardians should also be given both verbal and written instructions regarding post-operative pain management and what to do if problems arise.

5.12 Monitoring

The clinical condition of the anaesthetized child can deteriorate more rapidly and with less warning than that of patients in any other age group. It follows that careful and continuous monitoring is essential. While no piece of machinery will adequately replace the careful anaesthetist, a number of devices providing helpful information that cannot be gleaned by clinical means alone are available. The monitoring employed in any particular case depends on the physical status of the child and the surgical procedure to be undertaken.

5.13 Cardiovascular Monitoring

5.13.1 Precordial and Oesophageal Stethoscope

Although its use in paediatric anaesthetic practice has declined, the stethoscope is particularly valuable, allowing continuous monitoring of heart and breath sounds both cheaply and simply. In the neonate, the intensity of the heart sounds varies with the stroke volume so that an indication of cardiac output is provided. Use of a monaural earpiece greatly improves the comfort of the listener.

5.13.2 ECG

As myocardial ischaemia is uncommon in children the principal function of the ECG is to monitor heart rate and detect arrhythmias, especially bradycardia. Primary arrhythmias are uncommon except in those with congenital heart disease, but causes of secondary arrhythmias include hypoxia, hypercarbia and surgical stimulation, e.g. strabismus surgery. ECG monitoring may also detect inadvertent i.v. injection of local anaesthetics.

5.13.3 Blood Pressure

Routine non-invasive monitoring of blood pressure during anaesthesia and surgery is carried out with automated devices using oscillometry. The appropriate cuff size must be used in order to obtain accurate measurements. Direct intra-arterial monitoring is the most accurate measurement of blood pressure and provides a "beat to beat" assessment. Its use is generally restricted to very ill children or those undergoing major surgery. All the proximal and distal arteries of the arms and legs may be used.

5.13.4 Central Venous Pressure

Central venous pressure monitoring is useful in infants and children undergoing major surgery with anticipated large fluid shifts, if significant blood loss (and replacement) is expected, and during surgery for congenital heart disease. The right internal jugular vein is usually the simplest to cannulate. Monitoring of left atrial pressure and pulmonary capillary wedge pressure is rarely indicated in infants or children.

5.14 Respiratory Monitoring

5.14.1 Pulse Oximetry

Hypoxia is the most common critical incident in paediatric anaesthesia. As detection of cyanosis in infants and young children is difficult, the routine use of pulse oximetry is now mandatory. Thermal injury and pressure necrosis have been reported when sensor probes have been applied too tightly.

5.14.2 Capnography

The measurement of pCO_2 in inspired and expired gases is also mandatory. Capnography is not only a monitor of the adequacy of ventilation but also gives warning of disruption in gas supply, inadequate fresh gas flow and oesophageal intubation.

5.15 Temperature

Monitoring temperature is important in paediatrics because of the increased risk of both hypo- and hyperthermia. Common sites for temperature probes used perioperatively include the pharynx, oesophagus and rectum.

5.16 Neuromuscular Blockade

Monitoring neuromuscular blockade using a peripheral nerve stimulator is routine practice when non-depolarizing muscle relaxants have been administered.

5.17 Fluid Balance

Healthy children undergoing minor operations can reasonably be expected to tolerate oral fluids a short time after completion of surgery and do not require intraoperative i.v. fluids. The goal of intraoperative fluid management in those who are dehydrated pre-operatively or who are undergoing major surgery is to sustain homeostasis by providing the appropriate amount of parenteral fluid to maintain adequate intravascular volume, cardiac output, and, ultimately, oxygen delivery to tissues at a time when normal physiological functions are altered by surgical stress and anaesthetic agents. The composition of the administered fluid will vary according to the maturity of the child and pre-operative electrolyte and glucose levels. Because of the problems associated with hyperglycaemic states in infancy, care should be taken with the use of 10% dextrose infusions. Blood and fluid loss can be extensive and very difficult to measure during neonatal surgery. The former is best estimated by the use of small volume suction traps, by weighing small numbers of surgical swabs before they dry out, and by serial haematocrit measurements. During lengthy surgery, serum electrolytes and blood glucose should be measured at regular intervals. Urine output may be monitored by the use of adhesive collecting bags or bladder catheterization. Estimated third space loss may be replaced by continuous administration of lactated Ringer's solution at 3–5 ml/kg/h. The adequacy of volume replacement can be assessed by monitoring blood pressure, central venous pressure, peripheral circulatory state and urine output.

5.18 Special Considerations for the Premature Infant

Congenital defects occur more commonly in preterm infants, so that surgery is frequently required. Organs and enzyme systems are very immature and meticulous attention to detail during anaesthetic and surgical management is imperative if survival rates are to be high. The large body surface area and lack of subcutaneous fat make maintenance of body temperature very difficult, so that a high neutral thermal environment is essential. Respiratory fatigue occurs very easily and may be exacerbated by residual lung damage following mechanical ventilation, persistent fetal circulation and oxygen dependency. The response to exogenous vitamin K is less satisfactory than in term infants and there is an increased risk of bleeding. In addition, anaemia is common because of reduced erythropoiesis, a short erythrocyte life span and iatrogenic causes such as frequent blood sampling. Fluid and electrolyte management can be difficult—insensitive losses are high and hypoglycaemia and hypocalcaemia occur easily, while renal function and the ability of the cardiovascular system to tolerate fluid loads are reduced.

5.19 Anaesthesia for Specific Surgical Conditions

5.19.1 Oesophageal Atresia

Once a diagnosis of oesophageal atresia (with or without fistula) has been made, the blind upper pouch should be continuously aspirated using a Replogle or similar tube. In general, the operation may be safely delayed pending improvement of any aspiration pneumonia that has developed. Pre-thoracotomy bronchoscopy is practised in some centres and may influence subsequent management. Anaesthesia is similar to that for other neonatal procedures, but special care must be taken with positioning of the endotracheal tube, the tip of which should be located above the carina but below any fistula present. Surgical retraction during the operation may compromise either respiratory or cardiac function, so that close monitoring is essential. If serious contamination has not occurred and unless the surgeon deems the anastomosis to be especially tight, extubation is usually possible shortly after the conclusion of surgery.

5.19.2 Congenital Diaphragmatic Hernia

This condition was formerly regarded as one of the great emergencies of paediatric surgical practice, but it is now considered that the timing of repair should be based on the optimization of clinical parameters rather than a specific time period post-delivery. Pre-operative ventilatory and haemodynamic support along with correction of metabolic disturbance are almost invariably required. Inhaled nitric oxide, high frequency oscillation ventilation, liquid ventilation and extracorporeal membrane oxygenation may also be used. Positive pressure ventilation using bag and mask should be avoided prior to endotracheal intubation, as expansion of the viscera contained within the hernia will cause

further lung compression. Nitrous oxide should be avoided for the same reason. A reasonable anaesthetic technique includes controlled ventilation with fentanyl 0.01–0.02 mg/kg, intermediate-acting muscle relaxant and 100% oxygen or oxygen in air as required. Great caution should be exercised in the use of volatile anaesthetic agents. Airway pressures should be kept as low as possible. Should advanced ventilatory techniques such as the use high frequency oscillation be required in order to achieve pre-operative stabilisation, these may be safely continued during surgery. Most infants will require mechanical ventilation in the post-operative period.

5.19.3 Intestinal Obstruction

The various forms of neonatal intestinal obstruction account for approximately 35% of all surgical procedures in the newborn. The major anaesthetic problems are those of fluid and electrolyte imbalance (which must be corrected pre-operatively), abdominal distension (causing respiratory embarrassment) and the risk of regurgitation and aspiration of gastric contents into the lungs. Following decompression of the stomach, a rapid-sequence induction incorporating pre-oxygenation, propofol and succinylcholine with gentle cricoid pressure is advised. Anaesthesia is then continued in the usual way. The same principles apply to the management of those older infants with a diagnosis of intussusception who require operative reduction.

5.19.4 Exomphalos and Gastroschisis

Anaesthetic concerns include heat and fluid loss from the exposed bowel and the fact that primary closure of the abdominal wall defect may push the diaphragm cephalad, thus compromising respiratory function. Special care must be taken to keep heat loss to a minimum. Fluid requirements are much greater than in normal neonates. To maintain plasma oncotic pressure, at least 25% of fluid intake should be given as colloid. The extent of respiratory compromise can assist the anaesthetist in advising the surgeon whether or not primary closure is feasible. A proportion of infants, especially after repair of gastroschisis, require post-operative mechanical ventilation. The introduction of staged closure of gastroschisis using preformed silos has simplified anaesthetic and paediatric intensive care unit management.

5.19.5 Congenital Lobar Emphysema

This condition may cause severe respiratory distress in the neonatal period. Induction of anaesthesia for lobectomy should be as smooth as possible—struggling may trap large amounts of air in the affected lobe during violent inspiratory efforts. Nitrous oxide can also increase the volume of trapped air considerably and is contraindicated. Great care should be taken with controlled ventilation because of the risk of pneumothorax.

5.19.6 Myelomeningocele, Shunt (and Revision Shunt) for Spina Bifida

Surgery for myelomeningocele is carried out with the infant in the prone position and the chest and pelvis should be supported with pads so that the abdomen remains free from external pressure. If the defect is large, heat and fluid loss during surgery can pose problems and should be monitored as closely as possible. Endotracheal intubation may be difficult in the presence of hydrocephalus. Children who have had repeated shunt surgery and regular bladder catheterization may develop latex allergy and a latex-free anaesthesia technique should be used.

5.19.7 Tonsillectomy and Adenoidectomy

While most children presenting for these operations are comparatively healthy, some may have obstructive sleep apnoea syndrome, which can be associated with significant right heart strain and pulmonary hypertension, with the danger of perioperative upper airway obstruction and potential cardiovascular collapse. Sedative premedication is best avoided in this group because of the risk of causing complete upper airway obstruction. As far as is possible, short-acting anaesthetic agents that do not cause significant respiratory or cardiovascular depression

should be used. Extubation should not take place until the child is awake, and careful post-operative monitoring, preferably in a high dependency unit, is required.

5.19.8 Muscle Biopsy

This operation represents an example of a procedure that, although relatively minor and innocuous from the surgeon's viewpoint, may pose considerable problems for the anaesthetist. It is most frequently performed to either confirm or exclude a diagnosis of possible neuromuscular disease. Children presenting for muscle biopsy may have decreased respiratory and cardiac reserve, and be at increased risk of perioperative aspiration. They may also have metabolic derangements and can be prone to developing hypoglycaemia. Use of succinylcholine is absolutely contraindicated as it has been associated with lethal hyperkalaemia in this patient population, while there may be increased sensitivity to non-depolarizing muscle relaxants. Many paediatric anaesthetists also prefer to avoid volatile agents, thus necessitating the use of a continuous infusion anaesthetic technique, most commonly with propofol.

5.19.9 Herniotomy in the Ex-Premature Infant

Improved survival rates in premature and low birth weight infants have led to increased numbers of them presenting for inguinal hernia repair. While the surgical procedure may be relatively straightforward, these babies represent a considerable challenge for the anaesthetist. They must be managed by anaesthetists and surgeons with adequate training and ongoing experience in hospitals with appropriate facilities and personnel. Ex-premature infants up to 60 weeks post-conceptual age are at risk of life-threatening apnoea after anaesthesia and surgery. They should have respiratory monitoring for at least 12 h post-operatively and should not be managed as day cases. Intravenous caffeine 5 mg/kg given i.v. at induction appears to reduce the risk of apnoeic episodes, but respiratory monitoring is still required. Regional techniques also reduce, but do not eliminate, the risk of post-operative apnoea and may require supplementary sedation or light general anaesthesia.

5.20 Post-operative Analgesia in Children

There have been significant improvements in pain relief following surgery in children. In the past this was usually achieved by intramuscular injection of narcotics—many children suffered in silence, believing "the cure to be worse than the disease". Nowadays, a variety of different drugs and more effective and humane routes of administration are employed, which can and should be used to provide optimum post-operative analgesia for children. Prevention of pain whenever possible using multi-modal analgesia can be adapted for day cases, major surgery, the critically ill child and the very young. Most paediatric acute pain services use techniques of co-analgesia based on four classes of drugs, namely local anaesthetics, opioids, non-steroidal anti-inflammatory drugs (NSAIDs) and paracetamol (acetaminophen). For many day-case procedures opioids can and should be omitted altogether because combinations of the other three classes usually provide excellent pain control. In children's hospitals or other centres where significant numbers of children undergo anaesthesia and surgery, the establishment of a dedicated paediatric pain service is the desirable standard of care.

5.20.1 Local and Regional Anaesthesia

The use of regional anaesthesia reduces intraoperative anaesthetic requirements and provides excellent post-operative analgesia for infants and children. The incidence of major complications is extremely low even when central blocks, e.g. epidural analgesia, are used. Commonly used simple techniques include topical application of local anaesthetic gel as in the case of circumcision and direct instillation of local anaesthetic at the surgical site by the surgeon, e.g. for inguinal hernia repair or orchidopexy. Alternatively, the anaesthetist may perform either a penile or ilio-inguinal block for the same procedures. Numerous other local, regional and central anaesthetic blocks, often performed with ultrasound guidance, are used on an increasingly regular basis for virtually all types of surgery, including open cardiac surgery, and in many instances their efficacy in the post-operative period can be prolonged for as long as necessary through the use of continuous infusion techniques.

Until recently, the most widely used local anaesthetic agent for regional blockade was racemic bupivicaine. This has now largely been replaced by either ropivicaine or levobupivicaine, both of which appear to offer greater safety. However, it remains essential to adhere to published maximum dosage guidelines (2 mg/kg in infants, 2.5 mg/kg in children for single bolus injection with either drug). Use of some adjunctive agents, e.g. clonidine, ketamine with single dose or continuous epidural blockade, is increasingly popular as both the effectiveness and duration of blockade appear to be enhanced.

5.20.2 Opioids

Morphine remains the most widely used opioid for intra and post-operative analgesia in infants and children. Bolus injections of 0.1–0.2 mg/kg or infusions between 0.01 and 0.03 mg/kg/h provide adequate analgesia with an acceptable level of side-effects when administered with an appropriate level of monitoring. It should be noted that morphine elimination half-life is prolonged in the newborn when compared with older infants and children. Patients in this age-group are also more susceptible to the drug's respiratory depressant effects, Patient-controlled analgesia (PCA) is now widely used in children as young as 5 years and compares favourably with continuous infusion. Nurse-controlled analgesia (NCA) is useful in younger children or in those without the physical or mental capacity to use PCA successfully. Oral, sublingual, transdermal, intranasal and rectal routes of opioid administration have all been described and may have a role to play in specific cases. Use of the intramuscular route is no longer considered appropriate. Tramadol, oxycodone and pethidine may have some applicability as alternatives to morphine in the perioperative period. Fentanyl, alfentanil and remifentanil may have a role in intensive care practice after major surgery.

5.20.3 Non-steroidal Anti-inflammatory Drugs (NSAIDs)

These drugs are important in the prevention and treatment of mild to moderate pain in children. They are highly effective when used in combination with local or regional nerve blocks. They may also be used in combination with opioids, leading to a significant "opioid-sparing" effect, which not only reduces the opioid dose requirement but also lessens the incidence of opioid-related side-effects, e.g. ileus, urinary retention. NSAIDs, e.g. diclofenac in combination with paracetamol, produce better analgesia than either alone. They should be avoided in infants aged less than 6 months, children with aspirin or NSAID allergy, those with dehydration or hypovolaemia, children with renal or hepatic failure, coagulation disorders, peptic ulcer disease, or in those who are at significant risk of haemorrhage. Concurrent administration of NSAIDs with anti-coagulants, steroids or nephrotoxic agents is not recommended. NSAIDs may provoke bronchospasm in some asthmatic patients. However it is useful to check for past exposure to these drugs as many asthmatic children can take them with no adverse effects. There have been suggestions that they impair bone healing. The beneficial effects of their short-term use in most children undergoing orthopaedic surgery probably outweigh this possible risk but caution is recommended following some major orthopaedic surgery, e.g. spinal fusion, limb-lengthening procedures.

5.20.4 Paracetamol (Acetaminophen)

Paracetamol has both analgesic and antipyretic effects. Its analgesic potency is relatively low. On its own, it can be used to treat most mild and some moderate pain. In combination with NSAIDs or a mild opioid such as codeine, it can be used to treat or prevent most moderate pain. Oral formulations are widely available. Absorption from the rectum is slow and incomplete, except in neonates. Intravenous formulations have recently become available and may have higher analgesic potency. It is important to realise that the time to peak analgesia even after i.v. administration is 1–2 h. In younger infants and sick children, considerable downward dose adjustments are needed.

5.21 Day-Case Anaesthesia and Surgery

In many units, up to 75% of surgery in children is carried out on a day-care basis. The same standards of care apply whether surgery is carried out on in-patients or out-patients. Staff should have been trained in the care of children, the environment should be child-friendly and child-safe, and there should be free parental access to the conscious child. While many operations can be carried out as day cases, a number of procedures are not suitable. These include any operation following which there is a significant risk of post-operative haemorrhage, where there is a likelihood of post-operative pain requiring sophisticated control, and also body cavity surgery. Other factors that need to be considered include the age and maturity of the child, his or her overall medical condition, the presence of anaesthetic risk factors, and the family's social circumstances.

5.21.1 Preparation of Child and Parents

The child and parents should be provided with a clear verbal explanation of what will happen on the day of surgery and this should be reinforced by written information and guidance regarding pre-operative fasting. Pre-admission programmes, e.g. "Saturday Clubs" may be helpful.

5.21.2 Premedication

In many centres the majority of children presenting for day-case surgery are not routinely premedicated. Midazolam has for some years been the drug of choice but it has recently been suggested that clonidine may be preferable.

5.21.3 Anaesthetic Technique

The anaesthetic technique employed should be as simple and non-invasive as possible. Both inhalational and i.v. induction techniques may be used.

It is preferable to maintain spontaneous respiration during the maintenance period, although use of non-depolarizing muscle relaxants is not an absolute contraindication to day-case surgery. If possible airway control should be achieved with either a face-mask or laryngeal mask airway, with endotracheal tubes being reserved for cases where they are specifically required, e.g. upper gastrointestinal endoscopy.

5.21.4 Analgesia for Day Cases

Good pain control is critical to the success of paediatric day surgery. Opioids are associated with a higher incidence of post-operative nausea and vomiting (PONV) and should be avoided if possible. Local analgesia is effective and safe, and should probably be used as part of the analgesic regime in all cases where it is practical to do so. Peripheral nerve blocks are highly effective. Single-injection techniques are preferred, the most useful being penile block, ilioinguinal-iliohypogastric block and great auricular nerve block. Some also consider that single-dose caudal epidural block is appropriate for paediatric day-case surgery although motor block may be a problem. NSAIDs should also be used routinely unless specifically contraindicated. These may be given, by a number of routes, either as a component of premedication or after induction. Paracetamol may also be given. Oral analgesics are the mainstay of continuing pain relief at home after day surgery and it is vital to encourage parents to give analgesics pre-emptively for 24–48 h and before any local anaesthetic has worn off. They should also be advised on whom to contact if pain control problems arise.

5.21.5 Discharge Criteria

Prior to discharge the child should be fully conscious, pain-free and able to move normally. Vital signs should be normal. There should be no respiratory distress or stridor. The ability to drink and tolerate clear fluids is desirable, but adequately hydrated children can be allowed home prior to drinking if they meet other discharge criteria.

5.21.6 Reasons for Hospital Admission

Approximately one per cent of children undergoing day-case surgery ultimately require overnight hospital admission. The reasons include persistently abnormal vital signs or level of consciousness, persistent nausea and vomiting, surgical or anaesthetic problems (unexpectedly prolonged or difficult surgery, regurgitation, aspiration, allergic reactions), bleeding and difficulties with pain control.

5.21.7 Transport Home

The child should travel home in a private car or taxi and should be accompanied by a responsible adult. Use of buses or trains should be avoided and the total travelling time should not be excessively long.

5.22 Some Topics of Current Interest to Both Anaesthetists and Surgeons

5.22.1 Fasting Prior to Anaesthesia and Surgery

Pulmonary aspiration of acid gastric contents has long been recognized as a cause of morbidity and mortality in patients undergoing anaesthesia and surgery. While the precise incidence of this dreaded complication is unknown, there is evidence that children are affected more frequently than adults, with as many as 26% of deaths associated with paediatric anaesthesia being attributed to aspiration in one series. Of the various preventive measures that have been advocated to reduce the incidence of this complication one, the preoperative fast, has long since achieved universal acceptance with the result that patients of all ages have been required to abstain from food and drink prior to induction of anaesthesia. For decades, children were "fasted from midnight the night before". If surgery was delayed, fasting times became excessively long and apart from being uncomfortable for the child, there was the risk of hypoglycaemia and dehydration—there are obvious dangers involved in administering potent anaesthetic drugs to potentially hypovolaemic young children. Furthermore, fasting leads to children becoming hungry, thirsty and emotionally upset and it has been shown that inhalational induction of anaesthesia is accomplished with a reduced incidence of airway complications if children are calm and cooperative. It follows that the minimum "starve time" that will not

Table 5.1 Fasting guidelines prior to anaesthesia and surgery

Children scheduled for elective anaesthesia

Clear fluids: 2 h minimum

Breast milk: 4 h minimum

Other fluids and all solids: 6 h minimum

Children scheduled for emergency anaesthesia

All fluids and solids: 6 h minimum

Table 5.2 Guidelines regarding anaesthesia, surgery and immunization

1. Postpone all elective procedures requiring anaesthesia rather than immunization, especially in infants.
2. Opportunistic immunization during anaesthesia is inadvisable.
3. Postpone anaesthesia for 1 week after vaccination with inactive vaccines: diphtheria, tetanus, pertussis, inactive polio, Hib, Meningitis C.
4. Postpone anaesthesia for 3 weeks after vaccination with live attenuated vaccines: measles, mumps, rubella, oral polio vaccine and BCG.
5. Delay immunization for 1 week after surgery has taken place.

significantly increase the risk of regurgitation and aspiration of gastric contents should be used in institutions caring for the child undergoing surgery. Table 5.1 outlines some current recommendations.

5.22.2 Upper Respiratory Tract Infection

In the past, almost all children with evidence of upper respiratory tract infection (URTI) had their surgery postponed. While most studies agree that children with active or recent URTI are at increased risk of perioperative complications, these are for the most part manageable and without long-term sequelae. Most paediatric anaesthetists now agree that children with mild uncomplicated URTIs undergoing procedures that do not involve instrumentation of the airway can be safely anaesthetized without any significant increase in risk. Most also agree that any child with severe symptoms should have surgery deferred for at least 4 weeks.

5.22.3 Anaesthesia and Immunization

Anaesthetists are often faced with a child who has been recently immunized presenting for either elective or emergency surgery. Questions frequently asked include whether or not the anaesthesia or surgery will affect the response of the child to the vaccine in achieving seroconversion, or more seriously whether the vaccine might cause major adverse consequences in these circumstances. A recent international survey carried

out to ascertain the attitudes and practices of paediatric anaesthetists regarding anaesthesia in the child who had recently been immunized or who was scheduled for immunization in the near future revealed little consensus of opinion. It does seem prudent, however, to adopt a cautious approach where the timing of elective surgery is concerned, and guidelines issued as a result of this survey are summarized in Table 5.2.

Further Reading

Baum VC (2007) When nitrous oxide is no laughing matter: Nitrous oxide and pediatric anesthesia. Pediatr Anesth 17: 824–30

Llewellyn N, Moriarty A (2007) The national pediatric epidural audit. Pediatr Anesth 17:520–33

Lönnqvist P-A, Morton NS (2005) Postoperative analgesia in infants and children. Br J Anaesth 95:59–68

Moscuzza F (2003) Monitoring during paediatric anaesthesia. Anaesth Intens Care Med 4:19–21

Puri P, Höllwarth ME (eds) (2006) Pediatric Surgery. Springer, Berlin, Heidelberg

Short JA, Van der Walt JH, Zoanetti DC (2006) Immunization and anesthesia: An international survey. Pediatr Anesth 16:514–22

Stoddart PA, Lauder GL (2004) Problems in Anaesthesia: Paediatric Anaesthesia, Taylor & Francis, London

Tait AR, Malviya S (2005) Anesthesia for the child with an upper respiratory tract infection: Still a dilemma? Anesth Analg 100:59–65

Fluid, Electrolyte and Respiratory Management

6

Desmond Bohn

Contents

6.1 Introduction

Children who have undergone major surgical procedures frequently require admission to an intensive care unit or observation area for monitoring of vital signs, respiratory support, and for the management and replacement of fluid and electrolytes. This chapter will focus on the important aspects of postoperative ventilation and fluid management.

6.2 Fluid and Electrolyte Management

6.2.1 Body Water Distribution in Children

Body water content changes significantly with age in children (Table 6.1). Total body water (TBW) is high in the fetus and preterm infant. During early fetal life, TBW represents 90% of total body weight with 65% being in the extracellular fluid (ECF) compartment. By term, the ECF and the intracellular fluid (ICF) volume falls to 45% and 30% of TBW, respectively (Fig. 6.1). The preterm infant has a relative expansion of both TBW and ECF volume expansion, and a diuresis in the first few days of postnatal life is a common finding. Fractional excretion of sodium is inversely correlated with age in the preterm who is susceptible to sodium loss as well as sodium and volume overload. In addition, glomerular filtration rate is lower than in the term infant and water losses due to the large surface area to body weight ratio leads to considerable evaporative losses. Further discussion of fluid and electrolyte physiology in the preterm infant is beyond the scope of this chapter.

Significant changes occur in TBW over the first year of life from 75% of body weight at birth to 65% at

P. Puri and M. Höllwarth (eds.), *Pediatric Surgery: Diagnosis and Management,*
DOI: 10.1007/978-3-540-69560-8_6, © Springer-Verlag Berlin Heidelberg 2009

Table 6.1 Water content of body compartments in children

Age	TBW (% body weight)	Extracellular fluid (% body weight)	Intracellular fluid (% body weight)
Premature	80	45	35
Full-term newborn	75	40	35
12 months to 1 year	65	30	35
1–12 years	60	20	40
Adolescents			–
Males	60	20	40–45
Females	55	18	40

Table 6.2 Water losses in normal children (ml/100 kcals/24 h)

Source	Newborn to 6 months	6 months– 5 years	5–10 years	Adolescence
Insensible	40	30	20	10
Urine	60	60	50	40
Fecal	20	10	–	–
Total	120	100	70	50

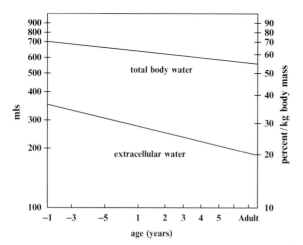

Fig. 6.1 Changes in total body water (TBW) with age. The intracellular water is represented by the difference between the two diagonal lines. (Adapted from Kooh and Metcoff 1963. With permission)

6 months and 60% at 1 year of life. Some of this is accounted for by an increase in body fat. By puberty, TBW is approximately 60% of body weight in males with a slightly lower percentage in females. Extracellular fluid volume decreases over the first year of life to 30% of TBW and decreases with age thereafter reaching adult values early in childhood. The relatively high ECF volume in infancy is largely due to the larger interstitial-lymph space. In contrast, the ICF volume remains relatively constant during childhood.

6.2.2   Fluid Homeostasis in Children

To achieve normal fluid homeostasis, fluid intake must balance losses. The latter consist of urine output and insensible losses (evaporation from the skin surface and respiratory tract) with the addition of fluid loss in the stool, which in the absence of diarrhea should be relatively small. Insensible losses are mainly in the form of electrolyte-free water (EFW) from the respiratory tract (15 ml/100 kcal/day). This loss is eliminated during positive pressure ventilation. Sweat contains mainly water with a small amount of sodium except in situations where sweat glands contain excessive amounts of sodium, e.g. patients with cystic fibrosis. Evaporative losses also increase with elevations in body temperature, and during thermal stress water losses may increase to as much as 25/ml/100 kcals/day (Table 6.2).

Obligate water excretion in the urine is dependent on solute load and the ability to concentrate and dilute the urine. The average osmolar excretion in newborn infants receiving infant formula is 16–20 mOsm/kg/day. Infants are somewhat disadvantaged compared to the older child and adult in that they cannot maximally dilute (infant 200 mOsm/l vs adult 80 mOsm/l) and concentrate the urine (infant 800 mOsm/l vs adult 1200 mOsm/l). In addition, the infant's high metabolic rate and the solute load from enteral feeding formula means that they require more water excretion per unit solute amount. The high solute load and the limited urine concentrating ability makes them prone to significant ECF contraction (dehydration) when there are excessive amounts of water loss. Typically this occurs in gastroenteritis where reduced oral intake is combined with excessive water and electrolyte loss in the stool.

Urine is the major source of electrolyte loss in the body except when there are fluid losses from the GI tract. The commonly used values for sodium (Na) and potassium (K) requirements in parenteral fluids in children are 2–3 and 1–2 mmol/kg/day (Table 6.3). This assumes that these are the amounts of cations needed for normal homeostasis. However, in critically ill children, urinary Na and K concentration may be much higher.

In the normal healthy individual, water intake is regulated by thirst stimulated via osmoreceptors in the

Table 6.3 Requirements for maintenance parenteral fluids based on the formula published by Holliday and Segar in 1957

Body weight	0–10 kg	10–20 kg	>20 kg
Water requirements	100 ml/kg/day	1,000 ml + 50 ml/kg/day for each kg > 10 kg	1,500 ml + 20 ml/kg for each kg above 20 kg

Table 6.4 Water and electrolyte content of commonly used intravenous fluids

Fluid type	Na$^+$ (mmol/l)	Cl$^-$ (mmol/l)	Osmolality (mOsm/kg)	Osmolality with 20 mmol KCl/l added	pH	Electrolyte free water/l
0.9 NaCl	154	154	308	348	5.5	0
0.45 NaCl	77	77	154	194	5.5	500
0.9 NaCl 5% dex	154	154	560	600	4	0
5% dex 0.45 NaCl	77	77	406	446	4	500
5% dex 0.2 NaCl	34	34	321	361	4	780
4% dex 0.18 NaCl	31	31	284	324	4	800
5% dex	0	0	252	292	4	1000
Ringers lactate	130	109	272	312	6.5	114
Ringers lactate 5%	130	109	525		6.5	114
3% NaCl	513	513	1027		5.5	0

hypothalamus. Infants and small children are unable to regulate their intake because they do not have access to water for the same reasons that apply in older children or adults in coma or with reduced levels of consciousness. When oral intake is replaced by parenteral fluids in children the amount of fluid (i.e., water) given depends on body weight and energy expenditure (Table 6.4). In 1957, Holliday and Segar published a formula that linked body weight to energy expenditure. An allowance of 116.7 ml/100 kcal/day was calculated with 66.7 100 kcal/day to replace urine output and 50 mls/100 kcal/day of insensible loss. Factoring in water of oxidation gain of 16.7 ml/100 kcal/day leaves a total of 100 ml/100 kcal/day for replacement of normal losses.

The estimates for Na (3 mmol/100 kcal/day) and K (2 mmol/100 kcal/day) requirements in maintenance fluids were calculated from the sodium and potassium concentration of cow's milk and breast milk.

The Holliday and Segar formula for prescribing iv fluid administration has been the standard reference text in pediatrics for 50 years. Although convenient and simple to use, the assumptions made about daily requirements for sodium, potassium, and electrolyte-free water (EFW) mandates the use of hypotonic intravenous solutions, which has been almost universal practice in pediatric medicine for almost 50 years. However, nonphysiological stimuli for antidiuretic hormone (ADH)

Table 6.5 Electrolyte composition of body fluids (mmol/l)

	Na$^+$	K$^+$	Cl$^-$	HCO$_3^-$
Sweat	50	5	55	
Saliva	30	20	35	15
Gastric juice	60	10	90	
Bile	145	5	110	40
Duodenum	140	5	80	50
Ileum	130	10	110	30
Colon	60	30	40	20

secretion, which inhibits the excretion of EFW (pain, anxiety, narcotics, positive pressure ventilation), are common in critically ill patients. It is therefore not surprising that mild degrees of hyponatremia are a common finding in pediatric patients receiving parenteral fluid therapy. Several studies have shown that children admitted to hospital with acute medical illnesses are frequently admitted with low sodium levels and plasma ADH levels that were higher than would be expected for that degree of hyponatremia. An increasing number of publications are now recommending the use of isotonic or near isotonic fluids for standard maintenance in pediatrics in order to avoid the administration of EFW, which is potentially hazardous in situations where ADH secretion is not inhibited. Hypotonic fluids should be reserved for patients with a demonstrated need for EFW (serum Na$^+$ > 145 mmol/l) (Table 6.5).

6.2.3 Perioperative Fluid Management

The standard practice in perioperative fluid management has been to replace intravascular volume loss with blood or colloid solutions and to use electrolyte solutions to provide for ongoing fluid requirements, replacement of losses from exposed serosal surfaces in open body cavities in thoracic and abdominal surgery and losses from third space fluid sequestration. Extra fluid is also frequently administered to treat hypotension due to the vasodilating effects of anesthetic agents. The preferred electrolyte solution used by most anesthesiologists for intraoperative fluid administration is now Ringer's lactate or isotonic saline because of concerns about the development of postoperative fluid retention and hyponatremia associated with elevated ADH levels. The potential for this is increased when hypotonic dextrose or saline solutions are used. This inability to excrete a sodium-free water load is amply illustrated in scoliosis surgery where patients seem to be particularly at risk for the development of hyponatremia. Two nonrandomized studies have now shown that the degree of hyponatremia is less when isotonic or near-isotonic solutions are used. In a nonrandomized trial comparing Ringer's lactate with 0.2 NaCl in a group of children undergoing scoliosis surgery, the investigators found that the postoperative plasma Na level fell in both groups but that the reduction was marked in those patients receiving the hypotonic fluid. Although at first glance the explanation for this is EFW retention due to nonphysiological stimulation of ADH secretion, it does not explain the reduction in plasma Na seen with Ringer's lactate. Further insights to explain this observation come from a study where plasma and urine Na were measured in adult patients undergoing elective surgery, all of whom received Ringer's lactate as their perioperative fluid. They found that the urine Na concentration was consistently above 150 mmol/l and as high as 350 mmol/l in some instances. This was associated with a significant positive water balance and a fall in the plasma Na, a process they termed postoperative "desalination". In a similar study of children undergoing elective surgery at the Hospital for Sick Children, all of whom received Ringer's lactate, we found similar levels of urinary Na loss (unpublished observations). We believe that this desalination process is consistent with the kidney's attempts to deal with a volume overload situation after the vasodilating effects of anesthetic agents are no longer present but ADH is still being actively secreted. In this situation it would be unwise to prescribed hypotonic fluids in the postoperative period and impose an extra burden of more EFW to be excreted by the kidney.

The prescription of postoperative fluids should be based on the individual patient's need for water and electrolytes. The wise assumption is that every postoperative patient will have nonphysiological secretion of ADH and will therefore be able to excrete dilute (hypotonic) urine. Indeed, all evidence points to the fact that the urine is hypertonic because of the high sodium content. In this situation the prescription of maintenance fluid for patients who are unable to take oral fluids should be an isotonic or near-isotonic solution, with added potassium to replace urinary losses. Fluid losses from the GI tract should also be replaced with isotonic saline with added potassium. Although dextrose is frequently added to solutions used during surgery and in the postoperative period because of concerns about hypoglycemia, there is no evidence that this is necessary except in newborns or in patients who were previously receiving preoperative solutions containing high concentrations of glucose. Patients should be prescribed iv fluids based on measurements of their serum electrolytes rather than theoretical considerations of the water and electrolyte requirements that have been calculated for healthy children. Hypotonic saline should only be administered to children who have a demonstrated free water deficit (PNa > 145 mmol/l).

6.3 Respiratory Management

Children require postrespiratory support for a variety of reasons. These include central respiratory depression due to the effect of anesthetic agents and narcotics or surgery or injury of the brain itself following neurosurgical procedures. There may also be compromise of the actual mechanics of respiration due to reduced respiratory system compliance from thoracic surgery or from abdominal wound closure. Prolonged surgical procedures with large amounts of blood loss may result in pulmonary edema secondary to large volume transfusion of blood products and electrolyte solutions. This is particularly true in the newborn where major abdominal or thoracic surgical procedures renders the infant particularly vulnerable to develop respiratory failure, as surgery frequently has an adverse effect on the mechanics of the respiratory system. Repair of congenital abnormalities such as gastroschisis or congenital diaphragmatic hernia (CDH) frequently result in rises in intra-abdominal pressure, upward displacement of the diaphragms, and a fall in total thoracic compliance. Normal tidal respiration in the infant occurs around the closing capacity and therefore any loss of lung volume will result in further atelectasis and hypoxemia. Also, the metabolism and elimination of inhalational anesthetic agents, narcotics, and muscle relaxants is slower in the neonate and their effects will extend well into the postoperative period.

The basic concept behind the original mechanical ventilators was to use positive pressure to both operate the ventilator and to generate a gas flow into the lung, sufficient to expand alveoli by overcoming the opposing forces generated by the elastic properties of the lung (compliance) and the endotracheal tube and airways (resistance). In the small child the ET tube is the site of greatest resistance in the circuit. Very few of these ventilators were specifically designed for use in children and the initial approach was to adapt adult ventilators to the child. Ventilator technology has improved significantly in the past 20 years and the currently available machines are adaptable enough to ventilate both adults and children. The most commonly used newer generation machines have a pneumatic system where oxygen and air are mixed at 50 psi. A microprocessor controls an inspiratory valve that, when opened, delivers heated humidified gas to the patient. The microprocessor also controls an expiratory valve that opens during expiration and filtered gas is vented to the atmosphere. The expiratory valve also controls the amount of PEEP applied at end-expiration.

The detailed descriptive characteristics of ventilators used in intensive care can be complex and are beyond the scope of this chapter. For the purposes of a general discussion on postoperative ventilation it is sufficient to know that all deliver positive pressure to the lung, the inspiratory and expiratory phases are time-cycled and the ventilator can be set to deliver gas either according to a preset pressure limit (pressure ventilation) or a preset tidal volume (volume ventilation). The number of breaths delivered by the ventilator is set by the operator while the duration of the inspiratory and expiratory time of each ventilator cycle can be altered by adjusting the inspiratory time. The machine cycles from inspiration to expiration when either the preset pressure or volume is reached.

6.3.1 Pressure Ventilation

In pressure ventilation a preselected pressure is set, defined as the peak inspiratory pressure (PIP), and is chosen depending on that required to deliver an adequate tidal volume, considering the compliance of the lung and the airway resistance. In uncomplicated postoperative ventilation, adequate tidal volume can be delivered at a PIP of 15–20 cmH$_2$O. This may increase significantly when resistance in the lung or airway distal to the ET tube connector rises or pulmonary or thoracic (lung and chest wall) compliance falls. The airway pressure at end-expiration (normally zero during spontaneous breathing) can be increased to 5–20 cmH$_2$O, depending on whether PEEP is required to maintain lung expansion. It is important to note that the tidal volume delivered by a pressure ventilator will change significantly according to conditions within the thorax. A fall in compliance or a rise in airway resistance results in the ventilator rapidly reaching its preselected inspiratory pressure. A reduction in delivered alveolar ventilation will inevitably follow, which can only be overcome by increasing the preset pressure. A large leak around the ETT may prevent the ventilator reaching its cycling pressure. With pressure ventilation, PIP is constant but tidal volume may vary.

6.3.2 Volume Ventilation

The alternative ventilation system is a time-cycled, volume preset respirator that will deliver a set tidal volume at a preselected rate. A tidal volume is chosen based on body weight and is usually in the range of 6–12 ml/kg, depending on the patient's resistance and compliance. In certain machines, the operator chooses the minute volume and ventilatory rate and the tidal volume can be calculated from these two settings. Alternatively, in other types of respirators the tidal volume and rate are selected and the minute volume calculated. The more modern machines have the ability to measure and display both the inspired and expired tidal volume. As with the pressure type respirator, the duration of the inspiratory and expiratory time can be adjusted according to conditions within the thorax. A fall in compliance or rise in airway resistance should not result in a fall in alveolar ventilation as the machine will merely increase the pressure in order to overcome these changes. However, PIP will rise. The respirator however will not compensate for leaks around the ET tube and a significant proportion of the preset volume will be vented around the tube when there is a large leak. In volume ventilation, the tidal volume is constant while PIP may vary. These ventilators are most commonly used for ventilating adult patients or older children where cuffed ET tubes are used and leaks around the trachea are not a concern. They can also be used effectively in smaller children as long as the leak is not large.

6.3.3 Triggering the Ventilator

The term "triggering" in mechanical ventilation refers to the process that results in the opening of the inspiratory valve and the initiation of inspiration. This can either be machine initiated in the pressure or volume control modes or patient initiated in assist and control, pressure support, or CPAP modes. The sensitivity of the inspiratory valve can be set by the operator. Patient-generated triggering is preferred because it facilitates weaning and allows the patient to use his respiratory muscles.

6.4 Respiratory Gas Exchange

6.4.1 Carbon Dioxide Elimination

Adequate CO_2 elimination depends on the ratio between CO_2 production (metabolic rate) and alveolar ventilation (tidal volume—dead space). In the normal spontaneous respiration, the two sides of the equation balance and normal CO_2 homeostasis is preserved. An increase in CO_2 production, as seen during a rise in body temperature or sepsis, can normally be met by increased alveolar ventilation and the child achieves this by increasing its respiratory rate. Similarly, abnormalities within the thorax will result primarily in an increase in respiratory rate rather than volume in order

to achieve the same alveolar ventilation. In mechanical ventilation, the $PaCO_2$ level can be controlled by adjusting both ventilator rate and the volume delivered by each respiratory cycle (alveolar ventilation = tidal volume—dead space × frequency). With a pressure preset ventilator, minute ventilation is increased by increasing the PIP and rate, while in the volume respirator $PaCO_2$ is controlled by adjusting rate and delivered volume.

6.4.2 Oxygen Uptake

The diffusion gradient for oxygen within the lung is high as the PO_2 in the pulmonary artery is 40 mmHg (5.3 kpa) compared to the alveolar PO_2 (PAO_2) of 105 mmHg (14 kpa) while breathing air. Despite this favorable gradient for oxygen diffusion, the alveoli must remain open for gas exchange to occur. In the normal lung, due to the hysteresis, the alveoli open during inspiration and remain open during most of expiration and only cease exchanging gas at end-expiration. In the diffusely atelectatic lung, of which the Acute Respiratory Distress Syndrome (ARDS) is a prime example, the alveoli become unstable and tend to collapse at low lung volumes. The degree of alveolar expansion depends to a large part on mean airway pressure (Paw), which is a measure of the average pressure that the alveoli are exposed to during the respiratory cycle. This in turn is determined by a combination of the PIP, PEEP, and the duration of the inspiratory phase of the respiratory cycle. Attempts to improve oxygenation are based on the manipulation of one or more of these variables in order to increase Paw. The simplest and most time honored of these measures is to increase the amount of PEEP, which was first introduced to improve oxygenation in lung disease of prematurity. Abnormalities within the lung that cause a large difference between PAO_2 and PaO_2 (A-a DO_2) may also be compensated for by increasing the FiO_2.

6.5 Setting Ventilator Parameters

Choosing the options in postoperative ventilatory management is in a large part determined by conditions within the patient. The objective is to maintain gases within a physiological range (PaCO$_2$ 5–6.5 kpa, 38–50 mmHg, PaO$_2$ 8–12 kpa, 60–100 mmHg,) using the lowest FiO$_2$, TV, and airway pressure compatible with that objective. This is consistent with a systemic oxygen saturation of >90%. This may be relatively simple where the lungs are normal, but may require a different strategy in the presence of abnormalities within the abdomen or thorax. Therefore, one must consider these when selecting ventilator settings. Generally speaking, children with normal respiratory system compliance and airways resistance on a pressure preset ventilator would require a PIP of 15–20 cmH$_2$O, a rate of 30–40/min, an FiO$_2$ 0.25–0.35, and an inspiratory to expiratory ratio (I:E ratio) of 1:2 or 1:2.5, and a minimum of 3–5 cmH$_2$O PEEP as a routine. Having selected the appropriate ventilator parameters, practitioners should ensure themselves of the adequacy of alveolar ventilation and oxygenation by observing chest rise during inspiration and the pulse oximeter saturation (SaO$_2$). This can then be verified by end-tidal CO$_2$ (PetCO$_2$) and blood gas measurements.

6.5.1 Weaning from Ventilation

Weaning from mechanical ventilation has been considerably simplified by the widespread use of IMV and other forms of ventilatory assist modes (Table 6.6). With these systems, the infant may take spontaneous breaths from a gas flow provided either through a demand valve or from a separate spontaneous breathing circuit. In this manner, the mandatory breaths are gradually reduced as spontaneous respiratory effort improves, until the child is breathing entirely spontaneously through a constant positive airway pressure (CPAP) system. The pace of weaning depends on the type of surgery and any additional pathology within the lung and is set by observing the spontaneous respiratory rate and the measured blood gas response to changes in ventilation settings. In order to tolerate the transition from CPAP to extubation, the patient should be on FiO$_2$ 0.4, PEEP 5 cmH$_2$O, with normal blood gases. A more recent innovation has been the introduction of pressure support ventilation where each

Table 6.6 Commonly used forms of positive pressure ventilation and terminology

Terminology	Descriptor	Comments
Volume ventilation or volume control ventilation	Preset TV. Patient cannot trigger the ventilator. Tidal volume is constant while PIP may vary	Most commonly used mode in adults and older children. Also effective in smaller children with minimal ET tube leaks
Pressure ventilation or pressure control ventilation	Preset pressure. Patient cannot trigger the ventilator. PIP is constant but tidal volume may vary	Commonly used in neonates. Increasing use in adults to prevent ventilator-induced lung injury in patients with ARDS
Continuous positive airway pressure (CPAP)	Spontaneous breathing mode with no mechanically delivered breaths and positive end expiratory pressure. High gas flow delivered by a demand valve	First introduced to treat preterm infants with lung disease of prematurity. Now commonly used as a pre-extubation mode of respiratory support
Assist control ventilation	Minimum rate and TV (or pressure) set. Patient may trigger inspiration at a more rapid rate	Common form of weaning from mechanical ventilation
Assisted ventilation	All breaths are patient triggered at the ventilator's set volume or pressure	Most commonly used as ***Pressure Support*** ventilation
Mandatory ventilation, intermittent mandatory ventilation (IMV), or synchronized intermittent mandatory ventilation (SIMV)	Machine generated breath that is triggered, limited, and cycled by the ventilator	Now commonly used
Noninvasive ventilation (NIV)	Positive pressure delivered by either nasal or face mask. Commonly used as a bilevel device with preselected inspiratory airway pressure (IPAP) and expiratory airway (EPAP) pressure (EPAP)	Increasingly used in patients with less severe lung disease and in premature infants. Avoids the need for intubation and risk of ventilator-associated pneumonia (VAP)

spontaneously initiated breath generates a positive pressure from the machine to a preset inspiratory level. This helps to overcome the fixed resistance of small endotracheal tubes.

6.6 Alternative Modes of Ventilation

6.6.1 Noninvasive Ventilation

An important advance in the management of respiratory failure in both newborns and older children has been the increasingly widespread use of noninvasive ventilation either in the form of a face mask or nasal cannulae. The high gas flow used in this system means that airway pressure remains positive throughout both the inspiratory and expiratory cycle. Functional residual capacity (FRC) is maintained, decreasing the work of breathing and preventing lung collapse. There is an additional potential advantage in that avoiding invasion of the airway reduces the risk of nosocomial lung infections. The system has proved effective in the treatment of lung disease of prematurity as a primary mode of therapy. It has also been used to avoid reintubation in patients who remain tachypneic with increased work of breathing following extubation. This mode of ventilation may be particularly effective in children with musculoskeletal disease who have undergone surgery for correction of scoliosis.

6.6.2 High-Frequency Ventilation

One of the major innovations in mechanical ventilation in children has been the use of high-frequency ventilation (HFV), which allows patients to be ventilated at tidal volumes well below anatomical dead space and very low airway pressures. HFV exists in two forms: either high frequency oscillatory ventilation (HFOV) or high frequency jet ventilation (HFJV). The former generates a high frequency sine wave that accelerates diffusion and elimination of CO_2 from the lung with very little in the way of bulk gas flow. Oxygenation is achieved by a high fresh gas flow into the circuit and, by adjusting this, the device is capable of generating mean airway pressures in excess of

$30\,cmH_2O$. High-frequency jet ventilation (HFJV) was first developed in clinical anesthesia to provide small tidal volume ventilation for procedures involving the larynx and the tracheobronchial tree where the ability to achieve a normal CO_2 with low airway pressures provided ideal operating conditions. In HFJV, the lung is ventilated by the rapid injection of gas into the airway at rates of 100–600/min with a supplemental air or oxygen gas flow entrained. Gas exchange occurs by a combination of very small amounts of bulk flow and enhanced diffusion.

Although HFJV and HFOV operate on the same physiological principles of very small tidal volumes delivered at high rates, they should not be considered as merely two variations on the same theme. Apart from the slower rates used in HFJV, the other major difference is that expiration is passive in the former while it is active in HFOV. Both techniques have the potential advantage of reducing the incidence of ventilator-induced lung injury and have been extensively used in newborn infants with lung disease of prematurity and meconium aspiration syndrome. There are several case series of the successful use of HFOV in the management of infants with CDH with reports of improved survival using a low mean airway pressure strategy to avoid lung distention. HFJV has been used successfully in pulmonary trauma associate with bronchopulmonary fistula where the low tidal volumes reduce the air leak from the lung (Table 6.7). However, there are some technical concerns about the adequacy of humidification in this system as well as reported cases of tracheal damage (necrotizing tracheobronchitis) in severely ill newborn infants. In addition, the airway pressures measured from the catheter within the trachea during HFJV probably represent a serious underestimate of true MAP because of the Bernoulli effect, and consequently there is likely to be a significant amount of auto-PEEP present.

6.7 Respiratory Monitoring

6.7.1 Blood Gas Measurement

Monitoring of respiratory function in the postoperative period requires measurement of gas exchange. The most reliable and accurate method is to measure PaO_2, $PaCO_2$, and pH from an arterial sample. The common sites for invasive arterial monitoring are umbilical artery (newborns) and radial or dorsalis pedis arteries in older children. In the newborn, a blood gas drawn from the right radial will measure preductal PaO_2 values, whereas the other sites will be postductal. On some occasions the left subclavian artery is juxta-ductal and will therefore measure similar values to the right. With the newer generation of automated blood gas machines, samples as small as 0.1 ml are sufficient for a full blood gas and pH profile. This is particularly important in premature infants in whom frequent sampling may necessitate "top up" transfusions. An alternative method of measuring $PaCO_2$, PaO_2, and pH is to use "arterialized" capillary blood taken from an area of skin that has been vasodilated by warming, usually the heel. This technique is generally reliable for $PaCO_2$ and pH. With arterial PaO_2 levels above 60–70 mmHg, accuracy drops off considerably.

6.7.2 Noninvasive Oxygenation and CO_2 Monitoring

The development of pulse oximetry has made it possible to measure arterial saturation and heart rate on a beat-to-beat basis and has proved to be a reliable and effective method of monitoring and trending oxygenation. The absolute values do not correlate well when measured at blood saturations of less than 70% and in low cardiac output states where there is inadequate perfusion for a pulse to be recorded by the probe. Careful sensor placement is important to prevent distorting by light and the probes are sensitive to light artifact. It is a useful monitor to record the rapid response of PO_2 to interventions such as suctioning and changes in ventilation. Due to the shape of the oxygen hemoglobin dissociation curve, high PaO_2 levels (>95 mmHg, 12.6 kpa) will not be accurately reflected by saturation measurements. In the premature neonate (<1,000 g), where high PaO_2 levels may predispose to the development of retinopathy of prematurity (ROP), the transcutaneous PO_2 ($TcPO_2$) probe is the preferred method of monitoring oxygenation as it indirectly measures the actual PaO_2.

The $TcPO_2$ technique uses a modified Clark electrode with a heating element that raises skin temperature to 41°C–44°C in order to augment cutaneous blood flow. These devices correlate well with arterial oxygen in small infants who have little subcutaneous tissue, and

are reliable where cardiac output and peripheral perfusion are adequate. However, quality declines in the older child and in low cardiac output states. Transcutaneous CO_2 ($TcPCO_2$) monitoring uses the modified Severinghous probe with a heating element, which heats the skin to 41–44°C. These have proved to be reliable in small infants. While transcutaneous PO_2 and PCO_2 monitoring are useful trending devices, absolute values should be occasionally checked against an arterial sample. Greater accuracy is obtained by careful maintenance of the probes and care in calibration and application to the skin. The risk of skin damage from the heating element requires that the measuring site be changed every 4–6 h.

6.7.3 End-Tidal CO_2 Monitoring

Capnography is the measurement and display of CO_2 concentration in the airway using an infrared technique and has recently become a standard fixture on most mechanical ventilators. In the normal capnogram, CO_2 is zero during inspiration and at the beginning of expiration as anatomical dead space gas is washed out. The concentration then rises as alveolar gas mixes with anatomical dead space gas and reaches a plateau with an upward slope when pure alveolar gas reaches the sensor. The end expiratory point of the plateau before the inspiratory cycle starts is the end-tidal pressure ($PetCO_2$) and approximates alveolar PCO_2 ($PACO_2$). This is usually approximately 5 mmHg less than the $PaCO_2$. The $PetCO_2$ provides useful information of the adequacy of alveolar ventilation in patients with normal lungs but in the presence of lung disease $PaCO_2$—$PetCO_2$ gradient widens.

6.8 Management of the Intubated Patient

6.8.1 Tube Size and Position (Table 6.8)

Newborns are commonly managed with nasotracheal tubes rather than oral tubes unless there is some congenital abnormality of or injury to the nasal area that precludes their use. They provide for greater patient comfort and acceptability and the tube may be more securely

Table 6.7 Characteristics of high-frequency ventilators

	HFOV	HFJV
Rate	180–900/min	100–600/min
VT	At high rates (>10 Hz) minimal TV. TV increases as rates decreases	TV 2–5 ml/kg
Expiration	Active	Passive
Gas movement	Diffusion	Diffusion plus bulk flow
Indications	Used in lung disease associate with low lung compliance (MAS, IRDS) as part of an open lung strategy. Also has been extensively used in CDH	IRDS, MAS, and bronchopleural fistula

VT: tidal volume, IRDS: infant respiratory distress syndrome: MAS: meconium aspiration syndrome: Hz: cycles per second

fastened to the face and upper lip. In older children oral tubes are satisfactory for brief periods of ventilation but nasal ones are frequently preferred. In terms of length, the tip of the tube should reach the level of the clavicles on the chest film. Tubes that extend lower may enter a main bronchus, especially during flexion or extension movements of the head. A routine chest film should be obtained immediately after intubation or change of tube position to ascertain correct placement. The proximal end of the tube should protrude sufficiently far from the nose so that the tube connector does not impinge on the external nares. Severe excoriation of nares and erosion of cartilage can occur with long-term intubation. In selecting a tube of correct diameter, the size should be sufficient to provide a small leak under positive pressure, but not large enough to provide an airtight seal. Tight-fitting tubes left in situ for prolonged periods will lead to tracheal stenosis and vocal cord granuloma formation, requiring tracheostomy and extended postoperative care. At the same time, too large a leak will make positive pressure ventilation extremely difficult. In the term newborn, 3, 3.5 or 4 mm tubes may be used depending on the size of the infant; 2.5 or 2 mm may be used in premature infants, but these are prone to block with secretions. Cuffed tubes in pediatric sizes are now available with low pressure inflatable cuffs that have been used successfully in small children and newborns.

6.8.2 Endotracheal Tube Suctioning

Routine suctioning to maintain the patency of the endotracheal tube and prevent atelectasis is of prime importance especially in newborns. However, even skillful suctioning can lead to a profound fall in PaO_2 and bradycardia, especially in patients who are already hypoxemic. Consequently, prior to suctioning, all patients should have their lungs inflated with 100% oxygen by manual hyperventilation. A catheter of a size that does not occlude the lumen of the endotracheal tube should be chosen so that the suctioning does not generate negative pressures large enough to cause atelectasis. End-hole catheters should be used rather that the side-hole type, which can trap and injure the respiratory tract mucosa. Suction should only be applied while the catheter is being withdrawn and for not longer than a few seconds. Between each suctioning, the patient should be ventilated with 100% oxygen. The onset of bradycardia during suctioning is an immediate indication to stop and ventilate with oxygen, as it is almost always indicative of hypoxemia.

Endotracheal suctioning should always be performed as a sterile procedure using surgical gloves and a sterile catheter. The objective should be to pass the catheter down as far as it will go to beyond the carina and down either one or the other main bronchus, at the same time stimulating the patient to cough. The catheter tip may be encouraged to pass down either one or the other side by rotating the head to the opposite side. The presence of unduly thick secretions in the respiratory tract should alert one to the possibility of inadequate humidification. Intrapulmonary hemorrhage increases the chances of endotracheal tube blockage substantially and indicates the need for more frequent suctioning.

6.8.3 Humidification

Humidification is one of the least emphasized but most important aspects of respiratory care. The small diameter

Table 6.8 Endotracheal tube size selection

Age	Endotracheal tube diameter (mm)
Term newborn	3.0 to 3.5
1 Month	3.5
1–6 Months	3.5 or 4.0
1 Year	4.0
3 Years	4.5
5 Years	5.0 or 5.5
10 Years	6.0 or 6.5
>13 Years	6.5 or 7.0

ETT size (diameter) formula—age in years/4 plus 4 mm

endotracheal tube in the newborn patient is notoriously prone to blockage from secretions, especially where they become inspissated due to inadequate humidification. Too much humidification leads to "rainout", as the inspired gas cools during its passage between the humidifier and the infant's airway and can lead to the absorption of considerable amounts of water.

The goal of optimal humidity is to deliver fully saturated gases (44 mg/l H_2O) at a temperature of 37°C to the peak of the airway. This can only be achieved with the heated water bath type humidifier as opposed to the nebulizer type. The temperature of the water bath must be raised above body temperature, to about 40°C, in order to deliver gases at 35–37°C at the ET tube. Between the humidifier and the endotracheal tube, considerable condensation of water vapor may occur as the gases cool, which may impede gas flow. This problem has been overcome to some extent with the newer humidifiers that have a heated electric coil inside the inspiratory line. This maintains a consistent temperature throughout the inspiratory line by means of a dual servo mechanism with temperature sensors in both the water bath and at the patient's airway. Therefore, there is less cooling of gases in the respirator tubing and inspired gas is delivered to the ET tube fully saturated and at 37°C.

The condenser humidifier or "Swedish nose" is also capable of supplying moisture and preventing heat loss from the respiratory tract. While obviously not as efficient as the water bath type, it is particularly useful for patient transport or for providing humidity to children who have been intubated for upper airway problems. As the condenser humidifier becomes increasingly saturated, the airway resistance tends to rise and they must be changed every 24 h.

Further Reading

Bohn D (2005) Fluids and electrolytes in pediatrics. In M Fink, E Abraham, J-L Vincent, PM Kochanek (eds). Textbook of Critical Care, 5th edn. Elsevier Saunders, Philadelphia, PA, pp 1131–7

Hess D, Kacmarek RM (1996) Essentials of Mechanical Ventilation. McGraw-Hill, New York

Kooh SW, Metcoff J (1963) Physiologic considerations in fluid and electrolyte therapy with particular reference to diarrheal dehydration in children. J Pediatr 62:107–31

Moritz ML, Ayus JC (2002) Disorders of water metabolism in children: hyponatremia and hypernatremia. Pediatr Rev 23(11):371–80

Moritz ML, Ayus JC (2003) Prevention of hospital-acquired hyponatremia: A case for using isotonic saline. Pediatrics 111(2):227–30

Paut O, Lacroix F (2006) Recent developments in the perioperative fluid management for the paediatric patient. Curr Opin Anaesthesiol 19(3):268–77

Puri P, Höllwarth ME (eds) (2006) Pediatric Surgery. Springer, Berlin, Heidelberg

Holliday MA, Segar WE (1957) The maintenance need for water in parenteral fluid therapy. Pediatrics 19:823–832

Sepsis

7

Christian J. Ochoa, Jeffrey S. Upperman,
and Henri R. Ford

Contents

7.1 Introduction Including Definition and Incidence

Sepsis from an infectious etiology is a major cause of morbidity and mortality in the United States. Despite recent advances in neonatal and pediatric critical care medicine, the number of children suffering from sepsis continues to rise. A review in the New England Journal of Medicine reported an 8.7% annual increase in the incidence of sepsis in the United States. A national survey of nearly 1.6 million hospitalized children, ages 19 years or younger, revealed 42,364 cases of sepsis per year. Infants were affected more often than older children.

Sepsis can be caused by a variety of insults, including infection or tissue injury. Invasive microbial infections often result from the inability of the intrinsic host defense mechanisms to combat certain virulence factors. The most frequent organisms identified in the pediatric and adult populations include *Escherichia coli*, *Pseudomonas aeruginosa*, *Klebsiella*, and *Bacteriodes* species. The most common pathogens in the neonatal population are group B streptococci and *E. coli*. These pathogens induce a localized inflammatory response in the host designed to destroy the microorganisms. Lack of control, over-exuberance of this inflammatory response, or inability of the host to eradicate the infection may lead to a clinical syndrome characterized by fever, inadequate tissue perfusion, organ dysfunction, and generalized edema. This constellation of symptoms is referred to as the sepsis syndrome or the systemic inflammatory response syndrome (SIRS). This may represent the final common pathway through which microbial infection or extensive tissue injury results in the demise of the host.

P. Puri and M. Höllwarth (eds.), *Pediatric Surgery: Diagnosis and Management*,
DOI: 10.1007/978-3-540-69560-8_7, © Springer-Verlag Berlin Heidelberg 2009

7.2 Risk Factors

7.2.1 Barriers to Infection

The human body is colonized by a variety of nonpatho-
genic organisms. These indigenous microbes normally
adhere to the epithelial lining and prevent attachment of
pathogenic microbes. There are other protective mechanisms, such as intestinal peristalsis and immunoglobulins, which help to limit microbial invasion (Table 7.1).
Oropharyngeal, nasopharyngeal, tracheobronchial, and
gastrointestinal secretions are rich in immunoglobulins,
which help to prevent bacterial attachment to the
epithelium—a critical step in the establishment of
infections. In particular, immunoglobulin A (IgA) binds
microorganisms at the epithelial surface, thereby
impairing their ability to attach to the epithelial lining.
Any breach in the mucosal barrier permits bacteria or
viruses to infiltrate the epithelial lining and elicit an
inflammatory response. Trauma, surgery, malnutrition,
burns, immunosuppression, shock, and reperfusion
injury following an ischemic event can cause gut barrier failure. Reperfusion injury allows the elaboration
of toxic reactive oxygen species, such as superoxide
(O_2^-) and hydrogen peroxide (H_2O_2), which damage the
epithelial lining and permit the translocation and internalization of microbes.

7.3 Pathophysiology of Sepsis

7.3.1 Bacterial Virulence

Establishment of a clinical infection in the host begins
with bacterial attachment to the epithelial surface
followed by subsequent internalization of the microbe.
The internalized microbe must elude the local cellular
and humoral host defense mechanisms in order to
cause infection. Evasion of the host immune system
allows the microbe to multiply, damage local tissue,
and elicit an inflammatory response; this process
depends largely on microbial virulence factors.

The process of microbial adherence requires interaction between specific cell surface receptors on the
host and key molecules on the bacteria, called adhesins.
Bacterial fimbriae or pili are known to promote bacterial adherence to mucosal surfaces. *E. coli* expresses

Table 7.1 Defense mechanisms against microbial invasion

Host defense	Actions
Gastric acid	Lower pH promotes a hostile environment for bacterial growth
Peristalsis	Coordinated movements sweep the bacteria downstream, limiting their attachment to the mucosa
Local flora	Indigenous microbial flora prevent the overgrowth of pathogenic Gram-negative bacteria
Immunoglobulin	IgA coats and aggregates bacteria and prevents their attachment to intestinal mucosa
Mucus	Intestinal mucus forms a thick barrier, which prevents bacterial attachment

different types of fimbriae that permit their attachment
to the D-mannose receptor on epithelial cells. Some
microbes also display adhesins that facilitate entry into
the host. Indirectly, the host secretes proteins that have
a common peptide sequence Arg–Gly–Asp, such as
fibronectin, laminin, collagen, and vitronectin, which
enhance bacterial attachment to the host.

Once the microbe has attached to the cell surface,
the organism may gain entry into the cell through a
process called internalization. This requires high
affinity binding between the microbe's pili and cell
surface receptors. The cell surface contains a receptor called integrin, which binds the bacterial pili.
The affinity of the pili for this receptor determines
whether the microbe attaches to the cell and becomes
internalized.

Once the bacteria have evaded the initial host
defense mechanisms and gained entry into the cell,
they must survive within the intracellular milieu in
order to establish an infection. Bacterial internalization takes place through phagocytosis. The internalized bacteria are transported in intracellular vesicles
known as endosomes or phagosomes. Fusion of the
cell's lysosome with the phagosome leads to acidifica-
tion of the phagolysosome complex and neutralization
of the internalized bacteria by specific toxins such as
hyaluronidase, collagenase, proteinase, deoxyribonu-
clease, and lecithinase. The bacteria may counterattack
by secreting exotoxins to help neutralize the host
defense mechanisms. For instance, *S. aureus* produces
catalase, which neutralizes hydrogen peroxide. Strepto-
lysin, a streptococcal exotoxin, can inhibit neutrophil

migration and impair phagocyte cytotoxicity. Thus, bacterial virulence is important not only for the microbe to gain entry into a host cell but also to avoid the host innate defense mechanisms such as neutrophils and macrophages. One of the most potent bacterial toxins is called lipopolysaccharide (LPS) (or endotoxin). It contains an O-specific side chain, a core polysaccharide, and an inner lipid A region. The lipid A region is a highly potent stimulator of the inflammatory response. This molecule may initiate septic shock by stimulating the release of inflammatory mediators such as arachidonic acid and leukotrienes, or through complement activation. Endotoxin alone is sufficient to induce shock when given experimentally to laboratory animals or to human volunteers.

7.3.2 Neutrophils

Neutrophils are terminally differentiated effector cells that constitute the first line of defense in response to infection or tissue injury. The neutrophil contains a plethora of proteolytic enzymes and reactive oxygen species that can cause local tissue damage when released into the extracellular matrix. After a 14-day development in the bone marrow, the neutrophils circulate in the bloodstream for 6–14 h. Nearly 50% of the circulating neutrophils attach or adhere to the vascular endothelium—a process known as margination. If there are no detectable infections, the neutrophils undergo apoptosis or programmed cell death in the liver or the bone marrow. The neutrophils that adhere to the vascular endothelium must leave the bloodstream through a process known as diapedesis to reach the tissues. There, they can survive for another 48 h performing critical functions such as phagocytosis and microbial killing. Adhesion molecules such as selectins, integrins, and the immunoglobulin superfamily govern the adherence of neutrophils to the vascular endothelium. (L)-selectin (CD62L) on the neutrophil surface binds to endothelium (E)-selectin and platelet (P)-selectin, which is upregulated when the endothelial cells are activated by injury, infectious agents, or by inflammatory mediators. Leukocyte or neutrophil rolling occurs when there is low affinity binding of L-selectin and P-selectin. Migration of the neutrophil to the site of injury is regulated by a class of molecules known as integrins, which are expressed on the neutrophil surface. Specifically, binding of β_2 integrin to intercellular adhesion molecule 1 (ICAM-1) on the endothelial cell directs neutrophil trafficking.

LPS can affect neutrophil adhesion and migration by stimulating the release of tumor necrosis factor-α (TNF-α), interleukin-1 (IL-1) and interferon-γ (IFN-γ), which are known to upregulate ICAM-1 and E-selectin. An acute phase reactant called lipopolysaccharide binding protein (LBP), a 58-kDa protein that is synthesized in the liver, enhances the sensitivity of monocytes and granulocytes to LPS by facilitating binding of LPS to the CD14 cell membrane molecule and to Toll-like receptor 4 (TLR-4) on the surface of neutrophils and monocytes. This interaction upregulates β_2 integrin CD11b/CD18 and enhances the neutrophil–endothelial interaction. Clinically, patients with leukocyte adhesion deficiency are susceptible to recurrent bacterial infections due to the lack of β_2 integrin receptor CD11b/CD18, which results in inability of the neutrophil to adhere to the endothelium and effect bacterial killing.

Once the neutrophil has adhered to the endothelium, then migration of the neutrophil to the site of tissue injury is governed, in part, by platelet endothelial cell adhesion molecule 1 (PECAM-1). It is expressed on the surface of blood vessels and maintains the vascular permeability barrier. Evidence suggests that the antibody to PECAM-1 causes leaky barriers and inhibits neutrophil transmigration and endotoxin-induced leukocyte sequestration in the lung, liver, and muscle. Also neutrophil egress requires a chemotactic gradient through the extracellular matrix. Important chemotactic peptides include monocyte chemotactic protein 1 (MCP-1), platelet-activating factor (PAF), leukotriene B_4, and interleukin 8. Small amounts of chemotaxins are required for the neutrophil to become responsive. A cascade of intracellular signaling pathways is activated when the neutrophil binds to the endothelium. These events eventually lead to conformational changes in the cytoskeleton of the neutrophil and permit its trans-endothelial egress and rapid movement toward the chemotactic gradient.

The neutrophil's primary objective is to destroy the microorganism; this is achieved through phagocytosis followed by intracellular killing. Specific immunoglobulins such as IgG enhance the phagocytic activity of the neutrophil, facilitate these events, and stimulate complement activation. Priming of the neutrophil or prior stimulation leads to more efficient killing. The fusion of the phagosome with the lysosome, which contains powerful antimicrobial agents, aids in the killing of the microbe.

Release of reactive oxygen intermediates, formed by the enzyme NADPH, is the principal oxygen-dependent mechanism involved in the killing of microbes in the lysosome. In the neutrophil, the respiratory burst catalyzes the reduction of molecular oxygen (O_2) to superoxide (O_2^-), which is subsequently converted to hydrogen peroxide (H_2O_2) by superoxide dismutase. Hydrogen peroxide can form a hydroxyl radical in the presence of iron or other metals and can also form hypochlorous acid (HOCl) in the presence of myeloperoxidase. HOCl is the chemical that accounts for the cytotoxicity of the neutrophil in the presence of nitrogen-containing compounds. Enzymes such as lysozyme, elastase, lactoferrin, cathepsin, and defensins, within the phagolysosome act synergistically to promote microbial killing.

7.3.3 Monocytes-Macrophages

Just like the neutrophil, the monocyte-macrophage also plays an important role in the eradication of infections. There are many similarities between the neutrophil and monocyte-macrophage complex. Both phagocytose and use lysosomes to kill the bacteria. Both produce reactive oxygen intermediates on stimulation by LPS and IFN-γ. The monocyte evolves from a precursor (promonocyte) in the bone marrow, which undergoes maturation by acquiring specific granules. The monocyte then migrates to various tissues and organs where it further differentiates into macrophages. Tissue macrophages are the principal effectors in the defense against intracellular pathogens. They can phagocytose and destroy many common bacteria, but with less efficiency than the neutrophil. Macrophages express adhesion molecules such as L-selectin and β_1 and β_2 integrins. This distinction is important since macrophages can still migrate to the site of inflammation in patients with leukocyte adhesion deficiency (lack of β_2 integrin). An important difference between the neutrophil and the macrophage is that the macrophage, after engulfing the bacteria, can present the antigenic fragments to the T lymphocytes in the context of major histocompatibility complex (MHC) class II molecules. This enhances the release of inflammatory cytokines and the microbicidal activity of the macrophage.

Similar to the neutrophils, macrophages produce reactive oxygen species; however, they also produce nitric oxide (NO), which has diverse biological properties. NO is the product of the conversion of arginine to citrulline by nitric oxide synthase (NOS). Three isoforms of NOS exist: neuronal NOS (NOS-1) and endothelial NOS (NOS-3) are expressed constitutively. Inducible NOS (NOS-2, or iNOS), found in the macrophage and other cells, is activated in response to inflammatory mediators. NO is relatively innocuous, but can react with reactive oxygen species to form cytotoxic molecules. For instance, peroxynitrite is an important reactive nitrogen intermediate that is formed by the reaction of NO with O_2^- in inflammatory lesions in vivo and is responsible for the cytopathic effects of NO. NO may also react with metalloproteins to form S-nitrosothiols. Sustained overproduction of these compounds may lead to cellular injury and multisystem organ dysfunction.

7.3.4 Lymphocytes

Lymphocytes and natural killer cells are the predominant effector cells against intracellular organisms. Lymphocytes originate from the bone marrow; however, some leave the bone marrow to undergo maturation or "education" in the thymus. Once mature, the T lymphocytes migrate to peripheral lymphoid organs such as the spleen, lymph nodes, and the Peyer's patches in the intestine, where they establish residence. Other lymphocytes mature in the bone marrow and become B cells, which produce immunoglobulins. The main job of T lymphocytes is to regulate cell-mediated immunity against intracellular pathogens. This requires recognition of the inciting antigen by MHC class II proteins, cellular activation, clonal expansion, and targeted killing. The MHC proteins on cell surfaces govern antigen presentation. Macrophages, dendritic cells, and B-lymphocytes can act as antigen-presenting cells. These cells phagocytose the microbe and digest it into smaller fragments or peptides that are then bound to the MHC class II proteins, and then presented to T helper cells. In addition, any cell that is infected can present microbial antigen on its cell surface using MHC class I molecules. CD8+ cytotoxic T lymphocytes then target these cells and release serine proteases to induce apoptosis or programmed cell death.

7.3.5 Immunoglobulins

Immunoglobulins or antibodies represent a class of proteins that are synthesized from mature B-lymphocytes or plasma cells. The primary role of antibodies is to prevent microbial attachment to, or invasion of, the host epithelium. There are five major classes of immunoglobulins: IgA, IgG, IgM, IgD, and IgE. The predominant immunoglobulins are IgG, IgM, and IgA.

IgM, with its short half-life of 5 days, initiates the first response to an infection in the blood stream. The levels of IgM then start to decrease while the levels IgG begin to increase. IgG, which is directed against bacteria and viruses, constitutes 85% of serum immunoglobulins found in the intravascular and extravascular compartments. The biologic potency of this protein resides in its ability to opsonize bacteria by binding the antigen to the neutrophil, monocyte, or macrophage.

Mucosal immunity is governed by IgA, which is synthesized by plasma cells within lymphoid tissue adjacent to the epithelial surface. Once secreted, IgA binds pathogenic microbes and prevents their attachment to the epithelial surface. All of the immunoglobulins play a role in mucosal immunity, especially during cases of congenital IgA deficiency.

7.3.6 Cytokines

There are specific glycoproteins called cytokines that orchestrate the interactions of immune cells with bacteria. Most of the immune cells, such as neutrophils, monocytes–macrophages, and B and T lymphocytes secrete these proteins in response to an inflammatory or antigenic stimulus. The proinflammatory cytokines include TNF-α, IL-1, IL-6, IL-8, IL-11, and IL-18. The earliest inflammatory cytokine to arrive at the site of injury is TNF-α. The principal anti-inflammatory cytokines are IL-10 and transforming growth factor-β, which help neutralize or modulate the production of inflammatory products from monocytes–macrophages.

7.3.7 Genetic Predisposition to Sepsis

Proteins that are expressed as part of the host response to sepsis or other inflammatory events vary in the population. Genetic predisposition of the host may influence morbidity and mortality due to infection. It is well established that the genetic makeup of an individual can alter the manner in which drugs are metabolized. Similarly, microbes, which use specific receptors to attach to the host, can have altered responses based on host genetic polymorphisms. Polymorphic genes consist of multiple alleles of a gene within a population, usually expressing different phenotypes at a frequency >1%. In sepsis, polymorphic genes encode for proteins that are involved with the receptors used for the microbe to invade the host (TLR4, Fcγ receptors, mannose-binding lectin), and in the generation of inflammatory mediators (tumor necrosis factor α, interleukins and heat shock proteins) in response to the microbe. A recent review of genetic polymorphisms in sepsis by Dahmer M et al., describes the emerging genes involved in the response to sepsis.

TLR4 is required for LPS to elicit a response in the host and a single amino acid modification can reduce its effectiveness. Association of TLR4 with Gram-negative infection and septic shock was demonstrated in single nucleotide polymorphism (SNP) that replaced an aspartic acid to glycine and threonine to an isoleucine amino acid. In a separate study of 94 patients with SIRS, a trend toward an increase in mortality was found in those with the glycine polymorphism. CD14, which is a component of the LPS receptor complex, contains a polymorphic site that can increase its transcriptional activity. However, clinical studies have failed to demonstrate a difference in mortality or morbidity due to this polymorphism. Mannose-binding lectin (MBL), which is primarily involved in the opsonization of bacteria and the activation of complement, can have genetic polymorphisms that lead to increased degradation and decreased levels of MBL. The consequence of this polymorphism is an association of recurrent respiratory infections in children that lead to hospitalization and an increase in susceptibility to infections in those afflicted with systemic lupus erythematosus.

Figure 7.1 summarizes the series of events that lead to SIRS and the immune elements that are required.

7.3.8 Neonates

As stated earlier, neonates are predisposed to bacterial infections secondary to an immature cellular and humoral (antibody-mediated) immune system. The pool

Pathogenesis of systemic inflammatory response syndrome (SIRS)

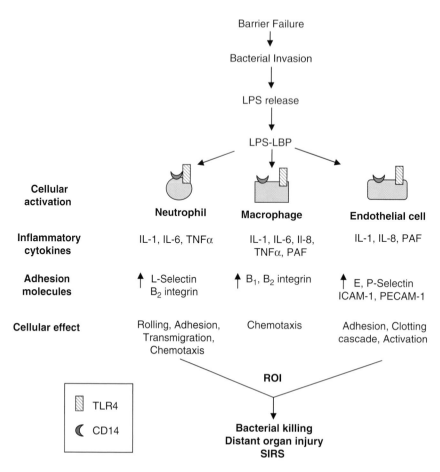

Fig. 7.1 Pathogenesis of systemic inflammatory response syndrome (SIRS). Bacterial invasion secondary to barrier failure leads to the local release of lipopolysaccharide (LPS), with consequent formation of an LPS-lipopolysaccharide binding protein (LBP)-CD14-Toll-like receptor 4 (TLR4) complex on neutrophils, macrophages, and endothelial cells, resulting in cellular activation. Inflammatory cytokines are released, upregulate adhesion molecules, and promote chemotaxis of neutrophils and macrophages. The activated cells release microbicidal agents typically designed for bacterial killing, but they may be injurious and promote distant organ injury and SIRS if the inflammatory process is "uncontrolled." ICAM, intercellular adhesion molecule; IL, interleukin; MCP, monocyte chemotactic protein; MIP, macrophage inflammatory protein; NO, nitric oxide; PAF, platelet-activating factor; PECAM, platelet-endothelial cell adhesion molecule; ROI, reactive oxygen intermediate (or species); TNF, tumor necrosis factor

of neutrophils in the neonate represents only 20–30% of the total adult pool and consists of 60% circulating leukocytes and 15% immature bands. Neonates have limited ability to increase the pool of circulating neutrophils in response to infections. This predisposes the neonate to severe neutropenia because it takes at least 5–7 days to increase the formation of myeloid progenitor stem cells (precursors of neutrophils) in response to infections. Neutrophils in the neonate

also demonstrate decreased adhesion to activated endothelium, decreased efficiency at phagocytosis due to deficiency in opsonins, and decreased ability to kill phagocytosed microbes by oxygen-dependent mechanisms.

T-cell mediated immunity is also different in the neonate compared to the adult. There is a decrease in T-cell mediated cytotoxicity, which is due to the lack of prior antigenic exposure, and a deficiency in cytokine production. In addition, B-cell function is reduced due to its relative immaturity. Immunoglobulin synthesis is different in the neonate. Immunoglobulin M is more abundant in neonatal secretions and the differentiation of the B cell into IgA- or IgG-producing plasma cell does not occur for months. The term neonate relies on maternal transfer of IgG during the third trimester and on the mother's breast milk, which is rich in IgG and IgA, for most of these immunoglobulins. By the fourth month, the neonate begins to increase production of IgG and the maternal IgG dissipates. As a result, they exhibit increased susceptibility to infections during this period.

In addition to a deficiency in cell mediated and humoral immunity, the neonate is also at risk for infection because of immaturity of the antibody-independent, complement system. The levels of key components of the complement system are decreased, which leads to diminished capacity to fight off gram-negative microbes (C9), decreased production of chemotactic factor C5a, and a decrease in functional opsonins due to a lack of efficient cross-linking (C3b).

7.4 Clinical Features and Diagnosis

Microbial invasion has different consequences in the neonate compared to the adult. The neonate's immune system is premature and its ability to ward off infection is dampened secondary to low levels of certain inflammatory mediators. The neonate can manifest the symptoms of the sepsis syndrome in a number of ways. The following criteria help to define these characteristics in the pediatric population. The criteria consist of:

1. Clinical evidence of sepsis with fever (rectal temperature > 38°C) or hypothermia (<35.6°C)
2. Tachycardia (heart rate > 95th percentile for age)
3. Tachypnea (respiratory rate > 95th percentile for age)
4. Hypotension (mean arterial blood pressure < 5th percentile for age)
5. Altered mental status, metabolic acidosis (arterial pH < 7.35 or base deficit > −5), oliguria (urine output < 1 ml /kg/h) or signs of poor peripheral perfusion, such as delayed capillary refill.

In addition, the diagnosis of SIRS includes most of the Bone criteria, but includes a white blood cell count greater than 12,000 cells/mm^3 or less than 4,000 cells/mm^3 or the presence of 10% bands. The use of white blood cell count in the neonate is of limited value since less than 50% of neonates with values greater than 20,000/mm^3 or less than 4,000/mm^3 are ultimately diagnosed with a bacterial infection. The ratio of immature to total neutrophils is useful in determining the likelihood of infection in the neonate. A ratio greater than 0.2 is a sensitive indicator of infection, while a ratio greater than 0.8 or severe neutropenia signifies severe bone marrow depletion and a poor prognosis. Thrombocytopenia is a nonspecific and late predictor of neonatal sepsis, but trends in platelet count are important for the clinician to address.

The most prominent clinical or physiologic changes that occur in SIRS are reduced vascular resistance and decreased peripheral extraction of oxygen. The pediatric patient must increase cardiac output and increase minute ventilation to achieve a higher delivery of oxygen to ischemic tissues. The inability to increase oxygen delivery causes marked anaerobic metabolism with the production of excess lactate.

The 2001 International Sepsis Definitions Conference proposed a purely biochemical or immunological, rather than clinical, criteria to identify the inflammatory response in children. C-reactive protein (CRP), interleukin 6 (IL-6), and procalcitonin (PCT) were mentioned as potential markers for use in the neonates and pediatric patients. PCT is secreted during gram-negative sepsis from an unknown extrathyroid source and can be used as a guide for antibiotic therapy. Maja Pavcnik-Arnol et al. performed a prospective observational study looking at potential biochemical markers that could diagnose bacterial sepsis in the neonate. In critically ill neonates less than 48 h old, LBP on the first day of suspected infection was a better marker of sepsis than IL-6 and PCT and was similar to CRP. In critically ill neonates older than 48 h and in children, LBP was a better marker than IL-6 and CRP and was similar to PCT. In culture confirmed sepsis, LBP had 91% sensitivity, 98% negative predictive value, 85% specificity, and 52% positive predictive value.

The objective in diagnosing the cause of sepsis in the neonate is to isolate bacterial or fungal organisms and then treat with appropriate antibiotics. Documentation of bacterial infection in suspected neonates is positive in only 10% of cases. Cultures should be obtained from peripheral blood as well as any indwelling intravenous lines. The presence of microorganisms in the blood is the initiating event, leading to fever and chills 1–2 h after the development of bacteremia. Blood cultures are frequently negative at the time of the temperature spike. Thus, blood cultures are ideally drawn prior to the onset of a temperature spike. In reality, however, this is not possible; therefore, spreading out the collection of blood cultures increases the likelihood of blood collection during bacteremia. It is therefore recommended that separate needle sticks be obtained from different venipuncture sites. Once bloodstream infection is identified, repeat or follow-up cultures are not necessary in most cases. Subsequent blood cultures may be justified, however, in patients who deteriorate clinically, or who fail to improve despite appropriate antibiotic therapy. In some cases bacteremia may be prolonged, necessitating further blood cultures during treatment. Urine cultures as well as lumbar puncture should be performed since up to one-third of neonates can have meningitis. Unfortunately, no single laboratory test can diagnose sepsis or SIRS in the neonate; however, the use of the physical exam and history may give insight into the cause of a patient's decline.

7.5 Management

As stated in the previous section, the most prominent feature of sepsis or SIRS is the increase in oxygen demand by end organs and a decrease in vascular resistance, which is manifested as a low blood pressure. In the treatment of sepsis or the early stages of SIRS, the goal is to increase oxygen delivery by aggressive fluid resuscitation, cardiovascular and respiratory support, and optimal management of fluids and electrolytes, hematologic, renal, metabolic, and nutritional needs. Initial fluid boluses of 20 ml/kg of normal saline are required to correct hypovolemia. Rapid fluid resuscitation in excess of 40 ml/kg in the first hour following emergency department presentation was associated with improved survival, decreased occurrence of persistent hypovolemia, and no increase in the risk of cardiogenic pulmonary edema in a group of pediatric patients with septic shock. The use of vasopressors is withheld until the child is adequately resuscitated. If vasopressors are to be used, then dopamine is chosen first because it stimulates dopaminergic receptors and potentially increases renal blood flow. The physician should monitor the urine output as a guide to end organ perfusion

and adjust the management accordingly (1–2 ml/kg/h). In addition, since respiratory failure is often seen in a septic neonate, mechanical ventilation may be important to help relieve the failing respiratory muscles. Adjustment to the respiratory rate or to the oxygen concentration on the ventilator is governed by arterial blood gas.

Source control with antimicrobial therapy is the cornerstone of treatment of presumed sepsis or infectious causes of SIRS. Broad-spectrum antibiotics should be started at the first signs of sepsis. Most patients with sepsis or infectious SIRS are diagnosed with Gram-negative infections such as *E. coli*, *P. aeruginosa*, *Klebsiella*, and *Bacteroides* species. In neonates or term infants, the most common organisms encountered are group B streptococcus, *E. coli*, and *L. monocytogenes*. The antibiotics should be tailored to the species and sensitivities identified in the blood, urine, or lumbar puncture. If fever persists despite empiric antibiotics and no source of infection has been identified, empiric antifungal therapy may be indicated if the patient has risk factors for candidal infection.

In severe sepsis or SIRS, activation of the inflammatory cytokine and coagulation cascades may lead to thrombin production and fibrin deposition in the microvasculature or microvascular thrombosis. During systemic Gram-negative and Gram-positive bacterial infections, activation of coagulation is mediated via the extrinsic tissue factor pathway. Activated protein C is an endogenous regulator of coagulation and inflammation and is a promising therapeutic target in patients with severe sepsis. The PROWESS (Protein C Worldwide Evaluation in Severe Sepsis) study was a large multicenter randomized double blind, placebo-controlled trial in patients with severe sepsis. The trial demonstrated a decrease in the 28-day mortality from all causes in adults with sepsis. An interim analysis of pediatric patients found an increase in the levels of protein C and antithrombin in addition to a 5% incidence of serious bleeding. More studies are needed to see if Activated protein C is a viable option in the pediatric population.

Sepsis or SIRS causes a release of inflammatory cytokines and hormones that lead to hyperglycemia. Increased peripheral insulin resistance is caused by a release of cortisol, TNF-α and IL-1. In addition, there is an increase in hepatic glucose production, which causes hyperglycemia. Elevated blood glucose causes an increase in microbial infections and increased mortality. A landmark study by van den Berghe and colleagues demonstrated that tight glycemic control with a blood glucose level of 80–110 mg/dl decreases in-hospital mortality by 34% in a mixed medical-surgical ICU (predominantly cardiac surgery patients) compared to patients with a targeted blood glucose level of 180–200 mg/dl. In septic neonates, hyperglycemia correlated with prolonged ventilator dependency and increased hospital length of stay. Adhering to strict glucose control can help neonates and infants decrease the mortality associated with sepsis or SIRS.

Nutritional support of the infant with enteral or parenteral feeding during sepsis is important to help provide necessary nutrients. The advantages of enteral as compared with parenteral feeding include gastric pH buffering, avoidance of the use of parenteral-nutrition catheters, preservation of gut mucosa with the avoidance of the introduction of bacteria and toxins from the gastrointestinal tract into the circulation, and a more physiologic pattern of enteric hormone secretion.

Further Reading

Alaedeen DI, Walsh MC, Chwals WJ (2006) Total parenteral nutrition-associated hyperglycemia correlates with prolonged mechanical ventilation and hospital stay in septic infants. J Pediatr Surg 41(1):239–244, discussion 239–244

Brown KA, Brain SD, Pearson JD, Edgeworth JD, Lewis SM, Treacher DF (2006) Neutrophils in development of multiple organ failure in sepsis. Lancet 368(9530):157–169

Dahmer MK, Randolph A, Vitali S, Quasney MW (2005) Genetic polymorphisms in sepsis. Pediatr Crit Care Med 6(3 Suppl):S61–73

Martin GS, Mannino DM, Eaton S, Moss M (2003) The epidemiology of sepsis in the United States from 1979 through 2000. N Engl J Med 348(16):1546–1554

Pavcnik-Arnol M, Hojker S, Derganc M (2004) Lipopolysaccharide-binding protein in critically ill neonates and children with suspected infection: Comparison with procalcitonin, interleukin-6, and C-reactive protein. Intensive Care Med 30(7):1454–1460

Puri P, Höllwarth ME (eds) (2006) Pediatric Surgery. Springer, Berlin, Heidelberg

Watson RS, Carcillo JA, Linde-Zwirble WT, Clermont G, Lidicker J, Angus DC (2003) The epidemiology of severe sepsis in children in the United States. Am J Respir Crit Care Med 167(5):695–701

Nutrition

Agostino Pierro and Simon Eaton

8

Contents

8.1 Introduction

The nutrition of neonates and children has significantly improved over the last 20 years. Most of the nutritional challenges in paediatrics are related to the first year of life. For this reason this chapter focuses on the nutrition of neonates and infants.

The newborn infant is in a "critical epoch" of development not only for the organism as a whole but also for the individual organs and most significantly for the brain. Adequate nutrition in the neonatal period is necessary to avoid the adverse effects of malnutrition on morbidity and mortality and to minimise the future menace of stunted mental and physical development.

The survival rate of newborn infants affected by isolated congenital gastrointestinal abnormalities has improved considerably and is now in excess of 90% in most paediatric surgical centres. The introduction of parenteral nutrition and advancement in nutritional management are certainly among the main factors responsible for this improvement.

8.2 Historical Background

Parenteral nutrition has progressed from numerous historical anecdotes in the 1930s with the first successful infusion of protein hydrolysates in humans, followed by the first report of successful total parenteral nutrition in an infant in 1944 and has been given a huge boost by the first placement of a catheter in the superior vena cava to deliver nutrients for prolonged periods. Using this system, Dudrick and Wilmore showed that adequate growth and development could be achieved in beagle puppies and in a surgical infant. Following these initial reports, Filler and co-authors

P. Puri and M. Höllwarth (eds.), *Pediatric Surgery: Diagnosis and Management*,
DOI: 10.1007/978-3-540-69560-8_8, © Springer-Verlag Berlin Heidelberg 2009

reported the first series of surgical neonates with gastrointestinal abnormalities treated with long-term total parenteral nutrition. During the 1970s and 1980s significant improvements were made in the technique itself and in the reduction of complications, and the last 10 years have seen considerable changes in the nutritional management of surgical neonates. Various investigators have highlighted the importance of introducing enteral nutrition as soon as possible in surgical neonates. The beneficial effects of minimal enteral feeding on the immune system, infection rate and liver function have been elucidated.

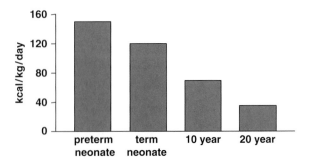

Fig. 8.1   Total energy requirement according to age

8.3 Body Composition

Newborn infants grow very rapidly, have lower caloric reserves than adults and therefore do not tolerate prolonged periods of starvation. The body composition of newborn infants is markedly different from that of adults. The total body water varies from 86% of body weight at 28 weeks of gestation to 69% at 40 weeks of gestation and 60% in adulthood. This decline in body water reflects also an increase in energy content of the body. The ratio between minimal metabolic rate to non-protein energy reserve is only 1:2 at 28 weeks of gestation, it decreases to 1:29 for term infants and 1:100 for the adult, which explains the urgent need for adequate caloric intake in very-low-birth-weight infants after birth. Full-term neonates have a higher content of endogenous fat (approximately 600 g) and therefore can tolerate few days of undernutrition.

8.4 Energy Metabolism

Newborn infants have a significantly higher metabolic rate and energy requirement per unit body weight than children and adults (Fig. 8.1). They require approximately 40–70 kcal/kg/day for maintenance metabolism, 50–70 kcal/kg/day for growth (tissue synthesis and energy stored) and up to 20 kcal/kg/day to cover energy losses in excreta (Fig. 8.2). The total energy requirement for a newborn infant fed enterally is 100–120 kcal/kg/day, compared to 60–80 kcal/kg/day for a 10-year-old and 30–40 kcal/kg/day for a 20-year-old individual. Newborn infants receiving total parenteral

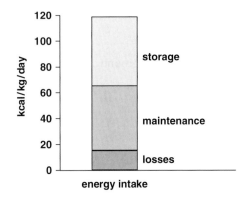

Fig. 8.2   Partition of energy metabolism in surgical newborn infants. (Adapted from Pierro et al. 1991)

nutrition (TPN) require fewer calories (80–100 kcal/kg/day). This is due to the absence of energy losses in excreta and to the fact that energy is not required for thermoregulation when the infant is nursed in a thermoneutral environment using a double-insulated incubator. Although energy expenditure may double during periods of activity, including crying, most surgical infants are at rest 80–90% of the time. Significant differences in resting energy expenditure (REE) have been reported among full-term surgical newborn infants (range 33.3–50.8 kcal/kg/day) and between premature and full-term babies. A full-term infant requires 100–120 kcal/kg/day and a premature infant 110–160 kcal/kg/day (Fig. 8.1). These variations in maintenance metabolism explain the different growth rates frequently observed in surgical neonates receiving similar caloric intakes, and probably represent differences in metabolically active tissue mass, i.e. organ and muscle size. Several equations have been published to predict energy expenditure in adults and equations have been developed to predict REE in stable surgical neonates, to which the major contributing predictors are body weight, heart rate (providing an indirect measure of haemodynamic and metabolic status) and post-natal age.

8.4.1 Operative Trauma

In contrast with adults, the energy requirement of infants and children undergoing major operations seems to be modified minimally by the operative trauma *per se*. In adults, trauma or surgery causes a brief "ebb" period of a depressed metabolic rate followed by a "flow phase" characterised by an increase in oxygen consumption to support the massive exchanges of substrate between organs. In newborn infants, major abdominal surgery causes a moderate (15%) and immediate (peak at 4 h) elevation of oxygen consumption and resting energy expenditure and a rapid return to baseline 12–24 h post-operatively. There is no further increase in energy expenditure in the first 5–7 days following an operation. The timing of these changes corresponds with the post-operative changes in catecholamine levels and other biochemical and endocrine parameters. It has been demonstrated that the post-operative increase in energy expenditure can, at least partially, result from severe underlying acute illness, which frequently necessitates surgery (i.e. sepsis or intense inflammation, see below). Interestingly, infants having a major operation after the second day of life have a significantly greater increase in resting energy expenditure than infants undergoing surgery within the first 48 h of life. A possible explanation for this may be greater secretion of endogenous opioids in the perinatal period blunting the endocrine and metabolic responses.

Resting energy expenditure is directly proportional to growth rate in healthy infants, and growth is retarded during acute metabolic stress. Studies in adult surgical patients have shown that operative stress causes marked changes in protein metabolism characterised by a post-operative increase in protein degradation, negative nitrogen balance and a decrease in muscle protein synthesis. However, changes in whole body protein flux, protein synthesis, amino acid oxidation or protein degradation do not seem to occur in infants and young children undergoing major operations, which led us to speculate that infants and children divert protein and

energy from growth to tissue repair, thereby avoiding the overall increase in energy expenditure and catabolism seen in the adult.

8.4.2 Critical Illness and Sepsis

Nutritional problems in infants and children requiring surgery are not unusual. The real nutritional challenge is not represented by the operation *per se* but by the clinical condition of the patient. Examples include intrauterine growth retardation in small-for-gestational age preterm infants, infants who have suffered massive intestinal resection for necrotizing enterocolitis and infants with motility disorders of the intestine following surgery for atresia, malrotation and midgut volvulus, meconium ileus or gastroschisis.

Nutritional integrity particularly in the neonatal period should be maintained regardless of the severity of the illness or organ failure due to the limited energy and protein stores in neonates. Infants and children require nutrition for maintenance of protein status as well as for growth and wound healing. One considerable challenge in paediatrics is represented by nutrition support during critical illness and sepsis. Keshen et al. have shown that parenterally fed neonates on extracorporeal life support are in hypermetabolic and protein catabolic states. These authors recommend the provision of additional protein and non-protein calories to attenuate the net protein losses.

Sepsis is an intriguing pathological condition associated with many complex metabolic and physiological alterations. Studies in adults have shown that the metabolic response to sepsis is characterised by hypermetabolism, increased tissue catabolism, gluconeogenesis and hepatic release of glucose. Energy is largely derived from fat, and increased protein catabolism provides precursors for enhanced hepatic gluconeogenesis. However, fat mobilisation is far greater than fat oxidation, implying considerable cycling, and in later stages of sepsis, oxidative metabolism and fat utilisation may become impaired.

The existing knowledge on the metabolic response to sepsis in infants is limited. There are conflicting reports on whether critically ill infants are hypermetabolic. However, recent studies suggest that infants with sepsis do not become hypermetabolic (Fig. 8.3) and that septic neonates with necrotizing enterocolitis do

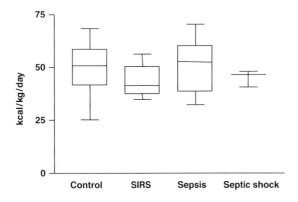

Fig. 8.3 Resting energy expenditure in critically ill infants and controls. Indirect calorimetry was performed on infants and children with systemic inflammatory response syndrome (SIRS), sepsis, septic shock and controls. Results are expressed as median, range and interquartile range. There were no significant differences between the groups (see Turi et al., 2001)

not show any increase in whole body protein turnover, synthesis and catabolism.

From these studies, it is clear that the metabolic rate and hormonal response to surgery, stress and sepsis in infants may well be different from that of adults and therefore it is not possible to adapt nutritional recommendations made for adults to the neonatal population. It is possible that neonates divert the products of protein synthesis and breakdown from growth into tissue repair. This may explain the lack of growth commonly observed in infants with critical illness or sepsis. Further studies are needed in this field to delineate the metabolic response of neonates and children to trauma and sepsis, to explore the relationship between nutrition and immunity and to design the most appropriate diet.

8.5 Parenteral Nutrition

8.5.1 Indications

Parenteral nutrition should be utilised when enteral feeding is impossible, inadequate or hazardous for more than 4–5 days. The most frequent indication in neonatal surgery is intestinal obstruction due to congenital anomalies. Frequently, after an operation on the gastrointestinal tract, adequate enteral feeding cannot be achieved for more than 1 week and parenteral nutrition becomes

necessary. This modality of therapy has significantly improved the survival rate of newborns with gastroschisis—a condition that requires intravenous administration of nutrients for 2–3 weeks. Parenteral nutrition is also used in cases of necrotizing enterocolitis, short-bowel syndrome and respiratory distress.

8.5.2 Components of Parenteral Nutrition

The parenteral nutrition formulation includes carbohydrate, fat, protein, electrolytes, vitamins, trace elements and water. The caloric needs for total parenteral nutrition are provided by carbohydrate and lipid. Protein is not used as a source of calories, since the catabolism of protein to produce energy is an uneconomic metabolic process compared to the oxidation of carbohydrate and fat, which produces more energy at a lower metabolic cost. The ideal total parenteral nutrition regimen therefore should provide enough amino acids for protein turnover and tissue growth and sufficient calories to minimise protein oxidation for energy.

8.5.2.1 Fluid Requirements

Any newborn infant deprived of oral fluids will lose body fluids and electrolytes in urine, stools, sweat and evaporative losses from the lungs and the skin. The insensible water losses from the skin are particularly high (up to 80–100 ml/kg/day) in low-birth-weight infants. This is due to the very large surface area relative to body weight, to the very thin and permeable epidermis, to reduced subcutaneous fat and to the large proportion of total body water and extracellular water. The preterm infant requires larger amounts of fluid to replace the high obligatory renal water excretion due to the limited ability to concentrate urine. In surgical newborns, it is not unusual to have significant water losses from gastric drainage and gastrointestinal stoma. In order to reduce the water losses, it is important to use double-walled incubators, to place the infant in relatively high humidity, to use warm humidified air via the endotracheal tube and in premature babies to cover the body surface with an impermeable sheet. However, overhydration is potentially a problem, leading to complications such as pulmonary oedema.

8.5.2.2 Energy Sources

Carbohydrates and fat provide the main energy sources in the diet, and this is reflected by their importance as a source of calories in parenteral nutrition.

Glucose is a main energy source for body cells and is the primary energy substrate in parenteral nutrition. The amount of glucose that can be infused safely depends on the clinical condition and maturity of the infant. The ability of neonates to metabolise glucose may be impaired by prematurity and low birth weight. Conversion of carbohydrate to fat (lipogenesis) occurs when glucose intake exceeds metabolic needs. The risks associated with this process are twofold: accumulation of the newly synthesised fat in the liver and aggravation of respiratory acidosis resulting from increased CO_2 production, particularly in patients with compromised pulmonary function.

Since the 1960s, safe commercial intravenous fat emulsions have become widely used. These preparations have a high caloric value (9 kcal/g of fat), prevent essential fatty acid deficiency and are isotonic, allowing adequate calories to be given via a peripheral vein. A number of studies in both adults and infants have shown that combined infusion of glucose and lipids confers metabolic advantages over glucose, because it lowers the metabolic rate and increases the efficiency of energy utilisation.

It has been shown that in surgical infants receiving parenteral nutrition there is a negative linear relationship between glucose intake and fat utilisation (oxidation and conversion to fat). Net fat synthesis from glucose exceeds net fat oxidation when the glucose intake is greater than 18 g/kg/day (i.e. in excess of energy expenditure) (Fig. 8.4). There is a significant relationship between glucose intake and CO_2 production. The slope of this relationship (i.e. increased CO_2 production) was steeper when glucose intake exceeded 18 g/kg/day than when glucose intake was less than 18 g/kg/day, indicating that lipogenesis results in a significantly increased CO_2 production. More recent studies on stable surgical newborn infants receiving fixed amounts of carbohydrate and amino acids and variable amounts of intravenous long-chain fat emulsion have shown that at a carbohydrate intake of 15 g/kg/day, the proportion of energy metabolism derived from fat oxidation does not exceed 20% even with a fat intake as high as 6 g/kg/day. At a carbohydrate intake of 10 g/kg/day this proportion can be as high as 50%. This study seems to indicate that during parenteral nutrition in surgical infants the majority of the intravenous fat infused is not oxidised but deposited.

Fat tolerance has been extensively studied by monitoring fat clearance from plasma. However, clearance from plasma does not imply that the fat is being utilised to meet energy requirements, since it may be being stored instead. Pierro et al. have studied intravenous fat utilisation by performing a "lipid utilisation test". This consisted of infusing lipid for 4 h in isocaloric and isovolaemic amounts to the previously given mixture of glucose and amino acids. Gas exchange was measured by indirect calorimetry to calculate the patient's O_2 consumption and CO_2 production, and net fat utilisation (Fig. 8.5). The study showed that within 2 h, more

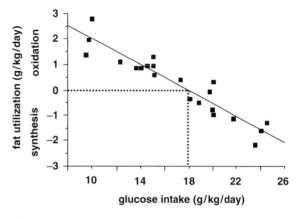

Fig. 8.4 Linear relationship between glucose intake and fat utilisation ($r = -0.9$; $p < 0.0001$). Lipogenesis is significant when glucose intake exceeds 18 g/kg/day. (Adapted from Pierro et al., 1993)

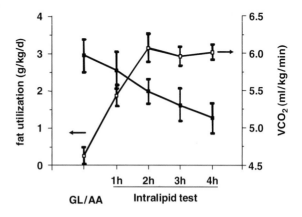

Fig. 8.5 Intralipid utilisation test: surgical newborn infants adapt very rapidly to the infusion of intravenous fat. The oxidation of exogenous fat is associated with a significant reduction in CO_2 production. Fat utilisation open symbols; CO_2 production ($V\dot{C}O_2$ closed symbols). (Adapted from Pierro et al., 1989)

than 80% of the exogenous fat can be oxidised and that CO_2 production is reduced during fat infusion as a consequence of the cessation of carbohydrate conversion to fat (lipogenesis).

Net fat oxidation seems to be significantly influenced by the carbohydrate intake and by the resting energy expenditure of the neonate. When the intake of glucose calories exceeds the resting energy expenditure of the infant, net fat oxidation is minimal regardless of fat intake. In order to use intravenous fat as an energy source (i.e. oxidation to CO_2 and H_2O), it is necessary to maintain carbohydrate intake below basal energy requirements. Glucose intake exceeding 18 g/kg/day is also associated with a significant increase in respiratory rate and plasma triglyceride levels. It is advisable therefore in stable surgical newborn infants requiring parenteral nutrition to not exceed 18 g/kg/day of intravenous glucose intake.

Commonly used fat emulsion for parenteral nutrition in paediatrics is based on long-chain triglycerides (LCT). The rate of intravenous fat oxidation during total parenteral nutrition could potentially be enhanced by the addition of L-carnitine and medium chain triglycerides (MCT) to the intravenous diet. L-Carnitine is required for the oxidation of long-chain triglycerides and although it is present in breast milk and infant formula, it is not present in parenteral feeds. Although some authors have found decreased carnitine levels in parenterally fed neonates and reported enhanced fat oxidation upon carnitine supplementation, carnitine levels have to fall extremely low before fatty acid oxidation is impaired and although supplementation has been recommended by some groups, a systematic review found no evidence to support the routine supplementation of parenterally fed neonates with carnitine. MCT are both cleared from the blood-stream and oxidised at a faster rate than LCT, and various studies have suggested that MCT–LCT mixtures in paediatric parenteral nutrition provide benefits over LCT alone. However, randomised controlled trials are necessary before MCT–LCT mixtures find routine use in parenteral nutrition of neonates. We have recently investigated the metabolic response to intravenous medium-chain triglycerides in surgical infants and found that, providing that carbohydrate calories do not exceed energy expenditure, partial replacement of LCT by MCT can increase net fat oxidation without increasing metabolic rate (Fig. 8.6).

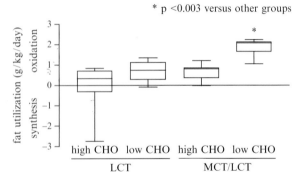

Fig. 8.6 Fat utilisation: a positive value represents net fat oxidation and a negative value represents fat synthesis from carbohydrate. LCT patients received a fat emulsion containing 100% long-chain triglycerides. MCT and LCT patients received a fat emulsion containing 50% medium-chain triglycerides (MCT) and 50% long-chain triglycerides. High carbohydrate (CHO) intake was 15 g/kg/day and low CHO intake was 10 g/kg/day (Reproduced with permission from Donnell et al. 2002)

8.5.2.3 Amino Acids

In contrast to healthy adults who exist in a state of neutral nitrogen balance, infants need to be in positive nitrogen balance in order to achieve satisfactory growth and development. Infants are efficient at retaining nitrogen, and can retain up to 80% of the metabolizable protein intake on both oral and intravenous diets. Protein metabolism is dependent on both protein and energy intake. The influence of dietary protein is well established. An increased protein intake has been shown to enhance protein synthesis, reduce endogenous protein breakdown and thus enhance net protein retention. The protein requirements of newborn infants are between 2.5 and 3.0 g/kg/day. The nitrogen source of TPN is usually provided as a mixture of amino acids. The solutions commercially available contain the eight known essential amino acids and histidine, which is known to be essential in children. Complications like azotemia, hyperammonaemia and metabolic acidosis have been described in patients receiving high levels of intravenous amino acids but rarely seen with amino acid intake of 2–3 g/kg/day. In patients with severe malnutrition or with additional losses (i.e. jejunostomy, ileostomy), protein requirements are higher.

The influence of non-protein energy intake on protein metabolism is more controversial. Protein retention can be enhanced by giving carbohydrates or fat, which are said to be protein sparing. Although some studies have suggested that the protein sparing effect of carbohydrate is greater than that of fat, others have suggested that the protein sparing effect of fat may be either equivalent to, or greater than, that of carbohydrate. The addition of fat calories to the intravenous diet of surgical newborn infants reduces protein oxidation, protein contribution to the energy expenditure and increases protein retention. In a further study, we compared protein metabolism in two groups of neonates receiving isonitrogenous and isocaloric total parenteral nutrition: one group received a high fat diet and the other, a high carbohydrate diet. There was no significant difference between the two groups with regard to any of the components of whole body protein metabolism: protein synthesis, protein breakdown, protein oxidation and excretion and total protein flux, thus supporting the use of fat in the intravenous diet of surgical newborn infants.

The ideal quantitative composition of amino acid solutions is still controversial. In a newborn infant, cysteine taurine and tyrosine seem to be essential amino acids. However, the addition of cysteine in the parenteral nutrition of neonates does not cause any difference in the growth rate and nitrogen retention.

8.5.2.3.1 Glutamine

Nutrients can modulate immune, metabolic and inflammatory responses. Of these nutrients, glutamine is of particular interest. Glutamine is the most abundant free amino acid in the body where it plays fundamental physiological roles. It is the predominant amino acid supplied to the fetus through the placenta and is normally present in the enteral diet. Glutamine can be synthesised in the human body in substantial amounts and therefore is usually considered to be non-essential. However, in patients with acute and long-term sepsis and trauma, glutamine stores decline. This may be due to a combination of reduced glutamine production, possibly reflecting low muscle glycogen levels, glucose intolerance and increased glutamine utilisation. During sepsis, the liver and the immune system become major glutamine consumers such that net glutamine utilisation exceeds production and glutamine becomes "conditionally essential". In rats, glutamine oxidation supplies a third of the total energy requirement of the gut. In humans who have sustained multi-system trauma or sepsis, glutamine concentration is 15% higher in arterial blood than in portal blood, confirming the selective uptake of glutamine in the gut.

Until recently glutamine has been excluded from parenteral nutrition because of low solubility and instability in solution. However, glutamine dipeptides with improved stability and solubility are now available making it possible to add glutamine to parenteral nutrition formulation. There are several reasons why glutamine may be beneficial for critically ill patients receiving parenteral nutrition. Firstly, glutamine supplementation has been shown to be beneficial, both *in vitro* and *in vivo*, for the immune system. The effect of glutamine supplementation on the prevention of infectious complications has been examined in randomised trials in *adult* patients receiving either glutamine-supplemented parenteral nutrition or isonitrogenous isocaloric parenteral nutrition. These trials included patients undergoing elective operation for colorectal cancer, patients with multiple trauma, critically ill patients and patients undergoing bone marrow transplantation. All these studies showed that parenteral glutamine administration does reduce infectious complications. Secondly, glutamine has multiple effects on gastrointestinal function. Glutamine deficiency leads to gut atrophy and bacterial translocation. Glutamine prevents deterioration of gut permeability, prevents intestinal mucosal atrophy and preserves mucosal structure in patients receiving parenteral nutrition. Reduced nitrogen loss has been demonstrated in adult patients receiving glutamine-supplemented parenteral nutrition after major abdominal operations.

Recent studies have shown that in a neonatal animal model, glutamine reverses the liver dysfunction caused by sepsis due to an increase in the production of glutathione, a major intracellular antioxidant, for which glutamine is an important precursor.

There have been several trials of glutamine parenteral nutrition supplementation in adults. However, a recent Cochrane systematic review has identified only two published randomised controlled trials of glutamine in neonates including one on parenteral nutrition supplementation. This trial did not identify any adverse effects attributable to glutamine. Glutamine administration was associated with a reduced duration of artificial ventilation, hospital admission and parenteral nutrition but effects on immunity or infection and its generalisability to other settings or patient groups remain unclear. The Cochrane Review highlighted the requirement for a large randomised controlled trial of glutamine supplementation in neonates requiring parenteral nutrition.

8.5.2.4   Vitamins and Trace Elements

Vitamins and trace elements are important cofactors or components of enzymes, and provision of adequate supplies is important for the growing neonate. Vitamins and trace elements are particularly important in maintenance of the body's antioxidant defences: vitamins C and E, selenium (for glutathione peroxidase), copper, zinc and manganese (all for superoxide dismutases) are all added to parenteral nutrition. However, vitamins and trace elements are particularly vulnerable to photoxidation and loss or to increase lipid peroxide production, and various studies have suggested photoprotection of parenteral nutrition bags in order to minimise losses and peroxide generation. Free radical production and lipid peroxidation will be considered in more detail below.

8.5.3   Complications of Parenteral Nutrition

8.5.3.1   Infectious Complications

In spite of significant improvement in the management of parenteral nutrition including the introduction of nutrition support teams, recently published infection rates from large children's hospitals indicate that between 5% and 37% of infants may develop sepsis while receiving parenteral nutrition. This may lead to impaired liver function, critical illness and removal of central venous catheters. It has always been assumed that the central venous catheter is the major portal of entry for micro-organisms causing septicaemia in patients on parenteral nutrition. However, studies in animals and surgical neonates have reported microbial translocation (migration of micro-organisms from the intestinal lumen to the systemic circulation) during parenteral nutrition. In a study on surgical neonates on parenteral nutrition, all but one episode of microbial translocation occurred in patients with elevated serum bilirubin (cholestasis). Pierro et al. have reported that almost half the surgical infants on parenteral nutrition develop abnormal flora and that all cases of septicae-

mia were preceded by gut colonisation with abnormal flora. Furthermore, it has been reported that parenteral nutrition itself impairs host defence mechanisms and contributes to the occurrence of infection in neonates. This may be due to individual components of the parenteral nutrition solution, such as lipid emulsion, or due to a lack of nutrients, such as glutamine, normally present in the enteral diet.

Important factors in reducing the incidence of septic complications are placing intravenous catheters under strict aseptic conditions, preparing the parenteral nutrition solutions in pharmacy in aseptic conditions and using meticulous care when the catheters are used. Sepsis should be suspected when infants on parenteral nutrition present clinical features of generalised inflammation including one or more of the following features: temperature instability, poor perfusion, hypotension, lethargy, tachycardia, respiratory distress and fever. In these neonates, blood culture should be performed from the central venous line and from a peripheral vein.

8.5.3.2   Metabolic Complications

The metabolic complications most frequently observed in newborn infants receiving parenteral nutrition are listed in Table 8.1. These complications are related to inappropriate administration of nutrients, fluid, electrolytes and trace elements or to the inability of the individual patient to metabolise the intravenous diet.

Hyperglycaemia occurs frequently during the course of parenteral nutrition, particularly while the glucose concentration of the infusate is being increased, but most patients will produce adequate endogenous insulin to metabolise the carbohydrate load within hours. The treatment of symptomatic hyperglycaemia is usually by reduction of the infusion rate. Hypoglycaemia usually results from sudden interruption of an infusion containing a high glucose concentration.

High doses of fat or an accidental rapid infusion of fat may lead to fat overload syndrome, characterised by an acute febrile illness with jaundice and abnormal coagulation. The intravenous administration of fat emulsion in premature infants seems to increase the incidence of bronchopulmonary dysplasia and retinopathy. Peroxidation in stored fat emulsions and the generation of free radicals during intravenous infusion of fat in premature infants have been reported.

Table 8.1 Metabolic complications of TPN

Carbohydrate administration
  Hyperglycaemia
  Hypoglycaemia
  Fatty infiltration of the liver
  Hyperosmolarity and osmotic diuresis
  Increased CO_2 production
Protein administration
  Hyperammonaemia, azotemia
  Abnormal plasma amino acid profiles
  Hepatic dysfunction
  Cholestatic jaundice
Fat administration
  Hyperlipidaemia
  Fat overload syndrome
  Displacement of albumin-bound bilirubin by free fatty acids
  Peroxidation and generation of free radicals
Fluid administration
  Patent ductus arteriosus
  Pulmonary oedema
Electrolyte imbalance
  Sodium, potassium, chlorine,
  calcium, phosphate
Trace element and vitamin deficiency

Table 8.2 Mechanical complications of parenteral nutrition

Extravasation of parenteral nutrition solution
Blockage of the central venous line
Migration of the central venous line
Breakage of the infusion line
Right atrium thrombosis
Cardiac tamponade (perforation of right atrium or vena cava)

The release of free radicals may overwhelm the endogenous protective mechanisms, resulting in cellular damage (see below).

8.5.3.3 Mechanical Complications

Mechanical complications related to the intravenous infusion of nutrients are not uncommon. Table 8.2 lists the mechanical complications reported in the literature. Extravasation of parenteral nutrition solution is a common complication of peripheral parenteral nutrition. Unfortunately, even a low osmolarity solution is detrimental for peripheral veins leading to inflammation and extravasation of the solution, which can cause tissue necrosis and infection. Intravenous lines may become clogged from thrombus formation, calcium precipitates or lipid deposition. There is disagreement on the ideal position of central venous lines (CVL) for parenteral nutrition in infants. Some authors advocate the atrium as the ideal position because this would give less chance of catheter dysfunction. Others believe that placement in the superior vena cava would reduce the risk of perforation. In a survey of 587 CVL inserted in neonates, cardiac tamponade was the cause of death in two neonates (0.3%). In most of the cases reported in the literature

of cardiac tamponade following CVL insertion, the perforation was thought to be in the right atrium.

8.5.3.4 Hepatic Complications

The hepatobiliary complications related to parenteral nutrition remain serious and often life threatening. The commonest hepatobiliary complication of parenteral nutrition in surgical neonates is cholestasis. The incidence of parenteral nutrition-related cholestasis varies widely from as low as 7.4% to as high as 84%. Although the frequency of this complication seems to be diminishing, this is probably related to the early initiation of oral feeding rather than to an improvement in the intravenous diet. The aetiology of cholestatic jaundice in infants requiring parenteral nutrition is still unclear. However, infants requiring long-term parenteral nutrition still develop progressive jaundice, commonly preceded by elevation of biochemical non-specific tests of hepatic damage, function and excretion.

Various clinical factors are thought to contribute to the development of parenteral nutrition-related cholestasis (Table 8.3). These include prematurity, low birth weight, duration of parenteral nutrition, immature entero-hepatic circulation, intestinal microflora, septicaemia, failure to implement enteral nutrition and number of operations. Parenteral nutrition-related cholestasis has a higher incidence in premature infants than in children and adults. This may be due to the immaturity of the biliary secretory system since bile salts pool size, synthesis and intestinal concentration are low in premature infants in comparison with full-term infants. Parenteral nutrition-related cholestasis is a diagnosis of exclusion without any specific marker yet available. Therefore, infants with cholestasis who are receiving or have received parenteral nutrition must have an appropriate diagnostic evaluation to exclude other causes of cholestasis. These include bacterial and viral infections, metabolic diseases and congenital anomalies. Gall bladder sludge, which can progress to

Table 8.3 Patient risk factors for the development of parenteral nutrition-related cholestasis

Age
Prematurity
Immaturity of biliary secretory system
Absence of oral or enteral intake
Septicaemia
Bacterial overgrowth in the small bowel
Short bowel length
Necrotising enterocolitis
Hypoxia
Major abdominal operations
General anaesthesia

"sludge balls" and gallstones, appeared in 18 neonates (44%) after a mean period of 10 days of parenteral nutrition. The cholestasis is progressive unless parenteral nutrition is ceased and enteral feeding introduced. Hepatosplenomegaly and severe jaundice are characteristic features of the advanced disease, and portal hypertension may develop. Although parenteral nutrition-related cholestasis resolves with time after discontinuation of parenteral nutrition, in a small percentage of cases it remains intractable and progresses to severe hepatic dysfunction and death.

The aetiology of parenteral nutrition-related cholestasis remains unclear. Possible causes include the toxicity of components of parenteral nutrition, lack of enteral feeding, continuous non-pulsatile delivery of nutrients and host factors. Most of the components of parenteral nutrition have been implicated in the pathogenesis of cholestasis. Hepatic damage from the components of intravenous diet may result from excessive nutrient administration, deficient nutrient administration, toxicity of by-products and abnormal metabolism in the neonate.

The clinical care of infants and children who require parenteral nutrition and develop progressive jaundice represents a real challenge, compounded by this lack of knowledge. Prevention of parenteral nutrition-related cholestasis is based on the early usage of enteral feeding and on the administration of intravenous feeding only when appropriate and necessary. In most patients the cholestasis resolves gradually as enteral feedings are initiated and parenteral nutrition is discontinued. It has been recently shown that minimal bolus enteral feeding (1 ml/kg) during parenteral nutrition in premature infants induces significant gall bladder contraction and after 3 days of starting minimal enteral feeds, the gallbladder volume returns to normal. Unfortunately, as a consequence of gut dysfunction, enteral feeding is often not feasible. It has been suggested that cycling the parenteral nutrition may diminish cholestatic hepatic changes in adults. This may explain the less frequent liver disease in children receiving their parenteral nutrition cyclically at home. Experience with this technique in premature infants is extremely limited but encouraging. Rebound hypoglycaemia is a common complication of this approach. Modification of the parenteral nutrition constituents has been proposed but no prospective trial has demonstrated any benefit in reducing or changing the intake of nutrients.

Several reports have described the attempts to use drug therapy to treat or prevent parenteral nutrition-related cholestasis. Cholecystokinin has been administered to diminish the gallbladder stasis and promote bile flow. It has been demonstrated in a randomised, double-blind controlled study in adults receiving parenteral nutrition that cholecystokinin given intravenously daily prevents stasis and sludge in the gallbladder. Rintala et al. reported the reversal of parenteral nutrition-related cholestasis in seven infants by intravenous administration of cholecystokinin; however, all the patients except one were completely weaned from parenteral nutrition before the treatment with cholecystokinin. Teitelbaum et al. conducted a prospective trial of cholecystokinin in the prevention of parenteral nutrition-related cholestasis; however, the patients were consecutive rather than randomised and there is a need for a randomized controlled trial of cholecystokinin in administration to neonates on parenteral nutrition.

Ursodeoxycholic acid can be used in infants and children on parenteral nutrition to correct the decreased secretion of endogenous bile acids. Ursodeoxycholic acid is non-toxic and acts as a natural bile acid after conjugation. Although there have been limited trials of the use of ursodeoxycholic acid in preterm neonates on TPN, results were inconclusive.

Cholecystectomy is the treatment of choice for patients with acute and symptomatic cholelithiasis and cholecystitis. Some authors proposed laparotomy and operative cholangiography followed by biliary tract irrigation in patients with progressive cholestatic jaundice not responding to medical treatment. In some patients the hepatic disease may progress to cirrhosis, portal hypertension and hepatic failure. In selected cases small bowel and liver transplantation have been used. The introduction of tacrolimus has allowed clinical intestinal transplantation to become feasible. However, infectious and immunological problems still cause significant morbidity and mortality, even 1–3 years after transplantation.

8.5.3.5 Free Radicals and Parenteral Nutrition

Free radicals are highly reactive short-lived species in possession of an unpaired electron, and are produced during many physiological processes. When neutrophils and macrophages engulf foreign particles, the particle is exposed to superoxide and hydroxyl radicals and a variety of other reactive compounds during the so-called "respiratory burst," which occurs as the white cell destroys the bacteria. Intracellular and extracellular antioxidants protect against uncontrolled free radical activity. These include enzymes (e.g. superoxide dismutase, catalase, glutathione peroxidase) and chemical antioxidants such as vitamins E and C. A pathologic increase in free radical activity may occur when the normal balance between free radical formation and protective antioxidant activity becomes altered and free radicals can then attack and damage cells and tissues. TPN may exacerbate free radical activity in newborn infants by providing (1) the substrates for free radical production (polyunsaturated fatty acids), (2) the initiators of free radical reactions (carbon centred radicals derived from fatty acids) and (3) the catalysts (transition metal ions) for chain reactions. However, TPN also provides (1) vitamins C and E (antioxidants), (2) metal ions that are important components of antioxidant enzymes (Cu, Zn Mn, Se) and (3) amino acids that are components of glutathione, and important intracellular antioxidant. An increased generation of free radicals during total parenteral nutrition (TPN) in premature infants was reported. Bronchopulmonary dysplasia and retinopathy in premature infants are associated with fat infusions, and these conditions have been linked to free radical-mediated cell damage. Reducing the exposure of premature infants to any unnecessary source of oxidative stress would be desirable. To this end it has been suggested that the use of intravenous fat infusion should be restricted; however, we have shown that a reduction in the carbohydrate to fat ratio in PN diet will result in increased oxidation of administered fat and a decrease in free radical-mediated lipid peroxide formation (Fig. 8.7). It is interesting to note that the decrease in MDA accompanying increased fat utilisation was of a similar magnitude to

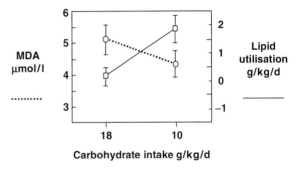

Fig. 8.7 Free radical production (assessed as plasma malondialdehyde, MDA, concentration) in response to different carbohydrate contents of PN (Data from Basu et al. 1999a)

that observed when the fat infusion was discontinued. Therefore, it is not necessary to discontinue the infusion of fat to reduce the production of oxygen-derived free radicals. Manipulation of the carbohydrate to fat ratio therefore may be a powerful tool in changing the metabolism of fat infusions to mitigate their toxic effects while allowing continued administration.

8.6 Enteral Nutrition

The energy requirement of an infant fed enterally is greater than the intravenous requirement because of the energetic cost of absorption from the gastrointestinal tract and energy lost in the stools. Even small amounts of enteral feeding allow the preservation of normal intestinal villi and the maintenance of the epithelial barrier function. Clinical and laboratory studies have shown that enteral feeding is associated with less infectious and immunological complications than parenteral nutrition. Patients receiving total enteral feeding experience significantly fewer septic complications than patients on parenteral and enteral nutrition. Kudsk et al. showed that enteral feeding improved survival after *Esherichia coli* peritonitis in both malnourished and well-nourished rats, compared with rats receiving total PN. The reason for these findings remains poorly understood. However, enteral feeding may act by stimulating more effective immune response. Enternal feeding in a rodent model maintains normal biliary concentrations of secretory IgA (S-IgA), which is an important component of mucosal immunity. In contrast, total parenteral nutrition decreases the biliary levels of this immunogloblin. Furthermore, it has been demonstrated that the level of

TNF-α in peritoneal lavage fluid was higher in enterally fed rats than in rats receiving total PN after 2 h peritoneal bacterial challenge. TNF-α, which is mainly produced by macrophages and lymphocytes, is an important factor in the activation of neutrophils, macrophages and lymphocytes and may therefore be required for effective eradication of bacterial infections.

In surgical infants, enteral feeding often results in vomiting, interruption of feeding, inadequate calorie intake and rarely in necrotizing enterocolitis. In infants with congenital gastrointestinal anomalies, exclusive enteral feeding is commonly precluded for some time after surgery due to large gastric aspirate and intestinal dysmotility. Therefore, appropriate calorie intake is established initially by total parenteral nutrition. Supplementary enteral feeding is introduced when intestinal motility and absorption improves. The percentage of calories given enterally is gradually increased at the expense of intravenous calorie intake. This transition time from total parenteral nutrition to total enteral feeding could be quite long. The presence of significant gastric aspirate often induces clinicians and surgeons not to use the gut for nutrition. However, minimal enteral feeding can be implemented early in these patients even if its nutritional value is questionable. Minimal enteral feeding may be all that is required to enhance some immunological function. This is supported by studies in animals and infants. Shou et al. reported that supplementation of parenteral nutrition with just 10% enteral calories as chew diet improved rat macrophage and splenocyte function, and the introduction of small volumes of enteral feed improved the impaired host bactericidal activity against coagulase negative staphylococci and the abnormal cytokine response observed during total parenteral nutrition. The increase in bactericidal activity against coagulase negative staphylococci after the addition of small enteral feeds in patients on parenteral nutrition was significantly correlated with the duration of enteral feeding. This implies that stimulation of the gastrointestinal tract may modulate immune function in neonates and prevent bacterial infection.

8.6.1 Feeding Routes

Oral feeding is the preferred modality of feeding with breast-feeding being the most physiological up to 6 months of age. Surgical infants do not always tolerate oral feeding due to prematurity, critical illness, abnormalities of the swallowing mechanism, oesophageal dysmotility, gastro-oesophageal reflux or gastric outlet obstruction. Alternative feeding routes in these clinical situations include naso-gastric or oro-gastric tubes, naso-jejunal tubes, gastrostomy tubes or jejunostomy tubes.

Gastric feeding is preferable to intestinal feeding because it allows for a more natural digestive process. In addition, gastric feeding is associated with a larger osmotic and volume tolerance and a lower frequency of diarrhoea and dumping syndrome. Neonates are obligatory nose breathers and therefore oro-gastric feeding is preferable over naso-gastric feeding in preterm infants to avoid upper airway obstruction.

In surgical infants requiring gastric tube feeding for more than 6–8 weeks, it is advisable to insert a gastrostomy tube. The tube can be inserted using an open, endoscopic or laparoscopic approach. In infants with significant gastro-oesophageal reflux, fundoplication with gastrostomy tube or enterostomy tube placement is indicated. In preterm infants with gastro-oesophageal reflux, enteral feeding can be established via a naso-jejunal tube inserted under fluoroscopy. Naso-jejunal feeding usually minimise the episodes of gastro-oesophageal reflux and their consequences. However, it is common for these tubes to dislocate back in the stomach. Regular analysis of the pH in the aspirate is essential to monitor the correct position of the tube. Feeding jejunostomy tubes can be inserted through existing gastrostomy or directly into the jejunum via laparotomy or laparoscopy.

8.6.2 Selection of Enteral Feeds

Breast milk is the ideal feed for infants because it has specific anti-infectious activities that protect them from gastrointestinal and respiratory diseases. In addition, breast milk has high content of non-protein metabolizable nitrogen notably urea. When breast milk is not available chemically defined formulae can be used. If malabsorption persists, an appropriate specific formula should be introduced. A soya-based disaccharide-free feed is used when there is disaccharide intolerance resulting in loose stools containing disaccharides. For fat malabsorption, a formula containing medium-chain triglycerides (MCT) should be used. An elemental formula may be indicated when there is severe malabsorption due to short bowel syndrome or severe mucosal damage as in necrotising enterocolitis. Infants recovering from neonatal necrotising enterocolitis pose a particular problem, as malabsorption may be severe and prolonged. These infants may have had small bowel resected, in addition to which the remaining bowel may not have healed completely by the time feeds are begun. Feeding may provoke a relapse of the necrotising enterocolitis and feeding should therefore be introduced cautiously. Elemental formula preparations contain amino acids, glucose and fats, including MCTs. Dipeptide preparations that include dipeptides as well as amino acids have the advantage of a lower osmolality, are well absorbed and have a more palatable taste.

For persistent severe malabsorption, a modular diet may be necessary. Glucose, amino acid and MCT preparations are provided separately, beginning with the amino acid solution and adding the glucose and then the fats as tolerated. Minerals, trace elements and vitamins are also added. These solutions have high osmolality and if given too quickly may precipitate dumping syndrome, with diarrhoea, abdominal cramps and hypoglycaemia. It is important therefore to start with a dilute solution and increase the concentration and volume of each component slowly. This may take several weeks and infants will need parenteral nutritional support during this period.

8.6.3 Administration of Enteral Feeds

Enteral feeds can be administered as boluses, continuous feeds or as a combination of the two. Bolus feeds are more physiological and are known to stimulate intestinal motility, enterohepatic circulation of bile acids and gallbladder contraction. They mimic or supplement meals and are easier to administer than continuous feeds since a feeding pump is not required. Bolus feeds are usually given over 15–20 min and usually every 3 h. In preterm neonates or in neonates soon after surgery, 2-hourly feeds are occasionally given.

Continuous feeds should be administered via an infusion pump. This modality of feeding is used in infants with gastro-oesophageal reflux, delayed gastric emptying or intestinal malabsorption. Infants with a jejunal tube should receive continuous feeds and not bolus feeds. Continuous feedings are usually given over 24 h. Term infants can tolerate a period of 4 h without feeds before hypoglycaemia occurs. This modality of tube feeding can be very advantageous; however, there is evidence to suggest that normal physiology may be altered when this approach is adopted. Continuous enteral feeding leads to an enlarged, non-contractile gallbladder in infants. Contraction is observed immediately after resuming bolus enteral feeds and gallbladder volume returns to baseline after 4 days. Therefore the mode of feeding has important bearings on the motility of the extrahepatic biliary tree. Studies in adults have reported biliary sludging in patients receiving continuous enteral nutrition, implying gallbladder stasis. In one study, the sludge cleared within 2 weeks of starting bolus oral feeds. This complication has not been reported in infants or children undergoing continuous enteral feeding. In preterm infants, continuous enteral feedings are associated with lower energy expenditure and better growth compared with bolus feedings.

8.6.4 Complications of Enteral Tube Feeding

Enteral tube feeding is associated with fewer complications than parenteral feeding. The complications can be mechanical including tube blockage, tube displacement or migration and intestinal perforation. Other complications involve the gastrointestinal tract. These include gastro-oesophageal reflux with aspiration pneumonia, dumping syndrome and diarrhoea. Jejunostomy tubes inserted at laparotomy can also be associated with intestinal obstruction. The use of hyperosmolar feeds has been associated with development of necrotizing enterocolitis, dehydration and rarely intestinal obstruction due to milk curds.

Further Reading

Basu R, Muller DPR, Eaton S, Merryweather I, Pierro A (1999a) Lipid peroxidation can be reduced in infants on total parenteral nutrition by promoting fat utilisation. J Pediatr Surg 34:255–259

Donnell SC, Lloyd DA, Eaton S, Pierro A (2002) The metabolic response to intravenous medium-chain triglycerides in infants after surgery. J Pediatr 141:689–694

Pierro et al (1991) Partition of energy metabolism in the surgical newborn. J Pediatr Surg 26:581–586

Pierro A, Jones MO, Hammond P, Nunn A, Lloyed DA (1993) Utilisation of intravenous fat in the surgical newborn infant. In Proceedings of the Nutrition Society. In vol 52, p 237A

Pierro A, Camielli V, Filler RM, Smith J Heim T (1989) Metabolism of infravenous fat emulsion in the surgical newborn. J Pediatr surg 24:95–101

Puri P, Höllwarth ME (eds) (2006) Pediatric Surgery. Springer, Berlin, Heidelberg

Turi RA, Petros A, Eaton S et al (2001) Energy metabolism of infants and children with systemic inflammatory response syndrome and sepsis. Ann Surg 233:581–587

Haematological Problems

9

Owen Patrick Smith

Contents

9.1 Haematological Basic Science

9.1.1 Blood Formation (Haematopoiesis)

The bone marrow is a mesenchymal derived tissue divided into irregular interconnective spaces by bone trabeculae. It consists of a complex haematopoietic cellular component that is extremely labile and continuously goes through self-replication and differentiation processes. These cells are supported by a micro environment composed of stromal cells (endothelial cells, fibroblast like cells, adipocytes), extracellular matrix and vascular structures.

- Embryonic haematopoeisis (which predominantly is associated with red cell development) begins in the yolk sac at the end of the 3rd week of gestation and declines to an insignificant level by the end of the first trimester.
- By the end of the first trimester, the liver is the dominant source of haematopoiesis producing all the haemopoietic elements. Hepatic haematopoietic activity reaches its maximum level at around the 3rd month and gradually declines from the 7th month until birth.
- Bone marrow haematopoiesis begins to occur at around the 5th month of gestation and continues to increase thereafter.
- Every day, in normal adult bone marrow, approximately 2.5 billion red cells, 1 billion granulocytes and 2.5 billion platelets are produced per kilogram of body weight.
- Haematopoiesis is regulated and sustained by a complex cellular interaction of haemopoietic and stromal elements and a network of cytokine growth factors including the interleukins and colony stimulating factors.

P. Puri and M. Höllwarth (eds.), *Pediatric Surgery: Diagnosis and Management,*
DOI: 10.1007/978-3-540-69560-8_9, © Springer-Verlag Berlin Heidelberg 2009

- All the cells of the haemopoietic system originate from a pluripotent haemopoietic stem cell (HSC). HSCs have the intrinsic capacity for self renewal and are low in number and divide infrequently. The committed progenitors are responsible for the massive amount of cell proliferation required to maintain blood cell production in numbers outlined above. The common lymphoid progenitors develop into T and B cells whereas the common myeloid progenitor gives rise to erythrocytes, megakaryocytes, monocytes and granulocytes.

9.1.2 Mechanisms of Haemostasis

Normal blood coagulation or haemostasis is a complex sequence of inter-related events by which the body prevents blood loss from the vascular tree. This is achieved by a multi-pathway interactive system with multiple negative and positive feedback loops, which ultimately ensure that blood is at all times fluid within the vasculature, but it also needs to be transformed into a clot when there is a breach in the integrity of the vascular tree. The protein (pro- and anticoagulants—outlined below) and cellular (endothelial cells, monocytes and platelets) components have also shown to be intimately involved in the inflammatory response, vasculogenesis, metastasis, cellular proliferation and tissue repair.

- Tissue factor, a cell surface glycoprotein is the principal biological initiator of blood coagulation.
- Exposure of circulating plasma VIIa to tissue factor triggers the coagulation cascade *in vivo*, which results in thrombin generation (Fig. 9.1).
- Thrombin converts soluble fibrinogen to a fibrin network, activates platelets and stimulates coagulation by positive feedback activators of cofactors, factors V and VIII and the zymogens II, VII, IX, X, XII and XIII.
- Under physiological conditions, pro-and anticoagulant (see below) mechanisms are balanced in favour of anticoagulation; however, at sites of vascular damage resulting from inflammation, trauma, etc, the anticoagulant system is down-regulated and thus procoagulant forces prevail.

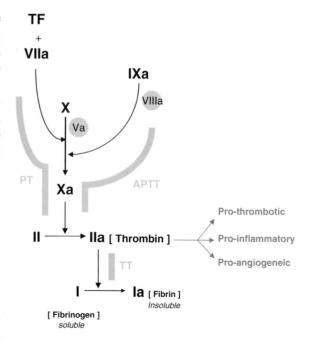

Fig. 9.1 Blood coagulation is initiated (initiation phase) when tissue factor (TF), expressed after injury to cell (endothelial, monocytic cells, etc.) wall, is exposed to FVIIa in the bloodstream. TF-FVIIa complex in turn activates FIX to FIXa and FX to FXa. FIXa with its cofactor FVIIIa in turn also activates FX to FXa (amplication phase). FXa with its cofactor FVa activates Prothrombin (II) to Thrombin (IIa) (propagation phase). Thrombin converts soluble fibrinogen to insoluble fibrin. Thrombin is not only pro-thrombotic but activates platelets and is proinflammatory and promotes new vessel formation. Shown in grey are three global coagulation screens prothrombin time (PT), activated partial thromboplastin time (APTT) and thrombin time (TT)

9.1.3 Natural Anticoagulation Control Mechanisms

Several natural anticoagulant mechanisms have been discovered that exert dampening effects upon procoagulation and in turn halt the generation of thrombin. The major anticoagulant inhibitors of blood coagulation include tissue pathway inhibitor, antithrombin and the Protein C pathway (Fig. 9.2). The protein C pathway regulates the amount of thrombin in the microcirculation whereas the tissue factor pathway inhibitor and the antithrombin exert more of an effect in the macro-circulation.

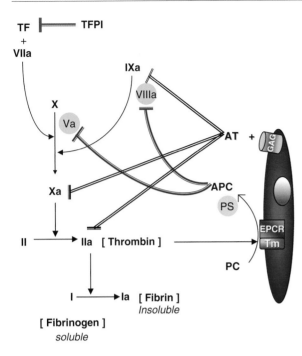

Fig. 9.2 The initiation phase of coagulation is controlled by inhibiting the complex of TF, FVIIa and FXa by tissue factor pathway inhibitor (TFPI). The amplification phase of coagulation is blocked by the protein C pathway. Protein C (PC) is activated by a complex of thrombin, thrombomodulin (Tm), and endothelial protein C receptor (EPCR) to APC which in association with protein S (PS) inactivates FVa and FVIIa. The thrombin formed in the propagation phase is controlled by antithrombin (AT)

Table 9.1 Platelet function disorders

- Storage Pool Disorders (SPD)
  - Dense granule storage pool disease (δ-SPD)
    - Hermanksy-Pudlak
    - Chediak-Higashi
    - Wiskott-Aldrich
    - Thrombocytopenia absent radii
    - May-Hegglin
  - Alpha granule storage pool disease (α-SPD)
    - Grey platelet syndrome
  - δ, α storage pool disease (δ,α-SPD)
- Release defects
  - Asprin-like syndromes
    - Cyclooxygenase deficiency
    - Thromboxane synthetase deficiency
    - Thromboxane A2 receptor defects
  - Drug-induced
    - Asprin
    - Other non-steroidal anti-inflammatory agents
    - Furosemide
    - Nitrofurantoin

9.1.4 Platelets

Platelets derived from megakaryocytes play an essenial role in thrombosis and haemostasis. Megarkaryopoiesis in the bone marrow is governed by a complex interaction of cytokines (e.g. thrombopoietin) and their receptors (e.g. c-mpl). Platelets play a major role in primary haemostasis (adhesion, aggregation and release). Platelets may also have functional defects and these can manifest as a diminished platelet response to weak agonists (storage pool defects and release defects or aspirin-like syndromes) (Table 9.1) or where there is an absence of platelet aggregation to all agonists as seen in Glanzmann's thrombasthenia, dysfibrinogenaemia or afibrinogenaemia. These disorders cause primary haemostatic bleeding ranging from mild to severe.

9.1.5 Blood Groups and Antibodies

There are 26 blood group systems corresponding to red blood cell (RBC) surface antigens. The ABO system is the most important. Antibodies against blood group antigens A and B occur naturally in people who lack these antigens, for example, patients who are Group A will have naturally occurring anti-B antibodies, while patients who are Group O will have anti-A and anti-B and so on. These antibodies are IgM, and so can cause complement activation and acute intravascular haemolysis. Other clinically important antibodies do not occur naturally and require exposure to an antigen—either by a blood product transfusion or *via* feto-maternal exposure. These antigens vary in their immunogenicity, e.g. the Rhesus antigen "D" and the Kell antigen are highly immunogenic.

9.2 Secelted Haemato-Surgical Case Scenarios

9.2.1 Haemophilia

Haemophilia A (factor VIII deficiency) is the second commonest inherited bleeding disorder with a frequency of approximately 1 in 500 male births. Haemophilia B (factor IX Deficiency) is approximately one-sixth as common as Haemophilia A.

Clinical Features

- Majority of severe and moderate (factor VIII levels <1% and 1–5%, respectively) cases present in the first few years of life.
- Haemophilia A and B are X-linked recessive disorders.
- One-third of cases of FVIII Deficiency have no family history (spontaneous mutations).
- When there is no family history, infants with moderate or severe disease usually present:

    - Post-circumcision bleeding (Fig. 9.3)
    - Bad "toddler bruising"
    - Soft tissue and muscle or joint bleeds at 6–18 months of age
    - Intracranial ilio-psoas, intra-abdominal haematuria are all rare

- Children presenting with bruising and severe bleeding, not uncommon for the first presumed diagnosis to be non-accidental injury.
- True coagulation defects need to be excluded. Normal coagulation screen does not exclude all significant coagulation disorders

Treatment

- Objectives of modern management include the following:

    - Prevention of chronic joint damage (Fig. 9.4)
    - Prevention of "life threatening" bleeds
    - To facilitate social and physical well-being and help children achieve their full potential
    - To provide a comprehensive service to the family

- Successful treatment involves prompt and sufficient intravenous replacement of FVIII/FIX to haemostatic levels.
- Prophylactic administration of factor concentrate converts a child who has severe or moderately severe disease to a child with mild disease. Because of the different plasma half-lives of coagulation factors, FVIII is given three times per week and FIX is given twice a week in prophylactic programmes.
- Prophylaxis usually requires a central venous access device (see below) to be placed in the child to facilitate regular intravenous administration.

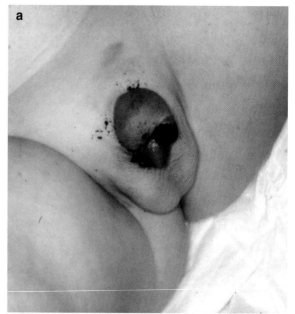

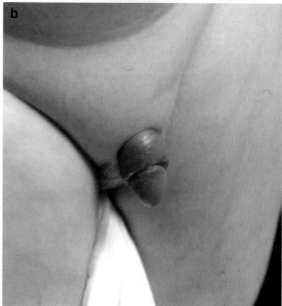

Fig. 9.3 Haemophilia A: (**a**) Post-circumcisional haematoma in an infant with no family history of haemophilia. Mutational analyses showed the presence of IVS 22 mutation. (**b**) Full haematoma resolution 1 week later following replacement with recombinant FVIII

- Recombinant factor concentrates are now the gold standard.
- Inhibitor formation to FVIII/IX is the single biggest complication in modern management of haemo-philia.

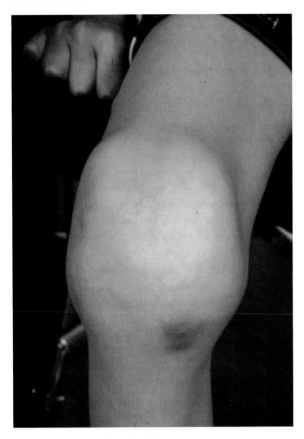

Fig. 9.4 Haemophilia B: chronic severe haemophiliac arthropathy of the right knee joint. The quadrecep muscle is severly wasted. This adolescent was only treated intermittently with plasma through out the first 5 years of life

9.2.2 Central Venous Access Devices

The intravenous administration of factor concentrate twice or three times per week is fraught with difficulty in the majority of young children when only using peripheral veins. Similarly, immune tolerance therapy (ITT) using large doses of factor concentrate, twice a day for 12–24 months for children with inhibitors to factor VIII/IX is almost impossible without regular venous access. These devices can be fully implantable (PortaCath™, Deltac USA) or partly externalised (single or double lumen Quintan™ Catheters). The use of a port is preferable to an external device because it causes fewer limitations to the child's lifestyle and it has been suggested that there is a lower infective risk. However, despite the obvious attractions of these devices, their routine use for prophylaxis and ITT has

not gained universal acceptance because of the potential risks of haemorrhage, thrombosis and infection both of which may lead to a high rate of morbidity and permanent removal of the device.

Infection is cited as the reason for removal of port in up to 70% of all port removals. The rate of infection is higher in children with inhibitors. In the best of hands, the patient with a port-a-cath, without inhibitors and on regular prophylaxis, will probably have a maximum of one catheter-related infection in approximately 10 years.

There is now a growing consensus that long-term indwelling devices are necessary to facilitate the modern intensive treatment of congenital coagulation disorders. There are complications, as outlined above, in particular infections, but with improved management of the perioperative period and regular, frequent re-education, particularly in those children with inhibitors, many of these complications may be avoided.

More recently the use of arteriovenous fistulae (AVF) as a reliable means of vascular access in children with haemophilia has been reported. Complication rates are reported to be minimal: bleeding complication rate at 16%, thrombotic complication rates at 3% and infection rate at 0%. The vast majority of children (>95%) achieved functional AVF that are still regularly used for home treatment over a median period of 29 months, suggesting that this approach, i.e. the creation of AVF as the first option for achieving permanent venous access in children with severe haemophilia, is warranted.

9.2.3 Platelet Disorders

The normal range of the platelet count in fetal life is similar to that seen in adult life, being about 150–400 $\times 10^9/l$. The causes of thrombocytopenia can be divided into two broad categories: those arising on the background of an established genetic defect ((inherited thrombocytopenia) and those that are acquired either around the time of birth (congenital thrombocytopenia) or those that occur later in childhood. Inherited thrombocytopenia can be accompanied with or without dysfunctional platelets (Table 9.1). It is important to remember to confirm that the low platelet count is genuine by careful inspection of the blood sample and smear before initiating further investigations. Once

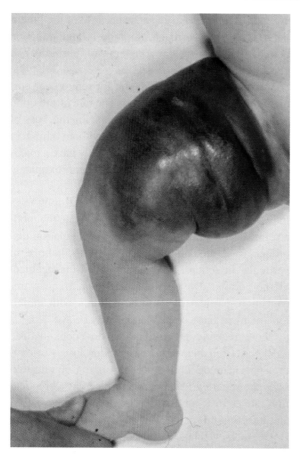

Fig. 9.5 Capillary haemangioma in a 2-month-old boy with Kasabackh-Merrit syndrome (KMS). The lesion involuted after 4 months of therapy involving vincristine, prednisilone and anti-platelet agents (asprin and ticlopidine)

established, the approach to the diagnosis of thrombo-cytopenia should be tailored to the individual child or infant and mother if dealing with neonatal thrombocy-topenia. For example, assessment of the child's gen-eral wellbeing is very important as healthy children usually have an immune or an inherited aetiology, whereas the presence of lymphadenopathy, hepatos-plenomegaly, mass lesions, hemangiomas (Fig. 9.5) bruits and congenital anomalies point towards a totally different spectrum of causes. In neonates, it should also be emphasised that obtaining a detailed maternal history, including bleeding problems, pre-eclampsia and drug ingestion in the present and past pregnancies and any history of viral infections (cytomegalovirus, rubella, herpes simplex and HIV) or connective tissue

disease (systemic lupus erythematosus [SLE]), will save time and unnecessary investigation.

Immune Thrombocytopenia Purpura (ITP), defined as thrombocytopenia purpura, without any other asso-ciated condition is the commonest form seen in childhood

Clinical Features

- Predominantly seen in children aged between 2 and 5 years
- Usually preceded by a viral illness or prodrome
- Usually seen in autumn and winter months
- Bleeding uncommon when platelet count > 50,000 /ml
- Spontaneous bleeding is frequent when the platelet count < 50,000/ml
- Diagnosis is one of exclusion in that the vast majority of children will have had a preceding viral infection or will have been vaccinated in the previous month

Clinical and Patho-physiology

- Examination usually normal with the exception of cutaneous bleeding.
- Most likely a heterogenous group of disorders, whose cardinal clinical feature is a low platelet count.
- Inappropriate immune response to several different stimuli.
- The antibody produced is cross reacting to platelet surface proteins such as GPIIb–IIIa.

Treatment

- Bone marrow examination is not required in the vast majority of disorders with ITP
- The majority of children will respond spontaneously
- If treatment is required then intravenous immuno-globulin (1 g per kg for 2 days) and prednisolone (2 mg per kg daily × 7 days with taper) are front line treatments.
- Majority of children will respond but may have side-effects.
- Children who fail to respond, therapeutic interven-tions include anti-D, Rituximab (anti CD20) Danazol, Cyclosporin A and azathioprine should be considered.
- A small number of children may develop a chronic form of ITP (thrombocytopenia lasting greater than 6 months) that can be symptomatic. Treatment can be problematic and hence **splenectomy** (see below) is worth considering.

9.2.4 Disseminated Intravascular Coagulopathy (DIC)

DIC is a clinico-pathological entity resulting in simultaneous and unregulated activation of the coagulation and fibrinolytic pathways. It is a syndrome of serious clinical consequences, which is encountered in all area of paediatrics particularly in the intensive care unit. DIC is not a primary disease entity; it is secondary to an underlying usually severe and most often systemic illness. DIC is a progressive, pathological process resulting in profuse thrombin formation and excessive activity of the fibrinolytic pathway and its most prominent clinical feature is a bleeding tendency.

- In DIC with haemorrhage, bleeding is typically from multiple sites, indicating the systemic nature of the process.
- Purpura fulminans seen in the majority of cases of disseminated meningococaemia, the skin lesions appear haemorrhagic; however, microthromboses are underlying histological findings (Fig. 9.6)
- Diagnostic features in DIC include prothrombin, PT, APTT, fibrinogen, D˙Dimer, platelet count, blood smear and natural anticoagulant factor levels.

Treatment

- Blood product replacement in the form of FFP, cryo-precipitate, fibrinogen concentrate and platelets is the first line of therapy.

- Other forms of intervention such as heparin, natural anticoagulant concentrates and anti-fibrinolytic agents may also have a defined role.
- Since DIC is not a primary disease entity, treatment should be directed towards the underlying process causing the consumption.

9.2.5 Thrombotic Disorders

Thrombotic disease in children is rare compared to adults. When seen in childhood it is either secondary to an acquired prothrombotic state or the child has an inherited gene defect predisposing to clot formation. When it does occur in childhood it can be fatal or associated with several sequlae such as amputation, organ dysfunction and post-phlebitic syndrome. The peak incidence of these thrombotic events is undoubtedly the neonatal period.

- Thrombotic tendency is seen in a number of clinical scenarios as outlined in Tables 9.2 and 9.3.
- Approximately 80% of these genetic disorders have lesions directly or indirectly affecting the Protein C natural anticoagulant pathway (Table 9.2).
- Homozygocity of these natural anticoagulant proteins are rare, common as being Protein C deficiency that causes purpura fulminans within the neonatal period.

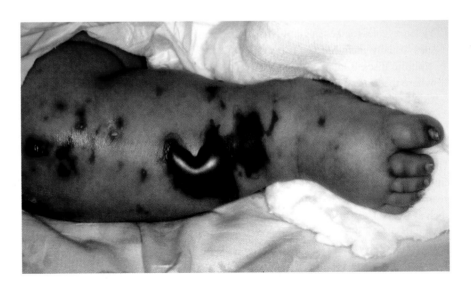

Fig. 9.6 Purpura fulminans secondary to severe acquired protein C deficiency in association with meningococcal septicaemia

Table 9.2   Acquired thrombotic tendency

- Indwelling vascular catheters
- Renal artery and vein thrombosis
- Acquired natural anticoagulant deficiency
  - Nephrotic syndrome → antithrombin deficiency
  - Purpura fulminans → varicella & protein S deficiency and meningococcaemia & protein C deficiency
- Necrotising enterocolitis (NEC)
- Respiratory distress syndrome
- Heparin-induced thrombocytopenia/thrombosis syndrome (HIT/HITTs)
- Maternal anticardiolipin antibodies (lupus anticoagulant)
- Extracorporeal membrane oxygenation (ECMO)
- Haemolytic uraemic syndrome/thrombotic thrombocytopenic purpura (HUS / TTP)
- Birth asphyxia

Table 9.3   Inherited thrombotic tendency

- Defects within the Protein C Pathway
  - PCR and FVR506Q (factor V Leiden)
  - Protein C Deficiency
  - Protein S Deficiency
  - FIIG20210A (prothrombin gene variant)
  - High circulating levels of FVIII
- Antithrombin Deficiency
- Hyperhomocysteinaemia
  - Cystathionine B-synthase
  - Methionine synthase
  - Thermolabile methylenetetrahydrofolate reductase
- Fibrinolytic Pathway
  - PAI-1 (4G/5G polymorphic status)
  - Plasminogenaemia
- Dysfibrinogenaemia
- Haemoglobinopathy
- Platelet defects

- Heterozygotes for these natural anticoagulant deficiencies usually manifest as being venous thromboembolic disease later in life, usually in the setting where these are further perturbation to the coagulation pathway, e.g. on the background of sepsis, immobility, dehydration etc

Treatment

The indications for use of anticoagulants in infants and children have changed dramatically over the past 20 years with major advances in tertiary paediatric care such as ECMO, cardio-pulmonary bypass, haemodialysis and the use of intra-arterial and intravenous indwelling catheters. The following should be considered:

- Choice of anticoagulant is dependent on the duration of anticoagulation.

- In the acute phase, heparins, either unfractionated or low-molecular-weight forms, are used.
- In the longer term, oral anticoagulants are the treatment of choice at the present time.
- In more specific disease states such as inherited or acquired protein C or antithrombin deficiencies, factor concentrate replacement as an adjuvant haemostatic support is used increasingly.
- Children who develop heparin-induced thrombocytopenia, recombinant hirudin or a heparinoid should be considered.

9.2.6   Asplenia or Hyposplenism

The commonest form of asplenia or hyposplenism is surgical splenectomy. The usual haematological indications for splenectomy include the following:

- Repeated splenic sequestration in children with sickle cell disease
- Thalassemia major with associated hypersplenism
- Hereditary spherycytosis
- Refractory immune cytopenias

Congenital absence of the spleen can be associated with multiple abnormalities including cardiovascular and visceral abnormalities and some of these have a genetic basis.

Loss of splenic substances as a result of infarction is seen in sickle cell disease and essential thrombocytopenia, the latter being extremely rare in children. These conditions are usually accompanied by functional hyposplenism.

- Assessment of splenic filtration function is usually made by examination of the peripheral blood for evidence of red cell inclusions, which are pitted out during filtration by the normally functioning spleen (Fig. 9.7). These inclusions include Howell Jolly bodies and "pits" in red cells. The presence of Howell Jolly bodies usually reflects significant splenic hypo-function and the risk of overwhelming infection.
- Immune-mediated conditions associated with functional hyposplenism include the following:

  - Chronic graft versus host disease (GvHD)
  - HIV/AIDS
  - Coeliac disease/Dermatitis herpetiforms
  - Rheumatoid arthritis/SLE
  - Thyroid disease
  - Ulcer colitis/Crohns disease

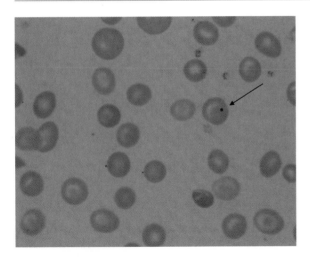

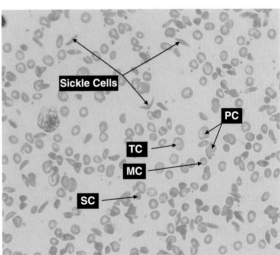

Fig. 9.7 The arrowed red cell shows a dark dense inclusion "Howell Jolly body". Howell Jolly bodies are most commonly seen in splenectomised (surgical or "auto") patients, severe forms of megaloblastic and haemolytic anaemias and haemoglobin-opathies

Fig. 9.8 A 9-year-old Nigerian boy with HbSS. The arrowed cells are markedly elongated with two pointed ends. Also note the other classic findings of target cells (TC), microcytes (MC), spherocytes (SC) and polychromatophilic cells (PC)

- In many of these diseases, there is not only functional hyposplenism but the spleen may also become atrophied. This is seen especially frequently in patients with coeliac disease, the majority of whom are adults.

9.2.7 Sickle Cell Disease

Sickle cell disease is common in people of African, Afro-Caribbean and Middle Eastern heritage. It is now the most common genetic disease in the UK. Sickle haemoglobin (HbS) results from a point mutation in the β-globin gene. HbS polymerises when it becomes deoxygenated, then polymerises into molecular bundles that interfere with RBC membrane structure and deformability. The distorted RBCs cannot traverse small blood vessels in the microcirculation and thus vaso-occlusion leading to ischaemia and local tissue damage occurs. The inheritance of one HbS gene ("Sickle Trait" or "HbAS") is a benign condition. Sickling disorders are seen when two HbS genes are inherited or when HbS is coinherited with certain other β-chain variants: HbC, HbE, HbD, HbO[Arab] and β-thalassaemia. The diagnosis is suspected by blood film examination that shows characteristic sickle cells and features of hyposplenism (Fig. 9.8). It should be remembered that the "Sickledex", a solubility test is unreliable in children under 6 months old or in those who have been recently transfused. High performance liquid chromatography confirms the diagnosis and Hb electrophoresis or Isoelectric Focussing may be required if there is doubt about the nature of the abnormal Hb.

Clinical Features and Management

- Vaso-occlusion is often precipitated by cold or dehydration or infection. Causes severe pain in the affected area. Most commonly seen in bones, GIT (**may mimic acute abdomen**), lungs (may result in ARDS-type picture: "chest crisis") and brain (stroke). Priapism may also be seen.
- Pain control is essential—opiates are frequently required.
- Patients should be well hydrated and antibiotics given if there is any suspicion of infection.
- RBC transfusion (top-up or exchange) may be required for chest crisis or stroke.
- Sequestration is usually seen in the under 5-year-olds. The spleen (or liver) becomes engorged by sickled RBCs and may cause rapid haemodynamic collapse and an RBC transfusion is usually required. The parents should be instructed on how to monitor spleen size.
- Aplasia is usually seen in association with Parvovirus B19 infection (suppresses erythropoieisis). This is usually suspected with inadequate reticulocyte count.

- Sepsis is not uncommon as a significant number of these patients are hyposplenic due to autoinfarction of spleen. The most common organism is Strep. pneumoniae and is treated with broad-spectrum antibiotics.
- All patients should take prophylactic penicillin and receive Pneumovax.

With repeated vascular occlusion events, chronic complications may arise that include the following:

- Pulmonary hypertension exacerbated by chronic intravascular haemolysis causing release of free Hb and scavenging of nitric oxide.
- Nearly all patients have hyposthenuria and chronic renal impairment may be seen.
- "Silent" infarction may contribute to intellectual impairment (Fig. 9.9).
- Chronic osteomyelitis or Avascular Necrosis (AVN).
- Proliferative retinopathy is more commonly seen in HbSC disease.
- Chronic leg ulceration in young adults.

Patients are usually placed on a transfusion programme if there is evidence of acute stroke or if they have an abnormal transcranial Dopplers (flow rates in cerebral vessels are increased if vessels are narrowed due to endothelial damage—strongly predicts stroke risk). Transfusion occurs every 3–4 weeks; suppresses and iron overload should be aggressively managed with chelation therapy.

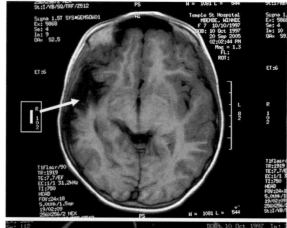

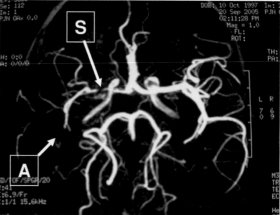

Fig. 9.9 About 25% of patients with SCD develop cerebrovascular complications and about 80 of these are under 15 years of age. The MRI Brain shows an area of infarction (I) secondary to vessel occlusion (stenosis (S) and absence (A))

9.2.8 Neutropenia and Typhilitis (Neutropenic Colitis)

9.2.8.1 Neutropenia

Neutrophils differentiate in the bone marrow for approximately 7 days and then circulate in the blood for approximately 6.5 h. Newborns often have neutrophilia for the first 2 weeks, mean count $11 \times 10^9/l$, whereas children between 1 month and 8 years have mean levels of $3.6 \times 10^8/l$. Above this age, counts are similar to adult levels.

- Neutropenia in children can have inherited or acquired causes and these are usually characterised as either transient or chronic. Sometimes the inherited neutropenia is part of a more complex syndrome (see below)

- The usual work up for a child with neutropenia requires documentation of the neutropenia over time, elimination of possible precipitating causes by history and bone marrow examination in those children in whom a clear cause is not found. Children with neutrophil counts of less than $0.5 \times 10^9/l$ are at increased susceptibility to bacterial infections.
- Acquired transient causes include infections (viral, bacterial), burns, drugs, haemodyalisis, haematinic deficiencies (B12 Folic Acid).
- Acquired chronic causes will include haematological malignancies, myelodysplasia, immune-mediated (allo-immune and auto-immune), hypersplenism, viral, bone marrow suppression and idiopathic.
- Isolated inherited causes include infantile genetic agranulocytosis (Kostmann's Syndrome), other chronic

congenital neutropenias such as cyclical neutropenia, benign chronic neutropenia, myelokathexis

- Those associated with complex syndromes include Cartilage Hair hypoplasia, Chediak-Higashi Syndrome, Dyskerytosis Congenita, primary immuno-deficiency (e.g. S linked hyper IGM Syndrome), Fanconi Anaemia, Shwachman Diamond Syndrome, Cyclical Dysgenesis and metabolic disorders such as Glyogen Storage Type 1B Disease.
- The genetic basis for the majority of these inherited disorders has now been elucidated.
- Treatment usually involves supported measures such as antibiotics, G-CSF therapy and in those cases associated with bone marrow failure, allogeneic bone marrow transplantation.

9.2.8.2 Typhilitis (Neutropenic Colitis)

Typhilitis (inflammation of the caecum due to Gram-negative bacteria of the gut flora) is a diagnosis unique to the neutropenic patient. Its diagnosis is relatively common in the haemato-oncology wards where intensive chemotherapeutic protocols are routinely used. Patients are febrile and usually have right-sided or generalised abdominal pain. It should be remembered that no clinical findings differentiate typhilitis from other abdominal diseases. CT and ultrasound imaging show distention and thickening of the caecum and bowel wall thickening with associated marked pseudopoly-poid formation of the mucosa, respectively. Neutrophil recovery is a good prognostic factor. Conservative management with broad-spectrum antibiotics and anti-fungals with or without bowel rest is the treatment of choice. Surgical intervention should be only be considered in the most severe cases

9.2.9 Blood Products

A list of blood products used in children in the surgical setting is shown below:

- *Red cell concentrate* (RBCs): Dose (ml) = (Desired rise in Hb) × 3 × recipient weight (kg)

The cross-match(ing of blood) is geared to ensure that an inadvertent exposure to a foreign antigen does not occur and consists of the following:

1. ABO and D grouping of the recipient
2. Antibody screen of the recipient (or mother in the case of neonatal transfusion)—serum is tested against a "panel" of commercially available RBCs that carry all clinically important antigens between them
3. A comparison of these results with any available historical record (a "group and screen" finishes at this point)
4. Testing of patient serum against the RBCs to be transfused

- *Platelets*: Dose = 15 ml/kg. Usual maximum dose is one pool ("adult dose") unless bleeding or specific target platelet count
- *Frozen Plasma* (FP): Usual dose 15 ml/kg, usually used as source of clotting factors in DIC, haemorrhagic disease of the newborn. Children born after 01/01/96 receive "pathogen-reduced plasma", which has undergone a viral inactivation process
- *Cryoprecipitate*: Obtained by thawing FP at 4°C, rich in fibrinogen, FVIII, VWF and FXIII. Main use is hypofibrinogenaemia (usually in DIC), usual dose 10–15 ml/kg.
- RBCs and platelets are leucodepleted to remove WBCs that can cause immune reactions and harbour infections (e.g. CMV)
- CMV negative and irradiated products are usually required for immunosuppressed patients—refer to local guidelines

There are recognised acute and long-term adverse events associated with blood product transfusions and are briefly highlighted below. The most serious reactions have similar presentations.

- Haemolytic reaction: fever, dyspnoea, back pain, haemoglobinuria (with intravascular haemolysis)
- Urticarial and anaphylactic reaction
- Bacterial contamination—usually seen with platelets (stored at 22°C)
- TRALI: Transfusion-related acute lung injury: occurs due to anti-WBC or HLA antibodies in donor or recipient. Causes ARDS-like picture
- In practice, all these possibilities need to be considered:

    (i) Stop the transfusion
    (ii) Assess haemodynamic stability—resuscitate if necessary

(iii) Check the patient identification against the blood product

(iv) Examine the product for abnormal appearance suggesting contamination

(v) Order full septic screen (include product if bacterial contamination is a possibility)

(vi) Order CXR if dyspnoea or hypoxia

(vii) Repeat cross-match, antibody screen and check indices of haemolysis

- Febrile non-haemolytic reaction: non-specific reaction to foreign antigen must be differentiated from more serious reactions
- Volume overload: deaths have been described in SHOT report. Must be differentiated from TRALI
- Delayed haemolytic reactions occur after 5–10 days—evidence of haemolysis and possibly renal impairment due to toxic effects of free Hb
- Infection can be bacterial, viral, protozoal (Chagas' disease), prion (vCJD Transmission reported in the UK)
- Iron overload seen with chronic RBC transfusion

- Post-transfusion purpura can occur especially in HPA-1a negative patients develop thrombocytopaenia 7–10 days post-platelet transfusion.
- Graft-versus-host disease is rare but universally fatal due to bone marrow suppression

Further Reading

Arcesi R, Hann IM, Smith OP (2006) Paediatric haematology, 3rd edn. Blackwell Publishing, Oxford, ISBN 1-4051-3400-3/9781405134002

Hutchinson RJ (2006) Surgerical implications of hematological disease. In JL Grosfeld, JA O'Neill, AG Coran, EW Fonkalsrud (eds) Pediatric Surgery. Mosby, Philadelphia, PA, pp 178–193

Luchtman-Jones L (2005) Blood. In KT Oldham, PM Colombani, RP Foglia, MA Skinner (eds) Principles of Practice of Pediatric Surgery. Lippincott Williams & Wilkins, Philadelphia, PA, pp 297–312

Puri P, Höllwarth ME (eds) (2006) Pediatric Surgery. Springer, Berlin, Heidelberg

Shaun McCann, Robin Foa, Owen Smith, Eibhlin Conneally (2005) Case-Based Haematology. Blackwell Publishing, Oxford, ISBN 4051-1321-9

Smith OP, Hann I (2002) Essential Paediatric Haematology. Martin Dunitz Publishers, London, ISBN 90-5823-179-8

Genetics

10

Andrew Green

Contents

10.1 Introduction

Genetic disorders are common in paediatric practice, and contribute to between 30% and 70% of hospital admissions for children. Some genetic conditions cause malformations and many others cause a range of clinical problems, including metabolic disorders, learning disability, or neurological disease. Almost every aspect of paediatrics will involve managing children with genetic disorders. Clinical geneticists can offer expertise both in diagnosing rare genetic disorders and advising families with known genetic disorders. This chapter will focus on an aspect of paediatric surgery, which is the diagnosis of congenital anomalies, and different forms of genetic disease which can cause congenital anomalies.

10.2 A Clinical Genetic Approach to Diagnosis of Malformation Syndromes

10.2.1 Definitions

One child in 40 (2.5%) is born with a significant major congenital anomaly. Congenital anomalies account for 20–25% of perinatal and childhood mortality. Most affected children have a single isolated major congenital anomaly, without any underlying syndrome. However, when a child has more than one congenital anomaly, with or without dysmorphic features, the possibility of an underlying syndrome should be considered.

It is also important to note that about 10% of the normal population will have a minor congenital anomaly, such as 5th finger clinodactyly or a single palmar crease.

P. Puri and M. Höllwarth (eds.), *Pediatric Surgery: Diagnosis and Management*,
DOI: 10.1007/978-3-540-69560-8_10, © Springer-Verlag Berlin Heidelberg 2009

Table 10.1 Examples of major congenital anomalies

Examples of major congenital anomalies	Birth incidence (per 1,000 births)
Cardiovascular	10
Ventricular septal defect	2.5
Atrial septal defect	1
Patent ductus arteriosus	1
Fallot's tetralogy	1
Central Nervous System	10
Anencephaly	1
Hydrocephalus	1
Microcephaly	1
Lumbosacral spina bifida	2
Gastrointestinal	4
Cleft lip/palate	1.5
Diaphragmatic hernia	0.5
Oesophageal atresia	0.3
Imperforate anus	0.2
Limb	2
Transverse amputation	0.2
Urogenital	4
Bilateral renal agenesis	2
Polycystic kidneys (infantile)	0.02
Bladder extrophy	0.03

In the absence of any other problems, such minor congenital anomalies are of no major significance.

There are many different congenital anomalies, some of which are extremely rare. Examples of the more common congenital anomalies, by the organ system affected and approximate birth incidence are shown in Table 10.1.

Awareness of the possibility of a genetic or syndromal association for anomalies is very important for management of the patient and for advising the whole family. A distinction has also to be made between several different forms of abnormality, with appropriate definitions.

A *disruption* can be defined as an anomaly which is caused by interference in the structure of a normally developing organ. A good example would be the digital constrictions and amputations caused by amniotic bands. Amniotic bands are strands of tissue which cross from one wall of the amniotic sac to the other and can constrict parts of the developing foetus.

A *deformation* can be defined as an anomaly which is caused by an external interference in the structure of a normally developing organ. An example would be talipes equinovarus caused by chronic oligohydramnios, perhaps from an amniotic leak.

A *malformation* can be defined as an anomaly which is caused by an intrinsic failure in the normal development of an organ. Common examples would

be congenital heart disease, cleft lip and palate, and neural tube defects.

A *dysplasia* is an abnormal organisation of cells in a tissue, often specific to a particular tissue. For example, achondroplasia is a skeletal dysplasia caused by a mutation in the FGFR3 gene. Most dysplasias are single gene disorders.

A *sequence* can be defined as a group of anomalies which arise due to one single event. An example would be Potter's sequence. Potter's sequence (see Fig. 10.1) is the group of anomalies consisting of pulmonary hypoplasia, oligohydramnios, talipes, cleft palate, and hypertelorism. All of these anomalies arise as a result of the failure of urine production in the foetus. The cause of Potter's syndrome and failure of urine production could be posterior urethral valves, dysplastic or cystic kidneys, or renal agenesis, all of which can have genetic, non-genetic or chromosomal origins. The Pierre-Robin sequence is the grouping of cleft palate, micrognathia and glossoptosis, which can have at least 30 different causes. A sequence therefore does not have a specific cause or inheritance pattern.

An *association* can be defined as a clustering of anomalies, which is not a sequence, which occurs more frequently than by chance, but has no prior assumption about causation. A good example is the association of VATER, whose acronym is made up from the grouping of vertebral anomalies, anal abnormalities, tracheo-esphageal fistula, and radial or renal anomalies. There is no clear cause for VATER, although it can rarely occur in people with chromosome 22q11 microdeletions, and can also rarely be mimicked by Fanconi's anaemia.

A *syndrome* is a description of a group of symptoms and signs, and a pattern of anomalies, where there is often a known cause or an assumption about causation. The looser definition of 'syndrome' to describe any anomaly should be avoided. The term can include chromosomal disorders such as Down's syndrome, or single gene disorders such as van der Woude syndrome which can cause cleft lip and palate with lower lip pits.

10.2.2 An Approach to Diagnosis

When a child is born with a congenital anomaly, several particular aspects of the history need to be explored. A good family history must be taken, with reference not only to a history of the same anomaly, but other

Fig. 10.1 Potter's sequence

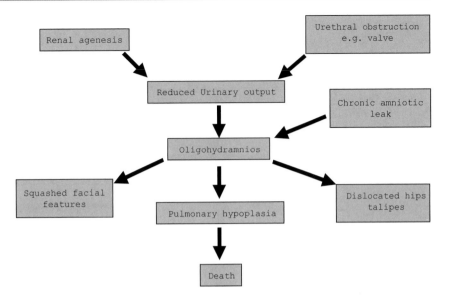

anomalies as well. The clinician should record medical details on sibs, parents, grandparents, uncles and aunts. A family history must include documentation of pregnancy losses, stillbirths and neonatal deaths. Any history of potential teratogens in the pregnancy should be looked for, considering the likely embryological timing of the anomaly. Teratogens can include medications, recreational drugs, maternal diabetes and prolonged maternal hyperthermia.

If a child has one congenital anomaly, a very careful examination should be carried out to check for any other more subtle abnormalities or for dysmorphic facial features, e.g. to check for hydrocephalus in an infant with a spinal meningomyelocoele. If there is more than one malformation, or significant dysmorphology, a chromosomal analysis should be requested, as chromosomal aneuploidy is a well-recognised cause of multiple malformations. A clinical genetic opinion should also be sought, as a clinical geneticist can often help greatly in achieving a diagnosis as well as in counselling parents about the likelihood of recurrence of similar problems in other family members.

A diagnostic approach to congenital anomalies is outlined in Fig. 10.2. Deformations and disruptions need to be excluded first. If the pattern of malformations fits into a well-described sequence, then a cause for that sequence should be sought. If the anomalies do not fit into a sequence, then a syndrome or association diagnosis should be attempted. If a syndrome diagnosis is achieved, it is important to remember that

syndromes can be caused by chromosomal disorders, single gene (monogenic disorders), or by environmental agents (teratogens).

The majority of congenital anomalies have a polygenic or multifactorial origin, and most are isolated (non-syndromal). The causes of congenital abnormalities are outlined in Table 10.2, and it is important to note that about 50% do not have any clear cause. Nonetheless, parents and families want an explanation as to the origin of their child's anomaly, and it is therefore worthwhile to pursue a diagnosis wherever possible.

10.3 Chromosome Disorders

Disorders of either chromosome number or chromosome structure affect about 6/10,000 births. There is a finite number of disorders of chromosome number, including Down's syndrome, Edward's syndrome, and Patau's syndrome. There are potentially thousands of disorders of chromosome structure, many of which are extremely rare or unique to a particular family. Many chromosome disorders, such as Down's syndrome, are usually new genetic events in the affected child. However, there is a small subset of chromosome disorders which can be inherited in the form of a balanced chromosome rearrangement called a translocation, present in one or other healthy parent. About 6% of all congenital anomalies is caused by a chromosome

Fig. 10.2 A diagnostic approach
to congenital anomalies

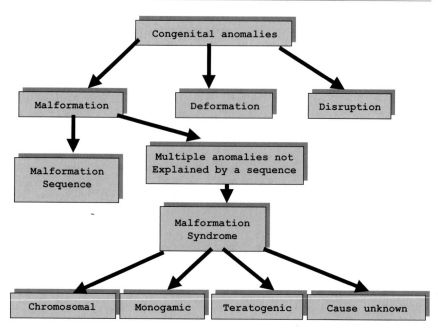

Table 10.2   Causes of congenital anomalies

Causes of congenital anomalies	Relative frequency (%)
Genetic	
Chromosomal	6
Single gene	7.5
Multifactorial/polygenic	20–30
Environmental	
Drugs, infections,	5–10
maternal illness	
Unknown	50
Total	100

disorder. Chromosome disorders are detected by cytogenetic analysis, analysing the structure and banding pattern of the 46 chromosomes within each cell nucleus, usually in white blood cells. More detailed analysis can use fluorescently labelled DNA probes, targeted to a particular chromosome region, hybridised to the patient's chromosomes, a technique called fluorescent in situ hybridisation (FISH).

10.3.1 Specific Chromosome Disorders

10.3.1.1 Down's Syndrome

Down's syndrome is the most common chromosome disorder, with an average incidence estimated at 1 in 700 births, and is characterised by the presence of an extra (third) chromosome 21. The most frequent congenital anomaly in children with Down's syndrome is congenital heart disease, usually an AV canal defect. However, children with Down's syndrome are also more prone to duodenal and jejunal atresias, and Hirschsprung's disease. Children with Down's syndrome will also have a varying degree of learning difficulty, and are also prone to deafness, hypothyroidism, and have a higher than average incidence of acute and chronic leukaemias. Over 90% of Down's syndrome arises as a new genetic event in the child, with a separate extra chromosome 21. Under these circumstances, there is no need to check parents' chromosomes. There is a rare translocation form of Down's syndrome, which can be readily distinguished on analysing the child's chromosome. For the rare translocation form, the parents can be offered chromosome analysis, as the translocation forms can run in families.

10.3.1.2 Patau's Syndrome

Patau's syndrome is caused by the presence of an extra chromosome 13, and is a condition that is usually lethal in the period just after birth. It occurs in about 1 in 5,000 births. Affected children have congenital heart disease, polydactyly, cleft lip and palate, microcephaly, and often a single frontal lobe in their brain (holoprosencephaly). Once recognised, despite the congenital anomalies, surgery is unlikely to alter the outcome for the infant. Like Down's syndrome, 95% are new genetic events. There are rare translocation forms which can run in families, and again the distinction between the common and rare forms can be identified on analysing the baby's chromosome.

10.3.1.3 Edward's Syndrome

Edward's syndrome is caused by the presence of an extra chromosome 18, and is a condition that is usually lethal in the period just after birth. It occurs in about 1 in 3,000 births. Affected children are usually extremely small, and have congenital heart disease, exomphalos, renal anomalies, and clenched hands and rocker bottom feet. Once recognised, despite the congenital anomalies, surgery is unlikely to alter the outcome for the infant. Over 95% are new genetic events in the affected infant.

10.3.1.4 Other Chromosome Disorders

Klinefelter's syndrome is a condition characterised by the presence of an extra X chromosome in a male—i.e. 47,XXY. Boys with the condition rarely present surgically in childhood. However, a significant number of boys with 47,XXY can have delayed puberty, and can also present with teenage gynaecomastia. Turner's syndrome is the presence of a single X chromosome in a female—45,X. Girls with Turner's are more prone to congenital heart disease, classically coarctation of the aorta, and also have renal anomalies. They have short stature and are very unlikely to go through puberty spontaneously due to ovarian dysgenesis. Children with a very small deletion of one of their two chromosomes 22, detectable by FISH, have a condition called Di George syndrome, or velocardiofacial syndrome. They can have a wide range of congenital anomalies, most commonly congenital heart disease, but also cleft palate, laryngeal anomalies, and renal anomalies. They can also have hypocalcaemia, learning difficulties, and, sometimes, immunodeficiency.

10.4 Single Gene Disorders

Single gene disorders are caused by an alteration in one or both copies of one specific gene. Such gene alterations are sufficient to cause the disorder. There

are over 4,000 single gene disorders described, and about 7.5% of all congenital anomalies are caused by a single gene disorder. Single gene disorders have one of three principal modes of inheritance: autosomal dominant, autosomal recessive, and X-linked recessive. Other rare forms of inheritance include X-linked dominant, and mitochondrial disorders, as well as disorders due to abnormalities of genetic imprinting.

10.4.1 Autosomal Dominant Inheritance

Autosomal dominant disorders are caused by a mutation in one of the two copies of a specific gene. Families will often have several generations affected, and usually males and females are equally affected. Each child of a person with an autosomal dominant disorder has a 50:50 chance of inheriting the gene responsible for the condition from its parent, and thereby being affected. The hallmark of autosomal dominant inheritance is father to son transmission. However, not all people with an autosomal dominant disorder have a family history of the condition. For some autosomal dominant conditions such as Marfan's syndrome or neurofibromatosis 1, the new mutation rate can be 20–30%.

There can often be variability in both *expression* and *penetrance* of autosomal dominant disorders. For example, neurofibromatosis 1, an autosomal dominant condition, will almost always manifest in someone who has an altered neurofibromatosis 1 gene. This means that the condition has almost complete *penetrance*. However, different people can manifest the condition in different ways, with some people showing mild skin lesions, and others with severe intracerebral complications. This means that the *expression* or *expressivity* of the condition is very variable. In contrast, only 80% of those who have a single altered gene for the rare hereditary form of retinoblastoma will actually develop an eye tumour. The penetrance in this situation is 80%, but the expression of the altered gene is consistent, as manifested by a retinoblastoma.

Autosomal dominant disorders are not commonly seen in neonatal surgical practice. In general paediatric surgical practice, a subset of children with Hirschsprung's disease, Beckwith Wiedemann syndrome and pyloric stenosis can have the condition as an autosomal dominant trait with reduced penetrance. Some forms of craniosynostosis and oro-facial clefting can also be caused by an autosomal dominant disorder. There are also rare childhood cancer predisposition syndromes such as polyposis coli, retinoblastoma, and Li-Fraumeni syndrome which have an autosomal dominant inheritance.

10.4.2 Autosomal Recessive Inheritance

When a child is diagnosed with an autosomal recessive disorder, both copies of a particular gene responsible for the condition are altered. Both its parents are therefore carriers for that condition, with one normal and one altered gene. Two of the child's four grandparents are also carriers, and it is likely that many of the child's relatives are, unknowingly, also carriers. In most cases, being a carrier for an autosomal recessive condition has no effect on that person.

When both parents are carriers for an alteration in the same gene, then there is a 25% or 1 in 4 chance for each of their children of being affected by the condition. The risk of a healthy carrier sib of having a child with the same condition depends on the chances of that sib's partner also being a carrier. A child of a person with an autosomal recessive disorder will automatically be a carrier. That child's chances of being affected will depend on whether its unaffected parent is a carrier for an alteration in the same gene.

Autosomal recessive disorders are commonly encountered in paediatric practice, and the nature of the disorder depends on the population being studied. Each regional population has its own recessive disorder, where the frequency of carriers for that disorder is highest. For instance, cystic fibrosis is a very common autosomal recessive disorder in Western Europe, whereas sickle cell anaemia is the most common autosomal recessive disorder in West Africa. Common examples of autosomal recessive conditions include cystic fibrosis, sickle cell anaemia, several of the mucopolysaccharidoses, beta-thalassaemia, spinal muscular atrophy and congenital adrenal hyperplasia. Direct genetic diagnosis is available for many of these conditions, and in a number of countries, newborn screening includes testing for a number of autosomal recessive disorders including galactosaemia, homocystinuria and cystic fibrosis. In some countries, carrier testing for some of these diseases is offered to couples planning a pregnancy, or to women in the early stages of pregnancy.

10.4.3 X-Linked Recessive Inheritance

X-linked conditions are caused by mutations in a gene on the X chromosome. Males only have one X chromosome, and therefore males with a mutated gene manifest the disease, as they have no normal gene. Females have two X chromosomes, and therefore, even if a female has an altered gene, the normal gene usually offsets the effect of the mutated gene. Females are therefore carriers, and only some females will manifest the disorder. The daughters of a man with an X-linked recessive condition are all obligate carriers, as they all inherit his X chromosome. The sons of a man with an X-linked condition are all normal, as they inherit his Y chromosome, and not his X chromosome. When a woman is a carrier of an X-linked condition, each of her sons has a 50:50 chance of being affected, and each of her daughters has a 50:50 chance of being a carrier. There can be a relatively high mutation rate for some X-linked recessive conditions, and affected boys may not have any family history of the condition. New mutations are responsible for muscular dystrophy in about one-third of boys with Duchenne. The classic examples of such conditions are haemophilia A and B, Duchenne and Becker muscular dystrophy, and Hunter's syndrome.

10.5 Polygenic Inheritance

Many paediatric disorders do not have a clear mode of inheritance, and can be classed as polygenic or oligogenic, where a disease may arise as a result of the effects of several genes and may also be influenced by several environmental factors.

A good example is cleft lip and palate, which usually occurs in the absence of a family history. However, monozygotic twins have a high concordance for cleft palate, suggesting a genetic influence. In addition, the likelihood of having a further child with a cleft lip or palate is increased, when a couple have already had one child with the condition, suggesting a genetic influence. However, the genetic influence does not follow the Mendelian or single pattern.

Other examples of polygenic disorders include neural tube defects, congenital heart disease, vesico-ureteric reflux, and coeliac disease.

Further Reading

Contact a Family is a UK charity for families with disabled children, which offers information on specific conditions and rare disorders. www.cafamily.org.uk

Flake AW (2006) Molecular clinical genetics and gene therapy. In JL Grosfeld, JA O' Neill, EW Fonkalsrud, AG Coran (eds) Pediatric Surgery Mosby, Philadelphia, PA, pp 11–29

Green A (2003) Genetics in neonatal surgical practice. In P Puri (ed) Newborn Surgery. Arnold, London, pp 157–172

OMIM, Online Mendelian Inheritance in Man, a database of human genes and genetic disorders developed by staff at Johns Hopkins. www.ncbi.nlm.nih.gov/Omim/

Orphanet—a database (in several languages) of genetic disorders, clinical information, clinic listings and research and diagnostic genetic testing for a wide range of disorders. www.orpha.net

Puri P, Höllwarth ME (eds) (2006) Pediatric Surgery. Springer, Berlin, Heidelberg

Understanding Gene testing—a website with information on basic genetic concepts, and the utility and limitations of genetic testing. http://www.accessexcellence.org/AE/AEPC/NIH/

Ethical Considerations in Pediatric Surgery

11

Benedict C. Nwomeh and Donna A. Caniano

Contents

11.1 Introduction

Pediatric surgeons are often confronted with clinical situations that involve decisions about the continuation of life-sustaining treatments for infants and children with critical illness. These difficult issues fall within the basic social commitment that defines the professional obligation of physicians to sustain life and relieve suffering. Ethics is the philosophic discipline concerned with questions of right and wrong. Medical ethics, also known as bioethics, outlines the standards, principles, and rules of conduct that govern physician behavior and the practice of medicine. It also seeks to inform and guide the resolution of moral dilemmas as they arise in patient care and within the broad context of societal healthcare.

Four major principles have been elucidated in medical ethics: *beneficence*, which exhorts physicians "to do or promote good;" *nonmaleficence*, which cautions physicians "to do no harm;" *autonomy*, which respects the right of competent persons to give informed consent for medical treatment and have control over their bodies; and *justice*, which involves the fair and equitable distribution of medical care to all persons. These principles focus on the action or actions that give rise to dilemmas, such as withdrawing life-sustaining treatment from a terminally ill patient. In contrast, virtue ethics emphasizes the agents (physicians) and the recipients (patients) of principle-based actions and decisions. It espouses several virtues that are necessary for the delivery of "good medical care," and is particularly relevant to the practice of pediatric surgery. These virtues include fidelity to trust, compassion, phronesis or common sense, fortitude, integrity, honesty, and self-effacement.

P. Puri and M. Höllwarth (eds.), *Pediatric Surgery: Diagnosis and Management,*
DOI: 10.1007/978-3-540-69560-8_11, © Springer-Verlag Berlin Heidelberg 2009

11.1.1 What Is a Moral Problem?

A moral dilemma is a type of moral problem that arises when two or more conflicting ethical principles support mutually inconsistent actions. An example of a moral dilemma in pediatric surgery is the conflict between the principles of autonomy and beneficence, when parents decide on a course of treatment for their child that does not align with the recommendations of the pediatric surgeon. Moral uncertainty and moral distress are additional types of dilemmas that may occur in pediatric surgery, especially when the prognosis is unclear for a given condition, when two or more equally valid treatment options are available, or when parents are in disagreement with each other and/or their physicians about the best medical decisions.

11.1.2 Resolution of Ethical Problems

When a moral problem arises in the context of decision making for a given pediatric surgical patient, the members of the healthcare team should work toward a resolution that promotes respect for all parties and all views. As we and others have noted, successful outcomes require that the team: (1) develop common moral language for the discussion of moral issues; (2) have training in how to articulate their views about issues; (3) have common experiences on which to base recommendations; and (4) agree on a moral decision making method for all to use in the course of their deliberations.

The following guidelines provide a framework for the effective resolution of difficult moral problems:

1. Identify the decision makers. For most cases in pediatric surgery, the decision makers will be the parents, unless the patient is a mature minor.
2. Ascertain "value data" from the parents and other relevant family members. These may include their views on the sanctity of life, spirituality and religious beliefs, cultural norms, and community values.
3. Collect all relevant medical information, including the prognosis. Clarify the areas of uncertainty and identify whether additional diagnostic testing would be of value in the decision making process.
4. Define all treatment options, including their benefits, risks, and chances of achieving the desired outcomes.
5. Provide the parents with a professional recommendation for the best treatment option.
6. Seek a consensus resolution that can be accepted by all participants.

In order for the above paradigm to be successful, the healthcare team must accept that rational people of goodwill may hold divergent views that are irreconcilable, even after extended discussions. The goal of reaching a consensus decision should be viewed as a successful outcome for all participants.

11.2 Informed Consent

The doctrine of informed consent is firmly embedded in contemporary medical practice and is based on the bioethical principles of respect for individual autonomy, nonmaleficence, beneficence, and justice as discussed previously.

Respect for patient's *autonomy* is the guiding principle for informed consent. Autonomy is paramount in mentally competent patients who can exercise the freedom to choose among alternative interventions based on full disclosure of the risks and benefits of these alternatives, and consistent with their beliefs, values, and goals. In children, autonomy is limited when the decision is made by proxies, including parents who are well meaning. Therefore, depending on the circumstances, the *assent* of the pediatric patient should be sought as appropriate to their development, age, and understanding. In addition, most legal jurisdictions have enacted minor consent statutes that seek to determine instances where children can give their informed consent. Apart from the ethical and legal obligation, it is clear that increasing patient autonomy and participation in care is also associated with better outcomes in some situations.

Because the exercise of autonomy is limited, beneficence and nonmaleficence assume greater relevance during the informed consent process in pediatric patients. Thus, pediatric surgeons assume significant responsibility for providing active guidance to parents in protecting the best interests of the child. Unfortunately, during this process conflict may arise between parents and caregivers. Justice is achieved when the tension between parental exercise of autonomy and the imperatives of beneficence is resolved in the best interest of the child.

11.2.1 Elements of Informed Consent

Four critical elements must be included in the informed consent process: (1) The physician provides adequate information with which to make a decision to (2) a competent patient or legal proxy who (3) indicates full understanding of the intervention, including the indications, risks, and possible alternatives and (4) voluntarily consents to the proposed intervention.

11.2.2 Exceptions to Informed Consent

There are several legitimate exceptions to the right of informed consent, including exceptions for medical emergency, public health emergency, the incompetent patient, and patient waiver of consent. The exceptions for emergencies and for patients unable to give consent are particularly relevant to situations requiring emergency surgery. In the case of children, any delay may also have significant negative long-term consequences for growth and development.

Although significant emphasis on the informed consent process has been made in the context of medical research and non-acute medical and surgical treatment, several professional societies have established guidelines for dealing with patients in emergency settings. When immediate action must be taken to prevent death or other serious harm to the patient, the emergency exception mandates that appropriate care not be delayed. Despite the urgency involved, quite often there is ample time for preoperative education of the family, which is essential for a truly informed consent.

11.3 Withholding and Withdrawal of Life-Sustaining Treatment

Life-sustaining treatments include all interventions that prolong a patient's life. These include "high tech" measures such as renal dialysis, ventilators, and organ transplantation, as well as less technically advanced modalities such as antibiotics, fluids and nutrition delivered through enteral tubes or intravenous means, and chemotherapy. Decisions to withhold life-sustaining treatment are generally made in advance and agreed upon by the parents and physicians. For example, a child with recurrent metastatic neuroblastoma who has already received maximal adjuvant treatment may be offered no additional chemotherapy and referred to hospice care. While many individuals believe it is "worse" to discontinue life-sustaining treatment than to never institute such treatment, ethicists, moral philosophers, and legal scholars find no ethical or legal distinction between not starting treatment and stopping treatment. There is also the very real concern that fear and reluctance about discontinuing life-sustaining treatment could keep some physicians from initiating therapy that may be beneficial for some patients with critical illness. In pediatric surgery, it is generally believed that life-sustaining treatment for an infant or child should be instituted, and it should be stopped if it proves to be of no benefit later.

11.3.1 The Surgical Neonate

"A 3 week old baby boy, born at 25 weeks gestation, develops perforated necrotizing enterocolitis. He has chronic lung disease and a grade 4 intraventricular hemorrhage. At laparotomy he has necrosis of all but 20 cm of jejunum and half of the colon. The bowel is resected and stomas are created. Postoperatively, he develops worsening lung disease and renal failure. The physicians discuss his poor prognosis with the parents and request withdrawal of life-sustaining treatment."

This case typifies an all too frequent ethical dilemma faced by pediatric surgeons when extremely premature infants with multiple medical problems develop necrotizing enterocolitis complicated by short bowel syndrome. When making decisions to prolong life or to discontinue life-sustaining treatment for an infant with critical illness, the *best interests standard* is generally used to focus on issues that are patient-centered and to assess the benefits and burdens of continued treatment for a *particular infant*. In this case the infant's best interests standard would include consideration of:

1. Severity of the medical condition
2. Availability of curative or corrective treatment
3. Achievability of medical goals
4. Presence of serious neurological impairments
5. All associated medical conditions
6. Life expectancy
7. Extent of suffering

8. Proportionality of treatment benefits to burdens in both the short and long terms

Parents of imperiled surgical neonates seek the counsel and advice of their infant's pediatric surgeon, who should make a recommendation based on the medical facts, the parents' values, and the infant's physiological condition. When, as in the present case, continued life-sustaining treatment is judged to prolong the dying process rather than to extend life, the pediatric surgeon should present her/his assessment with candor and compassion. It should be kept in mind that many neonates with extensive bowel loss will be candidates for prolonged total parenteral nutrition in the hope of eventual bowel adaptation and/or intestinal transplantation. Decisions to continue life-sustaining treatment for them should be based upon the pediatric surgeon's assessment of the benefits of such treatment, its likelihood of success, and the anticipated burdens of therapy. In cases where prognostic uncertainty about outcome is high, the parents should be accorded latitude in decision making, whether they choose to continue treatment or to stop life-sustaining measures.

11.3.2 Older Children and Adolescents

Life-threatening illnesses, such as terminal cancer, may impact the developmental understanding of pediatric patients by accelerating their grasp of serious illness and their own mortality and by promoting their wishes to control decisions about their healthcare. The stresses of their illness may "make them grow up faster" and make them wiser than their same-age peer group. For example, a 12-year-old child with terminal cancer may ask to discontinue chemotherapy or other unpleasant treatments and request to have "one final special vacation."

Because children cannot give morally or legally valid consent to or refusal of treatment, practice among physicians in the past was to shelter dying children from the truth of their dire circumstances. Current practice, favored by The American Academy of Pediatrics, acknowledges that these patients usually have a much more mature understanding of their situation than previously realized by their physicians and parents and that they should be told the truth about their prognosis and included in discussions about their care. These discussions should include the extent of desired life-sustaining treatments, whether a do-not-resuscitate (DNR) status is to be invoked, the role of palliative procedures in granting a better quality of life, and their desire for hospice services.

11.4 Multiculturalism

Cultural practices that are different from the norms of the majority can pose frustrating problems for pediatric surgeons, particularly when they affect parental acceptance of and compliance with recommended treatments. "Culture" is defined as the common and accepted way of thinking, feeling, and acting for a group of people. This includes the full range of accepted beliefs, values, attitudes, patterns of meanings, and behaviors that are held in common by a group of people. Culture is the mechanism by which people navigate and make sense of their world through their shared meanings and patterns of behavior. Because culture is so broad in scope, it cannot be defined solely by political borders, religious practices, or physical characteristics. It is important for pediatric surgeons to understand the importance that culture plays in healthcare because it may elucidate both *how* and *why* parents of a particular culture tend to behave as they do.

It should be emphasized that physicians are socialized by traditional values inherent in Western medical training, which are based on a set of assumptions and values about disease and well-being. For example, the traditional medical paradigm focuses on disease as a malfunction of a biologic process in the patient. In contrast, patients experience illness (including children and their parents) as represented by their personal, interpersonal, and cultural reactions to the disease. Therefore, it is important for the pediatric surgeon to be mindful of her/his own individual cultural beliefs as well as the unique culture within pediatric surgery. In meeting parents and children whose culture is different, the pediatric surgeon should inquire about their beliefs, goals of treatment, and their concerns. The pediatric surgeon should not automatically assume that an individual set of parents from a certain culture will hold all of their beliefs in common with their cultural group. For example, not all Chinese parents believe in or use traditional Chinese medicines or complementary practices.

Language barriers may pose additional difficulties in the multicultural medical setting, particularly when parents want to rely on a family member or older sibling of the patient for translation. The pediatric surgeon should utilize experienced medical translators to ensure accuracy of transmitted information both to and from the parents and child patient, to avoid translation bias, and to help in reading nonverbal and verbal cues about underlying concerns.

When different cultures meet in the pediatric surgical healthcare setting, some aspects of the encounter will include similar values (for example, the parents want good health for their child). However, it is also possible that some important values may be in conflict and have a different set of priorities (such as how the child will recover). The following strategies are useful in lessening cross-cultural conflicts: (1) asking questions about the parents' values and listening to their responses; (2) indicating to the parents that their views are important; (3) allowing enough time to deal with the parents whose culture is different; and (4) seeking assistance from "experts" who understand the parents' cultural beliefs when significant differences arise in the course of treatment.

11.5 Surgical Error

In recent times, the high incidence of medical errors and the significant impact they have on patient outcomes has been in the spotlight. Examples of errors encountered during surgical treatment include wrong diagnosis, wrong patient (or site) procedures, and retained foreign bodies. Pediatric surgeons have an ethical responsibility to inform parents of changes in diagnoses resulting from retrospective review of test results or any other information, even when surgical treatment or therapeutic options may not be altered by the new information. Full disclosure is imperative for errors that are harmful to patients. Nondisclosure has been described as "one of the deadly sins of medical ethics." Disclosure of errors is endorsed by most professional organizations and increasingly required by regulatory and governmental agencies.

Studies have revealed the difficulty that surgeons face in deciding whether and how to disclose harmful errors. Most parents desire an explicit acknowledgment that an error had occurred, what the error was,

how the error occurred, how the error will affect their child, and what efforts are being made to prevent occurrence of similar errors in the future. In addition, most parents desire an explicit admission of responsibility and an apology. Some physicians may feel reluctant to admit error, partly because risk managers routinely advise that error disclosure not include any statement that could constitute an admission of liability. Clearly, considerable skill and tact is often required in the disclosure of errors. However, concern regarding legal liability should not affect the pediatric surgeon's honesty with parents. To the contrary, failure or inadequate disclosure of errors might feed into parents' anger and mistrust, thereby increasing the likelihood of lawsuits.

11.6 Research and Innovation in Pediatric Surgery

Advancements in pediatric surgery have been brought about by research and development of innovative surgical techniques. While it is vital that research endeavors be encouraged, protection of research subjects is paramount. Current ethical standards for the conduct of clinical research in the United States are derived from several sources including the Nuremberg Code and the Belmont Report. Similar standards are in place in most progressive societies. Several of the bioethical principles previously discussed in the context of clinical practice were originally developed to protect subjects in research studies. These principles are applied using informed consent, risk/benefit assessment, the impartial selection of study subjects, and the protection of vulnerable subjects, especially children. Recent implementation of the Privacy Rule now requires the investigator to protect not only the safety but also the privacy of the research subject. In most institutions, compliance with these requirements is promoted by the Institutional Review Board (IRB). In addition, editors of most pediatric surgery journals have joined a growing coalition of medical journals requiring IRB approval prior to publication of results of research studies.

In contrast to clinical research where different approaches to treatment are being tested, surgical innovation entails application of new techniques or therapies, or modification of existing procedures, when deemed to be in the best interest of the patient. In most countries, drugs and medical devices are strictly regulated, but currently there are no clear regulations pertaining to innovative surgical procedures. Pediatric surgeons have been among the most notable surgical innovators, and many of the procedures beneficial to children today may never have passed the rigor of randomized clinical trials. Yet, too little regulation creates the potential for abuse and can be harmful and dangerous. For example, some operations that have now been abandoned, such as sympathetectomy for Hirschsprung's disease and jejunoileal bypass for morbid obesity, may never have been widely used under a stricter regulatory environment.

Parents and society expect pediatric surgeons to be conservative guardians in surgical innovation. A useful approach is to regard any new procedure as *non-validated*, a term that recognizes the ethical and medical hazard of novel operations, which may be obscured by the terminology of innovation. The concept of a non-validated operation is more transparent and honest because it embodies the fact that the proposed operation has not been subjected to rigorous investigation.

Ultimately, this awareness may nudge both parents and pediatric surgeons toward the ideal of multi-institutional clinical trials that seek to establish the best operations or treatment for children.

Further Reading

American Academy of Pediatrics Committee on Bioethics (1996) Ethics and the care of critically ill infants and children. Pediatrics 98:149–152

American Academy of Pediatrics Committee on Bioethics (1995) Informed consent, parental permission, and assent in pediatric practice. Pediatrics 95:314–317

Caniano DA (2004) Ethical issues in the management of neonatal surgical anomalies. Semin Perinatol 28(3):240–245

Ells C, Caniano DA (2002) The impact of culture on the patient-surgeon relationship. J Am Coll Surg 195(4):520–530

Morgenstern L (2006) Innovative surgery's dilemma. Surg Innov 13(1):73–74

Puri P, Höllwarth ME (eds) (2006) Pediatric Surgery. Springer, Berlin, Heidelberg

VanDeVeer D, Regan T (eds) (1987) Health Care Ethics: An Introduction. Temple University Press, Philadelphia, PA

Minimally Invasive Surgery in Infants and Children

12

Keith Georgeson

Contents

12.1 Introduction

The evolution of minimally invasive surgical techniques for adults has been among the most important surgical developments of the last century. Much of the morbidity, stress, and pain of an operation are due to the trauma of the access wound. By decreasing the size of the incision, the postoperative morbidity and pain should be diminished. The potential advantages of minimally invasive surgery (MIS) have been documented in many adult and animal studies.

The application of minimally invasive techniques to infants and children has advanced more slowly than in adults. This delay in development has multiple causes. Surgical instruments developed for adults are cumbersome and less safe when used in infants and children. No single procedure propelled the evolution of MIS in neonates like laparoscopic cholecystomy in adults. Medical practitioners have frequently underestimated the importance of pain and stress caused by surgical incisions in children who are less able to articulate their distress. The absolute length of an open surgical incision in a neonate is short and thought to be less traumatic. However, these incisions are proportionally as long as incisions for similar surgical procedures in adults. Due to the small size of neonates and young children, the intracavitary working space for endoscopic procedures is small, making procedures in this age group more technically difficult.

Development of smaller instruments and documentation of the safety of endoscopic techniques have allowed pediatric surgeons to apply thoracoscopy and laparoscopy to infants and children. Over the last 15 years, there has been a virtual explosion in neonatal minimally invasive surgical procedures. This chapter will outline the current procedures commonly performed

P. Puri and M. Höllwarth (eds.), *Pediatric Surgery: Diagnosis and Management*,
DOI: 10.1007/978-3-540-69560-8_12, © Springer-Verlag Berlin Heidelberg 2009

endoscopically in children. With the evolution of constantly improving surgical instruments and alternative devices for anastomosis, pediatric endoscopic surgery should continue to grow at a rapid pace.

12.2 Thoracoscopy

In the mid-1970s, thoracoscopy was first used for exploration and biopsy of intrathoracic lesions in children. With the advances in endoscopic technology, thoracoscopy has become an alternative to thoracotomy for many diagnostic and therapeutic procedures. Avoiding an incision has many advantages, as has been outlined earlier. Additionally, thoracotomy in the infant is associated with the development of scoliosis in about 30% of patients. It is hoped that thoracoscopy may diminish the postoperative development of scoliosis.

For thoracoscopy to be applied in children, appropriate anesthetic techniques play a central role. General anesthesia and positive pressure ventilation can impair visualization inside the pleural space during thoracoscopy due to lung expansion. Single lung ventilation by intubation of the contralateral mainstem bronchus is the most common technique used by pediatric anesthesiologists to partially collapse the ipsilateral lung for pediatric thoracoscopy. Double lumen tubes are not available in appropriate sizes for neonates and small children. Bronchial blockers, such as a Fogarty catheter passed through or beside an endotracheal tube, can be used to block ventilation in the ipsilateral lung. Low flow and low pressure ($<8\,cm\ H_2O$) infusion of CO_2 into the ipsilateral pleural space can help to partially compress the lung and to increase visualization of intrathoracic structures. This technique is well tolerated in most neonates. Potential complications of the technique, such as CO_2 embolism and hypotension due to impaired venous return, have not been reported in significant numbers. Stopping the infusion and relieving the pneumothorax can readily reverse hypercarbia and hypoxia due to intrapleural infusion of CO_2.

12.2.1 Diagnostic Thoracoscopy

Thoracoscopy for diagnostic purposes is used infrequently due to the advances in diagnostic imaging. In carefully selected patients, however, visualization of obscure structures or lesions in the thoracic cavity can be achieved using thoracoscopy. Additionally, biopsies of intrathoracic lesions are commonly performed thoracoscopically.

12.2.2 Lung Biopsy

Biopsy of lung lesions is one of the most common indications for thoracoscopy. Lung biopsies are obtained in infants and children with diffuse lung disease of undetermined origin or for specific pulmonary nodules of unknown etiology. The small segment of lung to be biopsied is encircled by a loop ligature. An adequate specimen of lung tissue is obtained by cutting away the tissue peripheral to the loop ligature. The tissue is removed through one of the trocar sites. Lung biopsies can also be obtained using stapling devices or sealing energy sources, which coagulate and seal the lung tissue. The biopsy is then taken using scissors to excise the sealed portion of the lung.

12.2.3 Pulmonary Resection

Lung resection using a thoracoscopic approach is being performed in some pediatric surgical centers. Cystadenomatoid malformations, intra-lobar and extra-lobar sequestrations, lobar emphysema, and bronchiectasis have been managed by thoracoscopic excision. Usually, the lungs are freed using sealing energy sources followed by stapling or ligation of the bronchus and major vessels. A trocar site is then enlarged for removal of the resected lobe.

12.2.4 Mediastinal Masses

Resection of mediastinal cysts and esophageal duplications are amenable to thoracoscopic approaches in children. Bronchogenic cysts usually have no discrete connections to other important structures in the chest. Esophageal duplications usually have a common wall with the esophagus and sometimes have a luminal communication. All mediastinal dissections should be performed with a Bougie in the esophagus. If there is a luminal communication between the esophagus and the esophageal duplication, the mucosa and muscle of the remaining esophagus can be closed using sutures placed thoracoscopically. Great care must be taken not to compromise the esophageal lumen during closure of the esophagus. Thoracoscopic biopsy of undefined mediastinal masses is a simple technique and avoids the large thoracotomy wound normally employed for such a biopsy.

12.2.5 Closure of Patent Ductus Arteriosus

Thoracoscopic clipping of a patent ductus arteriosus (PDA) is performed using three or four ports. The patient is placed in a semi-prone position to allow the lung to fall away from the posterior thorax. The ductus is carefully dissected, preserving the recurrent laryngeal nerve, which loops around the PDA. A clip applier can be passed directly through a small incision in the chest wall. The clip is then applied under endoscopic surveillance. The recurrent laryngeal nerve is observed while the clip is being applied to avoid injury to the nerve. Placement of a chest tube is optional, depending upon the surgeon's preference.

12.2.6 Esophageal Atresia

One of the most dramatic changes in pediatric surgery has been the use of thoracoscopy to divide and clip a tracheoesophageal fistula and to approximate the proximal and distal esophageal segments. Three or four trocars are used. The neonate is placed in a semi-prone position to induce the lung to fall away from the posterior mediastinum. The azygos vein is divided using energy sealing devices. The tracheoesophageal fistula is identified and clipped or sutured immediately adjacent to the trachea. The distal esophagus is divided. The proximal pouch is dissected thoracoscopically and the distal end of the proximal pouch is opened. A hand-sewn thoracoscopic anastomosis is fashioned with 10–15 sutures. The knots are tied either extracorporeally or intracorporeally. Suturing in this setting is tedious because of the very small working space in the posterior chest. Only experienced pediatric endoscopic surgeons are currently performing this procedure. With further evolution of alternative suturing devices, the practice of thoracoscopic repair of esophageal atresia should expand.

12.2.7 Repair of Diaphragmatic Hernias and Diaphragmatic Eventrations

Both Bochdalek and Morgani diaphragmatic hernias have been repaired using an endoscopic technique. Thoracoscopic repair of diaphragmatic hernias have been performed in stable patients but have not usually been attempted in infants with pulmonary hypertension and severe pulmonary hypoplasia. Diaphragmatic hernias have been repaired using a primary closure technique as well as by application of a patch graft. Repair of diaphragmatic hernia has been performed both thoracoscopically and laparoscopically. The author favors the laparoscopic approach. Eventration of the diaphragm and a high-riding paralyzed diaphragm are usually plicated with a thoracoscopic technique. If CO_2 infusion is used for enhancement of intrathoracic visualization, there is the added benefit of the diaphragm being pushed down by the pressure of the infused pneumothorax. This pressure enlarges the involved pleural space and aids the plication of the hemidiaphragm. The plicating sutures are placed and tied thoracoscopically.

12.2.8 Empyema

The treatment of empyema using thoracoscopic debridement has become a standard of care in the last few years. Children with a diagnosis of empyema should be examined by either ultrasound or CT scanning. Children with obvious fibrinous septi and loculation of the empyema should be treated by thoracoscopic debridement of the intrapleural space. This technique can be started using a chest tube to access the pleural space of an anesthetized child. If the chest tube does not sufficiently drain the purulent material in the chest, the next step should be thoracoscopic access of the pleural space followed by thoracoscopic debridement of the fibrinous septi within the pleural space. Once the pleural space has been accessed with a trocar, a suction device is used as a probe to separate the lung from the parietal pleura. CO_2 is infused to further develop this space. A scope is then placed through the original trocar and several other trocars are introduced. The fibrinous material within the pleural space is removed using grasping forceps. Usually, most of the fibrinous debris can be removed within 45 min to 1 h. The pleural space is irrigated with saline and aspirated using a suction device. One or two chest tubes are left in place to drain the pleural space. Using this technique, recovery from the empyema is usually much more rapid than following chest tube drainage alone or chest tube drainage with fibrinolytic agents to break up the fibrinous septi. The chest tubes are usually left in place for 3 or 4 days and then removed when drainage becomes minimal.

12.3 Laparoscopy

12.3.1 Pneumoperitoneum

Successful laparoscopy depends on adequate expansion of the peritoneal cavity for clear visualization of intra-abdominal structures. A pneumoperitoneum usually achieves this abdominal expansion. Although many gases have been utilized for maintaining a pneumoperitoneum, the most commonly used gas is carbon dioxide (CO_2). The physiological effects of CO_2 pneumoperitoneum may be more pronounced in infants and children than in adults. Neonates have a higher level of end-tidal CO_2 during carbon dioxide pneumoperitoneum. This enhanced absorption of CO_2 pneumoperitoneum can result in hypercapnia and respiratory acidosis.

Hypercapnia is usually overcome by increasing the minute ventilation and by blowing off the CO_2. Postoperatively, there is a risk that the child may be unable to maintain the increased ventilatory effort needed to ventilate off the CO_2.

Increased intra-abdominal pressure also has cardiovascular effects in the child. The younger the child, the greater the potential cardiovascular compromise. Pressures within the peritoneal cavity above 10 mmHg can lead to compression of the inferior vena cava with a reduced venous return to the heart and to secondary hypotension. The infants' sensitivity to intraperitoneal pressures greater than 10 mmHg must be carefully considered for safe laparoscopy.

12.3.2 Abdominal Access

Access to the peritoneal cavity can be obtained either by an open technique or with a Veress needle. Many operated neonates have retained umbilical stumps, making access through the umbilicus problematic. An open technique just below the umbilical stump, via an umbilical fold, is usually successful in giving rapid access to the peritoneal cavity. Although Veress needle access has been said to be more prone to induce unintended injury to intra-abdominal structures than open peritoneal access, the author has used a Veress needle access technique in over 1,000 neonatal and pediatric laparoscopies without significant injury.

Slippage of trocars can be a major problem, especially in pediatric laparoscopic surgery due to a thin abdominal wall. The problem can be managed in a variety of ways. Our preference is to use a radially expanding 5 mm trocar. With trocars 4 mm in diameter or smaller, the use of reusable trocars with a snugly fitting red rubber catheter sleeve around the outside of the trocar is our preference. The sleeve is sutured to the skin, allowing the trocar to be moved in and out without unintended slippage during operative manipulation.

12.3.3 Pyloromyotomy

Laparoscopic pyloromyotomy is performed using one trocar just below the umbilicus and 2 mm stab wounds in the right and left upper quadrants. The hypertrophied pylorus is incised with a retractable knife and the muscle is split. A pyloromyotomy spreader or pediatric small bowel grasper is used to widely spread the incised hypertrophied pyloric muscle. The operative times, postoperative stay, and complications are similar to the open pyloromyotomy technique. Laparoscopic pyloromyotomy is a technically unforgiving operation requiring at least 20 procedures to become proficient.

12.3.4 Fundoplication and Gastrostomy

Gastrostomy, with or without fundoplication, is a frequent procedure performed in children. Common indications include: primary aspiration, gastroesophageal reflux, profound neurologic impairment, and severe pulmonary and cardiac disease with failure to thrive or recurrent aspiration. Most infants and children needing fundoplication are excellent candidates for a laparoscopic approach. The fundoplication is performed using 3 mm trocars. The distal esophagus is mobilized and secured in the abdomen, and the crura are approximated behind the esophagus. The fundal wrap is formed loosely around the intra-abdominal esophagus.

Laparoscopic gastrostomy is usually performed by placing a gastrostomy button. If the gastrostomy is performed without fundoplication, an effort is made to site the gastrostomy at an appropriate distance from both the gastroesophageal junction and the pylorus. Adequate distance from the fundus is important in case a fundoplication is needed at a later date. The usual technique utilizes two large U sutures, passed through the abdominal wall, into the stomach, and back out through the abdominal wall. A Seldinger technique is used to obtain access to the gastric lumen, followed by dilation of the tract over a guide wire. The gastrostomy is completed by pushing the gastrostomy button into the stomach and tying the ends of the U sutures over the wings of the gastrostomy button. Many pediatric surgeons now prefer the laparoscopic gastrostomy to percutaneous endoscopic gastrostomy tube placement. With the laparoscopic approach, visualization of the entire left upper quadrant allows for selection of the site of gastric entry, helps in avoiding nearby structures such as the colon, and can easily be combined with the performance of other laparoscopic procedures.

12.3.5 Duodenal Atresia

Duodenal atresia repair is being performed using a laparoscopic approach with increasing frequency. The proximal and distal segments of the duodenum are mobilized and approximated with the placement and tying of anastomotic sutures intracorporeally. Alternatively, a duodenojejunostomy can be utilized which is easier to perform laparoscopically than duodenoduodenostomy and has similar outcomes.

12.3.6 Malrotation

Malrotation, with or without mid-gut volvulus, has been successfully repaired laparoscopically. The volvulus is detorsed, and a Ladd's procedure performed using three or four access trocars. Appendectomy can also be performed by exteriorizing the appendix through a 3 mm trocar site. There is some controversy as to whether the lack of adhesion formation after the laparoscopic technique is a flaw of the laparoscopic procedure.

12.3.7 Pull-Through for Hirschsprung's Disease

The management of Hirschsprung's disease has been radically changed by minimally invasive techniques. A pull-through is utilized after laparoscopic identification of ganglion cells proximal to the transition zone. Although the pull-through can be performed using a Duhamel or Swenson technique, the most common procedure performed endoscopically is an endorectal pull-through. Hirschsprung's disease is now managed by a single primary pull-through as opposed to the two- or three-stage procedures formerly used to correct the disorder.

12.3.8 Repair of Imperforate Anus

High imperforate anus is usually repaired by a posterior sagittal anorectoplasty. The alternative laparoscopic repair of a high imperforate anus starts by the dissection of the rectourethral or rectovesicular fistula transabdominally. The muscle complex is identified by muscle stimulation on the perineum. A tract is developed through the muscle complex by identifying the appropriate landmarks both perineally and transabdominally. This tract is sequentially dilated using a radially expanding trocar. The fistula is pulled down to the perineum through the tract and secured to the perineal skin with sutures. The laparoscopic repair of a high imperforate anus mimics the repair of a low imperforate anus where the fistula to the perineum is mobilized and pulled through the external sphincter. Continence after laparoscopic pull-through has not been fully assessed although the early results appear to be promising.

12.3.9 Inguinal Hernia Repair

Laparoscopic evaluation of a patent contralateral processus vaginalis is commonly performed around the world. A pneumoperitoneum is developed by way of the exposed hernia sac. An angled scope is then passed through the hernia sac, and the contralateral groin is visualized for patency. Laparoscopic repair of an inguinal hernia is also possible. Placement of a purse-string or figure-of-eight suture laparoscopically or transabdominally with laparoscopic surveillance closes the internal ring. A potential advantage of the laparoscopic-assisted inguinal hernia repair includes the avoidance of injury to the cord structures and testicles. In the classic open hernia repair, the hernia sac is stripped away from the vas deferens and testicular vessels. Many studies have suggested that this stripping of the cord structures may produce unintended permanent changes in the vas deferens and testicles.

12.3.10 Ovarian and Pelvic Pathology

A variety of treatment options for ovarian cysts can be pursued laparoscopically. These options include decompression, excision, fenestration, oophorectomy, and adnexal detorsion and fixation.

The use of laparoscopic dissection of the pelvic portion of a sacrococcygeal teratoma has been described by Bax and van der Zee. The author has also performed the pelvic dissection laparoscopically in two patients with sacrococcygeal teratoma and concurs with Bax that the intra-abdominal and pelvic portions of teratomas are expediently managed with laparoscopic assistance.

12.3.11 Appendectomy

Laparoscopic appendectomy has taken its place as the primary technique used to treat appendicitis in the Western world. In pediatric surgery centers with considerable laparoscopic experience, converting to an open operation after attempting laparoscopic appendectomy is a very uncommon event.

The laparoscopic procedure is utilized whenever appendectomy is indicated. It is usually performed with three trocars: one large trocar through the umbilicus, one small trocar placed suprapubically, and the other trocar in the left lower quadrant. The appendix is identified and separated from contiguous structures using blunt and sharp dissection. The mesoappendix is divided, usually with a hook cautery. The appendiceal stump is ligated with loop ligatures or with a stapling device. The appendix is delivered through the umbilical port site.

Results after laparoscopic appendectomy show a decreased incidence of wound infection when compared to the open approach. The incidence of a postoperative intraperitoneal abscess is about the same as after open appendectomy. Morbidity seems to be diminished with a more rapid discharge from the hospital being reported in several very large series. As previously mentioned, laparoscopic appendectomy has become the standard of care for children with appendicitis.

12.4 Conclusion

Minimally invasive surgical techniques are playing an expanding role in pediatric surgery. Despite the growing use of endoscopic surgery in children, the current literature supporting the safety and efficacy of thoracoscopy and laparoscopy in children is based on relatively small numbers of patients. It seems clear, even with these small numbers, that children tolerate minimally invasive techniques well but have specific sensitivities that must be recognized and respected to achieve safe results. With the further development in alternative devices for anastomosis, minimally invasive pediatric surgery should continue to grow at a rapid pace. Surely children deserve to enjoy the same benefits of incisionless surgery as their parents and grandparents.

Further Reading

Bax NM, van der Zee DC (1998) Laparoscopic treatment of intestinal malrotation in children. Surg Endosc 12:1314–1316

Bax NM, Ure BM, van der Zee DC et al (2001) Laparoscopic duodenoduodenostomy for duodenal atresia. Surg Endosc 15:217

Esposito C, Cucchiara S, Morrelli O et al (2000) Laparoscopic esophagomyotomy for the treatment of achalasia in children: A preliminary report of eight cases. Surg Endosc 14:110–113

Georgeson KE (2002) Laparoscopic-assisted total colectomy with pouch reconstruction. Semin Pediatr Surg 11:233–236

Georgeson KE (2002) Laparoscopic-assisted pull-through for Hirschsprung's disease. Semin Pediatr Surg 11:205–210

Georgeson KE, Fuenfer MM, Hardin WD (1995) Primary laparoscopic pull-through for Hirschsprung's disease in infants and children. J Pediatr Surg 30:1–7

Georgeson KE, Inge TH, Albanese CT (2000) Laparoscopically assisted anorectal pull-through for high imperforate anus: A new technique. J Pediatr Surg 35:927–931

Harmon CM, Barnhart DB, Georgeson KE et al (2004) Comparison of the incidence of complications in open and laparoscopic pyloromyotomy: A concurrent single institution series. J Pediatr Surg 39:292–296

Lin CL, Wong KKY, Lan LCL et al (2003) Earlier appearance and higher incidence of the rectoanal relaxation reflex in patients with imperforate anus repaired with laparoscopically assisted anorectoplasty. Surg Endosc 17:1646–1649

Meguerditchian AN, Prasil P, Cloutier R et al (2002) Laparoscopic appendectomy in children: A favorable alternative in simple and complicated appendicitis. J Pediatr Surg 37:695–698

Puri P, Höllwarth M (2006) Pediatric Surgery. Springer, Berlin, Heidelberg

Rescorla FJ (2002) Laparoscopic splenectomy. Semin Pediatr Surg 11:226–232

Rescorla FJ, West KW, Engum SA et al (1997) The "other side" of pediatric hernias: The role of laparoscopy. Am Surg 63:690–693

Schier F, Montupet P, Esposito C (2002) Laparoscopic inguinal herniorrhaphy in children: A three-center experience with 933 repairs. J Pediatr Surg 37:395–397

Birth Trauma

13

Thambipillai Sri Paran and Prem Puri

Contents

13.1 Introduction

Due to the intrinsic nature of the mechanical forces involved and the bony boundaries of the birth passage, the process of birth is naturally traumatic for the infant. Even under optimal conditions, injuries such as greenstick fracture of clavicle and subdural haemorrhages are seen in children born by normal spontaneous vaginal delivery. Furthermore, subdural haematoma has been documented in utero even before the initiation of labour. Added to this are the trauma caused by the mechanical forces applied by the obstetrician in delivering the baby. It is no surprise that the exact cause of a particular trauma in a newborn, with associated emotional and medico-legal sensitivities, may at times be far from clear or certain.

The risk factors for birth injuries include macrosomia, prematurity, instrumental delivery, breech and other abnormal presentations, prolonged second stage of labour and precipitous delivery. These risk factors are well recognised and efforts such as decreased use of forceps and more pre-emptive Caeserean sections have helped in reducing the incidence of birth trauma over the years. However, as mentioned above, due to the nature of labour itself, the overall incidence of birth injuries still remains at over 1% in most studies.

Birth trauma caused by intrinsic and applied mechanical forces during labour are discussed in this chapter, in order of anatomical location. We have focussed mostly on the diagnosis and management of the most common mechanical injuries reported during labour.

P. Puri and M. Höllwarth (eds.), *Pediatric Surgery: Diagnosis and Management,*
DOI: 10.1007/978-3-540-69560-8_13, © Springer-Verlag Berlin Heidelberg 2009

13.2 Head

Head trauma could be classified, according to its location, into three categories: extracranial, cranial or intracranial. Extracranial injuries include skin lacerations secondary to blood sampling, and haemorrhage in between various extracranial anatomical layers secondary to rupturing of blood vessels or bony fractures. Cranial injuries are usually related to fractures of skull bones, either linear or depressed. The most common intracranial injuries are those where veins are ruptured within the subdural space leading to subdural haematoma; epidural and subarachnoid haemorrhages are also seen, though less frequently.

13.2.1 Extracranial Haematomas

Extracranial haematomas can be classified according to their anatomical location. These include caput succedaneum, subgaleal haemorrhage and cephalhaematoma.

13.2.1.1 Caput Succedaneum

Caput succedaneum is due to rupture of blood vessels within the dense connective tissue underneath the skin and can be secondary to birth trauma itself or due to vacuum or forceps delivery. Purpura and ecchymosis of the overlying skin are common, and the suture lines do not restrict the swelling. The bleeding is usually minimal due to the tamponading effect of the dense connective tissue. These haematomas resolve spontaneously within a few days.

13.2.1.2 Subgaleal Haemorrhage

Subgaleal haemorrhage is secondary to rupture of emissary veins within the loose connective tissue between the galea aponeurotica and the periosteum. The bleeding can also sometimes result from a bony fracture. It is seen in up to 6.4 per 1,000 forceps deliveries, and the bleeding can continue for 2–3 days and result in significant loss of blood due to the lack of resistance by the loose connective tissue. Other risk factors include prolonged second stage of labour,

foetal distress and macrosomia. It presents as a firm to fluctuant mass that crosses the suture lines. It is estimated that each 1 cm increase in the head circumference correlates to 38 ml of blood loss. Treatment is largely supportive including serial blood tests and fluid replacement. A full blood count is necessary to establish the extent of blood loss and a coagulation screen is required following transfusion of blood and large volume of fluids. Bilirubin levels may increase due to reabsorption of large haematomas in neonates, and this needs to be monitored closely. The overall mortality is reported to be in the range of 14–22% when there is excessive blood loss, and surgery may be required in severe cases to cauterize the bleeding vessels.

13.2.1.3 Cephalhaematoma

Cephalhaematoma is by far the most common extracranial haematoma and is due to the rupture of blood vessels beneath the periosteum. It is seen in approximately 2.5% of newborns and is associated with forceps and breech deliveries. The swelling does not cross the suture lines due to the periosteal attachments to the bone, and purpura or ecchymosis is not a feature of cephalhaematoma. A small percentage (5%) is associated with bony fractures. Rapid expansion and excessive blood loss are rare, but can occur if the periosteum ruptures. Cephalhaematoma usually resolves over a few weeks and no treatment is necessary. However, if rapid expansion with signs of sepsis is noted, infection of the haematoma should be suspected; aspiration of fluid for diagnosis and treatment may be necessary in such situations (Fig. 13.1).

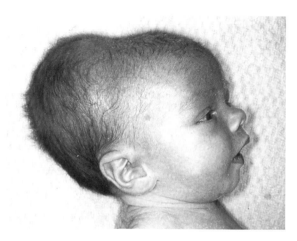

Fig. 13.1 Large cephalhaematoma

13.2.2 Cranial Injuries

Cranial injuries usually consist of linear fractures of parietal bones. As it is the case with most birth injuries, such fractures can occur even in uncomplicated spontaneous vaginal deliveries. Additional risk factors include forceps delivery and prolonged labour. Depressed fractures are seen infrequently, and such depressed fractures are mostly of the 'ping-pong ball' type that is due to inward buckling of the resilient neonatal calvarial bones. Again most of the cranial injuries could be managed conservatively. In the absence of neurological deficits or signs of raised intracranial pressure, surgery is not indicated for the treatment of depressed bony fractures. However, non-surgical interventions such as elevation of the depressed segment with digital pressure or a breast pump have been utilised successfully in the past. When there are signs and symptoms of raised intracranial pressure such as apnoea, seizures, focal neurological deficits, lethargy and hypotonia, neurosurgical intervention is necessary to evacuate any haematoma and to elevate the fractured segment.

13.2.3 Intracranial Haemorrhage

Intracranial haemorrhage is seen less frequently than extracranial haemorrhage and the prevalence of symptomatic intracranial haemorrhage in term infants is approximately 5–6 per 10,000 live births. Again, intracranial injuries have been documented in infants born by normal vaginal deliveries, but the incidence is higher with risk factors such as forceps delivery, prolonged labour and macrosomia. The most frequent intracranial haemorrhage is subdural haemorrhage (75%); epidural haemorrhage is rare and subarachnoid haemorrhage is usually associated with preterm infants and asphyxia.

13.2.3.1 Subdural Haemorrhage

Subdural haemorrhage is seen in 8–10 per 10,000 forceps deliveries and the prevalence has decreased over the years with the reduction in the use of forceps. It is seen in 6% of all uncomplicated vaginal deliveries and has even been documented in some infants before the initiation of labour. Subdural haemorrhage commonly results from the tearing of the tentorial and interhemispheric veins. Studies have shown that in asymptomatic children the haemorrhage resolves spontaneously within 4 weeks and results in no long-term developmental abnormalities. Significant bleeding can lead to volume depletion and raised intracranial pressure, and the infant exhibits the following symptoms: apnoea, seizures, focal neurological deficits, unequal pupils, eye deviation, bulging fontanelle, lethargy, hypotonia, drowsiness and coma. Though these symptoms are usually seen within 24 h of birth, on occasions it may take up to a few days to fully develop, as the bleeding can be slow and continuous. Cranial ultrasound is useful in the diagnosis of subdural haemorrhages, but is operator dependent. CT scan is the diagnostic procedure of choice in suspected cases, and MRI scan may be useful to gain added information in selected cases. Most children with subdural haemorrhage are asymptomatic and could be treated conservatively following diagnostic imaging. However, a small percentage will have symptoms; posterior fossa bleeds are more symptomatic and may lead to brain-stem compression. These symptomatic infants will require surgical evacuation of their haematoma. Progressive hydrocephalus is a well-known complication of subdural haemorrhage in some, and symptomatic and asymptomatic children must be monitored with serial head circumference measurements on a centile chart. When detected, ventriculoperitoneal shunt insertion is indicated to drain the Cerebrospinal fluid (CSF) into the peritoneal cavity. Though a majority of children with subdural haemorrhage meet their developmental milestones well, a significant proportion (up to 30% in one study) show mild to severe developmental delay as they grow older. When the bleeding is within the posterior fossa, developmental delay is seen in up to 50% of infants.

13.2.3.2 Subarachnoid Haemorrhage

Subarachnoid haemorrhage is caused by rupture of the bridging veins of the subarachnoid space in preterm infants. Though seen in 1 in 10,000 spontaneous vaginal deliveries, the prevalence increases to 3 per 10,000 in forceps deliveries. Symptoms are that of raised intracranial pressure in an infant seen within the first 1–2 days of life. Cranial ultrasound, CT scan and CSF sampling may all help in the diagnosis. As with subdural haemorrhage, most subarachnoid haemorrhages also resolve spontaneously with no long-term morbidity, and do not need surgical intervention. Progressive hydrocephalus is a known complication of subarachnoid haemorrhage and should be monitored for in the recovering infant. If seen, ventriculoperitoneal shunting is necessary. Hypoxic injury to the brain tissue must also be monitored for in those with large subarachnoid bleed.

13.2.3.3　Epidural Haemorrhage

Epidural haemorrhage is rare and is usually associated with cephalhaematoma or skull fracture. It is usually due to a direct injury to the middle meningeal artery, which is not protected within a bony groove in the newborns, and can on occasions be very large. Skull X-rays and CT scan are useful in the diagnosis of this injury. Unlike those with subdural haemorrhage, most infants with epidural haemorrhage are symptomatic and will need neurosurgical intervention. Aspiration of the haematoma, without surgery, has also been reported to be successful in the treatment of epidural haemorrhage.

13.3　Injuries to Peripheral Nerves

These injuries are usually caused by excessive traction or direct compression of nerves during the delivery. The nerves most commonly involved are the brachial plexus, facial nerve, and the phrenic nerve. The outcome of treatment from these injuries is usually good. This type of nerve injury was first classified by Seddon into three categories and was later expanded into the following five categories by Sunderland:

1. First-degree injury or neuropraxia—involves a temporary conduction block with demyelination of the nerve at the site of injury; complete recovery is normal and takes up to 12 weeks.
2. Second-degree injury or axonotmesis—severe trauma causing proximal and distal axonal degeneration. The endoneurial tubes are intact and the recovery is complete, with axonal regeneration occurring at a rate of 1 mm per day.
3. Third-degree injury—same as a second-degree injury but more severe, with disruption to the endoneurial tubes. As with second-degree, the regeneration is complete, but the regenerating axons may not reinnervate their original motor and sensory targets.
4. Fourth-degree injury—larger area of axon is damaged and this precludes any axons from advancing distally during regeneration. Surgery is necessary to restore neural continuity.
5. Fifth-degree injury—complete transection of the nerve, and surgery is again necessary for recovery of function.

13.3.1　Brachial Plexus Injury

Brachial plexus injury could either affect the entire plexus or some part of it. It is by far the most common injury and is reported in 0.1–0.3% of all live births. Risk factors include large birth weight (maternal diabetes), prolonged second stage of labour, forceps delivery, shoulder dystocia and malpresentation. It is believed to occur due to excessive downward traction on the head so as to dislodge an impacted shoulder. However, brachial plexus injury has been reported on the opposite side, in the posterior shoulder, in up to 40% of affected infants. It has also been reported after normal uncomplicated vaginal deliveries, and in infants born by elective Caesarean sections. The explanation for some of these injuries may lie in the overall traumatic nature of birth and the significant mechanical forces involved during normal labour, and may not simply be attributable to the techniques employed by the midwife or obstetrician during labour. Brachial plexus injury has been divided into three main types depending on the site of the injury within the brachial plexus: Erb's palsy, Klumpke's palsy and injury to the entire plexus.

13.3.1.1　Erb's Palsy

The upper brachial plexus injury was first described by Erb in 1874, and is by far the most common type (90%) of birth-related peripheral nerve injury. The injury is to the C5-C6 nerve roots resulting in the affected arm hanging limply adducted and internally rotated at the shoulder, and extended and pronated at the elbow with flexed wrist and fingers in the typical 'waiter's tip' posture (Fig. 13.2). This is the result of paralysis of the deltoid, supraspinatus, infraspinatus, brachioradialis and supinator brevis muscles. On the affected side the Moro, biceps and radial reflexes are absent, while the grasp reflex is preserved. Associated phrenic nerve injury should be excluded.

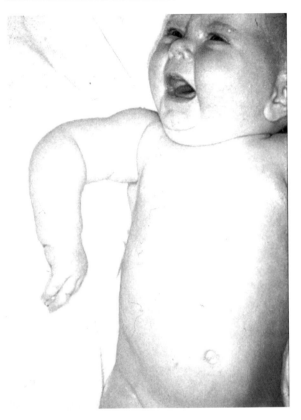

Fig. 13.2 Erb's palsy with 'waiter's tip position of the right arm

the intrinsic muscles of the hand and flexors of the wrist and fingers. The grasp reflex is absent. The same trauma that causes lower plexus injury may also lead to injury of the cervical sympathetic fibres. Injury to cervical sympathetic fibres may result in ipsilateral Horner's syndrome. Treatment is again conservative, but the recovery rates are poorer than for Erb's palsy. Again surgical exploration must be sought early, when no recovery is noted after 3–6 months of age. In all children considered for surgery, electrodiagnostic studies and CT or MRI scan must be carried out preoperatively. Advanced microsurgical techniques combined with nerve grafting from the dural nerve can improve the functional outcome in some children.

13.3.1.3 Injury to Entire Brachial Plexus

Injury to the entire brachial plexus results in flaccid arm with absence of sweating, sensation, and deep tendon reflexes. X-ray of the upper arm and shoulder should be performed to exclude the possibility of bony injuries. Children with injury to the entire brachial plexus have severe nerve disruption and get worse on conservative management. Early neurosurgical opinion and surgical exploration should be considered for these children as well.

Most neonates will make a complete or partial recovery on conservative treatment alone, as this type of nerve injury is mostly of the first and second degree according to Suderland's scale. Initial conservative treatment includes immobilization of the affected arm underneath the sleeve for 1 week. After 1 week of rest, the arm is put through passive range-of-motion exercises at the shoulder, elbow and wrist to prevent contractures. The prognosis is excellent when antigravity muscle movements are seen within biceps and shoulder abductors by 3 months of age. If by 3 months no movements are documented within these muscle groups, then specialised neurosurgical opinion should be sought, in view to reconstructive surgery. The recovery is somewhat guarded following surgical correction in children with Erb's palsy.

13.3.2 Facial Nerve Injury

Facial nerve injury is usually unilateral and is secondary to compression of the nerve against stylomastoid foramen or the ramus of the mandible. Compression could be either with forceps or against the sacral promontory. It is seen in approximately 0.06–0.7% of all live births. Most injuries are simple swelling of the axons secondary to the compression, and disruption of the axons is rarely seen. The affected side of the face would have absent or decreased forehead wrinkling, a persistently open eye, a decreased nasolabial fold and flattening of the corner of the mouth. Spontaneous complete recovery within a month is seen in >90% of infants. Therefore, the initial treatment consists of protecting the affected eye from drying out with application of artificial tears, until full recovery is documented. Because of the high incidence of spontaneous recovery, surgery should only be considered for those with no signs of recovery after 1 year.

13.3.1.2 Klumpke's Paralysis

Injury to lower plexus including C8-T1 nerve roots was later described by Klumpke in 1885. This lower plexus injury is uncommon. It results in paralysis of

13.3.3 Phrenic Nerve Injury

Phrenic nerve injury arises from C3–C5 nerve roots and is the motor supply to the ipsilateral diaphragm. Injury to this nerve usually results from excessive traction of the neck muscles, and leads to paralysis of the ipsilateral diaphragm. Most of these injuries (up to 75%) occur together with brachial plexus injury, or fracture of the clavicle, and are unilateral. The most common cause of phrenic nerve injury is a difficult breech delivery. Clinically, the infant may show respiratory distress and decreased air-entry on the affected side. Chest X-ray will show a raised hemidiaphragm with mediastinal shift to the opposite side (Fig. 13.3). Atelectasis of the lower lobe of lung on the affected side with pneumonia may be present. Ultrasound may confirm paralysis by demonstrating paradoxical movement of the affected hemidiaphragm. Treatment is again conservative with oxygen, physiotherapy and antibiotics when indicated. If the respiratory distress is significant, continuous positive airway pressure ventilation should be considered. Surgery is indicated when

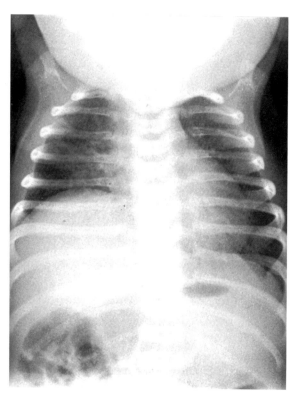

Fig. 13.3 Elevated right diaphragm due to phrenic nerve analysis

no improvement is seen after 2 weeks of mechanical ventilation or 3 months of conservative treatment. Surgical options include plication of the diaphragm or, rarely, excision and artificial patch repair of the diaphragm as employed in the repair of large congenital diaphragmatic hernias.

13.3.4 Spinal Cord Injury

This is an extremely rare injury. Due to the incomplete mineralisation of the vertebrae and lax ligaments in a newborn, the spine could potentially stretch more than the spinal cord, and thereby result in an injury to the cord. Damage to the upper cervical cord is common and is associated with rotation of the head during vertex delivery with forceps. Lower cord injury occurs during breech delivery, when the head is trapped secondary to cephalopelvic disproportion. Injury above the level of C4 will result in paralysis of the diaphragm due to phrenic nerve injury and cause apnoea. When the injury is below the level of C4, the following signs and symptoms will be present: absent spontaneous movement, absent tendon reflexes and lack of response to painful stimuli below the level of the injury. The bladder will be atonic and distended while the anal sphincter will be atonic and patulent. The outcome, in general, is very poor for these infants. Early management should consist of strict immobilization of the head, neck and spine. Ultrasonography and MRI scan will reveal the extent of injury and may help in determining the prognosis. X-rays alone are usually not helpful. Treatment should be supportive including ventilation and passive range of movements to prevent pressure ulcers and pain relief. The overall outcome in this group of children is poor resulting in early death, severe disability and ventilator dependency.

13.4 Abdominal Organ Injuries

Trauma to abdominal organs is uncommon during birth. The organs most commonly affected are the liver, spleen, adrenal gland and kidney. Risk factors include hepatosplenomegaly, breech presentation, macrosomia, prematurity and coagulation disorders. Proposed mechanism of injury to the liver and spleen include: direct trauma by the rib cage secondary to thoracic wall compression; thoracic wall compression causing a pulling effect on the ligamentous attachments to the liver and spleen with consequent tearing of the parenchyma; and trauma secondary to instrumental compression of the organs. Subcapsular bleeds are common, but organ rupture with intra-abdominal bleed is also seen. Clinical signs and symptoms are that of an intra-abdominal bleeding with pallor, shock, abdominal distension and abdominal discoloration. Adrenal haemorrhage may present as a flank mass. When suspected, abdominal ultrasound, CT and abdominal paracentesis could all help in the diagnosis. Blood tests should include full blood count, coagulation screen and cross match. Treatment is supportive with fluid replacement and/or transfusion as indicated by the severity of the blood loss. When supportive treatment fails or the infant becomes haemodynamically unstable, explorative laparotomy must be undertaken. In splenic injury, every attempt must be made to preserve the spleen before considering splenectomy to overcome the active bleeding.

Risk factors for adrenal haemorrhage include prolonged labour, asphyxia, prematurity, septicaemia, renal vein thrombosis and haemorrhagic disease of the newborn. The right side is involved in 70% of cases, with bilateral involvement seen in 5–10% of cases. The classical adrenal haemorrhage presents within the first 4 days of life as a flank mass with fever and jaundice or anaemia. Ultrasound is useful in the diagnosis, and a rim of suprarenal calcification may be seen on abdominal radiograph 2–4 weeks later. Management is the same as above with supportive transfusion followed by laparotomy in severe cases.

Renal traumas are rare and are usually seen in the background of congenital renal anomalies. Investigations such as renal ultrasound, CT scan, DMSA or MAG3 scan may be necessary to assess the injury and any underlying congenital abnormality, following supportive management for the bleeding. Long-term follow-up may be necessary as renal trauma could lead to scarring of the renal parenchyma.

13.5 Fractures

13.5.1 Fracture of Clavicle

This is the most frequently fractured bone during birth and is seen in 0.3–3% of newborns. The vast difference in the reported incidence is due to the fact that a

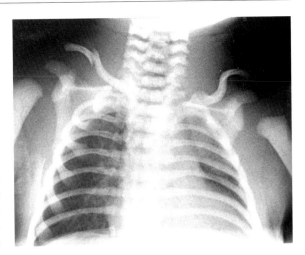

Fig. 13.4 Fractured right clavicle

majority of these fractures go unnoticed due to lack of external findings. A majority of these fractures are of the greenstick type are not even recognized at the time of discharge of the infant from hospital. Risk factors are the same as for most birth traumas, and are sometimes seen in uncomplicated normal deliveries as well. The most common finding is reduced movement of the affected arm, but discolouration and bony deformity are also seen infrequently. A normal X-ray will confirm the diagnosis (Fig. 13.4). Treatment is usually conservative for incomplete fractures. When complete fracture is noted, the arm should be immobilized for 7–10 days. Differential diagnoses include brachial plexus injury, fracture of humerus, and shoulder dislocation. Erb's palsy and phrenic nerve injury must be excluded. Recovery is complete in most infants.

13.5.2 Long Bone Fractures

Fractures of humerus and femur are uncommon, but are associated with breech presentation, low birth weight and traction during delivery. Swelling, pain and decreased movement of the limb may be present. A normal X-ray will confirm fracture of long bones. However, high index of suspicion of epiphyseal injuries must be borne in mind. These epiphyseal injuries will not show up on plain X-rays, and when suspected ultrasonography for accurate diagnosis must be done. Treatment consists of immobilisation and splinting of the joint. For displaced fractures, closed reduction and casting may be necessary. Proximal femoral fractures need Pavlik harness or spica cast for a period of time.

Further Reading

Noetzel MJ (2006) Perinatal trauma and cerebral palsy. Clin Perinatol 33:355–366

Piatt JH (2004) Birth injuries of the brachial plexus. Pediatr Clin N Am 51:421–440

Puri P (2003) Fetal and birth trauma. In P Puri (ed) Newborn Surgery. Arnold, London, pp 27–38

Puri P, Höllwarth M (2006) Pediatric Surgery. Springer, Berlin, Heidelberg

Sorantin E et al (2006) Neonatal trauma. Eur J Radiol 60(2): 199–207

Uhing MR (2005) Management of birth injuries. Clin Perinatol 32:19–38

Pediatric Thoracic Trauma

14

David E. Sawaya Jr. and Paul M. Colombani

Contents

14.1 Introduction

When treating pediatric trauma patients, many important differences must be considered when compared to adults. It may be difficult to have access to emergency vascular treatment especially in cases of shock or cardiac arrest. Interosseous access is an important option in all children and is more commonly implemented in the very young. Children have a smaller blood volume and a more insidious onset of hemorrhagic shock, commonly with tachycardia, as the only early warning sign.

Regarding thoracic injuries, children have a markedly compliant thorax making them vulnerable to intrathoracic injury without overlying bony injury. It is crucial to be vigilant while evaluating children with blunt trauma injuries. The pediatric mediastinum is also very mobile allowing it to be shifted with much less intrathoracic pressure. Susceptibility to tension pneumothorax or hemothorax is much greater and these injuries must be treated promptly. This mobility, however, does make it less susceptible to major vascular or airway injuries. Thoracic trauma in children is a marker for the presence of associated injuries, found in more than 50% of these children.

Children are much less likely to have concomitant systemic illnesses compromising their respiratory and cardiovascular reserves. This allows lower morbidity and mortality rates with aggressive medical therapy and faster recovery from injury.

14.2 Mechanism of Injury

Blunt trauma accounts for 85–90% of pediatric thoracic injuries. The majority of blunt thoracic injuries result from motor vehicle crashes. Children may be passengers

P. Puri and M. Höllwarth (eds.), *Pediatric Surgery: Diagnosis and Management*,
DOI: 10.1007/978-3-540-69560-8_14, © Springer-Verlag Berlin Heidelberg 2009

in the motor vehicle or, frequently, may be struck by the motor vehicle. Falls from various heights are the next most common causes of thoracic injuries. Isolated blunt thoracic trauma carries a 5% mortality rate. When associated with blunt traumatic brain injuries, the mortality rate rises to 25%. When associated with brain and abdominal injuries, the mortality rate rises to 40%.

Penetrating trauma represents only 10–15% of thoracic trauma but the incidence increases with age, especially for children over 12 years of age. Nearly 14% of children suffering from penetrating thoracic trauma die from thoracic injury. Associated injuries with penetrating thoracic trauma are less common.

14.3 Immediately Life-Threatening Injuries Found During Primary Survey

14.3.1 Airway Obstruction

Airway obstruction can prove to be fatal if it is not treated immediately. Securing the airway is the first task in patient management. This takes precedence over all other needs and requires immediate attention and redirection if a patient's airway is lost during evaluation. Complete airway obstruction presents with a total absence of air movement and breath sounds.

Partial obstruction presents with inspiratory stridor if the obstruction is above the vocal cords or expiratory stridor if the level of obstruction is below the vocal cords. Other signs and symptoms include agitation, diaphoresis, chest wall retractions, cyanosis, and bradycardia. Airway obstruction can occur from something as simple as a folding or closure of the normal hypopharynx, merely requiring a chin-tilt, jaw-thrust maneuver to reestablish a patient's airway. More serious causes of airway obstruction involve tracheal injury or foreign body aspiration. Unless an obstructed airway can be immediately cleared and ventilation reestablished, intubation is required. Non-cuffed endotracheal tubes are used and the size is determined by using the formula $(age + 4)/4$. If a child can be adequately ventilated with a bag-valve-mask, this allows for a more controlled intubation and repeat attempts if unsuccessful. If intubation cannot be achieved, a cricothyroidotomy must be performed. In children under 12 years, a needle cricothyroidotomy is accomplished by placing a large bore needle/angiocath through the cricoid membrane for temporary high flow oxygen administration followed by an immediate tracheostomy. In children 12 years or older an open cricothyroidotomy is done followed by a tracheostomy; after the patient is stabilized, other life-threatening issues are addressed and the secondary survey is completed. Foreign body aspiration requires airway control via endotracheal intubation followed by removal via rigid bronchoscopy (Fig. 14.1).

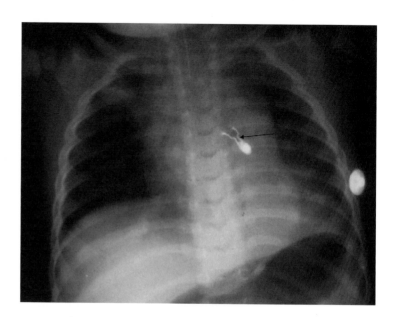

Fig. 14.1 Left bronchial foreign body

14.3.2 Tension Pneumothorax

A pneumothorax is caused by air entering the potential space between the visceral and parietal pleura resulting in air getting trapped in the hemithorax. This occurs following a tear in the pulmonary parenchymal due to rib fracture and laceration, deceleration injury, crush injury, or due to increased intrathoracic pressure causing pulmonary rupture. Signs and symptoms include chest pain, dyspnea, increased respiratory rate, and hyper-resonance on the injured side. A pneumothorax can quickly result in cardiovascular demise if tension within the hemithorax develops (Fig. 14.2). Findings of hyper-resonance, diminished breath sounds on the affected side, tracheal deviation, and hemodynamic instability indicate a potentially lethal tension pneumothorax requiring immediate intervention. Chest x-ray is not required to make this diagnosis and may waste valuable time. Needle decompression is the most efficient therapy for a tension pneumothorax; it is accomplished by placing a large bore angiocath in the second intercostal space along the mid-clavicular line just above the third rib. Alternatively, the decompression can be performed in the anterior axillary line just above the sixth rib. This should be followed by placement of chest tube. This results in the expansion of the lung and continued evacuation of air and fluid until the injured lung seals and air leak resolves.

14.3.3 Open Pneumothorax

An open pneumothorax is caused by a persistent or continuous communication between the environment and the chest cavity, and is sometimes referred to as a sucking chest wound. The negative intrathoracic pressure generated during inhalation results in air from the environment being sucked into the chest cavity and collapse of the lung on the affected side. Signs and symptoms include shortness of breath, chest pain, decreased breath sounds on the affected side, and sound of air being sucked into the chest cavity. This can result in respiratory arrest and cardiovascular collapse if not treated promptly. Treatment involves sealing or closing the hole in the chest wall. Vaseline gauze is commonly used. Placement of a chest tube evacuates residual air from the affected hemithorax and enables lung re-expansion. If there is an associated parenchymal injury, the chest tube is left in place until this air leak resolves.

14.3.4 Flail Chest

Flail chest is caused by multiple rib fractures or disarticulation of the ribs from the sternum resulting in an unstable segment of chest wall. The flail segment demonstrates paradoxical chest wall movement during the

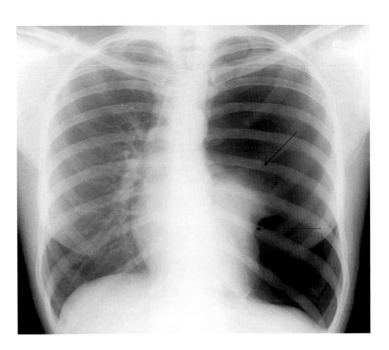

Fig. 14.2 Left tension pneumothorax with mediastinal shift

respiratory cycle and physical exam is diagnostic. Radiographic findings are only supportive. Treatment involves adequate analgesia, positive pressure ventilation, and possible rib fixation stabilizing the flail segment. Placement of chest tube may be required for associated pneumothorax or hemothorax. As with less complicated rib fractures, pain control and pulmonary toilet are essential.

14.3.5 Hemothorax

A traumatic hemothorax is the accumulation of blood in the hemithorax following blunt or penetrating trauma. Bleeding can result from rib fractures that lacerate the intercostal vessels, pulmonary parenchymal laceration, or, less commonly, great vessel injury. A massive hemothorax results from life-threatening exsanguination into the chest cavity requiring immediate intervention. Signs and symptoms include shock, hypotension, diminished breath sounds and dullness to percussion on the affected side, chest pain, shortness of breath, and oxygen requirement. This is a clinical diagnosis especially in the unstable child. In the stable child, a chest x-ray confirms the diagnosis (Fig. 14.3). Standard therapy includes large bore tube thoracostomy for evacuation of fluid and air providing for lung re-expansion. Resuscitation with intravenous fluid and possibly packed red blood cells is required. Thoracotomy is indicated for hemodynamic instability, loss of >25% total blood volume with initial chest tube placement, or persistent bleeding greater than 2 ml/kg/h.

14.3.6 Cardiac Tamponade and Commotio Cordis

Penetrating cardiac trauma quickly results in life-threatening injuries requiring surgical intervention. These are typically manifested by cardiovascular instability. Traumatic cardiac pericardial effusions and tamponade result from the accumulation of blood, fluid, or, rarely, air between the heart and the pericardium. This impairs cardiac filling during diastole. Signs and symptoms include muffled heart sounds, hypotension, distended neck veins (Beck's Triad), narrow pulse pressure, and pulsus pardoxus. Echocardiography in the Emergency Department (ED) is the radiologic test of choice and can help guide therapy. Emergency thoracotomy is required for cardiac repair and may be performed in the trauma bay for hemodynamic instability. Rib disarticulation from sternum may provide better exposure. A vertical pericardotomy is performed, with identification and repair of cardiac injuries with 5-0 nonabsorbable monofilament suture and pledgets. During pericardiotomy, care is taken to avoid the

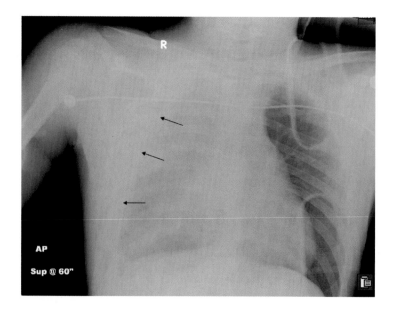

Fig. 14.3   Right hemothorax following a gunshot wound to the chest

phrenic nerve and the pericardium remains open after cardiac repair. In patients with equivocal signs and symptoms of pericardial effusion or tamponade, a sub-xyphoid pericardial window should be performed. This allows to assess the presence of blood or fluid within the pericardium. A note of caution to be ready for thoracotomy or sternotomy is warranted. Findings range from decompensation during pericardiotomy to finding blood in the pericardium (both necessitating thoracotomy) or a negative pericardiotomy. Pericardiocentesis is less commonly indicated but useful during resuscitation of an unstable patient with profound hypotension and suspected cardiac tamponade. A large bore needle/angiocath is inserted in the subxyphoid space at a 45° angle while aspirating with a syringe. If blood is obtained, the angiocath is left in the pericardial space while preparations for thoracotomy are made. Pericardiocentesis can be diagnostic and therapeutic but may result in further cardiac injury from needle instrumentation. Cardiac rupture due to massive blunt trauma is typically lethal.

Commotio cordis is a life-threatening arrhythmia resulting from a direct blow to the precordium. Several cases of precordial blows have been reported from sports such as baseball, softball, soccer, lacrosse, and karate. Commotio cordis triggers ventricular fibrillation or other fatal arrhythmias that quickly deteriorate. Defibrillation within 1–2 min results in 80–100% survival rates. Survivors have minimal to no identifiable laboratory abnormalities but usually have EKG abnormalities including S-T elevation or complete heart block.

14.4 Potentially Life-Threatening Injuries Found During Secondary Survey

14.4.1 Tracheobronchial Injury

Tracheal and bronchial injuries are uncommon in the pediatric population but have been reported following thoracic crush injuries and penetrating injuries. Signs and symptoms include chest pain, dyspnea, hypoxia, stridor, crepitance in the neck and chest wall, mediastinal air, tension pneumothorax, and hemoptysis. Placement of chest tube for pneumothorax results in identification of a large non-resolving air leak. Further diagnostic evaluation is best accomplished via rigid bronchoscopy for direct visualization of the injury and evacuation of blood and secretions. Eighty percent of these injuries typically occur within 2 cm of the carina in the trachea or mainstem bronchi and require early operative repair. Flap coverage of the repair with pleura or muscle reinforces and protects the repair.

14.4.2 Pulmonary Contusions

Pulmonary contusions are due to alveolar hemorrhage and parenchymal destruction. Pulmonary contusions, the most common injury found in children with thoracic trauma, can result from blunt or penetrating trauma. Only 40% of these patients have associated rib fractures. This low percentage is due to increased pediatric chest wall compliance. Signs and symptoms of pulmonary contusions include chest pain, shortness of breath, hypoxia, and, less commonly, hemoptysis. Pulmonary contusions may present insidiously during the first 24 h following thoracic trauma with worsening pulmonary symptoms and delayed radiologic findings. Chest x-ray remains the initial diagnostic exam and computer tomography is used for complicated cases when further imaging is required (Fig. 14.4). Treatment involves supplemental oxygen, fluid restriction as tolerated, chest physiotherapy to clear secretions and blood, as well as adequate pain control. Intubation and mechanical ventilation are infrequently required. The mortality rate due to isolated pulmonary contusions is low, and there are no long-term respiratory problems.

14.4.3 Myocardial Contusion

Substernal chest pain following blunt chest trauma is indicative of myocardial contusion. Other signs and symptoms include cardiac arrhythmias and hypotension. Myocardial contusion is the most common pediatric cardiac injury, accounting for 95% of blunt cardiac injuries. Motor vehicle accidents are the leading cause. Diagnostic evaluation reveals elevated cardiac enzymes and EKG shows S-T changes, arrhythmias, or heart block. Echocardiography may show wall motion

Fig. 14.4 Left pulmonary contusion due to blunt thoracic trauma

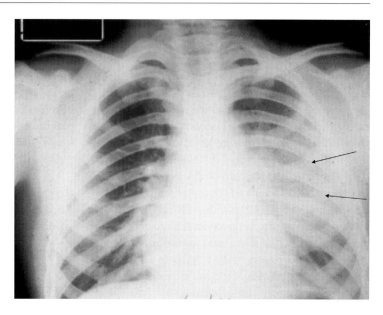

changes consistent with contusion or hematoma. Most injuries are self-limiting but can result in aneurysm formation and possibly cardiac rupture. Patients with myocardial contusions should be continuously monitored until free of arrhythmias for 24 h.

Primary surgical repair with nonabsorbable suture is most common; a patch is used if the defect is too large and not amenable to primary closure. Closure of larger defects with an intercostal muscle flap has also been accomplished.

14.4.4 Diaphragmatic Injuries

Diaphragmatic injuries are more commonly caused by penetrating trauma. Signs and symptoms include dyspnea, abdominal pain, vomiting, and decreased breath sounds. These injuries can be diagnostic dilemmas. The initial radiologic exam consists of chest x-ray with a nasogastric tube (NGT) in place. With a left diaphragmatic injury, the stomach may be herniated into the chest and the NGT confirmatory of the injury. Helical computer tomography is currently the most useful exam with 70–100% accuracy. MRI is as accurate but commonly not available in the acute setting and requires much more time. This is costly especially during the golden hour. Up to one-half of diaphragmatic injuries are not found upon initial diagnostic evaluation. Nearly one-third are found intraoperatively, either incidentally or with minimally invasive surgical techniques. Isolated diaphragmatic rupture from blunt trauma is more common in children and occurs more frequently on the left side (Fig. 14.5).

14.4.5 Esophageal Rupture

Esophageal rupture is a very rare injury resulting from rapid elevation of intraluminal pressure. In cases of esophageal rupture, this is relieved by laceration of the wall rather than intraluminal dissipation. Signs and symptoms include chest pain, fever, subcutaneous emphysema, and dysphagia. X-rays may reveal subcutaneous air (Fig. 14.6). The resulting mediastinal sepsis can prove to be fatal if not diagnosed and treated promptly. Esophageal debridement, closure, and drainage remain the primary course of treatment.

14.4.6 Great Vessel Injury

Great vessel injury in the pediatric population is uncommon but can be devastating when the injury is not promptly recognized and treated. Aortic rupture is suspected with rapid deceleration injuries from motor

Fig. 14.5 Left diaphragmatic rupture

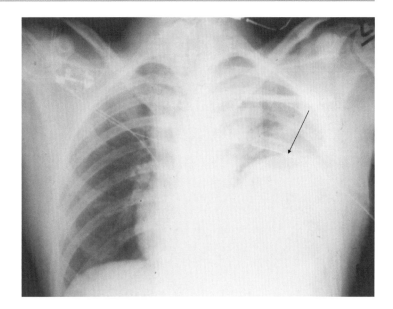

Fig. 14.6 Cervical soft tissue air and mediastinal air from esophageal rupture

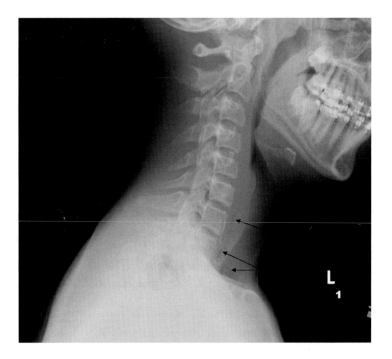

vehicle crashes and falls from great heights. The most common site is at the level of the ligamentum arteriosum. Signs and symptoms include chest pain and hemodynamic instability. Chest x-ray may reveal a widened mediastinum, elevated left bronchus, loss of the contour of the aortic knob, first rib fracture, and deviation of the esophagus demonstrated with a nasogastric tube in place (Fig. 14.7).

The diagnostic test of choice is arteriography but is commonly preceeded by helical computer tomography. Transesophageal echocardiography may also be useful. Treatment consists of aortic repair, commonly requiring cardiopulmonary bypass. Primary repair may be accomplished with nonabsorbable monofilament sutures with pledgets and vascular graft interposition

Fig. 14.7 Mediastinal widening and loss of aortic knob due to aortic rupture

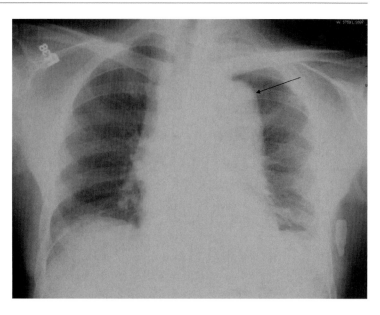

may also be required. Branches of the thoracic aorta can usually be repaired without cardiopulmonary bypass.

14.5 Non-Life Threatening Injuries Often Found on Physical Exam or Chest Radiograph

14.5.1 Simple Pneumothorax

A simple pneumothorax occurs when air gets accumulated in the chest cavity without putting it in any tension. Decreased breath sounds may be observed as well as chest pain and shortness of breath. Chest x-ray is diagnostic and placement of chest tube is therapeutic (Fig. 14.8). In rare cases, a pneumothorax may remain very small due to a transient air leak from the parenchyma that readily stops. In this situation, conservative management may prevail without the placement of chest tube.

14.5.2 Small Hemothorax

A small hemothorax is caused by minor bleeding in the chest cavity due to pulmonary parenchymal injury or chest wall injury. Only the placement of a chest tube is required for drainage if the lung volume is compromised.

14.5.3 Rib Fractures

Rib fractures in children are less common than in adults due to the increased compliance of the chest wall. Therefore, rib fractures are felt to be a marker of increased injury severity. Rib fractures are also commonly associated with child abuse. Nearly two-thirds of rib fractures in children under three years of age result from abuse. The most common cause of rib fractures in older children are motor vehicle crashes. Signs and symptoms include chest pain, dyspnea, and splinting on the side of the fracture which can result in atelectasis and pneumonia. Chest x-ray will confirm the diagnosis and more importantly evaluate for an underlying pulmonary injury, pneumothorax, or hemothorax. Rib fractures typically require no surgical therapy. Pain control and pulmonary toilet significantly reduce the risk of complications from these fractures. Children with first rib fractures should be evaluated for vascular injury.

14.5.4 Chest Wall Laceration

Chest wall lacerations occur from multiple different mechanisms but the treatment remains the same. Wound exploration, foreign body removal, control of bleeding, debridement, and wound closure are the basics of laceration management.

Fig. 14.8 Simple left pneumothorax

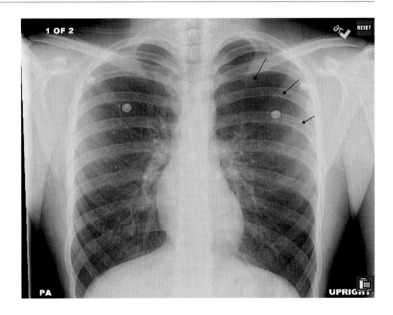

14.5.5 Traumatic Asphyxia (Perthes Syndrome)

Traumatic asphyxia is the inability to breathe due to compression of the thorax. Removal of the compressive force allows resumption of breathing and recovery. Commonly reported causes are compression from garage doors, motor vehicles, furniture, and other heavy objects. This results in global hypoxia most often rendering the patient unconscious followed by cerebral injury and death if the compression is not promptly relieved. Signs and symptoms include subconjunctival hemorrhage; facial, neck, and chest petechiae; and facial edema (Fig. 14.9). In hospitals, mortality rates are very low if these children survive the actual event.

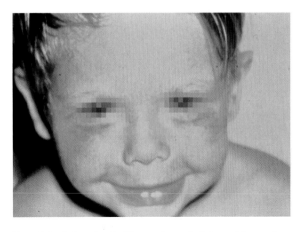

Fig. 14.9 Subconjuctival hemorrhage, facial petechiae, and edema from asphyxia

Further Reading

Bliss D, Silen M (2002) Pediatric thoracic trauma. Crit Care Med 30:s409–s415

Haxhija EQ, Nores H, Schober P, Hollwarth ME (2004) Lung contusion—Lacerations after blunt thoracic trauma in children. Pediatr Surg Int 20:412–414

Mendelson KG, Fallat ME (2007) Pediatric injuries prevention to resolution. Surg Clin N Am 87:207–228

Oldham KT, Colombani PM, Foglia RP, Skinner MA (2005) Principles and practice of pediatric surgery. Lippincott, Williams & Wilkins, Philadelphia, PA

Puri P, Höllwarth M (2006) Pediatric Surgery. Springer, Berlin, Heidelberg

Shehata S, Shabaan B (2006) Diaphragmatic injuries in children after blunt abdominal trauma. J Pediatr Surg 41:1727–1731

Wesson DE et al (2006) Pediatric Trauma. Taylor and Francis Group, New York and London

Westra SJ, Wallace EC (2005) Imaging evaluation of pediatric chest trauma. Radiol Clinic N Am 43:267–281

Abdominal and Genitourinary Trauma

15

Steven Stylianos, Barry A. Hicks, and Richard H. Pearl

Contents

15.1 Introduction

Who could have imagined the influence of James Simpson's publication in 1968 on the successful *nonoperative* treatment of select children presumed to have splenic injury. Nearly four decades later, the standard treatment of hemodynamically stable children with splenic injury is nonoperative and this concept has now been successfully applied to most blunt injuries of the liver, kidney, and pancreas as well. Surgical restraint has been the theme based on an increased awareness of the anatomic patterns and physiologic responses characteristic of injured children. Our colleagues in adult trauma care have slowly acknowledged this success and applied many of the principles learned in pediatric trauma to their patients.

Few surgeons have extensive experience with massive abdominal solid organ injury requiring immediate surgery. It is imperative that surgeons familiarize themselves with current treatment algorithms for life-threatening abdominal trauma. Important contributions have been made in the diagnosis and treatment of children with abdominal injury by radiologists and endoscopists. The resolution and speed of computed tomography (CT), screening capabilities of focused abdominal sonography for trauma (FAST), and the percutaneous, angiographic, and endoscopic interventions of non-surgeon members of the pediatric trauma team have all enhanced patient care and improved outcomes. Each section of this chapter will focus on the more common blunt injuries and unique aspects of care in children.

P. Puri and M. Höllwarth (eds.), *Pediatric Surgery: Diagnosis and Management,*
DOI: 10.1007/978-3-540-69560-8_15, © Springer-Verlag Berlin Heidelberg 2009

15.2 Diagnostic Modalities

The initial evaluation of the acutely injured child is similar to that of the adult. Plain radiography of the C-spine, chest, and pelvis are obtained following the initial survey and evaluation of A (airway), B (breathing), and C (circulation). Other plain abdominal films offer little in the acute evaluation of the pediatric trauma patient. As imaging modalities have improved, treatment algorithms have changed significantly in children with suspected intra-abdominal injuries. Prompt identification of potentially life-threatening injuries is now possible in the vast majority of children.

15.2.1 Computerized Tomography

Computerized tomography has now become the imaging study of choice for the evaluation of injured children due to several advantages. It is readily accessible in most health care facilities, it is noninvasive, it is a very accurate method of identifying and qualifying the extent of abdominal injury, and it has reduced the incidence of nontherapeutic exploratory laparotomy.

Use of intravenous contrast is essential and utilization of "dynamic" methods of scanning have optimized vascular and parenchymal enhancement. A head CT, if indicated, should first be performed without contrast, to avoid contrast concealing a hemorrhagic brain injury. Enteral contrast for enhancement of the gastrointestinal tract is generally not required in the acute trauma setting and can lead to aspiration.

Not all children with potential abdominal injuries are candidates for CT evaluation. Obvious penetrating injury often necessitates immediate operative intervention. The hemodynamically unstable child should not be taken out of an appropriate resuscitation room for a CT. These children may benefit from an alternative diagnostic study, such as a diagnostic peritoneal lavage, FAST, or urgent operative intervention. The greatest limitation of abdominal CT scanning in trauma is the lack of ability to reliably identify intestinal rupture. Findings suggestive but not diagnostic of intestinal perforation are pneumoperitoneum, bowel wall thickening, free intraperitoneal fluid, bowel wall enhancement, and dilated bowel. A high index of suspicion should exist for the presence of a bowel injury in the child with intraperitoneal fluid and no identifiable solid organ injury on CT scanning. Diagnosis and treatment of bowel injury will be reviewed in detail below.

15.2.2 Focused Abdominal Sonography for Trauma

Clinician-performed sonography for the early evaluation of the injured child is currently being evaluated to determine its optimal use. Examination of Morrison's pouch, the pouch of Douglas, the left flank to include the peri-splenic anatomy, and a subxiphoid view to visualize the pericardium is the standard four-view FAST exam (Fig. 15.1). This bedside exam may be useful as a rapid screening study, particularly in patients who are too unstable to undergo an abdominal

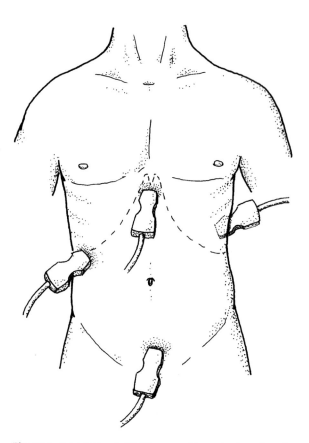

Fig. 15.1 Schematic of a FAST exam with emphasis on the subxiphoid, RUQ/Morrison's pouch, LUQ/left para-colic, and pelvic/Pouch of Douglas views
Source: Original illustration by Mark Mazziotti, MD

CT scan. Early reports have found FAST to be a useful screening tool in children, with a high specificity (95%), but a low sensitivity (33%) in identifying intestinal injury. A lack of identifiable free fluid does not exclude a significant injury. FAST may be very useful in decreasing the number of CT scans performed for "low-likelihood" injuries. The study may need to be repeated, dependent upon clinical correlation and the finding of free fluid in itself is not an indication for surgical intervention.

15.2.2.1 Laparoscopy

Large prospective trials in adults utilizing laparoscopy have demonstrated an increased diagnostic accuracy, decreased nontherapeutic laparotomy rates, and significant decrease in length of stay with attendant reduction in costs. Multiple studies have shown (principally in adults) the utility of laparoscopy in not only trauma evaluation but in definitive management of related injuries. Repairs of intestinal perforations, bladder ruptures, liver lacerations, diaphragmatic injuries, gastrostomy repair, splenic injuries, etc. have all been reported. The extent of operations feasible is directly related to the skill of the surgeon at advanced laparoscopic techniques and the overall stability of the patient. As with elective abdominal surgery, the role of laparoscopy in trauma will increase substantially as training programs and trauma centers redirect their training of residents to this modality and as more pediatric centers report outcome studies for laparoscopic trauma management in children.

15.3 Solid Organ Injury

15.3.1 Spleen and Liver

The spleen and liver are the organs most commonly injured in blunt abdominal trauma with each accounting for one third of the injuries. Nonoperative treatment of isolated splenic and hepatic injuries in stable children is now standard practice. Although nonoperative treatment of children with isolated, blunt spleen or liver injury has been universally successful, there has been great variation in the management algorithms used by individual pediatric surgeons. Controversy

also exists regarding the utility of CT grading and the finding of contrast "blush" as predictors of outcome in liver and spleen injury. Several recent studies have reported rates of contrast "blush" on CT between 7% and 12% in 365 children with blunt spleen injury. The rate of operation in the "blush" group approached or exceeded 20%. The authors emphasized that CT "blush" was worrisome but that most patients could still be managed successfully without operation. The role of angiographic embolization in pediatric spleen injury has yet to be determined.

Recently, the American Pediatric Surgical Association (APSA) Trauma Committee has defined consensus guidelines for resource utilization in hemodynamically stable children with isolated liver or spleen injury based on CT grading by analyzing a contemporary, multi-institution database of 832 children treated nonoperatively at 32 centers in North America from 1995 to 1997. Consensus guidelines on ICU stay, length of hospital stay, use of follow-up imaging, and physical activity restriction for clinically stable children with isolated spleen or liver injuries (Grades I–IV) were defined by analysis of this database (Table 15.1).

The guidelines were then applied prospectively in 312 children with liver or spleen injuries treated nonoperatively at 16 centers from 1998 to 2000. Patients with other minor injuries such as non-displaced, non-comminuted fractures or soft tissue injuries were included as long as the associated injuries did not influence the variables in this study. The patients were grouped by severity of injury defined by CT grade. Compliance with the proposed guidelines was analyzed for age, organ injured, and injury grade. The recovery of all patients was monitored for 4 months

Table 15.1 Proposed guidelines for resource utilization in children with isolated spleen or liver injury

CT Grade	I	II	III	IV
ICU days	None	None	None	1 day
Hospital stay	2 days	3 days	4 days	5 days
Pre-discharge imaging	None	None	None	None
Post-discharge imaging	None	None	None	None
Activity restriction[a]	3 weeks	4 weeks	5 weeks	6 weeks

[a]Return to **full contact, competitive sports** (i.e., football, wrestling, hockey, lacrosse, mountain climbing, etc.) should be at the discretion of the individual pediatric trauma surgeon. The proposed guidelines for return to unrestricted activity include **"normal" age-appropriate activities**.

Table 15.2   Effect of hospital-type and professional training on the probability of splenic operation

Database	Comparison	Number of Patients	Patient Distrib.	Adjusted Odds Ratio (95% CI)	P Value
Kid 2000—AHRQ	General hospital vs. children's hospital	2191	85:15	**2.85** (1.43, 5.69)	<0.003
New England Pediatric Trauma Database—UHDDS	General surgeon vs. pediatric surgeon	2631	68:32	**3.1** (2.3, 4.4)	<0.0001
Pennsylvania UHDDS	Adult or non-TC vs. pediatric TC	3145	85:15	**6.19** (4.43, 8.66)	<0.0001
CA, FL, NJ, NY UHDDS	Non-TC vs. TC	3232	34:66	**2.12** (1.45, 3.09)	<0.0001

Kid 2000—AHRQ: Agency for Healthcare Research and Quality's Hospital Cost Utilization Project State Inpatient Database for the Year 2000.
UHDDS: uniform hospital discharge data sets; TC: trauma center; CI: confidence intervals.

after injury. It is imperative to emphasize that these proposed guidelines assume hemodynamic stability. The extremely low rates of transfusion and operation document the stability of the study patients.

Not surprisingly, adult trauma services have reported excellent survival rates for pediatric trauma patients; however, analysis of treatment for spleen and liver injuries reveals alarmingly high rates of operative treatment (Table 15.2). This discrepancy in operative rates emphasizes the importance of disseminating effective guidelines as the majority of seriously injured children are treated outside of dedicated pediatric trauma centers.

15.3.2 Complications of Nonoperative Treatment

Nonoperative treatment protocols have been the standard for most children with blunt liver and spleen injury during the past two decades. The cumulative experience gained allows us to evaluate both the benefits and risks of the nonoperative approach. Fundamental to the success of the nonoperative strategy is the early, spontaneous cessation of hemorrhage. Transfusion rates for children with isolated spleen or liver injury have fallen below 10% confirming the lack of continued blood loss in the majority of patients. Despite many favorable observations, isolated reports of significant delayed hemorrhage with adverse outcome continue to appear. Shilyansky et al. reported two children with delayed hemorrhage 10 days after blunt liver injury. Both children had persistent right upper quadrant (RUQ) and right shoulder pain despite normal vital signs and stable hematocrits. The authors recommended continued in-house observation until

symptoms resolve. Recent reports described patients with significant bleeding 38 days after Grade II spleen injury and 24 days after Grade IV liver injury. These rare occurrences create anxiety in identifying the minimum safe interval prior to resuming unrestricted activities.

15.3.3 Sequelae of Damage Control Strategies

Even the most severe solid organ injuries can be treated without surgery if there is prompt response to resuscitation. In contrast, emergency laparotomy and/or embolization are indicated in patients who are hemodynamically unstable despite fluid and red blood cell transfusion. Most spleen and liver injuries requiring operation are amenable to simple methods of hemostasis using a combination of manual compression, direct suture, topical hemostatic agents, and mesh wrapping. In young children with significant hepatic injury, the sternum can be divided rapidly to expose the supra-hepatic or intra-pericardial inferior vena cava (IVC) allowing for total hepatic vascular isolation (Fig. 15.2). Children will tolerate periods of vascular isolation as long as their blood volume is replenished. With this exposure the liver and major peri-hepatic veins can be isolated and the bleeding controlled to permit direct suture repair or ligation of the offending vessel. While the cumbersome and dangerous technique of atrio-caval shunting has been largely abandoned, newer endovascular balloon catheters can be useful for temporary vascular occlusion to allow access to the juxtahepatic vena cava.

The early morbidity and mortality of severe hepatic injuries are related to the effects of massive blood loss

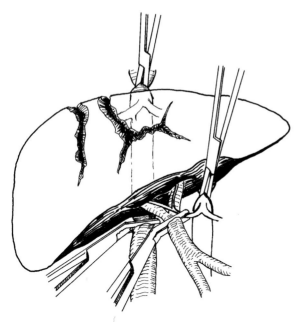

Fig. 15.2 Total hepatic vascular isolation with occlusion of the porta, supra-, and infra-hepatic inferior vena cava, and supra-celiac aorta (optional)
Source: Original illustration by Mark Mazziotti, MD

Table 15.3 "Damage control" strategy in the exsanguinating trauma patient

Phase 1	Abbreviated laparotomy for exploration
	Control of hemorrhage and contamination
	Packing and temporary abdominal wall closure
Phase 2	Aggressive ICU resuscitation
	Core rewarming
	Optimize volume and oxygen delivery
	Correction of coagulopathy
Phase 3	Planned reoperation(s) for packing change
	Definitive repair of injuries
	Abdominal wall closure

and replacement with large volumes of cold blood products. The consequences of prolonged operations with massive blood product replacement include hypothermia, coagulopathy, and acidosis. Maintenance of physiologic stability during the struggle for surgical control of severe bleeding is a formidable challenge even for the most experienced operative team, particularly when hypothermia, coagulopathy, and acidosis occur. This triad creates a vicious cycle in which each derangement exacerbates the others and the physiologic and metabolic consequences of the triad often preclude completion of the procedure. Lethal coagulopathy from dilution, hypothermia, and acidosis can occur rapidly. The infusion of activated recombinant Factor VII in patients with massive hemorrhage has been promising in several case reports.

Increased emphasis on physiologic and metabolic stability in emergency abdominal operations has led to the development of staged, multidisciplinary treatment plans including abbreviated laparotomy, peri-hepatic packing, temporary abdominal closure, angiographic embolization, and endoscopic biliary stenting. Trauma surgeons treating critically injured children must familiarize themselves with this life-saving technique. Abbreviated lapa-

rotomy with packing for hemostasis allowing resuscitation prior to planned reoperation is an alternative in unstable patients where further blood loss would be untenable. This "damage control" philosophy is a systematic, phased approach to the management of the exsanguinating trauma patient. The three phases of damage control are detailed in Table 15.3. Once patients are rewarmed, coagulation factors replaced, and oxygen delivery optimized the patient can be returned to the operating room for pack removal and definitive repair of injuries.

It is essential to emphasize that the success of the abbreviated laparotomy and planned reoperation depends on an early decision to employ this strategy prior to irreversible shock. Abdominal packing, when employed as a desperate, last-ditch resort after prolonged attempts at hemostasis have failed has been uniformly unsuccessful. Physiologic and anatomic criteria have been identified as indications for abdominal packing. Most of these have focused on intra-operative parameters including pH (~7.2), core temperature (<35°C), and coagulation values (prothrombin time > 16 s) in the patient with profuse hemorrhage requiring large volumes of blood product transfusion.

The optimal time for reexploration is controversial because neither the physiologic endpoints of resuscitation nor the increased risk of infection with prolonged packing are well defined. The obvious benefits of hemostasis provided by packing are also balanced against the potential deleterious effects of increased intra-abdominal pressure on ventilation, cardiac output, renal function, mesenteric circulation, and intracranial pressure. Timely alleviation of the secondary "abdominal compartment syndrome" may be a critical salvage maneuver for patients. Temporary abdominal wall closure at the time of packing can prevent the abdominal compartment syndrome. We recommend temporary abdominal wall expansion in all patients requiring packing until the hemostasis is obtained and visceral edema subsides.

A staged operative strategy for unstable trauma patients represents **advanced** surgical care and requires sound judgment and technical expertise. Intra-abdominal packing for control of exsanguinating hemorrhage is a life-saving maneuver in highly selected patients in whom coagulopathy, hypothermia and acidosis render further surgical procedures unduly hazardous. Early identification of patients likely to benefit from abbreviated laparotomy techniques is crucial for success.

15.3.4 Abdominal Compartment Syndrome

The abdominal compartment syndrome is a term used to describe the deleterious effects of increased intra-abdominal pressure. The "syndrome" includes respiratory insufficiency from worsening ventilation/perfusion mismatch, hemodynamic compromise from pre-load reduction due to IVC compression, impaired renal function from renal vein compression as well as decreased cardiac output, intracranial hypertension from increased ventilator pressures, splanchnic hypoperfusion, and abdominal wall overdistention. The causes of intra-abdominal hypertension in trauma patients include hemoperitoneum, retroperitoneal, and/or bowel edema and use of abdominal/pelvic packing. The combination of tissue injury and hemodynamic shock creates a cascade of events including capillary leak, ischemia-reperfusion, and release of vasoactive mediators and free radicals, which combine to increase extracellular volume and tissue edema. Experimental evidence indicates significant alterations in cytokine levels in the presence of sustained intra-abdominal pressure elevation. Once the combined effects of tissue edema and intra-abdominal fluid exceed a certain level, abdominal decompression must be considered.

The adverse effects of abdominal compartment syndrome have been acknowledged for decades; however, abdominal compartment syndrome has only recently been recognized as a life-threatening yet potentially treatable entity. The measurement of intra-abdominal pressure can be useful in determining the contribution of abdominal compartment syndrome to altered physiologic and metabolic parameters. Intra-abdominal pressure can be determined by measuring bladder pressure.

This involves instilling 1 ml/kg of saline into the Foley catheter and connecting it to a pressure transducer or manometer via a three-way stopcock. The symphysis pubis is used as the zero reference point and the pressure measured in cm H_2O or mm Hg. Intra-abdominal pressures in the range of 20–35 cm H_2O or 15–25 mm Hg have been identified as an indication to decompress the abdomen. Many prefer to intervene according to alterations in other physiologic and metabolic parameters rather than a specific pressure measurement. Anecdotally, decompressive laparotomy has been used successfully to reduce refractory intracranial hypertension in patients with isolated brain injury without overt signs of abdominal compartment syndrome.

Many materials have been suggested for use in temporary patch abdominoplasty including silastic sheeting, Goretex® sheeting, intravenous bags, cystoscopy bags, ostomy appliances, and various mesh materials (Fig. 15.3). The vacuum pack technique, used successfully in adults, seems promising.

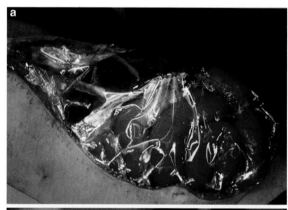

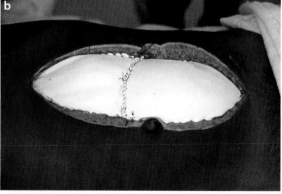

Fig. 15.3   a. Abdominal wall expansion with silastic sheeting. **b**. Abdominal wall expansion with goretex patch

15.3.5 Bile Duct Injury

Nonoperative management of pediatric blunt liver injury is highly successful but is complicated by a 4% risk of persistent bile leakage. Radionucleide scanning is recommended when biliary tree injury is suspected. Delayed views may show a bile leak even if early views are normal. Several reports have highlighted the benefits of endoscopic retrograde cholangio-pancreatography (ERCP) with placement of transampullary biliary stents for biliary duct injury following blunt hepatic trauma acknowledging that while ERCP is invasive and requires conscious sedation, it can pinpoint the site of injury and allow treatment of the injured ducts without open surgery. Endoscopic transampullary biliary decompression is a recent addition to treatment for patients with persistent bile leakage. The addition of sphincterotomy during ERCP for persistent bile leakage following blunt liver injury has been advocated to decrease intrabiliary pressure and encouraged internal decompression. It is important to note that endoscopic biliary stents may migrate or clog and require specific treatment.

15.4 Injuries to the Duodenum and Pancreas

In contrast to the liver and spleen, injuries to the duodenum and pancreas are much less frequent, reported as less than 10% of intra-abdominal injuries in children sustaining blunt trauma. Isolated duodenal and pancreatic injuries occur in approximately two third of cases with combined injury to both organs in the remainder of cases. The severity of the injury and other associated injuries determines the necessity for operative versus nonoperative management. The "protected" retroperitoneum both limits the chance of injury but increases the difficulty in early diagnosis. Added to this diagnostic dilemma is the frequency of associated intra-abdominal and/or multisystem injuries, which can mask subtle physical and radiographic diagnostic signs found in injury to the duodenum and pancreas.

15.4.1 Duodenum

A single-center experience in 27 children sustaining blunt duodenal injury (mean age of 7 years) revealed that 13 children had duodenal perforations (mean age = 9) and 14 sustained duodenal hematomas (mean age = 5). Associated injuries were seen in 19 (10 pancreas, 5 spleen, 4 hepatic, 2 long bone fracture, 1 CNS, 1 renal contusion, 1 jejunal perforation, and 1 gastric rupture). The median interval from injury to surgery was 6 h in those sustaining perforation. The clinical presentation, laboratory evaluation, and radiographic findings of those with duodenal hematoma versus perforation are summarized in Table 15.4. Most patients had abdominal CT scans performed with oral and IV contrast. A comparison of CT findings in these patient groups is

Table 15.4 Comparison of the presenting symptoms and signs in children with duodenal hematoma and duodenal perforation

Patient Characteristics	Duodenal Hematoma	Duodenal Perforation
N	14	13
Age (yr)	5	9*
ISS score	10	25*
Seat belt worn: n (%)	6 (100)	5 (71)
Presentation		
Pain or tenderness: n (%)	10 (71)	12 (92)
Bruising: n (%)	6 (43)	11 (85)
Glasgow coma scale	15	15
Associated injuries		
Pancreatic injury: n (%)	7 (50)	3 (23)
Lumbar spine injury: n (%)	1 (7)	4 (31)
Total: n (%)	11 (79)	8 (62)
Laboratory evaluation		
Hgb: (mg%)/Hct	12.3/0.36	12.1/0.37
Amylase: U (%)	678 (64)	332 (46)

*Statistically significant difference.

Table 15.5 Comparison of CT findings of children with duodenal hematoma and duodenal perforation

CT Findings	Duodenal Hematoma, $N = 10$ N (%)	Duodenal Perforation, $N = 9$ B (%)
Free air	1 (10)[a]	2 (22)
Free fluid	8 (80)	9 (100)
Retroperitoneal fluid	9 (90)	9 (100)
Bowel wall and peritoneal enhancement	2 (20)	4 (44)
Duodenal caliber change	4 (40)	3 (33)
Thickened duodenum	10 (100)	8 (89)
Mural hematoma	10 (100)	0
Retroperitoneal air	0	8 (89)
Retroperitoneal contrast[b]	0	4 (57)
Retroperitoneal air or contrast	0	9 (100)

[a]The child had an associated jejunal perforation.
[b]Enteral contrast was not administered in two children.

depicted in Table 15.5. These data demonstrate that the clinical presentation is strikingly similar in both groups with only age and ISS achieving significance statistically (but of little clinical relevance in individual patients). However, in comparing CT findings, extravasation of air or enteral contrast into the retroperitoneal, peri-duodenal, or pre-renal space was noted in every child with a duodenal perforation (9 of 9) and in none of 10 who had duodenal hematoma. The authors note that few previous reports in the literature describe these specific CT findings with duodenal injuries in general and no previous series of pediatric patients in particular with this data had previously been reported. The management of duodenal hematoma is expectant in most cases. The CT scans (or upper GI contrast studies in equivocal cases) showing duodenal narrowing, corkscrewing, or obstruction without extravasation was diagnostic in all. The experiences from Salt Lake City and Pittsburgh emphasize an alarming finding that a common cause of duodenal trauma was child abuse, especially in younger patients. Therefore, isolated duodenal injures should raise suspicion if the history and/or mechanism of injury described is inconsistent.

In all of these series, patients sustaining duodenal perforation were treated operatively in a variety of ways depending on the severity of the injury and surgeon's preference. We recommend primary closure of the duodenal perforation (whenever possible). Primary closure can be combined with duodenal drainage and either pyloric exclusion with gastro-jejunostomy (Fig. 15.4) or gastric drainage with feeding jejunostomy. These surgical options decrease the incidence of duodenal fistula, reduce the time to GI tract alimentation, and shorten hospital stay. An effective combination,

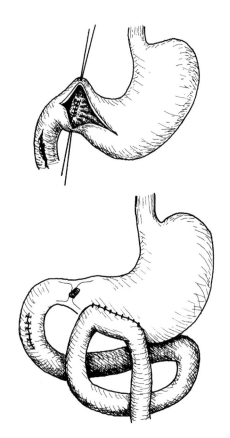

Fig. 15.4 Lateral duodenal injury treated by primary duodenal repair and "pyloric exclusion" consisting of closing the pylorus with an absorbable suture and gastrojejunostomy. Closed suction drainage of the repair is not depicted in this drawing
Source: Original illustration by Mark Mazziotti, MD

when faced with complicated duodenal trauma, is the "three tube technique": duodenal closure (primary repair, serosal patch, or anastomosis) with duodenal drainage tube for decompression (tube 1), pyloric exclusion with an absorbable suture via gastrotomy and gastric tube placement (tube 2), and feeding jejunostomy (tube 3). Several closed suction drains are placed adjacent to the repair. When the duodenum is excluded (via an absorbable suture for temporary closure of the pylorus), complete healing of the injury routinely occurs prior to the spontaneous reopening of the pyloric channel (Fig. 15.5). However, no matter what repair the surgeon selects, a summary of the literature demonstrates that protecting the duodenal closure (drain and exclusion) and a route for enteral feeds (gastrojejunostomy or feeding jejunostomy) reduces morbidity and shortens hospital stay. A summary of the surgical options are listed in Table 15.6 and illustrated in Figs. 15.4 and 15.5. Of note, a pancreaticoduodenectomy (Whipple Procedure) should rarely be required. Although occasionally reported in the literature, pancreaticoduodenectomy should be reserved for the most severe injuries to the duodenum and pancreas

Table 15.6 Surgical options in duodenal trauma

Repair of the duodenum
Diversion of the GI tract (pyloric exclusion or a duodenal diverticulization)
Gastric decompression (gastric tube insertion or gastrojejunostomy)
GI tract access for feeding (jejunostomy tube or gastrojejunal anastomosis)
Decompression of the duodenum (duodenostomy tube)
Biliary tube drainage
Wide drainage of the repaired area (lateral duodenal drains)

when the common blood supply is destroyed and any possibility of reconstruction is impossible.

15.4.2 Pancreas

Injuries to the pancreas are slightly more frequent than duodenal injuries with estimated ranges from 3% to 12% in children sustaining blunt abdominal trauma. Recently, two centers (Toronto and San Diego) reported their experience with divergent methods of managing blunt traumatic pancreatic injuries in a series of reports. A summary comparing the San Diego and Toronto protocols is depicted in Table 15.7. The striking differences in these series are: the 100% diagnostic sensitivity of CT scanning in Toronto versus 69% in San Diego and the 44% operative rate in San Diego versus 0% in Toronto. The authors of the Toronto protocol conclude that following nonoperative management of pancreatic blunt trauma, atrophy (distal) or recanalization occurs in all cases with no long-term morbidity. Important concepts include the efficacy of magnetic resonance cholangio-pancreatography (MRCP) as a diagnostic tool, early ERCP intervention for diagnosis and treatment with ductal stenting, and the use of somatostatin to decrease pancreatic secretions and promote healing.

These reports from major pediatric trauma centers are clearly in conflict. Some favor and document the efficacy and safety of observational care for virtually all pancreatic traumas to include duct disruption while others advocate aggressive surgical management with debridement and/or resections. Since proponents of each supply compelling data for these treatments algorithms individual hospital/surgeon preference will probably determine which treatment plan is selected. However, it is clear that with simple transection of the pancreas at or to the left of the spine, spleen-sparing distal pancreatectomy

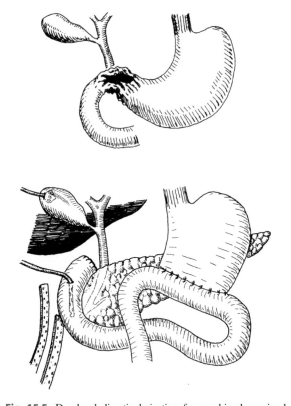

Fig. 15.5 Duodenal diverticularization for combined proximal duodenal and pancreatic injury. Resection and closure of the duodenal stump, tube duodenostomy, tube cholecystectomy, gastrojejunostomy, and multiple closed suction drains are depicted. A feeding jejunostomy should be strongly considered (not depicted) *Source*: Original illustration by Mark Mazziotti, MD

Table 15.7 A comparison
of protocols in the
management of blunt
pancreas injury in children

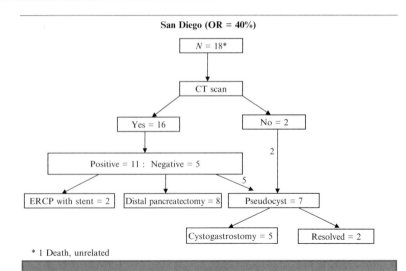

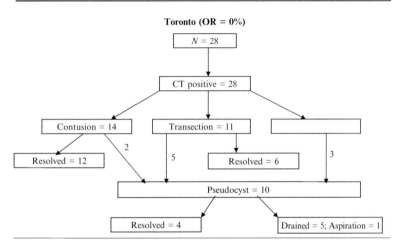

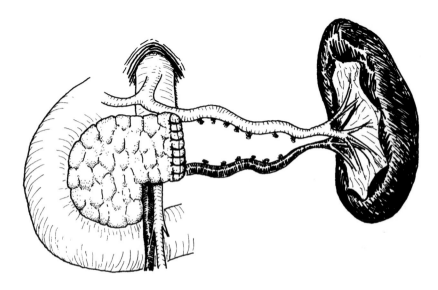

Fig. 15.6 Spleen-sparing
distal pancreatectomy
Source: Original illustration
by Mark Mazziotti, MD

can accomplish definitive care for this isolated injury with short hospitalization and acceptable morbidity (Fig. 15.6).

15.5 The "Seat Belt Sign"

Frequent physical exams and vigilance is required for the subset of injuries caused in children with lap belt restraints while passengers in high speed automobile crashes. These children present with visible "seat belt signs" on physical exam of the abdomen (Fig. 15.7). Multiple studies have documented increased abdominal injuries to both solid and hollow organs with this finding. An interesting triad of injuries have been noted with abdominal wall contusions/herniation, chance fractures of the lumbar spine, and isolated jejunal/ileal perforations. One report reviewed 95 patients all wearing seat belts admitted with abdominal trauma. In 60 of 95, there was an occurrence of "seat belt sign." The proportion of patients with intestinal injuries with and without the seat belt sign were 9/60 and 0/35, respectively. The more common injuries described above can distract both the patient and the trauma team causing delay in the diagnosis of serious vascular injuries involving the aorta and iliac vessels.

One in every nine children with an abdominal seat belt sign has a significant intra-abdominal injury. Therefore, although the seat belt sign is rare, CT scanning, admission, and serial examination is mandated when it is present. After adjusting for age and seating position, optimally restrained children were more than three times less likely as suboptimally restrained children to suffer an abdominal injury.

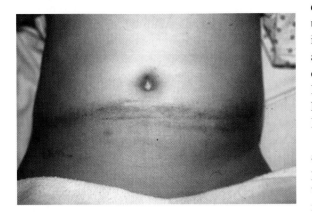

Fig. 15.7 Seat belt sign across lower abdomen

15.5.1 Imaging for Gastrointestinal Injury

Imaging of the GI tract has evolved over the past decade, with spiral CT and/or a FAST exam done by surgeons in the ER directly impacting our diagnostic accuracy and decision making. Some of the strengths and weaknesses of CT diagnosis have been discussed. However, our ability to diagnose and treat blunt abdominal trauma in children has been clearly enhanced by this modality. The significance of isolated free intraperitoneal fluid in the absence of solid organ injury has frequently been heralded as a sign of intestinal trauma. FAST was found to be useful as a screening tool with high specificity (95%), but unfortunately low sensitivity (33%) in evaluating intestinal injury. Clearly, as a screening tool, FAST can perhaps decrease the number of CT scans performed, but it will not allow for the diagnosis of specific abdominal organs injured. Finally, to come full circle, in a large study from Pittsburgh, 350 children with abdominal trauma were reviewed, with 30 requiring laparotomy (8.5%). There were 5 false negative CT scans (26%) in 19 patients who underwent delayed laparotomy (3.5 h or more post-injury). They concluded that serial physical examination and not CT scanning was the "gold standard" for diagnosing GI tract perforations in children. We concur!

15.6 Renal Trauma

The kidney is the most commonly injured organ in the urogenital system and children appear to be more susceptible to major renal trauma than adults. Several unique anatomic aspects contribute to this observation including: less cushioning from perirenal fat, weaker abdominal musculature, and a less well ossified thoracic cage. The child's kidney also occupies a proportionally larger space in the retroperitoneum than does an adult's kidney. In addition, the pediatric kidney may retain fetal lobulations, permitting easier parenchymal disruption.

Preexisting or congenital renal abnormalities, such as hydronephrosis, tumors, or abnormal position, may predispose the kidney to trauma despite relatively mild traumatic forces. Historically, congenital abnormalities in injured kidneys have been reported to vary from 1% to 21%. More accurate recent reviews have shown that incidence rates are 1–5%. Renal abnormalities, particularly hydronephrotic kidneys, may be first diagnosed after minor blunt abdominal trauma. Most often, these patients present with hematuria following blunt trauma. Others may present with an acute abdomen secondary to intraperitoneal rupture of the hydronephrotic kidney.

Major deceleration and flexion injuries can lead to renal artery or vein injuries due to stretching forces on a normally fixed vascular pedicle. This type of injury may be more common in children because of their increased flexibility and renal mobility. Posttraumatic thrombosis of the renal artery occurs secondary to an intimal tear. The intimal layer tears from the wall of the vessel because the media and adventitia of the renal artery are more elastic than the intima. The intimal tear produces turbulence, thrombosis, and eventual occlusion that then results in renal ischemia. A high index of suspicion must be maintained in order to identify these injuries.

15.6.1 Diagnosis of Renal Injury

Once the patient has been resuscitated and life-threatening injuries have been addressed, evaluation of the genitourinary system can be undertaken. Following any blunt injury, the presence of hematuria (microscopic or gross), a palpable flank mass, or flank hematomas are indications for urologic evaluations. Most major blunt renal injuries occur in association with other major injuries of the head, chest, and abdomen. Urologic investigations should be undertaken when trauma to the lower chest is associated with rib, thoracic, or lumbar spine fractures. It should also be undertaken in all crush injuries to the abdomen or pelvis when the patient has sustained a severe deceleration injury. Since a renal pedicle injury or ureteropelvic junction (UPJ) disruption may not be associated with one of the classic signs of renal injury, such as hematuria, radiologic evaluation of the urinary tract should always be considered in patients with a mechanism of injury that could potentially injure the upper urinary tract.

Gross hematuria is the most reliable indicator for serious urological injury. The need for imaging in the patient with blunt trauma and microscopic hematuria is not as clear cut. The degree of hematuria does not always correlate with the degree of injury. Renal vascular pedicle avulsion or acute thrombosis of segmental arteries can occur in the absence of hematuria while mild renal contusions can present with gross hematuria. Guidelines for evaluating the pediatric population are not as clearly defined. All children with any degree of microscopic hematuria after blunt trauma have traditionally undergone renal imaging. The presence of multisystem trauma significantly increases the risk for significant renal damage. It is reasonable to consider observation with no renal imaging in children with microscopic hematuria of <50 RBC/HPF that are stable and without a mechanism of injury that is suspect for renal injury.

CT scans are now used almost exclusively as the imaging study of choice for suspected renal trauma in hemodynamically stable adults and children. CT is both sensitive and specific for demonstrating parenchymal laceration, urinary extravasation, delineating segmental parenchymal infarcts, determining the size and location of the surrounding retroperitoneal hematoma, and/or associated intra-abdominal injury. CT also allows for accurate staging of the renal injury.

It is imperative to acknowledge that major renal injuries such as UPJ disruption or segmental arterial thrombosis may occur without the presence of hematuria or hypotension. Therefore, a high index of suspicion is necessary to diagnose these injuries. Nonvisualization of the injured kidney on intra-venous pyelogram (IVP), or failure to uptake contrast with a large associated perirenal hematoma on CT are hallmark findings for renal artery thrombosis. UPJ disruption is classically seen as perihilar extravasation of contrast with nonvisualization of the distal ureter.

15.6.2 Treatment of Renal Injury

In most patients, attempts should be made to manage all renal injuries conservatively. Minor renal injuries constitute the majority of blunt renal injuries and usually resolve without incident. The management of major renal parenchymal lacerations, although accounting for only 10–15% of all renal trauma patients, is currently controversial. Surgery is not always mandatory and many major renal injuries due to blunt trauma may be managed conservatively. When necessary, the goals of surgical renal exploration are to either definitively treat major renal injuries with preservation of renal parenchyma when possible, or to thoroughly evaluate a suspected renal injury. The need for surgical exploration is much higher in patients with penetrating trauma as opposed to blunt trauma.

The indications for renal exploration vary greatly between individual trauma centers. Most centers manage Grade I–III injuries with bed rest and observation, as expected. Controversies arise in the management of Grade IV–V injuries. The majority of blunt renal injuries sustained are contusions and lacerations that are minor in nature. Even in the presence of gross hematuria, most blunt renal injuries will not require exploration and will have excellent long-term outcomes. **Absolute indications** for renal exploration include persistent life-threatening bleeding, an expanding, pulsatile, or uncontained retroperitoneal hematoma, or suspected renal pedicle avulsion. Relative indications for exploration include substantial devitalized renal parenchyma or urinary extravasation. Urinary extravasation in itself does not demand surgical exploration. Matthews reported that in patients with major renal injury and urinary extravasation that are managed conservatively, urinary extravasation resolved spontaneously in 87%. Extravasation persisted in 13% and was successfully managed endoscopically. Incomplete staging of the renal injury demands either further imaging or renal exploration and reconstruction. Most commonly, these patients undergo renal exploration because they have persistent bleeding, or because they have an associated injury that requires laparotomy.

When conservative management is chosen, supportive care with bed rest, hydration, antibiotics, and serial hemoglobin and blood pressure monitoring is required for uneventful healing. After the gross hematuria resolves, limited activity is allowed for 2–4 weeks until microscopic hematuria ceases. Early complications can occur with observation within the first 4 weeks of injury and include delayed bleeding, abscess, sepsis, urinary fistula, urinary extravasation and urinoma, and hypertension. The greatest risk is delayed hemorrhage occurring within the first 2 weeks of injury and this may be life threatening. Immediate surgical exploration or angiographic embolization is indicated. Angiographic embolization is an alternative to surgery in a hemodynamically stable patient in whom persistent gross hematuria signifies persistent low grade hemorrhage from the injured kidney. Persistent urinary extravasation has successfully been managed by percutaneous drainage. Hypertension in the early post-trauma period is uncommon. Hypertension may develop in the ensuing months and in most instances is treated with medical management.

15.6.3 Renal Exploration and Reconstruction

If operation is required, early control of the vessels increases the rate of renal salvage. When proximal vascular control is initially achieved before any renal exploration, nephrectomy is required in less than 12% of cases. When primary vascular control is not achieved and massive bleeding is encountered, in the rush to control bleeding, a kidney that could have been salvaged may be sacrificed unnecessarily. The surgeon must carefully identify the kidney's relationships with the posterior abdomen and the posterior parietal peritoneum. The colon is lifted from the abdomen and placed on the anterior chest in order to allow mobilization of the small bowel. The inferior mesenteric vein and the aorta are identified at this point, and the posterior peritoneum is incised medial to the inferior epigastric vein. The aorta is dissected above the level of the ligament of Treitz, where the left renal vein is found crossing anterior to the aorta. Retraction of the left renal vein exposes both renal arteries beneath, which may now be isolated and controlled with vessel loops. Once vessel isolation is complete, an incision is made in the peritoneum just lateral to the colon. The colon is reflected medially to expose the retroperitoneal hematoma in its entirety and the kidney may be exposed. If significant bleeding is encountered, the ipsilateral renal vessels may be occluded. Warm ischemia time should not surpass 30 min.

Renal vascular injuries must be addressed promptly. Major lacerations to the renal vein are repaired directly by venorrhaphy. Repair of renal arterial injuries may require a variety of techniques, including resection and end-to-end anastomosis, bypass graft with autogenous vein or a synthetic graft, and arteriorrhaphy. Traumatic renal artery occlusion requires many of the same techniques for repair. However this must be performed in the first 12 h from the time of injury, otherwise, the kidney is usually nonviable following this length of ischemia.

Summary

Recent advances in the delivery of trauma and critical care in children have resulted in improved outcome following major injuries. It is imperative that pediatric surgeons familiarize themselves with current treatment algorithms for life-threatening abdominal trauma such as "damage control" and the consequences of the abdominal compartment syndrome. Important contributions have been made in the diagnosis and treatment of children with abdominal injury by radiologists and endoscopists. Clinical experience and published reports addressing specific concerns about the nonoperative treatment of children with solid organ injuries and recent radiologic and endoscopic contributions have made pediatric trauma care increasingly nonoperative. Although the trend is in this direction, the pediatric surgeon should remain the physician-of-record in the multidisciplinary care of critically injured children. *The decision not to operate is always a surgical decision!*

Further Reading

Acierno SP, Jurkovich GJ, Nathens AB (2004) Is pediatric trauma still a surgical disease? Patterns of emergent operative intervention in the injured child. J Trauma 56:960–966

Canty JG Sr, Weinman D (2001) Treatment of pancreatic duct disruption in children by an endoscopically placed stent. J Pediatr Surg 36:345–348

Chang MC, Miller PR, D'Agostino R et al (1998) Effects of abdominal decompression on cardiopulmonary function and visceral perfusion in patients with intra-abdominal hypertension. J Trauma 44:440–445

Hulka F, Mullins RJ, Leonardo V et al (1998) Significance of peritoneal fluid as an isolated finding on abdominal computed tomographic scans in pediatric trauma patients. J Trauma 44:1069–1072

Kushimoto S, Arai M, Aiboshi J et al (2003) The role of interventional radiology in patients requiring damage control laparotomy. J Trauma 54:171–176

Lenwand MJ, Atkinson CC, Mooney DP (2004) Application of the APSA evidence-based guidelines for isolated liver or spleen injuries: A single institution experience. J Pediatr Surg 39:487–490

Lutz N, Nance ML, Kallan MJ et al (2004) Incidence and clinical significance of abdominal wall bruising in restrained children involved in motor vehicle crashes. J Pediatr Surg 39:972–975

Mooney DP, Rothstein DH, Forbes PW (2006) Variation in the management of pediatric splenic injuries in the United States. J Trauma 61:330–333

Moss RL, Musemeche CA (1996) Clinical judgment is superior to diagnostic tests in the management of pediatric small bowel injury. J Pediatr Surg 8:1178–1181

Patel JC, Tepas JJ (1999) The efficacy of focused abdominal sonography for trauma (FAST) as a screening tool in the assessment of injured children. J Pediatric Surg 34:44–47, discussion 52–54

Puri P, Höllwarth ME (eds) (2006) Pediatric Surgery. Springer, Berlin, Heidelberg

Stylianos S, Egorova N, Guice KS, Arons R, Oldham KT (2006) Variation in treatment of pediatric spleen injury at trauma centers versus non-trauma centers: A call for dissemination of APSA benchmarks and guidelines. JACS 202:247–251

Tepas JJ, Frykberg ER, Schinco MA et al (2003) Pediatric trauma is very much a surgical disease. Ann Surg 237:775–781

Traumatic Head Injuries

16

Hans G. Eder

Contents

Head injuries are very common in children and account for most neurosurgical admissions to hospital. The majority are children with mild head injuries with a Glasgow coma scale (GCS) score of 13–15 without loss of consciousness or brief loss of consciousness for 5 min or less. About 10% of head injuries are severe as defined by a GCS score of 8 or less and the remaining are moderate head injuries with a GCS score of 9–13. The mortality rate of head injuries is five times higher than that of leukemia, which is the second most common cause of death in childhood and nearly 18 times higher than that of brain tumors. Only 20–30% of children with severe head injury require a neurosurgical operation.

Naturally, the etiology of traumatic brain injury varies according to age-specific activities of the child. As such, the most common cause of head injuries and skull fractures in small children are accidental falls whereas injuries in children older than 5 years are mostly a consequence of motor vehicle accidents. In some cases, children younger than 2 years of age are disproportionately affected by brain injuries from shaken baby syndrome.

In general, children have a lower mortality and better functional outcome than adults with similar injuries. The outcome in adolescents equals that of young adults whereas children of elementary school age do far better than very young ones.

The primary role of medical therapy is to prevent secondary brain injury from ischemia, increased intracranial pressure, focal brain compression, and brain edema. This therapy should begin with the initial resuscitation and continue throughout the child's stay at hospital.

P. Puri and M. Höllwarth (eds.), *Pediatric Surgery: Diagnosis and Management,*
DOI: 10.1007/978-3-540-69560-8_16, © Springer-Verlag Berlin Heidelberg 2009

16.1 Principles of Treatment

The primary injury occurs within a few milliseconds and damages the brain directly thus making it untreatable. Secondary injuries like brain ischemia are a significant and often preventable result from systemic hypotension or hypoxemia. Therefore, adequate pre-hospital care is crucial for these patients to avoid secondary injuries to the already injured brain and begins with the first aid at the accident scene. Hypoxemia is present in 30–45% of patients with severe head injuries, and even in 15% of patients with moderate head injuries.

When pre-hospital hypoxia and/or hypotension are present in patients with traumatic brain injuries, the mortality rate is significantly increased. Conversely, normotensive normoxic patients are associated with a good prognotis.

In addition to ischemia, increased intracranial pressure ICP due to epidural or subdural hematomas can lead to secondary injuries or focal swelling of the brain which often results in herniation syndrome without surgical intervention.

Initial clinical assessment, using either the GCS score or one of the modifications available for younger patients (children's coma score), is most important to identify the extent of head injury and the neurological status. The GCS score still remains a critical tool for grading the severity of neurological injury after traumatic brain injury and appears to correlate strongly with the outcome in children.

16.2 Management

16.2.1 Mild Head Trauma

Mild head trauma is defined as an injury to the head with a GCS score of 13–15. Depending on the child's age and the time after mild head trauma, most infants and small children will arrive alert or with minor alteration of consciousness. Young children are usually able to walk and respond well to verbal or painless stimuli. Vomiting is common. Neurological findings are typically normal. Older children complain of post-traumatic amnesia and intense headache. Clinical diagnosis should include examining the cervical spine, chest, abdomen, and limbs looking for other injuries. The vital signs of pulse rate, respiration, temperature, and blood pressure are recorded.

Most children with relatively mild injuries and a good clinical examination can be discharged from hospital and kept under observation by reliable family members at home.

For a child who has suffered loss of consciousness or amnesia, most neurosurgical departments will recommend admission for observation between 1 and 2 days and children with a skull fracture should be kept under observation for around 3 days. Children with intracranial lesions should be admitted to hospital for 5–7 days.

The appropriate evaluation of a child with apparent concussion is debatable. CT scans should be considered in all children with persistent symptoms or neurological findings. In the presence of localized scalp or penetrating injury, unconsciousness, or significant amnesia for over 10 min, CT scan should be obligatory. For children with mild or moderate head injuries, a follow-up CT scan should be performed prior to hospital discharge, if the initial CT scan showed intracranial lesions. A normal CT scan more than 6 h from the time of injury is sufficient unless the patient demonstrates neurological deterioration. An urgent follow-up CT scan should be performed for neurological deterioration, persistent vomiting, and seizures. If the initial CT scan reveals a nonoperative hematoma, repeat imaging should be performed within 24 h to ensure stabilization of the hematoma size.

CT scan is preferable to skull radiography because it provides more valuable information regarding anatomic evidence of brain injury and intracranial hemorrhage or raised intracranial pressure. Therefore, skull radiography is inadequate for assessing intracranial injuries because normal skull x-ray may occur despite significant intracerebral injury. Skull radiography was normal in 75% of minor head injury patients found to have intracranial lesions on CT scans and was only valuable in the treatment of 0.4–2% of patients. It is possibly useful for localizing a penetrating foreign body or in clinical signs suggesting an underlying fracture. Still, the increased probability of an intracranial injury in case of a skull fracture finally requires CT scan.

Skull x-rays are only recommended if CT scan is not available. MRI scans in trauma are usually not appropriate for acute head injuries. MRI may be helpful after the patient is stabilized to evaluate brain stem injuries or small white matter changes in the setting of a diffuse axonal injury. If the neurological status cannot be explained by CT scans alone, MRI is indicated for its higher sensitivity. However, in the acute phase of a trauma there were no surgical lesions demonstrated on MRI that were not evident on CT. Exact clinical examination before performing CT scan is of utmost importance because sedation for neuroimaging in very young children may disguise clinical assessment.

Once the child's clinical course demonstrates a return to baseline behavior and neurological function, discharge from hospital can be considered. Mild headaches or attention deficits for several weeks after injury may be expected. Guidelines for return to sports or other activities have not been standardized, but most authors suggest that the patients should at least be fully asymptomatic before returning to such activities.

Deterioration of neurological findings of a child who looks quite well initially includes several differential diagnoses such as iatrogenic sedation effects, seizures, expanding mass lesions, and brain swelling. Focal seizures especially followed by focal neurological deficits should be evaluated with neuroimaging. Early seizures after head injury are more common in children than in adults. However, posttraumatic epilepsy and delayed intellectual impairment occur with a very low incidence after mild head injury in children.

Contusions, intracranial hemorrhage, or extra-axial lesions can appear as a delayed complication although the majority of these are visualized within the first 6 h after injury.

Posttraumatic hyponatriemia commonly appears in moderate to severe injuries but has also been observed after mild head injury in rare cases. If untreated, it can lead to an impairment of consciousness and seizures due to cerebral swelling.

An unusual cause of neurological deterioration after relatively minor trauma is a carotid or vertebral dissection. Most children with this diagnosis have focal neck pain after injury. Deterioration is due to infarction at the affected artery distribution. The mechanism of injury is thought to be the stretching of the artery over the transverse processes of the upper cervical spine. Initially, there may be no neurological sequel; however, progressive thrombosis or embolic events may develop later.

16.3 Severe Head Injuries

Only 7–10% of head injuries are severe as defined by a GCS of 8 or less. These patients should be intubated and ventilated as soon as safely possible.

Intubation in patients with severe head injuries reduces the rate of aspiration and therefore the risk of pneumonia and helps to prevent respiratory insufficiency. Artificial ventilation should be adjusted to achieve an arterial saturation greater than 95%; pCO_2 should be kept between 30 and 35 mm Hg. Analyses have shown that the greatest reduction in ICP seems to occur when the pCO_2 is lowered to 35 mm Hg. Therefore, hyperventilation should only be used during actual ICP elevations and should not be lowered to 30 mm Hg. Recent data suggest that uncritical hyperventilation increases cerebral ischemia and worsens the patient's outcome.

Early and frequent measurements of the child's blood pressure are vital as hypotension is profoundly harmful to the child with a severe traumatic brain injury. Treatment of low blood pressure is needed to maintain a cerebral perfusion pressure (CPP) of at least 60 mm Hg. It should be kept in mind that the most common cause of hypotension is an extracranial injury.

Adequate sedation and analgesia are essential in patients with head injuries, especially if ventilated. Neurological assessment should ideally occur prior to the administration of these medications. Up to now no reliable drugs have been found to interfere with the molecular secondary injury or demonstrated any benefit.

CT scan of the head and usually upper spine to C3 and plane cervical spine radiographs are usually obtained. CT scan of the abdomen is done only if there is a possibility of abdominal trauma. Other radiographs will depend on the history and the examination. Approximately 20% of children with severe head injuries have mass lesions from hematomas that require evacuation.

The need and timing of repeat imaging depends on the findings of the initial CT scan and continuous clinical examinations. If the initial CT scan reveals a small hematoma, repeat imaging should be performed within 24 h to monitor the hematoma size. For stable patients, follow-up CT or MRI are usually obtained between 3 and 5 days after the injury and again between 10 and 14 days. An earlier MRI is recommended in patients presenting clinical deterioration which cannot be explained by a CT scan. Delayed imaging is indicated in children with diffuse axonal injury which occasionally results in posttraumatic hydrocephalus. External ventricular drainage may be necessary but permanent shunt placement is rarely required.

16.4 Intensive Care Unit

The aim of intensive care management is to minimize the degree of secondary brain injury by a tailored treatment strategy for each patient based on continuous monitoring of intracranial pressure, cerebral perfusion pressure, and hemodynamic parameters. To achieve this optimal care and treatment, a multidisciplinary team of neurosurgeons, critical care physicians, paediatric surgeons, anesthesiologists, and specially trained nursing staff is required.

All children with a GCS of 8 or less should receive an ICP monitor to guide management of intracranial hypertension as well as to detect an expanding mass lesion in an early stage. ICP monitoring by ventricular catheter is still considered the most accurate and reliable method. Beside ICP measurement, the ventricular catheter allows the therapeutic benefit of cerebral spinal fluid drainage for ICP control. Other acceptable methods include parenchymal fiber optic and microtransuser systems. Subarachnoid, subdural, or epidural monitors do not provide comparable accuracy and are not recommended.

Delayed rises in ICP are not uncommon 3–10 days after injury. Therefore, a longer period of observation may be warranted when the initial diagnosis is acute subdural hematoma or multiple contusions. Intraoperative ICP monitoring is also generally recommended in patients with moderate head injuries undergoing general anesthesia for extracranial injuries.

The risks of a ventricular catheter for ICP monitoring are quite small compared to the significant damage that could occur in patients with elevated ICP, and include intraparenchymal hemorrhage during placement and development of bacterial ventriculitis. The rate of intracerebral hemorrhage varies from 0% to 2% of placements. The placement of ventricular catheters should be avoided in patients with known coagulopathy or thrombocytopenia. Infection rate is approximately 7–11%. We do not routinely change the ventricular catheter before 10 days and recommend prophylactic antibiotics with periodic analysis of cultures and cell counts. The catheter should be replaced if there is a positive culture or increasing pleocytosis in the CSF.

16.4.1 Management of Increased Intracranial Pressure

Sedation and paralysis can lower ICP by minimizing the noxius stimulus of intubation, suction, patient agitation, and asynchronous ventilation.

Drainage of the CSF is the most effective treatment of ICP elevation. Either intermittent or continuous drainage can be performed. In case of intermittent drainage, the ventricular catheter is opened when ICP exceeds the treatment threshold. I personally prefer continuous ventricular drainage with a ventricular chamber at 5 cm above the level of the lateral ventricle to avoid sudden ICP fluctuations. We recommend tunneling the catheter subcutaneously as far from the borehole as possible to minimize a possible ventriculitis.

Beside CSF drainage through a ventricular catheter, the insertion of a lumbar drain is possible in selected cases to reduce ICP. However, this technique is quite controversial and is of unproven safety and efficacy.

Head elevation to 30° can lower ICP without significant changes in cerebral perfusion pressure (CPP) or cerebral blood flow (CBF) whereas further elevation decreases CBF.

Hyperventilation is recommended in the setting of clinical signs of herniation and may be used for brief periods. However, prophylactic hyperventilation is not supported in traumatic brain injury. We recommend maintaining pCO_2 between 30 and 35 mm Hg. Ventilation should be adapted to the clinical situation.

Mannitol is an excellent volume expander improving perfusion pressure. Additionally, it also removes extravascular water from the brain and reduces blood viscosity which improves CBF. Mannitol is usually administered intermittently as a bolus infusion every 4–6 h as necessary for ICP elevations. The use of mannitol is often reserved for the later treatment of head trauma 48 h after the event since there is little evidence of brain edema in the early stages and edema is the pathology for which mannitol seems most indicated.

Barbiturates produce a reduction in ICP via a reduction in cerebral metabolic rate which can be effective in the setting of refractory intracranial hypertension.

When barbiturates are used, the patient should be carefully monitored for reduction in cardiac output or inadequate systemic perfusion requiring vasopressors and fluid resuscitation. Some centers reserve this treatment as a conservative therapy of last resorts, although we often use barbiturate therapy in children after frustrane mannitol therapy to provide neuroprotection.

Moderate systemic hypothermia (30–34°C) has shown to be beneficial in the treatment of severe head injury. Seizure incidence was lower in the hypothermic patients and ICP was decreased during the hypothermic interval. For each degree Celsius drop in temperature there is an approximate 10% change in cerebral metabolism. Therefore, it is desirable to prevent fever or iatrogenic hyperthermia. However, a potential danger of hypothermia is interference with phagocyte activity and pulmonary ciliary function with resulting pneumonia. Therefore, in case of pulmonary contusion it may be safer to avoid hypothermia.

Decompressive craniectomy may result in a decrease of ICP and good outcome in selected patients with extremely refractory intracranial hypertension. However, specific recommendation or guidelines for this procedure have not been developed. We recommend aggressive surgical intervention only in children with severe head injuries with progressive edema, if the brain stem does not appear to be irreversibly damaged.

Antiepileptic drugs are necessary for repeated or prolonged posttraumatic seizures. Early posttraumatic seizures are seen in approximately 25% of patients with traumatic intracranial hematomas. Many of these seizures are often isolated events which do not always require medication. There are some centers that do use prophylactic anticonvulsants; however, no randomized studies have shown a clear effect from prophylactic anticonvulsant therapy in controlling the onset of late seizures.

16.5 Skull Fracture

Fractures are diagnosed either by plane radiographs or by CT with the use of bone window techniques. However, there has been conflicting literature concerning the usefulness of plane radiographs because children with a neurological deficit or with a GCS less than 13 should have a CT scan as the examination of choice. If a linear skull fracture is present, the occurrence of other lesions such as contusions and epidural hematomas (EDHs) is greatly increased. CT scan will not only detect skull fractures but also intracranial lesions. Therefore, if a patient with acute head injuries is found to have a skull fracture on the plane radiography, CT scan of the brain should be obtained to exclude possible intracranial lesions.

Children with head injuries who have linear skull fractures, normal CT scan of the brain, and normal neurological examinations do not need any treatment because they are less likely to have subsequent neurological deterioration. These children are usually discharged after an observation period of about 72 h. In infants or very young children, subgaleal hematomas due to subperiostal hemorrhage can result in symptomatic blood loss. Some children require blood transfusion.

16.6 Depressed Skull Fractures

Depressed skull fractures are usually the result of a very focal impact and represent approximately one-quarter of all skull fractures in children. Dural lacerations are reported in about 10% of patients. In newborns with a developing very thin skull, the undersurface of the depression is usually quite smooth resulting in so-called ping-pong fractures. Other common fractures are greenstick fractures where the bone remains connected and is fixed in its new abnormal position. Three-quarters of depressed skull fractures are located in frontal or parietal bones.

Location, degree of depression, and integrity of the scalp are important for the assessment of depressed skull fracture. If the depression of fractures is at least as deep as the thickness of the skull, surgical elevation should be considered, because fractures depressed more than 5 mm commonly tear the dura (Fig. 16.1a,b). In case of obvious compression of the brain or if CSF or brain tissue come through a laceration over the fracture, the fracture should be elevated and any dural tear repaired. Fractures without brain compression or tear of the dura have an excellent outcome with conservative therapy alone. In the young infant, especially, it has been suggested that there is no need for elevation because the skull will remodel itself.

Fig. 16.1 (**a**) An 8-year-old boy with laceration of the skin, CSF coming through the wound and a CT scan (bone window technique) revealing a frontal left depressed skull fracture; (**b**) after reconstruction of the bone fragments with absorbable sutures and closure of the dura

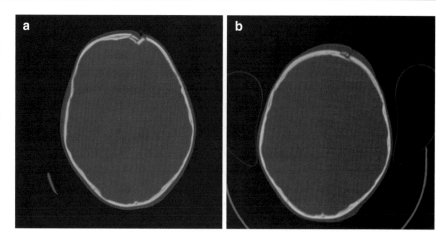

In some children, elevation of the skull fracture is necessary for cosmetic reasons, e.g., if the fracture is located on the forehead. This can be performed on an elective basis in the case of complete integrity of the scalp. More important than prophylactic antibiotics in open skull fractures is the early closure of the wound. If permanent closure is delayed for more than 48 h, the incidence of infection increases from approximately 5% to 37%. Regarding seizures, there are no clinical data that support elevating depressed skull fractures for seizure prophylaxis. Several investigators have concluded that if an epileptogenic focus develops, it occurs at the time of injury and not from depressed skull fracture.

Depressed bone fractures involving the dural sinus present a very high risk of death and morbidity to the patient undergoing surgery, because uncontrollable bleeding might occur and result in hypovolemic shock. The surgeon should keep in mind that the anterior one-third of the superior sagittal sinus tolerates ligation without neurological deficits whereas the posterior two-thirds does not.

Surgical techniques used for the elevation of depressed skull fractures vary from a simple borehole near the fracture to a more extensive craniotomy. In newborns, it might be possible to use a small borehole to lift the depressed fragment. In older children with more complex fractures, we prefer a more extensive craniotomy to have safe access to any dural and cortical injury.

Basilar skull fractures appear to occur more commonly in adults than in children. CSF otorrhea carries the same diagnostic importance as does CSF rhinor-

rhea and it is only present in 10% of cases. If the tympanic membrane remains intact, hematotympanum will be observed. The natural history of traumatic CSF leaks is that almost all will cease spontaneously with conservative management. CSF rhinorrhea is rare in children with basilar skull fractures, which sometimes requires lumbar CSF drainage. Another option is the detection of the CSF leak by fluoroscopy followed by the endoscopical sealing of the leak. The use of prophylactic antibiotics is controversial. The only randomized prospective study has not proven any beneficial effect of prophylactic antibiotics based on either the incidence or the severity of posttraumatic meningitis.

16.7 Leptomeningeal Cysts

Diastatic fractures to the skull in a growing child can result in the formation of a leptomeningeal cyst or growing skull fractures in less than 1% of cases. The leptomeningeal cyst is believed to develop due to a tear in the dura with subsequent enlargement of the bone caused by brain pulsation. CT scan or MRI will show both brain and meninges within the defect which delay the healing of the bone (Fig. 16.2a,b). The hallmark of a growing fracture is a palpable non-tender swelling in the area of a previous skull fracture. Surgical treatment includes watertight repair or replacement of the dura and closure of the skull defect. We prefer to use autogenous skull bone. Children under the age of 3 years

Fig. 16.2 (**a**) Skull film 8 months after linear skull fracture revealing enlargement of the bone defect; (**b**) MRI confirms the diagnosis growing skull fracture, showing brain and meninges within the bone defect

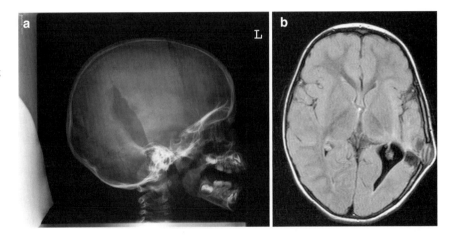

with a linear or diastatic skull fracture need a follow-up skull film at 6 months post-injury to detect a possible growing skull fracture early enough.

16.8 Penetrating Cerebral Injuries

CT scan remains the preferred initial imaging modality of penetrating cerebral injuries. In selected cases, plane films may help to delineate skull fractures and intracranial foreign bodies; however, the CT scan alone is generally sufficient. MRI is not indicated in the early evaluation period. In younger children, the side of injury is often around the face especially through the orbita. In cases of sharp instruments penetrating deep into the head and location of the foreign body to the major cerebral vessels, intradural and extradural exploration by craniotomy will maximize the comfort of safe removal of the foreign body. Rapid exploration should be possible if bleeding is to be expected during removal of the foreign body. Every effort should be made to remove the entire foreign body and to close the dura. Short courses of prophylactic antibiotics are generally indicated.

Gunshot wounds to the brain are operated on only if there is a chance of survival and recovery. A GCS score of 3–5 combined with nonreactive pupils or refractory hypotension has a mortality rate up to 100%. The decision whether or not to perform surgery in these patients is complex. The higher post-resuscitative GCS score of

5 is an indication for debridement of the wound and closure of the dura and the eventual placement of a monitoring device for ICP. There is no evidence that extensive parenchymal debridement or removal of deeply penetrating fragments of bullets or bone does prevent infection. Delayed complications include brain abscess, traumatic aneurysm formation, and wandering intracranial fragments.

16.9 Mass Lesions after Head Injury

Until proven otherwise, a child with an altered level of consciousness, pupillary dysfunction, and laterally extremity weakness should be suspected of having a mass lesion that may require surgery.

16.9.1 Epidural Hematomas (EDH)

Approximately 60% of patients with EDHs are below the age of 20. EDHs present differently from one age group to another. Neonates and infants present with a decrease in hematocrit, bradycardia, pallor, change in level of consciousness, bulging fontanelles, and focal neurological deficits (Fig. 16.3). These patients may be neurologically normal or have mild neurological abnormalities and then rapidly decompensate within hours or days after injury. The more common venous etiology

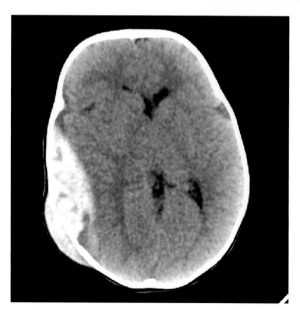

Fig. 16.3 Acute parietal EDH in a 6-month-old infant 4 h after falling 50 cm from the bench. Child presented initially without deficit at admission with vomiting, and pale and bulging fontanelles. Surgery due to visible mass lesion and increased intracranial pressure is indicated

accompanied with large cerebral spinal fluid spaces and open fontanelles allow a longer compensatory phase. In older children, EDHs usually originate from arterial bleeding that reduces the ability to compensate and lead to a more rapid progression of events. The lucid interval is shorter than in neonates. Another peculiarity of EDHs in children is its quite common location in the posterior fossa; however, the parietal and temporal regions are the regions that are most affected.

Not all EDHs are considered emergencies and need surgical intervention. There are some children with EDHs who are asymptomatic or minimally symptomatic with a relatively small hematoma without compression to the brain. In these patients, a nonsurgical approach is probably justified. Some of these hematomas show spontaneous regression followed by absorption within 4–6 weeks post injury. However, all patients with acute EDHs should be admitted to the intensive care unit for observation.

Appropriate preoperative planning is required in patients who need to undergo surgery because of the low incidence of finding the mass lesion only with the use of multiple exploratory boreholes. Therefore, there is rarely a reason for blind surgery unless a CT scan is unavailable and the child is deteriorating. In this case, boreholes are performed where the fracture is seen on

radiography and the location of which is compatible with the clinical picture of a possible EDH. Otherwise, the bone flap should be large enough to entirely expose and evacuate the blood clot. In children who were awake after trauma and then deteriorate to a GSC score of less than 8, ICP monitoring may not be required after rapid clot removal. On the other hand, children who have been unconscious from the time of injury, ICP monitoring should be placed after clot removal to allow appropriate treatment of the diffuse brain injury. In these children, EDHs may be associated with parenchymal injuries that are contributing to the coma. If preoperative CT scan reveals only the EDH, opening of the dura should be avoided to minimize the risk of injury to the underlying cortex.

16.9.2 Subdural Hematomas

Neonatal subdural hematomas (SDHs) are uncommon and can be caused by birth trauma related to vacuum extraction or forceps injury. In general, SDHs large enough to require surgery are also rare in children. SDHs in infants and young children are mostly associated with the shaken baby syndrome (Fig. 16.4a,b). These children are admitted with significant neurological injury and do not show much evidence of external damage. Every child who has minimal external signs of trauma with neurological damage, acute SDH, and retinal hemorrhages should be assumed to have been abused until proven otherwise.

SDHs usually are described as acute, subacute, or chronic in order to relate them to the time of initial hemorrhage. The etiology generally involves bridging veins from the cortical surface to the various venous sinuses that are disrupted secondary to force.

Acute SDHs usually present with sudden deterioration and compression of the brain or cerebellum and appear within a few hours of the injury. Patients present with varying degrees of loss of consciousness, pupillary dilatation, cranial nerve deficits, motor deficits, vomiting, and headaches.

Subacute SDHs develop a few days after the initial hemorrhage. During this time, more than one hemorrhage may occur as the hematoma enlarges and causes re-bleeding at the original site.

Three weeks to several months later, the SDH becomes a chronic SDH. This appearance often has multiple

Fig. 16.4 (a) MRI reveals subdural effusions over the right hemisphere due to shaken baby syndrome in a 2-month-old infant. Patient presented with signs of increased intracranial pressure. (b) MRI 1 month after subdural drainage for 5 days through a borehole on the right side

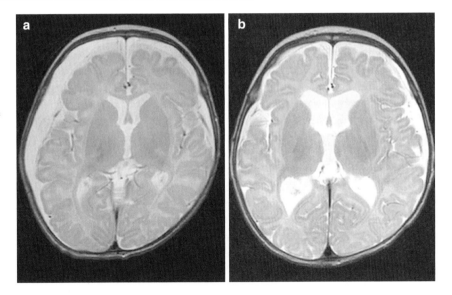

layers because of membrane formation and re-bleeding. Clinical symptoms in a chronic SDH are typically nonlocalizing and associated with vomiting, irritability, failure to thrive, and seizures. Chronic SDHs occur more frequently in children than acute SDHs.

SDHs commonly occur in the posterior fossa of neonates as the bridging veins of the cerebellum might be damaged during suction and forceps-assisted birth. Observation of posterior fossa SDH is the treatment of choice if there are no signs of brain stem compression or obstructive hydrocephalus.

The clinical presentation of an acute SDH in young infants is generally more diffuse. They appear pale with a full fontanelle and may or may not have a focal neurological deficit. In children with an open fontanelle, subdural collections are tapped only when intracranial pressure is elevated. Perinatal SDHs, especially small ones, may rather be managed conservatively because they may resolve within a few days. Acute SDHs are more commonly seen in older children. They are often associated with multiple trauma, cerebral contusions, and skull fractures. Patients presenting with impaired consciousness, signs of acute rise in ICP, and focal deficits need urgent surgical intervention. Large craniotomy extending close to the midline allows easier visualization of the bleeding site along the sagittal or sigmoid sinus. The goal of hemostasis is to find the cortical or bridging vein that has been torn by the trauma. Sometimes, acute SDHs may lead to diffuse edema and extensive swelling of the brain which make it necessary to leave the dura open for decompression of the brain. Intracranial pressure monitors are recommended for the treatment of subsequent cerebral swelling and in patients with a GCS score of 8 or less before operation. The outcome of patients with large acute SDH and a GCS score less than 8 is generally unsatisfactory. Prompt intervention in this setting may significantly improve the patient's outcome. Patients with minimal neurological deficits and a small SDH can be kept under observation. Small SDHs in association with diffuse brain injury or brain swelling are also rarely operated on since these hematomas play little or no role in the etiology of the coma.

Chronic SDHs are more common in infants than neonates. Unrecognized trauma may be the cause of these SDHs. These hemorrhages may often be managed nonsurgically because the infant cranium expands, which reduces the intracranial pressure, and small SDHs may resolve spontaneously. Larger chronic SDHs may need surgical intervention because of repeated bleeding of the fragile vessels of neo-membranes. The infants usually present with signs of a slow increase in ICP including nausea, vomiting, poor appetite, and irritability. Seizures may be seen in about 40% of these children.

16.9.3 Intracerebral Hematomas

Intracerebral hematomas (ICHs) in neonates are believed to be linked to the friction caused by the bony edges of the cranium during delivery. Bleeding can also occur due to arteriovenous malformations, hypoxia at birth, arterial emboli, or infarction. In older children, ICHs are more likely to occur from large angular acceleration–deceleration forces during injury. Characteristic findings of this trauma are small hemorrhages in the deep white matter, corpus callosum, and brain stem (diffuse axonal injury). The hallmark symptom of diffuse axonal injuries is immediate unconsciousness. Surgical intervention in this setting is usually not indicated and the patient can be treated conservatively.

Focal contusions after head traumas are usually limited to the cortex but they may expand into the white matter. It is rare for contusions to be considered as surgical lesions in children as the tissue often recovers. If the child is neurologically intact or has only minimal deficits, ICHs can be carefully observed. A large hematoma associated with significant midline shift and the deteriorating condition of a patient require craniotomy. A safe route to the hematoma should be taken to remove hemorrhage as much as possible. Areas that may be safely operated on without clear neurological sequel are the frontal and anterior temporal lobes in the nondominant hemisphere.

16.10 Conclusion

Although the majority of pediatric head injuries are mild and have no serious long-term sequel, it is important to identify children with severe head injuries. After prompt resuscitation and clinical evaluation, optimal management of intracranial hypertension under multimodal monitoring has to be done. ICP monitoring by ventricular catheter is considered the most accurate method and has the advantage of lowering the ICP by CSF drainage. Cerebral perfusion pressure of at least 40–50 mm Hg in infants and 50–60 mm Hg in children are probably reasonable goals. Surgical interventions may be necessary based on clinical assessment and morphology. Predictors of poor outcome for accidental injuries include multiple trauma and early hypoxia or shock. Other factors include low GCS scores. Mortality rates in children remain high, 40–60% for children with a GCS score of 3 or 4. Children with a GCS score of 5 or above have a mortality rate of less than 10%.

The developing brain in children absorbs the forces of traumatic impact leading to more diffuse injury and fewer mass lesions. Most mass lesions in children can be managed conservatively. However, mass lesions with neurological deficits, deterioration of the neurological status, and radiographic evidence of brain compression require urgent surgical intervention. Linear nondepressed skull fractures do not require any treatment. Most CSF fistulas in children due to skull base fractures cease spontaneously. The usefulness for prophylactic antibiotics remains unclear. The substantial number of neonatal depressed skull fractures reform spontaneously during the first few weeks after birth. Depressed fractures should be elevated in case of dural laceration or obvious compression of the brain. Growing skull fractures as a complication of large linear skull fractures usually associated with dural laceration always require surgical correction and can be detected on physical examination.

Optimal care of the infant or child with severe traumatic brain injury requires a multidisciplinary team in each phase of management. Treatment starts with the resuscitation at the scene of accident, extends over to the neurointensive care management including surgery, and ends with rehabilitation.

Further Reading

Albright AL, Pollack IF, Adelson PD (1999) Principles and Practice of Pediatric Neurosurgery. Thieme, New York

Bauer BL, Kuhn Th J (1997) Severe Head Injuries. Springer, Heidelberg

Choux M, Di Rocco C, Hockey A, Walker M (1999) Pediatric Neurosurgery. Churchill Livingstone, London

Section of Pediatric Neurosurgery of the A.A.N.S. (1994) Pediatric Neurosurgery, 3rd edn. Saunders, Philadelphia, PA

Puri P, Höllwarth ME (eds) (2006) Pediatric Surgery. Springer, Berlin, Heidelberg

Pediatric Orthopedic Trauma

17

Eva E. Fischerauer and Annelie M. Weinberg

Contents

17.1 The Basic Biology of Fracture Healing (Callus Formation)

The fracture healing process is divided into three phases:

1. Inflammation
2. Reparative phase
3. Remodeling

Inflammation describes the initial phase after a loss of integrity of the osseus structure. The haematoma formed due to ruptured blood vessels plays a central role. It fills the fracture gap, contains a lot of fibrin and inflammatory mediators that attract mesenchymal cells. Certain proteins are responsible for the differentiation of mesenchymal cells into chondroblast, osteoblasts, and angioblasts, a process that closely resembles the stages of bone development. Callus formation takes place in the reparative phase. Initially, the hard callus is formed by periostal cells that directly differentiate into osteoblasts which lay down bone by intramembranous ossification. In the centre of the fracture gap chondrocytes form the soft callus which serves as a scaffold for woven bone formed by endochondral ossification. The hard and the soft callus together represent the so-called provisional callus that provides temporary stabilization. Rigid stability that is necessary for full physical activity occurs when lamellar bone is laid down along the lines of stress and replaces the provisional callus. This remodelling phase can last months, even years in certain osseus structures.

P. Puri and M. Höllwarth (eds.), *Pediatric Surgery: Diagnosis and Management,*
DOI: 10.1007/978-3-540-69560-8_17, © Springer-Verlag Berlin Heidelberg 2009

17.2 Classification of Pediatric Injuries

17.2.1 Epiphyseal Injuries

They have been classified by many researchers. The most common classification of epiphyseal injuries was established by Salter and Harris in 1963, and is based on radiographic appearance of the fracture in relation to the growth plate.

This radiographic classification describes five types of epiphyseal fractures:

Type I This fracture is presented by a complete separation of the epiphysis and physis from the metaphysis. The fracture line goes through the hypertrophic zone of the growth plate (Fig. 17.1a).

Type II This type describes a fracture which in addition to type I includes a metaphyseal fragment on the compression side of the fracture, called the "Thurston-Holland sign" (Fig. 17.1b).

Type III This epiphyseal injury is composed of a physeal separation and a fracture through the epiphysis to the joint (Fig. 17.1c).

Type IV Type IV describes a fracture through the metaphysis, physis, and epiphysis into the joint (Fig. 17.1d).

Type V Type V is classified as a compression or crushing injury to the growth plate and occurs infrequently. On the initial radiograph it can be mistaken as a type I fracture, as its radiological appearance is similar. Though, this fracture is associated with severe soft tissue injuries including vascular lesions and is due to a considerable axial load.

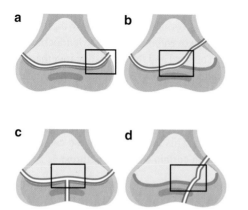

Fig. 17.1 (**a**) Salter-Harris type I, (**b**) Salter-Harris type II, (**c**) Salter-Harris type III, and (**d**) Salter-Harris type IV

17.2.2 Metaphyseal Injuries

Metaphyseal fractures including an epiphyseal separation with or without a metaphyseal part (e.g. Salter-Harris type I and II) can be further divided into a "buckle fracture", an incomplete fracture, a complete fracture, and a "muscular avulsion-fracture". *Buckle fractures* represent the most frequent fractures and are due to a compression failure of the bones. They are located in the metaphysis, as this part is of greatest porosity, in particular in younger children (Fig. 17.2).

17.2.3 Diaphyseal Fractures

Characteristics of a child's bone compared to an adult bone are the less density and the greater porosity. Furthermore, the cortex is pitted and can easily be cut, as the "Haversian canals" are larger and occupy a great part of the cortex. They are divided into different types according to their location and radiological appearance.

17.2.3.1 Greenstick Fractures

This fracture occurs when bones are bended beyond the limits. The fracture is due to a failure of the tension side—the compression side bends. As the fracture is incomplete the remaining bone undergoes plastic deformation. These fractures are characterized by the possibility of a refracture which is related to a consolidation failure of the convex site. The risk of a refracture can last for 8 months posttraumatically. This time depends on the localisation (the distaler the shorter the time of possible refractures) and on the patient's age (the younger the shorter the time of a refracture). Nevertheless, complete closure and realignment of the fracture can only be achieved by completing the fracture or overcorrecting the angulation.

17.2.3.2 Bending of Bones: Plastic Deformation

These plastic deformations can occur as a child's bone can tolerate a greater degree of deformation than an

Fig. 17.2 Buckle fracture

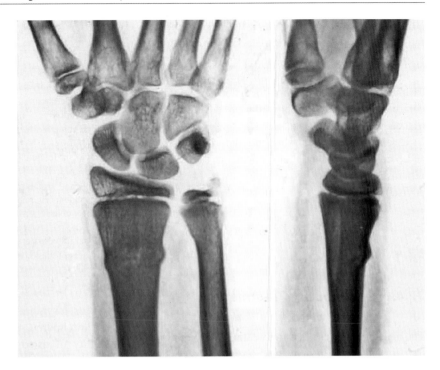

adult's bone before it breaks. This fracture can occur without any classical signs of a fracture, e.g. fracture gap. It can only be diagnosed by documenting a radiologically visible bending/curve of the bone.

17.2.3.3 Complete Fracture

These fractures are rarely comminuted in children due to the greater flexibility of a child's bone.

17.2.4 Toddler's Fracture

The isolated tibial fracture during childhood (until the age of 4) is named the "toddler's fracture". The typical feature of this fracture is that the child is unable to step on the foot and walk properly consequently, the infant is limping. A radiological diagnosis is often impossible. During check-ups, the fracture can be secondarily diagnosed by a radiologically detectable callus formation and decalcification of the fracture gap around the 10th day post trauma. As the fracture cannot be diag-

nosed at once, the child's leg is normally immobilized by an upper leg-cast. This treatment method will be prolonged for another 10 days by verification of the toddler's fracture 10–14 days later.

17.3 Diagnostic

Normally, the injury can already be diagnosed by observing a posttraumatic tumor and pain at the site of lesion. Approximately two thirds of injuries concern the upper limb and about one third concerns the lower limb. A manual palpable diagnostic is not necessary, as hereby pain is caused without the possibility to diagnose a fracture or observe its progressive course.

In most cases, x-ray photographs in 2 planes, AP-projection and lateral, are performed. One plane—x-ray examination is possible when a defective position is visible. Sometimes oblique x-ray photographs are indicated, e.g. the upper ankle or the knee. Basically, computer tomography (CT), or magnetic resonance imaging (MRI) are rarely indicated as progressive primary examinations to diagnose a fracture.

Nowadays, it is obsolete to take x-ray photographs of the opposite side in order to detect the plane of the growth plate.

Fractures which are treated conservatively with cast treatment and which imperil to dislocate should be controlled by x-ray examination on day 5–8 after trauma.

In elderly children, when no deformity can be accepted and the potential of spontaneous correction is diminished, an x-ray examination after 14 days is advisable.

17.4   Therapy

17.4.1   Conservative Treatment

The main aim of a conservative treatment is to diminish the pain and to minimize the risk of a secondary dislocation. Principle indications for conservative treatment should be considered. A cast reduces the possibility of secondary displacements and ensures healing by stabilising the fracture in a reduced position. Stabilisation can be provided by individual, appropriate kinds of casts.

17.4.2   Operative Treatment

In every case, the importance of a reduction has to be initially discussed. Meeting the criteria for reduction, the attending surgeon has to decide between an open or closed reduction, which is depending in particular on the fracture's morphology and on the surgeon's experience (Table 17.1).

Nowadays, in children, most fractures are closed reduced even when an osteosynthesis has to be performed. Joint fractures should be demonstrated (open or by arthroscopy), anatomically reduced and stabilized. However, open reductions are rarely indicated during childhood.

17.4.2.1   Methods of Osteosynthesis

During growth, a successful fracture osteosynthesis is based on a comprehensive knowledge about different

Table 17.1   Criteria for reduction

Criteria for reduction
No reduction:
• All stable, undislocated/undisplaced fractures of the upper and lower extremity independent of age
• Stable buckle fractures or metaphyseal fractures within the tolerated limits
• Unstable humeral fractures of initial tolerated angular deformity
• All clavicular fractures <12 years
Reduction:
• All stable and unstable fractures which do neither meet the age-dependent criteria, nor the localisation-dependent criteria for conservative treatment without reduction
• Fractures of the lower arm, as angular deformities can lead to functional impairment
• In fractures of the lower extremity it is important to obtain normal length, axis and rotation

kinds of osteosynthesis-techniques and their appropriate use in children, and is further depending on the availability of osteosynthesis-materials, suitable for children.

Since years the screw-, plate- and tension band wiring-osteosynthesis which is performed analogically to adults, has been displaced in operative pediatric orthopaedic trauma treatment and is now mainly performed in children over 12. In younger children, in most cases k-wire osteosynthesis, elastic-stable intramedullar nailing, cannulated screw-osteosynthesis or external fixator is performed.

- **Kirschner-wire (K-wire) osteosynthesis**

This osteosynthesis method represents a mere adaptation-osteosynthesis which enables maximal stability to movements but not to loading. This osteosynthesis requires additional cast immobilisation. The advantages of this method are the percutaneous performance and missing need for general narcosis for uncomplicated implant removals. Furthermore, K-wires are always and everywhere available (Fig. 17.3a).

- **Elastic-stable intramedullar nailing (ESIN)**

ESIN describes a minimal-invasive, minimal-traumatizing, sufficiently movement- and load-stable, biologically adapted, and appropriate osteosynthesis method for children. It can be performed in transverse, oblique, short-spiral, and diaphyseal fractures during infancy. The elastic-stable nails are made of steel or titan and are usable in every age. The aim of this biological, minimal-invasive fracture treatment is to achieve an

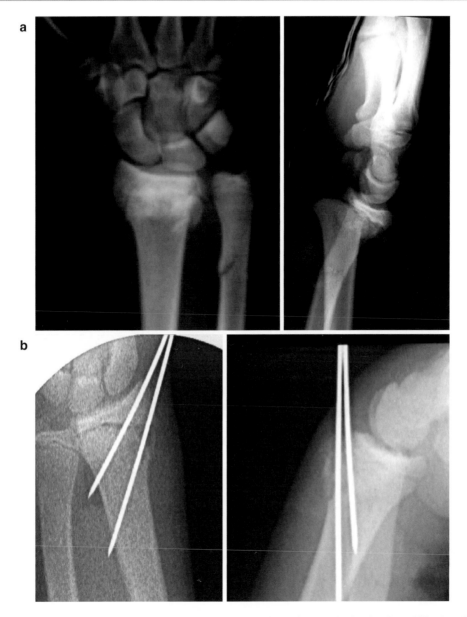

Fig. 17.3 (a)   **a**: Dislocated distal forearm fracture (ap and lateral view), **b**: Typical K-wire fixation for stabilisation of the reduced fracture

adequate reduction and stabilization. As this method represents a closed treatment procedure, it is only possible to achieve an axis-compatible position and no anatomical reduction.

The biomechanical principle of elastic-stable intramedullar nailing is based on the symmetric tension of two metaphyseal-inserted nails which have three intramedullar supporting-points. Optimal results are warranted by correctly symmetric-positioned nails (Fig. 17.3b).

- **Screw osteosynthesis**

This osteosynthesis method is another adaptation-osteosynthesis that additionally can bring the bone fragments under compression. Hereby the bone can be better stabilized although a cast is also required in most cases. Nowadays, spongiosa-screws are the standard and preferable self drilling, self cutting titan or steel screws are used in operative fracture treatment. They should further be back-cutting as this property eases

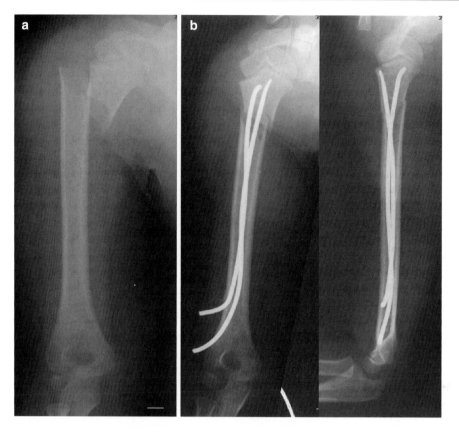

Fig. 17.3 (b)   a: Subcapital proximal humerus fracture, **b**: Osteosynthesis with ascending elastic-stable intramedullar nails

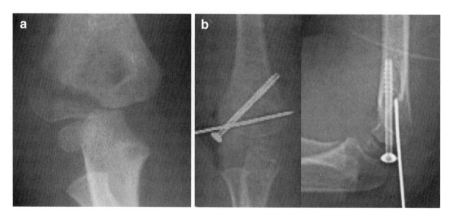

Fig. 17.3 (c)   a: Dislocated condylus redialis fracture of the elbow, **b**: Intraoperative canulated screw fixation (ap and lateral view)

the screw-removal. Furthermore, these screws are excellent for closed fixations, especially at the lower limb (Fig. 17.3c).

- **External fixator**

This method represents another frequently performed operative treatment for complex diaphyseal fractures during infancy. It is important to use adequate, appro-

priate fixators and implants for the child's age. Children do normally tolerate the external fixator quite well. Nevertheless, the child should not feel any pain during removal and may need sedation or a short narcosis.

The external fixator is a supplementing alternative method of the ESIN and is especially used in very instable fractures of an open angle of 3° and in older children (Fig. 17.3d).

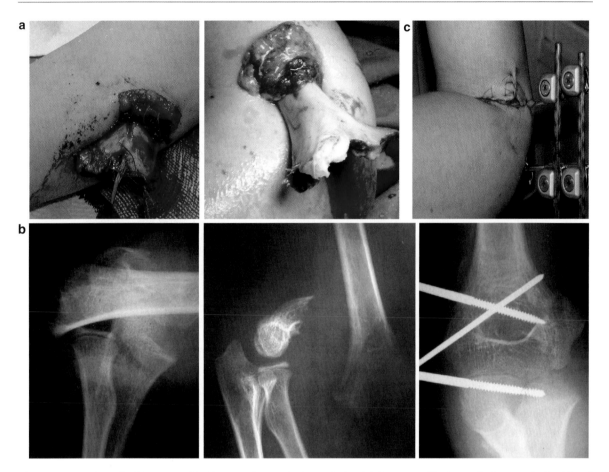

Fig. 17.3 (d)   a: Open distal (supracondylar) humerus fracture, before and after debridement and jet-lavage, **b**: Osteosynthesis with and external fixator, **c**: Clinical situation after surgery

17.4.2.2 Complications of Fracture Repair

Growth Disturbances

It has been recognized for a long time that growth disturbances occur in fractured bones. These growth disorders are divided into two kinds:

1. Overgrowth
2. Partial or complete growth arrest

Both growth disturbances concern the growth plate and only occur as long as the physis is open.

1. The overgrowth phenomenon

This disturbance is according to non Laer described as a posttraumatic stimulation of one or more growth plates in its overall size and must be expected in every fractured growing bone. The maximum stimulation is the biggest during growth years and occurs the least in the prematural age, as the growth stimulation leads to premature closure of the physis what eventually compensates the overgrowth. If the trauma takes place in the time of growth plate closure, the process is accelerated and results in bone shortening. This commonly means that under the age of 10 a growth stimulation with increased bone length is likely, whereas children over 10 probably have to deal with bone shortening.

Clinically it is important to avoid difficult reduction manoeuvres but to look for the best possible alignment of the fracture ends.

2. Partial or complete growth arrest

Growth arrest represents the worst complication during fracture repair. This growth disturbance occurs spontaneously and cannot be influenced by any treatment, consequently cannot be avoided. Supposedly, traumatic injuries of the soft tissues, severe contusions, or metaphyseal fracture, and operations, which interrupt the blood flow to the growth plate are the etiological causes and may lead to the formation of transient physeal bone-bridges, possibly resulting in premature ossification of the growth plate or even cartilage necrosis. Furthermore, premature closure of the growth plate can be a result of radiation, burning, infection, and long immobilisation, due to cast-treatment that may even force the child to stay in bed for a long period.

Clinically, it is important to know that every trans-epiphyseal lesion which either occurs post-traumatically or is due to the use of physeal-crossing implants is associated with the formation of physeal bone-bridges which could disrupt spontaneously during following growth. However, the final length alteration and the corresponding growth prognosis are dependent on the child's age at the time of bone trauma.

Spontaneous Corrections—Remodelling

A posttraumatic bone length discrepancy is stimulated by the process of bone remodelling of posttraumatic uncorrected angular deviations. Thus, it is important in upper leg and lower leg fractures to avoid angular deviations even if they would correct later on by remodelling processes. Conversely, length discrepancies caused by remodelling of angular deviations of the upper limb are not of the same importance. Therefore, the same angular deviations can be accepted due to spontaneous corrections of the proximal humerus, the radial head, and the distal forearm until the age of ten.

17.5 Pediatric Fractures of Consequences

17.5.1 Monteggia's Fracture

The "Monteggia lesion" describes the combination of an ulnar fracture in the proximal or middle third of the diaphysis with a radial head dislocation. Although this injury can easily be detected by x-ray examination, it is still frequently missed. Therefore, every ulnar fracture requires radiographs of the elbow joint (*in all views a line through the long axis of the radius should pass through the capitellum of the humerus*). These lesions are treated by anatomical reduction and stabilization of the ulnar fracture with correction of the radial head dislocation. In case of a greenstick or buckle fracture of the ulnar, conservative treatment (upperarm-cast-longuette in supination position of the lower arm and 90 degrees flexion in the elbow joint) can be performed (Fig. 17.4).

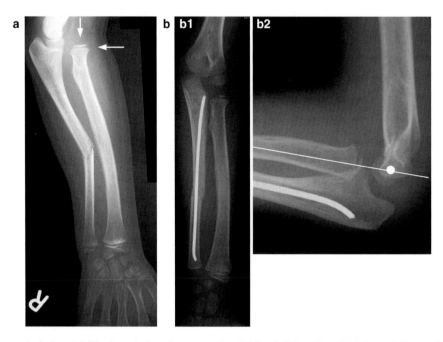

Fig. 17.4 Monteggia lesion. (**a**) Diaphyseal ulnar fracture and radial head dislocation, (**b**) Intramedullary nailing (**b1** ap, **b2** lateral view)

17.5.2 Supracondylar Humeral Fracture

This special fracture is the most frequent one during childhood and concerns especially children between 3 and 10 years. In 98% it represents an extension type fracture, in 2% a flexion type fracture occurs. According to Gartland, extension type fractures are classified into:

Type I: non-displaced fracture
Type II: minimally displaced fracture with intact posterior cortex
Type III: completely displaced fracture with no cortical contact

Displaced supracondylar humeral fractures can already be clinically distinguished from the undisplaced fracture by an elbow deformation and *functio laesa*. Every displaced fracture displays an emergency situation. Considering side-injuries, such as neurological defects, the neurovascular status has to be checked. Radiologically, extensional fractures display a dorsal displacement of the distal fragment, whereas flexional fractures show a ventral dislocation of the bone fragment.

Undisplaced stable fractures with at least partially intact periosteum, and without secondary injuries can be treated conservatively by a dorsal upperarm-cast-longuette in neutral position of the lower arm and 90 degrees flexion in the elbow joint or cuff and collar sling.

Displaced unstable supracondylar humeral fractures with torn periosteum require closed anatomical reduction and are mostly stabilized by K-wire or intramedullary nailing osteosyntheses. In case the closed reduction is impossible, an open reduction and stabilization is indicated (Fig. 17.5).

17.5.3 Fracture of the Lateral Condyle

Lateral condylar fractures represent Salter type IV epiphyseal injuries of the distal humerus. The complications of this fracture are malunion, resulting in stiffness and cubitus valgus, non-union because of immobilization, synovial fluid bathing the fracture, or soft tissue interposition, and growth arrest due to

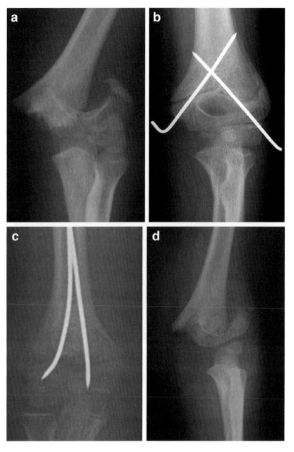

Fig. 17.5 Supracondylar humerus fracture. (a) supracondylar fracture, (b) K-wire osteosynthesis, (c) Intramedullary nailing, (d) Cubitus valgus because of displaced supracondylar humerus fracture

an accompanying growth plate lesion. "Milch's classification" is most frequently used for lateral condyle fractures:

Type I: the lateral trochlear ridge is attached to the main portion of the ridge
Type II: the lateral trochlear ridge is attached to the displaced fragment

Complications occur when an undisplaced fracture is overlooked. This can especially happen in the case of hairline fractures which can be missed on radiographs, or in very young children whose ossification center is very small leading to a misunderstanding of the nature of the injury. Clinically, the elbow displays signs of traumatisation including

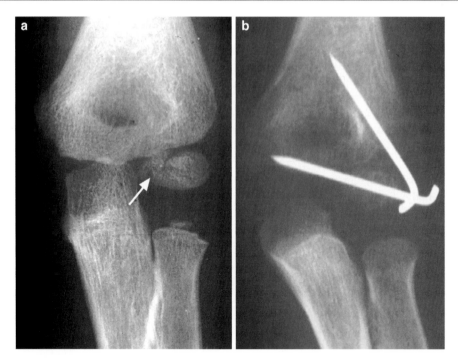

Fig. 17.6 Fracture of the lateral condyle. (**a**) Lateral condyle fracture, (**b**) K-wire osteosynthesis

pain and swelling, and a cubitus valgus which inevitably leads to ulnar nerve palsy. In contrast, displayed fractures of the lateral condyle are often accompanied by lateral subluxation of the ulna. Undisplaced fractures of the lateral condyle appear horizontal and are moderately stable due to an intact cartilage hinge. Normally, undisplaced fractures of the lateral condyle are treated by a long arm cast with the elbow at 90° for 3–4 weeks or by K-wire osteosynthesis. In the case of cast treatment, x-ray examinations are indicated for every 3–4 days for the first 2 weeks because of secondary displacement. Most undisplaced fractures heal well with cast immobilization, whereas displaced fractures require immediate open reduction and internal fixation to achieve excellent results (Fig. 17.6).

17.5.4 Metaphyseal Fracture of the Proximal Tibia

All metaphyseal tibial greenstick fractures are related to a temporary partial stimulation of the medial part of the proximal tibial growth plate, consequently leading to a valgus-deformation. In most cases, a slight valgus position is already pre-existing. An untreated gapping fracture is associated with a delayed consolidation, consequently leading to an increased stimulation of the medial physis. An enhanced medial growth intensifies the valgus deformation, resulting in an unilateral *genu valgum*. In order to avoid an exorbitant valgus deformation, it is important to correct the primary valgus position by compressing the medial (convex) fracture gap, either by wedging the cast or closed reduction and medial external fixator application. However, in young patients the valgus-deformation normally corrects spontaneously during following growth (Fig. 17.7).

17.5.5 Fracture of the Medial Malleolus

This fracture represents an intraarticular epiphyseal fracture of the distal tibia. It can occur with (Salter IV) or without (Salter III) an additional metaphyseal fragment. In case of a widely open growth plate, a premature partial growth arrest occurs in 20%, consequently resulting in a varus deformation. This growth disturbance is especially associated with a displaced

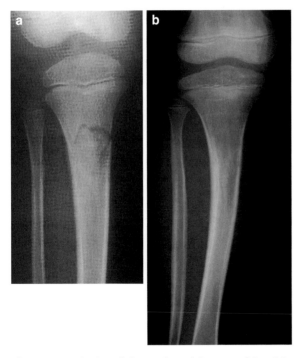

Fig. 17.7 Typical medial metaphyseal fracture of the tibia. (**a**) meta physeal greenstick fracture, (**b**) typical valgus deformity

fracture. However, in most cases the growth disturbance is not very distinctive due to the fact that fractures of the medial malleolus occur beyond the age of 10. Nowadays, undisplaced fractures are treated conservatively, while displaced fractures are treated by K-wire or screw osteosynthesis (Fig. 17.8).

Further Reading

Beaty JH, Rockwood CA, Wilkins KA (2005) Fractures in Children, 5th rev edn. Lippincott Williams & Wilkins, Philadelphia

Hefti F, Morscher E, Brunner R, Fliegel C (1997) Kinderorthopädie in der Praxis, 1st edn. Springer, Berlin

Laer Lv (2001) Frakturen und Luxationen im Wachstumalter, 4th rev. edn. Thieme, Stuttgart

Odgen JA, Hensinger RN, McCollough N (2000) Skeletal Injury in the Child, 3rd edn. Springer, New York

Puri P, Höllwarth ME (2006) Pediatric Surgery. Springer, Berlin, Heidelberg

Weinberg AM, Tscherne H (eds) (2006) Unfallchirurgie im Kindesalter. Springer-Verlag GmbH, Berlin Heidelberg, New York

Wilkins KE (2005) Principles of fracture remodeling in children. Injury 36(Suppl 1):A3–A11

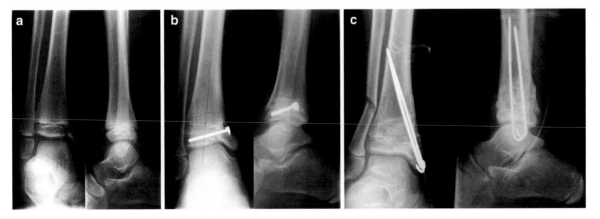

Fig. 17.8 Fracture of the medial malleolus. (**a**) Fracture of the medial malleolus (ap and lateral view), (**b**) Screw osteosynthesis (ap and lateral view), (**c**) K-wire osteosynthesis (ap and lateral view)

Injuries to the Tendons

18

Heidi Friedrich

Contents

18.1 Introduction

Tendon surgery only started in the early 16th century when one differentiated between nerves and tendons as, e.g., depicted by Leonardo da Vinci, Andreas Vesalius, and Rembrandt. The breakthrough, however, was only achieved in the 20th century with the advent of improved suturing material. Horsehair, linen, cotton, and silk threads used until then only poorly glided in the tendon sheath, such that as late as 1916 it was recommended to amputate an injured finger so as not to impair the finger or indeed the whole hand. Claude Verdan was the first to demonstrate a primary suture of a severed flexor tendon in 1961. Six years later Harold Kleinert was the first to successfully rejoin tendons in zone 2. In 1973, he furthermore recommended dynamic splinting of the finger generally leading to its full functional restitution. Later the secondary suture of the flexor tendon was abandoned and the delayed primary suture was introduced by Buck-Gramcko et al. (1983).

18.2 Flexor Tendons

18.2.1 Particulars of the Functional Anatomy

Tendon sheaths can be found wherever pressure is exerted on the tendons, such as on the palmar side of fingers and under the retinaculum flexorum and

P. Puri and M. Höllwarth (eds.), *Pediatric Surgery: Diagnosis and Management,*
DOI: 10.1007/978-3-540-69560-8_18, © Springer-Verlag Berlin Heidelberg 2009

extensorum. On the fingers, the tendon sheath reaches over three joints and is held in place by four pulleys ligaments (A1–A4) and by three cruciate ligaments (C1–C3). Damage to annular ligaments, notably A2 (over the base phalanx) and A4 (over the middle phalanx) leads to the "bow-string phenomenon," i.e., a protrusion of the tendon resulting in a reduced glide range and a reduced bending at the interphalangeal (IP) joint. The tendon sheath consists of the epitenon, which lies directly adjacent to the tendon and lines the tendon sheath canal and is also responsible for the blood supply. Vascularization within the tendon sheath is furthermore achieved to a large extent by the vincula tendinea, soft tissue sail-like structures containing arteries and veins, and therefore have to be handled with great caution. If they are destroyed by the injury, the tendons snap back into the palm. If, however, the vincula are preserved, the proximal tendon stumps can be found in the tendon sheath canal. Resection of the superficial tendons to enable the lower ones to glide more easily is considered an outdated method today (Fig. 18.1).

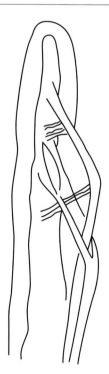

Fig. 18.1 Position of the vincula tendinea

18.2.2 Division into Zones

As with adults, the infantile hand is divided into the same injury zones that determine the required therapy.

The most common scheme applied is the one by Verdan and Michon (Fig. 18.2). Bunnell (1944) referred to zone 2 as a "no-man's-land." Due to the tightness in children's' hands in this region adhesion can easily occur.

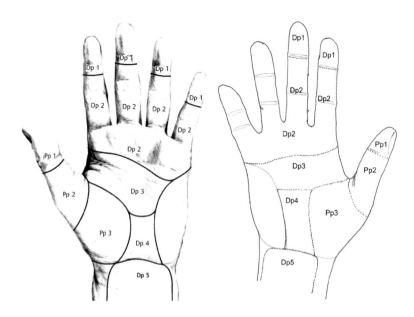

Fig. 18.2 Zone division according to Verdan (left) and Pechlaner et al. (right)

18.2.3 Evaluation

In small children, the function of the tendon cannot usually be tested such that the location of the injury and the position of the hand at rest are often the only clinical signs for a severed tendon. Cut injuries in toddlers are often caused by a fall while carrying a glass or falling into a glass pane, whereas older children hurt themselves while playing with knives.

18.2.4 Inspection of the Hand

If the end phalanx is extended, but not the base phalanx, the tendon of the m. flexor digitorum profundus (or of the flexor pollicis longus) is severed (Fig. 18.3).

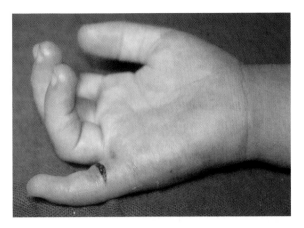

Fig. 18.4 Transsection of the tendon of the m. flexor digitorum superficialis

If the finger is only slightly bent, the tendon of the m. flexor digitorum superficialis is severed (Fig. 18.4).

If the finger is extended at the central and distal joints, both tendons are severed; this leads to a bending in the base joint caused by the mm. interossei and mm. lumbricales (Fig. 18.5).

Even if a flexor tendon is only partly transected, it must be surgically repaired (sutured) in order to pre-empt secondary ruptures.

18.2.5 Informative Dialogue

Before the operation, the child should be informed about the necessity of post-operative exercise therapy either by the doctor or by his/her parents. Most patients find it hard to believe that a 1 cm long injury can have such consequences and requires dedicated finger exercises for several months. But beyond subtle surgical techniques, only consistent training can ensure full recovery.

18.2.6 Surgical Management

A *primary* flexor tendon suture is one that is applied within 24 h; a *delayed primary* suture is one that is

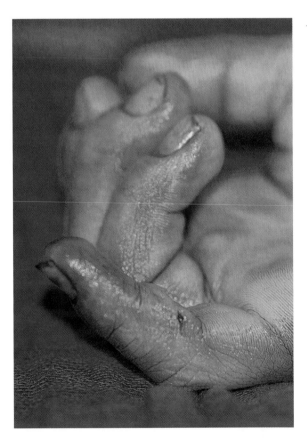

Fig. 18.3 Transsection of the tendon of the m. flexor digitorum profundus

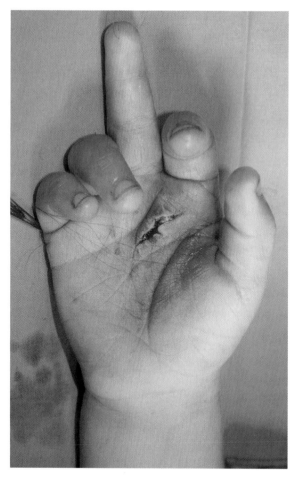

Fig. 18.5 Transsection of both tendons

18.2.7 Incision

In order to assess the extent and severity of the injury, the wound usually has to be opened on both sides to avoid any buttonhole surgery. To this end, one applies a Bruner incision (zigzag widening cut) as well as arc- and L-shaped palmar incisions. Longitudinal cuts on the finger should be avoided in children because they can lead to stringent scar formation and growth disturbances such as axial deviations. The skin flaps produced by the Bruner incision must not be too small to avoid problems with the blood circulation.

18.2.8 Suturing Technique

The more delicate the tendon, the more carefully the operation must be carried out: for example, the tendons must never be held with tweezers on the surface. A *Kirchmayr–Zechner* suture has turned out to be tear proof for children (Fig. 18.6). For the core suture, one uses a non-absorbable suture with a straight needle, doubly re-enforced. For the circular epidendinal adoption suture, an absorbable thread of gauge metric 0′7 (6-0) should be used in order to prevent bulging of the tendon stumps. The same suture can be used for the tendon sheath.

done within 2 weeks, or after the skin wound has healed. After the injury has healed, one refers to the flexor tendon suture as *secondary*, whereas operations in weeks 3–6 (*early secondary*) pose a high risk of complications. There is no rigid space of time for performing secondary sutures, but the chances for a successful reconnection of the tendon stumps—without an intermediary transplant— diminishes with time. For the operation under anaesthesia, a tourniquet and surgical loops and/or microscope are required. Duration of tourniquet inflation must not exceed 2 h. Beside general anaesthesia, a hand block or plexus anaesthesia is applied in order to keep the child free from pain during the first post-operative day which also helps with the occupational therapy.

18.2.9 The Kirchmayr–Zechner Suture

After fetching the stumps, a core suture is applied for which the thread is pierced four times. Moreover, one

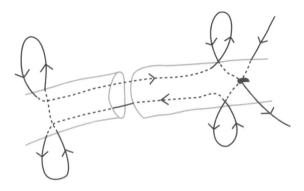

Fig. 18.6 Kirchmayr–Zechner suture

should also try to countersink the knots in children (according to Zechner) which may not always be possible due to the tiny diameters of the tendons. The circular adaptation suture should be a continuously overlapping helix-type suture. One has to pay attention to the pulleys ligaments A2 and A4; if they were to be damaged, they would have to be reconstructed so as to avoid the "bowstring phenomenon." Severed tendons often coincide with severed blood vessels and nerve bundles. If at all possible, not only the finger nerves, but also the arteries should be reconstructed. With only one finger artery, there is often a cold sensation of the finger.

18.2.10 Post-Operative Therapy

At the end of the operation, a forearm plaster or cast longuette is applied. For smaller children, one has to use an upper-arm longuette to ensure they do not become loose and are not stripped off at night. The injured finger is immobilized using a vessel loop, or with an extended rubber string attached to the fingernail with a suitable (first curing) glue. For children, the plaster cast longuette does not need to be in the original 40° position in the metacarpo-phalangeal joint or in the 50–60° position in the wrist joint, because children tend to maintain this extreme bent position after the removal of the plaster, unless they are constantly reminded otherwise. This effect does not occur if the wrist is bent by 5–10°. Furthermore, the longuette only extends to the metacarpo-phalangeal joint which greatly facilitates occupational exercising (Fig. 18.7). Occupational treatment commences on the first post-operative day; only in cases of extensive nerve repair one may begin a day later. The occupational therapist exercises five to six times a day in a playful atmosphere with the little patients and administration of a painkiller may often be helpful. These active and passive exercises are to be demonstrated to the parents so that they can be continued at home. In order not to risk losing the trust of the little patients, removal of the stitches is best done under general anaesthesia. After discharge, the children return two or three times a week for outpatient therapy and follow-ups. Using this modified bandage arrangement, the tendon itself and hence the suture is not under stress; this, of course, leads to synergistic relaxation of the flexor muscles. Adhesions which can occur at the injured area on the surface of the tendon and – in particular—in the tendon sheath can be pre-empted by daily multiple gliding move-

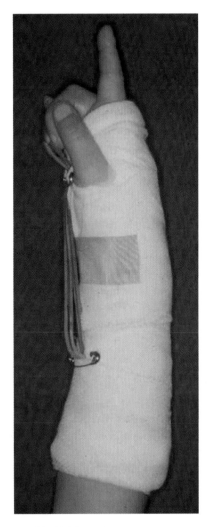

Fig. 18.7   Modified Kleinert plaster

ments to assure that the functioning of the tendon is not impaired. In children, the risk of adhesion is greater than in adults; on the other hand, secondary ruptures are more rare. Immobilization is limited to 5 weeks. Exercise therapy is sufficient if the PIP (proximal interphalangeal) joint is extended on the third post-operative day and if the finger can be fully extended within 10 days. Full recovery and mobility must be achieved within 3 months.

18.2.11 Follow-Up Treatment

Outpatient checks in increasingly larger intervals are strongly recommended and should be maintained until the end of adolescence. This is necessary because the injured area may not fully participate in a growth spurt; a resulting tendon shortening may require more occupational therapy.

18.3 Extensor Tendons

18.3.1 Functional Anatomy

The extensor tendons are more prone to injuries due to their location directly under the skin. The gliding ability of the extensor tendons is achieved by the paratenon, a loose soft tissue layer at the back of the hand and the distal forearm. In contrast to the flexor tendons, the extensor tendons change their shapes and their courses and consequently have to be attended differently. For this reason the extensor tendons are divided into zones (Fig. 18.8).

18.3.2 Diagnosis

One usually differentiates between open and closed (or subcutaneous) injuries of the extensor tendons; furthermore they may be fully or only partially ruptured. The latter injuries also have to be surgically repaired because poor nutrition and/or degeneration weakens the tendons and makes them prone to complete ruptures.

In adults and children, closed injuries above the distal interphalangeal joint are the most common tendon injuries and most frequently caused by impact with a solid object. Here the straight finger is compressed in its length and pressed in the palmar direction. This injury is also known as hammer-, dropping-, mallet-, or baseball-finger.

Classification of subcutaneous extensor tendon injuries (Fig. 18.9).

1. Rupture of the extensor aponeurosis (from the basis of the end phalanx) (Fig. 18.9a):

   The aponeurosis is avulsed from the Landmeer ligaments, the distal interphalangeal (DIP) joint is tilted by about 30°. The distal phalanx can no longer actively be straightened; clinically there is a slight swelling and redness combined with a moderate locally confined pressure pain.

2. Rupture of the extensor aponeurosis (proximal to the Landmeer ligaments) (Fig. 18.9b):

   This injury leads to a bending of the DIP joint by about 45°. This injury is also named "mallet-finger". If left untreated it leads to a "swan neck deformity".

3. Avulsion of the extensor aponeurosis together with a small dorsal bony fragment at the base of the distal phalanx (Fig. 18.9c):

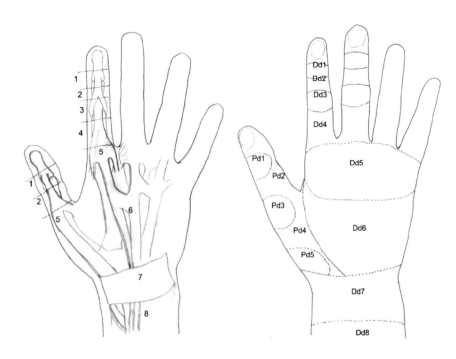

Fig. 18.8 Injury zones according to Verdan (left) and Pechlaner et al. (right)

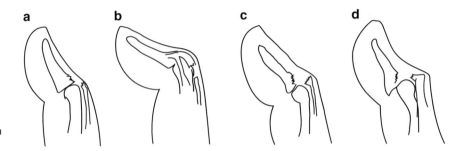

Fig. 18.9 Classification of subcutaneous extensor tendon lesions of zone 1

Here the DIP joint is bent by ~ 30°. Clinically there is a pronounced pressure pain. This chisel-(Busch-) fracture occurs when the end phalanx tends to give way in the dorsal direction.

4. Palmary luxation fracture with shearing of larger dorsal bony fragments from the base of the distal phalanx (Fig. 18.9d):

The DIP joint is unstable; it is only slightly bent and the end phalanx appears shortened and swollen (hyperextension injury).

18.3.3 History

In children, cuts and stab wounds can affect the extensor tendons. In ballgames or jamming injuries subcutaneous ruptures occur at the end phalanx, and are less frequent at the middle phalanx. Injuries at the proximal phalanx are always ominous for bite injuries; notably human bites – not uncommon in small children—are prone to severe purulent infections.

18.3.4 Physical Examination

Monitoring of the hand functions and the type of the injury can on occasions provide information pertaining to the diagnosis. The indication for a surgical inspection under general anaesthesia has to be generously applied particularly in infants and young and timid children.

18.3.5 Management

As in the case of injuries of the flexor tendon, suspected extensor tendon injuries in children have to be inspected under full anaesthesia, using a tourniquet and surgical loops and/or a microscope. The pressure of the tourniquet sleeve for children is between 180 and 230 mm Hg and the maximum duration of inflation must not exceed 2 h. If longer tourniquet intervals are required, a 20 min spell of blood circulation permits another 1 h of tourniquet use. Alternatively, one can apply "relative" bloodlessness, i.e., only the forearm is unwrapped and thus the residual blood facilitates to differentiate between nerves and blood vessels.

18.3.5.1 Injuries in zone 1 (at the distal interphalangeal joint)

Open Injuries

In children, open injuries need to be attended urgently.

ad a. Here the wound is widened in a zigzag manner and the joint stabilized in not more than 10° hyperextension by a K-wire (gauge 0.6–1 mm). This is to be applied obliquely to reduce the risk of infection. A manual drill or—for older children—an electric drill with low speed (to avoid overheating) is strongly recommended. Multiple trial drillings should be avoided so as not to damage the cartilage. The wire is bent above the skin level and can thus be removed without anaesthesia even in small children. The aponeurosis can thus be reconnected tension-free using interrupted 6/0 sutures. A Lengemann suture may sometimes be necessary for older children. Immobilization is achieved by means of a plaster-attached splint for 6 weeks which may be replaced after 4 weeks by a Stack splint. These splints must be cut to size for the children, but the PIP joint must also be immobilized. Although this is not desirable, it provides better stability for the small fingers. The splint may only be removed when drying the skin (to

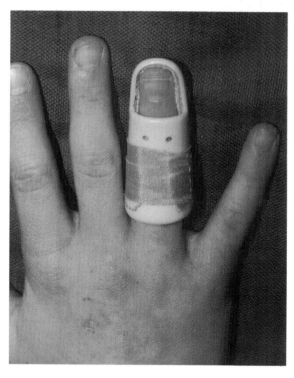

Fig. 18.10 Stack's splint

prevent maceration) without moving the end phalanx (Fig. 18.10).

ad b. as above: the aponeurosis is restored by means of a mattress suture line, but special care should be taken because the tendon stumps may easily tear. Again, the hand is immobilized for 6 weeks using a plaster-attached finger splint.

ad c. and ad d. In case of a bony avulsion or luxation fracture, the primary concern must be to carefully reposition the broken parts so that no unevenness remains at the joint surface. Here too the distal phalanx is temporarily stabilized by a K-wire supplemented by a Lengemann suture.

Closed Injuries

A closed, ruptured extensor aponeurosis in zone 1 can primarily be treated non-operatively. Given regular outpatient follow-up check-ups, the outcome is about the same as with primary surgical repair. In children, a plaster-attached splint is recommended initially since it can be better adapted than prefabricated plastic splints. After 4 weeks, the plaster splint has to be replaced by a Stack splint for another 4 weeks.

Inadequately reconstructed transsections of extensor tendons will lead to tendon callus formation at the tendon stumps, rendering the tendon too long to fully bend the distal interphalangeal joint. The tendon therefore has to be tightened or doubled. The same non-operative treatment is applied as with a bony avulsion of the extensor aponeurosis. After reducing the fragment into correct position, the quality of the reduction must be checked by X-ray. If the fragment cannot be reduced or held in that position, fixation must be accomplished surgically.

18.3.5.2 Injuries in zone 2 (at the middle phalanx)

As the extensor aponeurosis at the middle phalanx is laminar and thin, the suture may easily cut through the tendon tissue if tightened too hard. The injured distal phalanx can still actively be extended if only one of the side tracts remains. If both lateral ligaments are cut through, the distal phalanx can only partially be extended. If completely destroyed, a hammer-finger deformity develops. To check the extensor aponeurosis, the finger must be extended against a resistance applied at the level of the DIP joint. In case of doubt a surgical inspection is recommended.

Open Injuries

If only one side tract is affected, it must be restored using an absorbable suture (5/0 to 6/0). If both side tracts are affected they need to be adapted by some U-type sutures; in addition a temporary transfixation of the distal interphalangeal joint is required. Immobilization for 6 weeks in intrinsic-plus position is recommended (Fig. 18.11).

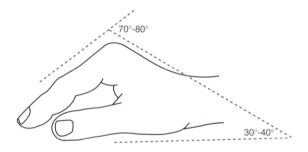

Fig. 18.11 Intrinsic-plus position

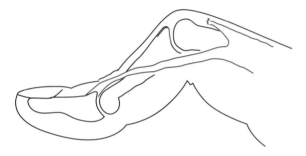

Fig. 18.12 Buttonhole deformity

Closed Injuries

In children closed injuries can also be treated non-operatively, but the injured finger must be immobilized for 8 weeks (3 or 4 weeks with a plaster-attached finger splint—in slight hyperextension of the DIP joint—and another 4 weeks with a Stack splint).

18.3.5.3 Injuries at zone 3 (at the proximal interphalangeal [PIP] joint)

The extensor aponeurosis at the PIP joint consists of a distal part of the tractus intermedius of the two side tracts of the musculi interossei and the musculus lumbricalis, as well as the fibres between the two. If the pars triangularis is affected, the PIP joint is bent. Tearing of the tractus intermedius is often overlooked as long as the side tracts and the ligamentum triangulare are intact. At the PIP joint, one finds a minor, pressure-sensitive spot and the joint cannot fully be extended. If left untreated the tractus intermedius retracts, the side reigns gradually slip down and the heads of the proximal phalanx protrudes as through a buttonhole (buttonhole deformity, boutonniere or, simply, buttonhole) between 10 and 14 days after the trauma (Fig. 18.12). In case of a full transsection of the extensor mechanism, the injured finger remains bent.

Open Injuries

In case of an injury directly above the PIP, a dorso–latero arch incision is used for surgical repair. After rinsing the joint thoroughly using sterile saline solution, the joint is closed using an absorbable suture (5/0 to 6/0 single-knot or U-sutures). A complete transsection of the tractus intermedius is treated similarly; conceivably, in older children an additional Lengemann

suture may be necessary. Smaller defects of the tractus intermedius are repaired after detaching it from the side tracts. This is achieved by temporarily transpositioning the tractus intermedius in distal direction and re-inserting the side tracts. In addition a 5-week immobilization is always required. For injuries in adults, a buttonhole splint is used, but this is not available for children. For repair of larger extensor tendon defects, there are several tendon replacement techniques available with the dip-over graft plasty technique being the most established.

Closed Injuries

The same surgical procedure is applied for closed injuries as with open injuries. Provided the side tracts are not affected, a rupture of the pars medialis of the tractus intermedius can be treated conservatively. In this case, it is necessary to maintain activity of the finger while the middle phalanx is passively extended.

18.3.5.4 Injuries at zone 4 (at the proximal phalanx)

In this rather rare case of a full transsection of the complete extensor apparatus, bones are always also affected. If only the central part is concerned, its function is compensated by the side tracts.

Open Injuries

Even if there is no functional deficiency, the severed central section of the extensor apparatus should definitively be surgically repaired in order to improve the results (similar arguments apply to severed side tracts). A Lengemann suture—as applied in adults—is generally not required for children. The tendon sheath must be carefully reconstructed to prevent adhesions. A severed tendon of the m. extensor pollicis longus tendon in a thumb renders it impossible to fully extend the interphalangeal joint. The tendons are joined using an U-suture, possibly with an additional semicircular absorbable suture (6-0) for adequate adaptation of the tendon stumps.

Closed Injuries

Injuries in zone 4 are rather rare in children, but should be surgically treated to ensure full functional restoration; the surgical intervention is to be followed by immobilization for 4 weeks using a plaster-attached finger splint in intrinsic-plus position.

18.3.5.5 Injuries in zone 5 (at the metacarpo-phalangeal joint)

In this case, the extensor tendons and/or the extensor caps are severed. The affected finger cannot be extended in the metacarpo-phalangeal joint, but both the proximal interphalangeal and the distal interphalangeal joints can be extended due to the unaffected palmar muscles (drop finger). If the tendons of fingers 2 and 5 are affected, extension is still possible by activation of the corresponding tendons of the m. extensor indicis proprius and m. extensor digit minimi, respectively. The cap of the extensor tendon is most commonly injured on the radial side leading to a slippage of the tendon towards the ulna when attempting to flex the fingers; this leads to a "snapping" phenomenon when clenching one's fist. The restoration at the radial aspect of the index finger is very important to provide a two-finger grip.

Open Injuries

Open injuries need to be repaired immediately, particularly if the joint is opened. After generous rinsing the joint is closed by fine absorbable sutures. Completely cut-through tendons are reconnected by U-sutures using a non-resorbable thread and an additional circular running type suture for adaptation. The post-operative therapy includes a molded plaster cast finger splint for 4 weeks.

Closed Injuries

Closed injuries are treated in the same manner as open injuries. Untreated injuries lead to the formation of tendon callus above the metacarpal heads resulting in a reduced range of motion of the joint and this should therefore be removed.

18.3.5.6 Injuries in zone 6 (at the back of the hand)

Owing to the intertendineous connections, these injuries only lead to partial loss of extension at the metacarpo-phalangeal joint.

Open Injuries

In children, the very thin and flat tendons at the back of the hand can be repaired using U-type sutures or, as in flexor tendon surgery, by modified Kirchmayr sutures. The surgical treatment is followed by 4 weeks of immobilization by a palmar plaster longuette.

The same procedure is applied for the tendons of the mm. extensor pollicis longus and brevis; the proximal stump may retract so much so that it can only be reached by a proximal additional incision.

Closed Injuries

Long extensor tendons of the thumb, as seen in adults—as a result of a radius fracture or a progressive-chronical polyarthritis, for example—practically never occur in children.

18.3.5.7 Injuries in zone 7 (wrist)

Due to the absence of a intertendineous connections, the proximal stumps of fully severed tendons slip far in a proximal direction, such that the affected finger can no longer be extended. On the other hand, adhesions occur more easily in the extensor sheath compartments of the wrist than at the at the distal forearm region.

Open Injuries

The flattened stumps of the extensor tendons of the long fingers should be adapted using U-type sutures; the rather more round tendons of the m. extensor carpi radialis and ulnaris, as well as the extensor pollicis longus allows to apply the flexor tendon surgery techniques for suturing. Post-operative treatment includes immobilization by a palmar plaster longuette for 3–4 weeks.

18.3.5.8 Injuries in zone 8 (distal forearm)

Severing of extensor tendons does not lead to a complete deficiency of the extensor function, but injury to the intertendineous connections may result in reduced strength.

Open Injuries

In this region, the tendon stumps are reconnected by U-sutures followed by 3–4 weeks of immobilization using a forearm-plaster cast longuette.

Further Reading

Buck-Gramcko D, Nigst H, Millesi H (1983) Verletzungen der Beugesehnen, Handchirurgie, 2nd vol. Verlag Thieme, Stuttgart, New York

Bunnell S (1944) Surgery of the Hand. Lippincott, Philadelphia

Doyle JR, Blythe W (1975) The finger flexor tendon sheath and pulleys: Anatomy and reconstruction. In A.A.O.S. Symposium on Tendon Surgery in the Hand. Mosby, St. Louis, pp 81–87

Friedrich H, Bäumel D (2003) Die Behandlung von Beugesehnenverletzungen im Kindesalter. Handchir Mikrochir Plast Chir 35:347–352

Kirchmayr L (1917) Zur Technik der Sehnennaht. Zbl Chir 44:906–907

Kleinert HE, Kutz JE, Atasoy E, Stormo A (1973) Primary repair of flexor tendons. Orthop Clin N Amer 4:865–876

Pechlaner S, Hussl H, Kerschbaumer U (1998) Operation satlas Handchirurgie. Thieme Verlag, Stuttgart, New York

Puri P, Höllwarth M (2006) Pediatric Surgery. Springer, Berlin, Heidelberg

Rockwell WB, Butler PN, Byrne BA (2000) Extensor tendon: Anatomy, injury and reconstruction. Plast Reconstr Surg 106:1592–1603

Snow JW (1973) Use of a retrograde tendon flap in repairing a severed extensor in the PIP joint area. Plast Reconst Surg 51:555–558

Stack HG (1969) Mallet Finger. Hand 1:83–85

Verdan C, Michon J (1961) Le traitement des plaies des tendons fléchisseurs des doigts. Rev Chir Orthop 47:285–425

Voigt C (2002) Sehnenverletzungen an der Hand. Chirurg 73:744–767

Burns

19

Jonathan Saul Karpelowsky and Heinz Rode

Contents

19.1 Introduction

Burns are defined as coagulative destruction of tissue by thermal, chemical or electrical injury.

This simplistic definition does however fail to incorporate the significant short and long term sequelae of these injuries, and the devastating social, functional and cosmetic consequences resulting from burn wounds.

A burn is one of the most devastating injuries with life-long consequences that can be inflicted upon mankind and, although many problems are still unresolved, substantial progress has been made. Guiding principles in the modern care of burns is a logical exercise in resuscitation, infection control, surgical wound care, nutrition and both psychological and physical rehabilitation.

Survival following severe burn injury has improved substantially over the last 40 years with a predictive 50% survival (LD50) of 98% total body surface area burned (TBSA) in children and 75% TBSA in adults in leading centres. These results are based on refinements in the early phase of fluid resuscitation, and inhalational burn management, in the latter phases by improved nutrition, bacterial control, and by a combination of early burn excision, and early coverage by auto-or allografting (cadaver skin), biological and synthetic skin substitutes and lastly by early and ongoing rehabilitation. Legislative requirements to reduce the hazards of thermal injury have also made an impact on the incidence and severity of burns.

19.2 Aetiology

The aetiology of burns varies according to age, activity and socio-economic circumstances. Children are more likely to be burned in conditions of social disruption, whether this takes the form of poor socio-economic infrastructure, poor adult supervision or blatant child abuse. It must be borne in mind that children are inquisitive by nature and their environmental exploration places them at risk for all types of burn injuries. In children, hot liquid accidents are responsible for 80% of patients, fire injuries for 18% and chemicals accidents for 2%. Electrical injuries are usually low voltage but can produce life threatening cardio respiratory complications and unique injuries. High voltage injuries are far less common and are usually associated with significant underlying muscle damage.

19.3 Pathology

The skin consists of two parts: the epidermis and the dermis. The epidermis is the superficial thinner layer responsible for limiting evaporation of water from the body, and is constantly replenished by cell division in the basal layer of the epidermis. The dermis is the deeper thicker layer providing strength and durability. It contains the adnexal structures which provide an epithelial reservoir from which partial thickness wounds can heal by a process known as reepithelialisation.

A burn wound is tri-dimensional in nature and pathologically consists of three concentric zones in surface and depth (Fig. 19.1).

The zone of coagulation represents irreversible tissue necrosis. The zone of stasis is an area of impaired circulation secondary to the release of vasoactive mediators and platelet aggregation, which given correct management, can be salvaged and needs to be protected, and optimised at all stages of resuscitation. The zone of hyperemia is caused by the release of inflammatory mediators and results in vasodilatation. It is this zone which causes much of the systemic fluid perturbation.

The evolution of the injury in a burn wound is a dynamic process and it may take up to 3–4 days for the size and eventual depth of cell death to become evident. This will depend on the effectiveness of treatment

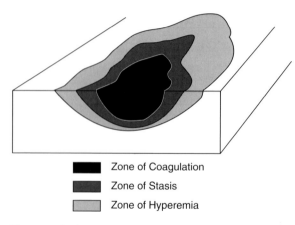

Zone of Coagulation
Zone of Stasis
Zone of Hyperemia

Fig. 19.1   Jackson's burn model

received and the potential salvage of the zone of stasis. Burn wounds from flames tend to be deeper and of a greater severity than scald burns.

No objective clinical methods are available to determine the depth of thermal injury and no standardized method has been adopted. Most burns are a combination of superficial and deeper burns and the best assessment can be made 3–4 days after the injury when wound evolution has been completed.

Burns are divided into various thicknesses, each of which relate to an anatomical level within the skin microstructure (Fig. 19.2).

(a) Superficial partial thickness: destruction of only superficial layers of the skin. There is enough preservation of dermal elements to ensure re-epithelisation. These wounds will, given the correct treatment, epithelialise spontaneously within 3 weeks.

(b) Indeterminate depth (deep dermal burn): destruction of epidermis and varying amounts of dermis. The dermis is affected and depending on the recovery of the zone of stasis may have enough remaining dermal elements to heal spontaneously but usually in a delayed manner. These wounds are difficult to assess during the first 3 days after injury due to the ongoing evolution within the burn wound which can be modulated by infection and dehydration.

(c) Unequivocally full thickness: total irreversible destruction of all elements of the skin with or without extension into the deeper tissues and structures. These wounds will not heal spontaneously within 3 weeks and have unsatisfactory functional and cosmetic results.

Fig. 19.2 Burn depth and skin structure

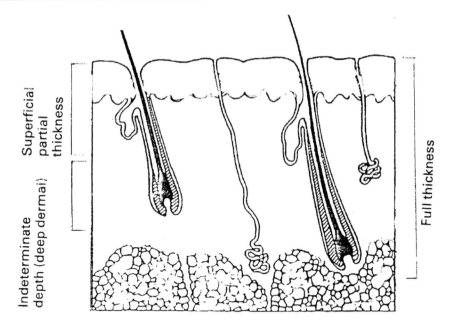

19.4 Pathophysiology

The initial burn wound may only appear to affect the integumentary system but the insult is widespread with a multi organ cascade of effects.

Haemodynamic changes: Thermal injury alters endothelial integrity and function. The subsequent systemic inflammatory response syndrome (SIRS) effects are mediated by the widespread release of inflammatory mediators, primarily from the zone of hyperemia. This results in obligatory isotonic fluid loss from the intravascular spaces into the burn area. The capillary changes occur very rapidly and are maximal within the first 3–12 h following small burns and up to 24–48 h after injury for larger burns. This fluid loss can be as much as 4.4 ml/kg/h. The fluid loss is not confined to the burnt area, but involves the whole body when the Total Body Surface Area (TBSA) >30%. This obligatory sequestration of fluid will lead to the formation of oedema with eventual loss of effective circulating fluid volume. If this loss is extensive, hypovolaemia and shock will develop. It remains a common cause of death.

Hypermetabolic response: Although a thermal insult occurs immediately, the systemic response to inflammatory mediators reaches a peak 5–6 days after the injury. Increased metabolic rates are often encountered in burns and may be as high as 50–100% above normal in major burns. This response is characterised by gluconeogenesis, severe protein catabolism, lipolysis and fat redistribution. Essential protein sources can be exhausted within 3–5 weeks, making nutritional supplementation essential either enterally or parenterally. Afferent stimuli from the burn wound i.e. pain cause the release of cytokines, tumour necrosis factor and thromboxane, which stimulate the hypothalamus to reset the core temperature. In addition, catabolic agents, i.e. glucagon and cortisol are increased and anabolic hormones (insulin and growth hormone) are uniformly decreased during the 1st period of the injury. These hormonal changes can significantly be ameliorated or abolished with early enteral feeding (less than 12 h post injury). Meticulous pain control and an ambient temperature maintained at 28–32°C to minimize metabolic expenditure for maintaining body temperature. Repeated insults secondary to hypovolaemia or infection result in an amplified response of mediators and can significantly intensify the systemic inflammatory syndrome.

Cardiovascular changes: Apart from hypovolaemia, the following changes are observed:

(a) Increased haemotocrit due to isotonic fluid loss from the intravascular space, erythrocyte heat damage, stasis and impaired microcirculation both in burned and unburned tissue, with ultimate compromise of substrate delivery and resultant propagation of the inflammatory cascade.

(b) Myocardial depression mediated primarily by Tumour Necrosis Factor (TNF) this is predominantly seen at burns exceeding >50% total body surface area.

(c) Increased systemic vascular resistance, catecholamine, both noradrenaline and adrenaline release with an increased sensitivity of peripheral vessels to adrenaline and acute phase reactants. This results in further compromise of essential substrate delivery.

Respiratory complications: Although the respiratory tree is well protected, there are several manifestations of respiratory burns. These are best assessed in several categories.

Supraglottic or central airway injury is usually a direct thermal injury resulting in progressive swelling of the airway and mechanical obstruction. This can result from the inhalation of steam or hot gases.

Infraglottic or peripheral airway injuries are usually secondary to a chemical injury due to incomplete products of combustion, i.e. hydrogenchloride/cyanide, aldehydes and acrolein. Clinically, patients present with three distinct phases. Firstly respiratory distress due to bronchospasm, necrotising tracheo-bronchitis and inflammation of the lower respiratory tree. This may result in pulmonary oedema and subsequent bronchopneumonia (bacterial).

Systemic pulmonary manifestations thus may result from acute respiratory distress syndrome (ARDS) in response to trauma, inhaled chemicals or sepsis, and manifests as significant hypoxia and bilateral pulmonary infiltrates on chest radiography.

The second systemic manifestation of an inhalational injury can be in response to intoxication by carbon monoxide or cyanide. Carbon monoxide is produced by incomplete combustion and has an affinity for haemoglobin 240 times that of oxygen for carboxyhaemoglobin (COHb). The resultant effect is that it displaces slowly taking about 250 min on room air and 40 min on 100% oxygen. In addition to haemoglobin binding, it combines with intracellular cytochromes disrupting cellular functioning leading to systemic aberration. This cytochrome bound carbon monoxide has a delayed washout which could result in delayed symptoms. Cyanide binds tightly to intracellular cytochromes disrupting oxidative phosphorolation and cellular respiration.

Renal failure: Several aspects may alter renal function, namely by a low perfusion state due to under or delayed resuscitation e.g. burn shock or alternatively due to electrical or extensive burns which may cause haemolysis, rhabdomyolysis with haemoglobinuria, myoglobinuria and renal failure.

Susceptibility to infection: The burnt patient is prone to micro-organism invasion because of impaired local defense mechanisms (loss of outer skin barrier, presence of dead tissue and impaired local blood flow) and impaired systemic immune defenses due to a decrease in phagocyte and lymphocyte function, compounded by impaired humoral and cell-mediated immunity. These factors together with an exposure to a high-risk environment for nosocomial infection and recurrent invasive procedures result in sepsis being the leading cause for delayed mortality in burns. Gram-positive organism infection predominate during the 1st week. Seventy percent of the wounds harbour organisms from an exogenous source (mostly Gram-positive) and 30% of the organisms are from an endogenous source predominantly the gastrointestinal tract, mostly gram negative organisms.

The common organisms encountered are as follows: Unfortunately many of them have become resistant to topical antiseptics.

1. *Staphylococcus aureus* 55%
2. *Pseudomonas aeruginosa* 20%
3. B-hemolytic Streptococcus 17%
4. *Acinetobacter baumannii* 10%
5. Mixed gram-negative flora 14%
6. Enterococcus 3%
7. *Candida albicans* 3%

The gastro intestinal tract: The bowel is very susceptible to injury during the periods of hypovolaemia and lack of enteral feeding. More than 60% of patients may have evidence of bowel ischaemic injury at autopsy. Release of stress hormones induces mesentric vasoconstriction and lead to decreased gut immune function and gut mucosal-integrity, predisposing the patient to bacterial and endotoxin translocation of endogenous flora into the systemic circulation. This process can be ameliorated by early aggressive enteral feeding and adequate circulatory resuscitation.

19.5 Clinical

19.5.1 Airway and Respiratory

The detection of respiratory insufficiency is paramount during the initial examination as it is a major cause of early mortality. Symptoms can be delayed for up to 48 h and may evolve over time thereby needing continued reassessment. Children, due to their relatively narrow airway and large tongue, are at greater risk for airway obstruction. Smoke inhalation is an important determinant of mortality in burns. The incidences vary from 2% to 35% and increases the mortality by 50% for any surface area burned. History of flame burns sustained in an enclosed space and loss of consciousness at the scene are good predictors of potential respiratory injury. Clinically the presence of burns on the face, either flame or hot water, carbonaceous sputum or nasal discharge, a hoarse voice, confusion, stridor and finally any of the routine signs associated with respiratory distress mandate very careful assessment, and early intervention. Signs of carbon monoxide intoxication range from nausea and fatigue to confusion, seizures and coma. These patients characteristically look "cherry red", a sign that is often absent, and with pulse oximetry readings misleading as carboxyhaemoglobin is mistaken for oxygenated haemoglobin giving normal oxygen saturation readings.

19.5.2 Cardiovascular

Perhaps the most significant cause of early morbidity is poor fluid resuscitation. Sole reliance on the blood pressure without the determination of end organ perfusion is a major pitfall during examination. Peripheral perfusion and pulses, mental state and importantly urinary output all must be continually assessed as a vital guide to the fluid status. There must be an active search for bleeding both external and internally which may be associated with concomitant trauma and this must be addressed.

19.5.3 Musculoskeletal

Two pitfall misassessments are: compartment syndrome either due to a constricting full thickness eschar or alternatively due to a swollen limb secondary to electrical injury and extensive underlying muscle damage or extensive fluid resuscitation; signs may be subtle and pre-emptive decompression escharotomies may be required. Absent pulses are an end-stage sign and action should be taken well before this point. Missed skeletal fractures from concomitant trauma necessitates close repeated clinical examination.

19.5.4 Burn Area

Accurate determination of the total burn surface area (TBSA) is essential in the assessment and management of the burn victim. All subsequent fluid administration, referrals and management will be based on the calculation of TBSA. Time taken to accurately plot the burned area rather than a cursory glance cannot be underestimated. Charts representing body area percentages are widely available but usually represent the adult "Rule of nines" where each part of the body is represented as a multiple of nine. The proportions of the child however are different and need to be modified depending on the age of the patient. Children will have proportionately bigger heads and smaller legs and hence the modifications made. The head in the infant is approximately 18% of the body surface area and each leg 14%. For each year of life above the first the head decreases in relative size by approximately 1% and each leg gains 1/2% in comparison with total body surface area. An alternative method for TBSA assessment will be to use the unstretched open hand representing 1% (Fig. 19.3).

19.5.5 Burn Depth

- Superficial partial thickness: Rarely cause functional or cosmetic defects or hypertrophic scars. They may never completely match the colour of the

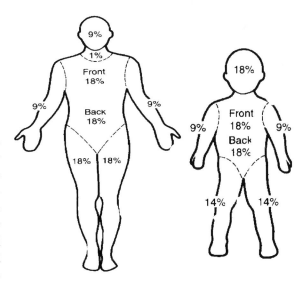

Fig. 19.3 Body surface area distribution

unburned surrounding skin. These wounds characteristically have an erythematous, moist, homogenous surface with blister formation, are painful and hypersensitive to touch, blanch readily and have a normal to firm texture on palpation.

- Indeterminate depth (deep dermal burn): The wounds present with a mottled pink and white dry surface and may blister. Capillary refill may be sluggish or absent after pressure is applied to the wound. Pain is perceived as discomfort and the wound is often less sensitive to pinprick than the surrounding normal skin. The burn is depressed in comparison with the surrounding skin and the healing time for these wounds may be variable. Hypertrophic scar formation is commonly encountered in the long term.
- Unequivocally full thickness: These wounds may mimic the appearance of an indeterminate burn and are usually mottled, white, red or charred and dry in appearance, insensitive to pain and leathery on palpation. Blisters are unusual and if present, are thin-walled and do not enlarge. Clotted superficial vessels may be visible. The surface of the burn is usually depressed relative to adjacent unburned skin and the appearance of the burn remains static with little change over the ensuing days.

19.6 Investigations

Investigations are directed toward monitoring the efficacy of resuscitation, and the multiple changes in the haematological, biochemical and bacteriological spheres during the emergent, acute and chronic phases of burn care.

If inhalational injury is suspected chest radiography should be performed. Other radiology will be required assessing concomitant trauma.

Laboratory investigations including, carboxyhaemoglobin levels, acid base status and lactate all of which will provide evidence of end organ perfusion. Urine examination for concentration, specific gravity and myoglobin will aid the resuscitation process.

19.7 Emergency Management

At the scene of the injury, smouldering hot clothing should be removed immediately and the adequacy and patency of the airway ensured. Hydrotherapy or burn cooling with tap water should be undertaken. Small burns (<25% TBSA) are immersed in cold water at 15–18°C or covered with cold, wet compresses for at least 30 min to reduce the depth of injury and relieve pain and discomfort. Larger burns may also undergo cooling hydrotherapy but caution must be exercised as hypothermia may develop. Alternatively burns can be covered with Melaleuca Hydrogel (Burnshield) which is a compact, easily transportable, light sterile dressing for a period of up to 24 h. A single application of Burnshield is as effective as cold water compressions. No oily substances should be used topically. Following hydrotherapy the wound should be covered with clean, dry dressings or antiseptic agent. Copious irrigation of the wound with water is indicated for chemical burns. Neutralising agents should not be used.

19.8 Transportation

Burn patients are usually stable immediately after injury and should be transported as soon as possible. Intravenous fluid therapy should be commenced if travel time is more than 1 h, or if transport is delayed. Children with major burns should be transferred only after fluid resuscitation has commenced, measures to maintain temperature have been instituted and the wound protected. All patient injured by electricity should have cardiac monitoring during transfer since dysrhythmias may occur. Oxygen should be administered to all major burns patients or when carbon monoxide poisoning is suspected.

19.9 Burn Resuscitation

Management of an inhalational injury should always take first priority. Humidified 100% oxygen should be provided to all major burns or those with carbon monoxide inhalation. If an airway injury is suspected, early intubation may be warranted as it will progress. A tracheostomy is seldom needed as airway oedema subsides in 5–7 days. Endoscopy is invaluable in confirming the diagnosis, determining severity and aiding in airway management. Intubation can be difficult and expertise should be sought if available. An additional 2 ml/% burn/kg weight is required to support the systemic circulation when considering fluid management. Ventilatory management should follow those of a protective lung strategy using low volume and pressure ventilation with the addition of positive end expiratory pressure. Despite the fact that 50% of inhalational injuries go onto develop pneumonia, prophylactic antibiotics and steroids are not indicated.

Cardiovascular and fluid management are the next priority. Any active bleeding need be sought, stopped and replaced. Thermal injury invariably leads to increased papillary permeability, the formation of obligatory burn oedema, hypovolaemia and shock. The initial therapeutic goal is the prompt restoration of vascular volume and preservation of tissue perfusion. The fluids administered to the burns patient have three components each vitally important but composed of different fluids, and each calculated in a different fashion. These are resuscitation fluid, fluid for ongoing losses and maintenance fluid.

Resuscitation fluid is used to correct any significant deficit causing poor end organ perfusion; it is usually given as fluid boluses (10–20 ml/kg) to restore circulating volume. This should continue until evidence of good perfusion has been restored i.e. slowing of pulse, improved capillary refill and good urine output.

Resuscitative fluids high in sodium of at least 130–150 mmol/l should be used, the most widely available and recommended fluid is Ringers Lactate/Hartman's solution/Plasmalyte B/Balsol. If there is bleeding from associated trauma the use of blood should be considered.

Ongoing losses should be administered according to the Parkland formula 4 ml/kg/% burn. This is the approximate amount of fluid that the child will need in the first 24 h following a burn. Half of this calculated volume is given in the first 8 h, and the rest over the next 16 h, starting from the time of injury.

Significant underestimation may occur in the infant less than 10 kg, so close monitoring of vital signs is essential. Urine output is a very good indicator of response to fluid therapy and should be 1 ml/kg/h and in small children 1.5 ml/kg/h.

Monitoring the effects of the resuscitation must be an ongoing and active process. It may be necessary to administer fluid boluses of 10–20 ml/kg/bolus of Ringer's lactate or increase the next hour's fluid administration to 150% of the calculated hourly rate to optimise urine output to > 1.5 ml/kg/h.

During the second 24 h following the burn, resuscitative fluid administration can be decreased as the inflammatory response subsides and are administered as 2 ml/kg/% burn. Finally maintenance fluid appropriate for the child's age should be administered in addition to the above.

Oral administration of fluids for burns <10% TBSA, is acceptable. The requirements for sodium are high at this time, so it is dangerous to give large volumes of fruit juices, tea or water, as this will lead to water intoxication and hyponatraemia. Nasogastric or preferably nasojejunal tubes can be invaluable for this purpose. Oral fluid administration should not proceed in the child with a significant ileus or in the haemodynamically compromised child. All these children should receive intravenous fluid therapy.

Additional fluid requirements will be needed in inhalational injury myoglobinuria, delayed resuscitation, associated trauma and electrical injury.

19.10 Pain Management

This is one of the most neglected components of management. Most analgesic requirements are for the first 48 h and subsequently for dressing changes and physical activities. Long-term pain management issues such as withdrawal and tolerance need to be looked for and managed in consultation with a specialised pain management team.

19.11 Nutrition

Patients with >20% TBSA require aggressive nutritional support and the calorie and protein requirements should be met from the 1st day to prevent impaired wound healing, cellular dysfunction and decreased resistance to infection.

Early enteral feeding within the first 12–24 h post burn decreases the release of stress hormones, improves nitrogen balance, maintains gut mucosal integrity, lowers the incidence of diarrhea and decreases hospital stay.

Due to high feed requirements patients often require tube feeds either via a nasogastric route or if not tolerated by a nasojejunal tube. The oral route is possible but difficult to sustain especially when combined with inter recurrent episodes of sepsis and theatre visits. Total parenteral nutrition has been associated with infections, metabolic and immunological complications.

The ideal enteral tube feed consists of 20% of the calories as protein, 30% as fat and 50% as carbohydrates. Immuno-modulating formulae may become important in the future. These formulae will deliver normal daily requirements and added needs for burns hypermetabolism and recovery.

- Protein: 3 gm/kg/bodyweight + 1 gm% burn
- Calories: 60 kcal/kg bodyweight + 150 kcal/kg/% burn
- Supplements: vitamins, zinc and iron

Another formula used for calculating nutritional requirements is (Galveston formula)

Age 0–12 months: $2,100 \text{ kcal/m}^2 + 1,000 \text{ kcal/m}^2$ burn

1–15 year: $1,600 \text{ kcal/m}^2 + 1,400 \text{ kcal/m}^2$ burn.

19.12 Prevention and Treatment of Wound Infection

Wound care is one of the pillars of burn care management with an ultimate goal of preventing and treating infection of the burn wound.

Initial management consists of gentle, but thorough cleansing, with removal of all debris left by combustion and the accident, debridement of loose non-viable tissue, as well as the application of a sterile dressing and topical therapy to prevent infection.

The patient should then be showered on a basis as determined by the chosen topical therapy, and the wounds cleaned with an antibacterial solution or soap. Smaller wounds may be done in the ward environment with appropriate analgesia but larger burns need be done in a warmed theater environment under general anesthetic.

External bacterial wound contamination should be controlled through environmental measures and monitoring bacterial presence and growth. Surface wound swabs are done 3 × weekly and quantitative wound biopsies: i.e. 1 biopsy/25 cm² eschar weekly. Wounds harboring >10⁵ org/g tissue signifies impending transeschar spread and septicemia. A strict antibiotic protocol should be followed with systemic antibiotics only

given in the presence of clinical burn wound sepsis, septicemia, B-hemolytic streptococci infections, and a bacterial count of $>10^5$ org/g eschar.

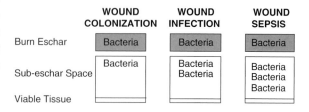

Wound sepsis: $> 10^5$ org/g tissue

Topical therapy has a dual purpose, prophylactic to control the microbial population and therapeutic to decrease counts to below 10^5 org/g. It is used to reduce bacterial and fungal proliferation but cannot sterilise a burn wound. Local organisms and sensitivity patterns need be monitored to establish the most effective topical application for the patient and unit involved.

Silver sulfadiazine has an excellent spectrum of activity, low toxicity, and ease of application with minimal pain; it is the most frequently used topical agent used. Its long half life ensures effectivity for at least 24 h. Problems experienced with the use of Silver sulphadiazine is frequently associated with the development of a "pseudo-eschar" within 2–4 days, owing to interaction of the drug with proteinaceous exudate in the wound, which can lead to error in the evaluation of burn depth by the inexperienced observer. There is also an emerging bacterial resistance to it in major burn units.

Povidone iodine—5% acts by destroying microbial protein and DNA. This antiseptic has excellent *in vitro* antimicrobial activity but is inactivated by wound exudate. It has a short half life and its clinical effectiveness is significantly decreased by bacterial resistance. Povidone iodine has not proven to be useful as a topical antimicrobial treatment for burn patients. Its adverse effects include systemic absorption of iodine, with resulting renal and thyroid dysfunction.

Mupirocin has excellent broad spectrum antimicrobial profile, predominantly against Gram-positive organisms and fungi. It is especially useful against Methicillin resistant Staphylococci (MRSA). It has no activity against *Pseudomonas* species.

Chlorhexidine acts through destruction of the bacterial cellular wall and precipitation of cellular content. It has a broad spectrum of antimicrobial action, especially with respect to Pseudomonas infection.

In combination with Mupirocin it often broadens staphylococcal cover. Its application can be difficult as it often melts becoming very liquid in nature.

Acticoat has had a major impact on the management of burns. It is a polyethylene mesh containing nanocrystals of metallic silver. In this nanocrystalline form, metallic silver exhibits pronounced antibacterial activity against a wide range of Gram-positive and Gram-negative bacteria including strains resistant to many types of antibiotics. It is also effective against clinically important strains of yeasts and fungi. This dressing appears to maintain antibacterial levels of silver ions in the wound for up to 5 days. Because Acticoat remains effective on the burn wound for this period, the patient is spared the pain associated with dressing changes, is nurse friendly, cost effective and easy to apply but must be kept moist by water, not saline application.

19.13 Definitive Management

19.13.1 Minor Burns

Initial therapy of minor burns should include administration of analgesics and cleaning of the wound. Dead tissue should be debrided and any tar removed with soft paraffin in a water base(Jelonet®) or mineral oil (Table 19.1). Topical antibacterial agents and occlusive dressings or an adhesive polyurethane sheet should be used to dress the wound (Omiderm) and tetanus toxoid administered. The patient should be encouraged to move the affected area. Local topical therapy is applied every 2–3 days until the wound is healed or Omiderm left undisturbed for 7–10 days or until the wound has healed. Prophylactic antibiotics are usually not required. The wounds should be examined regularly (daily/once a week) as necessary. Wounds that fail to heal with in 3 weeks will need to have a skin graft.

19.13.2 Major Burns

Management of major burns is a particularly time and energy intensive process and the requirement of a coherent multidisciplinary team cannot be underestimated.

Guiding principles of burn wound management are as follows:

- Surgery is an elective procedure in a stable patient.
- Superficial and partial thickness thermal injuries treated correctly will heal spontaneously within 3 weeks can be clinically identified and are best treated conservatively.
- Hot water (scald) burns in children are best left for 2 weeks to assess the need for operative intervention, thereby reducing the area for excision by >50%.
- Early excision and grafting should be considered the treatment of choice for all full thickness burns. Inadequate excision leads to skin graft loss. Exceptions might be ears, soles of feet, genitalia and face.
- The amount to be excised depends on the status of the patient, the burn size, availability of auto or

Table 19.1 Analgesics and anxiolytics

Acute management:	Morphine 10–40 mcg/kg/h infusion IVI		
	Tilidine HCl (Valoron) 0.5–1 mg/kg/dose		
	Paracetamol: 20 mg/kg/dose		
Sedation:	Trimeprazine (Vallergan)	2–3 mg/kg/dose (max 100 mg)	
	Droperidol (Inapsin)	0.1–0.2 mg/kg/dose (max 5 mg)	
	Hydroxyzine (Aterax)	0.5–1 mg/kg/day	
Anxiolysis:	Midazolam (Dormicum)	0.5 mg/kg/dose (max 15 mg)	
Dressing change:	Ketamine	→ IVI	0.25–0.5 mg/kg/dose
		→ IMI	1–2 mg/kg/dose
		→ Oral	0.5 mg/kg/dose
	Combination	Midazalam	0.5 mg/kg/dose
	(Orally)	Codeine	0.5–1 mg/kg/dose
		Brufen	5–6 mg/kg/dose
		Paracetamol	15–20 mg/kg/dose

allografts or skin substitutes and the volume of blood loss.

- Once the burn wound has been excised, immediate wound closure with autografts, allografts or biological alternatives is required.
- Non-life threatening burns in patients with severe concomitant diseases or injuries should only be excised when the patients are stable and the life-threatening processes controlled.
- Surgical excision can safely be done in the presence of inhalational injury.
- Beta-haemolytic *Streptococcus* infection, and heavily contaminated untreated wounds are a contra-indication to surgical excision and grafting until the infection has been eradicated.

19.14 Surgical Management

19.14.1 Decompression Escharotomies

Decompression escharotomies are emergency procedures done at the time of first assessment of the patient. Oedema accumulates under the rigid burned skin which acts as a tourniquet thereby obstructing normal circulation. Both arterial and venous blood flows are compromised. This is part of resuscitation and should be performed as soon as possible, to avoid irreversible ischemic and hypoxic damage of tissue, and or to permit adequate chest excursion and ventilation. Releasing decompression must be done where a circumferential deep burn is impeding circulation to more distal parts, especially round the arms, legs, or chest where respiration may be impaired. An escharotomy is the longitudinal incision of full thickness burned tissue thus permitting the expansion of the underlying viable tissue. The decompression incision must traverse the dead tissue as far into the subcutaneous layer or as necessary to encounter viable tissue, and must extend from nonviable through to viable tissue. Bleeding may be a problem (see haemostasis), especially if the incisions are too deep or performed over major vessels. Vital structures (e.g. nerves, blood vessels) may be damaged if the decompression is incorrectly sited. Transverse incisions in the limbs should not be made. Correct placement of these escharotomies is essential to avoid problems during the reconstructive and rehabilitation phases of treatment. Anaesthesia may not always be necessary for the decompression procedures, but monitor the response to surgery, and provide anaesthesia and analgesia if this becomes necessary.

19.14.2 Theatre Management

19.14.2.1 General

Vascular access must be adequate and secure. Large bore cannula access is preferred; a central venous catheter may often be the only available option. As the burn treatment progresses, the availability of venous access sites becomes extremely limited. Arterial lines are invaluable, and often provide the only continuous monitoring available during surgery on the child with major burns. It may be necessary to stitch these in place, as dressings may not adhere to burned tissue.

Temperature control is mandatory, as hypothermia is a significant problem. Preventable measures include an ambient theatre temperature of 28–32°C, warmed anaesthetic gases and intravenous fluids, the use of overhead radiant heaters, and a plastic-covered warming blanket on the operating table. Exposed areas may be covered with sterile plastic drapes.

Monitoring is a challenge. ECG electrodes may be placed on the chest, but it may be necessary to use the hands, feet, forehead, back or any other available dry surface. Surgical staples in the skin with crocodile clips attached are very useful. A urinary catheter is useful but it frequently crosses the field of surgery, and may be temporarily plugged off during the procedure.

19.14.2.2 Surgical Guidelines

The process of excision, grafting and progressive burn wound coverage must follow a predetermined progression. There will however need to be flexibility based on the healing process of the child.

The theatre procedure follows a set program:

- Administer analgesics
- Clean the wound with bland soap and water or detergent
- Remove any topically applied agents
- To be able to evaluate the extent of the burn, shave the hair where necessary
- Dead tissue should be debrided
- Joint and burn mobilisation with allied therapists

- The depth and extent of the burn wound will determine the surgical approach
- Excise and graft as per treatment plan
- Dress the wound with topical antibacterial agents, occlusive dressings, non- adhesive polyurethane sheet or temporary skin substitutes where indicted
- Routine antibiotics are not required

The amount to be excised at each procedure depends on the stability of the patient, the burn size, availability of auto- and allografts, the volume of blood loss incurred during the procedure and the adequacy of anaesthesia.

A practical guide to surgical excision is a follows:

- Burns <10% TBSA—Excision and autografting—meshed 1:1.5 or 1:2, side meshed or sheet grafts. The latter two are placed on all vital and visual areas (face, neck, chest, hands).
- Burns 10–30% TBSA—Excision and autografting—meshed 1:1.5 or 1:2 or sheet grafts. The latter is placed on all vital and visual areas (face, neck, chest, hands).
- Burns 30–40% TBSA—Sufficient donor sites are usually available to graft the excised bed despite the fact that about 30% TBSA is unavailable for donation (face, neck, hands, feet). The grafts should be meshed at 1:1.5–1:2, or temporary allografts used.
- Burns >40% TBSA—Donor sites are limited and it is impossible to cover all the excised wounds with autografts primarily. Preferred method is that of excision total or sequential (20% TBSA every alternative day). This is followed by skin cover with autograft 1:1.5, 1:2, 1:3 and/or autograft 1:3 with allograft 1:2 overlay and/or synthetic skin substitutes.

19.14.2.3 Excision

There are three types of surgical excision, i.e. removing eschar.

- Tangential or sequential excision entails the sequential excision of thin layers of burnt eschar until a viable bed is encountered. The appropriate level of excision or end-point is characterised by a shiny white surface with a brisk arteriolar or punctuate bleeding, or viable yellow non-haemorrhagic sub-cutaneous fat globules with bleeding vessels in all areas. Dark pink-brown haemorrhagic fat is non-viable and must be removed, as residual necrotic areas will jeopardise graft take. Tangential

excision is best done within the first 3–5 days, before hypervascularity and wound infections have become established. Blood loss may be substantial, and effective control of haemorrhage must be established. A maximum of ±20% TBSA should be excised at any one time. 30% TBSA surgery (debrided and donor area together) equates to one estimated blood volume loss. This will depend however on both patient stability and the anaesthetic and surgical expertise. Once excised to the appropriate level and haemostasis secured, an immediate split-thickness skin graft is performed. Sheet grafts are placed on important cosmetic and functional areas. To prevent desiccation of exposed and viable tissue, mesh grafts should not be expanded more than 1:1.5 or 1:2. If greater expansion is needed, temporary skin substitutes (cadaver or synthetic skin substitutes) should overlay the autograft.

- Fascial excision is generally reserved for very large, life-threatening, or deep full-thickness burns. The excision is performed using a combination of sharp dissection, traction, and haemorrhage control. The excision is preferably limited to approximately 10–20% TBSA at any one time. Fascial excision assures a viable bed for skin grafting with moderate blood loss, especially if done under tourniquet control, and excellent graft take may be expected if done within the first few days after injury. It is imperative to leave a thin layer of fat over the sub-cutaneous bony prominences and tendon sheaths. If a primary skin graft cannot be performed, consider vacuum assisted closure (VAC) or temporary skin substitutes. The former stimulates rapid granulation tissue formation that will cover the exposed tendons or joints. Complete haemostasis with electrocoagulation should substantially minimise blood loss, but bleeding often occurs from skin edges. Topical vasoconstrictor agents could be applied to the fascia as the dissection proceeds. At completion, the extremity is wrapped with a pressure bandage and elevated for 10 min. The excised area is covered with an expanded split thickness skin graft. If the ratio exceeds 1:2, if greater expansion is needed, temporary skin substitutes (cadaver or synthetic skin substitutes) should overlay the autograft. The major disadvantage of this method is that it causes damage to lymphatics, cutaneous nerves, loss of subcutaneous fat, long-term cosmetic deformity, and distal oedema.

- Delayed escharectomy is done after 1 week, or after spontaneous eschar separation has allowed for the formation of a bed of granulation tissue. Daily debridement by means of hydrotherapy (showering or bathing), or coarse mesh gauze dressings will hasten the eschar separation. The burn wound is ready for split skin grafting when there is a shiny, slightly granular, pinkish-red uniform bed of granulation tissue with no debris or evidence of infection. This method is most often used for old neglected burn wounds.

19.14.2.4 Haemostasis

Bleeding from excised areas should be minimized. Methods employed are local pressure for 10 min, diathermy or bipolar coagulation, suture ligation and the topical application of sponges soaked in 1:10,000/ 1:30,000 epinephrine (adrenaline) solution to the excised bed for 10 min.

19.14.2.5 Skin Grafting

Procured skin is grafted onto the recipient area at the time of eschar excision, directly from the mesh board. Grafts are placed with the shiny or cut surface facing the prepared bed, either longitudinally or transversely over joints. The edges should be approximated or slightly overlapping and secured with surgical clips, sutures, or fine mesh gauze. Alternatively, small to moderate sized skin grafts can be secured directly with adhesive dressings or glue and covered with a bandage. In general terms the recipient area is covered with an occlusive dressing to prevent infection, avulsion and desiccation of the graft, and to allow for graft vascularisation.

The donor site for skin grafts needs to be treated as a partial thickness burn. Initially, bleeding is stopped with epinephrine swab compression. Then dressings are placed with either antiseptics or occlusive dressings. Poorly cared for or infected donor sites can become deep and hence extend the total wound area.

19.14.2.6 Wound Closure

Early closure of full thickness burn wounds using split thickness autograft (i.e. from own skin) is optimal.

However, the autograft is an imperfect substitute for full thickness skin; it may be limited in quantity, and there may be morbidity associated with the donor site.

If the burned area is too large, with limited available donor site, temporary closure by another form of covering is indicated to provide a physiological and mechanical barrier while healing takes place.

Allograft or skin donated by another person/cadaver, is the most commonly used skin alternative. When applied to a clean excised wound, the tissue vascularises and provides cover until it is recognised as foreign by the host, resulting in graft loss approximately 2–3 weeks after application in most patients. It acts as physiological primary closure, conferring the following benefits to the wound: decreased losses from the surface, decreased pain and energy requirements and decreased infection. It may be replaced every 10–14 days if non healing persists or replaced by a definitive closure material (e.g. autologous skin) once the patient and wound are stable. Uses for allograft are:

- To cover excised wounds with deficient donor sites
- Testing graft take on non-epithelialised areas as a temporary biological dressing
- As a cover for a widely meshed autograft
- Occasionally as a permanent biological substitute

Temporary skin replacement products treat partial thickness burns while healing or for use as a temporary skin replacement for mid-dermal to indeterminate depth partial-thickness burns. It is also indicated as a temporary covering for surgically excised full-thickness and deep partial-thickness burns prior to auto grafting. The disadvantage is that it is extremely expensive.

Biobrane is a knitted nylon mesh that is bonded to a thin silicone membrane. The silicone membrane provides a barrier against bacteria invasion and water-vapor transmission. Biobrane has been used successfully in the treatment of superficial partial-thickness burns, especially in the outpatient setting and in the treatment of donor sites.

With TranCyte, the concept of Biobrane has been taken a step further. A human fibroblast-derived temporary skin substitute consisting of a polymer membrane and newborn human fibroblast cells cultured under aseptic conditions on a porcine collagen coated nylon mesh. The membrane is biocompatible and protects the burn wound surface from environmental insults. In addition, the membrane is semi permeable, allowing for fluid and gas exchange. As the fibroblasts proliferate within the nylon mesh, they secrete human dermal collagen, matrix proteins, and growth factors. Indications as above but due to cost should best be reserved for clean partial thickness burns to cosmetically and functionally sensitive areas.

Full thickness burns destroy the dermal layer and hence the functional elasticity of skin. Replacement of an autograft onto a full thickness burn thus usually results in a functionally stiff, poorly cosmetic wound. Alternative management would consist of replacing the dermis with a synthetic dermal replacement and the epidermis with an autograft. Integra is composed of a bilaminate membrane consisting of a bovine collagen-based dermal analogue and a temporary epidermal substitute layer of silicone. The outer silastic layer is porous to allow water vapour loss but no organism invasion, and inner collagen fibres which is highly porous (70–120 μm) to allow fibrovascular ingrowth from the host prior to it undergoing biodegradation, for strength and elasticity. The dermal component incorporates itself into the patient's cell-producing neodermis. After the neodermis has formed, the silicone layer is removed and a thin epidermal autograft may be applied. Take is 80%, and a major advantage is a low incidence of scarring. It is indicated in full thickness burns specifically those areas reliant on flexibility and cosmesis, e.g. joints, hands, face. It has also been used in delayed reconstruction.

19.14.2.7 Physical and Occupational Therapy

Involvement of therapists in the theatre team is essential. It provides an opportunity to maintain joint mobility, and apply and construct splints, which will be crucial to the long-term functional outcome of a patient. Early splinting in combination with pressure garments and goal directed physiotherapy will reduce complication rates and joint contractures that may limit rehabilitation.

19.15 Rehabilitation

Following a burn, a sequence of events is precipitated in the family and in the injured child. The family reacts with shock, anxiety, confusion and guilt. Eventually they take control of the situation which fluctuates between confidence, guilt, hope, doubt and often withdrawal and eventually come to terms with the consequences of emotionally drained and concerned about the future of their child. They are often doubtful and sceptical about the process and outcome of rehabilitation. This program can continue for more than 10 years and should only stop once all physical and psychological rehabilitation aspects have been completed. The involvement of psychologists, physical and occupational therapists and reconstructive teams are invaluable.

The success of any burn program should probably best be measured by the successful reintegration of its patients into society rather than its ability to preserve life.

19.16 Conclusion

The successful management of burns requires a dedicated multi-disciplinary team of individuals. Following the principles of early resuscitation and maximum tissue preservation completed by early wound coverage while supporting the patient systemically and psychologically can ultimately lead to a successful outcome in these potentially devastating injuries.

Further Reading

Barret-Nerin J, Herndon DN (eds) (2004) Principles and Practice of Burn Surgery. Informa Healthcare, New York

Chung DH, Sandford AP, Herndon DN (2006) In JL Grossfild, JA O' Neill, EW Fonkalsrud, AJ Coran (eds) Pediatric Surgery. Mosby, Philadelphia, PA, pp 386–399

Heimbach DM, Engrav' H (1984) Surgical Management of the Burn Wound. Raven, New York

Sheridan RL, Tompkins RJ (2005) In KT Oldham, PM Colombani, RP Foglia, MA Skinner (eds) Burns in Principles and Practice of Pediatric Surgery. Lippincott Williams & Wilkins, Philadelphia, PA, pp 487–507

Shields BJ et al., (2007) Healthcare resource utilization and epidemiology of pediatric burn-associated hospitalizations, United States, 2000. J Burn Care Res 2007, Nov–Dec

Puri P, Höllwarth ME (eds) (2006) Pediatric Surgery. Springer, Berlin, Heidelberg

Foreign Bodies

20

L.T. Nguyen

Contents

20.1 Introduction

Children can put just about anything they can grasp into their mouths or their noses and then swallow it or aspirate it. Foreign bodies (FB) of the aero-digestive tract, whether they are aspirated, inserted or ingested are potentially dangerous. If they are not diagnosed early and removed they can result in numerous complications, such as perforation, obstruction of the gastro-intestinal tract, tissue necrosis, fistula formation, ulcerations, massive bleeding, airway and lung infections.

These complications carry a significant morbidity and mortality. FB aspiration in the airways is the cause of 160 annual deaths in children younger than 14 years old in the United States. The 2001 Annual Report of the American Association of Poison Control Centers noted 115,320 cases of ingestion of a foreign body by children younger than 20 years. More than 70% of these children are younger than 6 years.

Food items such as peanuts, grains, seeds or pieces of meat compose 50–80% of FBs removed by endoscopy from children's aero-digestive tract. In 2001, the US Center for Diseases Control (CDC) reported an estimated 60% of choking episodes treated in Emergency Department were due to food items such as peanuts, seeds, candy, gum, pieces of fruit, vegetables and hot dogs. Another 30% were due to non food substances of which coins accounted for a significant portion. Other non food items are: plastic pieces, screws, pins and button batteries.

Sixty eight percent of the deaths in children younger than 14 years reported to the Consumer Product Safety Commission were due to non food substances. The remaining 32% of deaths were caused by household items. The majority of deaths occurred in children aged

P. Puri and M. Höllwarth (eds.), *Pediatric Surgery: Diagnosis and Management*,
DOI: 10.1007/978-3-540-69560-8_20, © Springer-Verlag Berlin Heidelberg 2009

3 years and older. The diagnosis of a foreign body in the aero-digestive tract may be challenging because of the difficulty in obtaining a reliable history from children, especially when they are very young.

In clinical practice, most children (80%) had been witnessed to choke on an identifiable object but only 52% of events of airway FB were diagnosed early.

An estimated 40% of foreign body ingestions are not witnessed, and in many cases, the child never develops symptoms. In a retrospective review, only 50% of children with confirmed foreign body ingestion were symptomatic.

Objects that have passed the esophagus, once they reach the stomach, do not cause symptoms unless complications occur. They are usually eliminated spontaneously—even sharp objects—with normal bowel movements. Therefore, one can imagine that a lot of ingested foreign objects are passed daily without notice because the child has never complained. Prior to the 1930s, the mortality associated with FBs was very high. Currently, it is about 1–2%. In recent years, the development of modern instruments and equipments has dramatically improved the techniques for the removal of foreign bodies, even in the small child. During the same period, the ability to make a better diagnosis of foreign body ingestion or aspiration and their complications has improved, reducing the mortality and morbidity in these children.

20.2 Airway Foreign Bodies

20.2.1 Ear

The child can place a multitude of relatively small objects in the ear canal. Tissue, foam or paper fragments are the most common FBs retrieved from the external ear canal followed by beads, round toys, fragments of food materials and erasers.

The majority of children with FBs in the ear canal were seen in the day of the accident (72%) but a good number (8%) were seen more than a week later. In the vast majority of cases, the child was asymptomatic. Some may complain of pain, ottorrhea, bleeding or decrease of hearing. FBs in the ear canal can be successfully removed by using small forceps or irrigation of the ear canal with gentle suction by using a small

suction tip. Removal of a FB in the ear canal is sometimes challenging. Without the cooperation of the child, it can be extremely difficult. In one study, retrieval by Emergency Room staff was successful in a small number of patients (7%). With the majority of cases referred to ENT specialists. General anesthesia was required when the child did not cooperate or the FBs were beads or solid objects which were difficult to remove without anesthesia.

20.2.2 Nose

Most of the nasal FBs may be visualized directly by using a rhinoscope or an otoscope. Common FBs placed in the nasal cavity are beads, pieces of paper, foam, tissue and food matter (nuts, seeds, dried beans, pieces of food). Other miscellaneous objects included stones, screws, button batteries, pellets and erasers. Nasal FBs, if not removed early, can cause foul smelling nasal discharge, air flow obstruction and rhinitis. In one study, 80% of patients present on the same day, 8% present the following day; 10% are discovered incidentally following the development of foul smelling nasal discharge.

Plastic and other inert materials may be tolerated for a relatively long period until reactive granulation tissue develops to produce a nasal obstruction. A delay in diagnosis of button batteries in the nasal cavity may lead to septal necrosis, with perforation and destruction of the cartilage causing deformity of the nose—saddle-nose deformity. Most nasal FBs can be removed in the Emergency Department by Emergency Physicians with good visualization and appropriate instrumentation. Long standing objects such as button batteries may be more complicated, requiring assistance from ENT specialists.

20.2.3 Throat

Throat FBs are most often encountered in children between 4 and 8 years of age. The most common presentation is local pain followed by dysphagia, vomiting, drooling, crying and hematemesis. Most throat FBs are fish bones. Other FBs include other bones (chicken, pork) and toys. Throat examination can successfully visualize the FB in the throat warranting its removal. Radiographs are indicated when the FBs cannot be found. A lateral view of the neck may be helpful to visualize and locate the FB. The percentage of positive radiographs is rather low, less than 10%. Often Emergency Physicians are able to remove FBs in the throat in Emergency Department setting. In a study, 23.4% of cases were discharged after successful removal of the FB in the Emergency Department, the rest being referred to ENT specialists.

20.2.4 Laryngeal FBs

Laryngeal FBs occur less frequently than bronchial foreign bodies. They may be large and bulky and present with acute, life-threatening obstruction. Smaller, thin, sharp or triangular-shaped objects are at risk of embedding in the laryngeal mucosa or of becoming caught between the vocal folds (Fig. 20.1). Some can wedge in the larynx and cause an inflammatory reaction, mimicking infectious disease or incomplete upper airway obstruction; non specific symptoms cause difficulty in making the diagnosis. An X-ray is not always helpful as plastic FBs are not always radio-opaque. Flexible fiberoptic laryngoscopy is indicated in any child suspected of having a laryngeal FB whether it is a life-threatening clinical picture or chronic upper airway symptoms.

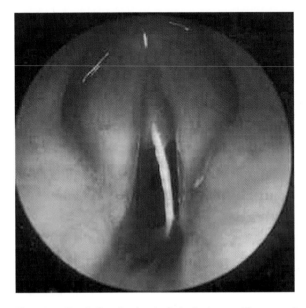

Fig. 20.1 Eggshell as foreign body in the larynx (Courtesy of Dr. J. Manoukian)

20.2.5 Tracheal and Bronchial Foreign Bodies

Children often play, run and laugh while eating and do not concentrate on chewing or swallowing. In addition to this, the mechanism that coordinates swallowing and respiration is still too immature to provide perfect control to avoid foods or other materials to enter the respiratory tract. Approximately 75% of tracheal and bronchial FBs in the pediatric group occur in children younger than 3 years. Most FBs are small enough to pass through the larynx and enter the trachea. Because the trachea is relatively large compared to the cricoid cartilage, only a small percentage of them (3–12%) lodge in the trachea.

Therefore most FBs will pass easily through the trachea and lodge in the primary or secondary bronchi. Among children aged 5 years or younger, aspiration of food items such as nuts, seeds and grains is more frequent than non food materials (79% versus 15%). In contrast, children older than 5 years are far less likely to aspirate food items (12%) than non food items (88%). In older children, pins, thumbtacks, paper clips and screws account for over half of the cases. Children have a tendency to put these objects in their mouth as a temporary repository while the hands are otherwise occupied (for example, holding a pen cap in the mouth while writing) the objects are then easily inhaled by accident. An accurate history and a good physical exam are the key factors in evaluating a child who has possibly aspirated a FB. A sudden *choking* episode, even not witnessed, is considered to be an important part of the history which may lead to a correct diagnosis of FBs of the airway. Choking alone may warrant a laryngo-bronchoscopy. It is the most sensitive clinical finding but its presence varies from one series to another (from 50% to 90%). The clinical triad which is considered to be diagnostic of FB aspiration consists of:

– *Wheezing*
– *Coughing*
– *Diminished or absent breath sounds*

Although each of the individual components of the triad may be present in 75% of the patients, all three are present in only 31% of cases, Kim noted that the triad was more often present in patients in which the discovery of the airway FB was late. The diagnosis of an airway FB is often delayed. Wiseman found that only 46% of patients were diagnosed on the 1st day. Pyman described six distinct types of clinical pictures depending on the degree of airway obstruction, location and duration of the FB:

1. Sudden wheezy breathing: most frequent
2. Cough alone with or without pyrexia
3. Hemoptysis
4. Stridor (seen only in cases of laryngeal and subglottic FB
5. Life-threatening asphyxia
6. Patient with no symptoms

Radiographic evaluation is helpful in a patient suspected of having an airway FB. It must consist of the following: anteroposterior and lateral views of the extended neck, anteroposterior and lateral views of the chest. Chest radiographs should be in both inspiration and expiration in order to appreciate air trapping which is present in 62% of patients when the bronchial FB acts as a one-way valve (Figs. 20.2a and b). Other X-ray findings include: Mediastinal shift, radiopaque objects, atelectasis. For late diagnosed airway FBs, X-ray may show signs of pneumonia, lung abscess, bronchiectasis, and empyema.

Wiseman found that X-ray findings were entirely negative in 18.5% of patients. However laryngo-bronchoscopy is the procedure of choice for both goals: diagnosis and removal of the FB.

In life-threatening asphyxia, laryngo-bronchoscopy is an emergency procedure. Otherwise, it should be well-planned. After induction of general anaesthesia the patient is placed in supine position with the head extended. A laryngoscope is first inserted to visualize and to expose the larynx for insertion of the bronchoscope. Great care is taken to protect the eyes, lips, teeth, tongue, and other laryngeal structures during the bronchoscopy. The bronchoscope is passed into the upper trachea, and ventilation is performed through the bronchoscope. The tracheobronchial tree is then completely inspected, and the FB removed.

Failure of bronchoscopic removal of FBs may result from:

– Inexperienced endoscopist
– Poor vision associated with bleeding, granulation tissue and edema
– Broken FB (especially nuts, vegetables) that migrate distally and become impacted.

Fragmentation of these FBs at the time of removal may be avoided by using Forgaty catheters instead of forceps. The Forgaty balloon is passed distally, the balloon is inflated, then withdrawn; the FB will be retrieved in the oropharynx.

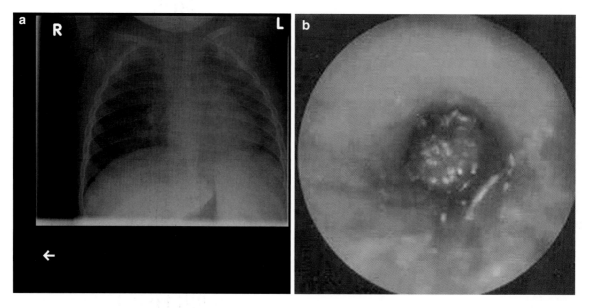

Fig. 20.2 (a) Hyperinflation of right lung secondary to a foreign body in the right mainstem bronchus. (b) Foreign body identified on bronchoscopy
Source: (Courtesy of Dr. J. Manoukian)

In other cases, a second procedure may be required. The second procedure may include repeated endoscopy, thoracotomy with bronchotomy or pulmonary resection.

20.3 Upper Gastrointestinal Tract Foreign Bodies

Ingestion of a FB is commonly encountered by physicians working in the Emergency Room. The management depends on the type of FB ingested, its location along the GI tract and the condition of the child. Eighty percent of all patients seen after ingestion of a FB are children. Children aged between 6 months and 3 years are the most affected. Most of ingested FBs pass spontaneously. An estimated 40% of foreign body ingestions in children are not witnessed, and in many cases, the child never develops symptoms. Objects with an irregular shape that are very sharp, that are unusually long or objects that can liberate toxic products like button batteries may require removal.

Complications of FB ingestion include: stenosis, perforation, tracheo-esophageal fistulae, bleeding and bowel obstruction. Although FB ingestion is less dangerous than FB aspiration, they are the cause of 1,500 deaths per year in the USA.

20.3.1 Esophageal Foreign Bodies

The esophagus has three naturally narrow areas: (1) the cricopharyngeous muscle, (2) the middle third of the esophagus at the level of the left mainstem bronchus, and (3) the lower esophagus. FBs tend to lodge in one of these three areas. Coins are by far the most frequent foreign objects swallowed by a child followed by fragments of food materials, metal, plastic, pins and bones. A significant geographic and cultural influence exists. For example, in Hong Kong, the most frequent FBs are fish bones. In one review from a Western Society, 89% of FBs were coins. The patients are most commonly between ages 18 and 48 months.

Twenty two percent of patients older than 5 years with esophageal FBs were noted to have anatomic abnormalities, such as a repaired esophageal atresia, a vascular ring, a cartilaginous rest, an esophageal stricture, and/or duplication cyst.

Most FB ingestions occur without symptoms and go unnoticed as the FB passes without complications through the GI tract. Clinical symptoms of a patient with a FB that obstructs the esophagus include:

– Sudden cough or sudden dysphagia
– Retrosternal pain
– Drooling, nausea, vomiting, choking
– Significant respiratory symptoms
– Bloodstained saliva

On the other hand, a small size FB lodged in the esophagus may be completely asymptomatic. Only 9.9% of patients with a button battery lodged in the esophagus were symptomatic in one study.

Radiographic studies are the simplest method to assess a child suspected of having a FB in the esophagus. The plain film should include the neck, the chest and the abdomen.

Radioopaque FBs can be easily seen on plain radiographs. If food materials or other radiolucent FBs are suspected as the cause of dysphagia and drooling, a barium esophagram is indicated. Obviously, in any suspected anomaly of the esophagus, barium swallows with or without other imaging studies is highly recommended.

Foreign bodies lodged in the esophagus, if not detected early can cause complications. Depending on the nature of the object and the duration of its presence, these include:

– *Button batteries*: esophageal burn, stricture, perforation aortoesophageal fistula, tracheoesophageal fistula, retropharyngeal abscess
– *Sharp objects*: perforation, abscess, retropharyngeal abscess mediastinitis
– *Others*: stricture, esophagitis

Therefore, foreign bodies in the esophagus should be removed promptly. Three main techniques have been described for removal of FBs in the esophagus:

– Extraction by using Foley catheter
– Bougienage
– Endoscopic retrieval

The first two techniques are limited to smooth objects such as coins. The choice between the three techniques depends on factors such as:

– Size and shape of the FB
– History of esophageal abnormalities
– How long the FB has been lodged in the esophagus
– Preference of treating physician

Foley catheter retrieval is generally successful for removing smooth objects like coins located in the upper two thirds of the esophagus. It can be performed in an outpatient setting with or without fluoroscopic guidance. Full resuscitation equipments should be available during the procedure. With the patient lying down in lateral decubitus and Trendelenburg, the Foley catheter is inserted into the esophagus through the mouth. Under fluoroscopy, the tip is passed further down, beyond the location of the FB. The balloon is inflated and carefully pulled back to bring the FB back into the mouth so it can be retrieved.

Success rate reported was excellent, up to 96%. This technique is not applicable for a coin that has been lodged in the esophagus for more than 2–3 days because it may be impacted.

Bougienage is a simple method for pushing smooth objects into the stomach with the expectation that they will then be eliminated spontaneously (up to 95%). Bougienage will be attempted in a selected group of patients:

– A single coin or impacted meat ingested less than 24 h since the ingestion
– No esophageal abnormalities
– No respiratory distress

Done under general anesthesia, endoscopic retrieval is the most thorough technique for safe removal of sharp or impacted objects in the esophagus with a success rate approaching 100%. At the time of the retrieval, the esophagus and its mucosa can be carefully inspected. Any esophageal stenosis can be dilated in the same setting.

For FBs that are present in the esophagus for an unknown duration, endoscopic removal is the only acceptable procedure.

Thoracotomy will be required to retrieve FBs in the mediastinum and to treat complications such as: aorto-esophageal fistula, tracheo-esophageal fistula, mediastinitis.

20.3.1.1 Disk or Button Batteries

Disk or button batteries can cause damage to the esophagus by direct corrosive effects, voltage burns and pressure necrosis. Injury to the wall of the esophagus may happen within few hours after the ingestion.

During the 7 year period from July 1983 to June 1990, the National Button Battery Ingestion Hotline in the USA reported 2,382 battery ingestions. Only 9.9%

of all patients were symptomatic but fatalities have been reported. Complications of esophageal button batteries include: pressure necrosis and burns to the esophagus leading to stenosis or perforation, aorta-esophageal fistula, tracheo-esophageal fistula.

Emergency endoscopic removal of all esophageal button batteries should be done because burns to the esophagus can occur as early as 4 h after ingestion. During the procedure, the esophagus is carefully inspected.

20.3.1.2 Coins in the Esophagus

Coins lodged in the upper two thirds of the esophagus will require removal as spontaneous passage is very rare.

However most esophageal coins are in the lower esophagus and these patients are usually asymptomatic. In asymptomatic patients with a coin in the lower esophagus, a conservative approach may be used for the first 24 h. This will consists of serial radiographs. Surprisingly, in up to 89% of patient, the coin passes spontaneously to the stomach (Figs. 20.3a and b)

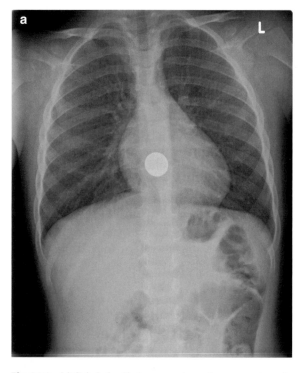

Fig. 20.3 (a) Coin lodged in lower esophagus in an asymptomatic patient

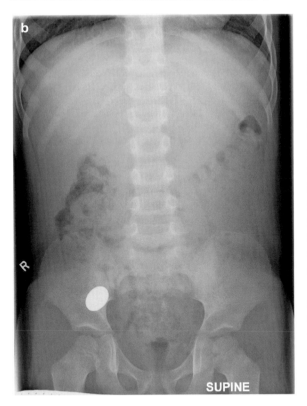

Fig. 20.3 (continued) **(b)** Spontaneous passage to the bowel after 24 h of observation

20.4 Sub-diaphragmatic Foreign Bodies

Smooth or blunt objects that reach the stomach will usually be evacuated spontaneously without complications. In one series of 1,259 children who had ingested FBs of all kinds in the subdiaphragmatic region, 97% of the FBs were passed spontaneously. Although the incidence of intervention for all ingested FBs is only about 1%, the rate for ingested sharp objects is 15–30%. These include toothpicks, bones, nails, pins, needles and sharp toys.

Objects longer than 5 cm tend to lodge in the stomach or duodenum because they can not negotiate through the C loop of the duodenum. Therefore they will need to be removed by endoscopy. For infants, objects larger than 2 cm in diameter can have difficulty traversing the pyloric channel and thus may require endoscopic retrieval. Bezoars are FBs that have accumulated over time in the GI tract and often occur in the stomach. They are commonly formed by plants and vegetable matters (phytobezoars), by hairs (trichobezoars) or by lactose (lactobezoars). These can cause obstruction symptoms, failure to thrive, vomiting, nausea and abdominal pain. Bezoars can be retrieved by endoscopy or eliminated by enzymatic fragmentation. Laparotomy may be necessary in very large bezoars.

For button batteries lodged in the stomach, the danger of leaking of battery content is less frequent than when it stays in the esophagus. Most of them can be followed by serial X-ray for 24 h. Gastroscopy with retrieval of the battery is indicated if the battery does not evacuate from the stomach within 24 h or if the patient experiences symptoms such as vomiting, nausea, or abdominal pain. The risk of complications increases when the battery is still charged. This will cause the batteries to adhere to the gastric wall and cause ulcerations.

Intestinal FBs rarely give complications. The only narrow place is the ileo-cecal valve. Most of the time, the FBs especially smooth objects, can be evacuated without difficulty. Sharp objects carry the risk of perforation. Therefore, they need to be followed by serial clinical examination and radiographs. Complications such as perforation and bowel obstruction have been reported. If after serial X-ray, the FB seems to stay in the same place, this FB may be lodged in a structure like appendix, a Meckel's diverticulum or another abnormal structure. Surgery may then be indicated.

20.4.1 Genitourinary Foreign Bodies

Vaginal FBs are most frequent between the age of 5 and 8 years old. Vaginal bleeding and blood-stained or foul-smelling secretions are the main clinical manifestations of foreign objects in the vagina. Most vaginal FBs are not radiopaque. Therefore, examination under anesthesia with a vaginoscope is essential. It allows for both diagnosis and for removal. The presence of vaginal FB may be an indication of a sexual abuse. In adolescents a vaginal foreign body may cause a vesico-vaginal fistula.

Self-insertion of FBs into the urethra and the bladder are extremely rare in children. However in adolescents and in young adult, especially in psychiatric patients, a multitude of objects have been found in the urethra and in the bladder such as needle, pin, piece of candle, a thermometer, a toothbrush, a metal hook. To avoid embarrassment, patients tend to seek treatment late, often waiting until the problem becomes symptomatic from urethritis, cystitis, or hematuria. Cystoscopy gives the diagnosis in difficult cases and allows the treatment.

Further Reading

American Association of Poison Control Centers (2001) Annual Report Vol.19; 5:335–395

Center for Disease Control (2004) 53 (SS07); 1–57

Chen MK, Beleri EA (2001) Gastrointestinal foreign bodies. Pediatr Ann 30:736–742

Kim IG, Brummitt WM, Humphry A et al (1973) Foreign body in the airway. Laryngoscope 83:347–354

Lelli Jr JL (2005) Foreign bodies. In KW Ashcraft, GW Holcomb III, JF Murphy (eds) Pediatric Surgery. Elsevier Saunders, Philadelphia, pp 137–145

Pyman C (1971) Inhaled foreign bodies in childhood. J Otolaryngol Soc Aust 3:170–180

Puri P, Höllwarth ME (eds) (2006) Pediatric Surgery. Springer, Berlin, Heidelberg

Stack LB, Munter DW (2006) Foreign bodies in the gastrointestinal tract. Emerg Med Clin N Am 14:493–521

Wiseman NE (1984) The diagnosis of foreign body aspiration in childhood. J Pediatr Surg 19:531–535

Physical and Sexual Child Abuse

21

Michael E. Höllwarth

Contents

21.1 Introduction

There are many aspects of child abuse, among them the most common forms are physical and sexual abuse, emotional or physical neglect and Munchausen by proxy syndrome. However, all aspects of intentional or unintentional malnutrition and hunger in childhood on the one side, as well as excess of everything possible on the other should be included in the list of child abuse. In this chapter we refer primarily to the symptoms, clinical signs, diagnostic procedures in children suspicious for physical or sexual child abuse and for the Munchausen by proxy syndrome.

The real incidence of child abuse is difficult to estimate due to the rather high number of unreported cases, especially when sexual abuse occurs. UNICEF has estimated that maltreatment leads to 3,500 death/year, and more than 800 are infants aged 0–11 months—resulting in an annual mortality rate of 6.1/100,000. The total number of cases of maltreatment is estimated to be 150–2,000 times higher than the number of deaths. A study of the US Department Health and Human Services estimated 903,000 children as victims of child abuse. Fifty-seven percent were neglected, 19% were physically abused, 10% were sexually abused, 7% were psychologically maltreated, and 2% experienced medical neglect. Parents were the perpetrators in 77% of child fatalities. The study showed that in 2001 approximately 1,300 death were attributed to child neglect or abuse. Of these deaths, 41% occurred in children under 1 year of age, and 85% occurred in children under 6 years of age. Factors which are typically associated with maltreatment are low socioeconomic status, violence in the family, breakdown of families, child morbidity, parental mental ill-health, and parents who were abused during their own childhood.

P. Puri and M. Höllwarth (eds.), *Pediatric Surgery: Diagnosis and Management,*
DOI: 10.1007/978-3-540-69560-8_21, © Springer-Verlag Berlin Heidelberg 2009

21.1.1 Physical Abuse

Physical abuse is not accidental but intentional and violent maltreatment caused either by harmful actions or by omission of helpful support by a person who is responsible for the child's welfare, leading to a temporary or permanent injury of a child under the age of 18.

In our Department, in three quarters of the cases the children are younger than 10 years with the highest incidence between 0 and 4 years (Fig. 21.1). The primary diagnoses in two thirds of the patients after admission to the hospital are injuries, while symptoms of somatisation or suicide are comparably rare—in contrast to patients with a history of sexual abuse (Fig. 21.2). Typical risk factors for child abuse in this age group are very young and inappropriate reacting mothers or fathers who have difficulties in coping with stressful situations, or parents overwhelmed with problems such as premature babies, handicapped children, constantly screaming babies or difficult living and social circumstances.

The history presented by the caregivers is often vague and may change from 1 day to the other or it is not consistent with the age of the child. It has been

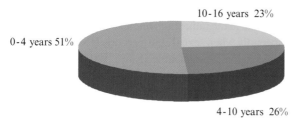

Fig. 21.1 Age distribution in children after physical abuse shows the highest incidence between 0 and 4 years

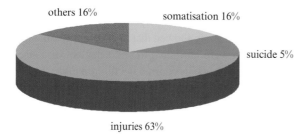

Fig. 21.2 The leading symptoms in patients with physical abuse are injuries while suicide or somatisation of symptoms is comparably rare

Table 21.1 It is of upmost importance to know which behaviour of caregivers or which posttraumatic findings should rise the attention towards physical abuse of a child

Suspicious behaviour of the caregivers
  Often change of doctors or hospitals
  Too late medical consultation
  Changing history presented from the caregivers
  Injury has not been observed at all and there is no explanation
  The demeanour of the caregivers is inadequate
Suspicious findings at the exam of the child
  Injuries not typical for the age of the child
  Several injuries of different age
  Formed injuries or marks
  Sudden and unexpected change of the behaviour of the child

shown that the absence of a history of trauma, changes in the history, or a history that blamed home resuscitative efforts is strongly associated with child abuse. Furthermore, our experience has shown that child abuse is likely when the reported trauma does not match with the severity, pattern, or localisation of injury. If an injury is suspicious to be caused by physical abuse a careful anamnesis by a person who is experienced in child abuse cases and has skills of interviewing is important. In Table 21.1 the most suspicious behaviours of caregivers and findings are listed.

21.1.1.1 Cutaneous Injuries

The most common manifestations of child abuse are cutaneous injuries. The physical examination of the patient may show multiple cutaneous injuries with swellings of the soft tissue or diffuse or formed bruises, abrasions, lacerations, petechiae and burns, often of different age (Figs. 21.3 and 21.4). Non intentional injuries in infants and children are usually localized around the prominent parts of the body—forehead, chin, hips, shins, and anterior or lateral parts of the extremities. Thus, suspicious injuries are localized on the side of the face, ears and neck, trunk, and inside or dorsal side of arms or legs, unless the history of the accident is appropriate.

In *bruises*, the inflicting instruments often may discern from the shape of the skin lesion. The human hand leaves parallel lines representing the spaces between the fingers. Cutaneous lesions of the upper arms or the thorax may result from hard pressure applied during violent handling.

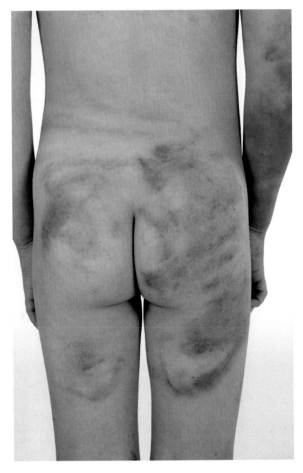

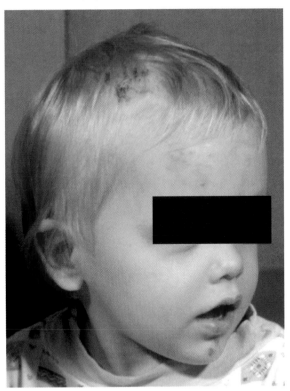

Fig. 21.4 Bruising on the frontal lateral side of the forehead. A punch of hear has been tuned out in this child

Fig. 21.3 Multiple cutaneous injuries and bruising with haematoma. The boy was beaten with a belt

In adult *bites* only one arch is often seen which usually reaches from one canine tooth to the other, while child bites can reach the second primary molar and involves both arches. Photographs should be taken and saline swabs should be used to pick up saliva for DNA analysis.

Ligatures cause typically lesions around the neck, the wrists or the ankles.

Burns represent around 10% of all physical abuse cases. The peak age of burn victims is from 13 to 24 months. Cigarette burns account for up to 5% of burns. They are round, often in clusters (Fig. 21.5). The classic lesions occur when the child is held in extremely hot water resulting in sharp demarcation lines on the margin of the hot water-skin contact line—e.g. stocking or glove immersion burns of the feet or hands. Immersion in the bath tub produces a typical doughnut lesion of the buttocks, sparing the parts, which are in direct contact with the basement of the tub. In contrast, if a child enters unintentionally a hot bathtub the resulting burn has no sharp edges and is unilateral.

21.1.1.2 Skeletal Injuries

Skeletal trauma is the second most common consequence of child abuse. A skeletal survey in children under 2 years is mandatory in all cases of suspected physical abuse. In older children we perform a bone scan to detect older skeletal injuries which may be not seen on plain radiographs. 80% of abuse fractures are seen in children younger than 18 months, 25% of them are skull fractures.

Fractures of the extremities occur in 44%. Accidental fractures in children under 2 years of age do occur, but are relatively rare in comparison with older children. Among them the most frequently injured long bones are the femur, the humerus and the tibia. Metaphyseal

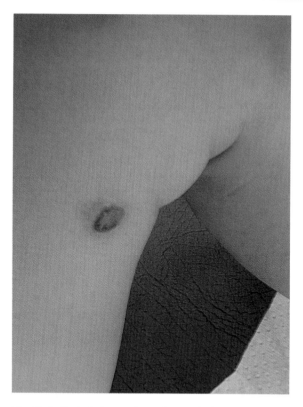

Fig. 21.5 Typical cigarette burn close to the breast

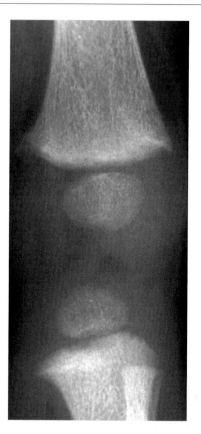

Fig. 21.6 Corner fracture at the distal metaphysio-epiphysial region of the femur

lesions of the long bones are highly suspicious signs of child abuse (Fig. 21.6). They occur very close to the growth plate and are known as bucket handle or corner fractures. Sites of predilection are the distal femur, proximal and distal tibiae and fibulae, and proximal humerus. They occur due to acceleration or deceleration forces during shaking the baby or twisting an individual limb –"the limbs are handles for mishandling the child".

Rib fractures may be diagnosed only coincidentally when chest radiographs are obtained for other reasons. In infants they are always caused by violence against the child unless the trauma has a consistent history, e.g. a severe car accident. These fractures in child abuse are often bilateral and usually localized close to the rib head or neck at the dorsal part of the thorax or in the lateral parts of the ribs (Fig. 21.7). It has been demonstrated that they are caused by anterior-posterior compression of the thoracic cage by placing the thumbs in front, the palms laterally and the fingers along the spine during shaking or other abusive acts.

Skull fractures can be simple or multiple and crossing suture lines. The latter fractures are more likely to be associated with abuse or caused by a high-energy injury. The explanation of the injury by the caregivers should be consistent with the type of the fracture, but—in contrast to metaphyseal fractures or rib fractures—it is a difficult task to decide whether or not it is a consequence of child abuse.

21.1.1.3 Shaken Baby Syndrome

The shaken baby syndrome (SBS) occurs in babies usually younger than 6 months, but it has also been described in significantly older children. The injury results from violently shaking the baby with or without

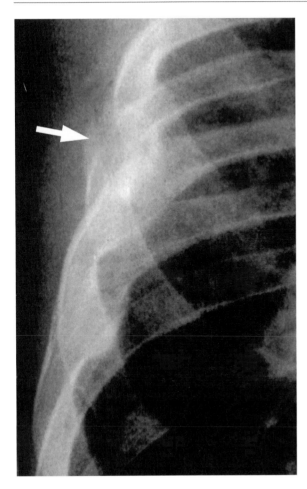

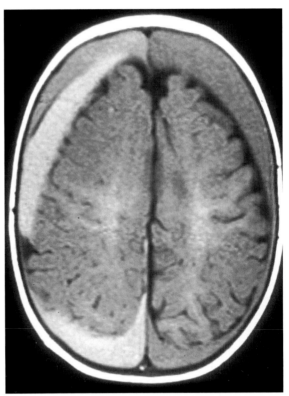

Fig. 21.8 Extensive subdural haematoma in a case of a shaken baby syndrome (SBS)

Fig. 21.7 Old rib fracture with a visible callus in an infant. This injury is typical for child abuse in infancy

additional impact. The usual trigger for shaking is inconsolable crying by the infant. A study has shown that in infants aged 6 months nearly 6% of parents reported taking at least one action to stop infants crying by smothering, slapping or shaking. One in five had taken more than one of these three actions and the cumulative rates rose steadily from 1 to 6 months and were highest for shaking. The risks were highest for parents from non-industrialized countries, those with either no job or a job with short working hours, and those who judged their infant's crying to be excessive.

The shaking results in a direct trauma to the brain, in tears of the subdural veins leading to a subdural hae-matoma or subarachnoid haemorrhages, in breaking of axons in deeper brain structures and in a reduced oxy-gen supply to the brain substance. The combined effects cause immediate brain swelling and an increase of the intracranial pressure leading to severe neuro-logical symptoms such as lethargy, irritability, convul-sions or even bradycardia and respiratory arrest. A CT-scan is the first imaging modality to prove intracra-nial lesions and skull fractures (Fig. 21.8). Associated injuries can be seen such as bruising of the thoracic skin and rib fractures. Retinal haemorrhages (RH) are the most commonly found additional lesions in SBS, characterized by extensive haemorrhages involving several layers of the retina. In contrast, vaginal delivery may cause fine preretinal petechiae which usually resolve without residuals within 10–14 days after delivery. Our current strategy is to confirm a SBS in babies with unexplained subdural haematoma—with or without a fracture—when a RH is present. However, there is a debate whether retinal haemorrhages can be caused by elevated intracranial pressure alone without a SBS. The main argument against this opinion comes from a study that has shown that RH were seen in only

2% of children under 6 years of age with unintentional head injuries while in 33% of the children with inflicted head injury.

21.1.1.4 Abdominal and Thoracic Injuries

Abdominal injuries are the second most common cause of fatality in child physical abuse. The history from the caregivers is usually very vague and they seek rather late for medical care. The injuries are more common in younger children and mortality is significantly higher (53%) when compared with unintentional accidents. The trauma results in most cases from violent hits with the fists or with the legs into the middle part of the abdomen. Therefore, injuries to hollow viscera in the midline (stomach, small bowel, and bladder) occur more often than injuries to solid organs, in contrast to other accidents.

Pharyngeal, hypopharyngeal and oesophageal injuries are rare manifestations of child abuse due to perforation with blunt instruments. Radiographs show subcutaneous or retropharyngeal or mediastinal emphysema. In half of the reported cases additional rib fractures have been present.

21.1.1.5 Prevention

An important prerequisite for effective prevention of physical child abuse is to recognize endangered persons or families. In those family systems, shown in Table 21.2, there exist an increased risk for child abuse. Early recognition allows to support the family

Table 21.2 Early support for endangered families may be helpful to prevent physical abuse of a child

Endangered families
- Families with hyperactive children
- Inconsolable infant crying
- Child abuse in the family history
- A very dominant family member
- Background of permissive violence
- Parental mental ill-health
- Low socioeconomic status
- Unemployment and financial problems
- Drug abuse
- Transcultural problems between family members
- Social isolation

and to strengthen its abilities for childrearing. Family doctors, paediatricians and gynaecologists are the professions which may recognize endangered families. At the time when a family has a new baby there is "a window of opportunity" to support parenting abilities. Many studies have documented the effectiveness of home visiting programs and early intervention which are performed in most countries by social worker organisations.

If a case child abuse has already occurred and has been documented in the children's hospital we try to establish a firm and trustful relation to the family. All children's hospitals in Austria must have by law a "Working group for abused children" which consists of paediatricians and paediatric surgeons, psychologists, paediatric nurses and social workers. The treatment strategies include education, paternal support, psychological help and community support programs. However, these programs only come into reality if the family accepts therapeutic measures and help, as well as control such as home visiting programs. If these programs turn out to be unsuccessful or if the family refuses to cooperate with the social system the appropriate State Organisations may look for an adequate and safe place for the child/children outside of the family.

21.1.2 Sexual Abuse

Sexual abuse is the encroachment of dependents in regard to their development immature children or adolescents for sexual actions which they cannot completely understand and are therefore not able to agree to because they have not yet the ability to understand the significance of consent and/or sexual actions which offend the family taboos.

In contrast to physical abuse, the average age of the victims is significantly older and the presenting symptoms of most of the patients are unspecific, such as sleep disturbances, abdominal pain, constipation, enuresis, weight loss and phobias (Figs. 21.9 and 21.10). Diagnosis and treatment of these children is a very difficult problem for the family doctor due to the involvement of family members. A single person is always overcharged with the circumstances around sexual abuse even if he/she is familiar with the problem and well trained in recognizing the subtle symptoms. Therefore, it is indicated in all suspicious cases of sexual

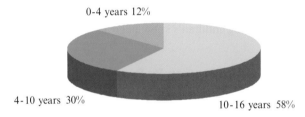

0-4 years 12%

4-10 years 30%

10-16 years 58%

Fig. 21.9   Age distribution in patients with sexual abuse

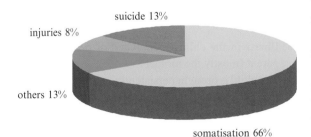

suicide 13%

injuries 8%

others 13%

somatisation 66%

Fig. 21.10   Typical complaints when a child is admitted after sexual abuse. Somatisation symptoms are leading

abuse to transfer the patient under a fake diagnosis to a specialized paediatric centre.

Evaluation of victims of sexual abuse involves careful questioning, individualized psychological techniques and tests, evidence collection procedures for forensic purposes, and specialized examination techniques which are best provided by a group of trained staff with expertise in the evaluation and treatment of these children.

Studies have provided evidence that up to 12–25% of girls and 8–10% of boys are victims of sexual abuse by 18 years of age. In USA in 2002, more than 88,000 children were confirmed victims of sexual abuse. Additionally, there is certainly a high number of so-called "hidden" abuse which never comes to the surface. Survey studies with large numbers of students and adult women came to the conclusion that 2–5% of girls up to 13 years of age have been victims of sexual abuse, numbers that would correspond in Austria to 10,000–25,000 cases of sexual abuse per year.

A careful evaluation of the patient's history and complaints will often yield important information. The interviews with the patient and the caregiver need a quiet environment and a good understanding of the child's needs appropriate to the age.

A full physical examination is always indicated when abuse or neglect is suspected. We recommend performing the examination of the anogenital region of children up to 10–12 years under anaesthesia, unless the patient agrees to have that examination under normal circumstances. The inspection of the genitalia should be done as gentle as possible. Various techniques and positions for visualizing genital and anal structures are described in the literature. Colposcopy and documentation with photographs is necessary, while speculum and digital examination are usually not required. It is important to know that in most of the abused children the anogenital aspects and findings are normal, which does not at all exclude sexual abuse. Signs of acute damage disappear rapidly and even tears in the posterior fourchette can heal with minimal scar tissue. Tears in the hymen can only be seen if penetration happened, but a recent study of pregnant adolescents showed that only 2 of 36 had evidence of penetration. Suspicious findings are vulvovaginitis, recurrent urinary tract infection and sexually transmitted diseases. The major causes for vulvovaginitis are poor hygiene and threadworms. However, the possibility of sexual abuse must be considered if vulvovaginitis is persistent or recurrent after adequate treatment. Similarly, most recurrent urinary tract infections are caused by anomalies of the urogenital tract.

Vaginal and perianal sampling of swab, blood tests and secretions is important. The presence of semen, sperm, acid phosphatase, or a positive culture for gonococci, Chlamydia trachomatis, or positive serologic tests for syphilis or HIV make the diagnosis of sexual abuse nearly certain. Positive findings for Trichomonas vaginalis, anogenital warts and papillomas—type HPV-6, HPV-11, HPV-16 and HPV-18—and genital localisation of herpes simplex are suspicious for sexual abuse.

When a child is sexually abused by a person outside the family there is outrage on the part of the parents with emphasis on the guilt and responsibility of the abuser. A difficult problem exists when parents are in the process of divorce and allege that their child is being sexually abused by the other parent during custodial visits. However, in most cases incest occurs in a seemingly normal family (Table 21.3).

The experience shows that in many situations the "non-offending" caregivers- most often the mothers—deny any knowledge of what was happening, sometimes for years. Thus, it seems likely that either subconscious forces block the ability to acknowledge what happened

Table 21.3 In most cases the sexual abuse occurs within the familiy by a relative, or a stepfather of the child

Perpetuator	n	%
Biological father	27	14
Adoptive father	1	1
Stepfather	15	8
Biological mother	1	1
Biological brother	23	12
Stepbrother	2	1
Biological sister	3	2
Biological grandfather	8	4
Step grandfather	3	2
Uncle	48	25
Male Cousin	30	16
Female Cousin	3	2
Brother-in-law	7	4
Other male Relative	15	8
Other female Relative	3	2
Total	189	

and may be dictated by the emotions and the shame which comes over the family—"that cannot happen in my family"—or the family members are under such massive pressure by the perpetrator that they don't dare to look at the reality. Denial of events is often the first defence. Thus, most often neither the nonoffending family members nor the child inform about suspected child abuse. Sometimes the child may start slowly to confide to one staff member on the ward and to tell him/her some secrets. But, as soon as the family is confronted with the suspicion they often begin to put the child under massive emotional pressure to call back everything that has been said. In cases where the results of the examinations are negative it is difficult to provide significant help to the child. Only regular "medical" controls may protect it from further abuse. When clear evidence exists involvement in the civil, juvenile, or family court system is necessary and the child must be protected in a safe environment.

In conclusion, cases of physical and sexual abuse belong to the most difficult problems- clinically and emotionally—in paediatric medicine. There is an absolute need that these children are treated by a team of experts, first to come to a definite diagnosis, and second to be able to help the child—together with or without the family. Prevention strategies include the early recognition of endangered families for physical abuse and appropriate school-based programs to teach the children recognizing impermissible kinds of physical touching, to fend off sexual advances, and to report abuse to a trusted person. These programs are effective in increasing children's knowledge and skills.

21.1.3 Muchausen By Proxy

Munchausen by proxy (MBP) is defined as a situation when the illness of the child is simulated by the caregiver and the child is presented several times to one or more different health care systems for medical assessment. This syndrome describes a strange form of child abuse and defines circumstances in which

(a) Illness of the child is simulated or produced by a parent (mostly the mother)
(b) The child is brought persistently for medical assessment and care, often resulting in multiple medical procedures
(c) Knowledge about the aetiology is denied by the perpetrator
(d) Acute symptoms and signs in the child abate when it is separated from the perpetrator

The difficulty comes from the problem to gather evidence that the illness of the child is simulated or faked. Careful evaluation of the findings and detailed notes in the charts are essential to formulate finally the diagnosis, when the case is brought to the court. A clear understanding of the parent's psychopathology is still not available and more information is needed about the long-term result of these children.

Further Reading

American Academy of Pediatrics (2003) Visual Diagnosis of Child Abuse (on CD-ROM), 2nd edn. American Academy of Pediatrics, Elk Grove Village, IL

Dubowitz H (2002) Preventing child neglect and physical abuse: A role for pediatricians. Pediatr Rev 23:191–196

Kellog N (2005) The evaluation of sexual abuse in children. Pediatrics 116:506–512

McCann J, Voris J, Simon M (1992) Genital injuries resulting from sexual abuse: A longitudinal study. Pediatrics 89:307–317

Paradise JE (2001) Current concepts in preventing sexual abuse. Curr Opin Pediatr 13:402–407

Puri P, Höllwarth M (2006) Pediatric Surgery. Springer, Berlin, Heidelberg

Reijneveld SA, van der Wal MF, Brugman E et al (2004) Infant crying and abuse. Lancet 364:1340–1342

Rubin D, Lane W, Ludwig St (2001) Child abuse prevention. Curr Opin Pediatr 13:388–401

Tenney-Soeiro R, Wilson C (2004) An update on child abuse and neglect. Curr Opin Pediatr 16:233–237

Choanal Atresia

22

Michael S. Harney and John Russell

Contents

22.1 Introduction

Infants are obligate nasal breathers for the first 4–6 weeks of life. Bilateral choanal atresia is therefore an airway emergency. Failure to recognize and promptly treat this condition may result in death by asphyxia. The condition was first described by Johann Roederer in 1755 and Emmert reported the first successful treatment of the condition in 1854. The posterior chaonae connects the nasal cavities to the nasopharynx. An image of the posterior choanae can be seen from Fig. 22.1 which shows the view from a 120° endoscope viewed through the mouth. It is an uncommon condition affecting 8:100,000 births. The rate of unilateral to bilateral atresia is 2:1. The atretic plate can be bony (30%) or bony and membranous (70%). The bony narrowing can arise from any combination of the sphenoid superiorly, pterygoid plates laterally, the vomer medially or inferiorly from the hard palate.

22.2 Embryology

The precise reason for the development of the atretic plate is not known. It may represent a persistence of the buccopharyngeal membrane, persistence of the nasobuccal membrane, medial outgrowth of the vertical or horizontal processes of the palatine bone, or a defect in neural crest migration.

22.3 Associated Conditions

Choanal atresia is a red flag condition. It is associated with additional anomalies in 50% of cases. It can be associated with CHARGE (25% cases), Treacher-Collins

P. Puri and M. Höllwarth (eds.), *Pediatric Surgery: Diagnosis and Management,*
DOI: 10.1007/978-3-540-69560-8_22, © Springer-Verlag Berlin Heidelberg 2009

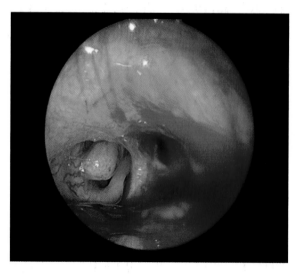

Fig. 22.1 Left choanal atresia viewed through 120° endoscope following puncture by small urethral sound

insensate larynx or a vocal cord palsy. They may have laryngomalacia or suffer from a laryngeal cleft. They may have oesophageal atresia or a tracheooesophageal fistula. Correspondingly the mortality rate in this group is higher; children with chaonal atresia with CHARGE association have a 20% perioperative mortality. A multidisciplinary pre-operative work-up is essential in these patients, with involvement of the cardiologists, ophthalmologists, geneticists, renal physicians, neonatologists and audiological scientists. Treacher-Collins is associated with retrognathia which may have additional implications for the newborn airway. Ten to fifteen percent of children with Treacher-Collins syndrome have choanal atresia.

22.4 Presentation

Obstruction can be unilateral or bilateral. Bilateral obstructions present in the early neonatal period. Infants are obligate nasal breathers as the tongue is in opposition to the palate. Attempts at inspiration results in sternal retraction and intercostal recession. A failure to adequately ventilate results in cyanosis. If the child starts to cry, the mouth opens and the apnea/cyanosis settles. Once the crying ceases the obstructed breathing pattern recommences. This *cyclical cyanosis* is typical of choanal atresia. This pattern may only become conspicuous during feeding. Occasionally the infant may present with failure to thrive secondary to an inability to maintain a satisfactory airway during feeding yet not present with cyclical cyanosis or choking during feeding. A unilateral atresia may not be detected during the neonatal period. It may present later in life with unilateral obstruction and discharge as the mucus that is produced on this side of the nasal cavity cannot be transported to the post nasal space.

syndrome, Aperts, Di George sequence, VATER syndrome or trisomy 18. CHARGE syndrome is a nonrandom association of **C**oloboma (of iris, choroid, and/or micropthalmia), **H**eart defects (septal defects and/or conotruncal lesion), choanal **A**tresia, mental or growth **R**etardation, **G**enito-urinary abnormalities (cryptorchidism, microphallus, and/or hydronephrosis) and **E**ar anomalies (hearing loss, external, middle or inner ear may be involved). In addition to these cardinal features additional minor characteristics include; characteristic face and hand dysmorphology, hypotonia, urinary tract abnormalities, orofacial clefting, deafness, dysphagia and tracheo-oesophageal abnormalities. A diagnosis of CHARGE syndrome requires the presence of at least three cardinal characteristics or two cardinal with three or more minor characteristics. The presence of bilateral choanal atresia indicates a poor prognosis in infants diagnosed with CHARGE. Choanal atresia is present in 57% of infants with CHARGE. CHARGE is inherited in an autosomal dominant fashion. Males and females are therefore equally affected. Several different genetic abnormalities have been identified in infants with CHARGE; most cases are due to a mutation or deletion of the chromodomain helicase DNA-binding protein-7 (CHD7) gene. Thirty percent of neonates with this condition will require a tracheostomy for airway difficulties in addition to choanal atresia. They may recurrently aspirate which can be from a number of different causes; glossopharyngeal or vagus parasthesias, causing an

22.5 Differential Diagnosis

The differential diagnosis represents all other causes of bilateral nasal blockage in the neonate, including; piriform aperture stenosis, encephalocoele, dermoid cysts, septal abnormalities, benign nasal tumours, nasolacrimal duct cysts and mucosal disease with turbinate hypertrophy.

22.6 Detection

Once the clinical picture is detected, the diagnosis is suspected if the child fails to mist up a stainless steel spatula or mirror that is held under the nose. Failure to pass a size 8 catheter 5.5 mm from the anterior choana is highly suggestive of atresia. Nasal airflow can usually be detected with the use of a stethoscope. The atretic plate can be visualized directly by nasal endoscopy. A computed tomography (CT) scan is usually performed to confirm the atresia; to outrule other diagnosis; to determine the proportion of membranous to bony narrowing and to determine the main sites of bony narrowing. The nose should be suctioned and decongested prior to performing the CT to avoid the presence of additional soft tissue shadowing.

22.7 Emergency Treatment

Prompt recognition is essential and can be quickly relieved by the insertion of an oropharyngeal airway which may need to be secured in place with a tape across the mouth. The oropharyngeal airway size can be measured by approximating the distance from the angle of the mandible to the centre of the two incisors. This airway can be left in for several weeks if necessary. A McGovern nipple is an alternative option. This is a nipple that has enlarged perforations at the tip which allows the child to breathe. Endotracheal intubation provides a safe and secure airway, though this will require an intensive care unit bed until definitive repair can be performed. Intubation may prove difficult in infants with retrognathia associated with Treacher-Collins syndrome. An orogastric tube is required for the child to feed until definitive surgical repair can be attempted.

22.8 Surgical Correction

The timing of surgery is controversial. Some authors suggest that the rule of 10s be adhered to; that the child is 10 lb, 10 weeks old and has 10 g of haemoglobin. Others suggest that correction should be performed as soon as the diagnosis is confirmed. Several different operative techniques have been described. They can be divided into endoscopic, trans-nasal, transpalatal, sublabial trans-septal and transmaxillary. The most popular approach is currently the endoscopic approach. The

transmaxillary approach is mainly of historical interest only and will not be discussed further here.

22.8.1 Endoscopic Technique

The author's technique of choice is the endoscopic approach. A tonsil (Boyle-Davis) mouth gag is inserted. A suture is placed through the uvula and clipped to provide retraction to the soft palate. A 120° endoscope is passed in to the nasopharynx and a view of the obstructed choanae obtained on the video monitor (Fig. 22.1). The nasal cavity is decongested with 1:10 000 adrenaline patties, and the atretic plate injected with 1% lignocaine with 1:200 000 adrenaline. The atretic plate is perforated with a small urethral sound using the 120° endoscope which is passed through the mouth to view the atretic plate at the time of perforation. The sound is passed to the medial and inferior aspect of the atretic plate to avoid inadvertent entry to the skull base or sphenoid. Even with thick atretic plates the sound can usually be passed without much force being required. Progressively larger sounds are introduced until the sound can no longer pass through the anterior choana. The drill is then inserted in through the nose until it reaches the nasopharynx. We use a specialized drill which has a protective sheath over the shaft preventing trauma to the nasal cavity. The drilling is performed medially over the vomer and laterally over the pterygoid plates. The posterior aspect of the vomer is then removed by inserting a back biting forceps into the nasopharynx and removing the posterior half of the vomer. This creates a common cavity posteriorly which minimizes the chance of restenosis. The repaired choana are soaked with mitomycin C (0.25 mg/ml) patties for 5 min at the end of the procedure. The area is then cleaned with saline soaked patties. Mitomycin C is an aminoglycoside which is produced by the bacteria streptomyces. It is a cytotoxic chemotherapeutic agent used in several oncology regimes. It crosslinks DNA leading to the induction of apoptosis. Fibroblasts are particularly sensitive to this action at the doses described above. This prevents fibroblast activation and reduces the propensity for future scar formation. While its role in subglottic stenosis and glaucoma surgery has been clearly demonstrated, its role in choanal atresia has yet to be defined. The role of stenting is controversial. Stents can cause several problems including; columellar necrosis, nasal vestibule excoriation, blockage and intranasal synechia. In addition, stents may act as a foreign body contributing to restenosis. We insert stents for 6 weeks. An oval shape is cut from the center of an endotracheal tube. The tube is inserted in to the right and left nasal cavities, through the posterior choanae, and the cut oval section over the columella to allow nasal breathing. These are secured in place with a 3.0 silk suture. Post-operatively the stents are kept patent with saline drops. Bethametason drops are used in the nasal cavities to minimize oedema, though benefit from their use has not been demonstrated. Some authors advocate the use of antibiotics for the duration of the stent placement to minimize risk of infection which may increase the risk of stenosis. The role of antibiotics however is also unclear. The child is anesthetized again in 6 weeks and the stents removed. Any granulations can be removed with the microdebrider. Dilatations are often required, with the largest reported series observing an average of 4.9 procedures being required per patient (Samadi et al., 2003). We perform all dilatations with the use of the 120° scope and the monitor. There are several variations on this technique described. The commonest variation is with all perforations, drilling and backbiting being performed using the 0° 4mm (or 2.5mm in neonate) nasal endoscope. This is the *transnasal technique*. This is acceptable, though the narrow nasal cavity of the newborn may result in difficulty using two instruments down one side of the nose. Some authors have described the use of the drill alone to refashion the posterior choanae. The sparing of mucosal flaps is also frequently described which are placed over raw surfaces at the end of the procedure to improve epithelialization. However, the author's experience is that these flaps are usually not viable by the end of the procedure. CT guidance systems are routinely used by certain authors. We feel this technology is not necessary in routine cases.

22.8.2 Transpalatal

The transpalatal technique involves making a U-shaped incision in the hard palate, 5 mm's from the dental arch and raising a posteriorly based subperiosteal flap to gain access to the nasopharynx. The blood supply to the flap is from the greater palatine arteries which enter posterolaterally. Care must be exercised in this area. The inferior aspect of the vomer is visualized and removed. The lateral atretic plates are then removed using a drill or a trucut forceps. The flap is closed using a two layered closure. This technique is useful if the nasopharynx is small and the skull base low which may be found in children with Treacher-Collins syndrome. The bony narrowing can be enlarged starting from a known safe area minimizing the chance of a skull base breach. There are several drawbacks to this technique however. The post-operative pain is higher, possibly requiring a longer hospital stay. Risks of palatal fistula and reduced growth of the midface have been described. This is felt to be secondary to resection of the palatine bone growth plate. Resulting dental malocclusion has been described in 50% of patients undergoing this technique. For these reasons, this technique should be reserved for children with difficult skull base anatomy.

22.8.3 Sublabial Transseptal

This technique is used by some authors in infants with abnormal intranasal anatomy or craniofacial anomalies. A sublabial incision is made through the perichondrium which is elevated over the premaxilla to expose the lower piriform aperture. The mucosa of the nasal floor and the mucoperichondrium from the septum is elevated. The posterior bony septum and the atretic plates laterally are then resected.

22.9 Conclusion

Prompt recognition of this condition is essential. Emergency airway management requires insertion of an oropharyngeal airway to stabilize the patient. There are several different techniques available to re-open the atretic plates. Revision surgery in the form of repeated dilatations is often required.

Further Reading

Gosepath J, Santamaria VE, Lippert BM, Mann WJ (2007) Forty-one cases of congenital choanal atresia over 26 years—Retrospective analysis of outcome and technique. Rhinology 45:158–163

Park AH, Brockenbrough J, Stankiewicz J (2000) Endoscopic versus traditional approaches to choanal atresia. Otolaryngol Clin N Am 33:77–90

Petkovska L, Petkovska I, Ramadan S, Aslam MO (2007) CT evaluation of congenital choanal atresia: Our experience and review of the literature. Australas Radiol 51:236–239

Puri P, Höllwarth M (2006) Pediatric Surgery. Springer, Berlin, Heidelberg

Samadi DS, Udayan K, Handker SD (2003) Choanal atresia: A twenty-year review of medical comorbidities and surgical outcomes. Laryngosocope 113:254–258

Thevasagayam M, El-Hakim H (2007) Diagnosing choanal atresia—A simple approach. Acta Paediatr 96:1238–1239

Thyreoglossal and Branchial Cysts, Sinuses and Fistulas

23

Michael E. Höllwarth

Contents

23.1 Introduction

Remnants of embryological structures in the neck derive either from the thyreoglossal duct or from the branchial arches and constitute the most common congenital anomaly in this anatomical region accounting for up to 60% of all excised neck masses in children.

Thyreoglossal duct cysts are slightly more common when compared with branchial cleft anomalies (55% vs. 45%) and present them as a midline neck mass below the hyoid bone. Sinuses drain into the foramen cecum of the tongue. Most commonly they cause clinical problems in the first decade of life and more than half of the cases are diagnosed before the age of 5. They rarely cause problems in older children.

Although branchial cysts and sinuses are most often operated in childhood, sometimes they are detected as a clinical problem not before adulthood. They are located along the anterior border of the sternocleidomastoid muscle, however they drain into very different regions depending on their origin from one of the branchial clefts. The knowledge of the embryology and the anatomical variants is crucial to avoid surgical mistakes, thereby creating nerve lesions and a significant morbidity.

23.2 Etiology

Thyreoglossal duct: The thyroid anlage is a part of the second branchial arch located in the midline floor of the pharynx. It descents as a pouch from the foramen cecum down to the neck during the third week of foetal live passing anterior, through or posterior to the hyoid bone. The cells differentiate at their final position into the thyroid gland anterior to the thyroid cartilage (Fig. 23.1). If duct cells persist they can form a cyst or a sinus, which is connected to the foramen cecum at the base of the tongue, but rarely a fistula with an external opening in the middle of the neck, only after perforation of a cyst.

Branchial cysts and sinuses: Five branchial arches form by condensation of the mesoderm five parallel ridges containing an artery, a nerve, a cartilage and a muscle anlage. They are separated outside by clefts and internally by four pharyngeal pouches. Congenital branchial cysts and fistulas are remnants of these embryonic structures, which have failed to regress completely. Treatment of branchial remnants requires knowledge of the related embryology. The first arch, cleft and pouch form the mandible, the maxillary process of the upper jaw, the external ear, parts of the Eustachian tube, and the tympanic cavity. The most common branchial cysts and fistulas derive from the second branchial pouch, which forms the tonsillar fossa and the palatine tonsils. The third arch forms the inferior parathyroid glands and the thymus, while the fourth arch migrates less far down and develops into the superior parathyroid glands.

Cysts, sinuses and fistulas result in persisting epithelial cells within the mesoderm and are lined by squamous or columnar epithelia. Between 75% and 90% of the anomalies derive from the second branchial cleft while 8–20% arise from the first cleft.

23.3 Pathology

Thyreoglossal duct remnants account for more than half of all congenital anomalies in the neck region. Three quarters present as cysts and 25% as sinuses with or without infection. Infected cysts form a red and tender tumor in the middle of the neck (Fig. 23.2). When elements of the duct persist after the descent of the thyroid most of them become clinically apparent before the age of 20. Ectopic thyroid tissue may be found in 25% in the wall of the cysts. In some cases the duct cysts may either contain papillary cancer or squamous cell carcinoma. In cases with papillary cancer additional nodes can exist within the thyroid gland and/or regional affected nodes may be present.

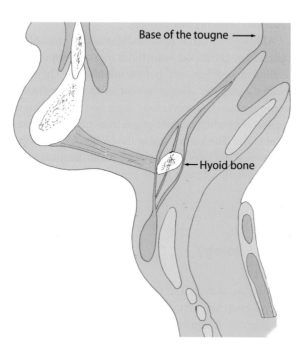

Fig. 23.1 Schematic drawing of a thyreoglossal cyst. The duct runs through, in front, or behind the foramen cecum to the base of the tongue

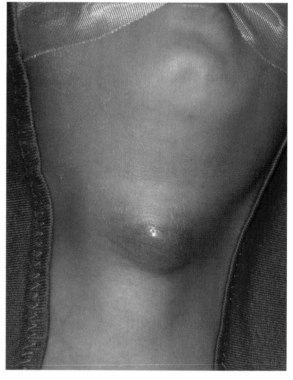

Fig. 23.2 Infected thyreoglossal cyst in the middle of the ventral neck side

Although *branchial cleft anomalies* are present at birth they may not appear until a fluid filled cyst is formed or becomes infected. Bilateral cysts or sinuses can be observed in 10–15% of patients. If a fistula of the second branchial cleft persists saliva is discharged periodically or continuously at the skin ventral to the sternocleidomastoid muscle. Although the majority of branchial anomalies are singular events, some cases of coincidence in families point to a genetically determined abnormality. Simple cystic remnants are present commonly in adolescence and adulthood, while sinuses and fistulas are usually diagnosed in infancy and early childhood. In principle, clinical manifestation – no matter at which age – should be taken as an indication for elective excision before infectious complications supervene.

23.4 Diagnosis and Differential Diagnosis

Thyreoglossal duct cysts are found in 60% of the cases in the midline at or below the hyoid bone. However, according to their origin 24% are located above the hyoid and 8% intralingual. In the latter case they can cause respiratory distress or even sudden infant death when located at the base of the tongue.

During palpation uninfected cysts are often ballotable and can be moved slightly from side to side, but not up or down. Due to their origin from the foramen cecum the thyroid cysts move upward during swallowing or when the tongue protrudes. However, this clinical sign is difficult to observe in small infants. The differential diagnosis includes complete ectopic thyroid gland or parts of the thyroid, dermoid cysts, lipomas, sebaceous cysts, submental lymphadenitis, thymus cysts or tumor. As mentioned above, the latter group of pathologies may be moved up and down with palpation but do not move during swallows unless the pathology is in close connection with the hyoid bone or the thyroid gland. Especially dermoid cysts may be located in close vicinity to the hyoid bone and should therefore be treated in a similar way as thyreoglossal duct cysts to avoid a recurrent pathology. An ultrasound investigation is often recommended as a preoperative workup to prove the cystic structure of the pathology. However, the information is limited because it is difficult to exclude other cystic pathologies such as infected or uninfected dermoid cysts or a lymph node abscess. If the ultrasound shows a solid structure, an ectopic thyroid gland may be present when the bilateral thyroid lobes are missing in their typical location. Some authors state categorically that a thyroid scan must be performed in all cases to exclude ectopic thyroid tissue, which would result in hypothyroidism if resected surgically. However, this anomaly is very rare and in the case of a seemingly solid tumor a frozen section during surgery may be diagnostic and prevent the resection of the gland.

Remnants of the second branchial cleft are typically located as a painless, smooth, slowly enlarging mass along the anterior border of the sternocleidomastoid muscle. The majority of the anomalies are cysts with or without an additional sinus tract; they may be painful and fluctuate in size from time to time. The diagnosis is easier when clear mucous or saliva or pus is discharged from an external opening (Fig. 23.3). The internal fistula enters the supratonsillar fossa and can be seen easily in adults. Injection of water-soluble contrast material into the neck fistula under X-ray control shows the extension of the tract up to the pharynx. From the supratonsillar fossa, the tract passes over the hypoglossal nerve and behind the bigastric muscle through the bifurcation of the carotid artery and in front of the superior thyroid artery. The most common complication is infection of the cyst leading to an abscess. More rare presentations are stridor, tumor feeling in the throat with dysphagia and hypoglossal nerve palsy. Differential diagnoses include suppurative lymphadenitis or dermoid cyst, vascular anomalies such as cystic hygroma, or subcutaneous haemangioma.

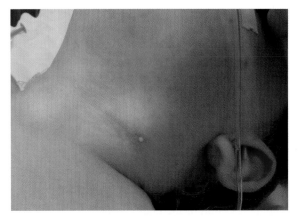

Fig. 23.3 Discharge of pus from the external opening of a second bronchial cleft fistula

Remnants of the first branchial cleft occur with an incidence of approximately 20%. They form small cysts at the posterior border of the parotid gland or a sinus anterior to the ear in close proximity to branches of the facial nerve. If a fistula is present it may drain into the external auditory canal or middle ear and a careful otologic examination is needed. Infection of the cysts or sinus is common and pus may be discharged from the ear. Diagnosis as well as surgical therapy are difficult and must avoid any damage to the facial nerve. Thus, either an ultrasound study or a MRI is recommended to demonstrate the course of the tract and the relation to the nerve. The remnants of the first branchial cleft need to be distinguished from the preauricular pits, cysts and sinuses which are remnants of the auditory tubercles. They are located anterior to the tragus of the ear, are often bilateral and tend to be inherited.

Remnants of the third and forth branchial cleft are uncommon. The external presentation of the former anomaly is similar as the remnants of the second branchial cleft, but the sinus tract passes between the hypoglossal and glossopharyngeal nerve and posterior to the carotid artery to end finally within the pyriform sinus. The epithelial tracts of the very rare remnants of the fourth branchial cleft enter also the pyriform sinus, but in nearly all cases on the left side. Typical symptoms are recurrent respiratory tract infection, hoarseness and painful swallowing. If the anomalies present as recurrent abscesses at the lateral side of the thyroid gland or in close vicinity to the pyriform sinus they may cause life threatening respiratory stridor in neonates and infants or acute unilateral thyroiditis in children and adults. The appropriate diagnosis is difficult and the cyst may evoke a false impression of acute thyroiditis. Most often these anomalies are treated, as they were harmless local lymphoid abscesses, a mistake that makes later surgical excision of the tract very difficult. MRI of the neck helps to identify the origin of such lesions. In an acute suppurative phase external pressure onto the mass may ensue in laryngoscopically visible evacuation of pus into the piriform fossa.

23.5 Therapy

Surgery of the *thyreoglossal cyst or duct* must always include resection of the middle part of the hyoid corpus whether or not the surgeon has the feeling that the duct ends at the bone (Fig. 23.4). In order to resect the hyoid bone, the upper and lower rim have to be freed from the straight neck muscles – omohyoid and sternohyoid muscle – and the middle 1–2 cm can be excised with a strong scissor. In some cases a clear continuity of the duct behind the bone can be seen which then has to be resected up to the base of the tongue including high ligature of the fistula. If the pathology presents primarily as an abscess, antibiotic therapy and a horizontal incision are recommended. The use of a drain depends on the size of the abscess. Some authors recommend antibiotic therapy alone or an additional needle aspiration of the pus in order to avoid seeding of ductal epithelium. We have not seen any disadvantage after a primary surgical incision of the abscess. The parents have to be informed that a second surgical procedure with excision of the duct will become necessary as soon as the local inflammation is under control. Recurrence only occurs when the middle part of the hyoid corpus has not been resected appropriately. Bleeding is minimal and rarely a small suction drain is needed. Reconstruction of the straight neck muscles is recommended to form the anterior aspect of the neck.

Surgery of the *lateral neck cysts or fistulas* starts in the case of a *remnant of the second branchial cleft* with the excision of the visible pathology at the anterior border of the sternocleidomastoid muscle. If an external opening exists a probe may be inserted and methylene blue can be injected to make the fistula easier to visualise (Fig. 23.5). The duct is then isolated carefully from the surrounding tissue avoiding any rough procedure, which could damage the carotid arteries within the bifurcation or the hypoglossal nerve (Fig. 23.6). In order to isolate and ligate the duct close to the supratonsillar region in older children it is useful to make a second stepladder incision 3–5 cm above the first incision. Drainage of the wound is rarely necessary. Recurrences only occur when the duct ruptures during the procedure and cannot be closed by ligature.

Surgery of the *first branchial cleft remnants* is difficult and only symptomatic forms need to be treated by local excision. At the beginning of the procedure it is essential to expose the facial nerve and all its horizontal and lower branches. The surgical procedure should start with the identification of the main trunk of the nerve by means of a retroauricular incision. The

Fig. 23.4 The surgical procedure of a thyreoglossal cyst and duct must include resection of the middle part of the hyoid bone

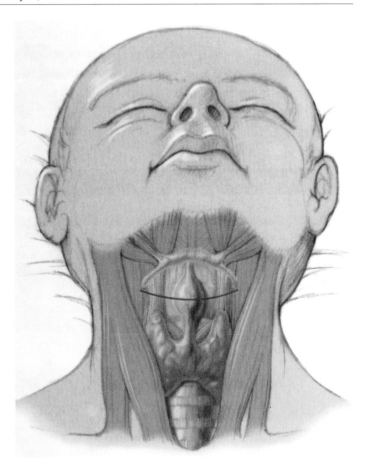

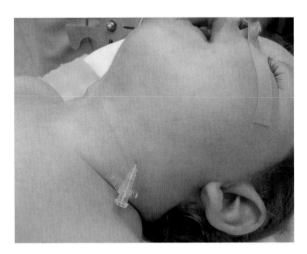

Fig. 23.5 If injection of methylene blue is possible the fistula is easily visible during surgery

Once the branches are isolated minor or major parts of the parotid gland must be resected to identify the tract. The opening of the fistula to the external ear canal should be included into the resection to avoid any recurrence. Rarely the duct opens to the middle ear or runs parallel to the Eustachian tube. The whole procedure is even more difficult in cases with a previous infection. Thus, it seems to be wise to perform this procedure in all cases together with specialists from the ENT-Department.

The special anatomy in the rare case of *remnants of the third and fourth branchial cleft* and the risk to damage the superior or the recurrent laryngeal nerve makes the surgical procedure difficult. Several approaches have been recommended, each of them bares its special risks. Recently, closure of the internal opening at the piriform sinus by injecting sclerosing material endoscopically into the tract has been recommended which may be an especially helpful solution after previous repeated infections.

exit of the nerve from the stylomastoid foramen can be found in a triangle formed by the sternocleidomastoid muscle, the bigastric muscle and the external ear canal.

Fig. 23.6 The fistula runs through
the carotid bifurcation and close to
the hypoglossal nerve. Therefore
dissection must be close to the fistula

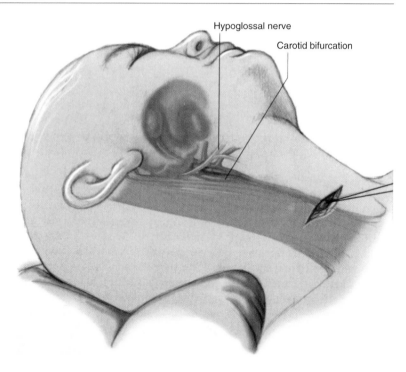

Hypoglossal nerve

Carotid bifurcation

Further Reading

Farrior JB, Santini H (1985) Facial nerve identification in children. Otolaryngol Head Neck Surg 93:173–176

Grosfeld JL, O'Neil JA Jr, Fonkalsrud EW, Coran AG (2006) Pediatric Surgery. Mosby–Elsevier, Philadelphia

Höllwarth ME (2006) Thyroglossal and Branchial Cysts, Sinuses and Fistulas. In P Puri, ME Höllwarth (eds) Pediatric Surgery, Springer Surgery Atlas Series. Springer-Verlag Berlin Heidelberg, New York, pp 3–18

Miller D, Hill JL, Sun CC et al (1983) The diagnosis and management of piriform sinus fistulae in infants and young children. J Pediatr Surg 18:377–381

Telander RL, Deane SA (1978) Surgery for thyreoglossal and branchial cleft anomalies. Am J Surg 136:348–353

Torsiglieri AJ Jr, Tom LW, Ross AJ et al (1988) Pediatric neck masses: Guidelines for evaluation. Int J Pediatr Otorhinolaryngol 16:199–210

Triglia JM, Nicollas R, Ducroz V et al (1998) First branchial cleft anomalies: A study of 39 cases and a review of the literature. Arch Otolaryngol Head Neck Surg 124:291–295

Tracheostomy

24

Thom E. Lobe

Contents

24.1 Introduction

Tracheostomy may be required for a number of congenital and acquired conditions of infancy and childhood. Thus, the well-trained pediatric surgeon should be comfortable in his or her knowledge of the current indications and should be able to perform this procedure under urgent or elective conditions.

While we occasionally encounter neonates that require urgent attention to their airway, most require a tracheostomy due to the need for long term ventilation. Pre-natal diagnosis now allows us to identify some infants at risk or requiring emergency airway access so that one can plan to attend the delivery in anticipation of requiring some sort of urgent intervention. Examples of this would be an infant with a congenital teratoma or massive cystic hygroma or laryngeal atresia. These are all cases of a Congenital High Airway Obstruction Syndrome or CHAOS, for which the pediatric surgical team is prepared to perform any necessary bronchoscopy, intubation or tracheostomy with the infant still connected to the placental circulation. A controlled situation then exists to allow ample time for accurate diagnosis and initial management, which may include a tracheostomy.

Otherwise, neonatology and technology have made great advances over the last few decades. Because of the routine use of surfactant and steroids, it is rare now to see a ventilator dependant infant from lung disease alone, and it is neither unusual nor unsafe to leave an infant on a ventilator with an endotracheal tube in place for months on end. Today nearly the only infants who need a tracheostomy do so because of an inadequate airway due to stenosis or laryngotracheo malacia. These infants otherwise are ready for discharged to go home or to a facility for technologically dependent children, but still require ventilatory assistance.

Older children are more likely to require a tracheostomy for acquired problems such as trauma or tumor management. The need for airway management in the course of trauma and burn care probably exceeds that required for the management of tumors. Some neurologically devastated children, regardless of the cause, also require a tracheostomy for optimal airway management.

This chapter will discuss the indications for and techniques for insertion and maintenance of a tracheostomy in infants and children.

24.2 Indications

The indications for tracheostomy in infants and children essentially fall into five main categories: airway immaturity, obstructing congenital anomalies, acquired obstructions, tumors and trauma.

The immature airway manifests itself as laryngomalacia, tracheomalacia or a combination of the two conditions. These infants present with inspiratory stridor, and some degree of nasal flaring and chest retractions. Other related conditions are congenital vocal chord paralysis, which is usually due to a central nervous system deficit, phrenic nerve injury, which may be associated with a difficult delivery, and recurrent laryngeal nerve injury after ligation of a patent ductus arteriosus.

Some patients with choanal atresia and Pierre Robin syndrome may be candidates for tracheostomy. Other craniofacial deformities such as Freeman Sheldon syndrome, Cerebro-costo-mandibular syndrome, arthrogyposis multiplex congenita and others also may require tracheostomies for airway maintenance.

Patients with a congenitally stenotic airway or tracheal agenesis may be special cases. In the case of agenesis, an emergency tracheostomy may be necessary incase the trachea reestablishes beyond the point of obstruction. Usually, however, these patients can be ventilated best using a mask as the bronchi come off the esophagus and a tube placed in the esophagus can cause obstruction.

There are a number of acquired conditions that require tracheostomy. Among them are infection, papillomatosis, neuromuscular failure, chronic aspiration and subglottic stenosis.

Occasionally the management of a tumor such as a cervical teratoma or sarcoma in infancy will mandate a tracheostomy. More likely a hemangioma or lymphangioma will compromise the airway to the extent that a more stable airway is needed and a tracheostomy will be performed.

And, rarely, trauma will prompt the surgeon to perform a tracheostomy in an infant. This can be birth related trauma, child abuse or accidental.

Older children rarely require a tracheostomy for a congenital problem but are more likely to need one due to some acquired condition resulting from infection, tumor or trauma. Some patients with severe papillomatosis require a tracheostomy for airway maintenance.

As a result of vascular accident, such as in the case of a patient with Sickle Cell Disease, or encephalopathy due to infection, patients who are neurologically devastated and have difficulty with ventilation and maintenance of their airway often require a tracheostomy.

Tumor patients with brain malignancies or with head and neck cancer comprise another group of patients who require a temporary or permanent tracheostomy.

And, trauma patients, whether as a result of head trauma or a high spinal cord injury, or burns typically make up the largest group of older children in need of a tracheostomy.

24.3 Pre-operative Evaluation

Most infants needing a trachestomy already have an endotracheal tube in place. Infants suspected of laryngotracheomalacia may require direct laryngoscopy and or bronchoscopy in the operating room.

The surgeon should make certain of the coagulation status, hemoglobin level and electrolyte status as indicated by the patient's condition. And, the nutritional status of the patient should be taken into consideration as poor nutrition will complicate nearly any condition in infancy and may be a factor in favor of an earlier tracheostomy than would otherwise be indicated.

When a child is not intubated, but is under consideration for tracheostomy because of suspected airway immaturity, the extent to which the child maintains oxygenation and demonstrates adequate ventilation as judged by the pCO_2 measured by transcutaneous monitoring will determine the need for a more direct assessment before a decision for tracheostomy is made.

Finally, patients with persistent aspiration, despite correction of any gastroesophageal reflux, may necessitate a tracheostomy to prevent severe pulmonary consequences.

Older children may or may not be intubated, depending on the circumstances. Most often, in the case of an elective procedure, the patient is already ventilator dependant and intubated. Regardless, it is best to perform direct laryngoscopy and bronchoscopy before you commit to a tracheostomy. We search for potential problems such as distal obstruction due to granulation tissue, stenosis or papillomatosis. As with any other operative patient, it is always wise to check for any coagulopathy or other condition that may add additional risk to the procedure.

24.4 Technique

The technique is slightly different for infant and older children and may be more different if done as an emergency in the case of burns or other trauma.

Infants are placed supine on the operating table, sufficiently toward the foot of the table so that the surgeon can easily access the infant's neck, but not so far down on the table that the anesthesiologist cannot reach the patient to manipulate the endotracheal tube so as to remove it from the airway at the appropriate time in the case.

These cases should be done under a general anesthetic unless the patient is so ill as to be unable to tolerate the drugs. Even so, an anesthesiologist or anesthetist should maintain control of the airway while the surgeon is exposing and manipulating the trachea.

The patient's cardiorespiratory status should be monitored during the case. This should consist of a cardiac monitor to monitor the heart rate, a blood pressure monitor, and ideally, a pulse oximeter to assess the infant's oxygenation. If there is any concern, an arterial line may be in order.

If there is any question as to the status of the airway, bronchoscopy should be performed to assure that the tracheal lumen will accept a tracheostomy cannula without difficulty. Special issues, such as a tracheostomy to stent an airway for severe tracheomalacia can be assessed by bronchoscopy to determine the proper length of the proposed cannula, which may have to be specially ordered. In this situation, it may be best to assess the airway by bronchoscopy and to use an endotracheal tube placed through the cervical incision and

secured to the skin of the neck until this temporary tracheostomy cannula can be replaced with the specially ordered device.

When positioning the infant on the operating table, the neck should be extended sufficiently so as to have complete access to the entire neck. Sometimes, on chubby infants, it is still difficult to see the entire neck, despite the best attempts. A roll can be placed under the infant's shoulders to facilitate the proper positioning.

The endotracheal tube should be secured in such a way that the anesthesiologist can easily remove the tube at the desired point in the case. This means that any tape should be loosened before hand. If there is a feeding tube in place, it may be best to remove it at this time so that it does not get in the anesthesiologist's way during endotracheal tube removal and manipulation.

When the infant is properly positioned and monitored, the entire neck from the lower lip to below the nipples should be prepped with a suitable surgical prep and drapped.

The superior surgical drape should allow easy access to the patient by the anesthesiologist.

Once prepped and drapped, the surgeon should carefully palpate the infant's neck to locate the trachea that hopefully is in the midline. The surgeon must keep in mind that the infant's trachea is quite mobile and compressible and may be difficult to palpate. If this is the case, asking the anesthesiologist to wiggle the endotracheal tube from above may be helpful.

We make our incision in the lower neck crease, about the width of one finger above the jugular notch. A transverse incision in this crease is preferable. If the incision is too low you will end up in the mediastinum and the cannula will end up too low in the trachea. We first score the skin with a scalpel, then use a needle-point electrocautery device to deepen the incision, taking care not to burn the skin. This incision is carried down through the subcutaneous fascia and platysma muscle, which is quite thin in the small infant.

It is helpful to insert two right-angled retractors in the corners of this incision to better expose the operative site.

Next, we use two atraumatic forceps to grasp the cervical fascia on either side of the midline and open this fascia in the midline. We extend this incision inferiorly to the jugular notch and superiorly to the thyroid gland.

The strap muscles, immediately beneath the anterior cervical fascia can be divided in a similar fashion.

Usually, there are few to no blood vessels in the dissection thus far. Occasionally, you will encounter a few small vessels that cross the midline. These should be cauterized and divided as they are encountered so that there will be no hemorrhage during the case.

Once these muscles are divided in the midline, we place the two retractors deep to the muscle edges and gently retract laterally to better expose the trachea below. Sometimes it may be necessary to free the muscle edges sufficiently to allow room for the blade of the retractor to gain a secure purchase.

At this point in the case, the trachea should be seen with ease. If it is not readily seen, then palpation in the wound with, perhaps, manipulation of the endotracheal tube by the anesthesiologist will help locate the trachea.

It is helpful to pause at this junction and select the proposed tracheostomy cannula. Once a cannula is selected, it should be opened and its outer diameter visually checked against the exposed trachea to judge the correctness of its size. If it seems that the initial selection was incorrect, then a tracheostomy cannula of a more appropriate size should be selected.

There will be some fascia surrounding the trachea. This should be scored with the cautery to coagulate any tiny vessels on the surface of the trachea in the midline. Again, the blades of the retractors should be deep in the wound, on either side of the trachea so that the trachea is easily exposed.

A suture of 4-0 Prolene or its equivalent is placed on either side of the midline scored anterior trachea. Each suture incorporates one or two tracheal rings. These sutures are not tied onto the tracheal wall, but can be tied at their ends, which should be left 6–8 cm in length. At the end of the case, the end of these sutures will be taped securely to the anterior chest wall and will be used to locate the tracheal incision in the event of a post-operative emergency in case the newly placed tracheostomy cannula dislodges. These sutures also can be used to hold open the edges of the tracheal incision for ease of placement of the tracheostomy cannula at operation.

The surgeon should request at this time that the endotracheal tube be loosened and prepared for removal. A vertical incision should be made in the trachea on the score mark, using a number 11 blade, below the thyroid gland, which can be quite large in the neonate. Two or three tracheal rings should be divided. Usually these are rings 2, 3 and 4. We do this

with the cautery to ensure hemostasis. The incision should be sufficiently deep so as to enter the lumen, but not so deep as to incise the endotracheal tube, which should still be in the trachea at this point. Rarely, it is necessary to divide the isthmus of the thyroid gland for proper tracheostomy positioning.

A transverse tracheal incision or removal of a tracheal ring is likely to result in a tracheal deformity and thus should be avoided.

Suction should be available in case blood or secretions get in the way of the surgeon's view of the tracheal lumen. The tip of the cannula to be inserted should be lubricated with a water soluble surgical lubricant and positioned over the incision, poised for insertion when the endotracheal is withdrawn.

The surgeon then requests the anesthesiologist that the endotracheal tube be withdrawn sufficiently to clear the lumen so that the tracheostomy cannula can be inserted into the lumen and directed caudally toward the carina.

One way to avoid misplacement of the cannula is to insert a suction catheter into the lumen and beyond the tip of the cannula. The suction catheter can be inserted into the tracheal lumen first and serve as a guide over which the cannula can be passed. This technique is also useful should the cannula become dislodged after the procedure.

If, for any reason, the tracheostomy cannula does not fit easily into the trachea, then the cannula should be removed and the endotracheal tube should be advanced beyond the tracheal incision so that ventilation will not be compromised. This might occur if the diameter of the tracheal lumen has been over estimated and the previously selected tracheostomy is too large to fit into the trachea. In that case, a smaller cannula should be selected and, after it is certain that the infant is well oxygenated, inserted as described above.

As soon as the cannula is in place, the obturator or suction catheter should be removed and the anesthesiologist should disconnect the ventilator hose from the endotracheal tube and connect it to the tracheostomy cannula. Once that is done, the anesthesiologist should administer several deep breaths to the patient to confirm that the cannula is in the proper place and that the infant can be ventilated satisfactorily. If it appears that, although the cannula width is appropriate, the cannula is too long and its tip rests on the carina, then several pieces of gauze can be used to build up the gap between the neck and the tracheostomy collar, thus backing the tip of the cannula away from the carina. Once adequate ventilation is confirmed, then the endotracheal tube can be removed completely.

Once the cannula is connected to the ventilator, the cervical wings of the body of the cannula need to be secured to the patient. We don't rely on the tie placed around the neck, but accomplish this with the aid of sutures.

On each wing, a suture of 3-0 silk or its equivalent is passed through the skin of the neck, then one edge of the wing of the cannula (midway between the midline and the end of the wing), through the other edge of the wing, then again through the skin. When this suture is tied, the skin will be drawn over the wing and will usually cover it. After you have placed these sutures, both wings will be securely fixed to the skin of the neck.

The two ties that were placed in the anterior tracheal wall are now taped securely to the anterior chest wall in such a fashion that their ends are easily accessible in case they are needed to reinsert the cannula.

Finally, the umbilical tape or tie that usually comes with the cannula is passed through the holes in the end of the wings and tied around the neck to further secure the cannula. A simple gauze dressing with some antibiotic ointment is placed underneath the cannula at the cervical incision to complete the procedure.

We send our infants to the intensive care unit for the first several days after a tracheostomy in case there is a problem.

Older children also are placed supine with their necks extended. Occasionally, this is not possible due to cervical injury. In that case, we do the best we can to clear the area of the proposed tracheostomy to facilitate the procedure. We still use a lower neck crease for the site of the incision, but the incision in children often seems higher in its placement. We palpate the thyroid cartilage and cricoid as landmarks for the site of the tracheostomy. In most instances we make our tracheotomy incision below the cricoid and perform the operation as described above.

There are some instances that become so urgent that they do not allow for careful planning. In cases of acute trauma or burns, when the airway is compromised, the concept of performing a tracheostomy if you even think you might need one holds true. In the case of burn injuries, the tissue swelling is so brisk and profound, the early one performs a tracheostomy, the easier it is. The converse also holds true. If one deliberates too long, it may be nearly impossible to perform a safe procedure.

Trauma to the head and neck often mandates urgent tracheostomy. This may be required at the time of injury in the form of a cricothyroidotomy. After the airway is established and the patient stabilized, it may be prudent to reassess the airway and convert the situation to something more stable and easier to care for.

Trachestomy performed in older children for tumor is usually elective and can be carried out in the operating room as described above.

24.5 Peri-operative Management

If the skin of the patient's neck is infected with a bacterial or fungal infection, then this should be cleared before any operation is undertaken unless emergency tracheostomy is required to save an infant's life.

In patients with short, fat necks, it may be necessary to place an infant in a position of neck extension to facilitate clearing any skin infection or breakdown that is due to chronic moisture. Simply exposing an infant's neck to air for drying often is sufficient to clear any problem.

Immediately after the cannula is secured, the roll under the neck should be removed and a radiograph of the chest should be reviewed before the patient is taken from the operating room. This is important to make certain that the tip of the cannula is sufficiently clear of the carina and will not become obstructed as the patient's neck is manipulated.

The newly placed tracheostomy should be left in place for about 10 days before it is disturbed. Once or twice each day, the gauze should be removed, the site should be cleaned with a cotton applicator soaked in a solution of hydrogen peroxide, and an antibiotic ointment should be applied to the incision site.

The sutures securing the tracheostomy should be left untouched for the initial 10 day period, after which they can be cut. The sutures to the edges of the tracheal incision are left until the tracheostomy is changed successfully for the first time.

If the patient is unusually agitated, or the ventilator tubing is so heavy that dislodging the cannula is highly likely, then sedation or paralysis may be helpful for up to 10 days until the wound has had some time to mature and reinsertion can be done more safely.

After the cannula is free and the umbilical tape untied, the cannula can be removed and replaced with a new cannula. Ideally, the parents or ultimate caretakers should observe the change, particularly if the patient is about to go home.

If a temporary endotracheal tube is being replaced with a specially ordered tracheostomy cannula, the new cannula should be inserted as described above.

Once it is clear that the cannula can be changed with ease and that after the change, the cannula is in the proper position and the patient can be ventilated, then the sutures to the edges of tracheal incision can be cut and removed.

Suctioning of the newly placed tracheostomy should be done as often as necessary, particularly immediately after the procedure. Care must be taken, however, to restrict the passage of the suction catheter to no further than the tip of the cannula. Routine suctioning beyond the tip of the cannula promotes the development of granulation tissue that may present a problem later on.

Most tracheostomies in infants are without balloons to prevent excessive air leaks. Older children, however, are more likely to require cannulae into which are incorporated soft balloons. It is imperative that caretakers understand that excessive pressure in the balloons can apply too much pressure to the tracheal wall and result in erosion, infection, hemorrhage or perforation. The balloon pressure should not exceed capillary pressure or 25 mmHg and should be checked at least three times a day to prevent these complications.

24.6   Home Instruction and Care

Patients should be discharged home with an extra tracheostomy cannula incase a problem occurs. They should be instructed and checked out on tracheotomy change, cuff pressure monitoring and cardiopulmonary resuscitation (CPR). They should know how to suction the cannula and be sent home with a suction machine. They should know how to use an Ambu bag for ventilation in conjunction with suctioning.

An air filter should be attached to the tracheostomy cannula if a ventilating device or some other moisturizing device is not otherwise connected. Of course, the family or caretakers must know how to use and trouble shoot all of these devices.

It is often helpful to arrange for home nursing visits until the family becomes familiar and comfortable with the new devices. This is especially true when it comes time for the first scheduled tracheostomy change if is to be done at home.

The physician may choose to do the first tracheostomy change in the office and take the opportunity to further instruct and reassure the family or caretakers.

24.7   Complications

Hemorrhage is an unusual complication. It can occur at the time of operation or as a delayed event.

When hemorrhage occurs at operation, it can be easily controlled with electrocautery or vessel ligation. Rarely, especially in the newborn, the thyroid gland is near the incision site on the anterior trachea and is inadvertently divided or lacerated. The resultant hemorrhage usually can be controlled with sutures or electrocautery.

Late hemorrhage often is more problematic and may be more serious. First, it must be ascertained whether the hemorrhage is from the tracheal lumen or from the incision. This can be accomplished by suctioning the cannula and inspecting the wound. Occasionally a small skin-vessel will bleed briskly but can be easily seen and controlled with a simple suture or even with an injection of lidocaine containing 1:100,000 epinephrine.

More problematic is the possibility of hemorrhage from one of the great vessels, such as the innominate vein or artery. This can occur from erosion of the vessels when the cannula fits too snugly in the thoracic inlet and partially compresses the vessels against the clavical. This type of hemorrhage often presents with a so-called "herald bleed" which starts briskly but stops, and usually requires a trip to the operating room to repair the damaged vessel.

Aside from hemorrhage, the cannula can become dislodged. We are compulsive about securing the cannula in place using the techniques described above in order to avoid this complication. Even so, despite our best efforts, a suture will pull loose or one of the plastic wings will tear allowing the cannula to dislodge.

Fortunately, we keep most of our infants and small children in the intensive care unit during the immediate post-operative period. We anticipate that if the cannula becomes dislodged, it will be noticed immediately by the nurse caring for the patient. Replacing the cannula in the immediate post-operative period can be a treacherous ordeal that under ideal circumstances should be done be someone familiar with cannula insertion. If a surgeon or intensivist is readily available, then one of them should replace the cannula and re-secure the device. The sutures to the tracheal incision should be taped in such a manner as to be easy to access, untape and retract to expose the tracheal lumen. Good lighting is essential to see well and the obturator should be inserted into the cannula before reinsertion is attempted.

The last thing you want to occur is for someone in a rush to force the cannula into an inappropriate position, outside the trachea perhaps. There are many important structures crammed into a small space. Care should be taken to assure that the cannula is in the trachea. This can be accomplished by administering a deep breath or two with an Ambu bag once the cannula is in place. If the chest does not rise immediately, chances are that the cannula is not in the proper place. In that case, it should be replaced.

Usually, it not necessary to use instruments to reinsert the cannula because the sutures attached to the edges of the tracheal incision should lead directly to the opening in the trachea. If difficulty arises, two small right-angled retractors should be sufficient to complete the job.

Infection is an unusual complication and should be treated with the appropriate antimicrobials according to culture results.

Injury to the vagus nerves or, more likely, the recurrent laryngeal nerves can occur. In experienced hands with a surgeon well versed in the anatomy of the infant's neck, this should be a rare injury.

Of course, great care should be taken initially to properly place the cannula in the tracheal lumen. While unlikely, it is possible to place the cannula in the esophagus. This can be accomplished if the trachea is retracted out of the field and the esophagus is entered in error.

If this occurs, then the esophagus should be repaired primarily and a drain should be placed. The tracheostomy cannula then can be inserted properly.

Endotracheal granulation tissue can result from the chronic irritation of the tip of the tracheostomy cannula against the tracheal wall or from the repeated suctioning of the trachea.

It is not unusual for granulation tissue to develop at the stoma. This can be exophytic at the level of the skin, or can be intralumenal. The exophytic granulation tissue at the skin should be cauterized as an outpatient with silver nitrate. This may need to be carried out every month or so if bothersome hemorrhage or chronic irritation with infection is present.

If the granulation tissue develops immediately within the trachea at the stoma, it usually can be left alone until it is time for decannulation. Only if the granulation tissue is so bulky that it interferes with routine tracheostomy changes should it be removed before decannulation is contemplated.

Granulation tissue developing at the tip of the cannula can present with obstruction, sometimes resulting in a "ball-valve effect with air trapping and difficulty with ventilation. This can be diagnosed by slipping a flexible bronchoscope through the cannula to visualize the tracheal lumen beyond the tip of the cannula. If the results of this diagnostic maneuver are unclear, rigid bronchoscopy may be necessary.

We believe that this type of granulation tissue is best removed with laser. Our preference is for the KTP/532 laser or an equivalent wavelength that operates using a flexible fiber. The technique for laser vaporization of granulation tissue is beyond the scope of this discussion.

24.8 Special Situations

Occasionally, there exist special circumstances, which require careful thought and planning. Such is the case in the infant with tracheal stenosis. Simple acquired subglottic stenosis is easily managed with a tracheostomy inserted as described with the only difference being the size of the endotracheal tube. In this case, a small endotracheal tube may be difficult to palpate and thus it may be difficult to locate the trachea as one makes the initial exposure.

In an infant with a particularly stenotic airway, it may not be possible to ventilate the patient with an endotracheal tube and mask ventilation may be the only way to maintain ventilation. In this situation, careful planning with the anesthesiologist is required. While the anesthesiologist ventilates the patient by mask, care is taken to carry out the operation as described above. Once again, the most difficult part of the case is locating the trachea without an indwelling endotracheal tube.

In patients with distal tracheal stenosis, a tracheostomy insertion may be inappropriate. While beyond the scope of this discussion, the infant should be carefully

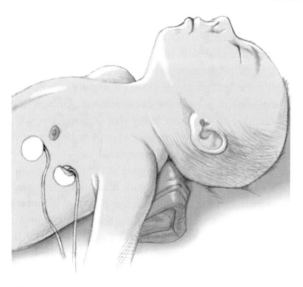

Fig. 24.1   The patient is placed supine on the operating table. The neck should be extended sufficiently to allow complete access to the neck.

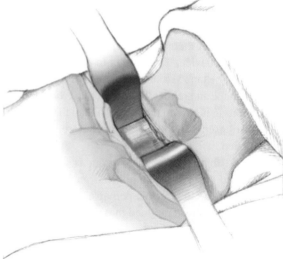

Fig. 24.3   The incision is extended through the tissue layer until the trachea can be visualised easily

studied if this diagnosis is suspected. Usually, plain radiographs of the chest may lead one to suspect the diagnosis. Computerized tomography or bronchoscopy may be required.

When the distal trachea is stenotic in an infant who is difficult to ventilate, a conventional tracheostomy cannula probably is inappropriate and may interfere with tracheal reconstruction.

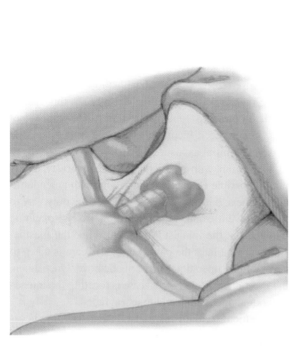

Fig. 24.2   Incision is made in the lower neck crease, about 1 cm above the jugular notch.

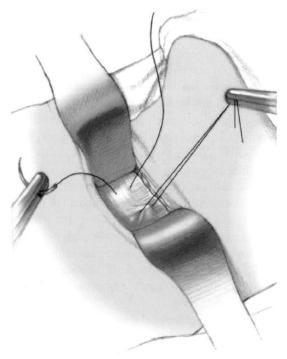

Fig. 24.4   A monofilament suture is placed on either side of the middle scored anterior trachea.

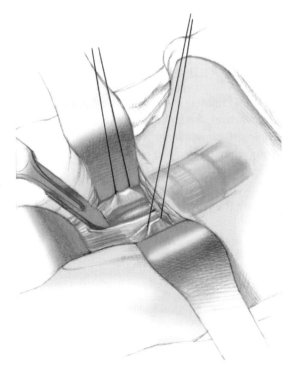

Fig. 24.5   A vertical incision is made throughout the tracheal wall.

Patients who are candidates for congenital heart surgery in whom the ultimate need for a tracheostomy is anticipated, may be best managed by completing the cardiac surgery before tracheostomy is performed. Otherwise, the sternal incision is so

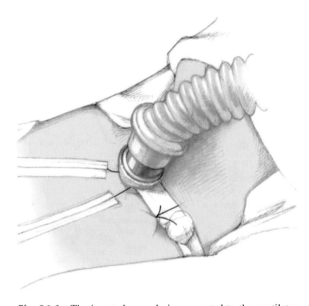

Fig. 24.6   The inserted cannula is connected to the ventilator and the cervical wings of the body of the cannula are secured to the patient.

close to the tracheostomy site that the risk of infection is greatly increased.

24.9 Decannulation

Decannulation usually is anticipated well in advance. It's timing depends to a large degree on the reason for the tracheostomy. Patients with severe subglottic stenoses may have their tracheostomy removed at the time of their laryngoplasty. The timing of this procedure, then, depends on the surgeon and may occur any time between 4 and 6 months and 2 years or later.

In patients whose tracheostomy was placed because of tracheomalacia, it would be unusual to attempt decannulation before the infant is a year of age. The infant should undergo periodic bronchoscopic examinations to assess the status of the malacia. Once it is certain that the airway is sufficiently mature as to be able to maintain a patent airway, decannulation can be attempted.

The first step is to make certain that the airway is mature and free of any potential obstructing lesions such as granulation tissue. This is best accomplished with rigid bronchoscopy performed in the operating room. Any residual malacia or granulation tissue can be seen and dealt with appropriately as needed.

At the time of attempted decannulation, we have the patient in the operating room, positioned as described above for insertion of the cannula with the neck extended and carry out the bronchoscopy. In order to assess whether malacia is present, the patient should not be paralyzed and the anesthesia should be light. This is to assure that the airway remains patent with the patient breathing without assistance.

Once committed to decannulation, the bronchoscope and neck roll are removed and the patient is observed for any difficulty such as severe chest retractions or deoxygenation that would suggest the continued need for the tracheostomy. If, on the other hand, the patient ventilates with ease, then the patient is fully awakened and recovered in a unit that permits careful observation.

We usually keep these patients in the hospital overnight, or longer if there is any question, to assure that the tracheostomy is no longer required.

Once the cannula is removed, a snug dressing of plain or petroleum jelly saturated gauze is secured over the tracheostomy stoma to occlude this opening and allow optimal ventilation through the trachea. The parents should be instructed how to change this dressing until the stoma closes completely.

Occasionally, we encounter a stoma that does not close on its own. If, after several months, the stoma remains open and appears unlikely to close and it is certain that the infant no longer is at risk for needing another tracheostomy, then operative closure of the stoma as an outpatient procedure can be performed. Usually, this is simply a matter of excising the stoma and placing a simple stitch in the anterior trachea. A larger persistent opening may require an anterior wedge excision for repair. This may necessitate admission to the hospital.

If, after the patient leaves the operating room decannulated, the infant fatigues or demonstrates other signs of not tolerating the decannulation, the dressing can be removed and another cannula should be reinserted. If it seems appropriate, a smaller cannula size can be inserted.

This technique often is used to serially wean a patient to progressively smaller sized cannulae until decannulation is nearly certain to be successful.

If, after decannulation, it is necessary to reinsert a trachestomy, the procedure should be done in the operating. While this is usually done with an endotracheal tube in place, there are some patients for whom it may be desirable not to insert an endotracheal tube which may further irritate the airway and possibly induce the airway to become stenotic. That being the case, the surgeon can inject a local anesthetic to anesthetize the stoma, dilate the stoma with Hegar dilators (or possibly make a small incision with a number 11 scalpel blade), and reinsert a cannula of an appropriate size. This maneuver should only be attempted if the anesthesiologist can maintain an adequate airway during the procedure.

Further Reading

Amin RS, Fitton CM (2003) Tracheostomy and home ventilation in children. Semin Neonatol 8:127–135

Cochrane LA, Bailey CM (2006) Surgical aspects of tracheostomy in children. Paediatr Respir Rev 7:169–174

Davis GM (2006–2007) Tracheostomy in children. Paediatr Respir Rev Suppl 1:S206–S209

Fiske E (2004) Effective strategies to prepare infants and families for home tracheostomy care. Adv Neonatal Care 4:42–53

Lobe TE (2006) Tracheostomy. In P Puri, ME Höllwarth (eds), Pediatric Surgery. Springer Surgery Atlas Series, Springer-Verlag Berlin Heidelberg, New York, pp 19–26

Wilson M (2005) Tracheostomy management. Paediatr Nurs 17:38–43

Chest Wall Deformities

25

Donald Nuss and Robert E. Kelly, Jr.

Contents

25.1 Introduction

Chest wall deformities may be congenital or acquired and may be divided into three categories. The most common category is the group of deformities in which there *is* rib overgrowth causing either a *depression (Pectus Excavatum)* (Fig. 25.1) or protrusion *(Pectus Carinatum)* (Fig. 25.2) of the anterior chest wall. The second category of deformities is due to *failure of normal development* (aplasia or dysplasia). The aplasia may be midline causing *bifid sternum*, in which there is partial or complete failure of midline fusion of the sternum resulting in *ectopia cordis* (Figs. 25.3 and 25.4). In addition to the sternum, there may be aplasia of the associated structures, such as the heart, pericardium, diaphragm and anterior abdominal wall *(Pentalogy of Cantrell)*. The aplasia may also be unilateral with an absence of ribs, pectoralis muscles and breast tissue as seen in *Poland's Syndrome* (Fig. 25.5). The third category of deformities is due to *trauma* or *pressure effects*. Too early and extensive rib resection for pectus excavatum may destroy growth centers and result in *acquired asphyxiating chondrodystrophy* (Fig. 25.6). Abnormal pressure effects and spasticity as seen in patients with severe cerebral palsy may result in very abnormal chest configuration.

Chest wall deformities are frequently *familial* with several members of one family affected. The incidence of *connective tissue disorders* such as *Marfan's Syndrome* and *Ehler's-Danlos Syndrome* is markedly increased in patients with chest wall deformities. As a result, systemic weakness of the connective tissues and poor muscular development of the thorax, abdomen and spine is common and *scoliosis* is present in up to 19% of these patients.

P. Puri and M. Höllwarth (eds.), *Pediatric Surgery: Diagnosis and Management*,
DOI: 10.1007/978-3-540-69560-8_25, © Springer-Verlag Berlin Heidelberg 2009

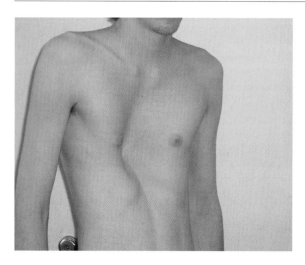

Fig. 25.1   Pectus excavatum

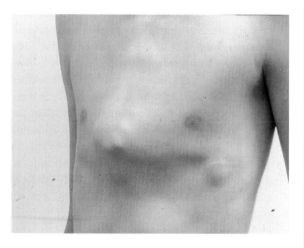

Fig. 25.2   Pectus carinatum

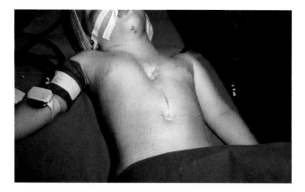

Fig. 25.3   Sternal fissure—Partial, superior

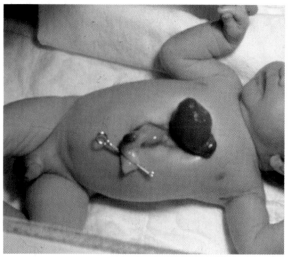

Fig. 25.4   Sternal fissure—Ectopia cordis

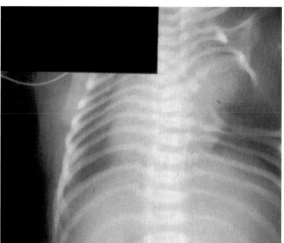

Fig. 25.5   Poland's syndrome showing rib dysplasia and aplasia

Emergency surgery in the newborn period is rare and only necessary for those conditions which are incompatible with life such as ectopia cordis and Pentalogy of Cantrell.

Surgical repair of the more common abnormalities such as pectus excavatum has changed dramatically over the last 20 years. Prior to 1990, the prevailing philosophy was extensive surgical resection in very young patients. The operation included bilateral rib cartilage resection, complete sternal

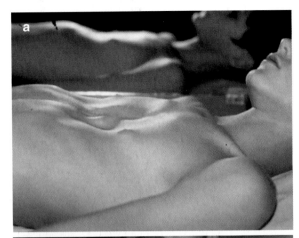

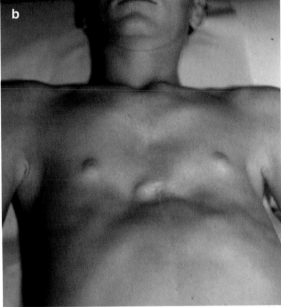

Fig. 25.6 (**a** and **b**) Acquired asphyxiating chondrodystrophy showing chest wall constriction after too extensive and too early open repair for pectus excavatum

mobilization and sternal osteotomy. This resulted in a significant number of patients developing asphyxiating chondrodystrophy because the growth centers were destroyed (Fig. 25.6a, b). However, during the 1990s it was recommended that patients be operated on after puberty and to perform minimal resection.

More recently still, a minimally invasive procedure with no resection, only internal bracing, has become the established procedure of choice. The new approach has resulted in many more patients presenting for treatment.

25.2 Pectus Excavatum

25.2.1 Introduction

Pectus excavatum is a depression of the anterior chest wall of variable severity, that may be mild, moderate or severe. In mild and moderate cases, the patients are usually asymptomatic, but in severe cases there is significant cardiac compression and pulmonary restriction leading to dyspnea on exertion, limited exercise tolerance and chest pain. The configuration of the deformity varies and may be localized and deep (cup-shaped) (Fig. 25.7), diffuse (saucer-shaped) (Fig. 25.8), eccentric (grand-canyon) (Fig. 25.9), or mixed excavatum/carinatum (horseshoe, horns of steer, pouter pigeon) (Fig. 25.10).

In approximately one third of the patients the deformity is present at birth. *Progression of the deformity* as the child grows occurs in a vast majority of patients, especially during times of rapid growth as occurs during puberty, when a mild deformity may become severe in as little as 6–12 months. Pediatricians often are unaware of this progression and mistakenly advise parents "not to worry because the deformity will resolve," thereby losing the opportunity to treat the condition non-operatively.

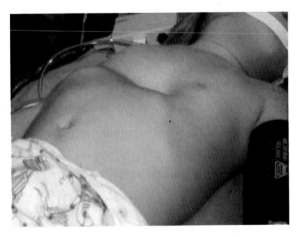

Fig. 25.7 Localized pectus excavatum (cup shaped)

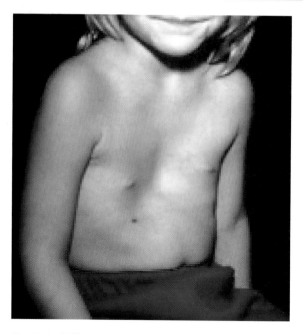

Fig. 25.8 Diffuse pectus excavatum (saucer shaped)

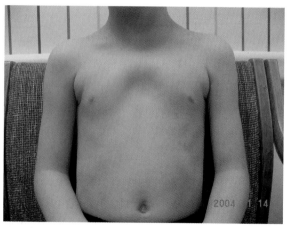

Fig. 25.10 Mixed pectus excavatum/carinatum (horseshoe, pouter pigeon or horns of steer shape)

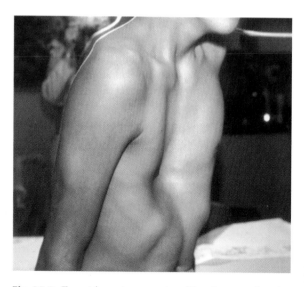

Fig. 25.9 Eccentric pectus excavatum (Grand canyon shape)

25.2.2 *History of Pectus Excavatum*

Bauhinus in 1594 described a patient with pectus excavatum who suffered from severe dyspnea and paroxysmal coughing. In 1820, Coulson noted the genetic predisposition of the condition in a family with three brothers who suffered from pectus excavatum. The first successful operation was done by Sauerbruch in 1913 on a patient who was severely incapacitated. He simply resected the depressed ribs and sternum to relieve the cardiac compression, thereby allowing the patient to return to work. Resecting the sternum caused flail chest and so in subsequent patients, he introduced the sternal osteotomy and rib cartilage resection procedure, later popularized by Ravitch. Sauerbruch used external traction post operatively, to keep the sternum from sinking back in. Ravitch did away with external traction, but to prevent recurrence, he recommended much wider and more radical resection of the cartilages and complete mobilization and osteotomy of the sternum. Since recurrence was still a problem even with wide resection, Wallgren and Sulamaa advocated internal bracing by passing a rod through the sternum and this was followed by Adkins and Blades who suggested passing the strut behind the sternum. This wide resection with or without a strut became the procedure of choice in the second half of the twentieth century and because it was easier to do in young patients, the 3- to 5-year old patients were the prime candidates. However, there were enough late complications for the pediatricians to become concerned and so they stopped referring patients for surgical correction. In 1990, Pena published a paper showing that asphyxiating chondrodystrophy developed in baby rabbits after early cartilage resection and in 1996 Haller drew attention to the risk of asphyxiating chondrodystrophy in a paper entitled "Chest Wall Constriction After Too Extensive and Too Early Operations for Pectus Excavatum." As a result, surgeons stopped operating on patients before puberty and reduced the amount of cartilage resected and introduced the concept of a "modified Ravitch procedure."

More recently Nuss, Kelly, et al. introduced the concept of a minimally invasive procedure which requires no resection and combined it with a deep breathing, posture and aerobic exercise program. This technique has now become the procedure of choice.

Other less invasive, but still experimental techniques include a suction device to elevate the sternum and implantation of a magnet under the sternum.

25.2.3 Incidence and Etiology

The incidence varies in different race groups but has been quoted to be anywhere from 1 in 300 to 1 in 1,000 children (see Table 25.1). It is more common in children of European and Asian descent and less common in children of African descent.

The exact cause is not known but the genetic predisposition was already noted in the 19th century. It is common to have several children in one family as well as other family members affected including parents, grandparents, cousins, etc. In our series of 1,500 patients, 40% have a positive family history. Of interest is that some family members have an excavatum deformity, while others have a carinatum deformity and others have a mixed deformity. In most series, boys out number girls 4 to 1, but when girls do have excavatum it is usually more severe and more frequently associated with scoliosis suggesting homozygous transmission. Other factors that suggest genetics plays a role are as follows: pectus patients usually are tall and asthenic resembling basketball players. They often have a delicate bone structure. The incidence of connective tissue disorders is much higher than in the normal population – 18% have associated scoliosis, 16% have features compatible with Marfan's Syndrome and 1% have Ehlers-Danlos Syndrome.

Table 25.1 Demographics of chest wall malformations at our institution, 2006

Incidence and Etiology	Number of patients
Total evaluated	1,574
Total with pectus excavatum	1,397 (88.8%)
Total with mixed pectus excavatum/Pectus carinatum	84 (5.3%)
Total with pectus carinatum	40 (2.5%)
Total with Poland's syndrome	11 (0.7%)
Total with other deformities	42 (2.7%)
Male-to-female ratio	4:1
Family history of pectus excavatum	39.8%
Incidence of scoliosis	18.9%
Incidence of Marfans	1.9%
Incidence of Marfanoid (presume Marfan)	14.0%
Incidence of Ehlers-Danlos	1.0%

25.2.4 Clinical Features

The most frequent symptoms are dyspnea on exertion, chest pain on exertion and lack of endurance resulting in exercise intolerance (see Table 25.2). Frequent respiratory tract infections and asthma may also occur. The presence and severity of symptoms is

Table 25.2 Preoperative symptoms of primary surgical patients (n = 865)

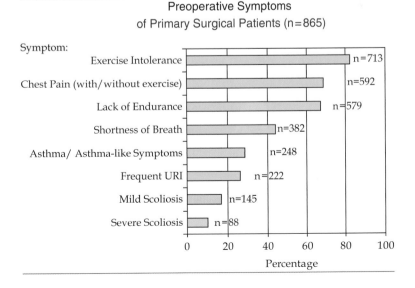

Preoperative Symptoms of Primary Surgical Patients (n=865)

directly related to the severity of cardiac and pulmonary compression and therefore to the severity of the deformity. Symptoms tend to be more prevalent in older children because teenagers have a deeper deformity and a more rigid chest, whereas younger children still have a very pliable chest wall, have significant cardiac and pulmonary reserves, don't participate in competitive sports, and the deformity has not progressed to its full extent.

Teenagers with pectus excavatum have a poor body image and because of their exercise intolerance they stop participating in team sports which leads to isolation and feelings of worthlessness. They hate and avoid situations where they have to take their shirt off in front of other children, therefore adding to their isolation and to a downward spiral of depression and suicidal thoughts.

On physical examination these patients have a classic "old age" or "pectus posture" that includes thoracic kyphosis, forward sloping shoulders, and a protuberant abdomen. They tend to be very asthenic, with long limbs, delicate bone structure and poor muscular development. The pectus deformity may be localized (cup-shaped) diffuse (saucer-shaped) eccentric (grand canyon) or mixed excavatum/carinatum (horseshoe, horns of steer, pouter pigeon). The sternum is frequently twisted so that it is at a 45% angle to the anterior chest wall.

Since the deformity may be mild, moderate or severe it is important to measure the severity objectively. The Haller CT index divides the internal transverse diameter

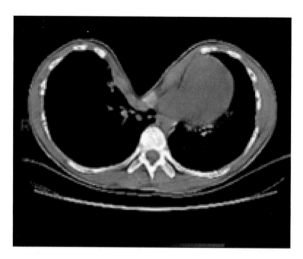

Fig. 25.11 CT showing CT index of 20 (Transverse diameter is 80 mm, AP diameter is 4 mm)

of the chest by the anteroposterior diameter. In normal patients the index is less than 2. An index greater than 3.25 is indicative of a severe depression (Fig. 25.11).

25.2.5 Cardiac and Pulmonary Effects

As the pectus excavatum may be mild, moderate or severe and may be localized, diffuse, eccentric or mixed and patients vary in age from newborn to adult, it is not surprising that there is controversy in the literature regarding the pathophysiologic effects of pectus excavatum. Some authors have shown significant compromise of cardiac and/or pulmonary function, whereas others have been unable to demonstrate any change. Numerous factors play a role when testing for cardio-pulmonary function and these include: the severity of the deformity, the age of the patient, the inherent physical fitness of the patient, associated medical conditions, (e.g., asthma) whether the studies are done supine or erect, whether they are done during exercise or at rest and a variety of technical factors, for example whether the study used uni-dimensional or two-dimensional echocardiography.

The cardiac compression has three main effects namely *decreased cardiac output, impaired valve function* and *arrhytmias*. Compression causes decreased filling, decreased stroke volume and therefore decreased cardiac output. This no doubt plays a significant role in causing the decreased endurance. The incidence of mitral valve prolapse varies from 15% to 65% in different series of patients, compared to only 1% in the normal pediatric population. Thirdly, arrthymias such as first degree heart block, right bundle branch block, and Wolff-Parkinson White Syndrome are noted in up to 16% of patients.

The pulmonary effects can be categorized into three groups as well, namely *restrictive lung disease, atelectasis and paradoxical respiration*. The thoracic restriction is demonstrated by stress testing which shows increased oxygen consumption for a given exercise. This increased work of breathing results in decreased endurance, despite the fact that these patients often compensate by increasing the diaphragmatic component of their respiration. Atelectasis results in frequent and prolonged respiratory tract infections which may also result in asthma. Paradoxical respiration causes decreased ventilation and therefore decreases exercise tolerance.

25.2.6 Evaluation and Indications for Operation

All patients are started on a deep breathing, aerobic exercise and posture program. The patients who have a mild or moderate deformity are re-evaluated at yearly intervals. The patients with a severe deformity who are symptomatic undergo testing to see if their condition warrants surgical correction.

Operation is indicated if two or more of the following criteria apply: (1) a chest CT showing cardiac and/or pulmonary compression and a CT index of 3.25 or greater; (2) a cardiology evaluation demonstrating compression, cardiac displacement, mitral valve prolapse, murmurs, or conduction abnormalities; (3) pulmonary function study showing restrictive and/or obstructive lung disease; (4) a failed previous repair.

Although the minimally invasive procedure may be done at any age, the ideal age is just before puberty because at that age the chest is still soft and malleable and the pubertal growth spurt will allow the chest to reconfigure to a normal contour and become more mature and rigid while the pectus support bar is in place.

25.2.7 Surgical Technique

The minimally invasive technique involves inserting one or two curved steel bars under the sternum in order to brace the anterior chest wall (Figs. 25.12 and 25.13). The bar is first bent into the convex shape to the required configuration and then under thoracoscopic control it is inserted into the chest through small lateral thoracic incisions with the convexity facing posteriorly. When the bar is in position it is rotated 180° thereby correcting the excavatum by pushing the depression outwards in an anterior direction. The bar is then stabilized and left in place for 3 years (Fig. 25.13). Two support bars may be placed in older patients.

The open technique involves making an anterior thoracic incision, taking the pectoralis muscles off the anterior chest wall, exposing the ribs and performing

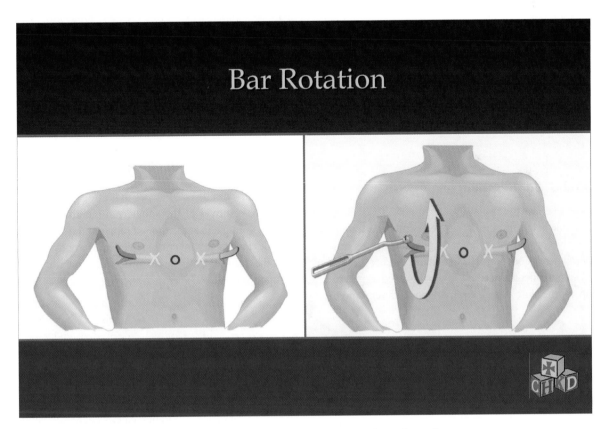

Fig. 25.12 Shows Bar Inserted under the Sternum and being rotated 180° in order to elevate the sternum

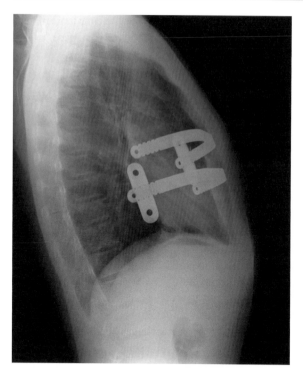

Fig. 25.13 Post op pectus repair showing two substernal support bars

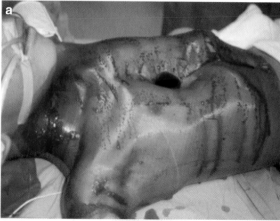

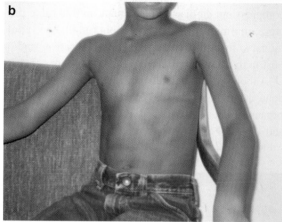

Fig. 25.14 (**a**) J.L. 8 year old patient with severe pectus excavatum; (**b**) J. L. 3 years post minimally invasive repair

subperiosteal cartilage resection. The sternum is widely mobilized and a wedge osteotomy is performed in order to elevate the sternum. A substernal bar may be inserted. The muscles and soft tissues are sutured back in place.

25.2.8 Bar Removal

The bar is left in place for 3 years after the minimally invasive procedure in order to give the tissues time to permanently reconfigure and mature. The bar is removed as an outpatient procedure. If a bar is used as part of the open procedure it is generally removed after 6 months.

25.2.9 Results

Results show that 95% of patients who undergo minimally invasive pectus repair have good to excellent long-term results (see Fig. 25.14a, b and Table 25.3).

Patients report marked improvement in their exercise capacity and parents report dramatic change in the child's self-confidence. Factors that affect a poor outcome are removal of the substernal bar in less than 2 years, young age at the time of repair and a sedentary lifestyle. Pulmonary function studies show improvement with the minimally invasive procedure but not with the open procedure.

25.2.10 Conclusion

Pectus excavatum is a progressive deformity during childhood and therefore these patients should be evaluated on a regular basis because of the risk of developing cardiac and pulmonary compression. Asymptomatic,

Table 25.3 Showing long-term results by age at time of surgery

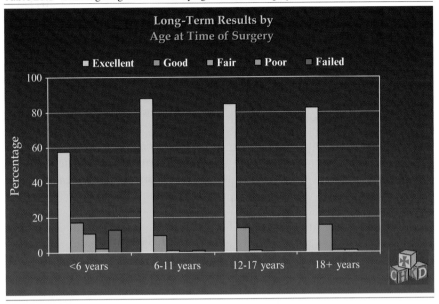

mild and moderately severe deformities can often be treated with a deep breathing, aerobic exercise and posture program. Severe and symptomatic patients should also be treated with the exercise and posture program but in addition they should be studied to see if they require surgical correction to decompress the heart and lungs.

25.3 Pectus Carinatum

Pectus carinatum is a ***protrusion deformity*** of the chest that is much less common than the excavatum deformity even though some patients have a mixed deformity and in some families one child may have pectus excavatum and another pectus carinatum (Fig. 25.2). The protrusion may involve the upper chest if the manubrium projects forward or it may involve the lower chest if the body (gladiolus) of the sternum projects forward. The protrusion may be unilateral, bilateral or mixed. It is more common in boys (4:1), and 25% have a positive family history.

Unlike excavatum, pectus carinatum usually appears in late childhood and progresses rapidly during puberty. Patients may complain of chest pain if pressure is applied to the anterior chest wall, as when lying on their stomachs. Unlike pectus excavatum there is no cardiac or pulmonary compression. Treatment is either by means of

application of a pressure brace or surgical resection. Application of a pressure brace has become popular over the last 10 years however the literature on the subject is still very limited. Resection of the deformed cartilages and sternal osteotomy have a long and successful history in patients with a severe deformity. However since the surgery is very invasive it should only be used in patients who have a very severe deformity which does not respond to orthostatic pressure management.

25.4 Poland's Syndrome

The condition was described by Alfred Poland and may include absence of all or some of the following: absent *ribs, pectoralis major, pectoralis minor, serratus anterior, rectus abdominus and latissimus dorsi muscles.* The *breast may be absent* (amastia) and there may be nipple deformities (Fig. 25.5). There may be associated limb deformities (syndactyly, brachydactyly), absent axillary hair and limited subcutaneous fat. The condition is usually unilateral and the etiology is unknown.

Surgical intervention is only required if the rib defect is large enough to cause a lung hernia or there are concerns regarding injury to the heart or lungs. Adolescent girls with amastia require breast reconstruction.

25.5 Sternal Defects

Sternal defects vary from the relatively benign *partial sternal cleft* to a *major deficiency* resulting in *ectopia cordis* (Figs. 25.3 and 25.4).

Sternal clefts are classified into partial or complete. Partial clefts may be superior or inferior. The superior clefts are most often isolated and relatively easy to repair in a newborn.

Inferior clefts are often associated with other anomalies in the adjacent organs including the heart, pericardium, diaphragm and anterior abdominal wall (omphalocele) giving rise to the Pentalogy of Cantrell. Survival depends on the severity of the various abnormalities.

Complete sternal fissure results in ectopia cordis where the heart has no covering and sits on the chest. The difficulty in repairing the defect arises from the fact that the chest is too small and cannot accommodate the heart. Closure is therefore not possible without causing heart failure.

25.6 Thoracic Insufficiency Syndrome Associated With Diffuse Skeletal Disorders

The Thoracic Insufficiency Syndrome may be defined as any *disorder that produces respiratory failure and prevents normal lung development* (Figs. 25.6a, b). It includes both congenital and acquired disorders such as asphyxiating thoracic dystrophy (Jeune's Syndrome), acquired asphyxiating osteochondrodystrophy (the result of damage to the growth centers by too early and extensive open pectus repair), spondylothoracic dysplasia (Jarcho-Levin Syndrome), congenital scoliosis with multiple vertebral anomalies and fused or absent ribs (jumbled spine) and severe kyphoscoliosis as a result of severe cerebral palsy or spina bifida.

These conditions are fortunately rare but repair requires complex surgical techniques if the patients exhibit respiratory insufficiency.

Further Reading

Nuss D, Kelly RE Jr et al (1998) A 10 year review of a minimally invasive technique for the correction of pectus excavatum. J Pediatr Surg 33(4):545–552

Croitoru DP, Kelly RE Jr, Nuss D et al (2002) Experience and modification update for the minimally invasive Nuss technique for pectus excavatum repair in 303 patients. J Pediatr Surg 37:437–445

Nuss D, Croitoru DP, Kelly RE Jr, Goretsky MJ (2005) Congenital chest wall deformities. In KW Ascheraft, GW Holcomb, JP Murphy (eds) Pediatric Surgery, 19th vol, 4th edn. Elsevier/W.B. Saunders, Philadelphia, PA

Shamberger RC (2006) Repair of pectus excavatum. In P Puri, ME Höllwarth (eds) Pediatric Surgery, Springer Surgery Atlas Series. Springer-Verlag, Berlin, Heidelberg, New York, pp 97–106

Shamberger RC, Nuss D, Kelly RE Jr (2006) Congenital chest wall deformities and the Nuss Procedure for pectus excavatum. In JL Grosfeld, JA O'Neill, EW Fonkalsrud, AG Coran (eds) Pediatric Surgery, 6th edn. Mosby, Philadelphia, PA

Breast Disorders in Children and Adolescents

26

Benno M. Ure and Martin L. Metzelder

Contents

Infants, children, and adolescents present with a wide spectrum of breast diseases. The underlying mechanisms include congenital and developmental factors, infections, trauma, endocrinological disorders, and benign and malignant tumors.

26.1 Congenital and Developmental Anomalies

26.1.1 Aplasia and Hypoplasia

Aplasia, or amastia, is defined as a complete absence of the breast. It is a rare condition and can be associated with diffuse ectodermal anomalies, such as congenital ectodermal dysplasia, and with Poland's syndrome, which is characterized by absence or hypoplasia of the breast, pectoralis muscles, and ribs, and occasionally the ipsilateral upper extremity. Several strategies of surgical breast reconstruction in Poland's syndrome at late or end of puberty have been suggested, including placement of a mammary prosthesis and flap techniques.

Bilateral hypoplasia is usually a familial condition. Absence of the nipple-areola complex with presence of breast tissue is named athelia. It can occur in accessory breasts and in the normal location, but is mostly associated with other malformations.

26.1.2 Breast Atrophy

Breast atrophy occurs in normally configured breasts, before and after normal development. Bilateral atrophy can be the result of eating disorders complicated

P. Puri and M. Höllwarth (eds.), *Pediatric Surgery: Diagnosis and Management,*
DOI: 10.1007/978-3-540-69560-8_26, © Springer-Verlag Berlin Heidelberg 2009

by hypoestrogenism, and of other conditions with high androgens and low estrogen. Specific hormone determinations to exclude thyroid and ovarian dysfunction, or hormone-producing tumors, should be performed in these patients. Unilateral atrophy can be the result of trauma or surgical procedures, such as chest tube placement, thoracotomy, or biopsy, mainly performed in prematures in whom it may be difficult to identify the nipple complex. In addition, the condition occurs after radiotherapy, severe burns, mononucleosis, and in scleroderma.

26.1.3 Polythelia and Polymastia

Accessory nipples are termed polythelia and occur along the milk line from the axilla to the pubis. They are most frequently located in the axilla or below a normally developed breast. The condition affects up to 2% of the population, of whom one third has more than one location of supernumerary breast tissue. Occasionally, a true accessory breast termed polymastia can develop. Ectopic breast tissue located outside the milk line is extremely rare and has been found in the perineum and the face. A possible association of polythelia with congenital malformations of the heart and urinary tract has been suggested, but is not generally accepted. Surgery for polythelia is performed for cosmetic reasons. Polymastia should be excised due to potential swelling during later pregnancy.

26.1.4 Macromastia and Breast Hypertrophy

Excessive enlargement of the breast is termed macromastia. Macromastia can be the result of virginal hypertrophy, tumors, exogenous or endogenous conditions leading to increased levels of estrogen and progesterone, and other rare conditions (Table 26.1).

Unilateral or bilateral virginal hypertrophy probably reflects a hypersensitivity of breast tissue to gonadal hormones in adolescents. Histologically, breast tissue appears with proliferation of glandular tissue as in gynecomastia. Serum levels of estradiol have been found to be normal. An occasional association with

Table 26.1 Macromastia in female children and adolescents: differential diagnosis and possible underlying disorders

Virginal hypertrophy
Breast tumors
Fibroadenoma
Hamartoma
Phyllodes tumor
Carcinoma
Sarcoma
Lymphoma
Metastasis of other tumors
Hormonally active tumors of other organs
Ovarian, adrenal, and pituitary gland tumors
Exogenous hormones
Estrogen, testosterone, corticosteriods, gonadotropins
Drugs
D-Penicillamine, marijuana

Hashimoto thyroiditis and rheumatoid arthritis suggests an autoimmune cause of juvenile hypertrophy. The growth of the breast can be excessive, leading to tissue necrosis and skin rupture. Therefore, there have been attempts to reduce growth using progesterone or antiestrogen during adolescence, when patients were still growing. However, after completion of breast growth reduction, mammoplasty is often indicated and has been reported to improve preoperative pulmonary function and complaints of short breath.

Hormonal stimulation of breast tissue with consecutive macromastia can occur due to hormonally active tumors of the ovary and the adrenal or pituitary gland. Exogenous hormones, such as corticosteroids, gonadotropins, estrogen, and testosterone, and other exogenous factors, including marijuana and D-Penicillamine, can also cause macromastia.

26.1.5 Gynecomastia

Gynecomastia is referred to as a benign proliferation of the male breast. The condition has been defined as any felt or seen enlargement and is exhibited by up to 70% of boys during puberty. It has been suggested that imbalances between estrogen and androgen levels contribute to the development of gynecomastia. A classification of gynecomastia has been suggested by Nydick et al. and defines stage 1 as limited to the subareolar area and stage 5 resembling a female breast (Fig. 26.1).

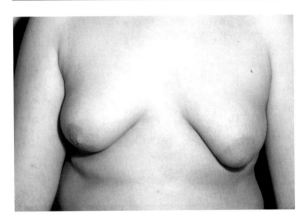

Fig. 26.1 Gynecomastia stage 5 resembling a female breast in a 16-year-old boy

Initially, a detailed history and clinical examination, including the testes, is performed. Gynecomastia combined with hypogonadism may indicate Klinefelter's syndrome. In cases without evidence of any of the known conditions associated with gynecomastia, in particular without evidence of tumor, follow-up every 6 months has been suggested. In patients with persistence of the condition for more than 1 year, endocrinologic and oncologic workup is proposed. The workup includes the determination of serum levels of human chorionic gonadotropin, luteinizing hormone, testosterone, and estradiol, and imaging studies in cases with suspected testicular or adrenal tumors.

In most instances, gynecomastia resolves spontaneously, although involution can take years. Psychosocial distress, despite psychological support, and pain or tenderness may necessitate treatment. Attempts to treat gynecomastia medically with tamoxifen, anastrazole, and other drugs have been made, but are limited by potential side effects. Surgical treatment includes subcutaneous mastectomy by a periareolar approach.

26.1.6 Mastitis/Abscess

Mastitis in the newborn period mostly affects term or near-term infants, and females more often than males. *Staphylococcus* represents the causative organism in nearly all cases, but occasionally infections with *Escherichia coli*, *Salmonella*, *Shigella*, and *Klebsiella* have been described. Clinically, the breast shows the typical signs of infection with induration, swelling,

occasional fluctuation, and excretion of pus. The therapy consists of immediate intravenous application of appropriate antibiotics. Small abscesses can be needle aspirated with ultrasonographic guidance. In cases with relevant fluctuance, incision and drainage is required. A decrease in breast size compared to the opposite side has been reported from a small series of adolescents who had undergone former drainage of a breast abscess. Therefore, the periareolar incision should be limited and can be placed radially to minimize lesion of the ducts. Breast abscess in the female adolescent is rare and may be attributed to nonpuerperal mastitis on infection of an epidermal cyst.

26.1.7 Nipple Discharge

Galactorrhea represents milky discharge and is a normal phenomenon in newborns. The neonatal breast responds to fetal prolactin, which peaks at birth. Galactorrhea beyond the neonatal period not related to pregnancy or breast feeding is most commonly associated with hypothyroidism. Numerous other causes of galactorrhea, such as neurogenic, hypothalamic, endocrine, drug-induced, and idiopathic conditions, have been identified. Chronic stimulation of the nipple, viral infections, and burns can lead to neurogenic lactation. Prolactinoma with failure of sexual maturation represents the most frequent hypothalamic cause in boys, and may also occur in girls. Drugs such as estrogens, opiates, catecholamine-depleting agents, and metoclopramide have been occasionally identified as causes of galactorrhea.

Other nipple discharge may include pus, cyst liquid, or blood. Benign dilatations of the ducts can lead to bacterial overgrowth with formation of abscesses and bloody discharge, requiring adequate antibiotic treatment. There is a high rate of spontaneous resolution of ductal ectasia, and surgical excision is only indicated in persisting cysts. Another cause of bloody nipple discharge is chronic irritation in athletic adolescents. Bloody discharge may also be caused by intraductal papillomas, which show ductal cells in the discharge and should be excised. However, in adolescents and young women, bloody nipple discharge remains a diagnostic dilemma, in particular when malignant sources have to be ruled out. Therefore, central duct resection has been recommended in these patients.

26.2 Breast Masses

26.2.1 Prepubertal Masses

Occasionally, breast development is asynchronic at the onset of puberty. In these cases, unilateral growth of one breast may appear as a mass under the areola weeks to months before growth of the other. This represents a physiological phenomenon and, therefore, biopsy is not indicated to prevent injury to the developing breast.

26.2.2 Adolescent Masses

26.2.2.1 Fibroadenomas

Fibroadenomas represent the most common breast mass in children and adolescents. Juvenile fibroadenomas can occur before the onset or at early puberty and mimic juvenile hypertrophy. Adult fibroadenomas occur in adolescence and are multiple in up to 25% of the patients. Clinically, fibroadenomas typically present as firm, mobile, painless, and easily palpable nodules, often located in the upper outer quadrant. A small proportion of fibroadenomas grow rapidly, whereas mostly there is an initial period of growth with subsequent stabilization and spontaneous resolvement in up to 40% of the patients.

Observation in presumed fibroadenomas with a stable size of less than 5 cm for 1–2 months has been recommended, due to the extremely low risk of malignancy. However, fibroadenoma, being a hyperplastic rather than a neoplastic process, has a wide range of differential diagnoses (Table 26.2) and can develop into phyllodes tumor. Therefore, biopsy is suggested in all growing fibroadenomas. Giant fibroadenomas are defined as being greater than 5 cm. The condition represents an indication for resection due to occasionally rapid growth and to problems in distinguishing them from phyllodes tumors by mammography or ultrasonography.

26.2.2.2 Phyllodes Tumors

Phyllodes tumors are fibroepithelial tumors classified histologically from benign to malignant. Phyllodes tumors can grow rapidly, metastasize, and recur. Although these tumors mostly occur in adults, they have been reported in prepuberty and adolescence. Clinically, phyllodes tumors cannot be differentiated from fibroadenomas; ultrasonographically they impose with heterogeneous echo pattern and lobulations. Occasionally, bloody nipple discharge is observed, and fine needle biopsy may not establish the diagnosis in all patients. Therefore, biopsy through excision is recommended.

The treatment of benign phyllodes tumors consists of the excision of the process with a 1–2 cm margin of normal breast tissue. Mastectomy is recommended in patients with malignant phyllodes tumors. However, other authors recommended wide resection or lumpectomy of clinically palpable masses, which can also be performed in adolescents with malignant phyllodes tumors. In cases of inadequate resection or chest wall infiltration, re-excision and radiation therapy has been suggested. In patients with local recurrence, which occurs in 20%, mastectomy is indicated. Phyllodes tumors can metastasize in lymph nodes, soft tissue, bone, pancreas, the lung, and the nerve system. The recurrence rate in benign tumors greater than 5 cm in diameter has been reported to be 39% compared to 10% in smaller ones. Malignant transformation has been observed in 20% of benign tumors with recurrence. However, the 5-year survival rate in adults with benign phyllodes tumors was 96%, in malignant tumors 66%, and the prognosis in adolescents has been suggested to be favorable. The role of adjuvant

Table 26.2 Unilateral breast masses in female children and adolescents: differential diagnosis and possible underlying disorders

Physiologic unilateral premature thelarche
Inflammatory conditions
Mastitis, abscess
Fibrosis
Necrosis
Breast tumors
Fibroadenoma
Hemangioma, lymphangioma
Cyst
Papilloma
Lipoma, neurofibroma
Phyllodes tumor
Carcinoma
Metastasis

radiotherapy for malignant phyllodes tumor in children is still under discussion.

26.2.2.3 Malignant Tumors

Primary carcinoma of the breast is extremely rare in children and adolescents. However, the condition has been described in children as young as 6 years of age. Primary breast cancer in female adolescents include histologic types seen in adults, such as invasive intraductal, invasive lobular, and signet ring tumors. Juvenile secretory carcinoma shows a lower grade malignant behavior with a better prognosis. The tumor has a capsule and may appear cystic on ultrasonography.

The treatment of primary carcinoma of the breast in children and adolescents is performed according to the national protocols for adult primary breast cancer, and according to histology, stage, and hormone receptors. However, the role of axillary node dissection and sentinel node mapping has not been determined in children.

Rhabdomyosarcoma and lymphoblastic non-Hodgkin's lymphoma of the breast are extremely rare in children. Other breast tumors include lyposarcoma, fibrosarcoma, lypomyosarcoma, and osteogenic sarcoma. Metastases in the breast have been reported in retinoblastoma, osteosarcoma, neuroblastoma, leukemia, lymphoma, and rhabdomyosarcoma.

Further Reading

Duflos D, et al (2004) Breast diseases in adolescents. In C Sultan (ed) Pediatric and Adolescent Gynecology, Karger, Basel Fruhstorfer BH, Malata CM (2003) A systematic approach to the surgical treatment of gynaecomastia. Br J Plast Surg 56: 237–246

Merlob P (2003) Congenital malformations and developmental changes of the breast: A neonatological view. J Pediatr Endocrinol Metab 16:471–485

Rogers DA, Lobe TE, Rao BN et al (1994) Breast malignancy in children. J Pediatr Surg 29:48–51

Sadove AM, van Aalst JA (2005) Congenital and acquired pediatric breast anomalies: A review of 20 years' experience. Plast Reconstr Surg 115:1039–1050

Sonmez K, Turkyilmay Z, Karabulut R et al (2006) Surgical breast lesions in adolescent patients and a review of the literature. Acta Chir Belg 106:400–404

Templeman C, Hertweck SP (2000) Breast disorders in the pediatric and adolescent patient. Obstet Gynecol Clin North Am 27:19–34

Puri P, Höllwarth ME (eds) (2006) Pediatric Surgery. Springer, Berlin, Heidelberg

Congenital Airway Malformations

27

Richard G Azizkhan

Contents

Congenital airway malformations comprise a broad spectrum of rare to common anomalies. These anomalies occur at various anatomic levels and manifest in a wide array of airway symptoms, with presentation significantly influenced by the level at which obstruction occurs as well as by the severity of obstruction. Given the distinctive anatomic features of the pediatric airway and the risk of airway symptoms rapidly progressing to life-threatening airway compromise, early recognition, diagnosis, and treatment of these anomalies are crucial.

This chapter provides an overview of congenital airway malformations, progressing from the larynx to the distal airway. In light of the comprehensive nature of this topic, many of these complex anomalies receive only cursory attention.

27.1 Patient History and Symptoms of Airway Obstruction

As an initial step in evaluating an infant with respiratory compromise, a clinician must thoroughly review the history of the child's airway symptoms. This review may provide information that helps in identifying the underlying etiology, which may determine or have an important impact on management strategy. Close attention should be paid to circumstances that trigger the onset of symptoms, the duration of symptoms, and symptom progression over time. Questioning parents about a history of dysphagia or feeding problems, the nature of their child's cry, and the possibility of foreign-body aspiration also can yield useful information. Additionally, any previous history of endotracheal intubation, trauma, or cardiopulmonary abnormalities should be carefully reviewed.

P. Puri and M. Höllwarth (eds.), *Pediatric Surgery: Diagnosis and Management,*
DOI: 10.1007/978-3-540-69560-8_27, © Springer-Verlag Berlin Heidelberg 2009

Airway obstruction may range from subtle to severe. Less severe airway compromise frequently manifests in subtle symptoms such as irritability, whereas more severe obstruction is likely to manifest in severe suprasternal and intercostal retractions, tachypnea, lethargy, and cyanosis. Stridor, a harsh sound caused by turbulent airflow through a partial obstruction of the airway, is the most important symptom of upper airway obstruction. Depending on the location of the obstruction in the upper airway, this symptom can be present during either the expiratory or inspiratory phase of the respiratory cycle or during both of these phases. The characteristics of stridor as well as its relationship to the respiratory cycle are generally helpful in establishing a differential diagnosis and in setting the priorities for diagnostic evaluation.

27.2 Diagnostic Evaluation

Conducting a complete and thorough endoscopic evaluation is the most critical part of airway assessment. This evaluation generally incorporates both flexible and rigid bronchoscopy. For the evaluation of certain types of lesions (e.g., tracheomalacia), airway assessment is performed with the patient awake or lightly sedated and spontaneously breathing. Clinicians should be aware of the fact that 17% of patients have a second airway lesion. Evaluation of the entire airway is thus essential. As up to 45% of children with congenital airway obstruction also have other significant nonairway anomalies, these patients require meticulous and complete overall investigation.

Complementary imaging studies are useful in both diagnosis and patient management. Computed tomography (CT) and magnetic resonance (MR) imaging studies provide a rapid and precise method of measuring the extent and length of airway narrowing or displacement. Additionally, they assist in identifying associated mediastinal and pulmonary anomalies. In particular, MR angiography is useful in assessing the relationship of mediastinal great vessel anomalies (e.g., vascular rings, pulmonary artery slings) to the airway. Newer computer software allows for three-dimensional image reconstruction and is helpful in planning surgical procedures. Echocardiography is primarily used to assess the presence of intracardiac defects and can detect the majority of

associated mediastinal vascular anomalies. Contrast swallow studies are valuable in assessing esophageal motility, aspiration, and some mediastinal lesions that impact the airway. Fiberoptic endoscopic evaluation of swallowing (FEES) is performed to evaluate structural and functional disorders of swallowing and to identify functional problems of the larynx, pharynx, epiglottis, and proximal esophagus.

27.3 Congenital Laryngeal Anomalies

27.3.1 Laryngomalacia

Laryngomalacia is characterized by laxity of both the glottic and supraglottic tissues, causing the epiglottis, arytenoids, and aryepiglottic folds to collapse and partially obstruct during inspiration. This malformation is the most common congenital laryngeal anomaly. It accounts for 60–75% of laryngeal problems in the neonate and also is the most common cause of stridor in the neonate. Stridor caused by laryngomalacia usually is evident soon after birth or within the first few days of life. It is generally mild but can be exacerbated by feeding, crying, and lying in a supine position. Fifty percent of children with laryngomalacia experience a worsening of stridor during the first 6 months of life. Children with severe laryngomalacia may have apnea, cyanosis, severe retractions, and failure to thrive. Cor pulmonale has been reported in cases that are extremely severe.

Diagnosis is confirmed by flexible transnasal fiberoptic laryngoscopy, which reveals short aryepiglottic folds, with prolapse of the cuneiform cartilages. Collapse of the supraglottic structures is seen on inspiration, and inflammation indicative of reflux laryngitis is also frequently seen (Fig. 27.1). Although symptoms spontaneously resolve by the age of 1 year, the infant with severe laryngomalacia may die of asphyxiation.

The need for surgical intervention and the type of surgery required is primarily based on the severity of symptoms. For severe symptoms, supraglottoplasty (also termed epiglottoplasty) is the operative procedure of choice. Both aryepiglottic folds are divided and one or both cuneiform cartilages also may be removed. If the aryepiglottic folds alone are divided, postoperative

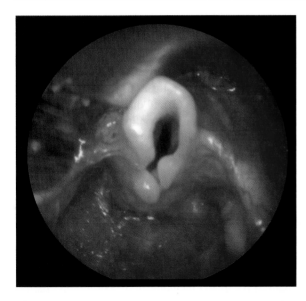

Fig. 27.1 Endoscopic view of laryngomalacia in an infant showing partial collapse of the supraglottic structures during inspiration

intubation is generally not required. Reflux management is useful in helping to minimize laryngeal edema. Patients are observed overnight in the intensive care unit. Occasionally, the infant's obstructive symptoms continue despite an adequate appearance of the larynx after surgery. Such cases are sometimes related to underlying neurologic problems and have a high likelihood of requiring tracheotomy placement.

27.3.2 Subglottic Stenosis

Subglottic stenosis (SGS) involves a narrowing of the subglottic lumen. This malformation may be either congenital or acquired, with the latter more commonly seen and generally a sequela of prolonged intubation during the neonatal period. In the full-term neonate, SGS is defined as a lumen of 4 mm or less in diameter at the level of the cricoid; in the premature infant, it is considered present when this lumen measures 3 mm or less. Congenital SGS may arise as an isolated anomaly or may be associated with other congenital head and neck lesions and syndromes such as a small larynx in a patient with Down syndrome.

It is thought to be caused by the failure of the laryngeal lumen to recanalize during embryogenesis. Incomplete recanalization results in various degrees

of stenosis that range from mild to severe; levels of severity are graded according to the Myer-Cotton grading system (Table 27.1). Mild SGS (no obstruction to 50% obstruction) may manifest in recurrent upper respiratory infections, which frequently are diagnosed as croup. More severe cases (71–99% obstruction) may present with acute airway compromise and require endotracheal intubation or tracheotomy placement at the time of delivery (Fig. 27.2). Many infants with severe obstruction may, however, remain asymptomatic for weeks or months. When stridor is present, it is initially inspiratory. As the severity of obstruction increases, stridor becomes biphasic.

Radiologic evaluation of the nonintubated airway can provide information regarding the location and extent of the stenosis. Useful studies include a chest X-ray, inspiratory and expiratory lateral soft-tissue neck films, and fluoroscopy to demonstrate the dynamics of the trachea and larynx. High-kilovoltage airway films are particularly important as they identify the characteristic steeple-like configuration seen in patients with SGS as well as possible tracheal stenosis. Flexible

Table 27.1 Myer-Cotton grading system for subglottic stenosis

Classification	Level of airway obstruction	
	From	To
Grade I	No obstruction	50% Obstruction
Grade II	51% Obstruction	70% Obstruction
Grade III	71% Obstruction	99% Obstruction
Grade IV	No detectable lumen	

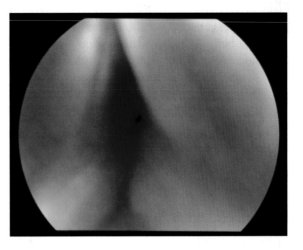

Fig. 27.2 Very high grade subglottic stenosis in a symptomatic neonate

and rigid endoscopy provide complementary methods of evaluating the airway. Flexible endoscopy documents the dynamics of the hypopharyngeal and laryngeal airways, whereas rigid endoscopy provides a clear image of the entire laryngotracheobronchial airway.

In patients with mild to moderate disease, congenital SGS improves with age. Less than 50% of these patients require tracheotomy placement to maintain their airway. For children with a minor degree of SGS and mild symptoms, endoscopic intervention (i.e., radial laser incision through the stenosis and laryngeal dilatation) may be useful. In contrast, children with significant airway obstruction are best managed with open airway reconstruction. Costal cartilage grafts are placed through either the anterior or posterior lamina of the cricoid cartilage or both. Stenting and placement of a temporary tracheostomy may be necessary. Recently, superior results for the management of severe SGS have been obtained by performing cricotracheal resection. Successful management depends on the presence of comorbidities such as gastroesophageal reflux (GER), eosinophilic esophagitis, and low-grade tracheal infection.

27.3.3 Vocal Cord Paralysis

Vocal cord paralysis is the third most common cause of neonatal stridor. This condition can be either congenital or acquired and can occur either unilaterally or bilaterally. Unilateral paralysis is usually an acquired condition caused by damage to the recurrent laryngeal nerve, whereas bilateral vocal cord paralysis usually is evident at birth. Although bilateral paralysis is generally idiopathic, it is frequently seen with central nervous system problems such as hydrocephalus and

Chiari malformation of the brainstem. Most children with bilateral paralysis present with significant airway compromise, though they do not aspirate.

The diagnosis is made by awake flexible laryngoscopy. Subsequent investigation for the underlying cause should then be carried out. Stabilization can be achieved with intubation, continuous positive airway pressure (CPAP), or high-flow nasal canula as an alternative temporizing measure. Most infants (90%) affected bilaterally require tracheotomy placement. Up to 50% of children with congenital idiopathic bilateral vocal cord paralysis experience spontaneous resolution of their paralysis by the age of 1 year. As such, decannulation is almost always delayed to allow time for this to occur.

A number of surgical procedures have been used for bilateral paralysis, including laser cordotomy, partial or complete arytenoidectomy, and vocal process lateralization (open or endoscopically guided). Each of these options is aimed at achieving an adequate decannulated airway while maintaining voice and preventing aspiration.

27.3.4 Posterior Laryngeal Cleft

Posterior laryngeal cleft is a rare congenital malformation that results from embryologic failure of the laryngotracheal groove to fuse. This malformation comprises five anatomic subtypes that differ with respect to involvement of the larynx and trachea (Fig. 27.3). Other associated anomalies, many of which affect the airway, are common. Such anomalies include tracheomalacia (always present in varying levels of severity), tracheoesophageal fistula (20%), laryngomalacia, vocal cord paralysis, SGS, and innominate artery compression.

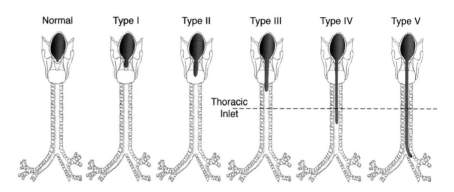

Fig. 27.3 Posterior laryngeal cleft classification

Associated conditions that do not involve the airway include GER, which is present in most children, cleft lip and palate, congenital heart defects, and hypospadias. The most common associated syndrome is Opitz-Frias syndrome, which is characterized by hypertelorism, anogenital anomalies, and laryngeal clefting.

Diagnosis can be extremely challenging and elusive, as presenting symptoms vary greatly and are not specifically diagnostic. Symptoms are often subtle and may mimic those of other disorders (e.g., GER). Some patients present early with feeding problems, choking, chronic coughing, wheezing, cyanotic spells, and apnea. There may be associated stridor either due to redundant mucosa on the edge of the cleft or a small cricoid ring. Severe tracheomalacia also may significantly compromise the airway, especially in children with an associated tracheoesophageal fistula. Although contrast swallow studies may demonstrate aspiration, definitive diagnosis requires rigid laryngotracheal bronchoscopy, with the interarytenoid area being specifically probed to determine if a posterior laryngeal cleft is present (Fig. 27.4).

In children who are symptomatic and do not have other more severe anomalies, repair of the posterior laryngeal cleft should be carried out as soon as possible to prevent chronic microaspiration with long-term pulmonary sequelae. Prior to repair, consideration should be given to whether the infant requires tracheotomy placement, gastrostomy tube placement, and Nissen fundoplication. Most type I and some type II clefts are amenable to endoscopic surgical repair, whereas clefts that extend into the cervical or thoracic trachea require open repair. A transtracheal approach is advised as it provides unparalleled exposure of the cleft while pro-

tecting the recurrent laryngeal nerves. A two-layer closure is recommended, with the option of performing an interposition graft if warranted. Type V clefts are often associated with multiple congenital anomalies. These long clefts are exceedingly difficult to repair and are prone to anastomotic breakdown. Success rates for cleft repair vary significantly (50–90%) depending on both the severity of the cleft and the presence of coexisting congenital anomalies and comorbidities.

27.3.5 Laryngeal Atresia

27.3.5.1 Congenital High Airway Obstruction Syndrome (CHAOS)

CHAOS is a life-threatening prenatally diagnosed condition caused by complete or near-complete obstruction of the fetal airway. This obstruction may be due to laryngeal atresia, tracheal atresia, or a laryngeal cyst. Atresia is sometimes an isolated anomaly but often is seen in associated with a spectrum of other anomalies, including hydrocephalus malformation of the Aqueduct of Sylvius, bronchotracheal fistula, esophageal atresia, tracheoesophageal fistula, syndactyly, and genitourinary, vertebral, and cardiac anomalies. Prenatal sonographic findings indicative of CHAOS include bilaterally enlarged echogenic lungs, dilated airways, and flattened or everted diaphragms with associated fetal ascites and nonimmune hydrops (Fig. 27.5). A fetus identified with these sonographic features is at significant risk of intrauterine death and faces a high likelihood of mortality should the pregnancy progress

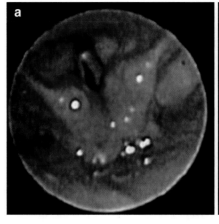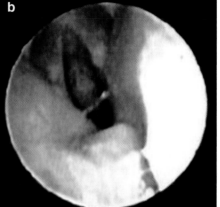

Fig. 27.4 Fiberoptic endoscopy demonstrating a type II laryngotracheal cleft. (**a**) Initial view of the larynx and the cleft is not readily apparent. (**b**) With gentle posterior probing of the interarytenoid region the cleft is now visible

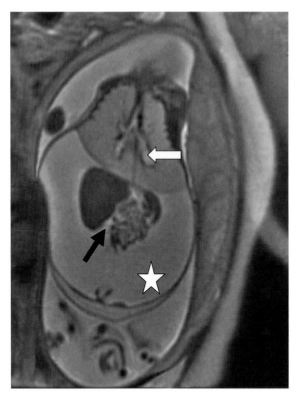

Fig. 27.5 Fetal ultrasonography demonstrating findings consistent with the diagnosis of congenital high airway obstruction: enlarged echogenic lungs, dilated airway (white arrow), flattened or everted diaphragms, and fetal ascites (white star) and hydrops. Fetal liver and intestines marked with a black arrow (Courtesy of Timothy Crombleholme MD, Cincinnati, Ohio)

to delivery. Diagnosis in the middle of the second trimester generally correlates with a poor outcome. A fetus presenting in the third trimester with CHAOS in the absence of associated anomalies or hydrops is likely to have incomplete obstruction. As such, this fetus is more likely to do well until delivery by the ex utero intrapartum technique (EXIT) procedure. This procedure maintains placental circulation to the fetus while securing the airway at the time of delivery. Instrumentation of the airway, including tracheostomy, may be accomplished at this time.

For the newborn diagnosed with CHAOS, securing and maintaining the airway are of utmost importance. Once the infant's cardiorespiratory status is stable and other critical or potentially life-threatening anomalies are ruled out, careful endoscopic evaluation of the airway precedes elective laryngotracheal reconstruction. Nevertheless, optimal timing for reconstruction

has not yet been determined. Although an adequate airway can be constructed, adequate speech may not be feasible.

27.4 Anomalies of the Trachea and Bronchi

27.4.1 Tracheal Agenesis and Atresia

Tracheal agenesis is a rare developmental abnormality that is almost always incompatible with life. Severe respiratory distress is present at birth, with the neonate attempting ventilation through bronchoesophageal communications. Although temporary ventilation may be possible with intubation of the esophagus, this generally cannot be sustained and results in neonatal demise. When a bronchoesophageal communication is not present, the fetus will have CHAOS.

27.4.2 Tracheal Webs and Stenosis

A broad spectrum of rare tracheal anomalies is classified as tracheal stenosis. Affected segments differ in the degree and extent of stenosis, ranging from gossamer thin webs to more severe long segments of stenosis that may involve the entire airway.

27.4.2.1 Tracheal Webs

Tracheal webs involve an intraluminal soft-tissue stenosis of the trachea. These webs may be membranous or composed of thick, inelastic tissue. Symptoms include biphasic stridor or expiratory wheezing, with severity dependent on the degree of tracheal narrowing. Thin webs can be readily managed by hydrostatic balloon dilatation alone. Thicker webs that are not associated with gross deformity of the underlying cartilage may be amenable to laser ablation. Lesions in the proximal trachea can be treated with the carbon dioxide (CO_2) or potassium-titanyl-phosphate (KTP) lasers; however, the KTP laser is preferred in the distal airway as it can be used through small fiberoptic cables. Children with a web greater than 1 cm in length or in whom the airway cartilage is suspected to be deficient or structurally abnormal are best managed by segmental tracheal resection or slide tracheoplasty.

27.4.2.2 Cartilaginous Ring Aplasia

Cartilaginous ring aplasia is an exceedingly rare anomaly in which a short segment of the trachea lacks cartilage. This creates a region that is both malacic and stenotic. The remainder of the trachea is normal and children generally do not have other congenital anomalies. Segmental resection of the trachea is usually curative.

27.4.2.3 Tracheal Cartilaginous Sleeve

Tracheal cartilaginous sleeve is an anomaly in which there are no discrete cartilaginous rings but rather a fused cartilaginous cylinder, with or without a membranous portion. This anomaly is often associated with craniosynostosis syndromes such as Apert, Pfeiffer, Crouzon, and Goldenhar. Patients present during the neonatal period with respiratory illness or in early infancy with acute respiratory symptoms, which may include biphasic stridor with respiratory distress, cough, and recurrent respiratory infections. Also, tracheal rigidity may cause difficulty in clearing secretions.

Bronchoscopy shows a smooth anterior tracheal wall without the normal appearance of tracheal rings. The membranous posterior tracheal wall may be normal, reduced, or absent. CT and MR imaging may assist in delineating the extent of the lesion. All patients require resection and repair; however, tracheotomy placement may be used as an initial stabilizing procedure.

27.4.2.4 Complete Tracheal Rings

Complete tracheal rings are an anomaly in which the trachea alone or both the trachea and bronchi are narrowed. In more than 50% of infants, a segmental stenosis is found. In such patients, the tracheal cartilage is abnormally shaped and forms complete rings (Fig. 27.6a, b). The clinical manifestations of complete tracheal rings vary from life-threatening respiratory distress at birth to subtle symptoms of airway compromise in older children. Many infants present with worsening of respiratory function over the first few months of life. Symptoms include stridor, retractions, cough, and alterations of cry. Atypical and persistent wheezing and rhonchi and sudden death can also occur. Over 80% of children with complete tracheal rings have other congenital anomalies, the most common of which are esophageal, cardiac, skeletal, and genitourinary. Fifty percent of children with complete tracheal rings also have a pulmonary artery sling or vascular ring.

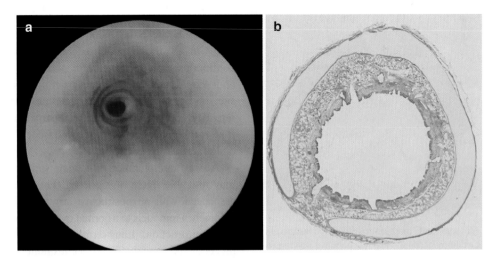

Fig. 27.6 Congenital tracheal stenosis. (**a**) Endoscopic view demonstrating complete tracheal rings. (**b**) Histology of tracheal segment demonstrating virtually complete tracheal cartilagenous ring

In some patients, placement of an endotracheal tube may exacerbate respiratory distress by causing acute swelling and inflammation. Partially obstructing tracheal lesions also may become life threatening following the onset of a respiratory infection. In an infant or child with an abnormal trachea, the cross-sectional area of airway can be decreased by one third to one half of its normal diameter with as little as 1 mm of edema. This accounts for the rapid progression of symptoms in some children who have acute inflammatory conditions superimposed on existent tracheal narrowing.

Expeditious diagnostic evaluation to define aberrant and normal tracheobronchial anatomy is required. Although an initial high-kilovolt airway film may show tracheal narrowing, the precise location and extent of the narrowing is best achieved by endoscopic techniques. CT scans provide a rapid and precise method of measuring the extent and length of airway narrowing or displacement. Visualization of the anatomic relationship between the airways and surrounding structures can be enhanced with intravascular contrast. Newer computer software allows for three-dimensional image reconstruction and is helpful in planning surgical procedures (Fig. 27.7). MR imaging is useful in assessing the relationship of the mediastinal great vessels to the airway. Echocardiography is primarily used to assess the presence of intracardiac defects and can detect the majority of associated mediastinal vascular anomalies.

Most children with complete tracheal rings require tracheal reconstruction. If a pulmonary artery sling or vascular ring is present, repair of such an anomaly should be undertaken concurrent with the tracheal repair. Segmental tracheal resection with end-to-end anastomosis is considered the treatment of choice for short-segment tracheal stenosis. Slide tracheoplasty is currently the procedure of choice for long segments of tracheal involvement, having replaced patch tracheoplasty (Fig. 27.8). This approach yields significantly less morbidity than other tracheal reconstruction techniques and is applicable to virtually all anatomic variants of complete tracheal rings. Slide tracheoplasty uses only autologous tracheal tissue and is performed by transecting the trachea into two equal segments. The anterior wall of the lower half of the trachea and the posterior wall of the upper trachea are incised. These segments are then slid over each other and anastomosed with 5-0 monofilament and absorbable sutures. Following surgery, the airway has four times the cross-sectional area and one half the length of its previous dimension. Airflow is increased 16-fold with this method of airway reconstruction.

Postoperatively, endotracheal intubation is required for 1 day to several weeks, though most patients are extubated within 48 h. To minimize the risk of damage to the newly reconstructed airway, unnecessary movements of the endotracheal tube or unplanned extubation must be avoided. Nasotracheal intubation is used preferentially because the endotracheal tube can be stabilized in position more securely. Patients require continuous monitoring, careful pulmonary toilet, and endoscopic removal of any obstructing granulation tissue. Just prior to and to ensure a safe extubation, the integrity and patency of the reconstructed airway are assessed by flexible fiberoptic endoscopy through the endotracheal tube.

Airway configuration following slide tracheoplasty may resemble figure of 8 trachea (Fig. 27.9) but is not associated with an obstructive airway. In most cases, the trachea remodels to a normal oval shape within 1 year of reconstruction. Long-term survival following this procedure is currently 90% in our institution. Mortality is usually associated with severe comorbidities such as cardiac disease rather than airway complications.

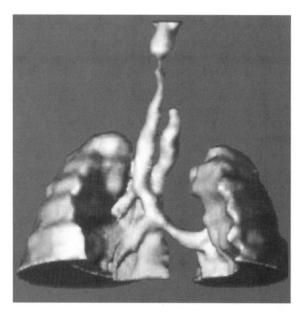

Fig. 27.7 CT scan with three-dimensional reconstruction to demonstrate anatomy of the trachea in a patient with congenital tracheal stenosis involving the proximal trachea. This patient had an aberrant tracheal bronchus and pulmonary artery sling surrounding the distal third of the trachea

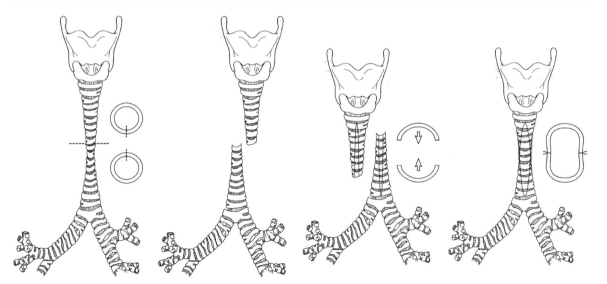

Fig. 27.8 Slide tracheoplasty procedure: The trachea is transversely divided at the midpoint of the tracheal stenosis. After proximal and distal tracheal mobilization, the posterior portion of the cephalic trachea segment and the anterior portion of the caudal tracheal segment are incised. The two tracheal segments are then overlapped and obliquely sutured together

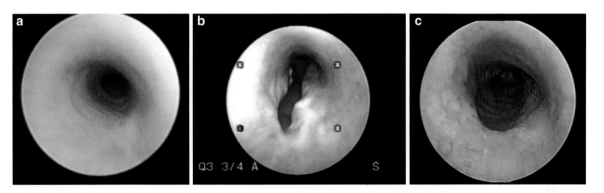

Fig. 27.9 Figure of 8 trachea following repair of complete tracheal rings: (**a**). Preoperative endoscopy documents complete tracheal rings; (**b**). Postoperative endoscopy at 6 weeks demonstrates the figure of 8 trachea—the patient had no airway symptoms; (**c**). Endoscopy at 2 years demonstrates significant remodeling of airway

27.4.3 Tracheal Diverticulum and Tracheal Bronchus

Tracheal diverticulum and tracheal bronchus are relatively common abnormalities of tracheal budding that occur during the third and fourth gestational weeks, when the trachea bifurcates and differentiates. Tracheal diverticula resemble a bronchus, though they originate from the trachea and end blindly or communicate with a rudimentary lung. Tracheal bronchi most often affect the right upper lobe bronchus and may connect to an isolated intrathoracic lung segment or the apical segment of an upper lobe. Both anomalies often are seen in children with other congenital defects. Diagnosis is established by airway endoscopy. Most children are asymptomatic and do not require treatment. Those who are symptomatic experience symptoms such as pneumonia and respiratory distress during the neonatal period. Additionally, they have an associated stenosis of the bronchus or other lung anomalies. Resection of involved lobe and bronchus in these patients is generally curative.

27.4.4 Tracheomalacia and Bronchomalacia

Tracheomalacia and bronchomalacia are conditions in which the structural integrity of the trachea or bronchi is diminished and the cartilaginous rings of the airway lack the necessary rigidity to prevent airway collapse during expiration. Malacia may occur in localized segments or diffusely throughout the airway. Tracheomalacia is the most common congenital tracheal anomaly. It may be idiopathic or associated with a number of conditions, including esophageal atresia or tracheoesophageal fistula, aberrant innominate artery, mediastinal masses, prolonged intubation for interstitial lung disease, or bronchopulmonary dysplasia. Premature neonates with bronchopulmonary dysplasia or children with chronic indwelling cuffed endotracheal or tracheostomy tubes are at particular risk for developing combined severe tracheal and bronchial malacia.

Presenting symptoms vary and depend on the severity, duration, and location of the malacia. Most children are either asymptomatic or minimally symptomatic and most cases involve posterior malacia of the trachealis, with associated broad tracheal rings. Other associated abnormalities include laryngeal clefts and tracheoesophageal fistulae. Presenting symptoms may include a honking cough, stridor, wheezing, respiratory distress when agitated, and cyanosis. Some children are misdiagnosed with allergic asthma and unsuccessfully treated with bronchodilators. Diagnosis is best established by rigid or flexible bronchoscopy, with the patient breathing spontaneously; this demonstrates dynamic distortion and compression of the trachea. Children who are minimally symptomatic are watched expectantly. Their symptoms often resolve by age 3. Children who experience a worsening of symptoms require more intensive medical or surgical intervention. Respiratory monitoring with nasal CPAP may be beneficial in some patients.

Segmental tracheal involvement is managed with endoscopic or open aortopexy, with thymectomy and anterior suspension of the ascending arch of the aorta to the posterior periosteum of the sternum. More diffuse malacia may require tracheotomy placement with positive pressure ventilation over a long period of time. The placement of intratracheal stents is used selectively in patients with severely problematic tracheomalacia or bronchomalacia that is unresponsive to nonoperative therapy or not suitable for surgical treatment. Major complications associated with this approach can occur, including stent collapse, dislodgement, or rarely, stent erosion into the great vessels. Additionally, stent removal can cause tracheal tearing or major hemorrhage.

27.4.5 Esophageal Bronchus

Isolated bronchial connection between the esophagus and the airway is extremely rare and occurs more frequently in females (2:1). Associated cardiac, genitourinary, vertebral, and diaphragmatic anomalies are common. This malformation is thought to develop from a supernumerary lung bud arising from the esophagus. Most commonly, a lower lobe is aerated by this ectopic bronchus, but an entire main bronchus and lung may be involved. As in pulmonary sequestration anomalies, the pulmonary vasculature in this anomaly may be abnormal, with the arterial supply coming off the aorta and venous drainage going into either the systemic or pulmonary veins.

Because of inadequate bronchial drainage, children usually have recurrent pulmonary infection; however, occasionally esophageal bronchus is not discovered until adolescence or adulthood. Although radiographic findings differ depending on the affected segment of the lung, collapse, consolidation, cavitation, and cyst formation within the pulmonary parenchyma are commonly seen. The diagnosis is confirmed by contrast studies of the esophagus, though occasionally false-negative results occur. Excision of the abnormal lung and closure of the bronchoesophageal fistula is the treatment of choice. Prognosis depends on early diagnosis and treatment and the severity of associated anomalies.

27.4.6 Tracheobronchial-Biliary Fistula

Congenital tracheobronchial-biliary fistulae are extremely rare and may arise from the distal trachea or either mainstem bronchus. All children with this anomaly have significant respiratory problems but the cardinal symptom is bile-stained sputum. The diagnosis is established either by bronchoscopy or endoscopic retrograde cholangiopancreatography (ERCP). Surgical division of the fistulous tract is the only effective therapy for this malformation.

27.4.7 Subglottic Hemangioma

Hemangiomas of infancy are benign congenital vascular tumors. These tumors are characterized by vascular endothelium that undergoes a phase of growth followed by slow, spontaneous involution that occurs over several years and is generally complete by the first decade of life. These tumors most commonly present cutaneously but can occur in any anatomic site. They usually become evident between 2 to 4 months of age and occur with a threefold female preponderance.

Of lesions that occur within the tracheobronchial tree, almost all are in the subglottis. The natural history of subglottic hemangiomas generally mirrors that of cutaneous lesions, and more than 50% of patients with a subglottic hemangioma also have cutaneous hemangiomas. As the hemangioma undergoes proliferation, progressive deterioration of the airway usually occurs. Presenting symptoms include biphasic stridor with retractions. The degree of obstruction varies and can be exacerbated by certain positions or crying, both of which increase venous pressure and lead to vascular engorgement. When airway obstruction is severe, apnea, cyanosis, and "dying spells" may occur. Diagnosis is based on medical history and findings on airway endoscopy. Lesions are typically asymmetric and may be covered by a normal smooth mucosa (Fig. 27.10). Because of the risk of hemorrhage, biopsy is not advised. Most patients require treatment and many treatment modalities are often combined. These include intralesional or systemic corticosteroids, chemotherapeutic agents such as vincristine for patients who are nonresponsive to steroids, laser ablation, and surgical excision. Depending on both the severity of the obstruction and the expertise of involved clinicians, early symptoms are managed with intralesional or systemic steroids. Some surgeons advocate laser fulguration or translaryngeal resection, whereas others place a tracheotomy below the lesion, with the expectation of removal following involution of the hemangioma.

27.4.8 Bronchogenic Cyst

Bronchogenic cysts result from abnormal budding of the bronchial tree in which a portion of the lung bud develops independently. The cyst walls frequently contain cartilage and are lined with ciliated columnar epithelium. These lesions tend to enlarge, thus causing airway obstruction. Infants with bronchogenic cysts most commonly present with respiratory distress. They also may have cough, chest pain, or wheezing. Although a plain chest X-ray may suggest the presence of a bronchogenic cyst, a CT scan and barium esophagram are useful in confirming this diagnosis. Open or thoracoscopic resection is curative (Fig. 27.11a, b).

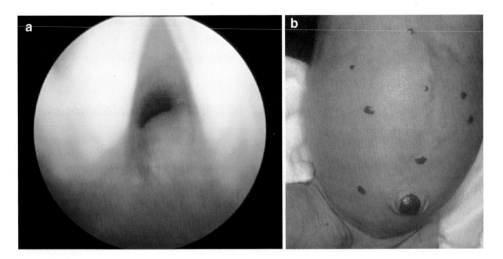

Fig. 27.10 Endoscopic view of a subglottic hemangioma (**a**) in a patient with multiple cutaneous infantile hemangiomas (**b**)

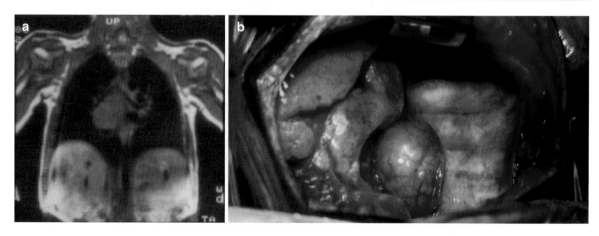

Fig. 27.11 Bronchogenic cyst: (**a**) Right hilar lesion seen on CT scan. (**b**) Operative photograph demonstrating the bronchogenic cyst in situ

27.4.9 Bronchial Atresia

Localized bronchial atresia is a rare anomaly in which the atretic bronchus obstructs the flow of secretions and air from the distal lung to the main tracheobronchial tree. This condition may simulate lobar emphysema or a mediastinal mass. At birth, the obstructed lung retains fluid, but eventually the affected lobe or segment becomes hyper-aerated as air enters through the pores of Kohn. Patients accumulate secretions proximal to the atresia and a mucocele forms. Emphysema of the segment may cause compression of the normal lung tissue and may be associated with wheezing and stridor. Plain chest radiographs often demonstrate a hilar mass with radiating solid channels surrounded by hyperaerated lung. A CT chest scan may indicate a cystic central mucocele and can help differentiate bronchial atresia from a bronchogenic cyst or lobar emphysema. Although children with bronchial atresia may be asymptomatic for long intervals, they are at risk of serious pulmonary infection when entrapped secretions become infected. When this anomaly is identified, resection is both indicated and curative.

27.4.10 Bronchial Agenesis

Congenital absence of a bronchus occurs more commonly than tracheal agenesis and in contrast to tracheal agenesis, this anomaly is compatible with life. Several possible anatomic variants have been described, including lobar, bronchial, and parenchymal agenesis. Specifically, there may be complete agenesis of the lung and its bronchus and blood supply; aplasia, in which there is a rudimentary bronchus and absent lung; or hypoplasia, in which there is a rudimentary bronchus and hypoplastic lung. As is common in children with airway malformations, children with bronchial agenesis also may have other congenital anomalies of the skeletal, cardiovascular, gastrointestinal, and genitourinary systems. Diagnosis is confirmed by chest radiographs and airway endoscopy. The majority of patients do not require surgical intervention. Nevertheless, these patients are important to identify as bronchial or lobar atresia may mimic other airway anomalies such as bronchial stenosis; extraluminal airway obstruction by tumors or masses; or complete intraluminal obstruction in which there is no aeration distal to the obstruction.

27.4.11 Bronchial Stenosis

Congenital bronchial stenosis is extremely rare, with reported cases caused by compressive vascular, cardiac, and congenital cystic lesions or soft tissue cartilaginous stenoses. Symptoms and treatment depend on the anatomic location of the lesion and its severity. By contrast, acquired bronchial stenosis is more common and is a major cause of morbidity and mortality in infants who require prolonged intubation and respiratory support. Most such cases can be managed endoscopically.

Further Reading

Austin J, Ali T (2003) Tracheomalacia and bronchomalacia in children: Pathophysiology, assessment, treatment and anaesthesia management. Paediatr Anaesth 13:3–11

Azizkhan RG (2005) Subglottic airway. In KT Oldham, PM Colombani, RP Foglia, MA Skinner (eds) Principles and Practice of Pediatric Surgery, 2nd vol. Lippincott Williams & Wilkins Philadelphia, PA, Chap 59

Bennett EC, Holinger LD (2003) Congenital malformations of the trachea and bronchi. In CD Bluestone, SE Stool, CM Alper, EM Arjmand et al (eds) Pediatric Otolaryngology, 2nd vol, 4th edn. WB Saunders, Philadelphia, PA, Chap 84

Gerber ME, Holinger LD (2003) Congenital laryngeal anomalies. In CD Bluestone, SE Stool, CM Alper, EM Arjmand, et al (eds) Pediatric Otolaryngology, 2nd vol, 4th edn. WB Saunders, Philadelphia, PA, Chap 83

Gustafson LM, Hartley BE, Liu JH et al (2000) Single-stage laryngotracheal reconstruction in children: A review of 200 cases. Otolaryngol Head Neck Surg 123:430–434

Lim FY, Crombleholme TM, Hedrick HL, Flake AW et al (2003) Congenital high airway obstruction syndrome: Natural history and management. J Pediatr Surg 38:940–945

Puri P, Höllwarth ME (eds) (2006) Pediatric Surgery. Springer, Berlin, Heidelberg

Rutter MJ, Azizkhan RG, Cotton RT (2003) Posterior laryngeal cleft. In MM Ziegler, RG Azizkhan, TR Weber (eds) Operative Pediatric Surgery. McGraw-Hill, New York, Chap 26

Rutter MJ (2006) Evaluation and management of upper airway disorders in children. Sem Pediatr Surg 15:116–123

Mediastinal Masses in the Children

28

S. J. Shochat

Contents

28.1 Introduction

Mediastinal masses in children represent a wide variety of congenital and neoplastic lesions that can present interesting diagnostic and therapeutic challenges. However, despite the heterogenous make-up of this group of lesions, an accurate pre-operative diagnosis can usually be established on the basis of the location of the mass within the mediastinum and age of the child at diagnosis.

28.2 Differential Diagnosis

The differential diagnosis of mediastinal masses in infants and children is simplified if the mediastinum is arbitrarily separated into three compartments (Fig. 28.1). For the purpose of this discussion the mediastinum will be partitioned as follows: the anterior mediastinum lies anterior to the heart and lung roots and contains the thymus, anterior mediastinal lymph nodes, and rarely a substernal extension of the thyroid and parathyroid. The middle mediastinum consists of the trachea, bronchi, mediastinal lymph nodes, heart, and great vessels. The posterior mediastinum lies behind the heart and lung roots and contains the oesophagus and intercostals sympathetic nerves. Anterior mediastinal masses include teratomas; thymic hyperplasia, cysts, or tumours; and cystic hygromas and lymphomas. Masses within the middle mediastinum include the lymphomas, bronchogenic cysts, and granulomatous infections within the mediastinal lymph nodes. Posterior mediastinal lesions include the tumours of neurogenic origin, enterogenous cysts, and the undifferentiated sarcomas.

P. Puri and M. Höllwarth (eds.), *Pediatric Surgery: Diagnosis and Management,*
DOI: 10.1007/978-3-540-69560-8_28, © Springer-Verlag Berlin Heidelberg 2009

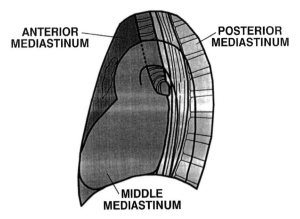

Fig. 28.1 Compartments of the mediastinum

The age of the patient at the time of diagnosis is extremely important, since certain masses have a predilection for younger infants and others are predominantly seen in older children and adolescents. In newborns and children under 2 years of age, the most common mediastinal mass is the neuroblastoma within the posterior mediastinum. In addition, thymic hyperplasia and bronchogenic cysts are seen predominantly in children less than 2 years of age. The various lymphomas are the most common mediastinal masses seen in children greater than 2 years of age. The mean age of children with mediastinal Hodgkin's disease is approximately 13 years of age and the mean age of children who present with non-Hodgkin's lymphoma is 11 years of age.

The presenting signs and symptoms in infants and children with mediastinal masses vary depending on the age.

- Acute respiratory distress
- Fever
- Cough
- Shortness of breath
- Cervical adenopathy
- Superior vena caval syndrome
- Horner's syndrome
- Asymptomatic

Infants under 2 years of age frequently present with signs of tracheal compression and acute respiratory distress. This is due to the smaller, softer, more pliable tracheobronchial tree in infants as well as the fact that they do not have a fixed mediastinum so that large mediastinal masses can cause a significant shift of the mediastinum with compromise of the contralateral

hemithorax. Older children will present with symptoms of fever, cough, and shortness of breath. Approximately half the children with mediastinal lymphomas will present with cervical adenopathy. Superior vena caval obstruction is rare in children, but is occasionally seen. Horner's syndrome may be the presenting finding in infants with neuroblastomas or neurogenic tumours of the posterior mediastinum. Asymptomatic mediastinal masses are seen in children of all ages and are frequently noted on a chest X-ray performed for a mild upper respiratory infection or are discovered incidentally following imaging studies for symptoms unrelated to the mediastinal mass.

28.3 Diagnosis

A systematic approach to the diagnosis of a mediastinal mass in children is imperative.

- Posteroanterior—lateral chest X-ray
- Barium swallow
- Ultrasonography
- CT scan
- MRI
- Bone marrow—lymph node biopsy
- Skin test—complement fixation
- Serum markers—α–FP, HCG
- Urinary catecholamines

The most helpful diagnostic technique in this age group is still the chest X-ray in the posteroanterior and lateral projections, in order to localize the position of the mass. Vertebral anomalies associated with a mediastinal mass in an infant should raise the suspicion of the so-called neuroenteric variety of enterogenous cyst that communicates with the meninges. Calcification within a posterior mediastinal mass suggests the presence of a neuroblastoma and anterior mediastinal teratomas frequently contain calcification. In cases of suspected enterogenous and bronchogenic cysts, the oesophagogram may be of value. Ultrasonography of the chest can be quite helpful in defining complicated mediastinal lesions and has been especially helpful in infants with suspected thymic hyperplasia. Echocardiography should be performed to delineate the heart and great vessels if lesions of these structures are suspected. A computed tomography scan should be used to delineate anatomical boundaries, as an aid to establish the correct diagnosis and in preparation for tumour resection. Magnetic resonance imaging is of help in differentiating masses of vascular origin from other mediastinal structures and may be helpful in infants with suspected thymic hyperplasia. In addition, magnetic resonance imaging should be considered in cases of posterior mediastinal masses in order to detect intraspinous extension of tumour (dumb-bell tumors).

Cervical lymph node biopsy should be considered in children with middle mediastinal lesions and suspected lymphoma. A bone marrow aspiration and biopsy should also be performed prior to other invasive studies in children suspected of having non-Hodgkin's lymphoma. Skin testing and complement fixation titres should be considered in children with middle mediastinal masses to rule out granulomatous infections. Alpha fetoprotein determination and HCG titres should be performed in children with anterior mediastinal masses if malignant teratomas are suspected. Urinary catecholamine metabolites should be evaluated in infants with posterior mediastinal masses both for diagnosis and for post-operative follow-up in children with suspected neuroblastomas.

28.4 Anterior Mediastinum

Thymic hyperplasia is the most common anterior mediastinal mass seen in infants (Fig. 28.2). This diagnosis is usually not difficult as there is frequently a characteristic "sail" sign on routine chest X-ray. Recently, ultrasonography has been very helpful in differentiating thymic hyperplasia from other mediastinal masses and should be considered in difficult cases. The use of steroids to help with the diagnosis of thymic hyperplasia in infants is mentioned only with historical perspective and is no longer indicated. Benign teratoma is the most frequent anterior mediastinal neoplasm seen in children under 2 years of age (Fig. 28.3). These masses are usually well encapsulated and can be treated by total excision through a posterolateral thoracotomy. Cystic hygromas also are observed in infants, but usually have a cervical or axillary component that makes this diagnosis obvious. Thymic cysts are extremely rare in children and only 20 thymomas have been reported in childhood. Germ cell tumours of the anterior mediastinum are usually seen in older children and adolescents and many have an endodermal sinus or yolk sac component with an ele-

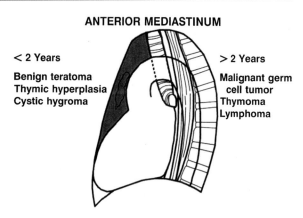

ANTERIOR MEDIASTINUM

< 2 Years

Benign teratoma
Thymic hyperplasia
Cystic hygroma

> 2 Years

Malignant germ
cell tumor
Thymoma
Lymphoma

Fig. 28.2 Anterior mediastinum

vated serum alpha fetoprotein. AFP and HCG levels should be performed in all older children with anterior mediastinal masses as these markers are helpful not only in diagnosis but in following response to therapy. These tumours are highly malignant lesions and total resection rarely is possible. Evaluation of these patients requires a multi-disciplinary approach with consultation between surgeon, paediatric oncologist, and radiation therapist. In the rare case where total excision is possible, this should be carried out and followed by multi-agent chemotherapy. However, radical resection is not indicated. When the tumor is non-resectable, a biopsy rather than partial resection is followed by chemotherapy and delayed primary excision. While isolated lymphomas of the thymus do occur, the majority of lymphomas of the anterior mediastinum will also have a major middle mediastinal component, which makes diagnosis straightforward.

28.5 Middle Mediastinum

Bronchogenic cysts may be seen in all age groups, but are the most frequent mass seen within the middle mediastinum in infants and children under 2 years of age (Fig. 28.4). Bronchogenic cysts are located in the subcarinal region and are frequently associated with a characteristic expiratory stridor due to accentuation of the obstruction of the lower trachea during expiration. Bronchogenic cysts are frequently difficult to diagnose on routine chest X-ray, but there is usually a characteristic displacement of the oesophagus on barium swallow (Fig. 28.5). Bronchogenic cysts occasionally are intimately attached to the membranous trachea and

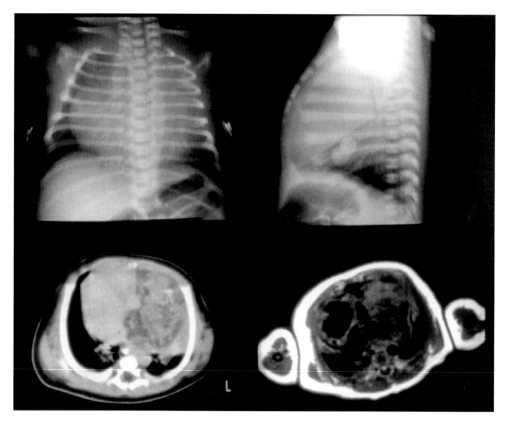

Fig. 28.3   Cardiac teratoma within anterior mediastinum

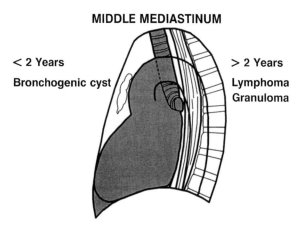

Fig. 28.4   Middle mediastinum

if this is the case a small portion of the cysts should be left attached to the trachea.

The most common mediastinal mass in individuals over 2 years of age is Hodgkin's or non-Hodgkin's lymphoma. Lymphomas are also the most frequent tumours involving the middle mediastinum. The initial diagnostic work-up in children with suspected lymphoma should include cervical or supraclavicular lymph node biopsy as well as bone marrow biopsy. Mediastinoscopy, anterior mediastinotomy, or CT-guided needle biopsy are the procedures of choice to establish a tissue diagnosis in the absence of cervical adenopathy. A formal thoracotomy is rarely indicated for diagnosis or treatment in children with lymphoma. Children who present with a large middle mediastinal mass, respiratory distress, and a suspected diagnosis of non-Hodgkin's lymphoma may be treated initially with steroids or localized radiotherapy prior to biopsy because of the dangers of acute respiratory decompensation on induction of anaesthesia. However, every attempt should be made to safely establish a diagnosis prior to the use of steroids or radiotherapy since even a brief course of therapy can make subsequent diagnosis difficult. A multi-disciplinary approach (surgeon, oncologist, radiotherapist) to the child with suspected mediastinal lymphoma is imperative and tissue obtained at the time of biopsy should be

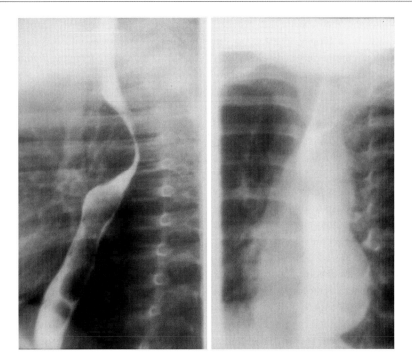

Fig. 28.5 Bronchogenic cyst showing displacement of oesophagus

placed in saline so that immunologic surface marker studies can be performed. These studies are extremely important in the classification and hence therapy of the various non-Hodgkin's lymphomas.

Granulomatous infections of the paratracheal, sub-carinal, or hilar lymph nodes are occasionally seen and can usually be diagnosed by appropriate skin tests and complement fixation titres. In the Midwest of the USA and other endemic areas, histoplasmosis seems to have a predilection for the azygous node with is charac-teristically enlarged in children with this infection. Diagnosis is confirmed by mediastinoscopy, mediasti-notomy, or rarely thoracotomy.

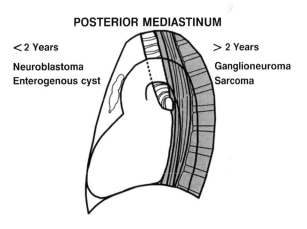

Fig. 28.6 Posterior mediastinum

28.6 Posterior Mediastinum

The most common mass of the posterior mediastinum and in fact the most common mass in newborns is a pos-terior mediastinal neuroblastoma (Fig. 28.6). Mediastinal neuroblastomas are interesting in that they seem to have a different biological behaviour than intra-abdominal tumours. The majority of mediastinal neuroblastomas are localized or low-stage disease and have a favourable outcome following resection. These tumours are more often occult and are diagnosed on X-ray examination for other complaints. Respiratory distress due to com-pression or deviation of the trachea is a feature in some cases, especially infants. Thoracic neuroblasomas with dumb-bell extension may present with neurological symptoms due to spinal cord compression. While the treatment of mediastinal neuroblastomas in children is total excision if at all possible, this does not mean radical chest wall resection. In the rare case of a massive mediastinal neuroblastomas that cannot be resected without a radical operation, a biopsy to establish the diagnosis is followed by chemotherapy and delayed primary excision. While this clinical situation is rarely seen, a tissue diagnosis can usually be obtained by a percutaneous core needle biopsy avoiding formal thoracotomy. Since Stages 1 & 2 neuroblastoma patients do not require chemotherapy this course of action should be critically assessed by a multi-disciplinary team. In children with disseminated neuroblastoma, thoracotomy and resection should be carried out after metastatic sites have responded to therapy. Despite impressive shrinkage of tumour following chemotherapy and complete delayed primary excision, the prognosis continues to be discouraging in these children.

Children with posterior mediastinal neuroblastoma can also present with unusual symptoms. The case in Fig. 28.7 presented with a 3-month history of diarrhoea. The mass turned out to be a large neuroblastoma that extended up into the cervical region. The tumour contained high concentrations of prostaglandin E, which was the aetiology of the diarrhea. Vasoactive intestinal polypeptide secreting neuroblastomas have also been described in children with profuse watery diarrhoea. Recently, Ratner and Pelton reported an infant who presented with progressively worsening laboured respirations and was found to have a neuroblastoma extending from the mediastinum, through the thoracic inlet, and into the neck.

Enterogenous cysts, while rare, represent an interesting spectrum of lesions. They may be intimately associated with the oesophagus and cause dysphagia or they can contain gastric mucosa that has been associated with peptic ulceration, perforation, and bleeding. Large cysts may have abdominal extensions and communicate with an intestinal duplication.

An interesting but rare variant is the so-called neurenteric cyst that communicates with the meninges through an intraspinous component. These infants present with a large mediastinal mass, respiratory distress, and rarely neurological symptoms. Characteristic deformities of the lower cervical and upper thoracic spine are always present on routine chest X-ray. During resection of these masses through a posterolateral thoracotomy, the communication between the thoracic and infraspinous component must be identified and ligated to prevent a spinal fluid leak and meningitis. These patients should be evaluated by an MRI scan, as the intraspinous cystic component may require laminectomy and excision.

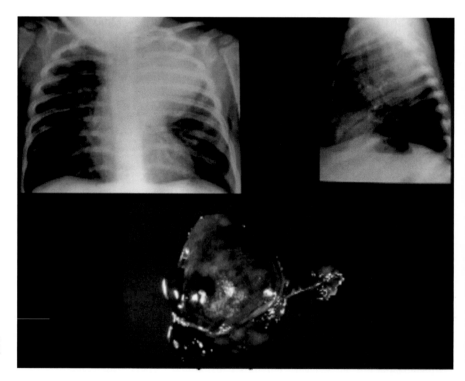

Fig. 28.7 Posterior mediastinal neuroblastoma. Total excision with cervical extension

28.7 Anaesthetic Management of Children with a Mediastinal Mass

Respiratory compromise on induction of general anaesthesia in children with large mediastinal masses is a well-recognized complication that must be considered in the pre-operative evaluation of any child with a mediastinal mass. Infants and small children have a small compressible airway, which is associated with significant increased airway resistance with even a modest degree of narrowing. In addition, infants do not have a fixed mediastinum and large masses can easily displace the mediastinal structures with compression of the tracheobrochial tree, superior vena cava, or right ventricular outflow tract. Cardiac output may also be diminished due to pressure on the great vessels. Induction of anaesthesia is associated with a decrease in the functional residual capacity, decrease in lung capacity, and an increase in lung retractile force. The above alterations are accentuated with the addition of paralysis. Narrowing of the trachea will also become more prominent when the patient changes from spontaneous to positive pressure ventilation. All of the above factors lead sometimes to critical decompensation that is associated with general anaesthesia in these patients.

The most important factor in preventing anaesthetic complications in children with a mediastinal mass is recognition of the above issue and the anticipation of a possible airway problem. A very thorough radiologic evaluation should be performed and CT examination to determine the tracheal cross-sectional area maybe of help especially in children with non-Hodgkins lymphoma. Once the pre-operative evaluation is completed the anaesthetic of choice can be determined depending on the procedure that will be performed. Pre-operative radiation therapy or chemotherapy may be required prior to primary excision or biopsy. Incisional biopsies or needle biopsies can be performed sometimes under local anaesthesia. In children with benign lesions one lung anaesthesia with placement of the endotracheal tube beyond the obstruction has been found to be helpful and occasionally ventilation through a rigid bronchoscope is necessary. While cardiopulmonary bypass or ECMO maybe required in selected cases these techniques are usually not necessary in the majority of patients.

A high index of suspicion, meticulous pre-operative evaluation, and a multi-disciplinary action plan decided upon by surgeons, anaesthesiology, radiation therapist, haematology or oncologist, and pathologist can usually advert the potential catastrophe associated with general anaesthesia in children with critical mediastinal masses.

28.8 Operative Technique for Removal of Mediastinal Neuroblastoma

The tumour is usually approached through a standard posterolateral thoracotomy at the approximate level of the tumour. The lung is retracted medially to reveal the tumour covered with pleura arising from the sympathetic trunk, and an assessment of it and obvious lymph node involvement in the vicinity is made. The pleura is incised around the tumour approximately 1 cm from it and the fascia and pleura mobilized towards the tumour. A plane of dissection can usually be developed superficial to the endothoracic fascia. The tumour is now mobilized from the ribs by sharp dissection, and intercostals vessels entering the tumour will need division. If the tumour extends far enough anteriorly, the azygos vein on the right side will need division between ties. Care is taken to avoid damage to the first thoracic nerve passing laterally across the first rib to join the brachial plexus. The superior intercostals artery normally descends between the first nerve and the sympathetic trunk. Other intercostals nerves may be sacrificed if they are intimate with the tumour.

Depending on how far the tumour has extended anteriorly, it will need to be dissected off the main structures in the superior mediastinum. This is most likely to be the oesophagus and the closely applied vagus nerve, but in a large tumour the trachea may be involved. It may prove useful to have a large size tube in the oesophagus to aid dissection. On the left side, the arch of the aorta with subclavian and carotid branches along with the vagus nerve will need protection. The thoracic duct should be identified and protected in lower tumours on the right and apiral tumours on the left in order to prevent a chylothorax.

It should now prove possible to dissect the tumour off the bodies of the vertebra and any extension into the intravertebral foramen should be carefully dissected out. Titanium clips may prove useful to control haemorrhage in small vessels, and these will not interfere with subsequent CT scanning. Any suspiciously involved lymph nodes locally should be considered for biopsy (staging). The chest is closed after leaving a chest drain.

Further Reading

Anghelescu DL, Burgoyne LL, Liu T et al (2007) Clinical and diagnostic imaging findings predict anesthetic complications in children presenting with malignant mediastinal masses. Paediatr Anaesth 17(11):1090–1098

Grosfeld JL, Skinner MA, Rescorla FJ et al (1994) Mediastinal tumors in children: Experience with 196 cases. Ann Surg Oncol 1:121–127

Hammer GB (2004) Anaesthetic management for the child with a mediastinal mass. Pediatr Anesth 14:95–97

Kang CH, Kim YT, Jeon SH, Sung SW, Kim JH (2007) Surgical treatment of malignant mediastinal neurogenic tumors in children. Eur J Cardiothorac Surg 31(4):725–730

Puri P, Höllwarth ME (eds) (2006) Pediatric Surgery. Springer, Berlin, Heidelberg

Saenz NC (1999) Posterior mediastinal neurogenic tumors in infants and children. Semin Pediatr Surg 8:78–84

Warnke RA, Link MP (1983) Indentification and significance of cell markers in leukemia and lymphoma. Annu Rev Med 34:117–131

Williams HJ, Alton HM (2003) Imaging of paediatric mediastinal abnormalities. Pediatr Respir Rev 4:55–66

Yaris N, Nas U, Cobanoglu U et al (2006) Brief report: Thymic carcinoma in children. Pediatr Blood Cancer 47:224–227

Pleural Effusion and Empyema

29

Klaas Bax

Contents

29.1 Introduction

The volume and composition of pleural liquid is governed by a number of interacting mechanisms that contribute to maintain the conditions for an efficient mechanical coupling between chest wall and lung. Under normal conditions there is only a thin layer of fluid present between the pleural surfaces. The composition of pleural fluid is essentially that of a plasma filtrate through two membranes with sieving properties. Pleural effusion means the accumulation of liquid in the pleural space. The nature of the fluid may vary: it may be blood, chyle, lymph, transudate, exudates, or pus. The distinction between a transudate and an exudate is mainly based on the different protein and cellular content. In general, transudates have protein content less than 30 g/L and a total leucocyte count less than 2,000/mm³. Lymph has a protein content that is intermediate between transudate and exudate and has a variable number of lymphocytes. Chyle is lymph drained from the intestinal tract. It is rich in lymphocytes and contains chylomicrons depending on nutrition containing long-chain triglycerides. Empyema means the accumulation of pus in a cavity of the body. When used without a descriptive qualifier it refers to thoracic empyema.

29.1.1 Fetal and Congenital Forms

Pleural effusions may arise antenatally. The estimated incidence of primary fetal hydrothorax is 1 in 10,000–15,000 pregnancies. Such an effusion may be secondary to a mediastinal tumor, adenomatoid tumor, pulmonary sequestration, infection, or chromosomal

P. Puri and M. Höllwarth (eds.), *Pediatric Surgery: Diagnosis and Management,*
DOI: 10.1007/978-3-540-69560-8_29, © Springer-Verlag Berlin Heidelberg 2009

anomaly. Primary pleural effusion has been called congenital primary chylothorax although no chylomicrons can be detected antenatally. Moreover the diagnostic value of a high lymphocyte count in the fetal aspirate remains controversial. So whether the term chylothorax should be used antenatally for a pleural effusion is debatable.

Rarely pleural effusions may arise in the context of lymphangiomatosis. Pleural manifestation may be present at birth or may become manifest later.

29.1.2 Acquired Forms

29.1.2.1 Hemothorax

A hemothorax is usually traumatic in origin and mostly associated with pneumothorax. It may occur as a complication of the central venous line catheterization.

29.1.2.2 Chylothorax

Chylothorax after thoracic operations is a well-known complication. Damage to the thoracic duct, disruption of accessory lymphatics, and an increased pressure in the systemic venous system, exceeding the pressure in the thoracic duct, have been proposed as possible causes. The incidence is on the rise from 1 to nearly 5%. The increased complexity of the procedures and possibly the earlier introduction of feeding after surgery are held responsible for the increased incidence. Procedures that predispose to increased systemic venous pressure are particularly at risk for causing chylothorax. Not only does the incidence increase after such a procedure but the duration of chylothorax also increases.

29.1.2.3 Hydrothorax

Iatrogenic

Hydrothorax in children may be iatrogenic or noniatrogenic in origin.

Several case reports of pleural effusion in children related to central venous catheter insertion have been described. Such a complication may not only occur early after insertion of the catheter but also later on.

Hydrothorax, especially on the right, may be caused by transdiaphragmatic fluid transport from the abdomen, e.g., in the context of peritoneal dialysis or ventriculoperitoneal shunting. The main mechanism seems to be transport through open communications between the abdomen and the chest. These can be observed thoracoscopically. Also, urine may enter the chest either retroperitoneally or through the diaphragm in case of urinary ascites.

Noniatrogenic

Transdiaphragmatic fluid transport may also occur in cases of hepatic ascites. Other noniatrogenic causes for hydrothorax are congestive heart disease, nephrotic syndrome, and malignancy, especially non-Hodgkin lymphoma, and metastatic disease also.

29.1.2.4 Pleural Exudate and Empyema

Pleural exudate and empyema may be the result of trauma to the chest, esophageal foreign body perforation, or surgical causes, such as leaking bronchial stump and esophageal anastomotic leak. Also, infradiaphramatic pathology may be responsible, e.g., retained gallstones after cholecystectomy, pancreatitis, and hollow viscus perforation, e.g., appendiceal perforation with peritonitis.

Parapneumonic effusion, meaning effusion between both leaves of the pleura due to pneumonic disease, once a rare complication of bacterial pneumonia in children, has become increasingly common both in the United States and in Europe. The prevalence of parapneumonic effusion in Utah USA was 14 in 100,000 children. Vaccination with heptavalent pneumococcal polysaccharide conjugate vaccine has not decreased the relative all over incidence of streptococcus pneumoniae infections but the relative incidence of the subtypes has changed. In contrast, the incidence of Haemophylus influenzae empyema has decreased. Recently Epstein-Barr virus has been implicated in the pathogenesis of pleural effusion.

In third world countries, Staphylococcus Aureus is the main causative infectious agent. In areas endemic for tuberculosis, the incidence of tuberculous effusion and empyema is high. Echinococcus is another causative agent for empyema in endemic areas.

29.2 Pathology

The aspect of the fluid in the thorax between both leaves of the pleura depends on the underlying pathology. It can be bloody as in case of a hematothorax or milky as in case of chylothorax. Chylous fluid looks relatively clear in the absence of enteral feeding. Clear fluid is seen when there is leakage of dialysis fluid or cerebrospinal fluid in case of a ventriculoperitoneal drain. The pleural space may be occupied with lymphatic cysts in lymphangiomatosis. In case of an exudate, the fluid looks cloudy.

In the event of an empyema, classically, three stages are distinguished

1. Exudative phase: thin pleural fluid with relatively few cells, lasting 24–72 h
2. Fibrinopurulent phase: accumulation of fibrinous material and loss of lung mobility, lasting 7–10 days
3. Organizing phase: formation of a pleural peal

29.3 Clinical Features

Pleural effusion interferes with lung expansion and can compress the heart. When present antenatally it can cause hydrops and pulmonary hypoplasia.

In the absence of infection, respiratory symptoms such as tachypnea, dyspnea, and orthopnea prevail. There is dullness of the chest on the affected side with diminished breath sounds. The dullness may vary depending on the most dependent position of the fluid accumulation. The heart sounds may be displaced to the other side. Depending on the underlying condition, the effusion may be bilateral, e.g., in congestive heart failure.

The presence of edema may suggest congestive heart failure, cirrhosis, or nephrotic syndrome. Lymphadenopathy may point in the direction of a malignant lymphoma.

Painless ascites may be the result of hepatic disease, peritoneal dialysis, or ventriculoperitoneal shunting.

In the event of inflammation, general signs such as fever, tachycardia, and lethargia are present in combination with severe local pain, exaggerating during respiration. The pain is often referred to the back and the shoulder. The patient lies on the affected side with the spine bent around the affected chest in bed. Respiration is fast and superficial. Local signs differ depending on the stage of the disease. In early pleurisy there may be a pleural friction rub. Breath sounds are diminished especially in the lower part of the chest when the patient is in a head up position. Dullness of the chest may vary depending on the most dependent position of the fluid but becomes fixed when loculation occurs. There may be bronchial breathing unless the effusion is very extensive. Heart sounds may be displaced to the contralateral side.

Abdominal pain may be referred pain from the chest. Alternatively abdominal pain and tenderness may point into the direction of an intra-abdominal process causative for the effusion.

29.4 Imaging

29.4.1 Plain Chest X-Ray in AP Position

Blunting of the costophrenic and cardiophrenic angles is an early sign of pleural effusion (Fig. 29.1). More extensive effusions cause a widening of the interlobar spaces. In the absence of organization, the fluid shifts depending on the position of the patient. The heart may be displaced to the contralateral side (Fig. 29.2a, b, 29.3a). When the effusion becomes organized, the fluid collection or collections become static. There is no need for a routine lateral X-ray.

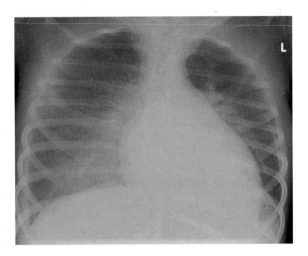

Fig. 29.1 Cardiac failure in a patient with Duchenne AP chest X-ray

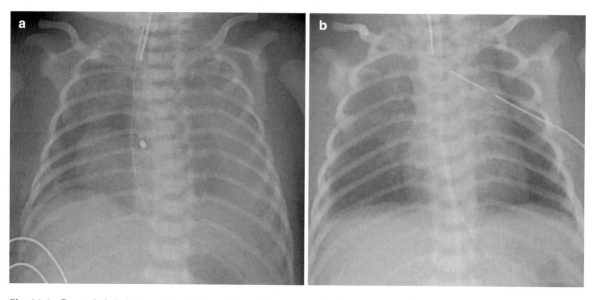

Fig. 29.2 Congenital chylothorax (**a**) AP chest X-ray. There is pleural fluid on the left. The lung is collapsed and the heart and mediastinum is displaced toward the right. (**b**) After drainage

29.4.2 Ultrasound

Ultrasound examination gives an idea about the amount of the pleural effusion and about the degree of organization (Fig. 29.3b). When organized, there is septation and no shifting of the fluid with changing patient position. Ultrasound is also helpful during the process of identification and actual puncture of a fluid collection to be drained.

29.4.3 CT and MR Scanning

CT or MRI scanning may be indicated for obtaining a complete picture of the chest (Fig. 29.3c). Collections of fluid or pus are identified. Thickening of the pleura points in the direction of inflammation. Underlying congenital or malignant pathology may be identified.

29.5 Diagnosis and Differential Diagnosis

From the history and clinical examination, a good idea about the pathology can be obtained in the majority of patients. Presence or absence of pain allows a rough separation of pleural transudate and exudate. Imaging provides information about the localization of the fluid, the degree of organization, and of potential underlying conditions. Blood tests are helpful in differentiating between infectious and noninfectious causes and may provide clues for malignant disease, e.g., malignant lymphoma. Blood cultures are essential when parapneumonic disease is suspected.

Analysis of the pleural fluid is essential in the treatment of pleural effusion and empyema. It allows for differentiation between transudate, exudate, and chyle, and for bacteriological examination. Several biological markers have been used to differentiate a transudate from an exudate in children but protein content in pleural fluid above 30 gL performs as well as any other individual test. If examined in patients under diuretic therapy, however, a serum minus pleural fluid albumin greater than 12/L rules out an exudative origin. Adenosine deaminase is raised in tuberculosis but may also be raised in pleural malignancies, lymphoproliferative diseases, and rheumatoid disease. Pleural biopsy, especially targeted biopsies, obtained during thoracoscopy, improves the diagnostic yield in tuberculosis.

Chylothorax is diagnosed when the fluid retrieved contains more than 1.1 mmol/L triglycerides with oral fat intake and has a total cell count equal or above 1,000 cells per μL. Cytology may be of help in diagnosing malignant pleural effusion in children, especially when associated with lymphoma or leukemia. Bacterial analysis of pleural fluid and blood should be

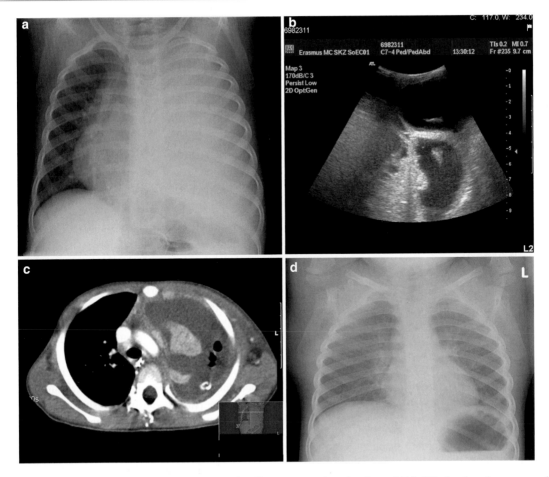

Fig. 29.3 (**a**) AP chest X-ray showing a parapneumonic effusion with displacement of the mediastinum to the right (**b**) Ultrasound examination of the same patient showing a collapsed lung with a fluid loculation below the lung (**c**) CT scan of the same patient showing turbid fluid in the pleural space around the lung and in between the lung lobes. The pleura is thickened. There are air bubbles. Posteriorly, a chest drain is seen (**d**) Complete resolution after 4 months

performed but the yield is rather low and reported to be about 40%.

29.6 Management

The management of pleural effusion depends on the underlying pathology.

29.6.1 Fetal Hydrothorax

Fetal hydrothorax may resolve spontaneously as the pregnancy progresses. Expectant management of stable and resolving effusions is therefore appropriate.

In contrast, in patients developing hydramnios or hydrops, thoracoamniotic shunting should be offered in the absence of underlying conditions such as chromosomal anomalies.

29.6.2 Congenital Chylothorax

Congenital chylothorax should be treated conservatively with mechanical ventilation, pleural fluid evacuation, and parenteral nutrition. Octreotide treatment has been suggested, but its efficacy remains difficult to prove especially against the background that most cases of congenital hydrothorax disappear during conservative treatment.

29.6.3 Pleural Effusion in the Context of Lymphangiomatosis

Treatment is largely symptomatic and by no means evidence based. Several treatment modalities have been suggested, e.g., feeding with medium-chain triglycerides, octreotide, interferon alpha, irradiation, surgical resection, ligation of the thoracic duct, pleuro-peritoneal shunting, and pleurodesis either surgically or with talc or other sclerosing agents.

29.6.4 Chylothorax after Thoracic Surgery

The treatment is basically conservative unless the thoracic duct was surgically damaged in which case ligation can be contemplated.

29.6.5 Pleural Effusion Related to Central Venous Catheters

Withdrawal of the catheter and evacuation of the fluid is all that is required.

29.6.6 Iatrogenic Hydrothorax

In case of peritoneal dialysis or ventriculo-peritoneal shunting, therapy may be directed at closing potential diaphragmatic holes. If not feasible pleurodesis may be an option.

29.6.7 Noniatrogenic Hydrothorax

In noniatrogenic hydrothorax, treatment should be directed at the underlying pathology. Puncture or drainage may increase patient comfort dramatically but rapid aspiration and reexpansion of the lung may lead to pulmonary edema. If treatment of the underlying disease is not possible, e.g., incurable malignant disease, pleurodesis may be an option.

29.6.8 Empyema

Underlying causes should of course be treated. For the treatment of the empyema itself, there is a lack of grade A evidence for best management practices. Treatment options include:

1. Antibiotics
2. Thoracocentesis
3. Tube thoracostomy
4. Intrapleural fibrinolytics
5. Decortication

   (a) Thoracoscopically
   (b) Through thoracotomy

There is no discussion on prompt initiation of antibiotic treatment. The type of antibiotics administered should depend on age, underlying medical condition, and suspected etiological agent. Of course, the antibiotic regimen should be adjusted according to culture results.

Repeat thoracocentesis is never recommended. When there is pleural infection, a drain should be inserted. For patient comfort, this should be done under general anesthesia. Moreover, general anesthesia offers the opportunity for a thoracoscopy allowing for inspection of the whole pleural cavity, aspiration of all fluid, and controlled chest tube placement. There is no evidence that large drains are better than smaller drains. Drains should not be inserted posteriorly as the intercostals spaces are narrower there.

There is no high grade evidence to support the utility of fibrinolytic therapy in the management of parapneumonic effusion or pleural empyema. In contrast, the British Thoracic Society advocates fibrinolytics.

When medical treatment fails, surgery is indicated but there is no consensus as to what failure of medical treatment entails. In general, however, there seems to be consensus that loculated empyema should be treated surgically.

Whether surgery should be done in an open or thoracoscopic way has not been clarified on a scientific basis, but when thoracoscopic expertise is available, the patient should have the less invasive approach.

Surgical treatment of empyema consists of decortication, which means removal of fibrin sheets and fibrous covering of the pleurae and the insertion of a drain (Fig. 29.4a–c).

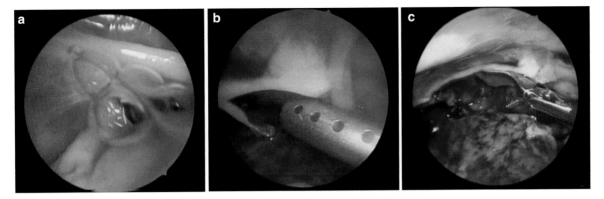

Fig. 29.4 Thoracoscopic pictures of an organized pleural empyema (**a**) The pleural space is covered with and bridged by fibrinous sheets. The thoracic wall itself is not visible (**b**) The fibrino-purulent material is being sucked away (**c**) Fibrinous sheets and strands are grasped and removed

29.7 Complications

The outcome after pleural effusion and empyema differs depending on potential underlying conditions.

The outcome of fetal hydrothorax is related to potential underlying conditions, and the progression to hydramnios and hydrops fetalis. Pleuroamniotic shunting has its owns complications such as premature rupture of membranes and possible trauma to tissues caused by the shunt. Postnatal chylothorax has usually a good outcome. The prognosis of lymphangiomatosis and especially of the Gorham Stout syndrome is not good.

The outcome of chylothorax after heart surgery is usually good, but depends on the underlying cardiac condition.

Long-lasting leakage of lymph and chyl predisposes for hypoproteinemia, lymphocytopenia, and infectious complications. Parenteral substitution of the losses and parenteral feeding are part of the treatment but have its own complications such as sepsis, thrombosis, and parenteral nutrition induced liver disease.

Pleural effusion due to central venous line malposition may cause a life-threatening condition but if resolved in time, the prognosis is good. The prognosis of an effusion due to malignant disease depends on the prognosis of the underlying disease.

The outcome in parapneumonic effusion and empyema is usually also good and long-lasting respiratory compromise is rare following any nonmedical treatment (Fig. 29.3d).

29.8 Etiology and Pathogenesis

The etiology and pathogenesis of pleural effusion can be subdivided into fetal congenital and acquired (Table 29.1).

Table 29.1 Etiology and pathogenesis

Antenatal and congenital pleural effusion
Fetal hydrothorax
Congenital chylothorax
Thoracic lymphangiomatosis
Acquired pleural effusion
Hemothorax
Chylothorax
Thoracic duct damage
Post cardiac surgery in the absence of thoracic duct damage
Hydrothorax
Iatrogenic
Central venous line malposition
Transdiaphragmatic hydrothorax
Peritoneal dialysis
Ventriculoperitoneal shunt
Noniatrogenic
Transdiaphragmatic e.g. hepatic ascites
Congestive heart disease
Nephrotic syndrome
Malignancy (non-Hodgkin lymphoma)
Pleural exudate and empyema
Traumatic or iatrogenic
Nontraumatic
Hydatid disease
Bacterial infections

Further Reading

Balfour-Lynn IM, Abrahamson E, Cohen G et al (2005) BTS guidelines for the management of pleural infection in children. Thorax 60:1–21

Bouros D, Tzouvelekis A, Antoniou K, Heffner JE (2006) Intrapleural fibrinolytic therapy for pleural infection. Pulm Pharmacol Ther 20(6):616–626, Doi 10.1016/j.pupt.2006.08.001

Byington CL, Spencer LY, Johson TA et al (2002) An epidemiological investigation of a sustained high rate of pediatric parapneumonic empyema: Risk factors and microbiological associations. Clin Infect Dis 34: 434–440

Chan S, Lau W, Wong WHS, Cheng L, Chau AKT, Cheung Y (2006) Chylothorax in children after congenital heart surgery. Ann Thorac Surg 82:1650–1657

Eastham KM, Freeman R, Kearns AM et al (2004) Clinical features, aetiology and outcome of empyema in children in the north east of England. Thorax 59:522–525

Klam S, Bigras J-L, Hudon L (2005) Predicting outcome in primary fetal hydrothorax. Fetal Diagn Ther 20:366–370

Light RW (2006) The undiagnosed pleural effusion. Clin Chest Med 27:309–319

Picone O, Benachi A, Mandelbrot L et al (2004) Thoracoamniotic shunting for fetal pleural effusions with hydrops. Am J Obstet Gynecol 191:2047–2050

Puri P, Höllwarth ME (eds) (2006) Pediatric Surgery. Springer, Berlin, Heidelberg

Congenital Malformations of the Lung

30

David M. Gourlay and Keith T. Oldham

Contents

30.1 Introduction

Congenital malformations of the lung are uncommon but extraordinarily diverse in their presentation and important to all physicians and surgeons who care for infants and children. The spectrum of presentation includes antenatal diagnosis of malformations to presentation in adulthood and ranges from asymptomatic to immediately life threatening. The most common congenital malformations such as congenital pulmonary airway malformations, pulmonary sequestrations, lobar emphysema, and bronchogenic cysts are themselves unique in their presentation and are considered below. Optimal management of congenital lung malformations requires an understanding by the surgeon of the embryology of lung development, respiratory physiology, and anatomy.

30.2 Pulmonary Embryology

During the 3rd week of gestation, the primordium of the respiratory systems develops from a diverticulum of the ventral wall of the foregut, immediately distal to the caudal pharyngeal complex. With the development of the esophagotracheal septum by the 4th week of gestation, the developing respiratory system and foregut are completely separated except at the larynx. The endodermal ventral diverticulum will become the epithelial lining of the larynx, trachea, bronchi, and alveoli. By the end of the 6th week of gestation, the trachea has undergone division into the right and left main-stem bronchi. Mesenchymal proliferation in the mediastinum provides the mesoderm that will eventually develop

P. Puri and M. Höllwarth (eds.), *Pediatric Surgery: Diagnosis and Management*,
DOI: 10.1007/978-3-540-69560-8_30, © Springer-Verlag Berlin Heidelberg 2009

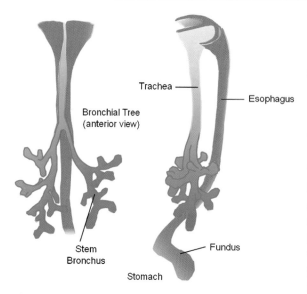

Trachea —

Esophagus

Bronchial Tree
(anterior view)

Stem
Bronchus

Fundus

Stomach

Fig. 30.1 Development of the trachea and bronchi. Anterior and lateral views at the beginning of the seventh week. The main lobar bronchial tree has developed and divided into five orders. (Modified from Skandalakis JE. Skandalakis' Surgical Anatomy: The Embryologic and Anatomic Basis of Modern Surgery. Paschalidis Medical Publications, Athens 2004; page 270)

into the cartilaginous, smooth muscle, and connective tissue of the lung. With progressive bronchial branching by the 9th week of gestation, segmental and lobar branching is complete and coincides with closure of the pleural peritoneal canal and the formation of the diaphragm (Fig. 30.1). By the 6th month of gestation, approximately 17 generations of subdivisions have been formed, giving rise to the respiratory bronchioles. Many of the congenital pulmonary malformations considered here are evident by this time. Considering the rapid expansion of pulmonary parenchyma during this period of development, one can understand how a congenital pulmonary lesion can have a severe negative impact on both fetal lung development and postnatal respiratory physiology. During the third trimester, development and maturation of the alveoli occur. Both the number and size of the alveoli increase during this time; however, it is important to recognize that this process is not complete until approximately 8 years of age. At birth, there are approximately 20 million alveoli, whereas an adult has approximately 300 million alveoli. Because of the continued development

of the alveoli after birth, pulmonary resection in infants and children is extraordinarily well tolerated with little long-term functional compromise in respiratory physiology.

30.3 Anatomy

The normal lobar and segmental anatomy of mature lungs and their relationship to adjacent mediastinal structures are demonstrated in Figs. 30.2 and 30.3. A detailed review of lung anatomy is outside the scope of this text, but several anatomic points of critical relevance in pediatric thoracic surgery deserve mention. In the term infant, the carina is located at the fourth or fifth vertebral body. The right main-stem bronchus is larger in diameter, shorter in length, and more vertical in direction than the left main-stem bronchus. This latter point accounts for the preference of aspirated material and deep endotracheal tubes to enter the right main-stem. In the infant and child, the hilum of either lung lies directly beneath the fifth intercostal space on the lateral chest wall. Thus, a thoracotomy incision through this space provides optimal exposure to the hilum for pulmonary resection.

30.4 Congenital Pulmonary Airway Malformations

30.4.1 Pathology

Congenital pulmonary airway malformations (CPAM), previously termed congenital cystic adenomatoid malformations (CCAM), are generally defined as benign hamartomatous or dysplastic tumors characterized by overgrowth of terminal bronchioles in a glandular or adenomatoid pattern. While relatively uncommon, CPAM constitute 10–30% of congenital lung malformations in most series, with a slight male predominance. Skandalakis et al. (2004) CPAM are thought to result from marked overgrowth of the terminal bronchioles at the expense of alveoli development. Histologically, CPAM are composed of disorganized cysts lined with ciliated cuboidal or columnar epithelium. Careful

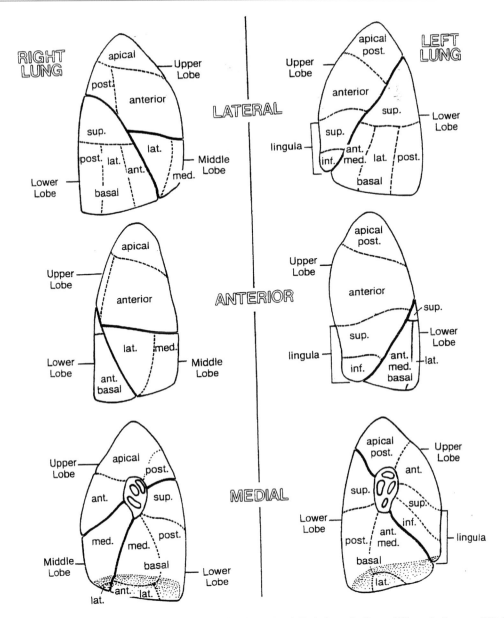

Fig. 30.2 The major bronchopulmonary segments. (Modified from Hood. Techniques in General Thoracic Surgery. WB Saunders Company, Philidelphia 1985; page 84)

pathologic dissection identifies a component of bronchial atresia in most CPAM lesions and may contribute to their pathogenesis. Involvement is generally unilobar with a slight predilection for the lower lobes, with right and left sides affected equally. Grossly, these lesions have both cystic and solid components. Typically, they have normal pulmonary arterial and venous blood supply and communicate with the tracheobronchial tree.

30.4.1.1 Diagnosis

Radiographic

Prenatal diagnosis by sonography is relatively common, which demonstrates an echogenic pulmonary mass with displacement of adjacent structures. Using antenatal sonography, Adzick and colleagues defined CPAM as

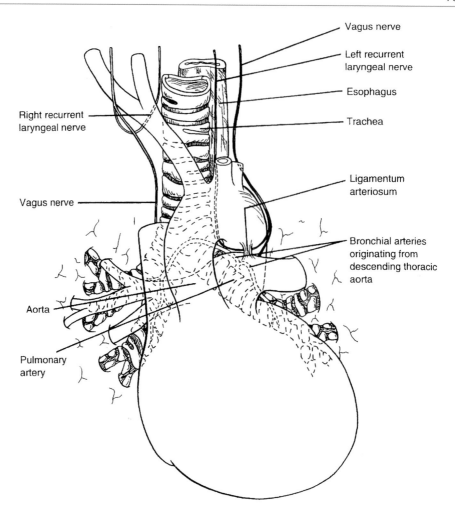

Fig. 30.3 Key anatomic relations of the structures of the pulmonsry hilum. (Modified from Oldham KT. Principles and Practice of Pediatric Surgery. Lippincott Williams & Wilkins, Philidelphia 2005; page 952)

either macrocystic (greater than 5-mm diameter cysts) or microcystic (solid or less than 5-mm diameter cysts), but as described below, the natural history of CPAM is determined more by overall size and degree of compression of adjacent structure than by their gross appearance. The prenatal differential diagnosis includes congenital diaphragmatic hernia, pulmonary sequestration, and bronchogenic cyst. Sonographic findings associated with CPAM include polyhydramnios, mediastinal shift, pleural effusions, and fetal hydrops. Fetal MRI has relatively high accuracy in differentiating CPAM from CDH; however, this is rarely necessary. Postnatal diagnosis can often be made by plain chest radiographs; however, in a stable patient, CT scans are often helpful to define anatomy and particularly to

identify aberrant systemic blood supply that is more suggestive of a pulmonary sequestration (Fig. 30.4). A CT scan is more accurate than plain chest radiography in confirming complete resolution of an antenatally diagnosed congenital pulmonary lesion that is not seen on postnatal plain chest radiography.

30.4.1.2 Clinical Features

The natural history of a CPAM diagnosed in the antenatal period is highly unpredictable and variable. While it is suggested that prenatal diagnosis is generally associated with a worse prognosis than postnatal diagnosis, this may reflect a significant selection bias.

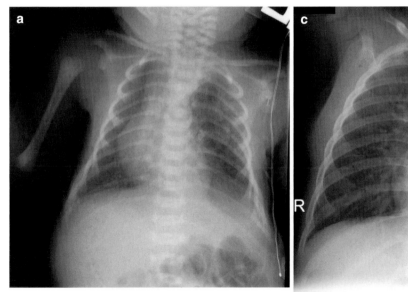

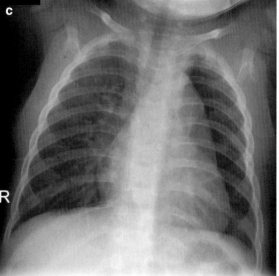

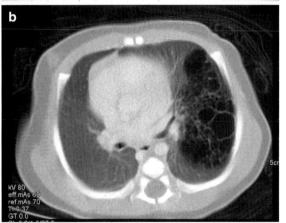

Fig. 30.4 Preoperative plain chest radiography (**A**) and CT scan (**B**) of a CPAM of the left upper lobe. A cystic pulmonary mass was identidies on prenatal US. Despite significant mediastinal shift and compression of adjacent normal lung parenchyma on both prenatal ultrasound and these preoperative images the infant was born at term and was asymptomatic. An elective resection was performed at two months. At the time of resection an associated extrapulmonary sequestration not seen on preoperative imaging was resected. **C**. Postoperative plain chest radiography three weeks postop demonstrating re-expansion of the left lower lobe and absence of mediastinal shift

In the antenatal and immediate postnatal period, the predominant physiologic consequences of a CPAM result from compression of the mediastinum and adjacent normal lung by the mass lesion. Because of the mass effect, polyhydraminos, mediastinal shift, pleural effusions, and fetal hydrops can be identified in the antenatal period. Fetal hydrops was identified in upwards of 40% of fetuses with CPAM and historically was an ominous finding, associated with a high risk of fetal or neonatal demise. In contrast, the mortality approaches zero for a fetus with a CPAM but without hydrops. In addition, spontaneous resolution in utero of an antenatally diagnosed CPAM is reported to occur in up to 15% of patients.

In order to help predict whether a fetus may be at risk of hydrops, Crumbleholme et al. developed and proposed sonographic determination of the CPAM volume ratio (CVR); CVR= (CPAM Length × Height × Width × 0.52)/head circumference. In particular, a CVR of ≤1.6 (excluding those with a dominant cyst) predicts a low risk (<3%) for the development of hydrops, whereas a CVR >1.6 predicts fetal hydrops in 75% of patients. In their series, postnatal intubation was required in fewer than 7% of patients with a CVR ≤ 1.6 and the survival rate was 94%. In contrast, for those with a CVR of >1.6, postnatal intubation was required in 88% of patients and survival was only 53%. Crumbleholme et al. also observed that the greatest increase in CVR occurred between 20 and 26 weeks gestation, and thereafter the CVR plateaus or diminishes with continued fetal growth. For these reasons, the authors suggested that surveillance ultrasounds of fetuses with a known CPAM, which are less than the estimated gestational age of 28 weeks, twice weekly if the CVR is greater than 1.6 and once weekly if the CVR is 1.6 or less, to evaluate for an increasing CVR or the development of hydrops.

Following delivery, the major risk to the newborn with a CPAM is respiratory distress as a consequence of compression of the adjacent normal lung and mediastinum by the CPAM. Rarely, emergent thoracotomy after birth is indicated due to severe respiratory embarrassment. Far more commonly, infants born with a CPAM either remain asymptomatic or have persistent mildly increased work in breathing that interferes with feeding. In those patients who require respiratory support or fail to thrive as a result of increased work of breathing, neonatal surgical resection is indicated.

There is little data regarding the long-term outcomes of patients with an untreated, asymptomatic CPAM. Most asymptomatic or undiagnosed CPAM will present with infectious complications during childhood or adolescence if not resected. In a small cohort of patients with unresected CPAM, Aziz et al found a 10% incidence of infectious complications by the age of 3 years. However, the long-term incidence of infections is likely higher. Pneumothorax and brochiectasis are reported in association with an untreated CPAM. Less commonly, a CPAM is diagnosed in a child or during adulthood in association with a pulmonary malignancy. More than 40 cases of CPAM associated with a brochioalveolar cancer, sarcoma, pulmonary blastoma, or mesenchymoma are reported in the literature.

30.4.2 Management

30.4.2.1 Fetal Therapy

One of the more controversial areas in pediatric surgery involves fetal treatment of surgical disease due to the high risk of complication and mortality for both fetus and mother. For congenital cystic pulmonary lesions, it is clear from the literature that provided the fetus does not experience hydrops or physiologic distress, treatment should be expectant management with

term delivery and postnatal evaluation. The type of treatment that should be offered to fetuses who demonstrate fetal hydrops or distress is less clear. As stated above, the previous published experience demonstrated universal fetal demise in fetuses with cystic pulmonary lesions and hydrops. More recent case series indicate that the development of hydrops in a fetus with a CPAM may not be uniformly fatal, and the risk of fetal loss may be further decreased if steroids are administered during the second trimester. In fetuses with ultrasonographic evidence of deterioration due to fetal hydrops, intervention should be considered (Fig. 30.5). Administration maternal steroids to any affected fetus less than the estimated gestational age of 34 weeks to help fetal lung maturation is reasonable. If hydrops develops during the third trimester, an EXIT procedure with thoracotomy and lobectomy using placental bypass can permit safe resection and avoid respiratory collapse. Hedrick et al. reported an 89% overall survival in nine patients in whom this approach was performed either because of fetal hydrops, extensive mediastinal shift, or persistently elevated CVR.[1] If the fetus is in the second trimester, several options exist for fetal intervention. Ultrasound-guided intrauterine thoracoamniotic shunting for a macrocystic CPAM with a large cyst has the best outcome with the lowest fetal and maternal risk. Of 23 such patients treated with this approach in one series, the volume reduction of the CPAM was 70% and survival through the neonatal period was 74%.[6] Open maternal-fetal surgery with pulmonary resection of a large CPAM yields a 50% probability of survival to discharge from the NICU, but given the technical complexity this should only be performed in a center with experience in open maternal-fetal surgery.

30.4.2.2 Postnatal Therapy

Prompt surgical resection should be performed in any symptomatic newborn. In those patients who remain asymptomatic in the newborn period, delaying resection until infancy is reasonable and allows somatic growth that may facilitate the ease of pulmonary resection. Delaying resection until later in infancy does not appear to pose an increased risk of complications and allows the opportunity for spontaneous resolution to occur. Complete spontaneous resolution of a CPAM identified on postnatal imaging is rare, but may occur in more than

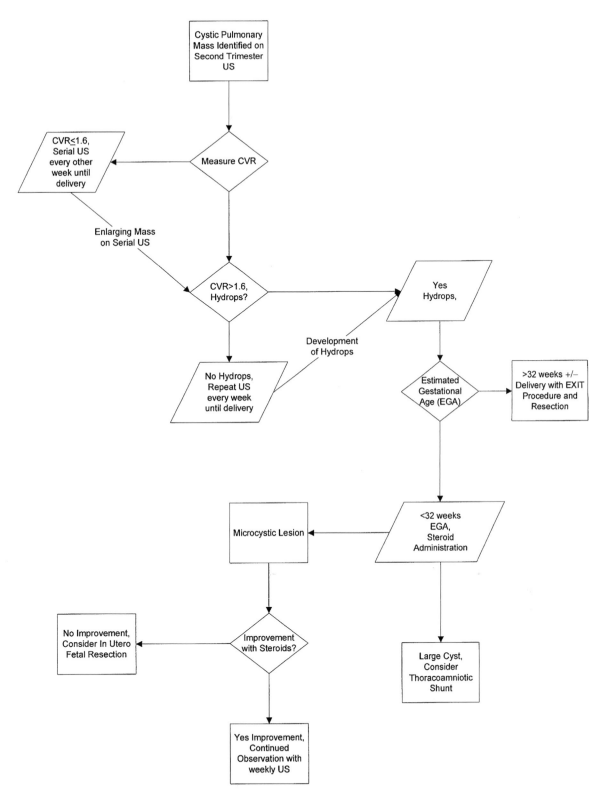

Fig. 30.5 An algorithym for the management of prenatally diagnosed congenital pulmonary malformations. Lesions with a CVR≤1.6 are at low risk for the development of hydrops and should expect to delivery at term with little respiratory compromise. Lesions with a CVR>1.6 are at high risk for the development of hydrops. The development of hydrops is associated with a high risk of fetal or neonatal demise due to the mass effect caused by the congenital pulmonary mass. Fetal intervention should be considered in fetuses who develop hydrops and the therapy tailored to the estimated gestational age and type of lesion

4% of patients. Because congenital pulmonary lesions may become undetectable by ultrasound (US) and plain radiograph, chest computed tomography (CT) is necessary to ensure complete resolution. Asymptomatic but persistent CPAM should be resected during infancy to prevent complications of recurrent infections or malignant degeneration.

Resection often includes formal lobectomy; however, for small CPAM, nonanatomical resection is reasonable. Traditionally, resection was performed through open thoracotomy but recent reports have demonstrated excellent outcomes for minimally invasive pulmonary resection.

30.5 Bronchopulmonary Sequestrations

30.5.1 Pathology

Pulmonary sequestrations account for roughly one third of congenital pulmonary malformations. Bronchopulmonary sequestrations are defined as either an intrathoracic or subdiaphragmatic mass of nonfunctional pulmonary tissue that lacks communication with the tracheo-bronchial tree of the normal lung. Histologically, pulmonary sequestrations demonstrate immature lung development, often resembling more peripheral lung parenchyma. Intrathoracic sequestrations are further categorized as either extralobar or intralobar, depending on whether the lesion is invested by its own pleura or that of the adjacent normal lobe, respectively. Typically, the arterial blood supply is anomalous, most commonly arising from the descending thoracic aorta. Venous drainage for intralobar sequestrations is most commonly via the pulmonary veins, whereas venous drainage for extralobar sequestrations is typically systemic via either the azygous or hemiazygous veins, inferior vena cava, or directly into the atrium. Extralobar sequestrations have anomalous blood supply from an infradiaphragmatic source in about 20% of patients.

The embryology of pulmonary sequestrations is not clear. Conflicting theories of embryogenesis exist and include abnormal budding of the tracheobronchial tree leading to an orphaned lobe, and accessory budding from the primitive foregut. In either case, pulmonary sequestrations occur as part of the spectrum of bronchopulmonary foregut malformations and extralobar sequestrations in particular are associated with other congenital anomalies in up to 40% of patients. Extralobar

pulmonary sequestrations are not infrequently associated with CPAM and congenital diaphragmatic hernias. Rarely, pulmonary sequestrations communicate with the esophagus or stomach.

30.5.1.1 Diagnosis

Radiographic

Extralobar sequestrations can be diagnosed by antenatal ultrasound and appear as an echogenic thoracic mass in the posterior mediastinum. Anomalous blood supply is often identified, using Doppler ultrasound, helping to differentiate these from a CPAM. Intralobar sequestrations appear similar, on prenatal ultrasound, to a CPAM. Pulmonary sequestrations can be associated with a pleural effusion, polyhydraminos, and nonimmune hydrops fetalis. They can be difficult to differentiate from a CPAM or CDH by prenatal ultrasound.

Postnatal plain chest radiography will occasionally be diagnostic for a sequestration. More commonly, plain films demonstrate a retrocardiac posterior mediastinal mass if extralobar, or a nonaerated mass within the lung if intralobar. Neither finding is specific for a sequestration and further axial imaging is warranted. CT and magnetic resonance imaging (MRI) are considered equivalent in making the diagnosis of either intralobar or extralobar sequestration (Fig. 30.6). The differential diagnosis often includes CPAM, CDH, and other posterior mediastinal masses such as neuroblastoma. CT and MR angiography have supplanted the need for conventional angiography to identify anomalous vasculature in differentiating pulmonary sequestrations from other diagnoses. Ninety percent of extralobar sequestrations are located in the left hemithorax within the posterior mediastinum. Sixty percent of intralobar sequestrations occur on the left side, most commonly involving the left lower lobe. A sequestration in the upper lobe occurs in only 10–15% of cases, and bilateral sequestrations are infrequent.

30.5.1.2 Clinical Features

Extralobar sequestrations are often identified on antenatal ultrasound or in infancy during surgery for other congenital anomalies such as CPAM or CDH. In contrast, most intralobar sequestrations present later in childhood due to recurrent pulmonary infections from inadequate tracheobronchial drainage, or less commonly

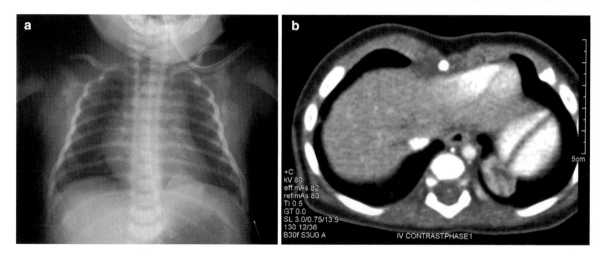

Fig. 30.6 Preoperative plain chest radiography (**A**) and CT scan (**B**) of an extrapulmonary sequestration. The prenatal ultrasound and the plain chest radiography after birth were interrupted as most likely consistent with a CPAM or small CDH. Chest CT nicely demonstrates a solid 2 cm mass in the left posterior mediastinum. Although no systemic blood supply could be identified by CT imaging this was felt to most consistent with an extrapulmonary sequestration since the diaphragm appeared intact and the mass was outside normal lung parachyma. The lesion failed to demonstrate signs of resolution on serial chest CT by four months of age and was resected at four months of age

with hemorrhage. Both intralobar and extralobar sequestrations can present in the newborn period with either respiratory distress due to mass effect or congestive heart failure because of arteriovenous shunting within the sequestration.

30.5.2 Management

Prenatal management is identical to that for CPAM as outlined above. Although a few observational studies of small cohorts of patients with unresected extralobar sequestrations followed over a short period of time appear to have a low risk of complications, in general postnatal resection of a sequestration is indicated. Both asymptomatic extralobar and intralobar sequestrations pose a risk of recurrent pulmonary infections or hemorrhage. The abnormally developed lung tissue is ineffective in gas exchange and therefore is not of benefit to the patient. Spontaneous involution of extralobar sequestrations has been described. In practice, extralobar sequestrations often present as a posterior mediastinal mass, and despite improvements in imaging, differentiation from solid tumors, CPAM, and CDH cannot be made short of surgical excision. Thoracoscopic resection of extralobar sequestrations is often technically straightforward because there is no attachment to the normal lung. The risk of complication from an unresected sequestration outweighs the risk of resection.

The goal of surgical resection is to remove only the abnormal portion of lung. For an extralobar sequestration, this is often easily achieved unless there is inflammation due to previous infection or hemorrhage. For intralobar sequestration, particularly if previously infected, this often necessitates lobar resection.

30.5.3 Congenital Lobar Emphysema

30.5.4 Pathology

Congenital lobar emphysema (CLE), or congenital lobar overinflation, is characterized by expiratory air trapping within the affected lobe. The air trapping leads to overdistension of the affected lobe and compression of the adjacent lung and mediastinal structures. While the lung parenchyma is typically normally developed, bronchial collapse is commonly seen due to a focal deficiency or absence of the cartilaginous components of the lobar bronchus. This causes air trapping within the affected lobe. Other potential etiologies for lobar emphysema include endobronchial obstruction due to secretions, granulation tissue, ingested foreign bodies, or endobronchial tumors that lead to air trapping. In addition, extrinsic compression can occur as a result of mediastinal lymphadenopathy, an aberrant or enlarged pulmonary artery, ductus arteriosus, and a mediastinal cyst or tumor. Rarely, an apparent CLE is associated with proliferation of normal alveoli within the affected lobe without bronchial obstruction. This is termed polyalveolar morphology.

30.5.4.1 Diagnosis

Radiographic

The diagnosis of CLE is rarely made by antenatal US or MRI as the process of air trapping occurs postnatally. This diagnosis can be difficult to differentiate from a microcystic CPAM as both may appear as an echogenic mass prenatally. Most commonly, the diagnosis of CLE is made by plain chest radiography in a

newborn with respiratory distress. Shortly after birth, a lobe affected by CLE may appear consolidated on chest radiography as a result of inadequate clearance of amniotic fluid from the affected lobe. Subsequent, classic radiographic findings include hyperinflation of the affected lobe, mediastinal displacement to the contralateral side, atelectasis of the adjacent lung, and flattening of the ipsilateral hemidiaphragm (Fig. 30.7). Tension pneumothorax and macrocystic CPAM are important in the differential diagnosis. Tension pneumothorax should be marked by complete collapse of the entire ipsilateral lung into the hilum, in contrast to CLE where some compressed aerated normal lung is seen on the affected side. CLE most often affects the left upper lobe (40–50%), followed by the right middle lobe (30–40%), the right upper lobe (20%), lower lobes

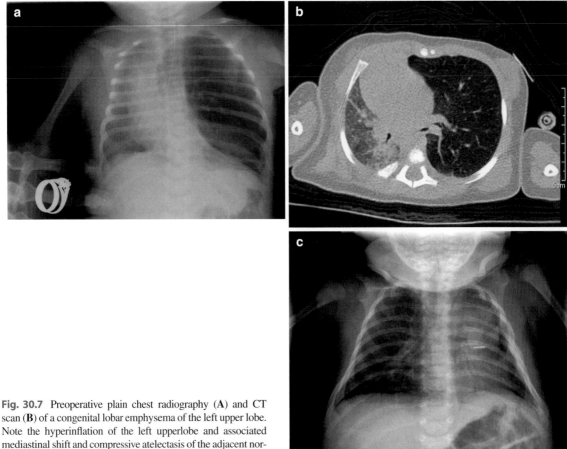

Fig. 30.7 Preoperative plain chest radiography (**A**) and CT scan (**B**) of a congenital lobar emphysema of the left upper lobe. Note the hyperinflation of the left upperlobe and associated mediastinal shift and compressive atelectasis of the adjacent normal lung parenchyma. Postoperative plain chest radiography (**C**) following resection. Note the re-expansion of the remaining lung parenchyma and absence of mediastinal shift

(1%), and multiple sites in the remainder. Further imaging beyond plain chest radiography is seldom necessary in newborns and infants. CLE is associated with congenital heart disease in approximately 15% of patients and therefore screening echocardiography is recommended. In older children, CT, MRA, and bronchoscopy are helpful to evaluate for reversible causes of lobar emphysema.

30.5.4.2 Clinical Features

CLE is most commonly found in term infants, but acquired emphysema can occur in premature infants as a result of barotrauma, oxygen toxicity, and lung immaturity. After birth, respiratory distress typically follows an insidious course. Most affected CLE infants do not demonstrate signs of respiratory distress at birth. However, spontaneous respiration leads to progressive over distension of the affected lobe and compression of normal lung. This process can be exacerbated by the need for positive pressure ventilation. Half of the affected infants will demonstrate signs of respiratory distress in the first few days of life; the remainder develop symptoms within the first few months or years of life. Rapidly progressive respiratory failure occurs in up to 10–15% of newborns and may require emergency thoracotomy. Occasionally children presenting with recurrent chest infections are subsequently identified to have a CLE.

30.5.5 Management

Lobar resection is indicated in any symptomatic patient with CLE. This is safely achieved by either traditional open thoracotomy or with video-assisted thoracoscopy. Emergent thoracotomy with delivery of the affected lobe can be life saving in a newborn with severe respiratory distress as a result of CLE. Although generally unnecessary in infants, children should undergo bronchoscopy preceding thoracotomy to evaluate for reversible endobronchial lesions not requiring pulmonary resection. Extrinsic compression is generally associated with a focal cartilaginous defect such that relief of the extrinsic compression alone is rarely adequate to relieve the bronchial obstruction. While bronchoplasty is theoretically attractive, the size of the bronchus in an infant or child poses an impractical obstacle to achieve an adequate result.

Rarely, a CLE is identified in an asymptomatic or minimally symptomatic child. There are no long-term data to support a decision not to remove a CLE. A few studies with short-term follow-up on a small cohort of selected patients who have not undergone resection suggest that there is a low incidence of progression of disease. While the long-term outcome of these patients with untreated CLE remains unknown, the long-term outcome after surgical resection for CLE is excellent and is detailed later in this chapter.

30.6 Bronchogenic Cysts and Congenital Lung Cysts

30.6.1 Pathology

Bronchogenic cysts are included in the spectrum of bronchopulmonary-forgut cystic malformations. Bronchogenic cysts are typically thick walled, unilocular cysts that originate from either the trachea or bronchus. The cyst wall is composed of smooth muscle, cartilage, elastic tissue, and mucous glands lined by pseudostratified ciliated columnar or cuboidal epithelium. While bronchogenic cysts arise from the airway and often remain intimately attached, they typically have lost their communication with the airway during development. Bronchogenic cysts are believed to occur as a result of abnormal budding of the tracheobronchial tree; therefore, they can be found anywhere along the conducting airways depending on the point in development of the airway when the anomalous budding occurred. Bronchogenic cysts are most often located within the lung parenchyma, mediastinum, or in the neck; but ectopic bronchogenic cysts have been reported in paravertebral, paraesophageal, pericardial, subcarinal, and subcutaneous locations.

Congenital lung cysts are included in this section since the clinical significance and treatment are similar. In contrast to bronchgenic cysts, congenital lung cyst arises from more distal airways, including the alveoli, or they may be pleural in origin. Differentiation of the cysts tends to be difficult short of resection. Although collectively these are rare, infection of these cysts is not uncommon as a result of their communication with the airways.

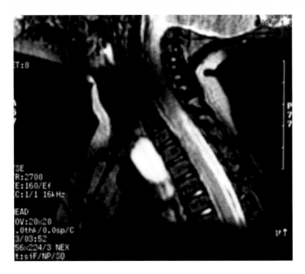

Fig. 30.8   Preoperative MRI of a bronchogenic cyst

30.6.1.1 Diagnosis

Radiographic

Plain chest radiography most commonly demonstrates a smooth, spherical mass in either a paratracheal or hilar location in the posterior mediastinum (Fig. 30.8). If infected or if the cyst communicates with the airway, an air fluid level may be present. CT and MR will demonstrate these as cystic lesions without calcification and help to differentiate bronchogenic cysts from neuroblastomas. A contrast-enhanced study will demonstrate a nonenhancing mass lesion; this also helps to differentiate bronchogenic cysts from an aberrant pulmonary artery (pulmonary sling). CT and MR also define additional anatomic relationships to adjacent mediastinal structures, in particular the spine, to help differentiate bronchogenic cysts from neuroenteric cysts. An esophagram can be helpful in selected cases to evaluate for foregut communication. Foregut duplication cysts, pericardial cysts, and lymphoma are included in the differential diagnosis depending on the location.

30.6.1.2 Clinical Features

Many bronchogenic cysts are asymptomatic and are discovered incidentally by chest radiography in the child or less commonly by antenatal ultrasound in the fetus. The symptomatology of bronchogenic cysts varies with age. Most infants present with wheezing, tachypnea, dyspnea, and cyanosis or less commonly, failure to thrive as a result of compression of adjacent mediastinal structures. Older children typically present with infectious complications. Rarely does enlargement of the cyst cause such mediastinal displacement that they lead to cardiopulmonary compromise. Rare cases of malignancies within bronchogenic cysts have been reported.

30.6.2 Management

Resection is typically indicated to alleviate symptoms, prevent future infection, and to provide pathologic identification. Generally, simple local resection can be accomplished with preservation of adjacent normal lung parenchyma. Resolution of active infection prior to attempted resection is helpful to minimize unnecessary pulmonary resection. Occasionally formal pulmonary resection is required either due to the anatomic location of the cyst or inflammation from previous infections. Rarely, it is not possible to remove the cyst in its entirety without sacrificing vital structures; in such instances, partial cyst resection with fulguration of the remaining cyst wall can be performed. Long-term follow-up is necessary as late recurrences have been reported for partially resected bronchogenic cysts. As with the other previously described congenital pulmonary malformations, this can often be accomplished with a minimally invasive approach.

30.7 Complications and Long-Term Outcomes

Pulmonary resection even in the newborn is generally very well tolerated. Most contemporary pediatric surgical series of pulmonary resection for congenital pulmonary malformations in the absence of diffuse lung disease cite a mortality rate of <2%. Increased mortality from pulmonary resection can be anticipated in newborns with nonimmune hydrops fetalis, significant mediastinal shift, pulmonary hypertension, or other associated anomalies. Short-term complications following resection are infrequent and include prolonged air leak, pneumothorax, hemorrhage, and infectious complications. Whether done by an open or a minimally invasive approach, the frequency of short-term complications does not appear to be higher in infants compared to older pediatric patients.

Because of, in part, the continued lung development that occurs well into childhood, pediatric pulmonary resection is associated with an excellent long-term functional outcome. Most patients who undergo pulmonary resection as an infant or child in the absence of other associated illness will have normal growth in both height and weight. Laros et al. demonstrated that several decades after pneumonectomy for tuberculosis or bronchiectasis, the loss in total lung capacity was almost fully compensated by the remaining lung if resection occurred in children less than 5 years of age. The compensatory response was inversely related to the age at the time of resection. Total lung capacity 30 years after pneumonectomy was 96%, 87%, and 70% if the pneumonectomy occurred at 0–5, 6–10, or 31–40 years of age, respectively. McBride et al. demonstrated similar adaptation of lung volume (total lung capacity and vital capacity) in 15 infants who underwent lobectomy for congenital lobar emphysema. They also observed evenly distributed pulmonary blood flow between the operated and nonoperated sides, suggesting compensatory growth of the pulmonary vascular bed. Despite normalization of lung volume and pulmonary blood flow, McBride et al. noted a decrease in expiratory flow rates and airway conductance. These later findings have been validated subsequently by others. Yet, despite the decreased expiratory flow rates and airway conductance, Frenckner et al. demonstrated normal $PaCO_2$ and PaO_2 at rest and following intense exercise in 16 patients who underwent lobectomy during infancy or childhood for either congenital lobar emphysema or CPAM. During intense exercise, these individuals achieved normal work load, heart rate, and oxygen uptake. Similarly, 3–20 years after partial pulmonary resection for congenital cystic pulmonary lesions in

infancy and early childhood, Warner et al. found that the decreased expiratory flow rates did not appear to impact exercise endurance. After excluding patients with other associated anomalies all of the patients in their series performed at or above the 25th percentile and half were above the 50th percentile for age in a treadmill endurance test.

In aggregate, whether this occurs through further lung development or simply by compensation by the remaining lung, these data demonstrate the excellent functional outcome associated with pediatric pulmonary resection.

Further Reading

Cano I, Anton-Pacheco JL, Rothenberg S et al (2006) Video-assisted thoracoscopic lobectomy in infants. Eur J Cardiothorac Surg 29:997–1000

Davenport M, Warne SA, Nicolaides K et al (2004) Current outcome of antenatally diagnosed cystic lung disease. J Pediatr Surg 39:549–556

Grethel EJ, Wagner AJ, Lee H et al (2007) Fetal intervention for mass lesions and hydrops improves outcome: A 15-year experience. J Pediatr Surg 42:117–123

Laberge JM, Puligandla P, Flageole H (2005) Asymptomatic congenital lung malformations. Semin Pediatr Surg 14:16–33

Langston C (2003) New concepts in the pathology of congenital lung malformations. Semin Pediatr Surg 12:17–37

Mei-Zahav M, Konen O, Langer JC et al (2006) Is congenital lobar emphysema a surgical disease? J Pediatr Surg 41:1058–1061

Oldham KT, Pinkerton HJ (2005) Lung In KT Oldham, PM Colombani, MA Skinner et al (eds) Principles and Practice of Pediatric Surgery, Lippincott Williams & Wilkens Philadelphia, 951

Swenney BT, Oldham KT (2006) Pulmonary Malformations In P Puri, ME Höllwarth (eds) Pediatric Surgery, Springer Surgery Atlas Series. Springer-Verlag, Berlin, Heidelberg, New York, pp 107–114

Wilson RD, Hedrick HL, Adzick NS et al (2006) Research review: Cystic adenomatoid malformation of the lung. Am J Med Genet 140:151–155

Congenital Diaphragmatic Hernia

31

Prem Puri and Nana Nakazawa

Contents

31.1 Introduction

Congenital Diaphragmatic Hernia (CDH) is a common malformation characterized by a defect in the posterolateral diaphragm, the foramen of Bochdaleck, through which the abdominal viscera migrate into the chest during fetal life. The incidence of CDH ranges from 1 in 2,500–5,000 births in recent population-based studies. Approximately 80% of posterolateral diaphragmatic hernia occurs on the left side and 20% on the right side. Bilateral CDH is rare. The size of the defect varies from small (2 or 3 cm) to very large, involving most of the hemidiaphragm.

The incidence of associated anomalies has been reported to be about 40% in most series. The most common abnormalities associated with CDH are cardiovascular anomalies, followed by skeletal, central nervous system, genitourinary, gastrointestinal, craniofacial, abdominal wall defects, and chromosomal and syndromic defects.

Despite significant advances in neonatal resuscitation and intensive care, newborn infants with CDH continue to have high mortality, which is assumed to be even higher when it includes "hidden mortality." Infants with associated anomalies have much lower survival rates than those with isolated CDH. The high mortality and morbidity in CDH is mainly attributed to pulmonary hypoplasia and persistent pulmonary hypertension.

31.2 Etiology and Embryology

The etiology of CDH is still unknown. Although it is generally considered to be sporadic, some familial cases have been reported. This appears to be multifactorial

P. Puri and M. Höllwarth (eds.), *Pediatric Surgery: Diagnosis and Management*,
DOI: 10.1007/978-3-540-69560-8_31, © Springer-Verlag Berlin Heidelberg 2009

inheritance, in which case the expected recurrence risk in a first degree relative would be 1 in 45 or approximately 2% based on an incidence of 1 in 2,000 births. A number of syndromes are associated with CDH. In some syndromes, such as Fryns syndrome and Donnai-Barrow syndrome, CDH is present in a high percentage of affected individuals. Others include Beckwith-Wiedemanch, Simpson-Golabi-Behmel, Coffin-Siris, and Denys-Drash syndromes. CDH has also been reported with trisomies 9, 13, 18, 21, and 22.

Nongenetic factors have also been incriminated in the etiology of CDH. Thalidomide, quinine, phanometrazine, and nitrofen have been mentioned as possible agents. A vitamin A deficient diet has been shown to produce CDH in rats.

Embryogenesis of CDH has been described as a failure of the closure of the pleuroperitoneal canal, which occurs during gestational week 8. Consequently, the abdominal viscera herniates into the thorax, which is thought to cause pulmonary hypoplasia by compression of the growing lung. However, experimental studies have suggested that the classical view of embryogenesis of CDH may have to be revised. Kluth et al. have shown that pleuroperitoneal canals are not wide enough to allow herniation of gut loops in rats. Furthermore, a toxicological nitrofen model of CDH has shown that abnormalities in the contralateral lung as well as the ipsilateral side are present even before the diaphragm starts to develop.

31.3 Clinical Features and Diagnosis

Widespread use of obstetrical ultrasonography has led us to an increased frequency of antenatal diagnosis of CDH. Displacement of the mediastinum, the absence of a stomach bubble in the abdomen, and the presence of abdominal organs in the chest are the signs of fetal diaphragmatic hernia. Incidence of pregnancies with polyhydramnios associated with CDH ranges from 15% to 75%. The presence of abdominal contents intrathoracically in a transverse sonographic scan at the level of a four-chamber view of the heart is required for diagnosis. A right-sided CDH is more difficult to identify because the echogenicity of the fetal liver is similar to that of the lung. Identifying the gallbladder in the fetal chest may be the most reliable sign in these cases.

Prenatal diagnosis offers the advantage that the mother can be referred to an institution with maternity services and a neonatal intensive care unit where the baby can be electively delivered, resuscitated, and undergo surgery by a fully prepared team of neonatologists and surgeons. Advanced ultrasound examination will discriminate the condition from other intrathoracic lesions, and other malformations will be looked for. Prenatal magnetic resonance imaging has been shown to be effective in confirming the diagnosis of CDH and detecting additional information that may affect prognosis.

If lethal congenital anomalies are also detected, prenatal diagnosis may lead to termination of pregnancy. In selected cases, in utero intervention may be possible.

The onset and severity of symptom depends on the amount of abdominal viscera in the chest and the degree of pulmonary hypoplasia. The most severely affected infants present with respiratory distress at birth. Other infants with CDH develop cyanosis, tachypnea, and grunting respirations within minutes or hours after birth. Physical examination reveals a scaphoid abdomen, an increased anteroposterior diameter of the thorax, and mediastinal shift. Breath sounds are absent on the affected side. Associated congenital anomalies may also be seen or revealed on further examination.

The definitive diagnosis of CDH is made postnatally by plain radiography of the chest and abdomen by demonstration of air-filled loops of the bowel in the chest and a paucity of gas in the abdomen (Figs. 31.1, 31.2). The diaphragmatic margin is absent, there is a mediastinal shift to the opposite side, and only a small portion of lung may be seen on the ipsilateral side.

31.3.1 Late Presentation

Although most CDH infants present in the first 24 h of life, 10–20% of the affected infants present later. The symptoms and signs of those patients are nonspecific and include recurrent chest infections, vomiting, abdominal pain, diarrhea, anorexia, failure to thrive, or an abdominal chest X-ray in an asymptomatic patient. Some children present acutely with volvulus or strangulation or acute respiratory distress. Chest X-ray with an in situ nasogastric tube is reliable for the diagnosis. Even if the hernia is asymptomatic, it should be repaired to prevent complications.

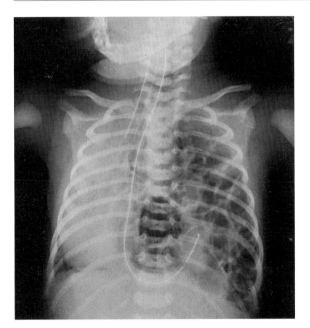

Fig. 31.1 X-ray of the chest in a newborn showing large left-sided Congenital Diaphragmatic Hernia with Mediastinal shift to the right

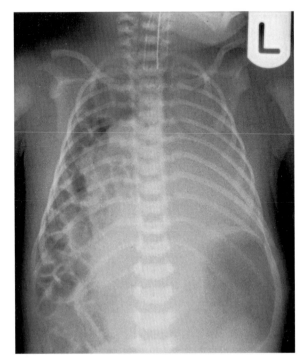

Fig. 31.2 X-ray of the chest and upper abdomen showing large right-sided diaphragmatic hernia

31.4 Differential Diagnosis

Differential diagnosis includes cystic lung disease (e.g. cystic adenomatoid malformation) and mediastinal cystic lesions (e.g. cystic teratoma, neuroenteric, bronchogenic, and thymic cysts). A congenital lung cyst in the neonate may produce a radiological picture mimicking that of diaphragmatic hernia but can be distinguished from CDH by the presence of outline of the lung and the diaphragm on chest X-ray and by the presence of a normal intestinal gas pattern on abdominal X-ray. The diagnosis of CDH can also be confused with other congenital thoracic conditions, such as eventration of the diaphragm, anterior diaphragmatic hernia of Morgagni, congenital esophageal hiatal hernia, and primary agenesis of the lung.

31.5 Prognostic Factors

Polyhydramnios, right-sided CDH, and intrathoracic stomach and liver have all been proposed as predictors for poor prognosis. Other studies suggest that there is no evidence to support these proposals. The determination of lung-to-head ratio (LHR), first described in 1996, has been suggested to be predictive of postnatal survival. LHR < 1.0 is reported to be correlated with poor outcome, whereas LHR > 1.4 equates with a better outcome. However, these reports have been contradicted by other investigators who found no correlation.

31.6 Management

31.6.1 Preoperative Management

An infant with respiratory distress requires endotracheal ventilatory support. Mask ventilation should be avoided as it will distend the stomach and further compromise respiratory status. These babies should be paralysed and sedated to prevent swallowing and noncompliance with ventilation and to minimize stressful stimuli that cause pulmonary vasoconstriction. The concept of "gentle" ventilation and permissive hypercapnia was proposed to minimize barotraumas by strictly limiting the peak inflation pressure.

Inhaled nitric oxide (iNO) induces pulmonary vaso-dilatation without systemic hypotension and can be beneficial in the context of pulmonary hypertension. However, a prospective randomized trial has revealed that the benefit was not seen in patients with CDH.

High-frequency oscillatory ventilation (HFOV) is a mode of ventilation that can be effectively used in CDH infants to maintain preductal oxygenation while avoiding hyperventilation and barotraumas. It has been reported that HFOV may be a more effective mode of ventilatory support than conventional ventilation in CDH when used as the initial therapy. Infants who fail to respond to optimal therapy may be placed on ECMO. This is a life support system that employs partial heart-lung bypass providing rest to the lungs for long periods of time during which it is hoped that the lung and, in particular, the lung vasculature will mature. Although the criteria for selection of ECMO vary in different centres, in general, candidates for ECMO are expected to have reversible cardiopulmonary process, with a predictive mortality greater than 90%.

31.6.2 Timing of Surgery

The timing of surgical repair has gradually shifted from an emergency repair to a policy of stabilization using a variety of ventilatory strategies prior to operation. However, recent studies concluded that there is no clear evidence to support delayed surgery over emergency surgery. Nevertheless, one should consider allowing time until the other parameters that influence survival in patients of CDH are optimized. Thus, our current recommendation is to adopt a conservative approach and delay surgical repair of the CDH until the infant stabilizes from a homodynamic and respiratory point of view.

31.6.3 Surgical Technique

The most commonly preferred approach is abdominal. This offers good exposure, easy reduction of the abdominal viscera, and recognition and correction of associated gastrointestinal anomalies. A subcostal transverse muscle cutting incision is made on the side of the hernia.

The contents of hernia are gently reduced in the abdomen. On the right side, the small intestine and the colon are first reduced and the liver is withdrawn last. After the hernia is reduced, an attempt is made to visualize the ipsilateral lung. This is usually done by retracting the anterior rim of the diaphragm. Often, a hypoplastic lung can be observed at the apex.

Most diaphragmatic defects can be sutured by direct sutures of the edges of the defect. Usually the anterior rim of the diaphragm is quite evident. However, the posterior rim may not be immediately apparent and may require dissection for delineation. The posterior rim of the diaphragm is mobilized by incising the overlying peritoneum.

The defect is closed by interrupted nonabsorbable suture (Figs. 31.3, 31.4). Occasionally, the posterior rim is absent altogether, in which case the anterior rim of the diaphragm is sutured to the lower ribs with either periostial or pericostal sutures.

If the defect is large, it may not be possible to repair it using direct sutures. Various techniques have been described and include the use of prerenal fascia, rib structures, the lastissimus dorsi muscle, rotational muscle flaps from the thoraco-abdominal wall, and prosthetic patches. The operations involving muscle flaps are too long and complex for critically ill patients and can lead to unsightly chest deformities. Prosthetic materials have been advocated for repair of large

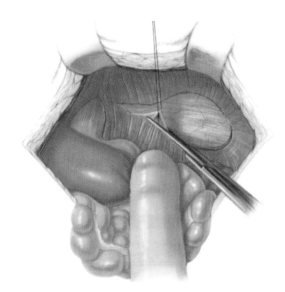

Fig. 31.3 Posterio rim of the diaphragm is mobilized by incising the overlying peritoneum

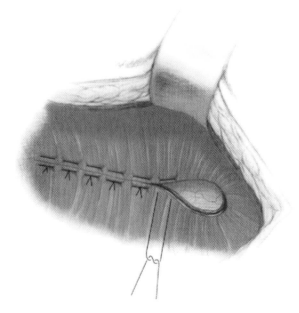

Fig. 31.4 The defect is closed by interrupted nonabsorbable sutures

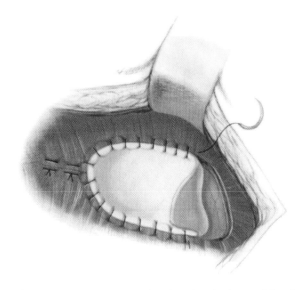

Fig. 31.5 Large diaphragmatic defect closed using surgisis soft tissue graft

defects. The most commonly used prosthetic material presently is surgisis soft tissue graft, which is incorporated into the adjacent tissue (Fig. 31.5). If the abdominal cavity is small, gentle stretching of the abdominal wall will enable safe closure in most of the patients. The use of a chest drain is controversial. The argument against the use of a chest drain is in avoidance of barotraumas as it increases the transpulmonary pressure gradient.

31.6.4 Postoperative Management

The infant is transferred to the intensive care unit, kept warm, and given maintenance requirements of intravenous fluids. The vital signs are monitored closely with regular blood gas analyses and monitoring of preductal and postductal oxygenation. Ventilatory support should be continued postoperatively. Some infants show improvement in oxygenation in the immediate postoperative period, the so-called honeymoon period, but deteriorate 6–24 h later. This deterioration is due to pulmonary hypertension and persistent fetal circulation with an increase in pulmonary artery resistance, elevated pulmonary artery pressure, and right-to-left ductal and preductal shunting leading to hypoxemia. Pulmonary hypertension is probably caused by multiple factors, such as increased abdominal pressure with impaired visceral and peripheral perfusion, limited diaphragmatic excursion, overdistension of the alveoli in the hypoplastic lungs with diminished alveolar-capillary blood flow, release of vasoactive cytokines, and deterioration in pulmonary compliance after surgical repair. Sudden deterioration in the patient's oxygenation status should raise the suspicion of pneumothorax, and a chest tube should be inserted if the diagnosis is confirmed. Infection complication, including pneumonia and septicemia, are not uncommon.

31.7 Long-Term Follow-Up

Recent improvement in the treatment of infants with CDH has increased the survival of more severely affected infants. Long-term follow up of those patients has led to the recognition of pulmonary and extrapulmonary morbidities that were not previously recognized.

Pulmonary morbidity, including pulmonary hypoplasia, bronchopulmonary dysplasia, persistant pulmonary hypertension, reactive airway disease, and limited postnatal alveolar growth, is the most common and significant problem in CDH infants surviving beyond the neonatal period. Neurodevelopmental abnormalities have been frequently described in CDH survivors. Developmental delay and abnormalities in both motor and cognitive skills have been documented. Nutritional and growth-related problems are common in CDH patients. Gastroesophageal reflux, which is one of the possible causes of this issue, has been frequently found in CDH survivors. Sensorineural hearing loss is also a well-described morbidity in CDH patients. Generally accepted risk factors for hearing loss in neonates include hyperventilation, ototoxic medications, severe hypoxemia, prolonged mechanical ventilation, and ECMO therapy. Musculoskeletal abnormalities have been also described in CDH survivors. Chest asymmetry and pectus deformity are the most commonly documented, followed by vertebral deformity. Recurrence of hernia has been reported more frequently in CDH patients repaired with a prosthetic patch. Because of significant morbidity in survivors with CDH, it has been suggested that these patients should be cared for in multidisciplinary follow-up clinics.

31.8 Congenital Eventration of Diaphragm

Eventration of the diaphragm has been described as an abnormally high or deviated position of all or part of the hemidiaphragm. Eventration may be congenital or acquired as a result of phrenic nerve palsy. Congenital eventration is a developmental abnormality that results in muscular aplasia of the diaphragm, which initially has fully developed musculature, and becomes atrophic secondary to phrenic nerve damage and disuse. Although this section deals with congenital eventration, the clinical features and principles of the management are similar in congenital and acquired forms of eventration.

31.8.1 Clinical Features

Clinical features range from being asymptomatic to severe respiratory distress. Patients may present later in infancy with repeated attacks of pneumonia, bronchitis, or bronchiectasis. Occasionally, patients present with gastrointestinal symptoms of vomiting or epigastric discomfort later in childhood. In patients with phrenic nerve palsy, there may be a history of difficult delivery. They may present with tachypnea, respiratory distress, or cyanosis. Physical examination reveals decreased breath sounds on the affected side mediastinal shift during inspiration and a scaphoid abdomen.

31.8.2 Diagnosis

The diagnosis of eventration is usually made on a chest X-ray. Frontal and lateral chest X-rays will show an elevated diaphragm with a smooth, unbroken outline. Fluoroscopy is a useful investigation for differentiating a complete eventration from a hernia. Paradoxical movement of the diaphragm is seen if complete eventration is present. Ultrasonography is the most useful study in the diagnosis of eventration of the diaphragm and for identification of abnormal organs underneath the eventration.

31.8.3 Management

Asymptomatic patients without a significant underlying pulmonary abnormality may be treated expectantly. Also, those patients with incomplete phrenic nerve palsy without paradoxical movement should be treated conservatively as normal function will usually return.

Symptomatic patients, especially those with respiratory distress, need prompt supportive care with endotracheal intubation and ventilation with humidified oxygen to minimize the diaphragmatic excursions. A nasogastric tube is passed to decompress the stomach, and intravenous fluids are commenced. Surgery is undertaken once the patient's condition is stabilized.

31.8.4 Operative Repair

Plication of the diaphragm has been used for many years to treat eventration (Fig. 31.6). Plication increases

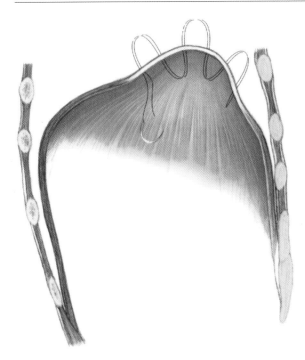

Fig. 31.6 Eventration repaired by plication of the diaphragm

both tidal volume and maximal breathing capacity and has been successful in many clinical series. An abdominal approach through a subcostal incision is preferred for left-sided eventratin but a thoracic approach through a posterolateral incision via the sixth space may be used for right-sided lesions. The transabdominal approach allows good visualization of the entire diaphragm from the front to back and easier mobilization of abdominal contents. Plication can also be accomplished by either a laparoscopic or thoracoscopic approach.

31.8.5   Outcome

The prognosis of patients with eventration of the diaphragm without underlying pulmonary hypoplasia is usually excellent. Mortality is related to pulmonary hypoplasia. Postoperative complications include recurrence and renal insufficiency.

Further Reading

Almendinger N, West SL, Wilson J (2006) Congenital diaphragmatic hernia. In MD Stringer, KT Oldham, PDE Mouriquand (eds) Pediatric Surgery and Urology: Longterm Outcomes. Cambridge University Press, Cambridge, pp 150–157

Bohn D (2002) Congenital diaphragmatic hernia. Am J Respir Crit Care Med 166:911–915

Downard CD, Jaksic T, Garza JJ et al (2003) Analysis of an improved survival rate for congenital diaphragmatic hernia. J Pediatr Surg 38:729–732

Granrholm T, Albanese CT, Harrison MR (2003) Congenital diaphragmatic hernia. In P Puri (ed) Newborn Surgery. Arnold, London, pp 309–314

Puri P (2006) Congenital diaphragmatic hernia. In Puri P, Höllwarth M (eds) Pediatric Surgery. Springer, Berlin, Heidelberg, pp 115–124

Sydorak RM, Harrison MR (2003) Congenital diaphragmatic hernia: Advances in prenatal therapy. Clin Perinatol 30:465–479

Extracorporeal Membrane Oxygenation

32

Joey C. Papa and Charles J.H. Stolar

Contents

32.1 Introduction

Extracorporeal Membrane Oxygenation (ECMO) is a life-saving technology that uses partial heart and lung bypass for extended periods. It is not a therapeutic modality, but rather a supportive tool that provides sufficient gas exchange and perfusion for patients with acute, reversible cardiac or respiratory failure. This affords the patient's cardiopulmonary system time to rest, sparing them from the deleterious effects of traumatic mechanical ventilation and perfusion impairment.

The Extracorporeal Life Support Organization (ELSO) was formed in 1989 by a collaboration of physicians, nurses, perfusionists, and scientists with an interest in ECMO. The group provides an international registry that collects data from almost all ECMO centers in the United States and throughout the world. At the end of 2005, ELSO registered nearly 30,000 neonatal and pediatric patients treated with ECMO for a variety of cardiopulmonary disorders with an overall survival rate of 66%.

32.2 Patient Selection Criteria

Neonates are the patients who benefit most from ECMO. Cardiopulmonary failure in this population can arise from meconium aspiration syndrome (MAS), congenital diaphragmatic hernia (CDH), persistent pulmonary hypertension of the newborn (PPHN), as well as several congenital cardiac diseases. For the pediatric population, the most common disorders treated with ECMO are bacterial and viral pneumonia, acute respiratory failure, ARDS, sepsis, and cardiac disease. The experience with pediatric cardiac ECMO

P. Puri and M. Höllwarth (eds.), *Pediatric Surgery: Diagnosis and Management*,
DOI: 10.1007/978-3-540-69560-8_32, © Springer-Verlag Berlin Heidelberg 2009

has been increasing over the past few years. Its use for treating postcardiotomy patients who are unable to wean from bypass as well as cardiac failure with bridge to transplantation have expanded greatly in the last decade. Some indications for ECMO that are not yet established clinically include emergency cardiopulmonary bypass and ECMO during CPR (ECPR) respiratory failure second to mediastinal compression (mass effect), smoke inhalation, severe asthma, or rewarming of hypercoagulopathic and hypothermic trauma patients (see Fig. 32.1).

The selection of patients as potential ECMO candidates continues to remain controversial. The selection criteria are based on data from multiple institutions, patient safety, and mechanical limitations related to equipment. The risk of performing an invasive procedure that requires systemic heparinization of a critically ill child must be weighted against the estimated mortality of the patient with conventional therapy alone. A predictive mortality of greater than 80% despite maximal medical management is the criterion most institutions use to select patients for ECMO. ECMO is indicated when a reversible disease process is present, tissue oxygenation requirements are not being met, and ventilator treatment is causing more harm than good. All ECMO centers must develop their own criteria and continually evaluate their patient selection based on ongoing outcomes data. A discussion

of generally accepted selection criteria for using ECMO follows.

Reversible Disease Process: The underlying principle of ECMO relies on the premise that the patient has a reversible disease process that can be corrected with either therapy or "rest" within a relatively short period of time. Exposure to high pressure mechanical ventilation with high concentrations of oxygen will frequently lead to the development of bronchopulmonary dysplasia (BPD). BPD can result from as little as 4 days of high-level ventilatory support. The pulmonary dysfunction following barotrauma and oxygen toxicity from mechanical ventilation can take weeks to months to resolve. Therefore, patients who have received aggressive ventilation for greater than 10–14 days are not considered ECMO candidates due to the high probability of established, irreversible lung injury.

Gestational Age: The gestational age should be at least 34 weeks. Significant morbidity and mortality related to intracranial hemorrhage (ICH) is associated with infants less than 34 weeks gestational age. In preterm infants, ependymal cells within the brain are not fully developed, thus making them susceptible to hemorrhage. In addition, the systemic heparinization necessary to maintain a thrombus-free ECMO circuit also increases the risk of hemorrhagic complications (Fig. 32.2).

a **Neonatal Respiratory Runs**

Diagnosis	Runs
Meconium Aspiration Syndrome	6,663
CDH	4,629
PPHN/PFC	2,996
Sepsis	2,396
RDS	1,388
Pneumonia	268
Air Leak Syndrome	97
Other	1,264

Pediatric Respiratory Runs

Diagnosis	Runs
Viral Pneumonia	747
Acute Respiratory Failure, non- ARDS	608
ARDS, not post-op/trauma	286
Bacterial Pneumonia	309
Aspiration Pneumonia	170
ARDS, post-op/trauma	72
Pneumocystis Pneumonia	22
Other	720

b **Cardiac Runs by Diagnosis**

Diagnosis	0 - 30 days	31 days - < 1yr.	1 yr. - 16 yr.	> 16 yrs.
Congenital Defect	2,119	1,366	769	77
Cardiomyopathy	73	65	204	75
Myocarditis	29	35	99	47
Cardiac Arrest	27	27	52	45
Cardiogenic Shock	24	12	34	15
Other	185	168	276	312

Fig. 32.1 Total number of ECMO runs reported by the ELSO registry at the end of 2005. (**a**) Respiratory diagnoses. (**b**) Cardiac diagnoses

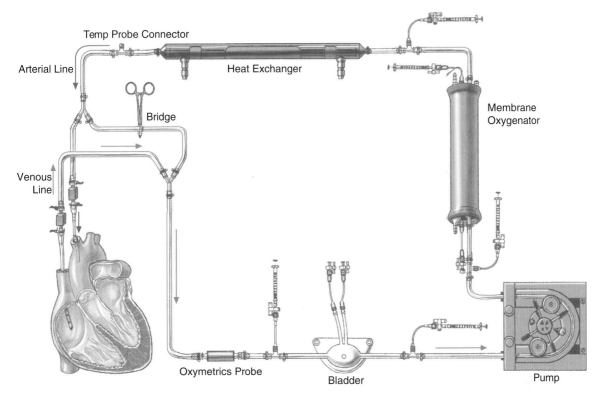

Fig. 32.2 Schematic of the ECMO circuit

Birth Weight: Technical consideration and limitation of cannula size restrict ECMO candidates to a birth weight of 2,000 g. The smallest single lumen ECMO cannula is 6 French (Fr), and flow through the tube is related to the radius of the tube by a power of 4. Babies that weigh less than 2 kg provide technical challenges in performing cannulation and in maintaining adequate flow through small catheters.

Bleeding Complications: Babies with ongoing, uncontrollable bleeding or an uncorrectable bleeding diathesis pose a relative contraindication to ECMO. Coagulopathy should be corrected before initiation of ECMO as the circuit requires continuous systemic heparinization.

Intracranial Hemorrhage: Patients who pose a high risk for ICH are those with previous history of seizures, intracranial bleed, cerebral infarction, prematurity, coagulopathy, ischemic central nervous system injury, or sepsis. Consideration of these patients for ECMO should be individualized.

In general, candidates for ECMO should not have an ICH. A preexisting ICH may be exacerbated by the use of heparin and the unavoidable alterations in cerebral blood flow while on ECMO support. Patients with small intraventricular (Grade I or II) or intraparenchymal hemorrhages can be successfully treated on ECMO by maintaining a lower than optimal activated clotting time (ACT) between 180 and 200 s. These patients should be closely observed for extension of intracranial bleeding with frequent neurologic exams and daily cranial ultrasonography.

Coexisting Anomalies: The patient should have no congenital anomalies that are incompatible with life. However, many lethal pulmonary conditions such as congenital alveolar proteinosis, alveolar capillary dysplasia, and overwhelming pulmonary hypoplasia may present as reversible diseases. Every effort should be made to establish a clear diagnosis before the initiation of ECMO as it is not intended to delay an inevitable death. Other treatable conditions, such as total anomalous pulmonary venous return and transposition of the great vessels, may initially manifest with respiratory failure but should be diagnosed with preoperative echocardiography.

Failure of Medical Management/Risk Assessment: ECMO candidates are expected to have a reversible cardiopulmonary disease process with a predictive mortality of greater than 80% despite maximal medical management. The pharmacologic agents that comprise part of the medical management include vasoconstrictive, inotropic and chronotropic agents, sedatives, and analgesics. Ventilatory management usually begins with conventional support but may also include the administration of surfactant, inhaled nitric oxide, inverse inspiratory–expiratory (I/E) ratios, or high-frequency oscillation.

Because of the invasive nature of ECMO and the potential life-threatening complications, investigators have worked to develop an objective set of criteria to predict which infants and children have 80% mortality without ECMO. Pulmonary insufficiency with associated hypoxia, hypercarbia, and acidosis is not an indication for ECMO unless tissue oxygen requirements are not being met, as evidenced by progressive metabolic acidosis, decreased mixed-venous oxygen saturation (SvO_2), and early evidence of multiple organ failure.

The two most commonly used measurements for respiratory failure are the alveolar-arterial oxygen gradient ($AaDO_2$) and the oxygenation index (OI), which are calculated as follows:

Alveolar-Arterial Oxygen Gradient

$$AaDO_2 = (P_{ATM} - 47)\,(FiO_2) - [(PaCO_2)/0.8] - PaO_2$$

Where P_{ATM} is the atmospheric pressure and FiO_2 is the inspired concentration of oxygen.

Oxygenation Index

$$OI = \frac{MAP \times FiO_2 \times 100}{PaO_2}$$

Where MAP is the mean airway pressure.

Although institutional criteria for ECMO vary, it is generally accepted that for neonates with an $AaDO_2$ greater than 625 mmHg for more than 4 h, an $AaDO_2$ greater than 600 for 12 h, or an OI greater than 40 establishes both relatively sensitive and specific predictors

of mortality. Other criteria used by many institutions include a preductal PaO_2 less than 35–50 mmHg for 2–12 h or a pH of less than 7.25 for at least 2 h with intractable hypotension. These are sustained values measured over a period of time and are not accurate individual predictors of mortality.

Older infants and children do not have such well-defined criteria for high mortality risk. The combination of a ventilation index

$$\frac{Respiratory \times rate\ PaCO_2 \times Peak\ inspiratory\ pressure}{1,000}$$

greater than 40 and an OI greater than 40 correlates with a 50–70% mortality risk. A mortality of 60–80% is associated with an $AaDO_2$ greater than 580 mmHg and a peak inspiratory pressure (PIP) of 40 cm H_2O.

Indications for support in patients with cardiac pathology are based on clinical signs of decreased peripheral perfusion, including hypotension, despite the administration of fluid resuscitation and inotropes, oliguria (urine output < 0.5 ml/kg/h), an elevated arterial lactate, and a decreased SvO_2.

Special mention should be made of infants with CDH who develop respiratory failure. Before ECMO is initiated in an infant with CDH, the infant must first demonstrate some evidence of adequate lung parenchyma. This includes maintaining a preductal oxygen saturation ≥ 90% for a sustained period of at least 1 h and at least one recorded $PaCO_2$ of less than 50 mmHg.

32.3 Methods of Extracorporeal Support

The goal of ECMO support is to provide oxygen delivery. Many different cannula configurations are possible, but the three most commonly used clinically include venoarterial (VA), venovenous (VV), and double-lumen venovenous (DLVV).

Veno-venous (VV), including single cannula, dual-lumen VV (DLVV): DLVV is used in neonates, infants, and children less than 15 kg due to limitations of flow based on cannula size. The catheter is inserted into the RIJ, with the tip in the RA. VV ECMO bypass is established by draining the RA via the RIJ, with reinfusion into a femoral vein. The advantages of VV and DLVV over VA ECMO include avoidance of arterial cannulation and permanent ligation of the carotid artery, maintaining pulsatile flow to the patient, continued blood flow to the lungs, and avoiding arterial emboli. A major limitation of DLVV ECMO is that there is mixing of unsaturated and saturated blood in the RA, because blood is both withdrawn and returned to the right atrium (RA). In addition, a fraction of the reinfused, oxygenated blood reenters the pump, called recirculation. Recirculation artificially raises the SvO_2 measurement on the pump and may limit oxygen delivery at higher flow rates.

Veno-arterial (VA): VA ECMO offers the ability to replace both cardiac and pulmonary function. Venous blood is drained from the RA through the right internal jugular vein (RIJ) and oxygenated blood is returned via the right common carotid artery (RCCA) to the ascending aorta. There are many potential disadvantages associated with VA ECMO. A major artery must be cannulated and therefore sacrificed. The risk of gas and particulate emboli being introduced into the systemic circulation is substantial. A decrease in the preload and an increase in the afterload may reduce cardiac output, resulting in nonpulsatile flow. Pulmonary perfusion is reduced and the coronary arteries are largely perfused by hypoxic left ventricular blood.

Veno-arterial (VA) via open chest: Transthoracic cannulation is the preferred mechanism of support for cardiac surgery patients who are unable to wean off bypass postcardiotomy or in cases of cardiac arrest in the immediate to early postoperative period. The venous cannula is placed directly into the right atrial appendage and the arterial cannula in the ascending aorta. The chief disadvantages to open-chest cannulation include significant risk of hemorrhage and infection (mediastinitis).

Patients with left heart or bi-ventricular failure are at risk of left ventricular distention. Left heart decompression is needed to reduce pulmonary edema, prevent pulmonary hemorrhage, and reduce ventricular distention that may aid in recovery of function. This can be avoided with a surgically created atrial septostomy or a cannula placed directly in the left atrium via open chest cannulation; patients with a preexisting atrial septal or ventricular septal defect (ASD or VSD) do not need further surgical intervention. At our institution, all patients with cardiac failure receive prophylactic atrial septostomy to prevent left-sided dilation and potential worsening cardiac function.

32.4 Cannulation

With proper monitoring, cannulation can be performed in the neonatal or pediatric intensive care units under adequate sedation and intravenous anesthesia. The child is positioned supine with the head at the foot of the bed. The head is turned to the left and the neck is hyperextended over a shoulder roll. After local anesthesia is administered over the incision site, a transverse cervical incision is made along the anterior border of the sternocleidomastoid muscle, one fingerbreadth above the right clavicle. The platysma muscle is divided, the sternocleidomastoid muscle is retracted laterally, and dissection is carried down to the carotid sheath. The sheath is opened and the internal jugular vein, common carotid artery, and vagus nerve are identified. The vein is dissected first and isolated with vessel loops. The common carotid lies medial and posterior, contains no branches, and is mobilized in a similar fashion. The vagus nerve should be identified only to protect it from injury.

Once the vessels have been isolated, the patient is given a bolus of 100 U/kg of heparin sulfate, which is allowed to circulate for 2–3 min. An ACT level should be drawn and should be greater than 300 s. For VA bypass, the arterial cannula is placed first. The carotid artery is ligated distally and once proximal control is obtained with a vessel loop a transverse arteriotomy is made near the distal ligature. Stay sutures can be placed in the artery to retract and to help prevent intimal dissection. The saline-filled cannula is inserted to its premeasured position (tip at the junction of the brachiocephalic artery and the aorta) and secured in the vessel with 2-0 silk ligatures. Additionally, a small piece of vessel loop may be placed under the ligature on the anterior aspect of the carotid to protect the vessel from injury during decannulation.

The patient must be paralyzed with succinylcholine before venous cannulation to inhibit spontaneous respiration and prevent air emboli. The jugular vein is then ligated and a venotomy is made close to the ligature. The saline-filled venous catheter is passed to a measured level of the RA and secured as described above. Any bubbles are aspirated from the cannulas, which are then connected to the preprimed ECMO circuit and bypass is initiated. The cannulae should then be secured to the patient's skin above the wound and the skin closed in layers to ensure meticulous hemostasis.

For VV and DLVV bypass, the procedure is exactly as described above, including dissection of the artery with the placement of a vessel loop to facilitate conversion to VA ECMO should the need arise. The venous catheter tip should be positioned in the mid-right atrium with the arterial portion of the DLVV catheter oriented medially to direct the flow of oxygenated blood toward the tricuspid valve. The cannula position is confirmed by chest radiography and transthoracic echocardiogram and readjusted as needed.

32.5 ECMO Circuit

Venous blood is drained from the infant or child by gravity into a small reservoir or bladder. An in-line oxymetric probe is located between the venous return cannula and the bladder to continuously monitor the SvO_2 saturation. The bladder is a 30- to 50-ml reservoir that acts as a safety valve. In the event venous drainage does not keep up with the arterial flow from the pump, the bladder volume will be depleted, the pump will be automatically shut off, and an alarm will be sounded. This serves to limit the potential for injury to the RA, RIJ, or cavitation of air and high negative pressures within the circuit. Hypovolemia is one of the common causes of decreased venous inflow into the circuit, but kinking with occlusion of the venous line should be suspected first. In addition, the height of the patient's bed can be raised to improve venous drainage by gravity.

A displacement roller pump pushes blood through the membrane oxygenator. The roller pumps are designed with microprocessors that allow calculation of the blood flow based on roller-head speed and tubing diameter of the circuit. In other words, the speed at which the pump is set determines what proportion of the patient's cardiac output will be diverted into the circuit and is adjusted according to how much support the patient requires. The pumps are connected to continuous pressure monitoring throughout the circuit and are servoregulated if pressures within the circuit exceed preset parameters. Another safety device, the bubble detector, is interposed between the pump and the membrane oxygenator and will stop flow if air is detected within the circuit.

The blood enters the membrane lung, after exiting the pump. The oxygenator consists of a long, two-compartment chamber composed of a spiral-wound silicone membrane and a polycarbonate core. This provides a large surface area across which blood and gas come into close contact, with blood flowing in one direction and gas flowing in the opposite direction. Oxygen diffuses through the membrane into the blood circuit and carbon dioxide and water vapor diffuse from the blood into the sweep gas. The size (surface area) of the oxygenator chosen is based on the patient's weight and size.

The blood emerges from the upper end of the oxygenator and passes through the countercurrent heat exchanger returning to the body at physiologic temperature into the RA (via DLVV cannulation) or the aortic arch via the RCCA.

32.6 ECMO Management

Prime Management: The tubing of the ECMO circuit is initially circulated with carbon dioxide gas. This is followed by the addition of crystalloid and 5% albumin solution. The albumin coats the tubing to decrease its reactivity to circulating blood. The carbon dioxide gas dissolves into the fluid. Approximately two units of packed red blood cells are required for initial priming of the pump, which displaces the crystalloid and colloid in the circuit.

The initial pH, oxygen content, and carbon dioxide content of the circuit are then measured and adjusted to physiologic parameters. If the prime blood is acidotic, this may exacerbate the infant's condition; or if the primed circuit has low carbon dioxide content, this may cause metabolic problems for the neonate. Additionally, a heat exchanger warms the prime to normal body temperature. In sum, the primed circuit must be physiologically compatible with life prior to initiating ECMO to maximize support and prevent initial worsening of the child's condition.

Pump Management: The goal of ECMO is to maintain adequate pump flow, which will result in good oxygen delivery to the tissues and organs. Oxygen delivery to the infant is dependent on the speed or rotations per minute (RPM) of the roller pump. Full bypass support is considered 100 cc/kg/min on VV ECMO and 150 cc/kg/min on VA ECMO. To increase a patient's oxygen level on ECMO, one can either increase the flow rate (~cardiac output) or increase oxygen carrying capacity with transfusion of PRBC to maintain a hemoglobin level of 15 g/dl (~oxygen content).

With VA ECMO, adequate perfusion and oxygen delivery can be monitored by the pH and pO_2 of a mixed venous blood sample (pre-oxygenator blood sample). The flow of the roller pump should be adjusted to maintain a mixed venous pO_2 of 37–40 mmHg and SVO_2 of 65–70%. With VV ECMO, the mixed venous sample may not be a reliable indicator of perfusion as recirculation may produce a falsely elevated pO_2. Therefore, other indicators of poor perfusion should be followed, such as persistent metabolic acidosis, oliguria, seizures, elevated liver function tests, and hypotension. If oxygen delivery is found to be inadequate, then the RPM of the pump may need to be increased to improve perfusion.

Roller pumps roll against the tubing to propel the blood towards the oxygenator. This area of contact is at risk of tubing rupture over time. To reduce the risk of rupture, the raceway is advanced every 5–7 days after temporarily stopping the pump flow. Tubing rupture is a rare event because of modern materials such as Supertygon (Norton Performance Plastics Corp., Akron, OH), a chemically altered polyvinyl chloride (PVC). The tubing should be inspected daily and all connections secured properly and replaced if defective. When a raceway rupture does occur, the pump must be turned off immediately, the patient must be ventilated and perfused with conventional methods (increased ventilator pressures and FiO_2), and CPR performed if necessary. The raceway tubing is then replaced or the entire circuit can be changed.

Oxygenator Management: The silicone membrane (envelope) oxygenator (Avecor, Inc., Minneapolis, MN) is critical to the success of ECMO and long-term bypass. The mechanism of gas exchange occurs when blood in the tubing enters a manifold region and is distributed around the envelope of a silicone membrane lung. Oxygen, which is mixed with a small amount of carbon dioxide to prevent hypocapnea, flows through the inside of the membrane envelope in a countercurrent direction to the flow of blood. Oxygen diffuses across the silicone membrane into the blood as carbon dioxide is eliminated. The oxygenated blood drains into a manifold and is returned to the infant via a heat exchanger.

Thrombus may form in the oxygenator over time. As the thrombus extends, the membrane surface area decreases, resulting in decreased oxygenation, increased carbon dioxide retention, and increased resistance to blood flow. Signs of clot formation can be detected by direct visualization of the top or bottom of the membrane, but the extent of the clot cannot be determined. Another sign of clot formation within the oxygenator is progressive consumption of clotting factors such as platelets and fibrinogen.

The gaseous portion of the oxygenator may also develop obstructions, which may lead to air emboli. Long-term use may wear out the silicone membrane resulting in blood and water in the gas phase causing water condensation. Therefore, the oxygenator should be replaced when the postoxygenator pO_2 decreases to <200 mmHg or pre-oxygenator circuit pressures increase to over 400 mmHg at flow rates required to support the patient. In addition, a larger oxygenator may also be required if the gas and blood flow rating of the old oxygenator are exceeded in order to maintain adequate perfusion.

Volume Management: While on ECMO, maintenance fluids for a term newborn under a radiant warmer are estimated at 100 cc/kg/day. Water loss through the oxygenator may approach $2 cc/m^2/h$. For a 3 kg baby, this would be about 13 cc/kg/day. Fluid losses from urine, stool, chest tubes, nasogastric tubes, ostomies, mechanical ventilation, radiant fluid loss, and blood draws should be carefully recorded and repleted. Fluid management may become difficult in the ECMO baby as fluid extravasates into the soft tissues during the early ECMO course. Therefore, meticulous recordings of the net fluid balance should be maintained on ECMO. Classically, the weight increases in the first 1–3 days as the patient becomes increasingly edematous. Starting the third day on ECMO, diuresis of the excess edema fluid begins, and can be facilitated with the use of furosemide. This diuretic phase is often the harbinger of recovery. In the event of renal failure on ECMO, hemofiltration or hemodialysis can be added to the ECMO circuit for removal of excess fluid and electrolyte correction.

Respiratory Management: Once the desired flow is attained, the ventilator should be promptly weaned to avoid further oxygen toxicity and barotrauma. Such "rest settings" have been studied and debated. At our institution, we decrease the FiO_2 to 0.4, PEEP to 5 cm H_2O, PIP to 20–25 cm H_2O, a rate of 12 breaths/min, and inspiratory time of 0.5 s if the infant's arterial and venous oxygenation are adequate.

If the baby remains hypoxic despite maximal pump flow, then higher ventilator settings may be temporarily required. Alternatively, hypoxic neonates on VV ECMO may need to be converted to VA ECMO for full cardio-respiratory support. On occasion, the chest X-ray will worsen in the first 24h independent of ventilator settings and will improve after diuresis. As the patient improves on ECMO and the pump flow is weaned, ventilator settings are then modestly increased to support the baby off ECMO.

In addition, during the course of ECMO, pulmonary toilet is essential to respiratory improvement and includes gentle chest percussion and postural drainage. Special attention should be paid to the ECMO catheters and to keep the head and body aligned. Endotracheal suctioning is also recommended every 4h and as needed based on the amount of pulmonary secretions present.

Medical Management: After the initiation of ECMO, vasoactive medications should be quickly weaned down if the blood pressure remains stable. Low-dose dopamine (5 mcg/kg/min) can be administered for renal protection, although its use is controversial. In the event of seizures, phenobarbital is usually given and maintained to prevent further seizures. In addition, gastrointestinal prophylaxis with an H2-blocker, such as ranitidine, is instituted. Fentanyl and midazolam is usually administered for mild sedation; however, the use of paralytics should be avoided as muscle activity is not only important for fluid mobilization but also to monitor neurologic activity.

Infectious prophylaxis is provided by the use of ampicillin and gentamicin, which covers most common bacterial infections. With the use of gentamicin, attention should be directed to renal function. For this reason, cefotaxime may be used for gram-negative coverage instead of gentamicin. Because of the cannula and manipulation of the circuit at stopcocks, the risk of infection is a constant concern; therefore, strict observance to aseptic technique when handling the ECMO circuit should be maintained. Daily routine blood, urine, and tracheal cultures should be obtained to monitor for infection.

Caloric intake on ECMO should be maximized using standard hyperalimentation. For a newborn, total parenteral nutrition (TPN) should be started at 100 kcal/kg/day. Normally, this should be supplied as 60% carbohydrates (14.6 gm/kg/day) and 40% fat (4.3 gm/kg/day). Intralipid infusions may be used as a fat source,

although there is some controversy with its use in the setting of severe lung disease. As a result, the percentage of fat in the hyperalimentation may be lowered. Amino acids may be added but must be considered in the setting of poor renal function and increasing BUN levels. With normal renal function, approximately 2.5 gm protein/kg/day should be provided in the TPN mixture. Electrolytes should be closely monitored with potassium, calcium, and magnesium repleted as necessary.

While on ECMO, the patient's hemoglobin is maintained at 15 gm/dl to maximize the oxygen carrying capacity of the blood. Platelet destruction during ECMO is anticipated and is secondary to the flow through the oxygenator. In order to reduce the risk of bleeding during ECMO, the platelet count should be kept above 100,000/mm. We recommend using "hyperspun" platelets in neonates to avoid the excess administration of fluid, and thus prevent further problems with volume overload and edema.

Heparin is initially administered as a bolus (50–100 mg/kg) followed by constant heparin infusion (30–60 mg/kg/h) to maintain a thrombus-free circuit. The level of anticoagulation is monitored hourly by the activated clotting time (ACT). The heparin infusion is adjusted to maintain an ACT of 180–220 s. After decannulating, the heparin infusion is stopped and not reversed with protamine sulfate.

Operative Procedures on ECMO: Surgical procedures, such as CDH repair, may be safely performed while the child remains on bypass. However, care must be taken to obtain meticulous hemostasis to avoid hemorrhagic complications. Before any invasive procedure, platelets should be transfused to a level greater than 150,000/mm^3 and the ACT level dropped to 180–200 s. The fibrinolysis inhibitor aminocaproic acid is administered as a 100 mg/kg bolus 30 min prior to incision and maintained at a continuous drip at 30 ml/kg/h for 72 h postoperatively.

Weaning and Decannulation: As the patient's underlying process improves, less blood flow is required to pass through the ECMO circuit in order to maintain adequate tissue oxygenation. The flow rate may be weaned slowly (10–20 ml/h) as long as the patient maintains oxygen saturations with evidence of adequate perfusion. The most important guide to weaning on VA ECMO is the SvO_2 and for VV ECMO, the SaO_2. When flow levels have decreased until they approximate 10% of the patient's cardiac output

(~30–50 cc/kg/min), the patient is usually ready for decannulation. As flow levels are decreased, the heparin drip should be increased for an ACT of 200–220 s to prevent thrombotic complications. Ventilator settings can be increased moderately if saturations drop during weaning, but should not revert to pre-ECMO settings. If the child continues to tolerate low flow, all medications and fluids should be switched to vascular access on the patient side and the cannulas can be clamped and flushed with heparanized saline (2 U/ml). Flow is maintained within the circuit with the bridge open as the possibility that the child may not tolerate clamping and may need to be placed back on bypass remains. Once the cannulas are clamped, the child is observed for 2–4 h. If he or she remains hemodynamically stable, with adequate saturations and does not become acidotic during this period, decannulation can safely be accomplished. Decannulation is performed in the ICU using a near-identical manner as cannulation. This should be done under sterile conditions in the Trendelenburg position using a muscle relaxant to prevent air aspiration into the vein. Once the cannula is withdrawn, the vessel is ligated, the wound irrigated, and closed over a small drain.

32.7 Complications

Complications on ECMO can be divided into technical, mechanical, or pump-related and patient-related. The most common technical complications include vessel injury or dissection during cannulation, cannula malposition and kinking, accidental decannulation, and limb ischemia from occlusion of distal flow. Most technical complications can be avoided with proper surgical technique and securing of the cannulas. Limb ischemia can be avoided with the placement of a distal perfusion catheter when signs of ischemia develop (loss of pulse, cool, mottled, or swollen extremity).

Mechanical complications include oxygenator failure, tubing rupture in the raceway (both described above), clot formation within the circuit tubing, and the introduction of air into the circuit. If clot is detected on the venous or pre-oxygenator side of the circuit, it can often be observed or segments of tubing can be selectively replaced. Clots on the arterial or postoxygenator side of the circuit are cause for concern as they can break off and cause emboli with pulmonary and neurologic complications. When a clot is detected on the arterial side, the entire circuit should be exchanged for a fresh preprimed circuit.

The introduction of air into the circuit is possible during the initial cannulation as well as through several connectors, tubing stop-cocks, and the membrane oxygenator. Prevention of air embolism is vital; when setting up the circuit, all air must be removed and all connections made tight and thoroughly inspected and the circuit must be continuously monitored. If air is detected on the venous side, it can often be aspirated from one of the ports without coming off bypass. Air on the arterial side is an emergency and requires the patient to be taken off bypass immediately until it can be safely aspirated. In the event that an air embolism reaches the patient, ECMO should be stopped, the patient placed in Trendelenburg position, and an attempt should be made to aspirate any air out of the arterial cannula. If air enters the coronary circulation, inotropic support may be necessary.

The most common patient complications are bleeding (cannula site 6.2–9.4%, surgical site 6.1–15.6%, intracranial 4.9–5.8%, GI 1.7–4.0%, tracheal, urinary) and coagulation disorders (hemolysis 12%, DIC 1.4%). Contact of blood with the foreign surface of the circuit activates the coagulation cascade. Platelets are consumed by the circuit and their function is also affected. Constant monitoring for signs of bleeding include observing for tachycardia, hypotension, a decreased hematocrit, or inadequate venous return are signs of hemorrhage. Treatment includes replenishing lost blood products, including platelets and coagulation factors, if necessary.

Patients on ECMO may also have hemodynamic compromise, including hypotension or hypertension. According to the 2005 ELSO registry, 13.2% of neonates and 43% of pediatric patients treated with ECMO for respiratory failure required the use of inotropes while on bypass. Hypotension can be from volume depletion (including blood loss) as well as decreased myocardial function from hypoxia prior to the initiation of ECMO support. Inotropes are often easily weaned when hypoxia is reversed, but euvolemia and adequate HCT should be maintained. Hypertension requiring the use of vasodilators was reported in 12.6% of neonates and 11.8% of pediatric patients. The patient should be assessed for reversible causes of hypertension such as pain, hypercarbia, and hypoxia. Hypertension should be aggressively treated due to the increased risk of intracerebral hemorrhage in ECMO patients.

Neurologic complications including intracerebral hemorrhage (ICH), infarct and stroke, and seizures can occur with an overall incidence of 20–25%. Seizures are widely reported among ECMO neonates, ranging from 20% to 70%. However, only 2% had a continued diagnosis of epilepsy at 5 years of age. Seizures in the neonatal ECMO population are associated with neurologic disease and poorer outcomes, including epilepsy and cerebral palsy. The incidence of ICH and infarct is recorded at 14% in neonates and 8% in pediatric patients on ECMO. As stated earlier, the risk is increased in low birth weight infants and premature infants <34 weeks gestation. Patients with small interventricular (Grade I or II) or intraparenchymal hemorrhages can be successfully treated on ECMO by maintaining a lower than optimal activated clotting time (ACT) between 180 and 200 s. These patients should be closely observed for extension of intracranial bleeding with frequent neurologic exams and daily cranial ultrasonography. Any progression or change in neurologic status requires cessation of anticoagulation and thus removal from ECMO support.

Oliguria and a slight rise in creatinine are common in ECMO patients and are often seen during the first 24–48 h. The capillary leak seen after placing a child on ECMO may cause decreased renal perfusion, or it may be due to the nonpulsatile nature of blood flow seen in VA ECMO. Once the patient is adequately volume resuscitated, furosemide can be used to improve urine output. The incidence of acute renal failure was 10% in neonates and 14% in pediatric patients on ECMO for respiratory support, with 10–15% requiring hemofiltration or dialysis. Continuous hemofiltration can be easily added in-line to the ECMO circuit and provides assistance with fluid balance, hyperkalemia, and azotemia, which is often not needed after ECMO support is withdrawn. Hemofiltration removes plasma water and dissolved solutes while retaining proteins and cellular components of the intravascular space.

The incidence of acquiring a nosocomial infection on ECMO has been reported at 26–30%. Associated risk factors include the duration of the ECMO run, the length of hospitalization, type of cannulation (open chest vs neck), and surgical procedures performed before or during ECMO. Fungal infections and sepsis carry a significantly higher morbidity and mortality rates. In addition, because of the large volume of blood products transfused into ECMO patients, the risk of developing a bloodborne infectious disease is significant. One study states that approximately 8% of children who were treated with ECMO as neonates were seropositive for antibodies to the Hepatitis C virus.

32.8 Results and Outcomes

There has been a decline in the use of ECMO for neonatal respiratory failure secondary to improved medical management (permissive hypercapnea and spontaneous ventilation, iNO, surfactant, and HFOV). Inhaled nitric oxide (iNO), a selective pulmonary vasodilator, improves oxygenation and has significantly contributed to the recent decrease in the need for extracorporeal membrane oxygenation (ECMO) in neonates with respiratory failure. In addition to iNO, high-frequency ventilation, the adjunct use of surfactant therapy, and improved cardiovascular support have recently been shown to decrease the need for ECMO in this patient population. According to a 10-year retrospective review of the ELSO registry data published in 2000, the use of surfactant, high-frequency ventilation, and inhaled nitric oxide in patients with respiratory failure who required ECMO increased from 0% in 1988 to 36%, 46%, and 24%, respectively, in 1997. The proportion of neonates with CDH requiring ECMO increased from 18% to 26%, while the proportion with respiratory distress syndrome decreased from 15% to 4%.

In contrast, the number of cardiac cases had steadily increased over 15 years with a peak in 2002; however, there was a notable decline in 2003 and 2004. This could be due to decreased use secondary to the poor overall survival reported, increased organ procurement and transplantation, or use of other methods of support, including the Berlin Heart Excor (Berlin Heart®, Berlin Heart AG, Berlin, Germany), LVAD, and BiVAD. In a recent study at our institution, we reviewed all transplant-related use of ECMO in patients who were placed on extracorporeal life support as a bridge to cardiac transplantation. The aggregate survival of these patients was 29% (6/21) but those who were successfully bridged to a cardiac transplant (i.e., survived on ECMO until transplanted) had 60% (6/10) survival.

Overall survival to discharge for neonates and pediatric patients treated with ECMO is dependent again on initial diagnosis. Higher survival rates are seen in neonates with respiratory diseases (77%) than cardiac diseases (38%). Within the neonatal population, newborns with MAS that require ECMO have the highest survival rate at 94%, whereas survival for infants with CDH is 52%. The pediatric population of ECMO patients represents a diverse group with regard to patient age as well as diagnosis. Over double the number of cardiac cases have been reported in the pediatric population compared to the respiratory cases (6,135 vs 2,934 at the end of 2005). Higher complication rates exist with the pediatric patients, reflecting the more complicated disease states as well as the longer duration of bypass required for reversal of the respiratory or cardiac failure.

Common long-term problems in ECMO-treated infants and children include feeding and growth sequelae, respiratory complications, and neurodevelopmental delays.

These children are at increased risk for complications both as a consequence of ECMO itself and from antecedent hypoxia, acidosis, and reperfusion injury. Approximately, one-third of infants treated with ECMO have feeding problems. The possible causes are numerous and include tachypnea, generalized central nervous system depression, poor hunger drive, postsurgical neck soreness (possibly from compression of the vagus nerve), and poor oral-motor coordination. CDH babies have a higher incidence of feeding difficulties as compared with infants with MAS secondary to foregut dysmotility, which leads to significant GERD and delayed gastric emptying. Respiratory compromise and chronic lung disease compound the problem.

Normal growth is most commonly reported in ECMO-treated patients; yet these children are more likely to experience problems with growth than age-matched normal controls. Head circumference below the fifth percentile occurs in 10% of ECMO-treated children. Growth problems are most commonly associated with ECMO children who have suffered from CDH or residual lung disease.

Neonatal ECMO survivors have a relatively high incidence of respiratory abnormalities initially with 15% requiring supplemental oxygen at 28 days of age and 25% having at least one episode of pneumonia by the age of 5 years as compared with controls (13%). These children with pneumonia are more likely to require hospitalization, and pneumonia occurs at a younger age, with over half diagnosed in the first year of life. CDH infants, in particular, have been found to have severe lung disease after ECMO and may require supplemental oxygen therapy at home.

Probably the most serious post-ECMO morbidity is neuromotor handicap. Most studies show approximately 20% (18–25%) ECMO survivors exhibit some type of handicap, with an 8–9% incidence of moderate-to-severe cognitive delay. Auditory defects are noted in over one-fourth of ECMO neonates at discharge, with sensorineural hearing loss in ~5%, speech and language delay in ~6% with roughly 10–15% requiring speech and language therapy.

Further Reading

Brown KL, Ridout DA, Shaw M et al (2006) Healthcare-associated infection in pediatric patients on extracorporeal life support: The role of multidisciplinary surveillance. Pediatr Crit Care Med 7(6):546–550 [Epub ahead of print]

Extracorporeal Life Support Organization (2005) International Registry Report of the Extracorporeal Life Support Organization. University of Michigan Medical Center, Ann Arbor, MI

Frischer J, Stolar CJ (2005) Extracorporeal Membrane Oxygenation. In KW Ashcraft, GW Holcomb III, JP Murphy (eds) Pediatric Surgery, 4th edn. Elsevier Saunders, Philadelphia, PA, pp 64–77, Chap 6

Hamrick SE, Gremmels DB, Keet CA et al (2003) Neurodevelopmental outcome of infants supported with extracorporeal membrane oxygenation after cardiac surgery. Pediatrics 111(6 Pt 1):e671–675

Kim ES, Stolar CJ (2000) ECMO in the newborn. Am J Perinatol 17(7):345–54

Puri P, Höllwarth ME (eds) (2006) Pediatric Surgery. Springer, Berlin, Heidelberg

Rozmiarek AJ, Qureshi FG, Cassidy L et al (2004) How low can you go? Effectiveness and safety of extracorporeal membrane oxygenation in lowbirth-weight neonates. J Pediatr Surg 39(6):845–7

Esophageal Atresia and Tracheoesophageal Fistula

33

Michael E. Höllwarth

Contents

33.1 Introduction

The term congenital atresia of the esophagus describes a large group of variant malformations that share a defect of the esophageal continuity with or without a fistula to the trachea or to the bronchi. It is one of the most life-threatening anomalies in a newborn baby and the quality of survival depends on early diagnosis and appropriate therapy. The first successful surgery of a 12-day-old female baby was performed by Cameron Haight at the University of Michigan in 1941. Now an adult, this patient gave birth to a newborn that suffered again from esophageal atresia that was successfully operated on at the same institution by Arnold Coran.

The history of surgical therapy of babies with esophageal atresia after Cameron Haight is a story of success starting with survival rates around 50%, but reaching nearly 100% today when associated life-threatening malformations are excluded. The mainstays of this success are appropriate diagnosis and preoperative therapy, reconstruction of the esophageal continuity with closure of an existing fistula, or esophageal replacement if necessary.

The incidence of an esophageal atresia with or without a fistula is approximately 1 in 3,000 to 4,500 births with a slight preponderance of males in the ratio of 3:2. Most cases occur sporadically. The high number of associated anomalies points to a very early disturbance of the developing embryo. A number of risk factors such as environmental teratogens are discussed in the literature including exposure to thalidomide, contraceptive pills, hormones, and endocrine diseases of the mother. Additionally, there is ample evidence that the anomaly can be genetically determined in some cases: first, chromosomal anomalies occur in 6–10% of all cases including Trisomy 13 and 18;

P. Puri and M. Höllwarth (eds.), *Pediatric Surgery: Diagnosis and Management*,
DOI: 10.1007/978-3-540-69560-8_33, © Springer-Verlag Berlin Heidelberg 2009

second, a large number of different syndromes have been reported in association with esophageal atresia; and finally the recurrence risk in a second child of parents with one affected child is around 0.5–2.0%, and the risk for a newborn born from an affected parent is around 3.0–4.0%. However, since most of the esophageal atresia occur sporadically, there is most likely a heterogeneous and multifactorial pathogenesis involving different or multiple genes and signalling pathways.

33.2 Etiology

The normal foregut embryology is still controversial. Within the fourth week of gestation, the separation of the esophagus and the trachea takes place by folding of the primitive foregut. The theories include malformation of a septum dividing the foregut from the airways, deviation of the septum in one or the other direction resulting in esophageal or tracheal atresia, and the failure of esophageal recanalization or vascularization. Recently, impaired tracheal development with the foregut developing into the trachea rather than the esophagus has been proposed. Experimental results of some authors lead to the hypothesis that the distal esophago-tracheal fistula arises as a blind ending duct from a trifurcation of the trachea and joins the stomach anlage only later, but these findings have not been confirmed by others. Today, a convincing theory of the embryology of the foregut and the atresia is still missing.

Significant insights have been provided by the Adriamycin-induced rat model of esophageal atresia. There is strong evidence of a close relationship between an abnormal notochord and disturbed somatic segmentation resulting finally in vertebral anomalies, cardiac malformation, and foregut anomalies such as esophageal atresia. Further experiments have shown a major role of the Sonic hedgehog (Shh) signalling pathway and it seems to be obvious that the Shh gene and the signalling glycoprotein are involved in the normal morphogenesis of organ systems such as notochord, vertebra, and differentiation of the trachea and esophagus. From these experiments one must conclude that there is either a primary gene related defect or an exogenous pathogenic insult that would have occurred within the first 10 days of pregnancy causing notochord dysfunction and leading to the manifestation of anomalies such as esophageal atresia or anorectal atresia, renal malformations, and others.

33.3 Associated Malformations

Due to the early embryogenesis, it is only logical that babies with esophageal atresia suffer from a high number of associated malformations in a range of 50–80%. For a successful treatment strategy, it is important to consider a detailed diagnostic workup that has significant impact on the treatment strategy. The most frequent associated anomalies are musculoskeletal malformations (20–70%), followed by cardiovascular (20–50%), genitourinary (15–25%), gastrointestinal (15–25%), and chromosomal anomalies (5–10%). The wide range of percentages given in the literature comes from differences in the diagnostic work-up. A careful X-ray of the whole vertebral spine, counting the ribs and vertebra in the different segments will show in up to 70% associated skeletal malformations and numerical variations in patients with esophageal atresia.

The most common cardiac anomaly is the ventricular septal defect (19%), which is associated with an up to 16% mortality rate. Other common anomalies include atrial septal defect (20%), tetralogy of Fallot (5%), and coarctation (1%) or right-descending aorta (4%). It is important to realize that some of these cardiac defects lead to a clinically evident heart insufficiency only a few days after delivery. Therefore, all patients with esophageal atresia should have an early echocardiography as well as ultrasound exams of the renal tract and the brain. The most common gastrointestinal associated anomaly is anorectal atresia (9%) followed by duodenal atresia (5%), malrotation (4%), and other intestinal atresia (1%). Further associated malformations may involve nearly all organ systems leading to omphalocele, neural tube defects, diaphragmatic hernia, and other anomalies. As mentioned above, association with at least 18 different syndromes are described in up to 10% of patients including Holt-Oram syndrome, DiGeorge syndrome, Goldenhair syndrome, trisomy 13, 18, 21, or the CHARGE association (**c**oloboma, **h**eart defect, **a**tresia of the choana, **r**etardation, **g**enital hypoplasia, and **e**ar deformities), and many others.

The pattern of common associated anomalies led to the creation of the acronym VATER association (vertebral anomaly, anal atresia, tracheoesophageal fistula, esophageal atresia, and renal anomaly) or VACTERL association (additionally: cardiac anomaly and limb malformation). The incidence of these associations is around 20% in the esophageal atresia population, but two or more anomalies occur in nearly half of the patients.

33.4 Classification

Classifications usually take their orientation on occurrence and type of tracheoesophageal fistula. The commonly used systems are those described by Vogt (1929) and Gross (1953). Vogt's extremely rare type 1 characterized by a more or less total lack of the esophagus is not included in Gross' classification. An isolated tracheoesophageal fistula (H-type fistula) is classified as type 4 or E, although it may belong to a different spectrum because the esophagus is patent. In Gross' classification, congenital esophageal stenosis constitutes type F (Table 33.1, Fig. 33.1). A complete list of all published variations of esophageal atresia is summarized in the dissertation work of Kluth in 1976.

In addition to the anatomical classification there are risk classifications based on birth weight, cardiac anomalies, and pneumonia, which allow comparing the results of different institutions. Associated cardiac malformations have still a significant influence on the survival rate of patients. The best-known classification is named after Waterston from 1962; however, a classification adapted to the recent progress in neonatal surgery and medicine has been published by Spitz in 1994 (Table 33.2).

Table 33.1 Anatomical classification

	VOGT-types	GROSS-types	%
Absent esophagus	1	–	–
EA without fistula	2	A	8.5
EA with fistula			
Proximal	3a	B	1.0
Distal	3b	C	85.0
Proximal and distal	3c	D	1.5
H-type fistula without atresia	4	E	4.0

33.5 Diagnosis

33.5.1 Clinical Features

The earliest symptom of esophageal atresia is a polyhydramnion in the second half of pregnancy. Polyhydramnion is an unspecific manifestation of swallowing disorders or of disturbed passage of fluid through the uppermost part of the intestinal tract of the fetus. Prenatal ultrasound may further reveal forward and backward shifting of fluid in the upper pouch and, in cases without a lower fistula, a paucity of fluid in the stomach and small intestine. Recently, fetal magnetic resonance imaging (MRI) has gained more attention for prenatal diagnosis of congenital anomalies.

Postnatal presentation is characterized by drooling of saliva, choking, coughing, and cyanotic attacks. A feeding trial is contraindicated with these symptoms because it causes early aspiration and pneumonia. The next diagnostic step is to pass a 12 F (firm and X-ray visible) feeding tube into the stomach. If this is not successful, esophageal atresia is almost certain. However, small tubes must be avoided because they may curl up in the upper pouch thereby giving the illusion that they have been pushed forward into the stomach (Fig. 33.2). If an esophageal atresia is suspected, a physical examination of the entire body is performed to detect further associated malformations.

33.5.2 Radiological Diagnosis

The next step is to perform a plain X-ray including the neck, the thorax, and the abdomen. The approximate length of the upper pouch can be estimated by the length of the X-ray visible tube in it. Air below the diaphragm can be seen in the presence of a lower tracheoesophageal fistula and additional fluid levels indicate a duodenal or intestinal atresia. A gasless abdomen indicates a pure esophageal atresia without a lower fistula (Fig. 33.3). A long distance between the segments is to be expected, but a tiny or secondary occluded fistula may be present extremely rarely. The translucency of the lungs provides the first information on whether aspiration pneumonia—either from the saliva or from the refluxed gastric acid through the lower fistula—is present. Some researchers inject 0.5–1.0 ml water-soluble

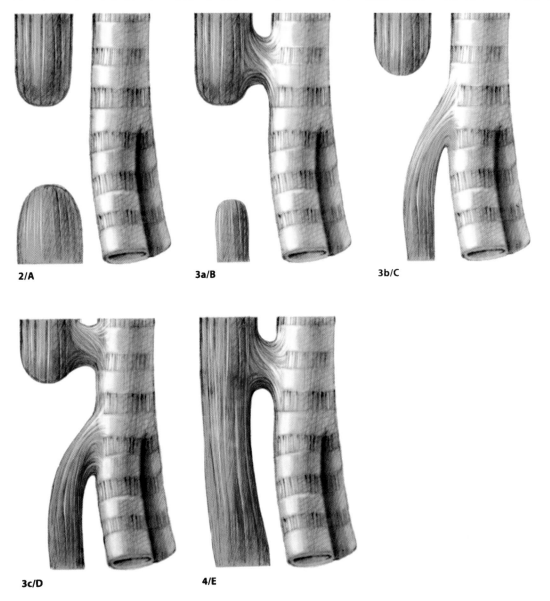

2/A   3a/B   3b/C

3c/D   4/E

Fig. 33.1 The most common different forms of esophageal atresia

contrast material (we see no need for barium contrast material) through the tube into the upper pouch under additional fluoroscopic control to detect a proximal tracheoesophageal fistula. Cardiologic assessment, including echocardiography forms a part of routine preoperative workup in order to recognize associated congenital cardiac anomalies or the presence of a right-descending aorta, which is important for the surgeon. Abdominal and urogenital ultrasound is performed routinely. Finally, one should first look for whether or not structural or numerical anomalies exist along the vertebral column or the ribs. Chromosomal analysis is performed only if the external aspect of the baby is suspicious for a genetic defect.

The history of a patient with an H-type fistula is different: there is no passage problem but the leading symptoms are recurrent coughing and cyanotic attacks during feeding due to aspiration through the fistula. Presentation is usually more protracted and sometimes delayed beyond the first year of life.

Table 33.2 Risk classification

	Waterstone	Survival (%)
Birthweight > 2.500 g otherwise healthy	A	100
Birthweight 2.000–2.500 g or higher mild pneumonia or moderate cardiac anomalies	B	85
Birthweight < 2.000 g or higher, severe pneumonia or severe associated cardiac anomalies	C	65
	Spitz	Survival (%)
Birthweight > 1.500 g otherwise healthy	I	97
Birthweight < 1.500 g or major cardiac anomaly	II	59
Birthweight < 1.500 g major cardiac anomaly	III	22

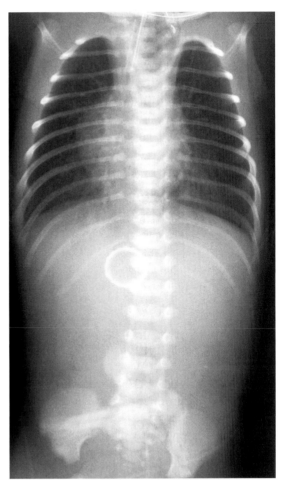

Fig. 33.3 Esophageal atresia without lower esophageal fistula indicating a long distance between esophageal segments

Diagnosis is made by esophagography with water-soluble contrast material that shows the spillage of parts of the contrast material through the fistula into the trachea. Tracheoscopy confirms the diagnosis.

33.6 Management

33.6.1 Preoperative Management

The babies are nursed in the ICU. Immediate surgery is rarely required; hence, all the above-mentioned investigations can be performed step by step. An oro- or naso-esophageal insertion of a double-lumen Replongle tube is mandatory for continuous or intermittent aspiration

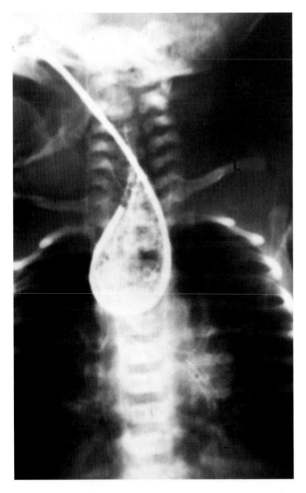

Fig. 33.2 In this case, a very small feeding tube was used to diagnose esophageal atresia. It resulted in a curling up in the upper esophageal pouch misleading to the diagnosis of a normal esophagus. Therefore, a rather firm and thicker tube has to be used for this procedure

of saliva in order to prevent aspiration. The baby should be positioned upright to minimize gastroesophageal reflux into the trachea and lungs via the lower fistula. Intubation and ventilation is necessary only in cases of respiratory distress, severe pneumonia, or severe associated malformations demanding respirator therapy. In these cases, the endotracheal tube should be possibly positioned beyond a distal tracheoesophageal fistula to avoid insufflation of gas into the stomach. Broadspectrum antibiotics, intravenous fluid therapy, and vitamin K analogue is administered before surgery. If severe pneumonia exists, surgery has to be postponed until the lung recovers. In the case of severe associated malformations (e.g. diaphragmatic hernia or cardiac malformation), a decision should be taken on the type of surgical procedure to be performed first or whether they should be performed in one step.

33.6.2 Operative Management

33.6.2.1 Esophageal Atresia with Distal Tracheoesophageal Fistula (85%)

Surgical repair is performed under general anaesthesia with endotracheal intubation. As mentioned above, the endotracheal tube is advanced close to the tracheal bifurcation and the infant is ventilated manually with rather low inspiratory pressure and small tidal volumes. We advice to start the procedure routinely with a *tracheo-bronchoscopy* using a rigid 3.5 mm endoscope. The trachea and the main bronchi are briefly inspected, and the fistula to the esophagus is localized, which is usually 5–7 mm above the carina. Exceptionally, it may be found at the carina or even in the right main bronchus indicating a short lower segment, and most likely a long esophageal gap. The next step is to look for an upper fistula. The dorsal membranous region of the tracheal wall is inspected carefully up to the cricoid's cartilage. Small upper fistulas can be missed. To avoid this pitfall, irregularities of the dorsal tracheal wall are gently probed with the tip of a 3 F ureteric catheter passed through the bronchoscope. If a fistula is present, the catheter will glide into it.

The goal of the surgical procedure is to divide the fistula, to close it on the tracheal side, and to perform an end-to-end anastomosis between the esophageal

segments. The essential surgical part is to ensure a very careful and non-tissue traumatizing procedure. The standard approach is through a right-sided extrapleural latero-dorsal thoracotomy via the fourth interspace. Recently, some authors published successful thoracoscopic repair of the atresia, but this is certainly a very demanding procedure and needs great experience in endoscopic surgery. If a right aortic arch is diagnosed preoperatively, a left-sided approach is recommended unless there is a double aortic arch. However, if an unsuspected right-descending aorta is encountered, the procedure can be continued in most cases, establishing the anastomosis to the right of the aortic arch. The azygos vein is divided between ties and the fibers of the vagal nerve are preserved as good as possible. The fistula is closed near the trachea, avoiding any narrowing of the airway. The anastomosis of the esophagus is performed with 6/0 absorbable sutures. The upper pouch mucosa often retracts and can be missed if the surgeon does not take particular care with the anastomosis. To facilitate the identification of the upper pouch, the Replongle tube can be pushed forward by the anaesthetist. Once the posterior wall is sutured, a 5 F feeding tube is introduced into the stomach with one end and back to the mouth with the other end to allow early postoperative feeding. In most cases with a distal fistula the goal of a tension-free anastomosis can be achieved. If the tension appears to be too much despite extensive mobilization of the lower esophagus and the upper pouch, further length may be gained with a circular myotomy (Livatitis method) (Fig. 33.4). However, some authors described the formation of problematic pseudodiverticula after this procedure. Another way to reduce inappropriate tension to the anastomosis in some cases is to fashion a mucosa-muscular flap from the upper esophageal

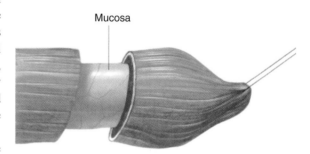

Fig. 33.4 The circular myotomy according to Livadatis can lengthen the upper esophageal pouch by 0.5–1.0 cm

Fig. 33.5 If a very large upper esophageal pouch is present, a flap can be fashioned to bridge the distance to the lower esophagus

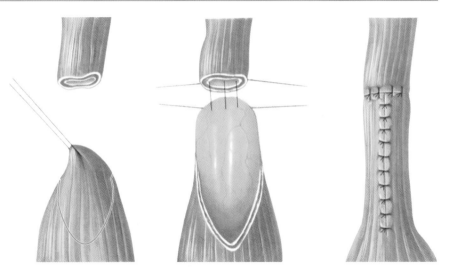

pouch (Fig. 33.5). At the end of the procedure, the thorax is closed. The use of a drain depends on the preference of the surgeon, but it should be away from the anastomosis to avoid any mechanical complication.

33.6.2.2 Esophageal Atresia with Proximal and Distal Tracheoesophageal Fistula (1.5%)

As mentioned above, a careful endoscopic examination of the dorsal tracheal wall using a 3 F ureteric catheter enables the surgeon to detect an upper fistula that can be as high as the cricoid cartilage. The catheter can be left in the fistula to facilitate the identification when the upper pouch is separated from the trachea. Any damage to the trachea should be carefully avoided. The recurrent laryngeal nerve runs in the groove between the trachea and the esophagus and must be identified and protected. The fistula is closed flush to the trachea and esophagus with 6/0 sutures.

33.6.2.3 Esophageal Atresia with a Proximal Tracheoesophageal Fistula Only: A Long Gap Problem (1%)

In the above-mentioned case, a long gap between the upper pouch and the lower esophagus has to be expected; therefore, a primary thoracotomy is not indi-

cated. The first step is to perform a gastrostomy and to insert a radio-opaque tube into the lower esophagus. The X-ray shows either a rather short lower esophageal pouch with a long distance between the segments, or even a tiny anlage of esophagus that cannot be used for an anastomosis. The gastrostomy is needed for feeding the baby and, depending on the choice of the surgeon, for the longitudinal bouginage (see later in this chapter).

The upper fistula can be approached and identified via a right neck incision. A 3 F catheter that has been inserted during tracheoscopy allows easy identification of the fistula, which is then divided and closed on both sides. The recurrent laryngeal nerve should be identified and preserved. The Replongle probe allows continuous suction from the upper pouch until the final procedure is performed.

33.6.2.4 H-Type Fistula (4%)

The fistula is identified by endoscopy and a 3 F ureteric catheter is passed across the fistula into the esophagus. Most H-type fistulas can be approached from the right side of the neck because they are usually situated at or above the level of the second thoracic vertebra. Palpation of the ureteric catheter facilitates the identification of the fistula. Again the upper laryngeal nerve must be identified and carefully preserved.

33.6.2.5 Isolated Esophageal Atresia: The Long Gap Problem (8.5%)

An airless abdomen on thoraco-abdominal X-ray leads to suspicions of an esophageal atresia without a lower fistula. An anastomosis is usually not possible in these cases due to the long distance between the esophageal pouches. Therefore, the primary procedure consists of the placement of a gastrostomy tube to allow early enteral feeding. During the operative procedure, the distance between the pouches can be estimated radiologically by inserting a radio-opaque tube in the upper pouch and across the gastrostomy in the lower pouch. A distance of three to four vertebral bodies on a chest film is considered as a long gap, and a distance of five or more vertebral bodies is an ultra long gap

Two basic surgical strategies are available in cases of long-gap esophageal atresia: either the preservation of the patient's own esophagus with delayed repair or esophageal replacement. All efforts should be directed to salvage the child's own esophagus because the ideal graft does not exist. Concerning the preservation of the native esophagus, three strategies exist: the first is to await spontaneous growth, which is more pronounced in the upper pouch—it needs 12–16 weeks on average

until a safe anastomosis is feasible; second, one can attempt to promote elongation of the upper esophageal segment by longitudinal stretching twice a day; third, approximation may be further accelerated by additional bouginage of the lower pouch through the gastrostomy. With the latter method, overlapping segments can be achieved within 3–5 weeks (Fig. 33.6). Recently, a modification of the old Rehbein's traction technique by using external traction forces has been described by Foker, but his results are controversially discussed and approval from other centers is still pending. In any case, it is essential to prove that a lower esophageal segment truly exists and is significantly different from a tiny nubbin at the upper end of the stomach. In the latter case, elongation procedures are useless and esophageal replacement should be planned primarily.

For esophageal replacement there are five options: reverse or isoperistaltic gastric tube, colon interposition, jejunal interposition, and gastric pull-up. There is no agreement on a single organ or a single route. While gastric tubes or free and pediculed jejunal tubes are used in some centers only, the most common techniques are colon interposition or gastric transposition. With the former technique the isoperistaltic transverse colon segment on the left colic vessels is the preferred

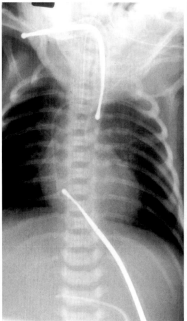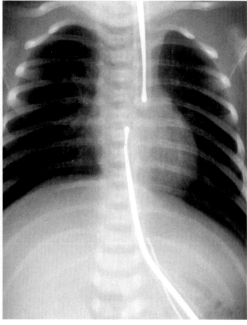

Fig. 33.6 Longitudinal bouginage of the upper and the upper and lower esophageal pouch (metal probes within plastic tubes). A near overlapping of the esophageal segments was achieved within 3 weeks

method of esophageal replacement. The colon is pulled up to the neck either substernally or through the hiatus and the posterior mediastinum. Unfortunately, the colon loses its own peristalsis with the procedure and the passage of ingested food is entirely by gravity. Typical complications are a leak of the upper anastomosis on the neck, intrathoracic redundant colon with delayed emptying and unpleasant stasis of ingested food, and graft necrosis in the worst case.

The gastric transposition is technically not so demanding because the organ has an excellent blood supply and the procedure involves only a single anastomosis in the neck. Typical complications are again anastomotic leaks or strictures and ulcers, delayed gastric emptying, and occasionally dumping syndrome.

33.6.3 Complications

Despite excellent long-term survival rate, there are a large number of early and late complications that need special care and attention.

33.6.3.1 Early Complications

The incidence of early complications has been reduced significantly in the last few decades. Today, a newborn with esophageal atresia is diagnosed in most centers shortly after birth by the probe test thereby preventing early pneumonia and aspiration after milk feeding. Additionally, surgical techniques have been refined and the quality of the suture material is significantly better than in the past. Finally, the progress in pre- and postoperative care as well as with the anesthesia techniques and pain control contribute largely to the excellent outcome rates in the Waterston A and B groups. An early but fortunately rare complication is the recurrence of the tracheoesophageal fistula (3%), which usually occurs following a significant anastomotic leak. Air bubbles out of the drain and a pneumothorax and a more or less extensive shadow can be recognized on the thoracic X-ray. A spontaneous closure cannot be expected; thus, the therapy consists of a rethoracotomy and surgical closure of the fistula and the anastomosis. This procedure is not easy because the local inflammatory process causes edema and a reduced tissue quality. Fibrinogen glue may be

helpful, including the use of a large pleural flap from the mediastinum or a vascularized pericardial flap interposed between the trachea and the esophagus.

The incidence of an isolated *anastomotic le*ak should be lower than 10% if no tension was on the anastomosis. In most of these cases the defects are small and clinically insignificant. We perform an esophagogram with water-soluble contrast material seven days after the procedure—it may show a tiny fistula from the anastomosis indicating the anastomotic leak. If the patient's conditions are stable we may even start oral feeding because spontaneous closure of the fistula can be expected. The early sign of a large fistula is the excretion of saliva through the thoracic drain. In these cases, oral feeding is postponed until the radiological control shows the closure of the fistula.

An anastomotic stenosis is a common finding. The esophagogram often shows a narrow anastomosis due to the differences in calibre of the esophageal segments. This finding is different from a true stenosis and in most cases oral feeding is tolerated without symptoms. A true cicatriceal stenosis does not improve spontaneously and causes a significant feeding problem sooner or later. Minimal stenosis can be treated successfully with one to three careful dilatations—to avoid esophageal rupture. A chronic esophageal stenosis results often when significant tension is on the anastomosis and it is aggravated by acidic gastroesophageal reflux. In the first line, several dilatations as well as proton pump inhibitor therapy are needed; in the long run, a fundoplication is necessary in most cases.

Tracheomalacia is a common finding after esophageal atresia patients with lower fistula. The weak part of the trachea is in the region of the former fistula. It causes a typical barking cough and an inspiratory stridor, which is in most cases self-limiting after a few months. However, severe forms of tracheomalacia may lead to respiratory insufficiency, apneic spells, and to sudden infant death syndromes. In these cases an aortopexy is the most often performed procedure, either by an open approach or by thoracoscopy. We used a Palmaz stent to stabilize the trachea (Fig. 33.7) in several cases. The stent is introduced endoscopically and the respiratory problems are normalized immediately. However, if the stent is not dilated sufficiently, recurrent granulation tissue is a typical complication due to the movements of the stent relative to the trachea. In contrast, if the stent is in firm contact with the trachea, the mucosa tends to grow over, and removal after the

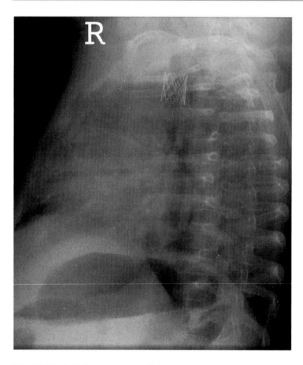

Fig. 33.7 A Palmaz stent used for severe tracheomalacia with life-threatening spells. The stent stabilized the trachea immediately and was removed after 8 months

period of a few months may be difficult. Different types of stents are available today, but experience is still poor.

33.6.3.2 Late Complications

The most common late complication is *gastroesophageal reflux* causing feeding problems, vomiting, reduced weight gain or dystrophy, and recurrent respiratory tract infections. Reflux is very typical when the lower segment of the esophagus has to be pulled-up to be able to perform a primary anastomosis. In contrast to otherwise normal babies, there is no chance for spontaneous maturation of the disturbed esophageal function. Chronic exposure of the anastomosis to refluxed gastric acid is a well-known cause of recurrent stenosis or Barrett's esophagus. Furthermore, the propulsive peristalsis in the lower segment of the

esophagus is missing and clearance time for acidic refluxes is significantly longer when compared to children with pathological reflux but without esophageal atresia. Therefore, nearly half of all patients with esophageal atresia need a fundoplication, which should be performed as soon as significant clinical problems occur.

Common long-term problems are recurrent respiratory tract infections due to microaspirations or some kind of swallowing disorders due to the missing or abnormal peristaltic activity of the lower segment. However, most patients learn to cope with this problem and are used to drinking fluids along with their meals as soon as they feel that a bolus does not pass easily through the esophagus.

In conclusion, neonates with esophageal atresia have an excellent prognosis if no severe additional malformations are present. However, problems still exist in babies with long-gap atresia. The use of the patient's own esophagus at each prize—e.g. with the Foker method—causes significant long-term problems due to the abnormal peristalsis, recurrent anastomotic stenosis, and severe gastroesophageal reflux. Although esophageal replacement strategies are well-established methods, they have also a number of short and long-term complications; thus, the ideal method has not been found yet.

Further Reading

Grosfeld JL, O'Neil Jr JA, Fonkalsrud EW, Coran AG (2006) Pediatric Surgery. Mosby–Elsevier, Philadelphia

Höllwarth ME, Zaupa P (2006) Oesophageal Atresia. In P Puri, ME Höllwarth (eds) Pediatric Surgery, Springer Surgery Atlas Series. Springer-Verlag Berlin Heidelberg, New York, pp 29–48

Kluth D (1977) Die Mißbildungen des Ösophagus und der Trachea. Dissertation, Medical University of Lübeck

Merei JM, Hutson JM (2002) Embryogenesis of tracheo esophageal anomalies: A review. Pediatr Surg Int 18:319–326

Puri P (2003) Neonatal Surgery. Arnold, London

Spitz L (2006) Esophageal atresia. Lessons I have learned in a 40-year experience. J Pediatr Surg 41:1635–1640

Spitz L, Kiely EM, Morecroft JA, Drake DP (1994) Oesophageal atresia: At-risk groups for the 1990s. J Pediatr Surg 29:723–725

Gastroesophageal Reflux Disease

34

Keith Georgeson

Contents

34.1 Introduction

Vomiting and regurgitation are common occurrences in childhood. Seventy percent of 4-month-old infants regurgitate daily but only 25% of their parents consider it a problem. The challenge for physicians is to differentiate the symptoms that are physiologic and will resolve spontaneously from those that need medical or surgical intervention. Gastroesophageal reflux disease (GERD) is defined as the pathologic consequences of the involuntary passage of gastric contents into the esophagus. In adults, GERD is primarily concerned with peptic esophagitis and its complications, including heartburn, esophageal stricture, and the formation of Barrett's esophagus. In children, pathologic reflux is considerably more complex. Gastroesophageal reflux is most commonly seen in children with neurologic dysfunction. Neurologically impaired children with GERD often have associated swallowing disorders, failure to thrive, primary aspiration, spasticity, increased intraabdominal pressure, and central mechanisms for inducing gagging and retching. Additionally, they often have associated delayed gastric emptying, dysmotility of the esophagus and upper gastrointestinal tract, and a hiatus hernia. Neurologically normal infants and children have reflux-associated reactive airways disease, aspiration, aspiration pneumonia, laryngeal symptoms, and apnea. Sometimes this apnea is prolonged and life-threatening. Children with GERD also have digestive symptoms including frequent regurgitation with failure to thrive, irritability, food rejection, heartburn, hematemesis, melena, dysphagia, and Barrett's esophagus.

P. Puri and M. Höllwarth (eds.), *Pediatric Surgery: Diagnosis and Management,*
DOI: 10.1007/978-3-540-69560-8_34, © Springer-Verlag Berlin Heidelberg 2009

34.2 Etiology

The precise mechanisms that predispose infants and children to gastroesophageal reflux are unknown. A high-pressure zone in the lower portion of the esophagus plays an important role in the prevention of gastroesophageal reflux. A critical length of intraabdominal esophagus is necessary to prevent GERD. Anatomical defects that affect the high pressure zone of the gastroesophageal junction and interfere with rapid clearing of physiologic gastroesophageal reflux are associated with significant reflux pathology.

34.3 Pathophysiology

GERD occurs when refluxed contents produce clinical symptoms or result in histopathologic alterations. Symptoms of GER can develop when a combination of dysfunctional esophageal peristalsis, esophageal clearance, abnormally low esophageal sphincter pressures, the presence of a hiatus hernia, delayed gastric emptying, increased intraabdominal pressure, and underlying congenital problems such as esophageal atresia or diaphragmatic hernia impact the mechanisms responsible for preventing or clearing GER. As mentioned previously, neurologically impaired children have many of these factors working in combination.

34.4 Diagnosis

There are few objective studies that compare the value of the various techniques used for the diagnosis of GERD in children. Tests for GERD are individually useful in documenting different aspects of GER and are valuable only when used in an appropriate clinical context.

History and physical examination: The history and physical examination are the most important components of the evaluation of an infant or child with GERD. Reflux-related symptoms such as failure to thrive, recurrent coughing, reactive airways disease, stridor, apnea, recurrent aspiration pneumonia, irritability, heartburn, abdominal pain, and dysphagia are all seen in patients with symptomatic GERD. In general, infants and children are high volume refluxers.

Recurrent vomiting is a common clinical event reported in these children.

An upper gastrointestinal contrast series is not specific or sensitive for the diagnosis of GER in children. It does show the patient's anatomy and can rule out other causes of vomiting such as pyloric stenosis, malrotation, duodenal outlet obstruction, and esophageal stricture. Esophageal pH monitoring measures the duration and frequency of acid reflux episodes. It should be used in conjunction with regular daily activities such as eating and sleeping. A reflux episode is defined as an esophageal pH of less than 4 for a period of 15–15 s. It should be noted that reflux is more common in the first year of life than in adults; hence, adult indices are not applicable to children. This is especially true in infants who have a much higher percentage of total reflux time than children or adults.

Recently, impedance technology has been described, which detects all types of reflux into the esophagus. Impedance technology may be very important in the workup of children with GER because more than half of their reflux episodes are nonacid events. Further investigation is needed to determine how impedance technologies can be useful in the diagnosis of GERD in infants and children.

Endoscopy and biopsy are useful in determining the presence and degree of esophagitis in patients with GERD. Histologic assessment of the esophageal lining is much more accurate than the endoscopic appearance. Pathologists then grade the level of esophagitis and can also detect the presence of Barrett's esophagus. Barrett's esophagus is the presence of columnar epithelium replacing the squamous epithelium of the normal esophagus. Barrett's esophagus is a premalignant disorder, especially as the cells become progressively more dysplastic.

Nuclear scintigraphy scanning is commonly used to detect delayed gastric emptying in children with GER. Many children with GER show delayed gastric emptying. However, the difficulty in standardizing the technique and the questionable benefit of performing a gastric outlet procedure limit the value of this test.

In summary, the appropriate steps of the evaluation of a child suspected of having GER are controversial. The workup must include a careful history and physical examination. An upper GI study to look for abnormalities, a 24-h pH probe monitoring study or an impedance study, and in some cases endoscopy with biopsy of the distal esophageal mucosa are often indicated as part of the workup.

34.5 Differential Diagnosis

An upper GI study can often help differentiate the presence of achalasia or duodenal stenosis from GER. Esophageal biopsies can detect eosinophilic esophagitis. A good history will usually define cyclical vomiting as opposed to GER.

34.6 Treatment

Medical management. Most infants and children who have symptoms of gastroesophageal reflux can benefit from changes in life style. Smaller, frequent feeding is encouraged in babies instead of larger feedings at infrequent intervals. Thickened feedings may be helpful. Infants and children with poor weight gain can be fed diets with higher caloric density. Hypoallergenic feedings can also be given to infants who may be vomiting due to a reaction to a particular formula. Although esophageal pH monitoring has demonstrated that infants have significantly less GER in the prone position than in the supine position, prone positioning has been associated with a higher rate of sudden infant death syndrome (SIDS). Therefore, nonprone positioning should be utilized during sleep for small infants. Prone positioning is acceptable if the baby is awake, in the postprandial period. In older children, conservative treatment includes weight loss if the patient is overweight, and avoidance of large meals, caffeine, chocolate, and spicy foods. The addition of proton pump inhibitors (PPIs) or histamine-2 receptor antagonists (H2RA) have been shown by randomized studies to be helpful in treating GERD in children. There have been no randomized studies documenting the clinical usefulness of prokinetic agents such as erythromycin and metoclopramide.

34.7 Interventional Therapies

There have been few reports of the benefits of endoluminal treatments in children. Most of these endoluminal treatments use instruments that are too large for application in small children. The use of endoluminal radiofrequency ablation of the distal esophageal mucosa has been reported but is not currently available for clinical use and has never been used in small children. Endoluminal suture plication of the GE junction has also been reported in a small number of children as a treatment for GE reflux. Similar suture plication studies in adults have shown mixed results with a high incidence of recurrence.

34.8 Surgical Management

Surgical management is indicated for children in the following circumstances:

1. Failure of medical therapy
2. Presence of an associated anatomical defect such as a hiatal hernia, malrotation, or diaphragmatic hernia
3. Esophageal stricture secondary to GERD
4. Postesophageal atresia repair with a recurrent stricture that does not respond to medical treatment
5. Neurologically impaired children who have difficulty feeding and have serious reflux-associated symptoms

The aim of surgery in GER is to prevent episodes of reflux while avoiding complications such as dysphagia and the inability to burp and vomit. Many operative techniques have been described for children. They can be divided into complete wrap procedures and partial wrap procedures. All of these techniques attempt to achieve a physiologic high-pressure zone at the distal end of the esophagus that will prevent reflux. Most studies report a higher incidence of recurrent GER after a partial wrap technique. However, some papers have reported a higher incidence of dysphagia, the inability to burp and vomit, and increased flatulence after a complete wrap fundoplication. Both complete and partial wrap fundoplications continue to be advocated by various pediatric surgery groups.

The Nissen fundoplication is the most commonly performed surgical procedure to correct GER in children (Fig. 34.1). The fundus is fitted around the esophagus for 360° for a distance of 1.5–2 cm. The wrap is performed over an appropriate-sized bougie to prevent the creation of a tight wrap.

The Thal fundoplication is a 180–270° anterior wrap of the fundus around the distal esophagus. Results after this technique are variable with some surgeons reporting a very high degree of success in relieving GER in children (Fig. 34.2).

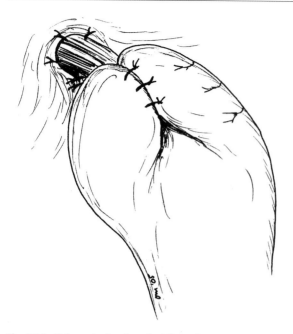

Fig. 34.1   Schematic drawing of a Nissen fundoplication. Note that the dilated esophagus must be pulled down into the abdominal cavity

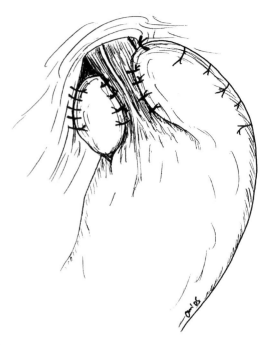

Fig. 34.3   The Toupet technique is characterized by a 270° wrap of the fundus dorsal of the esophagus.

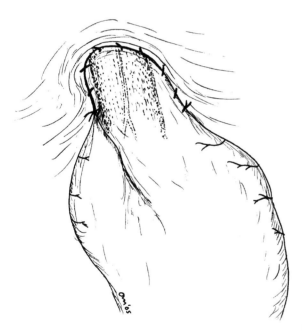

Fig. 34.2   The Thal procedure consists of a 270° wrap of the fundus ventral to the esophagus

The Toupet fundoplication is a 270° posterior partial wrap. As with the Thal fundoplication, it seems to be less effective than a complete wrap in preventing

GER. However, several large series have been reported with excellent results (Fig. 34.3).

All of these procedures were initiated using open access. However, the open approach has generally been replaced by the laparoscopic access. Laparoscopic fundoplication has now become the standard of care with results equivalent to the open technique. One difference between the techniques is that recurrent reflux often occurs after herniation of the wrap into the chest following laparoscopic fundoplication, whereas breakdown of the fundoplication wrap is the more common cause of recurrent reflux after open fundoplication.

34.9 Complications of Antireflux Procedures

Complications may be classified according to their occurrence—early or late after surgery. Early complications include dysphagia, which usually resolves within a few weeks. If the patient is having serious difficulty swallowing, a nasogastric tube can be passed and the patient fed through this tube for about 2 weeks followed by removal of the tube and normal feeding. Long-term dysphagia is more commonly caused by overzealous tightening of the hiatus during the fundoplication procedure.

Recurrent reflux is also a common complication after a fundoplication in children. It is most often related to postoperative retching and gagging. It can also be caused by overzealous feeding through a gastrostomy tube. Other less common complications include gas-bloat syndrome and postoperative dumping. Gas-bloat can be managed by removing the air in the stomach prior to feedings through the gastrostomy button. Dumping can be treated by smaller, more frequent feedings or drip feedings.

34.10   Outcome and Results

The success rates of open and laparoscopic antireflux procedures are excellent. In a multicenter review of more than 7,000 children over a 20 year period, good to excellent results were achieved in 95% of neurologically normal children and 85% of neurologically impaired children. As mentioned earlier, partial wrap fundoplication seems to be associated with a higher rate of recurrent reflux, but may be associated with less gas-bloat symptoms or the inability to vomit. Children at high risk for recurrent reflux should be treated with a primary biologic hiatal patch. Children with recurrent reflux due to herniation of the wrap into the chest should also be treated by reinforcing the hiatus with a biologic patch.

34.11   Gastrostomy

Gastrostomy is often performed in children with swallowing disorders, food refusal, and the chronic failure to thrive. Children with a short-term need for enteral feeding are benefited by nasogastric or nasojejunal tubes. However, patients with a long-term need for enteric feeding are best served by gastrostomy or jejunostomy.

It is controversial whether patients who need gastrostomy placement should undergo a workup for GER. Some authors contend that no workup is needed. They feel that most patients with a gastrostomy will tolerate feedings without significant reflux. However, other pediatric surgeons strongly recommend a workup for GER in children before a gastrostomy tube is placed. Those children identified with significant reflux should have a fundoplication in addition to the gastrostomy according to this school of thought. A third option is selectively performing a workup for GER in patients scheduled for gastrostomy if the patient has a history of significant vomiting. The history seems to be more important than the physiologic parameters identified by a workup. Often, the best test is to use a nasogastric tube for feeding purposes for 1 or 2 weeks, prior to placement of the gastrostomy. If the child tolerates installation of feeds into the stomach without significant vomiting, the patient will likely tolerate gastrostomy feeds without the need for a fundoplication.

Further Reading

Georgeson K (2002) Results of laparoscopic antireflux procedures in neurologically normal infants and children. Semin Laparosc Surg 9:172–176

Gibbons TE, Gold BD (2003) The use of proton pump inhibitors in children: A comprehensive review. Paediatr Drugs 5:25–40

Gremse DA (2002) Gastroesophageal reflux disease in children: An overview of pathophysiology, diagnosis, and treatment. J Pediatr Gastroenterol Nutr 35:S297–S299

Hunter JG, Smith CD, Branum GD et al (1999) Laparoscopic fundoplication failures: Patterns of failure and response to fundoplication revision. Am Surg 230:595–604

Georgeson KE (2006) Gastro-oesophageal Reflux and Hiatus Hernia. In P Puri, ME Höllwarth (eds) Pediatric Surgery, Springer Surgery Atlas Series. Springer-Verlag, Berlin, Heidelberg, New York, pp 49–60

Paterson WG (2001) The normal antireflux mechanism. Chest Surg Clin N Am 11:473–483

Rothenberg SS (2002) Laparoscopic Nissen procedure in children. Semin Laparosc Surg 9:146–152

Rudolph CD, Mazur LJ, Liptak GS et al (2001) Guidelines for evaluation and treatment of gastroesophageal reflux in infants and children. Recommendations of the North American Society for Pediatric Gastroenterology and Nutrition. J Pediatr Gastroenterol Nutr 32:S1–S31

Vandenplas Y (1994) Reflux esophagitis in infants and children: A report from the working group on gastro-oesophageal reflux disease of the European Society of Paediatric Gastroenterology and Nutrition. J Pediatr Gastroenterol Nutr 18:413

Achalasia

35

Paul K.H. Tam and Kenneth K.Y. Wong

Contents

35.1 Introduction

Achalasia is a disorder of esophageal motility characterized by esophageal aperistalsis and failure of the lower esophageal sphincter relaxation. The disease is progressive, resulting in gradual dilatation of the esophagus above the sphincter. Successful treatment of the disease by repeated esophageal bougienage was first described by Willis in 1674. Cardiomyotomy, the basis of modern surgical treatment for achalasia, was introduced by Heller in 1914. Despite advances in its treatment, the initiating factors and the underlying mechanisms of achalasia are still not well understood.

Achalasia is a rare condition that affects boys and girls equally. Achalasia may be primary (idiopathic) or secondary. Secondary achalasia shares clinical features with primary achalasia, but there is an identifiable cause. Primary achalasia has an estimated prevalence of 0.5–1 per 100,000 per year without a clear age predilection. Only less than 5% of all cases present before the age of 15 years. Epidemiology studies have revealed a small incidence peak in the 20–40 years age group. These, together with the rare occurrence of familial cases and syndromic associations, have led to the postulation of a possible hereditary factor for the disease. Recent work has also suggested a role for changes in neurotransmission and cell signaling in the lower esophagus as a possible pathophysiological mechanism.

35.2 Etiology

The most common cause of secondary achalasia is Chagas' disease, which is prevalent in Central and South America and is caused by *Trypanosoma cruzi*

P. Puri and M. Höllwarth (eds.), *Pediatric Surgery: Diagnosis and Management*,
DOI: 10.1007/978-3-540-69560-8_35, © Springer-Verlag Berlin Heidelberg 2009

infection. Pseudo-achalasia may be caused by neo-plasm or by infiltrative diseases such as amyloidosis and sarcoidosis. Neoplasms lead to pseudoachalasia most commonly by direct involvement of the esopha-gus (e.g. esophageal leiomyoma in children) or by a paraneoplastic phenomenon in malignancies not directly infiltrating the lower esophageal sphincter (LES). An achalasic picture may also be mimicked by complica-tions of surgery such as a fundoplication or vagal injury. Rarely, achalasia-like esophageal dysmotility is found in patients with esophageal atresia.

Early hypotheses for primary achalasia suggested chronic obstruction and neuronal degeneration as the possible etiological factors. However, the only consistent finding from histological specimens appears to be the inflammatory reaction with the decrease and loss of the myenteric inhibitory ganglion cells in the distal esopha-gus and the LES. The degree of the pathological changes seems to correlate with disease severity. There is a gen-eral consensus that there is a loss of inhibitory nitrergic neurotransmission in achalasia. However, the underlying triggering factor for the inflammation is unknown.

35.2.1 Infection

A clearly defined secondary achalasic syndrome that occurs in Chagas' disease has given support to an infec-tive cause for primary achalasia. Although viral infec-tions such as measles, VZV, and HSV-1 have been suggested, because the inflammatory infiltrates are of lymphocytic nature, no study has so far established a causal link. This however may be due to the destruction and absence of the myenteric ganglia, a reservoir for neurotrophic viruses, in late-stage achalasia patients.

35.2.2 Genetic Predisposition

In children, achalasia can be part of the Allgrove's (Four "A") syndrome, characterized by achalasia, alacrima, autonomic disturbance, and adrenocorticotrophic hormone resistant adrenal insufficiency. Allgrove's syndrome has been linked to mutations in the AAAS gene on chromo-some 12q13.8. However, this is a very rare cause of acha-lasia. Recent observations also suggest that achalasia is more frequent in Down's syndrome. There is little evi-dence from the studies available that achalasia is a genetic disease, except in the case of Allgrove's syndrome. The findings of HLA types that are found more frequently in achalasic patients than in the general population supports a genetic link, but this may be a predisposition to disease rather than a direct cause.

35.2.3 Immune-Mediated

An autoimmune etiology is supported by the presence of circulating autoantibodies against the myenteric plexus, the presence of inflammatory T-cell infiltrates in the myenteric plexus, and the increased prevalence of HLA class II antigens.

The HLA associations were first noticed after the discovery of a correlation of the class II HLA antigen DQw1 and achalasia. Subsequent immunotyping stud-ies showed that the DQw1 antigen conferred a relative risk of 3.6–4.2 for development of achalasia.

An autoantibody responsible for an immune-mediated destruction of esophageal neurons is also a possibility. The evidence stems from the occurrence of achalasia as a paraneoplastic phenomenon with the presence of doc-umented antineuronal antibodies and also as a secondary consequence of an autoimmune autonomic neuropathy with acetylcholine receptor antibodies.

35.3 Pathophysiology

The coordinated peristaltic wave that moves the food bolus through the esophagus depends on excitatory and inhibitory input from local enteric reflexes in the enteric nervous plexus and from the vagus nerve. Relaxation of the LES requires coordinated interaction of these nerves, smooth muscle, interstitial cells of Cajal (ICC), and gas-trointestinal hormones. The complex physiology high-lights the multiple potential pathological targets that could give rise to the clinical picture of achalasia.

Esophageal body aperistalsis, characteristic of acha-lasia, occurs over time in most patients. The pathologic characteristic of achalasia is the loss of myenteric neurons in the LES and esophageal body, accompa-nied by an inflammatory infiltration. However, a spec-trum of histopathologic changes can be found in achalasic patients, suggesting either different stages of a continuum or different etiologies. Interstitial fibrosis, endoneurofibrosis, fibrosis of the smooth muscle layer, and myopathic changes of the smooth muscle cells have also been observed. In patients with long-standing achalasia, myenteric ganglion cell bodies are markedly diminished or absent. On the other hand, a subset of patients with the so-called vigorous achalasia and a hypertensive LES show little or no myenteric ganglion cell loss and fibrosis.

Most data now strongly suggest that the major inhibitory neurotransmitter governing relaxation of the esophageal smooth muscle is nitric oxide (NO). The role of the loss of nitrergic neurons in the pathophysiology of achalasia is highlighted by studies on mice selectively lacking neuronal nitric oxide synthase (nNOS). These mice have manometric findings that mimic those in achalasia in the human. Nonetheless, the loss of nitrergic inhibitory enteric neurons is not selective in achalasic patients and appears to occur prior to the loss of cholinergic neurons. Other inhibitory neurotransmitters including vasoactive intestinal peptide (VIP) may also play a role.

Recently, immunohistochemical techniques have consistently demonstrated the presence of a CD8 lymphocytic infiltrate and collagen deposition within the myenteric plexus. These findings suggest an immune-mediated destruction of myenteric neurons. The exact stimulus initiating this autoimmune response or the antigen targeted remains to be identified.

35.4 Diagnosis

35.4.1 Clinical Features

In children, the net result of the motor abnormalities is that saliva and food will be retained in the esophagus leading to the typical symptoms of achalasia: dysphagia for solids and liquids, regurgitation of undigested food, respiratory complications (nocturnal cough and aspiration), chest pain, and weight loss. In infants, these symptoms mimic gastroesophageal reflux with occasional emesis and invariably failure to thrive.

The early symptoms of achalasia may be subtle and nonspecific and, indeed, the mean duration of symptoms before presentation is 2 years. The diagnosis often takes much longer because the symptoms are often attributed to gastroesophageal reflux disease or other disorders.

Rarely, achalasia is familial and can be associated with Allgrove's syndrome, microcephaly, cerebral palsy, and other congenital anomalies such as duodenal atresia, esophageal atresia, or myopathy. In clinical practice, the diagnosis is made preferably by manometry, after exclusion of organic causes of dysphagia. Endoscopy is diagnostic in about one-third and radiology in about two-thirds of the patients; diagnostic certainty is provided by manometry in over 90% of cases.

35.4.2 Radiology

A chest X-ray may show an air-fluid level in the posterior mediastinum, and a soft tissue mediastinal shadow in the left hemithorax corresponding to a dilated lower esophagus. Chronic aspiration may lead to pneumonic changes. A barium esophagram is usually the first definitive investigation performed in the evaluation of dysphagia. The classical appearance of achalasia on a barium study is the smooth tapering of the gastroesophageal junction ("bird's beak", or "rat-tail" deformity) with a column of contrast often mixed with retained food in the dilated proximal esophagus (Fig. 35.1).

Detailed fluoroscopic evaluation may also reveal aperistalsis, with failure to clear the barium from the esophagus.

35.4.3 Upper Endoscopy

Endoscopic evaluation is used to rule out other conditions that may mimic achalasia. The characteristic appearance is an atonic, dilated esophagus with a tightly closed LES that does not open with insufflation (Fig. 35.2) but provides little resistance to the advancing endoscope that can be admitted through with a "pop". Food residues, retained secretion, and an inflamed mucosa are often noted in the esophagus. Complications such as ulceration and yeast esophagitis, and suspicion of malignancy are indications for esophageal biopsies. The diagnosis of pseudo-achalasia is usually difficult and requires meticulous endoscopic inspection. In children, it is important to exclude tracheobronchal remnants in the distal esophagus mimicking as achalasia. Endoscopic ultrasound examination is useful for the differentiation.

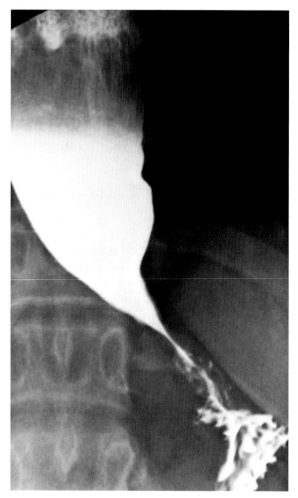

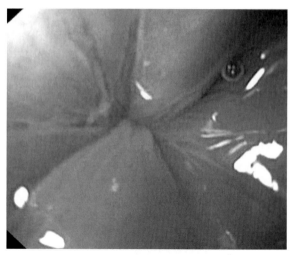

Fig. 35.2 Endoscopic view of the lower esophageal sphincter in a patient with achalasia, showing the constricted lumen

Fig. 35.1 A barium esophagram showing the typical radiological appearance of a "bird's beak" in achalasia

35.4.4 Esophageal Manometry

Manometry is the gold standard for confirming the diagnosis of achalasia. The resting LES pressure is usually elevated (>45 mmHg), and sometimes pressure in the esophageal body exceeds that in the stomach. The LES fails to relax completely with swallowing. Complete absence of peristalsis in the esophageal body is the sine qua non of achalasia. The waveforms are usually simultaneous and of low amplitude (Fig. 35.3). A subset of patients who have "vigorous achalasia" are found to have high-amplitude, long duration, and uncoordinated esophageal body contractions. In patients who have a dilated and tortuous esophagus, the LES may be difficult to intubate, requiring fluoroscopic guidance for manometry catheter placement. In the patient who will not tolerate esophageal manometry, nuclear scintigraphy can be used to evaluate esophageal transit.

35.5 Differential Diagnosis

Although achalasia is a rare condition in the pediatric population, the number of children presenting with signs and symptoms of dysphagia has increased during the past 2 decades. It has been reported that approximately 25% of children will experience some type of feeding difficulty. When facing a patient with the symptom of dysphagia, the complexity of pediatric swallowing disorders and the difficulty in classifying patients has to be considered. Other conditions that have similar symptoms to achalasia include diffuse esophageal spasm, gastroesophageal reflux with peptic stricture, pseudoachalasia, paraesophageal hiatal hernia, esophageal diverticulum, congenital esophageal stenosis, and gastric volvulus.

35.6 Management

The treatment of children with achalasia is largely comparable to that of adults. It is aimed at improving bolus transport across the LES by reducing the pressure

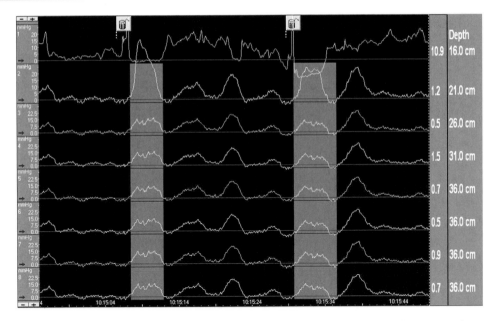

Fig. 35.3 Manometric recordings of an achalasic esophagus showing low amplitude and nonpropulsing contractions

at the LES. At present, treatment options in achalasia are pharmacotherapy, injection of botulinum toxin, pneumatic dilatation or surgery.

35.6.1 Pharmacotherapy

Although several adult studies have reported some degrees of success using calcium channel blockers or nitrates, these types of treatment are only useful in less severe types of achalasia. They are associated with cardiovascular side effects and peripheral edema.

Relief from these agents is inconsistent and generally short-lived, with most patients showing continued progression of their disease. Their usefulness is limited in children.

35.6.2 Botulinum injection

Local injection of botulinum toxin reduces pressure at the LES. The toxin binds to the cholinergic fibers and temporarily blocks the release of acetylcholine from excitatory motor neurons at the level of the LES. Typically, 100 units of toxin are injected into the four

quadrants of the LES (25 units/quadrant) endoscopically. While the initial rate of symptomatic benefit may be comparable to that of pneumatic dilatations, the effect wears off quickly in many patients. Also, the response seems to diminish with repeated injections. A series of 23 children with achalasia using botulinum toxin has been reported with similar results as in adults—83% with initial response, a median duration of effect for 3 months, and all patients require additional procedures to remain asymptomatic on follow-up. The major advantages of this therapy are its technical simplicity and relative safety and the procedure can typically be performed under minimal conscious sedation. It would appear that botulinum toxin should be used only in children who are poor candidates for either pneumatic dilation or surgery.

35.6.3 Pneumatic dilatation

Pneumatic dilatation aims at disruption of the LES circular muscle by balloon-insufflation. The procedure can be performed under sedation or general anesthesia (young children) as a day procedure. The esophagus should first be emptied. A wire-guided or incorporated balloon catheter is introduced via videoendoscope across the LES. The maximum insufflated size of the balloon should be no greater than the patient's own thumb. The balloon is inflated under fluoroscopic control until the "waist" disappears.

Follow-up studies in adults have indicated that the best predictor for a long-term remission is a post-treatment sphincter pressure less than 10 mmHg. Pneumatic dilatation yields good-to-excellent results in 70–90% of patients but on long-term follow up more than 40% of patients require additional treatment for recurrent symptoms. A similar response rate is reported in children. Pneumatic dilatation is associated with a small but significant risk (1–5%) of perforation. Moreover, patients who eventually undergo Heller myotomy after previous endoscopic therapy experience more intra and postoperative complications, and a higher failure rate than when no preoperative therapy has been used.

35.6.4 Surgery

Cardiomyotomy can achieve symptomatic relief in 90–95% of patients. It also provides more long-lasting effect than pneumatic dilation.

Traditional open approach is associated with a large incision and prolonged postoperative stays. Recent developments in minimally invasive techniques now allow performance of cardiomyotomy laparoscopically. The reduction in postoperative pain and morbidity, as well as improved cosmesis, has made this surgical option the treatment of choice for most patients. The advantages of laparoscopic cardiomyotomy include excellent visualization of the distal esophagus and the stomach, so that an extended gastric myotomy and a concomitant antireflux procedure may be performed.

The setup for laparoscopic Heller myotomy is the same as that for a Nissen fundoplication. The patient is placed in a modified lithotomy position with a large-bore nasogastric tube in situ. Standard five-port placement is the norm. An extensive anterior and lateral hiatal and mediastinal esophageal dissection is performed to maximize the length of the myotomy, taking care not to breach the pleura proximally. The gastric fundus and short gastric vessels are then mobilized to minimize tension on the subsequent fundoplication. The anterior vagus nerve is identified and protected from injury during the esophagogastric myotomy.

Myotomy is achieved by using the hook electrocautery device. The longitudinal muscle fibers are divided first, exposing the inner circular muscle, which is then separated until the submucosal plane is reached. The myotomy should be done as proximal as safely as possible to the level of the dilated esophagus (4–6 cm) and 1–2 cm onto the stomach. The GE junction is identified by the overlying fat pad and the "collar-like" circular muscle. On completion of the myotomy, the esophagus is insufflated to demonstrate the mucosal bulge. Accidental mucosal perforations should be repaired with fine absorbable sutures.

An antireflux procedure, either Dor or Toupet fundoplication, is then performed to prevent postoperative GERD.

35.6.4.1 Extent of the Esophageal Myotomy

While there is a general agreement that the proximal extent of the myotomy should reach 6 cm above the GE junction, the distal extent of the myotomy is controversial.

In adults, an extended gastric myotomy of 3 cm resulted in less dysphagia. Nonetheless, the length required may be less for children. Some authors recommend myotomy from the dilated esophagus where it is crossed by the anterior vagus from the right to the left proximally, to the transverse esophageal vessel over the gastroesophageal junction distally.

35.6.4.2 Antireflux Procedure

Some authors would not advocate an antireflux procedure after a Heller's cardiomyotomy.

With an extended gastric myotomy, an antireflux procedure is prudent in most cases due to a higher incidence of postoperative GERD.

A partial fundoplication (Dor or Toupet) is the best option and each has its own merits. An anterior (Dor/Thal) 180° fundoplication is easier to perform and theoretically preserves more of the antireflux barrier. Also, the anterior wrap can potentially cover any undetected mucosal injuries. A posterior (Toupet) 270° fundoplication is the preferred partial fundoplication when indicated for GERD and it can hold the myotomy edges apart.

35.7 Complications

35.7.1 Dysphagia

35.7.1.1 Inadequate Myotomy

An insufficient myotomy is one of the most important and preventable complications of surgery for achalasia and will lead to poor esophageal emptying and recurrent dysphagia. Even with an incomplete myotomy, patients often have some symptomatic improvement in their dysphagia, when compared to the preoperative state.

A postoperative barium study provides information on the adequacy of esophageal emptying. A successful myotomy will show complete (90–100%) emptying by the 5-min film. The most common cause of an inadequate myotomy is failure to carry the myotomy sufficiently far onto the stomach. Pneumatic dilation can be effective as secondary treatment of residual achalasia.

35.7.1.2 Myotomy Site

The location of the myotomy may be an important factor due to the asymmetrical muscle thickness around the gastroesophageal junction. Consequently, the best location for a myotomy would seem to be on the left side of the esophagus extending down across the angle of His onto the fundus of the stomach. A myotomy in this location would disrupt the longitudinal and circular muscular fibers of the esophagus as well as the oblique gastric fibers while preserving the clasp fibers along the lesser curve side of the stomach.

35.7.1.3 Postoperative Stricture

The development of a scar band at the myotomy site may lead to impaired esophageal emptying. It is thus important that the edges of the myotomy be widely separated. Performing a Toupet fundoplication may aid in distracting the muscle layers and has a theoretical advantage in preventing this type of recurrence.

35.7.1.4 Excessive Fundoplication

Long-term follow-up of patients who received a Nissen 360° fundoplication showed that recurrence of dysphagia was common. Thus, a complete fundoplication is inappropriate.

35.7.2 Postoperative Gastroesophageal Reflux

Gastroesophageal reflux can be a significant problem in a patient who has achalasia because the aperistaltic esophagus clears refluxed material poorly. Although the traditional Heller myotomy does not include an antireflux operation, most surgeons have adopted a partial fundoplication in addition to the myotomy as the standard surgical procedure for achalasia. One reason to add an antireflux procedure is that it allows the myotomy to extend well onto the stomach to be certain it is adequate. Further, the addition of an antireflux procedure has been shown to reduce esophageal acid exposure. A randomized trial comparing myotomy alone with myotomy and Dor fundoplication demonstrated that gastroesophageal reflux was significantly reduced by the addition of a Dor fundoplication. The incidence of pathologic reflux was 48% in those without a Dor fundoplication and 9% in those with a Dor fundoplication. The merits of a Toupet fundoplication versus a Dor partial fundoplication are debated.

An advantage of the Dor procedure is that typically no short gastric vessels need to be divided and no dissection needs to be done around the hiatus posteriorly. Further, because the Dor fundoplication is placed over the myotomy, it buttresses the mucosa and is useful in case a mucosal perforation occurs during the creation of the myotomy. The Toupet fundoplication, on the other hand, may lower the incidence of postoperative recurrent achalasia or stricture.

35.7.3 Esophageal Perforation

Perforation is one of the more common complications during surgical myotomy. The risk increases with previous treatment for achalasia, such as pneumatic dilatation or botulinum toxin injection. Mucosal perforations or tears discovered at the time of operation are amenable to laparoscopic repair using interrupted monofilament sutures. Typically perforations occur at or near the gastroesophageal junction. The mucosa in this region is very thin and tears easily; hence, a small perforation can quickly extend into a large one. Mucosal integrity can be reinforced by using fundoplication to cover the myotomy. Postoperatively a water-soluble contrast study is recommended before initiating oral feeding.

35.7.4 Postoperative Leak

A leak from the myotomy site should be suspected if the patient develops fever, chest pain, or clinical signs consistent with sepsis postoperatively. A water-soluble contrast study should be part of the routine postoperative investigation as described previously.

Endoscopy is a sensitive test and may be used with caution when contrast study fails to confirm leakage in a persistently septic patient. Most leaks are small and can be managed with intravenous antibiotics, fasting, and parenteral nutrition. Surgical drainage and repair may be necessary if sepsis persists despite medical treatment.

35.7.5 Malignancy

Patients who have achalasia are reported to be at increased risk for squamous cell carcinoma of the esophagus. The increased risk comes from chronic esophagitis. It is not known if this risk is decreased by an effective myotomy.

35.8 Long-Term Outcome

In terms of immediate improvement, it is clear that the treatment modalities of pneumatic dilatation, botulinum toxin, and cardiomyotomy all report early benefit in around 80–90% or more of patients. However, for botulinum toxin, the relief is temporary and only about two thirds of patients continue to have a sustained response. This holds true despite repeated injections. Further, the majority of patients will relapse within 6–12 months of the first treatment.

Surgical myotomy holds the most promise for a permanent solution to an elevated LES pressure. The

enthusiasm for laparoscopic Heller myotomy is clearly justified by the significant reduction in morbidity and hospitalization. Long-term results from various studies show that about two-thirds of patients are considered to have an excellent or good response after 10 years.

Since both pneumatic dilatation and botulinum toxin injections cause inflammation and fibrosis and have been shown to give rise to difficulties in the myotomy dissection and subsequent lower response rate, they should only be offered to patients who are at high risk for surgery.

We can conclude that laparoscopic myotomy should be the treatment of choice in younger patients. As we still do not fully understand the natural history of achalasia, long-term follow-up including the use of pH monitoring and esophageal manometry is recommended.

Further Reading

Babu R, Grier D, Cusick E, Spicer RD (2001) Pneumatic dilatation for childhood achalasia. Pediatr Surg Int 17:505–507

Hurwitz M, Bahar RJ, Ament ME et al (2000) Evaluation of the use of botulinum toxin in children with achalasia. J Pediatr Gastroenterol Nutr 30:509–514

Hussain SZ, Thomas R, Tolia V (2002) A review of achalasia in 33 children. Dig Dis Sci 47(11):2538–2543

Kraichely RE, Farrugia G (2006) Achalasia: Physiology and etiopathogenesis. Dis Esophagus 19:213–223

Mattioli G, Esposito C, Pini Prato A et al (2003) Results of the laparoscopic Heller-Dor procedure for pediatric esophageal achalasia. Surg Endosc 17:1650–1652

Mehra M, Bahar RJ, Ament ME et al (2001) Laparoscopic and thoracoscopic esophagomyotomy for children with achalasia. J Pediatr Gastroenterol Nutr 33:466–471

Tam PKH (2006) Achalasia. In P Puri, ME Höllwarth (eds) Pediatric Surgery, Springer Surgery Atlas Series. Springer-Verlag, Berlin, Heidelberg, New York, pp 61–66

Smith CD, Stival A, Howell DL, Swafford V (2006) Endoscopic therapy for achalasia before Heller myotomy results in worse outcomes than Heller myotomy alone. Ann Surg 243(5):579–586

Vane DW, Cosby K, West K, Grosfeld JL (1988) Late results following esophagomyotomy in children with achalasia. J Pediatr Surg 23(6):515–519

Zerbib F, Thetiot V, Richy F, Benajah DA, Message L, Lamouliatte H (2006) Repeated pneumatic dilations as long-term maintenance therapy for esophageal achalasia. Am J Gastroenterol 101:692–697

Esophageal Perforations and Caustic Injuries in Children

36

Alaa F. Hamza

Contents

36.1 Esophageal Perforations

36.1.1 Introduction

Esophageal perforations are not common in children; they include spontaneous perforations (Borhaave's syndrome) that are extremely rare, iatrogenic perforations in the neonate due to passage of the nasogastric tube or after endotracheal intubation, perforations after esophagoscopy and dilatation, and perforations due to ingestion of foreign bodies or caustic materials. The incidence is about 1% after endoscopic dilatation of the esophagus and slightly higher in prematures after tube insertion.

36.1.2 Pathogenesis and Etiology

Perforations due to expiration against closed glottis or Borhaave's syndrome are extremely rare and there are about 26 cases reported in the literature; they affect older children and the injury is due to perforation in the lower esophagus with resulting pneumothorax, mediastinal emphysema, and shock. The same perforation could happen after significant blunt trauma to the chest wall especially after crushing accidents.

Neonates, especially low birth weight infants, are prone to cervical esophageal perforation after endotracheal intubation or passage of nasogastric tubes; extension of the neck during instrumentation and compression of the esophagus by the cervical vertebrae predispose to injury. In these patients a linear tear in the esophagus usually occurs with passage of a

P. Puri and M. Höllwarth (eds.), *Pediatric Surgery: Diagnosis and Management,*
DOI: 10.1007/978-3-540-69560-8_36, © Springer-Verlag Berlin Heidelberg 2009

nasogastric tube. Through the tear, a false passage is created. A misdiagnosis of esophageal atresia occurs due to the inability to pass the nasogastric tube.

Esophageal perforation also occurs after endoscopic dilatation especially if there is esophageal stricture. Upper esophageal perforations occur on the right side and may lead to a right hydropneumothorax. Mid and lower esophageal perforations present on the left side. After dilatation there may be small linear mucosal tears, which might not be symptomatic but with insufflations of air during endoscopy the tear gets bigger and transmural perforation occurs into the thoracic cavity.

36.1.3 Diagnosis

In the neonate, excessive salivation, respiratory distress, and occasionally cervical swelling and crepitus may occur. Failure of passage of the nasogastric tube could be the first manifestation of cervical perforation and there are reports of cases explored for a false diagnosis of esophageal atresia. Lateral neck radiographs may demonstrate air in the facial planes early in cases of cervical perforations. A simple X-ray with tube in place may show the abnormal position of the tube, and if a dye is injected through the tube it will demonstrate a localized dye collection that may resemble an upper pouch of esophageal atresia (Figs. 36.1 and 36.2).

In cases of thoracic perforations, the patient usually presents with respiratory distress, tachycardia, and sweating. If there is tension pneumothorax, shock and death may occur if the tension is not promptly relieved.

A simple chest X-ray will show the pneumothorax. After insertion of a chest tube and improvement in the patient's condition, a water-soluble radio-opaque contrast may be instilled in the esophagus to identify the precise location of the leak (Fig. 36.3). A chest radiograph should be done after any esophageal dilatation to look for pneumo-mediastinum or pneumothorax. If there is any doubt, a contrast esophagogram should be

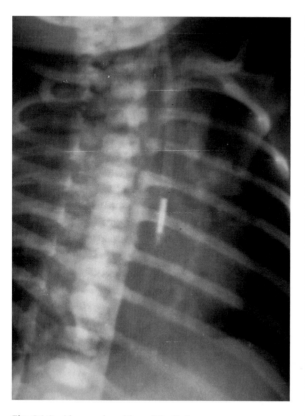

Fig. 36.1 Abnormal position of the Ryle

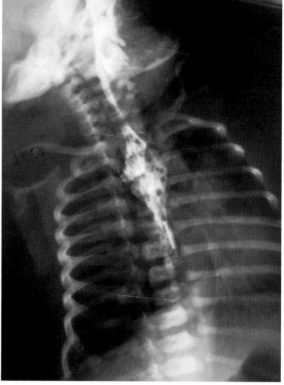

Fig. 36.2 A dye in the false passage mimicking esophageal atresia

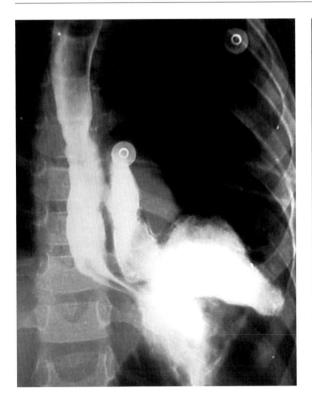

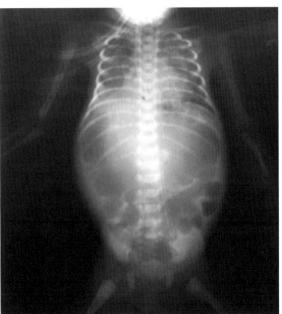

Fig. 36.4 A nasogastric tube in the pelvis after perforation of the abdominal esophagus

Fig. 36.3 Perforation of the esophagus with contrast in the thoracic cavity

done, especially if an increase in the airway pressure is noticed by the anesthetist. After routine dilatation the patient should be observed for at least 6 h and if there is any deterioration in the general condition, a delayed perforation should be suspected and rapid X-ray of the chest should be obtained. A widened mediastinum on the chest radiograph is also very suspicious of esophageal perforation. Sometimes the first sign would be cervicofacial emphysema, i.e., swelling of the face with crepitus.

36.1.4 Management

In contrast to adult patients, primary repair with tissue reinforcement is unnecessary in children. In cases of tension pneumothorax, a chest tube should be inserted immediately followed by reassessment of the patient.

In premature infants, the injury is usually cervical but sometimes the tube may have been advanced well into the chest cavity and rarely even to the pelvis if the perforation is in the abdominal esophagus (Fig. 36.4).

A passage of the nasogastric tube to the stomach under fluoroscopic guidance is one of the important steps in all esophageal perforations. It allows deflation of the stomach, thereby decreasing gastroesophageal reflux. Later feedings could be started through the tube with elevation of the patient's head. If reflux of enteral nutrition occurs and comes through the chest tube, then advancing the enteral feeding tube to the duodenum or the first part of the jejunum should be performed.

Chest drainage and nasogastric tube in the stomach are usually sufficient to heal most perforations in the neonates or prematures. Cervical injuries rarely need drainage of any collections. It usually takes from 1 week to 10 days for complete healing, which a radio-opaque swallow could verify. These lesions generally do not lead to any esophageal stenosis and further follow up is not needed.

Injuries to the thoracic esophagus after instrumentation or trauma also heal after chest drainage. However, in some traumatic cases, exploration and surgical closure of the tear should be done if the patient presents

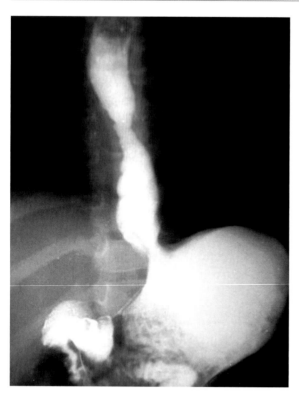

Fig. 36.5 Perforation healed completely by conservative measures

36.2 Caustic Injuries of the Esophagus

36.2.1 Introduction and Etiology

Although recently it has become much less common, caustic injuries of the esophagus and stomach still occur in some areas of the world. Some countries such as Egypt, India, Turkey, South Africa, and some eastern European countries see a high number of these injuries. The injury occurs in young children 2–4 years of age, more in boys than girls, with an incidence of 3:1 and is due to accidental swallowing of caustic material due to its resemblance to milk or water. The injury can also rarely occur in adolescents due to suicidal attempts. The causative agents are either alkalies or acids and they are usually in the liquid form but occasionally we have seen some injuries due to swallowing of crystal forms. The alkalies are usually potassium hydroxide (Potash) or sodium hydroxide. Acids are hydrochloric acid or sulfuric acid; drain cleaners also contains acids. When these substances are not placed in childproof containers they are extremely dangerous. Lithium batteries can also cause injuries to the esophagus especially if they are big enough to lodge in the cervical esophagus. If not promptly removed, it may lead to leakage of contents that usually causes severe esophageal injury with perforation.

early enough and has a large perforation. In cases after esophageal dilatation, the tear is usually linear and healing occurs after 10–15 days (Fig. 36.5).

In late presenting cases or after failure of conservative measures, exclusion of the esophagus by cervical esophagostomy and a gastrostomy should be done. A lateral esophagostomy for drainage of the saliva and a jejunostomy for feeding or a gastrostomy are other alternatives that could preserve the native esophagus.

Total parentral nutrition is started early in these cases to supply these children with their caloric needs till the time of enteral feeding is reestablished.

If the perforation occurs during a dilatation, dilatations should not be resumed until there is verification of healing by esophageal contrast study. Dilatation could be restarted, if needed after a period of healing, to the esophagus and with very careful under image control dilatation.

Some of these cases will eventually need esophageal replacement in those with severe injuries or after exclusion.

36.2.2 Pathology

The injury depends on the amount swallowed, the concentration, and the type of agent. Alkalies cause liquefactive necrosis of the esophagus and it usually most profoundly affects the areas of the esophagus that have slower transit of the bolus during swallowing. These include the cervical part, at the level of the carina, and just above the diaphragm. The injury may penetrate through the muscle layer and extend into the mediastinum, especially when high concentrations of the caustic agent are ingested. Healing occurs by resorption of the necrotic tissue and fibrosis. This leads to stricture formation, which is complete approximately 6 weeks following the injury Fig. 36.6.

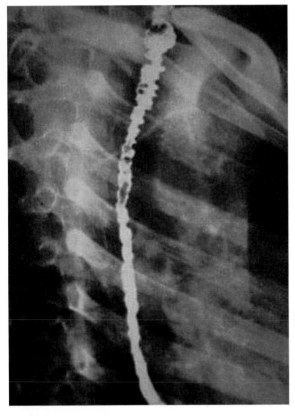

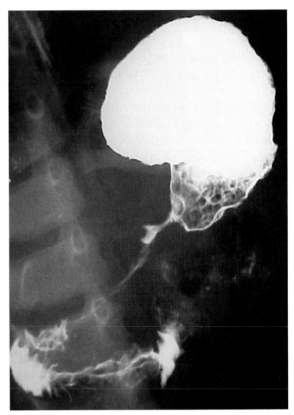

Fig. 36.6 Caustic esophageal stricture

Fig. 36.7 Pyloric obstruction due to acid injury

Acids are usually neutralized by the saliva and pass rapidly into the stomach. The acids may induce severe pyloric spasm that retains the ingested material in the antral area. This then leads to coagulative necrosis. Very severe injuries lead to perforation and necrosis and even milder acid ingestions may lead to pyloric and antral obstruction usually within 2–3 weeks (Fig. 36.7).

Acids may also lead to esophageal injury but this is less frequent than injuries to the stomach. Ingestion of very concentrated acids leads to necrosis of the whole esophagus and stomach.

36.2.3 Diagnosis and First Aid Measures

History of corrosive intake by the family is the first clue. If no history is available but there is hyperemia of the mouth with excessive salivation, suspicion of caustic ingestion should be placed at the top of a differential diagnosis. In cases of crystal ingestion, the crystals may adhere to the mucus membrane of the mouth resulting in ulcers and bleeding. Airway injuries may also occur in some severe cases and tracheostomy may be needed for airway stabilization. First responders should avoid dilution of the caustic agent by giving the patient water. Furthermore, any attempts to induce vomiting may expose the esophagus to a second injury. Caustic agents may induce pylorospasm and thus augment the risk of vomiting and further esophageal injury.

I.V. fluids, antibiotics, antacids, and urgent endoscopy are important tools as first aid measures. Steroids do not prove to be effective in the management of acute injuries of the esophagus, but it is very useful in airway edema and injuries. Fibro-optic endoscopy gives an idea about the degree of injury and the extent of lesions; some centers manage without endoscopy in mild alkali cases, as the management will not differ in mild and superficial injuries.

36.2.4 Management

Acids usually cause the most severe cases and if endoscopy has shown necrosis of the esophagus and stomach, then total esophagogastrectomy is needed urgently but fortunately this is very rare (Fig. 36.8).

For the usual injuries, patients are kept on I.V. fluids until they can swallow fluids orally, which usually occurs after healing of the mouth lesions. Children who cannot swallow are kept on TPN for 2–3 weeks and then a gastrostomy is established for enteral feeding and for retrograde esophageal dilatation.

In cases of pyloric obstruction several methods are available: antrectomy, pyloroplasty, and gastrojejunostomy depending on the lesion and extent of fibrosis.

Dilatation of caustic strictures can be started as early as the 3rd week but better results have been achieved if dilatations starts after the 6th week when complete healing is established. Balloon dilators, retrograde Tucker dilators through the stomach, or antegrade Savary-Guillard dilators have all been used successfully, but the best results in our hands has been with Savary antegrade dilators.

Dilatation is repeated every 2 weeks for a total of 6 weeks, then the patient is followed up by a contrast study. If swallowing of meat and solid food is satisfactory and the contrast esophagogram findings are encouraging, then the spacing of the dilatation procedures can be done and complete cure can occur in about 6 months–1 year. In cases of localized strictures,

Triamcinolone local injections lead to less frequent dilatation.

Antacids (proton pump inhibitors) should be used in these patients as injury of the cardiac sphincter with reflux usually occurs due to the caustic effect.

Contraindication to dilatation includes tortuous and very long strictures or multiple strictures and cases of tracheoesophageal fistula.

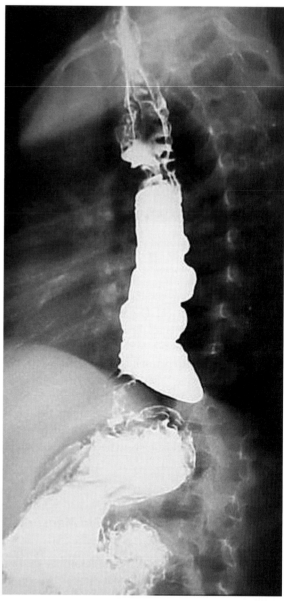

Fig. 36.9 Barium swallow showing colon replacement of the esophagus

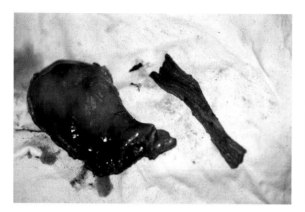

Fig. 36.8 Total gangrene of esophagus and stomach with esophagogastrectomy

Esophageal replacement is required when there is failure of dilatation because there is no improvement in swallowing, or discontinuation of dilatation is indicated because there is too rapid re-stricture formation, significant proximal dilatation of the esophagus with pouch formation, and in cases of perforation.

Esophageal sleeve resection can be done for very localized strictures but this is very uncommon as most of them respond to dilatation. Replacement of the esophagus is indicated in cases of failure or contraindication of dilatation. The stomach, gastric tube, jejunum, and the colon are all substitutes for the injured esophagus, but colon has proved to be better in cases of corrosive injuries (Fig. 36.9). Replacement is done when the child's physiological condition permits. The less the delay the better as swallowing solid food is essential for mouth and teeth development in children.

Further Reading

Hamza A (2006) Colonic replacement of the oesophagus. In P Puri, ME Höllwarth (eds) Pediatric Surgery, Springer Surgery Atlas Series. Springer-Verlag, Berlin, Heidelberg, New York, pp 67–76

Hamza AF, Abdelhay S, Sherif H et al (2003) Caustic esophageal strictures in children: 30 years experience. Overseas Guest Lecture. J Pediatr Surg 38(6):828–833

Panieri E, Millar AJ, Rode H, Brown RA, Cywes S (1996) Iatrogenic esophageal perforation in children: Patterns of injury, presentation, management, and outcome. J Pediatr Surg 31(7):890–895

Sapin E, Gumpert L, Bonnard A et al (2000) Iatrogenic pharyngoesophageal perforation in premature infants. Eur J Pediatr Surg 10(2):83–87

Weber T (2006) Esophageal rupture and perforation. In J Grosfeld, J O'neill, E Foncalsrud, A Coran (eds) Pediatric Surgery, 6th edn. Elsevier Mosby, Philadelphia, PA

Infantile Hypertrophic Pyloric Stenosis

37

Takao Fujimoto

Contents

37.1 Introduction Including Definition and Incidence

Infantile hypertrophic pyloric stenosis (IHPS) is a common surgical condition encountered in early infancy, occurring in 2–3 per 1,000 live births. It is characterized by hypertrophy of the circular muscle, causing pyloric narrowing and elongation and producing partial or complete luminal occlusion. The incidence of the disease varies widely with geographic location, season, and ethnic origin. Boys are affected four times more than girls.

The causes of hypertrophic circular muscle of the pylorus are still obscure and various hypotheses have been advocated.

Since Ramstedt introduced the extramucosal pyloromyotomy in 1912, a variety of approaches to the pylorus have been described.

37.2 Etiology

There is evidence of a genetic predisposition to the development of this condition. IHPS has been associated with a number of inherited syndromes (e.g., Smith-Lemli-Opitz and Cornelia de Lange syndromes) and with a variety of chromosome abnormalities. Nonsyndromic IHPS shows familial aggregation. Siblings of patients with IHPS are 15 times more likely to suffer the condition than children who have no family history of IHPS. The classic studies of Carter and Evans defined the disease as a paradigm for multifactorial, sex-modified threshold model of inheritance. The cause of hypertrophic circular muscle of the pylorus in IHPS is thought to result from the failure to relax

P. Puri and M. Höllwarth (eds.), *Pediatric Surgery: Diagnosis and Management*,
DOI: 10.1007/978-3-540-69560-8_37, © Springer-Verlag Berlin Heidelberg 2009

the sphincter smooth muscle. IHPS may be a developmental abnormality in which the pyloric muscle hypertrophies after birth. There are sound data showing that the dimensions of the pyloric muscle at birth are the same in normal infants as in those destined to develop IHPS. On the contrary, there have been a number of reports that have diagnosed this condition at birth, even in utero. Various hypotheses have been advocated including abnormal peptidergic innervations, abnormalities of extracellular matrix proteins, abnormalities of smooth-muscle cells, and abnormalities of intestinal hormones. The last decades shed some light on the immunohistochemical studies on the enteric nervous system to clarify the pathogenesis of IHPS. A decrease in immunoreactivities of the neurotransmitter such as substance-P, somatostatin, and neuronal structural proteins of S-100, GFAP, and D7 have been reported. In addition, recent studies implicate the cytokines epidermal growth factors (EGF), glial-derived growth factors (GDGF), transforming growth factor alpha (TGF-α), platelet-derived growth factor subtype BB (PDGF-BB), Platelet derived endothelial cell growth factor (PDEGF), and insulin-like growth factor-1 (IGF-1) in the pathogenesis of IHPS.

Most recently it has been proposed that disease susceptibility may be associated with an altered expression of neuronal nitric oxide synthesis, which is the major mediator of smooth muscle relaxation. In particular, NOS1, the gene encoding neuronal nitric oxide synthase, has been implicated in the disease pathogenesis by expression studies, animal models, and genetic analysis of small IHPS data sets. On the other hand, the changing rates of IHPS, which have been reported in several areas and countries, have highlighted the importance of environmental factors. The debate over a genetic or environmental origin of IHPS has not yet reached a final conclusion.

37.3 Pathology

The characteristic gross pathological feature in IHPS consists of thickening of the antropyloric portion of the stomach ("Olive like mass") and crowding of redundant and edematous mucosa within the lumen. Abnormally circumferentially thickened antropyloric muscle (thickness; 4–6 mm, length; 16–20 mm) separates the normally distendable portion of the antrum from the duodenal cap. It stops abruptly at both the ends. The rigid antropyloric canal is unable to accommodate the redundant mucosa, which protrudes into the gastric antrum. These anatomical abnormalities cause obstruction to the passage of gastric contents. Histologically, IHPS is characterized by thickened, hypertrophied, and edematous mucosa and its relationship to the underlying hypertrophied musculature, primarily involving the circular muscle. Various results of immunohistochemical studies in relation to the enteric nervous system in IHPS were described in the part of "etiology".

37.4 Diagnosis

The diagnosis of IHPS is usually based on clinical history, physical examination, and imaging studies such as ultrasonography and barium meal study.

37.4.1 Clinical Features

The usual onset of symptoms occurs between 2 and 8 weeks of age with peak occurrence at 3–5 weeks of age. It has been rarely reported in premature infants, especially extremely low birth weight infants, and these premature infants with IHPS present the signs and symptoms 2–4 weeks later as compared to normal term infants. The clinical features vary with the length of symptoms. Initially the vomiting may not be frequent and forceful, but over several days it progresses to every feeding and becomes forceful nonbilious vomiting described as "projectile". The emesis consists of gastric contents, which may become blood tinged with protracted vomiting and likely related to gastritis, with "coffee-ground" appearance (17–18% of cases). Infants with IHPS do not appear ill or febrile in the early stages. A significant delay in diagnosis leads to severe dehydration and weight loss due to inadequate fluid and calorie intake. Severe starvation can exacerbate diminished glucoronyl transferase activity and jaundice associated with indirect hyperbilirubimemia as seen in 2–5% of infants with IHPS. Associate anomalies are seen in 6–20% of patients.

37.4.2 Physical Examinations

It should be possible to diagnose IHPS on clinical features alone in 80–90% of infants. The important diagnostic features are visible gastric peristaltic waves in the left upper abdomen and a palpable enlarged pylorus ("olive" like mass). Physical examination requires a calm and cooperative infant with a relaxed abdomen. It would be easy to observe the gastric peristaltic waves after test feeding in a warm environment. However, to obtain successful palpation of the hypertrophic pylorus, it will be very difficult if the stomach distends. Aspiration using the nasogastric tube facilitates the successful palpation of an enlarged pylorus. After the edge of the liver has been identified with the finger tip, applied gentle pressure deep to the liver and progress caudally to reveal an enlarged pylorus. In most cases, an enlarged pylorus located just above the umbilicus at the lateral border of the rectal muscle below the liver edge.

37.4.3 Diagnostic Imaging

Ultrasonographic examination has become the most common imaging study for the diagnosis of the IHPS and is easily carried out without any sedation. The examination should be carried out with a high-frequency linear transducer (between 6 and 10 MHz). Ultrasonographic examination is preferably carried out by placing the patient in a right oblique position, permitting the fluid to gravitate to the antrum for adequate evaluation. In patients with IHPS, longitudinal ultrasonography shows a variable degree of hypertrophied muscle and the intervening mucosa that protrudes into the fluid-filled antrum. Cross-sectional study shows circumferential muscular thickening surrounding the central channel filled with mucosa (Fig. 37.1). The diagnosis of IHPS by ultrasonography is made by identifying these findings, and the most commonly used criteria are pyloric muscle thickness of 4 mm or more and pyloric channel length of 16 mm or

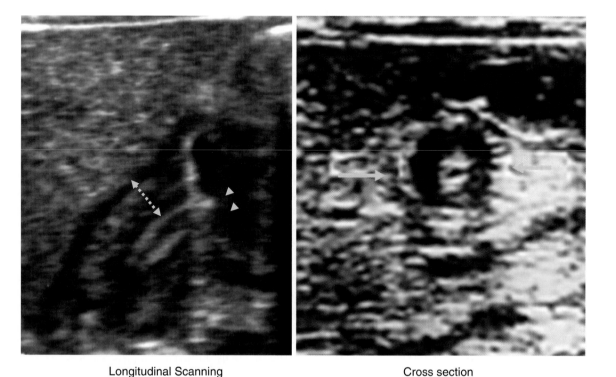

Longitudinal Scanning   Cross section

Fig. 37.1 Ultrasonographic findings of IHPS. Longitudinal ultrasonography shows variable degree of hypertrophied muscle (*arrow*) and intervening mucosa that protrudes into the fluid-filled antrum (*arrow head*)

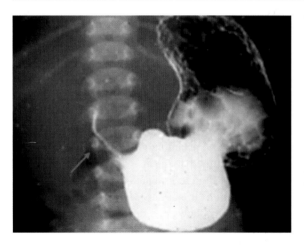

Fig. 37.2 Barium meal study of IHPS. Narrowed elongated pyloric canal giving a "string" or "double track" sign caused by compressed invaginated folds of mucosa in the pyloric canal (*arrow*)

more. Barium meal study is still a highly sensitive examination for the diagnosis of IHPS. The characteristic radiological feature of IHPS is a narrowed elongated pyloric canal giving a "string" or "double track" sign caused by compressed invaginated folds of mucosa in the pyloric canal (Fig. 37.2). However, barium meal study provides indirect information about the antropyloric canal status. Failure of the relaxation of the antropyloric lesion, known as pylorospasm, demonstrates the same findings as those of IHPS. The emptying speed of the barium meal to the distal bowel will be important to differentiate these two conditions.

37.5 Differential Diagnosis

Several conditions must be considered if the patient demonstrates nonbilious vomiting. Table 37.1 gives the list of Common differential diagnosis. Patients with

Table 37.1 Differential diagnosis of IHPS

Surgical conditions	Medical conditions
Phlorospasm	Gastroenteritis
Gastroesophageal Reflux	Increased intracranial pressure
Gastric volvulus	Metabolic disease
Antral web	
Preampullar duodenal stenosis	
Duplication cyst	
Ectopic pancreas within the Pyloric muscle	

bilious vomiting do not have IHPS and are not directed to an initial ultrasonographic examination. Pylorospasm and gastroesophageal reflux (GERD) give similar clinical findings and may be difficult to differentiate them from IHPS without further evaluation. However, both conditions are more easily excluded with ultrasonography than barium meal study because of the ability of the former to detect and measure the antropyloric muscle thickness. Herniation of gastric fundus and regurgitation of gastric contents in patients with GERD can also be identified by ultrasonography. Other surgical causes of nonbilious vomiting include gastric volvulus, antral web, preampullar duodenal stenosis, duplication cyst of the antropyloric lesion, and ectopic pancreatic tissue within an antropyloric muscle, which are all far less common than IHPS. Common medical causes of nonbilious vomiting are gastroenteritis, increased intracranial pressure, and metabolic disorders.

37.6 Management

Once the diagnosis of IHPS has been confirmed, surgical referral is made rapidly.

37.6.1 Preoperative Management

Recurrent and persistent vomiting in these patients results in chloride and potassium depletion with metabolic alkalosis. Estimation of serum electrolyte level, urea nitrogen level, hematocrit, and blood gases must be carried out to determine the state of dehydration and acid–base abnormalities. Fluid resuscitation should be based on the degree of dehydration and the extent of electrolyte abnormalities. Nowadays, many babies with IHPS do not show any clinical evidence of dehydration and electrolyte abnormalities on admission. If the infants develop mild dehydration and hypochloremic alkalosis, maintenance fluid with 5% dextrose in 0.45% normal saline containing 20–40 mEq/l of potassium chloride can be administrated. Most of the patients with IHPS should be able to be resuscitated within 24 h. The operation for IHPS is not an emergency and should never be undertaken until serum electrolytes level and acid–base balance have returned to normal.

There has been a debate in terms of preoperative placement of the nasogastric tube. Most infants with IHPS do not have complete gastric outlet obstruction and can tolerate their gastric secretion. An nasogastric tube removes additional fluid and hydrochloric acid from the stomach.

37.6.2 Operation

Pyloromyotomy for IHPS has been practiced by surgeons for over a century, and the most commonly used technique is that described by Ramstedt in 1912. The Ramstedt's pyloromyotomy for IHPS is well-established, universally accepted, and the safest procedure. The standard approach is the right upper quadrant transverse incision. Another incision that is commonly used is an umbilical fold incision. The hypertrophied antropyloric lesion is delivered by gentle traction through the surgical wound (Fig. 37.3a). Then a longitudinal serosal incision

is made on the antero-superior aspect of the pylorus beginning approximately 1–2 mm proximal to the duodenum and extended into the nonhypertrophied antrum. The blunt end of the scalpel handle is used to initially disrupt the muscle fiber. The hypertrophied circular muscle is then further disrupted down to the mucosa using the Benson spreader (Fig. 37.3b). When the pyloric muscle is adequately split, the mucosa can be seen to be bulging (Fig. 37.3c).

Recently, laparoscopy has been used as an alternative access for pyloromyotomy.

37.6.3 Nonoperative Treatment

Although the Ramstedt's pyloromyotomy is the gold standard therapy for IHPS, many studies with nonoperative medical treatment for IHPS have been reported over the past 50 years. However, medical treatment with oral anticholinergic drugs such as

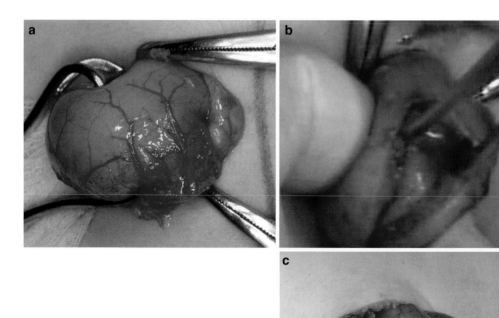

Fig. 37.3 Operative findings of hypertrophied antropyloric lesion. (**a**) Hypertrophic antropyloric lesion is delivered through the surgical wound. (**b**) After spreading the pyloric muscle. Loose prolapsing of intact mucosa is evidence of satisfactory myotomy. (**c**) Prolapsing mucosa after pylorus myotamy

atropine sulphate or methyl scopolamine nitrate have not worked consis-tently and been virtually abandoned since 1960. Recently, researchers from Japan have revived this medical treatment with reports of a new method using methyl atropine nitrate intravenously and have obtained successful results. Atropine is administrated intravenously at a dose of 0.01 mg/kg six times a day, 5 min before feeding.

37.7 Complications

The major postoperative complications are wound infection, mucosal perforation, and inadequate pyloromyotomy. Mucosal perforation may occur in 1–2% and incidence of wound infection has been reported in 1%–5% of the cases. The need for reoperation after

pyloromyotomy because of recurrent vomiting is reported with an incidence of up to 4%. With improvements in techniques, the incidence of complications after pyloromyotomy is extremely low at present.

Further Reading

Fujimoto T (2006) Hypertrophic Pyloric Stenosis. In P Puri, ME Höllwarth (eds) Pediatric Surgery. Springer Surgery Atlas Series, Springer-Verlag Berlin Heidelberg, New York, pp 171–180

Fujimoto T (2006) Pyloromyotomy. In A Najmaldin (ed) Pediatric Endoscopy & Endoscopic Surgery. Hodder Arnold, New York, pp 231–234

Hernanz-Schulman M (2003) Infantile hypertrophic pyloric stenosis. Radiology 227(2):319–341

Puri P (2003) Hypertrophic pyloric stenosis. In P Puri (ed) Newborn Surgery. Arnold, London, pp 389–398

Gastrostomy and Jejunostomy

38

Michael W.L. Gauderer

Contents

38.1 Gastrostomy and Jejunostomy

The establishment and care of long-term enteral access presently occupies a significant segment of pediatric surgical practice. Although pediatric surgeons have become more selective in the use of gastrostomies and jejunostomies for congenital malformations, during the last decades there has been a marked increase in the placement of feeding stomas in infants and children without associated surgical conditions. This has come about mainly because of the ever increasing survival of patients with inability to swallow secondary to central nervous system disorders and children who require feeding supplementation, special diets, and frequent administration of multiple medications. Refinements in the traditional access procedures and the addition of newer and simpler endoscopically, radiologically, ultrasonographically, and laparoscopically aided techniques have enhanced the safety and expanded the applicability of these upper intestinal stomas. Additionally, the use of softer, minimally irritating materials in the manufacture of traditional catheters and, more importantly, the development of skin-level devices have greatly reduced complications and facilitated the long-term use of these enteral routes.

Although these developments are clearly beneficial, the indication of a long-term feeding stoma can be quite difficult, often involving serious ethical considerations. The most desirable outcome is usually achieved by a team approach including parents, primary physicians, gastroenterologists, nutritionists, nurses, and other professionals who will be involved with the management of the child.

Gastrostomies and jejunostomies are generally considered basic surgical procedures. However, both have a significant potential for early and late morbidity and an occasional mortality. Therefore, attention to procedure selection and execution, as well as careful follow-up, is essential. Because gastrostomies and jejunostomies have slightly different indications, techniques, and complications, they will be addressed separately.

38.2 Gastrostomy

38.2.1 Introduction

This operation, initially performed over 100 years ago, is one of the oldest abdominal interventions in continuous use and some of the first patients were children who had swallowed corrosive materials. Gastrostomy is also closely associated with the early days of pediatric surgery, as it was commonly employed in conjunction with operations on the alimentary tract of newborns. Fortunately, lye strictures are now uncommon and advances in perioperative care, notably parenteral nutrition, have decreased the need for neonatal gastrostomies. On the other hand, because of the above-mentioned changes in the referred pediatric patient population, the placement of feeding stomas, particularly gastrostomies, is now at an all time high and continues to grow. A major contributor to this trend was the introduction of the gastrostomy without laparotomy in 1980. The original procedure, the percutaneous endoscopic gastrostomy or PEG, was in fact initially developed for high risk children. Along with its modifications, it is still the most widely employed technique for long-term enteral access. PEG has had an even greater impact on the adult patient population, where the simplicity of this gastric stoma has created the potential for overutilization. Not surprisingly, the extraordinarily large numbers of PEG placements, particularly in the end-of-life setting, have generated sizeable concerns reflected in numerous debates and publications on the ethics of long-term enteral feeding.

38.2.2 Indications

In infants and children, the main indications for gastrostomy are long-term feeding (including the administration of special diets and medications), decompression, or a combination of both. Other pediatric applications include gastric access for the insertion of trans-pyloric jejunal feeding tubes and esophageal bougienage. Gastrostomies are placed either as the sole procedure or in conjunction with other intra-abdominal interventions such as antireflux operations, correction of congenital intestinal lesions, or procedures associated with the management of major intestinal loss (e.g., midgut volvulus, necrotizing enterocolitis).

Feeding gastrostomies have two prerequisites: the upper gastrointestinal tract must be functional and the need for enteral feedings must be extended, at least a couple of months. For children requiring shorter spans, nasogastric or nasojejunal feeding tubes should be considered. Children benefiting from a feeding gastrostomy can be divided into two broad categories: (1) those unable to swallow and (2) those unable to consume adequate nutrients orally. The first group is the largest and is composed primarily of patients with neurologic disturbances. The second group encompasses patients with a variety of conditions in which the central nervous system is intact: failure to thrive, complex bowel disorders (e.g., short gut syndrome, malabsorption, inflammatory bowel disease), malignancy and other debilitating illnesses, and various congenital or acquired diseases interfering with growth. In selected patients, a gastrostomy is the most effective means of *administering a nonpalatable diet* (e.g., that used in chronic renal failure) or *ensuring compliance with medication* (e.g., cholestyramine in Alagille syndrome, antiretroviral medications in children with HIV).

Decompressing gastrostomies can be useful in cases of lengthy paralytic ileus, pseudo-obstruction, or for palliative care in the management of unresectable abdominal malignancy.

Decompressing-feeding gastrostomies are employed when the stoma is placed in conjunction with another intra-abdominal procedure such as a fundoplication or repair of duodenal atresia. The combination of gastrostomy and trans-anastomotic jejunal feeding tube was often used in newborns with high intestinal obstruction prior to the advent of parenteral nutrition. This set-up can still be employed advantageously today. It permits the evacuation of gastric contents, while providing intrajejunal feedings in these infants in whom the proximal dilated bowel segment causes delayed functioning of the anastomosis.

Gastrostomies as an adjunct in children with specific congenital or acquired surgical lesions should be considered if they will substantially facilitate perioperative or long-term care. In addition to the examples above, gastrostomies are employed in neonates with complex esophageal atresia, select abdominal wall defects in which prolonged ileus is anticipated, and in some cases of extensive intestinal loss. Examples of indications in older children include severe esophageal stricture, complex foregut trauma, malignancy, and extensive adhesive bowel obstruction.

38.2.3 Work-up

When a gastrostomy is performed in conjunction with another intra-abdominal procedure, the work-up depends on the type of surgical pathology being managed. If an abnormal epigastric anatomy is suspected, an ultrasonographic examination or an upper gastrointestinal contrast study may prove useful.

If the main purpose of the gastrostomy is feeding, the work-up should center on the question: *gastrostomy only or gastrostomy and an antireflux operation?* Neurologically impaired children, the main candidates for this intervention, frequently have foregut dysmotility and associated gastroesophageal reflux. Because gastrostomies can unmask reflux, these children should be evaluated prior to placing a stoma. This is usually done with an upper gastrointestinal contrast series and a pH probe study. Endoscopy with biopsy, manometry, and gastric-emptying studies may be added if deemed necessary. Unfortunately these studies, in addition to being time consuming and expensive, are not particularly helpful in predicting postgastrostomy reflux. For this reason, our routine approach is based on a trial of nasogastric tube feeding for 1–2 weeks. If these are well tolerated, we place a gastrostomy only. If, on the other hand, they are not, an antireflux operation is done in conjunction with the gastrostomy. The majority of children will fall in the first category. In our experience even patients with significant reflux, who tolerate the nasogastric test-feedings, can be managed well with only a gastrostomy. If the need to control reflux surgically arises later, an antireflux operation can be added, usually without taking down the gastrostomy. Several factors were considered when we developed this simplified approach over two decades ago. Among these are the increased risk associated with fundoplications and their high failure rate in the neurologically impaired child, the advent of more effective pharmacological

options, and the observation that, in many instances, once these children improve their nutritional status, they also tend to have improved gastric emptying.

38.2.3.1 Choice of Procedure

A wide variety of techniques for constructing a gastrostomy are now available. In spite of their apparent differences, the commonly used stomas can be divided into three basic types: (1) formation of a serosa-lined channel from the anterior gastric wall to the skin surface around a catheter; (2) formation of a tube from the full thickness gastric wall to the skin surface, a catheter being introduced intermittently for feeding; and (3) percutaneous techniques, in which the introduced catheter holds the gastric and abdominal walls in apposition. With certain adaptations and modifications, each of these interventions can be performed by minimally invasive techniques. A comparison of the most commonly used gastrostomies is depicted in Table 38.1.

38.2.3.2 Channel Formation Around a Catheter

In the first group of techniques, the catheter may be placed parallel to (Witzel technique) or perpendicular to the stomach (Stamm technique) with a laparotomy. The stomach is usually anchored to the abdominal wall with sutures. The essence of the Stamm-type gastrostomy is the use of concentric purse-string sutures around the gastrostomy tube, producing an invagination lined with serosa. This traditional procedure is versatile, safe, and reliable. It is commonly used when a gastrostomy is performed in conjunction with another "open" intra-abdominal procedure. This access is also invaluable in the management of complex esophageal lesions (Fig. 38.1).

38.2.3.3 Gastric Tube Brought to the Surface

The tube is constructed of a segment of gastric wall and then brought to the skin surface either as a direct conduit (Depage, Beck-Jianu, Hirsch, and Janeway methods) or interposing a valve or torsion of the tube to prevent reflux (Watsudjii, Spivack techniques). The main appeal of the Janeway-type stoma is that the patient does not need a catheter between feedings. The use of automatic

Table 38.1 Comparison of the most commonly used gastrostomies

	Serosa-lined channels	Gastric tubes	Percutaneous endoscopic techniques	Percutaneous Imaging guided "radiological" techniques	Laparoscopic and laparoscopically assisted techniques
Catheter/stoma device continuously in situ	Yes	No	Yes	Yes	Yes
Laparotomy	Yes	Yes	No	No	No
Laparoscopically feasible	Possible	Yes	Yes	N/A	Yes
Need for gastric endoscopy	No	No	Yes	No	No
Need for abdominal relaxation during operation	Yes	Yes	No	No	Yes and insufflation
Procedure time	Short	Moderate	Very short	Short	Short
Postoperative ileus	Yes	Yes	No	No	Some
Potential for bleeding	Yes	Yes	Remote	Remote	Small
Potential for wound dehiscence/hernia	Yes	Yes	No	No	No
Potential for early dislodgement of catheter	Yes	No	Rare	Yes	Small
Potential for gastric separation	Possible	Possible	Yes	Yes	Possible
Potential for infection	Yes	Yes	Yes	Yes	Yes
Potential for gastrocolic fistula	Low	No	Yes	Low	Low
Incidence of external leakage	Moderate	Significant	Low	Low	Low
"Permanent"	No	Yes	No	No	No
Suitable for passage of dilators for esophageal stricture	Yes	No	No	No	Possible
Limited diameter of catheter	No	N/A	No	Yes	No
Interferes with gastric reoperation (e.g. fundoplication)	No	Yes	No	No	No
Suitable for infants	Yes	No	Yes	Yes	Yes

stapling devices, including those designed for laparoscopic use, has greatly facilitated the construction of the tube from the anterior gastric wall. Although the lack of an abdominal wall feeding device is appealing, these gastrostomies are more complex to construct, significantly decrease the size of the pediatric stomach, have a tendency to leak and render subsequent operations such as a fundoplication much more difficult.

38.2.3.4 Percutaneous Techniques

In this third group, the catheter is placed with endoscopic or laparoscopic assistance without a laparotomy. The percutaneous endoscopic gastrostomy (PEG) is the most widely employed in this group. Depending on the method of introduction of the catheter, PEG may be performed using a "pull" (Gauderer-Ponsky technique), a "push" (Sachs et al. technique) in which a semi-rigid catheter guide is advanced over a Seldinger-type wire instead of being pulled into place by a string-like guide from inside the stomach to the skin, or the "introducer" (Russel et al. technique) in which a Foley balloon-type catheter is advanced through a removable sheath from the skin level into the stomach. Although basically in the same general category, radiologically (fluoroscopy or CT) and ultrasonographically guided gastrostomies are a little different in that the diameter of the inserted catheters is smaller and some form of gastric fixation is usually added to prevent accidental dislodgement. The large choice of procedures attests to their broad appeal and versatility (Fig. 38.2). Hybrid approaches combining the insertion of PEG type catheters with a mini-laparotomy can be useful in special instances.

38.2.3.5 Laparoscopic Techniques

Laparoscopically assisted gastrostomies are modifications of the above types allowing surgeons numerous options either as single interventions or associated with other intracavitary procedures. Many variations have been described and new ones are still being introduced

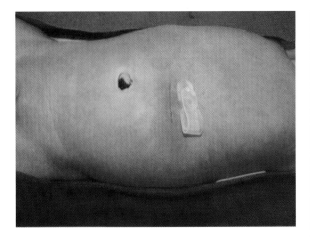

Fig. 38.1 One-week-old infant with esophageal atresia. The atresia with typical distal tracheoesophageal fistula was repaired on the first day of life. At 5 days of age, a routine contrast study showed an associated, previously unsuspected, lengthy stricture of the distal esophagus. Because oral feedings were not well tolerated and an initial balloon dilatation of the stricture was unsuccessful, an open, Stamm-type gastrostomy was placed. The photo, taken at the completion of the procedure, shows the button exiting through a counter incision

attesting to the creativity possible with the newer available technologies.

The choice of procedure and the technique employed depends on several factors, including the purpose of the gastrostomy, the child's age, anatomical particularities, and the experience of the surgeon, gastroenterologist or radiologist with the intervention, as well as the setting available for the necessary follow-up.

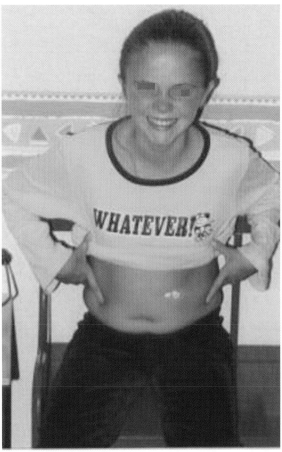

Fig. 38.2 Thirteen-year-old patient with cystic fibrosis. The percutaneous endoscopic gastrostomy, placed 8 years earlier, is used for supplemental feedings and medications, including pancreatic enzymes

38.2.4 Choice of Access Device

There are several types of commonly used gastrostomy tubes. The "traditional" long catheters are characterized by the mode of retention (semi-rigid intragastric portion and inflatable intragastric balloon). The skin-level devices or "buttons" are modifications in which the intragastric retention mechanism is similar to those of the long tubes. A comparison of the devices is shown in Table 38.2. Most are manufactured of silicone rubber or polyurethane to avoid the possibility of an allergic reaction to latex. Of the conventional, long tubes, the Foley or balloon catheters are the easiest to insert, but have the disadvantage of balloon deflation leading to dislodgement. Additionally these catheters are prone

to distal migration with possible intestinal obstruction. The de Pezzer and PEG-type catheters are less prone to dislodgement, but are a little harder to insert. The Malecot-type catheters, with its relatively soft winged tip, are easier to insert but also more prone to dislodgement. Although all types of catheters can be used for long-term care, the skin-level devices, introduced in 1984 with the original "button", are best suited for this purpose. The three most commonly employed skin-level devices are depicted in Fig. 38.3.

The original button has the lowest external profile and tends to last considerably longer than the other devices. In fact, many children have had the same button in place for several years. Its main disadvantages are the possibility of tract damage with discomfort when change is needed, and wearing out of the site of

Table 38.2 Comparison of commonly used gastrostomy devices

	PEG-type, De Pezzer, Malecot, T-tube	Foley (balloon type)	Skin-level ("button" type)
Suitable for initial insertion	Yes	Yes	Yes
Suitable for decompression	Yes	Yes	Yes[a]
Tendency for accidental dislodgement or external migration	Moderate[b]	Moderate	Very low (except balloon type)
Tendency for internal (distal) migration	Moderate	High	None
Tendency for peristomal leakage (particularly large tubes)	Moderate	Moderate	Low
Balloon deflation	No	Yes	Yes, with balloon type
Reinsertion	Easy to moderately difficult	Easy	Easy to moderately difficult
Long-term (particularly ambulatory patients)	Adequate	Adequate	Best suited
Overall complication rate	Significant	Significant	Low

[a]With special adaptor
[b]High with Malecot

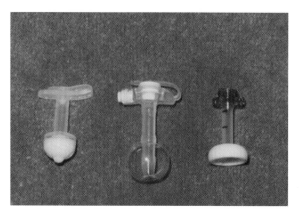

Fig. 38.3 Three types of skin-level enteral access devices. From left to right: the original button, a balloon-type device, and the changeable skin-level port-valve. The button has a very low external profile and a flat, one-way valve at the gastric end of the shaft. The balloon-type design permits easy device change. It has a duck bill, one-way valve at the skin level of the shaft. The skin-level port-valve is designed to permit conversion of a previously placed gastrostomy catheter to any desired length. It also allows subsequent changes, again without removal of the originally placed catheter

the connection with the feeding adapter, leading to possible disconnection. A combination PEG catheter-button for primary insertion is commercially available. However, judging the appropriate button length prior to insertion can be difficult and once the button is deployed, it cannot be changed.

The balloon type skin-level devices have the advantages of greater ease in the changing process and a feeding adapter is more securely connected. Disadvantages include a shorter life span because of balloon deflation and a slightly taller external profile. Additionally the balloon occupies more intragastric volume, and in some earlier models the protruding tip produced erosions on the posterior gastric wall.

The third type is a device with a changeable external port-valve. The greatest advantage of this concept is that an originally placed long gastrostomy tube can be converted to a skin-level device by simply cutting the tube to the desired length above the skin and placing the valve in the shaft. The tract is not disturbed, thus eliminating the possibility of gastric separation. The conversion can be done either immediately after the gastrostomy catheter insertion or any time thereafter. The main disadvantage in the present model is late valve failure. However, if this occurs, the external port-valve is changed, again without removal of the initially placed catheter. Because the valve can be applied at any level on the shaft of the tube, this skin-level device becomes specific for each patient. An additional advantage is that inventory is markedly simplified as the need for multiple catheter lengths is eliminated.

The diameter of the long tubes and the skin-level devices depends on the size of the child and the purpose of the gastrostomy. For infants and small children 14–16 F tubes are appropriate. For older children sizes 18–20 F are well suited. Because most children are given commercially available liquid formulas, smaller tubes can be used. However, there is a greater chance of plugging, particularly with certain medications. If the patient is to receive a home-made blenderized diet, larger diameter access devices are better suited for this purpose. Several different catheter models are available for the "pull" PEG. When choosing one of these, it is important to check the compressibility of the retaining intragastric "tulip" or disk, because if these are too large or stiff, they can damage the esophagus as they are pulled into place.

A special operative challenge is the placement of a gastrostomy tube in an infant with esophageal atresia without fistula or a small premature child. The stomach in these babies is extremely small and does not accommodate most commercially available gastrostomy tubes. For this reason we have used a 10 or 12 F "T" tube with the horizontal, transverse limbs cut close to the vertical portion.

38.2.5 Technical Aspects

Important points related to the stomas most commonly used by surgeons are highlighted here. For details the reader is referred to one of the atlases of surgical technique.

38.2.5.1 Stamm Gastrostomy

The stomach is approached through a short, left, transverse supraumbilical incision (Fig. 38.1). A vertical incision may be used for children with a high lying stomach or a narrow costal angle. The catheter exit site should be approximately at the junction of the lower two thirds and the upper third of a line from the umbilicus to the mid portion of the left rib cage, over the mid-rectus muscle. In general, catheters should not be brought out through the incision because this increases the complication rate, particularly leakage. The gastrotomy should be approximately in the mid body of the stomach. Placing the gastrostomy in the antrum can lead to gastric outlet obstruction by the tube and predispose to leakage. The fundus, the splenic hilum, and the greater curvature should also be avoided. A purse-string suture, using synthetic absorbable material, is placed around the gastrotomy site, the gastric wall is incised, the catheter is introduced into the stomach, and the suture tied. The

traditional second purse-string suture is modified so that it produces a water-tight approximation of the stomach to the abdominal wall. To do this, a continuous monofilament suture is used with the stitches alternating between the gastric serosa and the parietal peritoneum. The catheter is secured with monofilament sutures and a small cross bar is slipped over the catheter shaft and brought close to the skin level. Once the immobilizing sutures are removed after 1–2 weeks, this cross bar prevents the distal migration of the catheter. The procedure can be modified slightly to accommodate the placement of a skin-level device (Fig. 38.1).

38.2.5.2 Percutaneous Endoscopic Gastrostomy ("Pull" Technique)

Older children and those able to tolerate endoscopy without compromising the upper airway receive sedation and local anesthesia. Younger children require general endotracheal anesthesia, primarily because of possible difficulties with the airway management. A single dose of a broad-spectrum intravenous antibiotic is administered shortly before the procedure. The approximate site of the stoma is marked on the skin, using the above-mentioned guidelines. The stoma site should be away from the rib cage to allow placement of an incision if a fundoplication becomes necessary in the future. Additionally, gastrostomies too close to the rib cage are uncomfortable and tend to leak because of excessive motion with respirations. The gastroscope is inserted and the stomach insufflated. Under-insufflation as well as over-insufflation should be avoided to minimize the possibility of accidentally piercing the transverse colon. Insufflation of the small intestine tends to push the transverse colon in front of the stomach and should thus be avoided. Digital pressure is applied to the proposed gastrostomy site, which usually corresponds to the area where transillumination is brightest.

Transillumination and clear visualization of the anterior gastric wall indentation are key points. Without these, an open or laparoscopically aided gastrostomy should be employed. A long-lasting local anesthetic is drawn into a syringe and the proposed PEG site injected. The needle is advanced further and continuous aspirating pressure is applied to the plunger. Air bubbles should be visible in the remaining fluid when the tip of the needle is seen by the endoscopist. If air bubbles are noticed before the needle tip is in the stomach, the colon or other intestinal loop may be interposed between the stomach and the abdominal wall. This mishap will lead to a gastroenteric fistula.

An incision of 8–10 mm is made in the skin and a hemostat applied to maintain the intragastric indentation. The endoscopist then places a polypectomy snare around the indentation "mound." The intravenous cannula is placed in the incision between the slightly spread prongs of the hemostat and then firmly thrust through the abdominal and gastric walls, exiting through the tip of the "mound" into the loop of the polypectomy snare. The snare is partially closed, but not tightened around the cannula. The needle is removed and the looped steel wire inserted through the cannula. The polypectomy snare is allowed to slide away from the cannula and is tightened around the wire. An alternative method is to retrieve the wire with an alligator or biopsy forceps. The wire is then pulled back with the endoscope through the stomach and esophagus, exiting through the patient's mouth. A guiding tract is thus established. The catheter is attached to the guidewire by interlocking the two steel wire loops. Traction is applied to the abdominal end of the wire, guiding the catheter through the esophagus and stomach and across the gastric and abdominal walls. The tapered end of the catheter exits through the abdominal wall before the gastric retainer enters the patient's mouth, allowing complete control of the catheter during placement. Traction is continued until the gastric and abdominal walls are in loose contact. We routinely reendoscope to confirm the position of the catheter and to examine the esophagus.

The external cross bar is slipped over the catheter and guided to the skin level. Excessive tightening must be avoided to prevent pressure of the intragastric retainer on the mucosa and the cross bar on the skin. If the gastric and abdominal walls are "sandwiched" too tightly, this can give rise to pressure necrosis and the burying of the internal retainer or "bumper." The catheter is cut to the desired length and the feeding adapter attached. No sutures are used, and the feeding adapter is attached to a small, clear plastic trap.

38.2.5.3 Laparoscopic Gastrostomy

Several methods for establishing laparoscopic gastrostomy have been developed. In addition to the videoscopically controlled PEG, the two commonly employed methods are based on adaptations of the Stamm gastrostomy and modifications of the "push" PEG using the Seldinger technique. Our preference is for the latter, because in order to place a purse-string suture through the exposed segment of the anterior gastric wall, the trocar site must be sufficiently enlarged. This enlarged opening may predispose the site to leakage. In order to temporarily anchor the stomach to the abdominal wall, different approaches may be employed such as T fasteners or U-stitches.

The most suitable site for the gastrostomy is selected in the left upper quadrant and marked. As in the other types of gastrostomies, it should be away from the costal margin and the midline. A nasogastic tube is inserted. Pneumoperitoneum is established in the usual age-appropriate manner and a 30-degree laparoscope introduced at the umbilicus. The previously marked site is infiltrated with a long-lasting anesthetic. The needle is then pushed through the abdominal wall and the appropriate relation between the anterior gastric wall and the stoma site established. A small skin incision is made and a 5-mm trocar inserted. A grasper is introduced and the stoma site on the anterior gastric wall lifted toward the parietal peritoneum. A U-stitch is passed through the abdominal wall, through the anterior gastric wall, and back out through the abdominal wall. A second U-stitch is passed parallel to the first one, 1–2 cm apart. The sutures are lifted, maintaining the stomach in contact with the abdominal wall. The grasper and the trocar are removed. The stomach is insufflated with air through the nasogastric tube and a needle is inserted through the trocar site into the gastric lumen, between the two U-stitches. A Seldinger type guidewire is passed through the needle into the stomach. The tract is dilated over the guidewire to the size required to insert either a Foley type catheter or a balloon-type skin-level device. These are placed over the same guide-wire. The previously placed U-stitches are tied over the wings of the "button." If a long tube is placed, a pair of bolsters is employed.

38.2.5.4 Percutaneous Gastrostomy Guided by Fluoroscopy, Computer Tomography, or Ultrasonography

These techniques are, in many ways, similar to the previously described methods of creating an approximation of the anterior gastric wall to the parietal peritoneum and inserting a self-retaining tube. For the fluoroscopic and computerized tomography-guided procedures, the stomach is insufflated with air. In the ultrasonographic guided gastrostomy, the stomach is filled with saline. In some techniques the stomach is approximated and held in place by T-fasteners, prior to insertion of the catheter in an "introducer" PEG variation, whereas in others a pig-tail catheter is used to gain access and retention. In both cases, a Seldinger-type technique is employed, followed by dilatation of the tract, and catheter insertion. A fluoroscopically guided "pull" PEG can also be performed.

38.2.6 Postoperative Care and Catheter Change

Following open gastrostomies, enteral feedings begin once the ileus has resolved. After minimally invasive procedures, feedings may be started on the same day or on the following day. The latter has been our routine. The dressing is removed after 24 h, the wound is examined, and the tension on the external immobilizers adjusted in order to avoid excessive pressure that could lead to tissue damage. Our preference is to leave the stoma uncovered. We avoid harsh antiseptic solutions and, after a few days, use simply soap and water for cleaning. Granulation tissue forms after a couple of weeks and is controlled with gentle application of silver nitrate. If granulation tissue becomes excessive, it leads to leakage and needs to be excised. A local anesthetic containing epinephrine decreases the bleeding, which is then controlled with silver nitrate. We have observed good results with the application of triamcinolone and antifungal combination to prevent the recurrence of granulation tissue. Once the tract becomes epithelialized, no medication should be used.

A commonly asked question is: "When can a gastrostomy catheter safely be changed?" This depends on the type of procedure and the healing ability of the patient. For procedures in which the stomach is not anchored to the abdominal wall with sutures, we have arbitrarily recommended 3 months, although shorter periods may suffice. For children with cyanotic heart disease or those on steroids, impaired healing may necessitate further delay.

Once the feeding stoma is established, it is not uncommon for some children, particularly the neurologically impaired, to receive excessive calories and rapidly gain weight. It must be kept in mind that most of these patients, not being active, have far lower nutritional requirements than those recommended in pediatric manuals.

38.2.7 Complications and Their Management

Problems related to gastrostomies can be divided into those related to (1) operative technique, (2) care, and (3) catheters. Serious technique-related complications include separation of the stomach from the abdominal wall leading to peritonitis, wound separation, hemorrhage, infection, injury to the posterior gastric wall or other organs, and placement of the tube in an inappropriate gastric position. Separation of the stomach from the abdominal wall is a serious and potentially lethal complication. It is usually due to inadvertent premature dislodgment of the tube or a disruption during catheter change. The latter occurs when a new tube is inserted into a tract that is either not well formed because of incomplete adherence of the stomach to the abdominal wall or is damaged during removal of the old tube. This mishap requires immediate attention. If suspected, a study with water-soluble contrast is promptly done. The disruption is generally managed with a laparotomy, although in select cases a laparoscopic correction is possible. Most complications can be avoided by careful choice of the procedure and stoma device, considering a stoma placement a major intervention, and using meticulous technique. Other important points are approximation of the stomach to the abdominal wall, exiting the catheter through a counter-incision in open procedures and avoiding tubes in the midline where the abdominal wall is thinner, and keeping a reasonable distance from the rib cage to avoid excessive motion of the tube and discomfort. In the teaching setting, adequate supervision is essential.

One of the most serious long-term complications is the so-called "buried-bumper syndrome." The external migration of the dome of the catheter into the abdominal wall becomes apparent when there is difficulty with the administration of feedings that may also be associated with pain. This problem can be avoided by always allowing sufficient "play" between the skin-level device or external bumper on the catheter and the skin. Caregivers must be instructed to check this frequently, particularly if the patient has gained significant weight. The opposite problem, internal migration, does not occur with "buttons," but is occasionally seen with long tubes, particularly the balloon-type devices. The balloon advances into the duodenum and beyond and can produce intestinal obstruction. This mishap can be avoided by instructing the caregiver to make sure the external length of the tube is unchanged and the external bumper is properly adjusted. Additional caution is needed when a long Foley or balloon-type catheter is introduced in the stomach. If the shaft is advanced too far, the balloon may be in the esophagus or duodenum. Inflation can then seriously damage these organs.

Few complications will interfere with quality of life more than leakage. This problem is initially managed using conservative measures. If the patient has a long tube, this should be changed to a skin-level device. One of the most common factors leading to leakage in this setting is enlargement of the stoma created by the pivoting motion of the longer catheters. Two of the most common mistakes in handling leakage are applying traction to the tube and exchanging the leaking tube for a larger one. Traction will eventually shorten the tract and increase leakage. A larger tube will increase the diameter of the stoma and compound the problem. A better approach is to switch to a smaller tube and let the stoma "shrink" and then replace the catheter with a skin-level device. At times, it may become necessary to remove the device completely and let the stoma close partially. If these measures fail, the stoma may be relocated using a simple, nonendoscopic variation of the PEG. A new stoma site is selected and a small incision is made. A large curved needle is placed through the leaking stoma, through the gastric lumen, exiting through the new site. The suture is pulled through, establishing a tract. The catheter follows the tract, entering through the newly established one. Once the catheter is in place, the leaking stoma is closed extraperitoneally.

38.2.8 Gastrostomy Closure

When a stoma is no longer needed, the catheter is simply removed. If the gastrostomy has been in place for less than 6–12 months, the tract will usually close spontaneously. If this does not occur, operative closure may become necessary. This is done as an outpatient procedure under general anesthesia. The tissue around the stoma is infiltrated with a local anesthetic containing epinephrine and the stoma tract dissected down to the deepest possible extra-peritoneal level. The tract is then closed in layers using absorbable sutures.

38.3 Jejunostomy

38.3.1 Introduction

Direct operative access to the small bowel for feeding purposes is almost as old as that approach to the stomach. However, jejunostomies are not used as frequently as gastrostomies because they are more difficult to place and maintain, are more complication prone, and less physiologic (Table 38.3). Several traditional, as well as modified, approaches to the upper small bowel have been used in children.

Jejunostomies can be divided roughly into short-term, medium-term, and long-term access, regarding their expected length of use. They can also be divided

Table 38.3 Comparison of gastrostomy and jejunostomy

	Gastrostomy	Trans-pyloric tube jejunostomy	"Direct" jejunostomy
Physiologic feeding	Yes	No	No
Bolus feedings	Yes	No	No
Continuous feedings	Yes	Yes	Yes
Stoma/placement catheter	Many options	Imaging or endoscopy needed	Several options
Tube plugging	Low	High	Moderate (except Roux-en-Y)
Long-term maintenance	Simple	Difficult	Moderately difficult
Complication rate	Low	Moderate	High

into indirect and direct jejunal access, depending on how the catheters are placed. Nasojejunal catheters are a good example of short-term, indirectly placed jejunal tubes. These are usually well tolerated for a few weeks. Trans-gastric jejunal feeding tubes, with or without a gastrostomy, are examples of medium-term, indirectly placed catheters. Although they are better tolerated, they are not suitable for long-term use because they tend to become dislodged and plugged. Additionally, replacement usually requires endoscopic or radiologic manipulation. With both of these transpyloric tubes, duodenogastric reflux has been observed. Needle-catheter jejunostomies are examples of short-term direct jejunal access. They are usually placed for a defined period of time because plugging and the difficulty in replacement preclude their long-term use. For long-term, direct jejunal access, two approaches are commonly used: placement of a catheter directly in a loop of jejunum brought to the abdominal wall, or the more complex method of constructing a Roux-en-Y and introducing the catheter into the proximal segment of the distal, partially excluded loop.

38.3.2 Indications

In recent years, there has been an increased interest in the use of jejunostomies in the pediatric age group, mainly because children with more complex medical problems, unable to use a gastrostomy, have been referred for long-term enteral access (Fig. 38.4). These are mostly neurologically impaired patients, including children with severe foregut dysmotility, failed fundoplications, and gastric paresis. Many have had previous operations, including a gastrostomy. Jejunostomies are also employed in children who have had a gastric transposition for esophageal replacement or microgastria. In all of these children, the main indication is *feeding*. A less common use is the *administration of medication* (e.g., pancreatic enzymes in patients with cystic fibrosis). A combination *decompressing–feeding* jejunostomy is the Rehbein technique using a dual purpose catheter in infants with jejunal atresia. The larger lumen provides decompression of the proximal dilated bowel, while the thinner, trans-anastomotic tube permits early feeding.

38.3.3 Choice of Procedure

38.3.3.1 Needle Catheter Jejunostomy

Although this approach can be employed as an adjunct during other intra-abdominal interventions, it offers limited advantages. Because these catheters easily plug, are nearly impossible to change, and are associated with several serious complications, they are seldom employed.

38.3.3.2 Catheter Placement Directly into the Jejunum

The traditional technique is the formation of a Witzel-type channel. This method has two disadvantages: if the tube becomes dislodged or plugged, it is difficult to change, and in small children the formation of a channel substantially reduces the diameter of the lumen. We have had good results with direct jejunal access placing the feeding device with a Stamm-type technique.

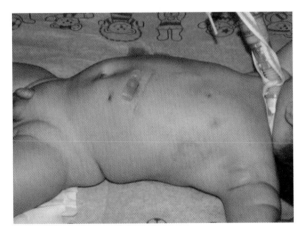

Fig. 38.4 Five-month-old child with complex myelodysplasia, hydrocephalus, and Arnold-Chiari malformation. Because of the inability to swallow, a nasogastric feeding tube was placed shortly after birth. The combination of small stomach and pronounced gastroesophageal reflux necessitated the insertion of a nasojejunal feeding tube. Respirator dependency required a tracheostomy. At 2 months of age, an antireflux procedure was done, and a gastrostomy as well as a jejunostomy was added. As the gastric size gradually increased, and emptying improved, feedings could be switched from the jejunal to the gastric route. Two months thereafter, the 12 F "T" tube jejunostomy tube could be removed

Although leakage was a concern, this has not been a significant problem in our experience. Catheter changes were not a problem either.

38.3.3.3 Catheter Placement in a Partially Excluded Loop

The main appeals of the Roux-en-Y feeding jejunostomy are the decreased likelihood of leakage and the possibility of safe catheter change. However, this approach is more complex and increases the possibility of early and late bowel-related complications.

38.3.4 Choice of Access Device

For direct jejunal access we employ a nonballoon button in older children and a T-tube in infants. The T-tube is then converted to a skin-level device with the external port-valve. Balloon catheters should not be used because they will occlude the lumen. Any of the gastric access devices will work in the Roux-en-Y set-up.

38.3.5 Technical Aspects

Except for the Roux-en-Y, the techniques are similar to those employed for gastrostomies. However, the thinner intestinal wall and the narrower lumen require adaptations and greater precision in execution. One of the most important aspects is the proper identification of the proximal jejunal loop. The safest way to do this is by clearly visualizing the ligament of Treitz. The access device should be placed at a short distance from the fourth portion of the duodenum to minimize reflux of feedings into the stomach. In the Roux-en-Y technique, the jejunum can be transected a little closer to the ligament of Treitz. Depending on the age of the child, the excluded bowel segment should be between 10 and 20 cm in length. The access device can be placed either in the end or the side of the loop that will form the feeding conduit. As in the other types of stomas, it must be securely attached to the parietal peritoneum. An attempt should be made to position the intestinal loops in such a manner that the possibility of internal hernias is minimized.

38.3.6 Postoperative Care

Although care following a jejunostomy is similar to that after a gastrostomy, feeding should be started at a much slower rate because of ileus and to decrease the possibility of diarrhea. As a rule, feedings are administered continuously by a pump. Following a period of adaptation, the regimen can be modified to allow for "windowing." Some patients may tolerate a limited amount of bolus feeds.

38.3.7 Complications

Overall, jejunostomies have more complications than gastrostomies. A contributing factor to this is that they are generally employed in more complex patients with preexisting problems. Specific jejunostomy-related complications include intestinal volvulus around the stoma, internal hernia, and adhesive bowel obstruction.

38.3.8 Follow-up of Children with Feeding Stomas

All children with gastrostomies and jejunostomies should be carefully followed to prevent long-term, catheter-related complications. Patients with gastrostomies need to be monitored for manifestations of foregut dysmotility, particularly gastroesophageal reflux. An important goal in children with feeding stomas is that, whenever possible, every effort should be made to institute or resume oral feedings (Figs. 38.5 and 38.6).

Placement of a gastrostomy or a jejunostomy in a child should be carefully planned and considered a major intervention. A problematic stoma can complicate the management of even a simple, temporary condition. On the other hand, a well indicated and properly placed stoma will contribute significantly to the child and the caregiver's quality of life.

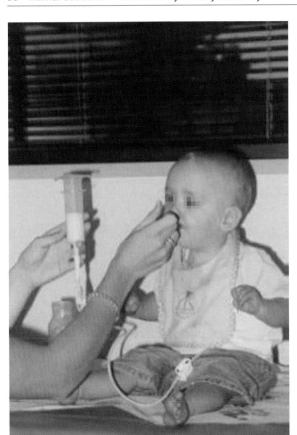

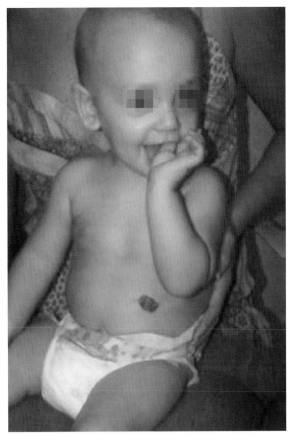

Fig. 38.5 Ten-month-old child receiving simultaneous oral and gastrostomy feedings. Shortly after birth, respiratory distress and drooling were observed. A large cervical neuroblastoma was diagnosed and resected. The swallowing difficulty was initially managed with a nasogastric tube. Because lengthy oropharyngeal incoordination was expected, a percutaneous endoscopic gastrostomy was placed at the age of 1 month. Aggressive oral feeding rehabilitation allowed the removal of the gastrostomy at the age of 16 months

Fig. 38.6 Same infant with a Genie™-type, skin-level port-valve depicted one month prior to gastrostomy removal. This photo illustrates one of the most important features of a skin-level device: the increased independence for the child

Further Reading

DeCou JM, Shorter NA, Karl SR (1993) Feeding Roux-en-Y jejunostomy in the management of severely neurologically impaired children. J Pediatr Surg 28:1276–1280

Gauderer MWL (2002) Percutaneous endoscopic gastrostomy (PEG) and the evolution of contemporary long-term enteral access. Clin Nutr 21:103–110 [Historical perspective]

Gauderer MWL, Abrams RS, Hammond JM (1998) Initial experience with the changeable skin-level port-valve: New concept for long-term gastrointestinal access. J Pediatr Surg 33:73–75

Gauderer MWL, Stellato TA (1986) Gastrostomies: Evolution, techniques, indications and complications. Curr Prob Surg 23:661–719 [Monograph]

Gauderer MWL (2006) Gastrostomy. In Puri P, Höllwarth ME (eds) Pediatric Surgery. Springer Surgery Atlas Series, Springer-Verlag Berlin Heidelberg, New York, pp 181–196

Puri P (2003) Newborn Surgery. 2 edn. Arnold, London [Textbook]

Puri P, Höllwarth M (2006) Pediatric Surgery. Springer, Berlin, Heidelberg [Atlas]

Sampson LK, Georgeson KE, Winters DC (1996) Laparoscopic gastrostomy as an adjunctive procedure to laparoscopic fundoplication in children. Surg Endosc 10:1106–1110

Stellato TA, Gauderer MWL (1989) Jejunostomy button as a new method for long-term jejunostomy feedings. Surg Gynecol Obstet 168:552–554

Duodenal Obstruction

39

Yechiel Sweed

Contents

39.1 Introduction Including Definition and Incidence

Congenital duodenal obstruction (DO) is a frequent cause of congenital intestinal obstruction in the newborn, occurring in 1 per 5,000–10,000 live births, and affecting boys more commonly than girls.

DO is the result of either intrinsic or extrinsic lesions. Figure 39.1 shows the various types of DO. Intrinsic DO may be caused by duodenal atresia, stenosis, diaphragm, perforated diaphragm, or a 'wind-sock' web. The wind-sock web is a duodenal membrane that balloons distally as a result of peristalsis from above. Extrinsic DO may be caused by annular pancreas, malrotation, or preduodenal portal vein. Although the annular pancreas forms a constricting ring around the second part of the duodenum, it is not believed to be the cause of DO and there is usually an associated atresia or stenosis in patients with an annular pancreas (Fig. 39.2).

The obstruction at the level of the duodenum may be complete or incomplete. Duodenal atresias cause complete bowel obstruction. They are classified into three types: Type I defect, the most common (65%) is represented by a mucosal web with normal muscular wall (Fig. 39.1e); Type II, by a short fibrous cord connecting the two atretic ends of the duodenum (18%) (Fig. 39.1c); and Type III, by a complete separation of the atretic ends with a mesenteric defect (18%) (Fig. 39.1a). Most of the unusual biliary duct anomalies coexist with this type of defect.

39.2 Etiology

Duodenal atresia, web, and stenosis usually occur in the second part of the duodenum, close to the area of intense embryological activity involved in the develop-

P. Puri and M. Höllwarth (eds.), *Pediatric Surgery: Diagnosis and Management*,
DOI: 10.1007/978-3-540-69560-8_39, © Springer-Verlag Berlin Heidelberg 2009

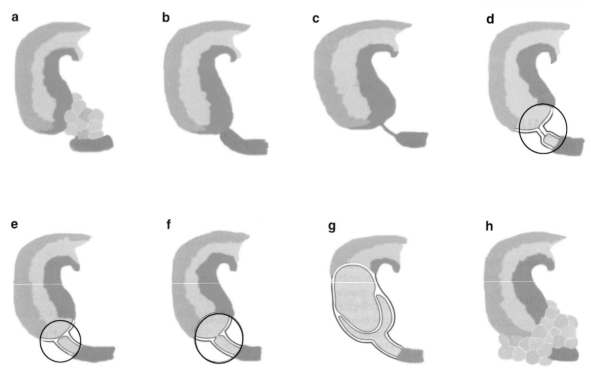

Fig. 39.1 Various types of duodenal obstruction. (**a**) Blind ends separated by a gap. (**b**) Two ends in apposition. (**c**) Ends joined by a fibrous cord. (**d**) Duodenal stenosis. (**e**) Complete duode-

nal membrane. (**f**) Perforated diaphragm. (**g**) "Wind-sock" web. (**h**) Annular pancreas

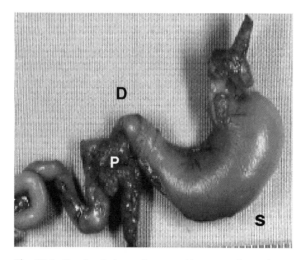

Fig. 39.2 Duodenal obstruction caused by an annular paricreas associated with duodenal stenosis in a post mortem of a 14-week old fetus with a diagnosis of down syndrome. S—stomach, D—duodenum, P—pancreas

ment of the biliary and pancreatic structures. Causative theories of congenital duodenal obstruction include abnormalities of pancreatic development, vascular disruption, and failure of recanalization of the duodenal

lumen from its solid cord stage. The last of these theories is currently the most popular. It has been demonstrated that from the fifth to the tenth week of gestation, endodermal lining of the duodenum proliferates rapidly, obliterates the lumen, and the duodenum becomes a solid cord. Later, the duodenal lumen is recanalized and is formed by vacuoles that coalesce. Duodenal atresia results from failure of vacuolization and recanalization. Duodenal stenosis and web result from incomplete recanalization of the duodenum. An annular pancreas results when the anterior and posterior anlage of the pancreas become fused to form a ring of pancreatic tissue that surrounds the second part of the duodenum (Fig. 39.2).

39.3 Associated Malformations

More than 50% of patients with duodenal atresia or duodenal stenosis have associated congenital anomalies, especially Down syndrome, which occurs in about 30% of patients (Table 39.1). The associated malformations in order of frequency are Down syndrome, annular pancreas, congenital heart disease, malrotation, esophageal atresia, urinary tract malformation, anorectal anomalies, other bowel atresias, vertebral anomalies, and musculoskeletal anomalies. Other rare anomalies include biliary atresia, choledochal cyst, anomalous bile duct communication between the proximal and distal ends of the duodenum, Feingold syndrome, deLange syndrome, and gastric antral web. Abdominal situs inversus has also been reported as an extremely rare association with congenital DO.

Table 39.1 presents the overall prevalence and distribution of associated anomalies reported in 1,759 patients, taken from 12 published articles in the English literature between 1969 and 1996.

These associated malformations have an impact on the morbidity and mortality of these patients. The most lethal of these abnormalities are cardiac anomalies that occur more frequently in children who have Down syndrome. It has been reported that 80% of patients born with DO and Down syndrome have an associated cardiac malformation.

The mortality rate is even higher in neonates born with three or more anomalies of the VACTERL association with an overall survival rate of 40–70%. The VACTERL association is an acronym describing the occurrence of specific congenital anomalies that occur in a greater-than-random frequency without hereditary factors. The anomalies include V, vertebral or vascular defects; A, anal malformation; C, cardiac anomaly; TE, tracheoesophageal fistula with esophageal atresia; R, renal anomalies; and L, radial limb anomalies. Duodenal atresia, which is not included in the VACTERL association, is seen in 6.3% of babies born with this spectrum of anomalies.

The incidence of combined esophageal and duodenal atresia varies between 3% and 6% and is associated

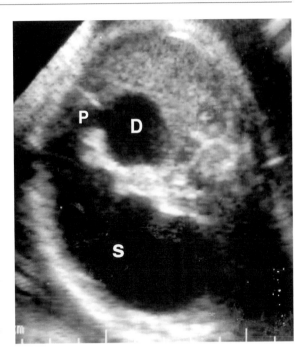

Fig. 39.3 Ultrasonography (transverse view) of 24-week gestational age fetus showing the "double bubble" sign. S—stomach, P—pylorus, D—duodenum

with significant morbidity and mortality (67–94% in various series). This high mortality is attributed to the failure to recognize the second abnormality preoperatively.

39.4 Prenatal Diagnosis

Duodenal obstruction is being increasingly diagnosed prenatally. The prenatal sonographic diagnosis of DO relies on the demonstration of the "double bubble" sign, which is due to the simultaneous distension of the stomach and the first portion of the duodenum. The dilated stomach and duodenum appear side by side across the midline of the upper fetal abdomen (Fig. 39.3). The "double bubble" has been observed as early as 12 weeks of gestation; however, the majority of cases are diagnosed during the 7th to the 8th month of gestation. The main reason for the late appearance of the "double bubble" sign is probably related to the hydrostatic pressure needed to dilate the duodenum and the degree of obstruction.

Table 39.1 Incidence of associated congenital anomalies (%) (N = 1,759 patients)

Associated anomaly	%
Down syndrome	28.2
Annular pancreas	23.1
Congenital heart disease	22.6
Malrotation	19.7
Esophageal atresia tracheoesophageal fistula	8.5
Genitourinary	8.0
Anorectal	4.4
Other bowel atresia	3.5
Others	10.9

Maternal polyhydramnios is also a common ultrasonographic finding observed in 20–75% of cases with duodenal atresia, mainly in the second half of pregnancy. In all cases of combined polyhydramnios and "double bubble" sign, a detailed evaluation for other associated anomalies, especially cardiac anomalies, should be undertaken. Amniocentesis for chromosomal analysis is helpful for counseling.

39.5 Diagnosis

The diagnosis of DO is usually based on prenatal ultrasonography, early clinical symptoms, physical examination, and plain radiographic abdominal films.

39.6 Clinical Features

About half of these patients are premature and of low birth weight. Vomiting and intolerance of attempted feedings are the most common symptoms and are usually present on the first day of life. Since 80% of the obstructions are located in the postampullary region of the duodenum, vomitus in the majority of cases is bile-stained. In supra-ampullary atresia, it is nonbilious. There is no abdominal distention because of the high level of obstruction. Infants may pass some meconium in the first 24 h of life and thereafter constipation may develop. Dehydration with weight loss and electrolyte imbalance soon follows if fluid and electrolyte losses have not been adequately replaced.

Incomplete duodenal obstruction (e.g., duodenal membrane with a central aperture) usually leads to the delayed onset of symptoms, which may appear a few months or years after birth.

39.7 Radiological Diagnosis

The diagnosis of the duodenal atresia is confirmed on X-ray examination. An abdominal radiograph will show a dilated stomach and duodenum, giving the characteristic appearance of a "double bubble sign" (the stomach and the proximal duodenum are air filled), with no gas beyond the duodenum (Fig. 39.4).

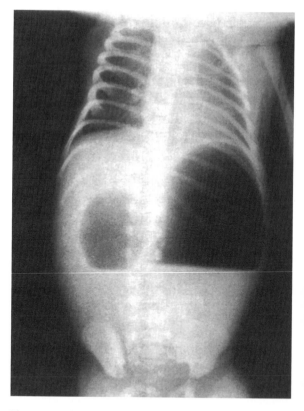

Fig. 39.4 Abdominal erect radiograph showing distended stomach and duodenum with a "double bubble" sign with no air beyond the duodenum

In partial duodenal obstruction, a plain film of the abdomen will show a "double bubble" appearance but there is usually some air in the distal intestine. Radiographic findings in the annular pancreas are usually indistinguishable from duodenal atresia and stenosis.

In some cases of partial duodenal obstruction, plain films may be normal and the upper gastrointestinal tract contrast radiography is indicated in these patients to establish the cause of the incomplete duodenal obstruction (Fig. 39.6). Occasionally, a duodenal diaphragm may be stretched and ballooned distally giving the wind-sock appearance on contrast study (Fig. 39.7).

39.7.1 Differential Diagnosis

All the various conditions of upper gastrointestinal obstruction should be included in the differential diagnosis of DO (Table 39.2). The most important ones for the pediatric surgeon are DO caused by

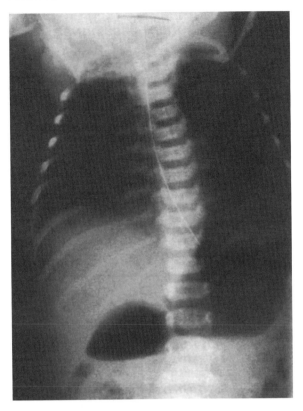

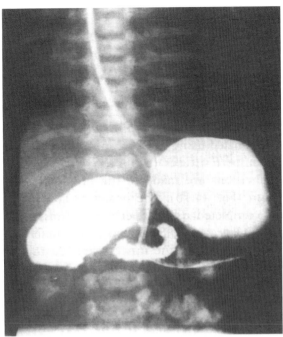

Fig. 39.6 Contrast study showing marked distension of the duodenum terminating with narrow caliber distally. A perforated diaphragm was found at operation

Fig. 39.5 Duodenal stenosis. Erect abdominal X-ray demonstrating a "double bubble" sign but with air beyond the duodenum

malrotation resulting in extrinsic compression related to Ladd's bands across the duodenum and volvulus of the midgut loop (Fig. 39.8a and b).

39.7.2 Malrotation

Malrotation may appear as acute and complete, most often seen in infancy, or as chronic and partial in older children. Clinical presentation of malrotation in the neonatal period may be either (1) recurrent episodes of subacute obstruction with intermittent bilious vomiting or (2) strangulating intestinal obstruction as a consequence of midgut volvulus. The infant presents with bile-stained vomiting that may contain altered blood, abdominal distention, and tenderness; the passage of dark blood per rectum; and shock. As the strangulation progresses to gangrene, perforation, and peritonitis, edema and erythema of the anterior abdominal wall becomes evident. Upper gastrointestinal contrast study is the procedure of choice showing the abnormal

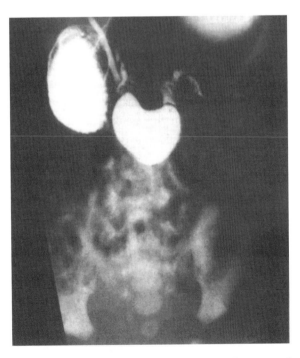

Fig. 39.7 "Wind–sock" web. Dilated duodenum demonstrated with duodenal membrane ballooned distally, giving characteristic "wind-sock" appearance

configuration of the duodenum, the duodenojejunal junction to the right of the midline, and small bowel located on the right side of the abdomen. The diagnostic investigation should be done urgently followed by an emergent operative intervention.

39.7.3 Pyloric Atresia and Prepyloric Antral Diaphragm

Pyloric atresia and prepyloric antral diaphragm are rare congenital malformations causing gastric outlet obstruction. They present shortly after birth with persistent nonbilious vomiting. In pyloric atresia, a plain X-ray of the abdomen will show gas in the dilated stomach—single gas bubble sign—and no gas beyond the pylorus.

39.7.4 Gastric Volvulus

Gastric volvulus is a rare congenital anomaly. Plain abdominal and chest radiographs are essential and will show a distended stomach in an abnormal position. Contrast studies clarify the anatomy and the site of obstruction.

39.7.5 Pyloric Stenosis

Clinical presentation of infants with hypertrophic pyloric stenosis is nonbilious vomiting usually occurring at 2–8 weeks of age. The diagnosis is based on the clinical history, palpable "pyloric tumor" found by physical examination, and ultrasonographic scanning of abdomen that reveals a typical hypoechoic ring with echogenic center of increased muscle thickness.

Table 39.2 Differential diagnosis of duodenal obstruction

Upper bowel obstructions
Malrotation
Pyloric atresia
Prepyloric antral diaphragm
Gastric vovulus
Pyloric stenosis
Jejunal-ileal atresia and stenosis
Preduodenal portal vein
Duodenal duplication cyst
Choledochal cyst
Superior mesenteric artery syndrome

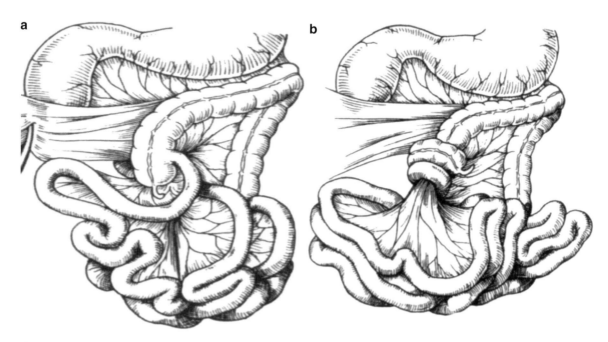

Fig. 39.8 A. Duodenal obstruction caused by (**a**) congenital adhesions—Ladd's bands. (**b**) Duodenal obstruction caused by volvulus

39.7.6 Jejuno-Ileal Atresia and Stenosis

This type of obstruction presents with abdominal distention and bile-stained vomiting. Diagnosis is confirmed on supine and erect abdominal radiographs that reveal distended small bowel loops and air-fluid levels.

39.7.7 Preduodenal Portal Vein

Preduodenal portal vein is a rare anomaly causing DO, and is often impossible to diagnose prior to surgery.

Duodenal duplication cyst, choledochal cyst, and superior mesenteric artery syndrome are rare causes of incomplete DO in infancy and are usually diagnosed in childhood or adolescence.

39.8 Preoperative Management

A wide variety of additional congenital anomalies that are often severe make preoperative diagnosis imperative. Anterior–posterior and lateral chest and abdominal radiographs, ascertaining visualization of the entire spine, should be made. Soon after the X-ray, cardiac and renal ultrasound should be carried out routinely in all these babies. A micturating cystourethrogram should be performed in babies with abnormal urogenital ultrasound or an associated anorectal anomaly.

Once the diagnosis is established, the infant should be prepared for early surgical exploration. Preoperative preparation consists of nasogastric decompression and fluid and electrolyte replacement. Care is taken to preserve body heat and avoid hypoglycemia since many of these newborn patients are premature and furthermore, small for date. Very low birth weight infants or those with respiratory distress and associated severe anomalies, e.g., congenital heart disease, will need special preparation such as resuscitation and ventilation.

39.9 Management

For patients with duodenal atresia, stenosis, and annular pancreas the recommended surgical procedure would be to bypass the obstruction by duodenoduodenostomy. Duodenoduodenostomy can be performed in either side-to-side fashion (Fig. 39.9) or proximal transverse to distal longitudinal (diamond shape) anastomosis as described by Kimura et al. (1977) (Fig. 39.10). In both surgical techniques, the downstream duodenum patency should always be demonstrated by passing a catheter or infusing saline to examine the distal bowel for other associated atresia or luminal

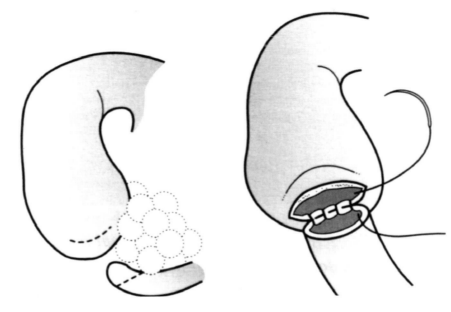

Fig. 39.9 Side-to-side duodenoduo denostomy

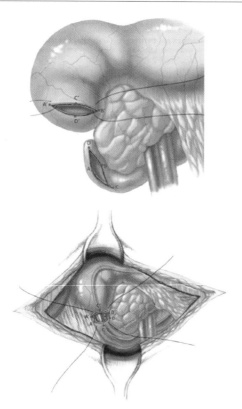

Fig. 39.10 Diamond-shaped duodenoduodenostomy

obstruction. Duodenal webs are excised through a longitudinal duodenotomy that is performed in the anterior duodenal wall at the site of the "transitional zone" connecting the wide and narrow segments of the duodenum. The membrane usually is localized in the second part and occasionally in the third part of the duodenum. The web can be excised as long as the ampulla of Vater is identified and preserved. The ampulla may open directly into the medial part of the membrane or proximately close to it. The mandatory identification of ampulla of Vater, to avoid injury, can be found by applying pressure on the gallbladder and seeing where the bile exits.

In the case of wind-sock duodenal web, it must be clearly identified because the visible transition from the distended proximal duodenum to the small downstream duodenum may be several centimeters distal to the base of the web. Traction applied at the apex of the web deforms the duodenum at its point of attachment and allows complete excision at the base after careful examination and identification of ampulla of Vater. In both duodenal web and "wind-sock," the duodenum is closed transversely.

The endoscopic surgical treatment of the duodenal membrane by either endoscopic incision or by laser ablation has also appeared in several reports in the literature, but subsequent surgery may be needed because of scar formation that may result in stenosis.

In recent years, with advances in minimally invasive surgery, laparoscopic duodenoduodenostomies are being performed in neonates but the evaluation of distal internal webs is more difficult to accomplish laparoscopically. Laparoscopic-assisted management provides excellent visualization, minimizes disfiguring and morbid upper abdominal incisions, and may decrease the risk of future adhesions. However, further clinical experience is necessary to establish the outcome of this technique.

39.10 Postoperative Care

Postoperatively, patients have a prolonged period of bile-stained aspirate through the nasogastric tube, mainly due to the inability of the markedly dilated duodenum to produce effective peristalsis. Some surgeons use a transanastomotic feeding tube to start early feeding and others use short-term intravenous nutrition.

39.11 Complications

Early complications are rare (except for missed anomalies) but late complications are reported to occur in 12–15% of patients with an associated 6% late mortality rate.

In a series of 138 patients, Dalla Vecchia et al. reported on a low early complication rate including anastomotic obstruction in 3%, congestive heart failure in 9%, prolonged adynamic ileus in 4%, pneumonia in 5%, and wound infection in 3% of cases.

Late complications include adhesive bowel obstruction in 9%, megaduodenum with duodenal dysmotility that required tapering duodenoplasty in 4%, and duodenogastro esophageal reflux (GERD) requiring surgery in 5% of cases. Blind loop syndrome, pancreatitis, cholecystitis, and cholelithiasis are rare complications.

Megaduodenum may occur up to 18 years postoperatively. It is associated with poor weight gain, frequent vomiting, abdominal pain, and blind loop syndrome. Megaduodenum can be avoided or corrected with an antimesenteric tapering duodenoplasty or by plication of the dilated atonic proximal duodenum. Blind loop syndrome occurs only in cases in which duodenojejunostomy is performed, but this procedure is rarely performed today.

A long-term follow-up study over 30 years by Escobar et al. reported that 20 of 169 patients required additional abdominal operations (e.g., fundoplication, 13, ulcer surgery, 4, and adhesiolysis, 4). Sixteen of 169 underwent revision of their original repair (tapering duodenoplasty or duodenal plication, 7, conversion of duodenojejunostomy to duodenoduodenosotmy, 3, and redo, 5). Ten late deaths were caused by complex cardiac malformations in 5, central nervous system bleeding in 1, pneumonia in 1, anastomotic leak in 1, and multisystem organ failure in 2 cases.

The late complications indicate that long-term follow-up is essential for infants treated for duodenal atresia and stenosis, particularly those with associated annular pancreas, GERD, delayed gastric emptying, peptic disorders, and megaduodenum.

Early operative mortality after correction of duodenal atresia has been reported to be as low as 4–5%. Long-term survival rate is excellent at 86–90%. Children with Down syndrome or other associated congenital anomalies, especially complex cardiac defects, have a higher long-term mortality rate. Five of the 10 late deaths (50%) in the series of 169 patients with DO occurred in patients with complex congenital heart diseases.

Overall, however, there has been significant improvement in the survival rate of patients with DO during the last three decades, resulting from early and appropriate surgical intervention, combined with advancements in neonatal intensive care, anesthesia, nutritional support, and early evaluation to identify associated anomalies.

Further Reading

Dalla Vecchia LK, Grosfeld JL, West KW et al (1998) Intestinal atresia and stenosis: A 25-year experience with 277 cases. Arch Surg 133:490–497

Escobar MA, Ladd AP, Grosfeld et al (2004) Duodenal Atresia and Stenosis: Long-term follow-up over 30 years. J Pediatr Surg 39:867–871

Sweed Y (2003) Duodenal obstruction. In P Puri (ed) Newborn Surgery. Arnold, London, pp 423–433

Sweed Y (2006) Duodenal Obstruction. In P Puri, ME Höllwarth (eds) Pediatric Surgery, Springer Surgery Atlas Series. Springer-Verlag, Berlin, Heidelberg, New York, pp 203–228

Intestinal Malrotation

40

Mark D. Stringer

Contents

40.1 Introduction

This spectrum of congenital anomalies is due to aberrant intestinal rotation and fixation occurring in early gestation. The incidence of malrotation is difficult to determine but symptomatic intestinal malrotation has an incidence of about 1 in 6,000 live births. The clinical effects of intestinal malrotation may manifest at any age but most cases present in infancy. Malrotation is an important cause of intestinal obstruction in the newborn. Failure to diagnose and treat the condition promptly can result in fatal midgut volvulus. In 1936, the North American surgeon, William Ladd, emphasized the importance of surgical treatment and his operation (Ladd's procedure) remains the definitive treatment today.

40.2 Embryology

The embryonic period in the developing human extends to the end of the 8th week of gestation (56 days) after which the fetal stage of development begins. The midgut of the human embryo receives blood supply from the superior mesenteric artery and is destined to become that part of the bowel extending from the second part of the duodenum to two thirds of the way along the transverse colon. In the embryo, the midgut forms a loop, the apex of which is continuous with the narrowing stalk of the yolk sac (vitellointestinal duct). During the 6th week of gestation, the midgut loop and its dorsal mesentery elongate rapidly and temporarily herniate into the extraembryonic celom in the umbilical cord. Umbilical herniation occurs because the developing liver and kidneys are relatively large and there is not enough room in the abdomen for the rapidly growing midgut. The proximal (cranial) limb of the midgut loop grows rapidly to form the small intestine while the distal (caudal) limb changes little except for the development of a cecal diverticulum.

During the stage of physiological herniation, the midgut rotates 90 degrees counterclockwise around the axis of the superior mesenteric artery so that the proximal limb comes to lie on the right side while the distal limb lies on the left side (Fig. 40.1). The midgut returns to the abdominal cavity between the 10th and 12th weeks of gestation. The proximal limb (small bowel) reenters first and passes behind the superior mesenteric artery. As the large bowel returns, it undergoes a further 180 degree counterclockwise rotation leaving the cecum on the right side of the abdomen. With continuing fetal growth, the ascending colon elongates and the cecum takes up its normal position in the right iliac fossa.

As each part of the gut achieves its definitive position during fetal life, mesenteric attachments are modified and fixed. Some mesenteric attachments shorten and others such as those associated with the duodenum and the ascending colon become retroperitoneal by fusion of the peritoneal layers. In the early embryo, the bowel mesentery is attached to the median plane of the posterior abdominal wall, but with gut rotation and growth the fan-shaped mesentery of the small intestine eventually originates along a line extending from the duodenojejunal flexure (ligament of Treitz) to the ileocecal junction (Fig. 40.2). This broad base of the small bowel mesentery helps to prevent axial rotation and volvulus of the gut.

Malrotation is the result of abnormalities of rotation and fixation of the intestine, most notably during the phase of midgut return. The etiology of malrotation is poorly understood. Defects of laterality, in general, just as much as abnormal ciliary mechanisms may be involved. Reports of familial malrotation indicate a genetic predisposition in some cases.

40.3 Pathology

There is confusion about the terminology, particularly with regard to nonrotation.

40.3.1 Incomplete Rotation

In this classic form of malrotation, the cecum lies in the epigastrium and the duodenojejunal flexure is sited inferiorly and to the right of the midline (Fig. 40.3). Peritoneal bands pass from the right upper quadrant lateral to the duodenum to the cecum and ascending colon (Ladd's bands). Whether these bands by themselves commonly cause duodenal obstruction is controversial; duodenal obstruction is most often due to associated midgut volvulus. The most hazardous element in incomplete malrotation of the gut is the narrow pedicled base of the midgut between the cecum and the duodenojejunal flexure, which predisposes to axial midgut volvulus. Lesser degrees of incomplete rotation are relatively common but the key feature dictating management in these cases is the width of the base of the small bowel mesentery i.e., the risk of midgut volvulus.

40.3.2 Non-Rotation

In its purest form, this is a rare and less hazardous form of intestinal malrotation. Failure of counterclockwise rotation of the midgut loop around the superior mesenteric artery leaves the bowel mesentery originating along a line close to the median plane of the posterior abdominal wall.

40.3.3 Other Abnormalities of Rotation and Fixation

In reverse rotation, a rare variant, the midgut rotates in a clockwise rather than in a counterclockwise direction around the axis of the superior mesenteric artery.

Thus, the third part of the duodenum is anterior to the superior mesenteric artery that in turn lies anterior to the transverse colon. The transverse colon may become obstructed by the superior mesenteric artery or the ileocecal region can undergo volvulus.

Mesocolic hernias are rare sequelae of malrotation and malfixation. A right-sided mesocolic hernia can

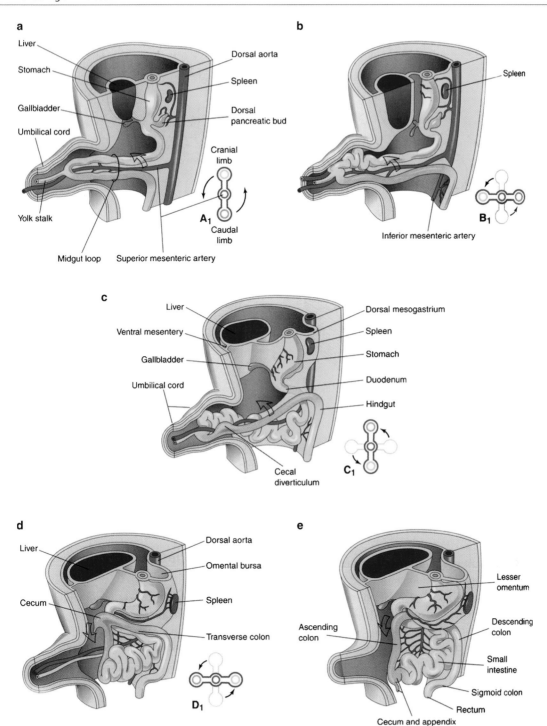

Fig. 40.1 Rotation of the midgut, as seen from the left. (**a**) Around the beginning of the 6th week, showing the midgut loop in the proximal part of the umbilical cord. A1 Transverse section through the midgut loop, illustrating the initial relationship of the limbs of the loop to the artery. (**b**) Later stage showing the beginning of midgut rotation. B1 Illustration of the 90-degree counterclockwise rotation that carries the cranial limb of the midgut to the right. (**c**) About 10 weeks, showing the intestines returning to the abdomen. C1 Illustration of a further rotation of 90 degrees. (**d**) About 11 weeks, after return of intestines to the abdomen. D1 Illustration of a further 90-degree rotation of the gut, for a total of 270 degrees. (**e**) Later fetal period, showing the cecum rotating to its normal position in the lower right quadrant of the abdomen (Reproduced with permission from Moore and Persaud. *The Developing Human*. 7th edn. Elsevier, 2003, p 270)

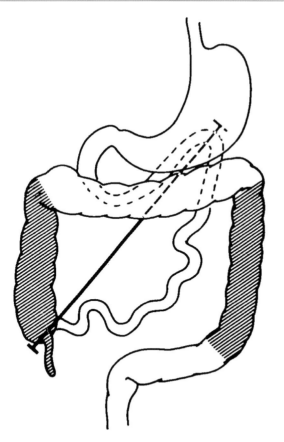

Fig. 40.2 Normal attachment of the small bowel mesentery. The normal broad base of mesenteric attachment extends from the ligament of Treitz to the ileocecal junction. Both ascending and descending colon are fixed retroperitoneally (Reproduced with permission from Filston and Kirks, *J Pediatr Surg* 1981; 16: 616, Figure 2)

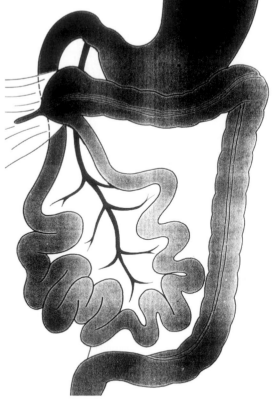

Fig. 40.3 Classical intestinal malrotation with a high central cecum, the duodenojejunal flexure to the right of the midline, and Ladd's peritoneal bands crossing the duodenum

develop as a result of nonrotation or reverse rotation of the proximal midgut (duodenum and jejunum) in association with clockwise rotation of the distal (colic) limb. The cecum becomes attached to the retroperitoneum in the right upper quadrant and the small intestine becomes trapped within a hernia sac created by the mesocolon of the cecum and the ascending colon. A left-sided mesocolic hernia occurs when the duodenum and the jejunum rotate normally behind and to the left of the superior mesenteric artery but then invaginate into a sac formed by the left mesocolon. These internal hernias are a rare cause of intestinal obstruction and strangulation.

Sometimes, rotation occurs normally but fixation is defective, resulting in a mobile cecum. This may predispose to intussusception or cecal volvulus.

40.3.4 Associated Anomalies

Intestinal malrotation is associated with a wide range of other congenital malformations. Nonrotation is seen in association with gastroschisis while various degrees of incomplete rotation are commonly found with congenital diaphragmatic hernia and exomphalos. Other less common associations are shown in Table 40.1. Some cases of small bowel atresia are associated with intestinal malrotation while others are caused by intestinal malrotation resulting in prenatal volvulus and infarction of the intestine.

An intrinsic duodenal obstruction (duodenal stenosis or atresia) is found in a small proportion of newborns with intestinal malrotation and this must be excluded at subsequent surgery.

Table 40.1 Other congenital anomalies associated with intestinal malrotation

Commonly associated

Abdominal wall defects (gastroschisis, exomphalos)

Congenital diaphragmatic hernia

Well-recognized but less frequent associations

Duodenal stenosis and atresia

Intestinal atresia

Biliary atresia splenic malformation syndrome

Meckel's diverticulum

Hirschsprung's disease

Anorectal malformations

Congenital cardiac disease

Esophageal atresia

Prune belly syndrome

Complete situs inversus (heterotaxia)

Rarer associations

Intussusception (Waugh's syndrome)

Megacystis-microcolon syndrome

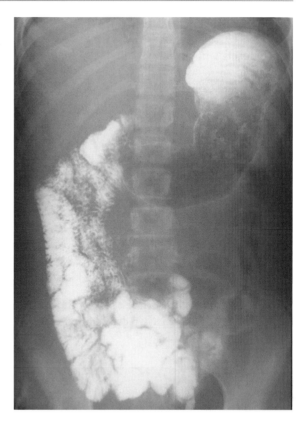

Fig. 40.4 Upper gastrointestinal contrast study in a boy with recurrent abdominal pain and vomiting due to intestinal malrotation. Note that the duodenojejunal flexure and the small bowel lie to the right of the midline

40.4 Clinical Features

Nearly 90% of symptomatic patients present during infancy, most of these in the newborn period. The newborn infant with intestinal malrotation is at greatest risk of life-threatening midgut volvulus, although this complication can occur at any age. The most common presentation of malrotation is bilious vomiting. In most cases, this is due to duodenal obstruction from intermittent midgut volvulus rather than compression by Ladd's bands or kinking of the duodenum. ***Bilious vomiting in the newborn is a sign of intestinal obstruction until proved otherwise***. If the acute midgut volvulus is intermittent or incomplete, the infant is well between attacks of vomiting although there may be evidence of failure to thrive. Abdominal examination at such times shows no abnormalities. However, if the acute midgut volvulus becomes established, then a strangulating closed loop obstruction of the midgut ensues. The infant becomes progressively sicker with the development of bloodstained stools, abdominal distension, and tenderness. Late and ominous features are shock, metabolic acidosis, sepsis, and multiorgan failure.

Other presentations that should be considered are as follows:

Prenatal—midgut volvulus can be a cause of intestinal atresia that may be first detected as dilated bowel during fetal ultrasound assessment. Compression of the duodenum by Ladd's bands in utero may also explain the association between malrotation and some cases of duodenal atresia or stenosis.

Child—beyond infancy, the child with malrotation may present with recurrent abdominal pain and chronic or intermittent vomiting, which may or may not be bilious (Fig. 40.4). There may be poor weight gain. Malabsorption and diarrhea, perhaps with occult blood loss, arising from chronic vascular and lymphatic congestion of the gut are occasional presenting features of chronic midgut volvulus.

Adult—rarely, intestinal malrotation is first diagnosed in adults when it may present with midgut volvulus.

Incidental—in some patients, malrotation is discovered incidentally during radiographic studies or at laparotomy undertaken for other indications.

40.5 Radiological Diagnosis

Stable infants with a history of bilious vomiting (and older children in whom bilious vomiting is a major symptom) should undergo an urgent upper gastrointestinal contrast study. If a midgut volvulus is demonstrated urgent surgery is required.

The plain abdominal radiograph in an infant with intestinal malrotation may be normal. In acute midgut volvulus the radiographic appearances can be notoriously variable and may include:

– A relatively normal bowel gas pattern
– A dilated stomach and duodenum ("double bubble" appearance) with a paucity of gas distally (Fig. 40.5)
– Multiple dilated loops of bowel
– A nearly gasless abdomen (Fig. 40.6)

An upper gastrointestinal contrast study performed by an experienced radiologist typically shows a duodenojejunal flexure to the right of the midline below the level of the pylorus (Fig. 40.7). Proximal small bowel loops are also seen to the right of the midline. In the presence of a midgut volvulus, there is incomplete duodenal obstruction often in the third part of the duodenum (Fig. 40.8) with a "beaked" or "corkscrew" appearance (Fig. 40.9). Delayed films typically show an abnormally sited cecum.

A barium enema is inferior to an upper gastrointestinal contrast study and, by itself, cannot be relied on to exclude malrotation. This is because a high and mobile cecum can be present in some healthy individuals without malrotation, and malrotation can occasionally occur despite the presence of the cecum in the right lower quadrant.

An ultrasound scan by an experienced sonographer can be helpful in diagnosis particularly if there is a midgut volvulus. Normally, the superior mesenteric vein (SMV) lies to the right of the superior mesenteric artery (SMA) but in malrotation this relationship is

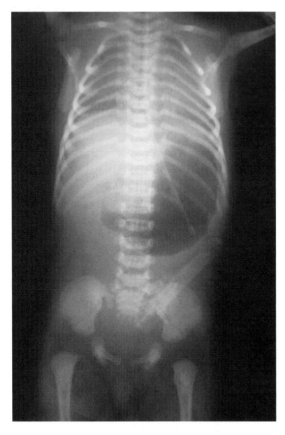

Fig. 40.5 A plain radiograph in a neonate with bilious vomiting showing a dilated stomach and duodenum with a paucity of gas distally. The baby had malrotation and a viable midgut volvulus

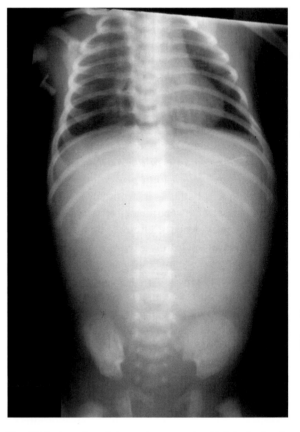

Fig. 40.6 A gasless abdomen in a neonate with intestinal malrotation and midgut volvulus

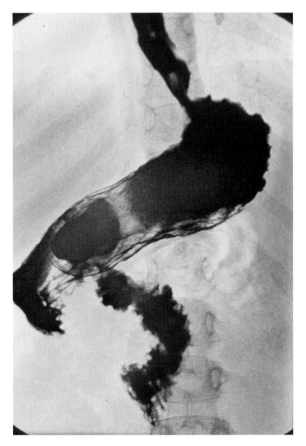

Fig. 40.7 An upper gastrointestinal contrast study showing the duodenojejunal flexure to the right of the midline in a child with symptomatic intestinal malrotation

reversed, i.e., the SMA is to the right of the vein (Fig. 40.10). Lesser degrees of inversion of these vessels (where they lie anteroposterior to one another) are less diagnostic. In midgut volvulus, color Doppler examination may show a "whirlpool" flow pattern of the SMV around the SMA together with a distended fluid-filled proximal duodenum. However, a normal anatomic relationship between the SMA and SMV does not exclude malrotation and an upper gastrointestinal contrast study remains the gold standard investigation.

40.6 Differential Diagnosis

In neonates with bilious vomiting, a surgical cause is found in almost 50% and intestinal malrotation accounts for a significant proportion of these. Other causes of bilious vomiting include intestinal obstruction from other causes such as intestinal atresia, meconium ileus, and Hirschsprung's disease. No surgical cause for bilious vomiting is found in some babies but intestinal malrotation must always be excluded.

40.7 Treatment

Operation should not be delayed once the diagnosis is made, although the degree of urgency depends on the presence of midgut volvulus. A well child with malrotation but no evidence of midgut volvulus should undergo surgery as soon as practically possible. An infant with volvulus requires urgent resuscitation and surgery. Delay increases the risk of potentially fatal catastrophic intestinal infarction. Resuscitation should therefore proceed while making arrangements for emergency surgery. Preoperative resuscitation should consist of adequate volume replacement, nasogastric decompression, correction of electrolyte and acid–base disturbances, and the administration of broad-spectrum intravenous antibiotics.

Asymptomatic patients with incidentally discovered classical malrotation (found at radiography or surgery) should, regardless of their age, have prompt corrective surgery if a narrow base to the midgut mesentery is suspected. However, minor degrees of incomplete rotation are relatively common and the management of these patients is controversial, e.g., a child with minor non-specific abdominal pain who is investigated by an upper gastrointestinal contrast study and found to have a duodenojejunal flexure in a low midline position and a cecum in the right lower quadrant. The risk of volvulus in this case is very low and surgery is unlikely to be beneficial. Some older patients with atypical and chronic symptoms do not benefit from correction of nonclassical malrotation. In some of these, malrotation is probably the consequence of a primary abnormality in gut motility rather than the root cause of symptoms.

40.7.1 Ladd's Procedure

The operation is conventionally performed through a transverse right upper quadrant abdominal incision. Laparoscopic approaches have been used successfully

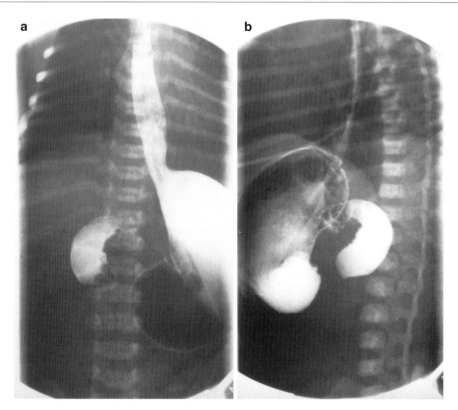

Fig. 40.8 (**a**) Anteroposterior and (**b**) lateral views of an upper gastrointestinal contrast study in intestinal malrotation with volvulus showing obstruction of the third part of the duodenum

in elective cases. Ladd's procedure consists of the following operative steps designed to relieve intestinal obstruction and prevent the risk of recurrent volvulus:

1. Reduce any volvulus—volvulus occurs in a clockwise direction around the SMA and thus reduction is achieved by gentle counterclockwise derotation of the gut (Fig. 40.11). The entire gut must be gently delivered from the abdomen in order to examine its orientation and fixation adequately.
2. Divide Ladd's bands (Fig. 40.12a), mobilize and straighten the duodenum, and check for any intrinsic duodenal obstruction (usually by passage of a large-bore nasogastric tube or balloon catheter).
3. Widen the base of the small bowel mesentery by carefully dividing overlying peritoneal adhesions (Fig. 40.12b).
4. Position the small bowel on the right side of the abdomen and the large bowel on the left so that the duodenojejunal flexure and the ileocecal junction

are wide apart. Because the cecum and the appendix now lie in the left upper quadrant, most surgeons perform an inversion appendicectomy.

If there is midgut volvulus, the viability of the derotated bowel must be carefully assessed (Fig. 40.13). As much bowel as possible should be preserved, but clearly infarcted gut should be resected. The decision regarding primary intestinal anastomosis or stoma formation will depend on the condition and length of the residual bowel and the stability of the infant. If there are long segments of small bowel with dubious viability, a planned second-look laparotomy 24 h after derotation is a useful strategy. In some cases, the entire midgut is infarcted when options are limited to resection and consideration of eventual small bowel transplantation or palliative care only. These are complex decisions depending primarily on the wishes of the parents.

Reverse rotation and mesocolic hernias are also corrected by dividing peritoneal attachments to free up the bowel. Elements of Ladd's procedure are necessary

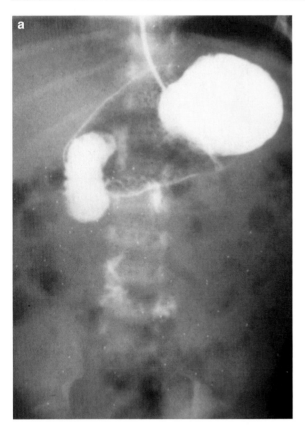
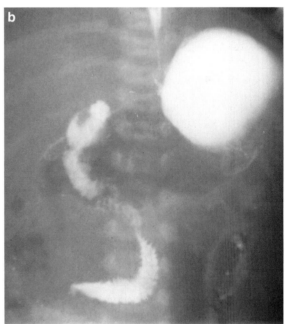

Fig. 40.9   a. and **b.** Upper gastrointestinal contrast studies showing examples of the "corkscrew" or "twisted ribbon" appearance of the duodenum and proximal jejunum in infants with intestinal malrotation and midgut volvulus

to minimize any future risk of volvulus. Care should always be taken to avoid injury to the mesenteric vessels during these dissections.

40.8 Complications

The outcome of children operated on for intestinal malrotation has steadily improved. Once the postoperative ileus has resolved, the vast majority recover uneventfully and have no further symptoms. A few have one or more of the following specific complications:

Intestinal infarction—this accounts for most of the 2–6% overall mortality associated with surgery for intestinal malrotation and midgut volvulus. Some of these patients have residual short bowel syndrome and require chronic parenteral nutrition with its attendant risks and the prospect of small bowel transplantation. Delay in recognizing and treating midgut volvulus is a major adverse determinant of outcome.

Recurrent midgut volvulus—this occurs in fewer than 2% of patients after surgery and is either due to failure to carry out the steps of Ladd's procedure adequately or due to lack of sufficient postoperative adhesion formation. Although fixation procedures have been devised to overcome the latter, these are rarely, if ever, necessary if Ladd's procedure is performed correctly.

Adhesive small bowel obstruction—this is a relatively common and often underestimated risk, occurring in approximately 8–10% of patients after Ladd's procedure. Parents should be warned of this complication.

Intestinal dysmotility—a small proportion of patients have ongoing gastrointestinal symptoms after successful surgery for malrotation and intestinal dysmotility appears to be the cause. These are more often older children in whom the primary indication for surgery was less clear cut abdominal symptoms.

Intussusception—postoperative small bowel intussusception is a rare cause of recurrent intestinal obstruction within the 1st or 2nd week after surgery.

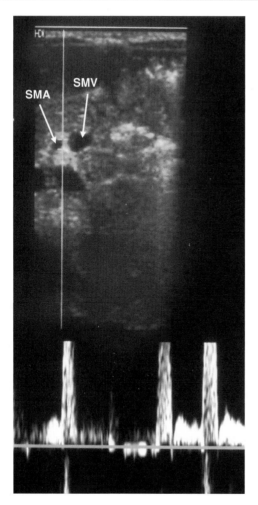

Fig. 40.10 Ultrasound scan of the abdomen in an infant with intestinal malrotation showing the reversed relationship of the superior mesenteric artery (SMA) and vein (SMV). The Doppler arterial waveform confirms the position of the SMA. (Kindly provided by Dr William Ramsden, St. James's University Hospital, Leeds)

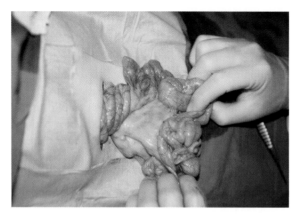

Fig. 40.11 Chronic midgut volvulus in a 3-year-old child with recurrent abdominal pain and vomiting. Note the thickened small bowel mesentery and patchy venous congestion

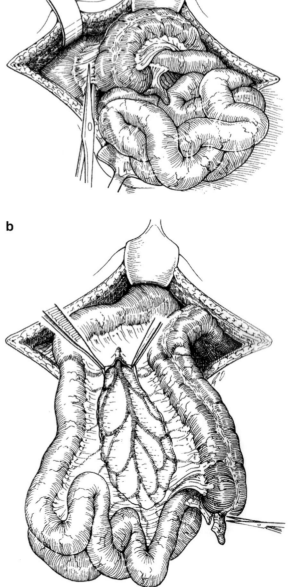

Fig. 40.12 (**a**) Division of Ladd's bands that extend from the cecum and ascending colon across the duodenum to the posterior peritoneum below the liver. (**b**) Splaying the root of the small bowel mesentery by dividing fibrous peritoneal bands and the anterior peritoneal layer crossing the superior mesenteric vessels (Reproduced with permission from Spitz, Malrotation. *In Newborn Surgery*. 2nd edition. Arnold, London, 2003, p. 438, Figures 45.7 and 45.9)

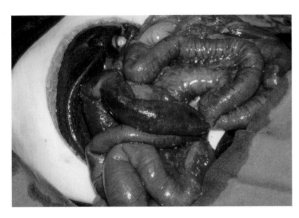

Fig. 40.13 Patchy small bowel infarction visible after derotation of the intestine in an infant with midgut volvulus associated with biliary atresia

40.9 Conclusions and Controversies

Intestinal malrotation is commonly encountered by pediatric surgeons. Bilious vomiting in infancy demands appropriate investigation and exclusion of malrotation. Children with classical intestinal malrotation are at risk of life-threatening midgut volvulus and

should be diagnosed and treated promptly. Ladd's procedure is an effective operation for treating the condition. However, several controversies and uncertainties remain: the importance of Ladd's bands in causing duodenal obstruction; the optimum treatment of minor degrees of incomplete malrotation; and the best strategy for infants with complete midgut infarction.

Further Reading

Pierro A, Ong EGP (2006) Malrotation. In P Puri, ME Höllworth (eds) Pediatric Surgery, Springer Surgery Atlas Series. Springer-Verlag, Berlin, Heidelberg, New York, pp 197–202

Filston HC, Kirks DR (1981) Malrotation—the ubiquitous anomaly. J Pediatr Surg 16:614–620

Moore KL, Persaud TVN (2003) The developing human, 7th edn. Saunders (an imprint of Elsevier), Philadelphia, PA, p 270

Puri P, Hollwarth ME (eds) (2006) Pediatric Surgery, Springer Surgery Atlas Series. Springer-Verlag, Berlin, MA, pp 135–145

Spitz L (2003) Malrotation. In P Puri (ed) Newborn Surgery, 2nd edn. Arnold, London, pp 435–439

Stringer MD, Oldham KT, Mouriquand PDE (2006) Pediatric Surgery and Urology: Long Term Outcomes, 2nd edn. Cambridge University Press, New York, pp 305–314

Jejuno-Ileal Atresia

41

Heinz Rode and A. Numanoglu

Contents

41.1 Introduction

Mural defects causing anatomical discontinuity of the small bowel can morphologically be divided into either atresia or stenosis and represent the most common cause of neonatal intestinal obstruction. Atresia refers to complete occlusion of the intestinal lumen and accounts for 95% of cases while stenosis is defined as a partial intra-luminal occlusion resulting in incomplete obstruction.

Jejuno-ileal atresia has a prevalence rate of approximately 1:330–1:1,500 live births, with a third of infants either born prematurely or small for date. Hereditary forms and familial patterns of atresia are exceptionally rare and may be on a basis of autosomal recessive or dominant transmission. A genetic basis however has been established for type III (b) and IV multiple atresias. Associated chromosomal and extra abdominal anomalies (7%) are well documented but not as common as in duodenal atresias.

Following surgical correction of the anomaly, the majority of children grow and develop normally, the end result influenced by the length and absorptive function of the residual bowel, associated anomalies and the successful management of the short bowel syndrome.

41.2 Etiology and Pathogenesis

Significant changes in surgical techniques and outcome of intestinal atresia and stenosis have occurred since Spriggs (1912) postulated that strangulation of a segment of fetal gut was most likely the causative factor producing intestinal atresia. Clinical and morbid anatomical data was presented by Louw in 1952 and subsequently proven by Barnard and Louw in canine experiments which produced anomalies identical to congenital intestinal atresia in humans. A localized intrauterine vascular accident can cause ischemic necrosis, liquefaction of tissues and subsequent resorption of the affected devitalized segment(s). The ischemia hypothesis is further supported by additional evidence supplied by incarceration or snaring of bowel in an exomphalos or gastroschisis, and the result of fetal events such as intussusception, midgut volvuli, trans-mesenteric internal herniation and thromboembolic occlusion resulting in atresia. Meconium ileus and Hirschsprung's disease should also be considered as possible underlying etiological factors in ileal atresia.

Additional hypothesis based on careful clinical observations, morphological studies and experimentation include Tandler's concept of failure of recanalization of the solid- cord stage of intestinal development, obliterative embryological events at Meckel's point with excessive resorption of the vitelline duct with adjacent ileum, epithelial occlusions and fetal inflammatory diseases. The localized nature of the defect would explain the low incidence of coexisting abnormalities of the extra-abdominal organs.

The clarification of the vascular hypothesis directly influenced and brought change to the surgical approach from: exteriorization or side-to-side anastomosis, to liberal back resection of the proximal blind ending bulbous end and primary end-to-end anastomosis. This resulted in elimination of blind-loop syndromes and anastomotic dysfunction with an immediate reduction in mortality rates from 69% to 33% at Great Ormond Street and 90–28% at the Red Cross Children's Hospital in 1955. Subsequent technical advances, improvement in neonatal care, anaesthesiology and nutritional support have further impacted upon and improved current day survival to over 90%.

41.3 Classification

The morphological classification of jejuno-ileal atresia into types I–IV has significant prognostic and therapeutic implications. The most proximal atresia determines whether it is classified as jejunal or ileal. Although single atresias are most commonly encountered, 6–12% of infants will have multiple atretic segments and up to 5% may have a second colonic atresia. The appearance of the atretic segment is determined by the type of occlusion, but in all cases maximum dilatation of the proximal bowel occurs at the site of the obstruction where the bowel is often dysperistaltic and of questionable viability when treatment is delayed. In rare instances jejuno-ileal atresias have been found to coexist with oesophageal, duodenal, colonic or rectal atresias.

- **Stenosis** (11%) is characterized by a short localized narrowing of the bowel without discontinuity or a mesenteric defect. A "wind-sock" effect can be created when increased intraluminal pressure in the proximal bowel bulges the membrane into the distal collapsed bowel creating a conical transition zone. The bowel is of normal length.
- **Atresia type I** (23%) is represented by a transluminal septum or short atretic segment. The dilated proximal bowel remains in continuity with the collapsed distal bowel, there is no mesenteric defect and the bowel is of normal length (Fig. 41.1).
- **Atresia type II** (10%) has two blind-ending atretic ends connected by a fibrous cord along the edge of the mesentery. There is no mesenteric defect and the bowel length is not foreshortened.
- **Atresia type III(a)** (15%) is similar to type II except that the fibrous connecting cord is absent and there is a V-shaped mesenteric defect. The bowel length may be foreshortened. Cystic fibrosis is commonly associated with this variety.
- **Atresia type III(b)** (19%) (Apple peel or Christmas tree) consists of a proximal jejunal atresia often with associated malrotation, absence of most of the superior mesenteric artery and a large mesenteric defect. The distal bowel is coiled in a helical configuration around a single perfusing artery arising from the right colic arcades. Occasionally, additional type I or type II atresias are found in the distal bowel. There is always a significant reduction in intestinal length. A familial incidence and atresias amongst siblings and identical twins point to a more complex genetic transmission with an overall recurrence rate of 18% (Fig. 41.2).
- **Atresia type IV** (22%) represents multiple segmental atresias like a string of sausages or a combination of types I–III. Bowel length is always reduced. The terminal ileum is usually spared; up

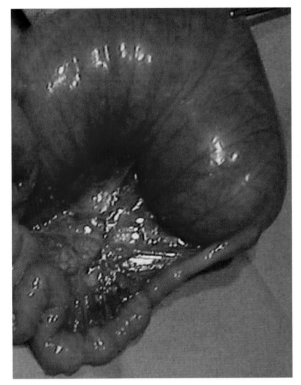

Fig. 41.1 Typical clinical picture of Jejunal atresia type 1

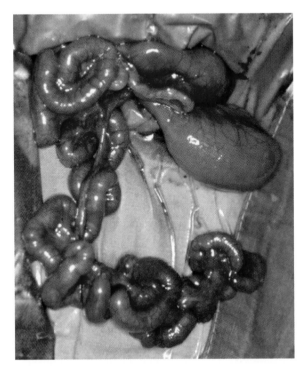

Fig. 41.2 Type III(b) (apple peel) atresia

Table 41.1 Types of intestinal atresias seen at Red Cross Children's Hospital 1959–2007

Type	Jejunum	Ileum	Total (%)
Stenosis	21	13	34 (10.7)
Type I	57	15	72 (22.7)
Type II	18	13	31 (9.7)
Type III(a)	28	24	52 (16)
Type III(b)	59	0	59 (18.6)
Type IV	56	14	70 (22)
Total	239	79	318

to 25 atretic sites have been encountered. A rare autosomal recessive pattern of transmission has been documented and pathological findings could support the concept that a developmental process early on, could have affected the whole bowel (Table 41.1).

41.4 Clinical Presentation and Diagnosis

Delay in diagnosis may lead to impairment of bowel viability or frank necrosis and perforation, fluid and electrolyte abnormalities and an increase incidence of sepsis (Figs. 41.3 and 41.4). The differentiation between atresia and other forms of intrinsic and extrinsic bowel obstruction due to volvulus or internal hernia, is the most important consideration that requires early exclusion. Many cases of intestinal atresia are now diagnosed prenatally by ultrasonographic investigation of the fetus, showing dilated intestine with vigorous peristalsis, suggesting obstruction, particularly so in pregnancies complicated by third trimester polyhydramnios. Intestinal atresia is also suspected in fetuses with gastroschisis and evidence of intestinal dilatation. However, prenatal ultrasound has a relatively poor predictive value for bowel abnormalities (31–42%). MRI imaging may prove to be more accurate in the prenatal diagnosis of bowel atresia. A positive family history will help identify hereditary forms. As the prognosis of intestinal atresia is excellent, there is no need for intrauterine intervention.

Postnatally, intestinal atresia or stenosis can present early with large intragastric volumes at birth (>25 ml gastric aspirate) followed by persistent bile stained vomiting, although in 20% of children, symptoms may

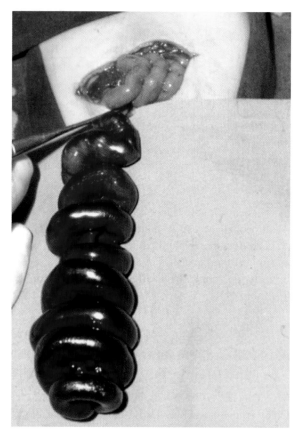

Fig. 41.3 A gangrenous type III(b) (apple peel) jejunal atresia due to volvulus

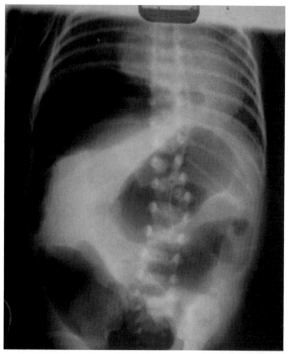

Fig. 41.4 Abdominal radiograph of a newborn showing a pneumoperitoneum due to proximal bowel perforation

be delayed for more than 24 h (Fig. 41.5). Abdominal distension is frequently present at or soon after birth; the more distal the obstruction the more generalized the abdominal distension. Visible loops of bowel may be observed but peristaltic activity is an inconsistent finding. Proximal jejunal atresia often presents with gastric distension, one or two loops of visible bowel in the upper abdomen decompressable by nasogastric tube aspiration in an otherwise gasless abdomen. Although the classic first stools passed by these patients are small, gray and mucoid, normal meconium can occasionally be passed. With delay in detection increasing intra-luminal pressure and/or secondary torsion of the proximal atretic distended bowel can lead to ischemia, perforation and peritonitis, precipitating abdominal tenderness, with oedema and erythema of the abdominal wall. One third of infants can have biochemically determined nonhemolitic jaundice.

The diagnosis is confirmed by radiological examination of the abdomen and chest by ordering a so-called "Baby Gram" (Fig. 41.6). Erect and supine whole body chest/abdominal radiographs done after birth will reveal distended air-filled small intestinal loops proximal to an obstruction in a gasless distal abdomen. In some instances, the first abdominal radiograph can reveal a completely opaque contrastless abdomen due to fluid-filled obstructed bowel. By emptying the stomach via a Replogle nasogastric tube and the injection of a bolus of air will demonstrate the obstruction.

The more distal the obstruction the greater the number of air–fluid filled and distended loops of bowel (Fig. 41.7). The bowel proximal to the site of obstruction may have the appearance of a large air-fluid filled loop. A prone lateral view could distinguish between low small and colonic obstructions. Occasionally scattered intraperitoneal or scrotal calcification or a large meconium pseudocyst or hydrocele may be encountered or seen radiographically, signifying

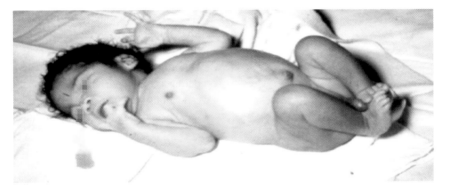

Fig. 41.5 Bile stained vomiting due to jejunal atresia

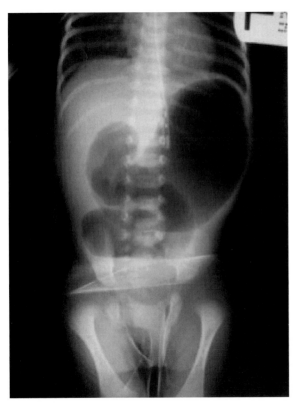

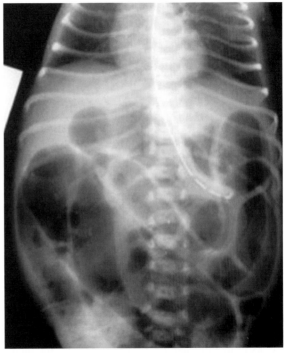

Fig. 41.7 Abdominal radiograph of a newborn with distal small bowel stenosis showing large air filled intestinal loops

Fig. 41.6 Abdominal radiograph of a newborn with jejunal atresia showing a few dilated proximal small bowel loops

intrauterine bowel perforation, meconium spill and dystrophic calcification.

In the presence of a radiologically determined complete obstruction, a contrast enema can be performed to confirm the level of obstruction (small or large bowel), document the calibre of the colon, exclude an associated colonic atresia, and locate the position of the caecum as an indication of malrotation (Fig. 41.8). Care must be taken not to rupture the microcolon, as the latter signifies an unused never filled colon with the obstruction located in the small bowel. Where the atresia is formed late in intrauterine life, the bowel distal to the

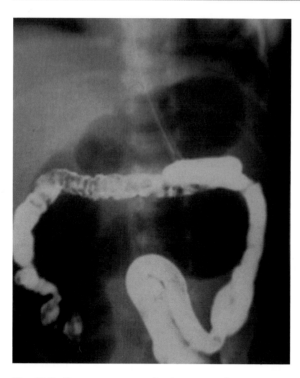

Fig. 41.8 Contrast enema confirming a normally rotated and patent colon with evidence of proximally dilated small bowel loops

atresia has a more normal calibre. With incomplete proximal small bowel obstruction an upper gastrointestinal contrast study or "aerogram" is indicated to demonstrate the site and nature of the obstruction and to exclude midgut volvulus.

The clinical and radiological presentation of jejunoileal stenosis will be determined by the level and degree of stenosis. The diagnosis is often delayed for several weeks to months and investigations may be inconclusive due to subclinical symptoms and findings.

41.5 Differential Diagnosis

A spectrum of other diseases can present with symptoms and signs of neonatal intestinal obstruction closely mimicking jejuno-ileal atresia. These include; those in the **wall of the bowel**-duodenal and colonic atresia and Hirschsprung's; those **in the bowel lumen**-meconium ileus and meconium plug syndrome; **external factors**-midgut volvulus and incarcerated hernia; and **non mechanical (functional) causes** such as

sepsis, necrotising enterocolitis and lastly **pregnancy related**, i.e. birth trauma, prematurity, and maternal medications.

Unfortunately these conditions can overlap, thereby rendering a correct presurgical diagnosis difficult. Special investigations may be needed to secure a correct diagnosis thereby avoiding unnecessary surgical intervention.

41.6 Treatment

These babies must be stabilized before transfer. Preoperative management is directed at optimizing the status of the infant, which apart from the atresia could be compromised by delayed diagnosis, fluid and electrolyte imbalance, associated abnormalities, prematurity, obstetrical related complications, transfer related, systemic sepsis, compromised bowel, and hypothermia. Basic factors required include: a warm humidified environment, gastric decompression to prevent aspiration, fluid management (maintenance, replacement of deficits and ongoing losses) correction of haematological and biochemical abnormalities and prophylactic antibiotics.

41.7 Anaesthesia

Neonates tolerate surgery well provided their special needs, physiological limitations and diseases processes are duly taken into account. The major anaesthetic considerations are related to prematurity, fluid and electrolyte homeostasis, abdominal distension, the risk of aspiration and associated life threatening congenital anomalies. Invasive monitoring is indicated in sick or unstable infants and a central line may be required for intravenous feeding postoperatively. The anaesthetic management is dictated by the condition of the infant and the available facilities. Light general and epidural anaesthesia may avoid the need for postoperative ventilation.

41.8 The Operation

The operative management of intestinal atresia is individualized and determined by the pathologic findings, associated abnormalities, the length of the undamaged bowel and the general condition of the infant.

41.8.1 Standard Surgical Procedure

A supra-umbilical transverse incision provides excellent exposure of the entire gastrointestinal tract. The bowel is exteriorized to determine the site and type of atresia and to exclude further downstream atresias or stenoses and associated lesions such as incomplete rotation or meconium ileus. The appearance of the atretic segment depends upon the type of occlusion, but in all cases maximum dilatation and hypertrophy of the proximal bowel occurs at the point of obstruction. This segment is often aperistaltic and of questionable viability, while the bowel distal to the obstruction is collapsed, tiny and wormlike in appearance. The intestinal content is milked backwards into the stomach from where it is aspirated. This must be a strictly controlled/co-ordinated maneuver with the anaesthetist; as aspiration is an ever-threatening complication. If a volvulus is present it should be derotated. Other distal small and large bowel atretic segments should be excluded by injecting and milking normal saline down the lumen of the distal bowel. These can occur in 6–21% of cases. The total length of small bowel is then accurately measured along the antimesenteric border as it has prognostic significance and will determine the method of reconstruction. If total usable bowel length is deemed adequate (>80 cm + ileocaecal valve), the bulbous hypertrophied proximal bowel is back resected (5–15 cm) alongside the mesenteric border in order to preserve maximal mesentery for later use, until normal diameter bowel has been reached. An atraumatic bowel clamp is then placed across the bowel a few centimetres proximal to the elected site for transaction. Failure to do so may result in functional obstruction and dysmotility in the retained bulbous proximal atretic bowel. The bowel is then divided at right angles leaving an opening of approximately 0.5–1.5 cm in width. The blood supply should be adequate to ensure a safe anatomosis. If however an extensive cut-back resection is contraindicated, the bulbous portion alone or any compromised bowel should be resected. The proximal bowel should then be tapered obliquely (GIA stapler) leaving the distal bowel opening the same size as the prestretched distal bowel lumen to facilitate an end-end primary anatomosis.

Proximal bowel resection is followed by very limited distal small bowel resection over a length of 2–3 cm. The resection line should be slightly oblique towards the anti-mesenteric border (fish-mouth) to ensure that the openings of the proximal and distal bowels are of approximately equal size to facilitate easy end-to-end or rarely an end-to-back (Dennis-Brown) single layer anatomosis; 5/0 or 6/0 absorbable suture material is used (Fig. 41.9). Alternatively an extra mucosal anastomosis can be performed, which is very difficult to achieve. The mesentry is approximated with interrupted stitches, which may be difficult with large mesenteric defects. A side-to-side anatomosis must not be performed as it can lead to a blind-loop

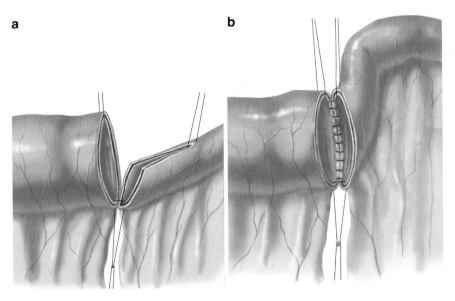

a   b

Fig. 41.9 End to end or end to back single layer bowel anastomosis

syndrome. There is no place for routine gastrostomy or transanastomotic tubes where TPN facilities are available and IV feeding is practiced.

41.8.2 Special Considerations

Atresia type I and stenosis are best dealt with by primary resection and end-to-end anastomosis. Procedures such as simple transverse enteroplasties, excision of membranes, bypass techniques or side-to-side anastomosis are no longer utilized. They fail to remove the abnormal dysfunctional segments of intestine thus increasing the risk of the blind loop syndrome and dysmotility

Atresia type II and IIIa are managed in the same manner as type I with back resection and primary end-to-end anastomosis. Conservation of bowel length is mandatory.

Multiple Membranous Diaphragms (type I atresias) can sometimes successfully be perforated by transluminal bouginage done along the entire length of the affected small bowel.

High jejunal atresia: With type IIIb or high jejunal atresia, the proximal bowel should be derotated, the ligament of Treitz, if present, taken down and resection of the bulbous portion may be extended well into the third part of the duodenum without jeopardizing the ampulla of Vater. This is followed by an **antimesenteric tapering duodenoplasty or inversion plication**. Bowel tapering can safely be done over a length of between 2 and 35 cm. The duodenoplasty is done to conserve bowel length, to reduce disparity in anastomotic size and to improve prograde duodenal peristaltic function. An intestinal autostapeling device may aid in this procedure. At completion the bowel is left in a position of derotation with the duodenum-jejunum dependent, the mesentery broad-based and the caecum lying anterior, to the left of the midline, in the upper abdomen. These additional maneuvers induce rapid prograde intestinal function return and the neonates are usually on graded to full oral intake within 14 days.

The distal 'apple peel' component of type III atresias may require the division of avascular restricting mesenteric bands along the free edge of the distally coiled narrow mesentery thereby releasing kinking and interference with the bowel blood supply. The large mesenteric defect is usually left open but where

associated with proximal bowel resection, the conserved mesentery can be used to obliterate the defect. Furthermore to prevent kinking of the marginal artery after completion of the anastomosis, the bowel is replaced carefully into the peritoneal cavity in the position of non-rotation.

Multiple type IV atresias, present in 20% of cases, are often localized to a segment facilitating an en-bloc resection with a single anastomosis in preference to multiple anastomosis. It is always important to ensure preservation of maximum bowel length and avoid the short bowel syndrome; for this reason the following techniques may be necessary.

Tapering or plication/inversion enteroplasty is indicated when: the ischemic insult has resulted in an atresia with markedly reduced intestinal length (<80 cm); where long length resection of abnormal or multiple atretic segments are required; to equalize disparity in anastomotic lumen size; for correction of a failed inversion plication procedure and to improve function in a persistently dilated non-functioning mega duodenum following surgery for upper jejunal atresia.

The plication enteroplasty method has the advantage of reducing the risk of leakage from the anti-mesenteric suture line, conserving mucosal surface area and may even facilitate return of bowel peristalsis (Fig. 41.10). More than half of the anti-mesenteric bowel circumference may be enfolded into the lumen over an extended length without causing an obstruction. The drawback of this method is that the holding suture-line can unravel within a few months, precipitating persistent duodenal motor dysfunction. As an alternative, antimesenteric seromuscular stripping combined with inversion plication may prevent this complication and preserves maximal mucosal surface for absorption.

Intestinal atresia and gastroschisis: The intestinal peel, often encountered in gastroschisis, hinders the detection and surgical management of an associated atresia. Three options are available; primary resection of the atretic segment with immediate anastomosis is only indicated if this can be done with safety, or, initial exteriorsation and delayed repair (very seldom done), or if identification of the atretic segment is difficult, the best approach is to reduce the eviscerated bowel with the atresia left undisturbed, awaiting resorption of the peel until a safe primary resection and anastomosis can be performed. This is usually delayed for 14–21 days.

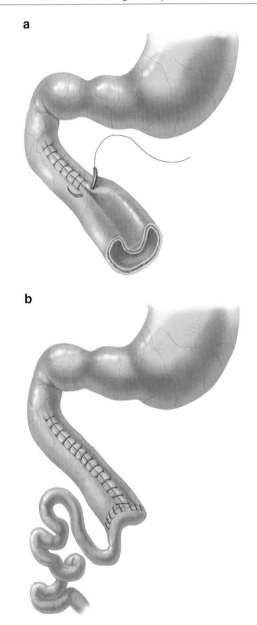

a

b

Fig. 41.10 **(a)** Plication Enteroplasty infrequently performed. **(b)** Antimesenteric tapering, duodenojejunoplasty for conserving length in high small bowel atresia

41.8.3 *Exteriorization or Stomas*

Although primary anastomosis is always preferred, a temporising proximal stoma or chimnied anastomosis (Bishop-Koop method) or a second look exploration 48–72 h later may be advisable when the vascular integrity of the intestine is questionable. This may be relevant in cases with late diagnosis, type III (b) atresias or with gross intraperitoneal faecal contamination.

41.8.4 *The Short Bowel Syndrome*

Insufficient bowel length either as a result of the primary injury, excessive removal of residual bowel, or an ischemic insult to the remaining bowel as a postoperative complication, can lead to the short bowel syndrome with long term sequelae for growth and development.

Bowel lengthening procedures are not indicated and have no place during the initial surgery. Three currently applicable techniques are: longitudinal intestinal lengthening method (Bianchi), serial transverse enteroplasty or step technique (Kim) and the myoenteropexy method of Kimura. Although they theoretically increase intestinal length and absorptive capacity, outcome ultimately depends on residual small bowel length and any complicating associated (liver) disease. Maximal bowel adaptation must be attained utilizing both TPN and enteral feeding as adjunctive methods of therapy before these additional surgical methods are contemplated.

41.9 Postoperative Care

Standard methods are used. Nasogastric decompression is usually required for 4–6 days after the operation (longer for high jejunal atresias). Therapeutic antibiotics are continued for 5–7 days or longer and an oral antifungal agent is given prophylactically. Graduated oral intake is commenced when the neonate is alert, sucks well, and there is evidence of prograde gastrointestinal function, i.e. clear gastric effluent of low volume, a soft abdomen, or when flatus or feces have been passed.

Surveillance for alimentary dysfunction should continue until the infant has established and stabilized normal gastrointestinal function. If at any time there is a suspicion of a leak at the anastomosis (suggested by sudden collapse, abdominal distension and vomiting), a plain erect or decubitis radiograph of the abdomen

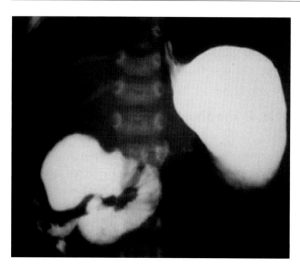

Fig. 41.11   Upper GIT contrast study indicating anastomotic stricture following repair for jejunal atresia

Table 41.2 Survival rates improved with change in surgical technique as well as improved anaesthetics and postoperative care of neonates

Authors	Years of study	N	Survival(%)
Evans	1950	1,498	9.3
Gross	1940–1952	71	51
Benson et al.	1945–1959	38	55
De Lorimer	1957–1966	587	65
Nixon and Tawes	1956–1967	62	62
Louw	1959–1967	33	94
Martin & Zerella	1957–1975	59	64
Cywes et al.	1959–1978	84	88
Danismead et al.	1967–1981	101	77
Smith & Glasson	1961–1986	84	61
Vecchia et al.	1972–1997	128	84
Rode et al.	1959–2007	318	92
	1990–2007	115	94

should be taken. If this reveals free air in the abdomen more than 24 h after operation, laparotomy should be performed immediately and the leaking site sutured, or the anastomosis redone. Other complications encountered include wound sepsis and dehiscence, anastomotic kinking, ischaemia with late onset anastomotic stenosis, adhesive obstruction and the short bowel syndrome (Fig. 41.11).

After massive intestinal length loss, TPN or other forms of enteral support should be continued with until maximum bowel adaptation is reached. It is imperative that graduated enteral feeding should be introduced as soon as possible to stimulate and enhance this process, which can take many months.

41.10 Outcome

Quality of life and functional status is usually not affected by intestinal atresia although cystic fibrosis, the short bowel syndrome and TPN induced liver failure may alter prognosis. Factors contributing to the <10% mortality rate include the type of atresia, proximal bowel infarction with peritonitis, anastomotic dysfunction, missed distal atresias, the short bowel syndrome, pneumonia, sepsis and associated abnormalities (Table 41.2).

Further Reading

Rode H, Millar AJW (2006) Jejuno-ileal Atresia. In P Puri, ME Höllwarth (eds) Pediatric Surgery, Springer Surgery Atlas Series. Springer-Verlag, Berlin, Heidelberg, New York, pp 213–228

Louw JH, Barnard CN (1955) Congenital intestinal atresia. Lancet 269:1065–1067

Rode H, Millar AJW (2003) Jejunoileal atresia. In P Puri (ed) Newborn Surgery. Arnold, London, pp 445–456

Rode H, Millar AJW (2006) Jejunoileal atresia. In P Puri, M Höllwarth (eds) Pediatric Surgery. Springer, Heidelberg, pp 213–228

Spriggs NI (1912) Congenital intestinal occlusion. Guy Hosp Rep 66:143–218

Wales PW (2004) Surgical therapy for short bowel syndrome. Pediatr Surg Int 20:647–657

Wax JR, Hamilton T, Cartin A (2006) Congenital jejumoileal atresia: Natural prenatal sonographic history and association with neonatal outcome. J Ultra sound Med 25:337–342

Meconium Ileus

42

Massimo Rivosecchi

Contents

42.1 Introduction

Meconium ileus is the earliest clinical manifestation of cystic fibrosis (CF) and occurs in 8-10% of patients with CF at birth. The clinical features are mainly due to the presence of abnormal, inspissated and viscid mucus of intestinal origin. In neonates affected by this condition, the impacted meconium produces an intraluminal obstruction occurring in the midileum, leading to a progressive distension. About 40% of patients with meconimu ileus are complicated by intestinal volvulus, atresia, gangrene and necrosis, perforation, peritonitis with abdominal calcifications and, finally, meconial pseudocyst.

42.2 Historical data

Intestinal occlusion, both associated with inspissated meconium and gross pathologic pancreatic changes, was first reported by Landsteiner in 1905 and subsequently confirmed by Kornblith and Fanconi. In 1936, Fanconi and Uehlinger described this complex and lethal newborn condition as "cystic fibrosis of the pancreas". In the mid 1900s, the Bodian's description of an abnormal sticky intestinal mucus, with a lower content of water, was the basis for the modern treatment using enemas and later intraoperative saline irrigations, thus avoiding excessive small bowel resections. Mikulicz, Gross, Bishop and Koop, Santulli and others were responsible, in later years, for the development of various surgical techniques including distal or proximal enterostomies. More recently relief of the intestinal obstruction has been obtained by irrigating the intestine with various solutions such as normal saline,

P. Puri and M. Höllwarth (eds.), *Pediatric Surgery: Diagnosis and Management,*
DOI: 10.1007/978-3-540-69560-8_42, © Springer-Verlag Berlin Heidelberg 2009

1% N-acetylcysteine, hyperosmolar Gastrografin enema, surfactant, and DNase. With respect to different types of surgical and medical efforts, the survival rate at 1 year increased from 10 to 90%, and the operative morality is drastically decreased to 15–23% of the treated newborn.

42.3 Incidence

Meconium Ileus accounts for 9–33% of all neonatal intestinal obstructions (300 new cases in Italy each year), with an incidence of 1:2500 newborns, representing the third most common cause of neonatal small bowel obstruction after ileal and duodeno-jejunal atresia and malrotation. Polyhydramnios is the most frequent feature observed in prenatal diagnosis of complicated forms of Meconium ileus. The presence of fetal hyperechogenic bowel on the ultrasound, associated with dilated bowel and/or ascites could be indicative of an intestinal obstruction. A family history of CF is clearly evident in almost 25% of these patients. Meconium Ileus is uncommon in premature infants (5–12%), and associated congenital anomalies are rare.

42.4 Pathogenesis

Meconium ileus is always associated with CF, which is the most common lethal autosomal recessive disorder in the caucasians population, and is characterized by dysfunctional chloride ion transport across epithelial surfaces. Parents are not affected, but both are heterozygotes carrying the abnormal gene(s). Intestine, pancreas, lungs, sweat glands, liver, salivary glands are all involved, as a result of an abnormal exocrine gland activity. However, these organs are affected differently during the course of life, the pancreas being the first, because the progressive retention of secretions and the atrophy of acinar cells starts during fetal life. On the contrary, the lungs of these patients are generally normal at birth, with the mucous plugging of the distal airways becoming responsible for progressive pulmonary insufficiency during adolescence. Interestingly, meconium ileus is not associated with CF in premature infants, suggesting that the associated intestinal abnormalities occur during the latter stages of fetal development.

Although recurrent lung infections and pulmonary insufficiency are the principal causes of morbidity and death, gastrointestinal symptoms commonly precede these findings and lead to this diagnosis in infants and young children. The gastrointestinal manifestations of CF result primarily from abnormally viscous luminal secretions within hollow viscera and the ducts of solid organs. As a result, bowel obstruction may be present at birth due to meconium plug syndrome. Early biochemical studies of this altered meconium has shown a lower content of carbohydrate, increased level of protein, the 'mucoproteins' and albumin, which has previously been used as a screening test. In more recent years, meconium ileus was found to be a result of abnormal intestinal secretions, and not so closely related to a sweat electrolyte defect (high levels of sodium and chloride) as was previously thought. In actual fact, the impermeability of CF epithelia to chloride ions has not been found to be correlated to the severity of intestinal involvement, and the pancreatic lesions are thought to play a secondary role. The sweat test is the main laboratory test used for the diagnosis but, since the 1990s, genetic analysis is commonly used for diagnostic as well as prognostic purposes. Cystic Fibrosis Transmembrane Conductance Regulator (CFTR) is the gene defective in CF, and was first identified in 1989. This gene is normally located in the apical membrane of the epithelial cells from the stomach to the colon: a mutation of CFTR on chromosome 7 is responsible for CF. The most common mutation is ΔF-508 and can be identified using DNA testing in affected neonates as well as in family members, who are considered possible carriers of this gene.

The CFTR gene codes for a 1480 amino acid protein that acts as a chloride channel, regulated by cyclic AMP. In the small intestinal wall, the clinical expression of CF depends largely on the decreased secretion of fluid and chloride ions, the increased permeability of the paracellular space between adjacent enterocytes and the sticky mucus cover over the enterocytes. As a rule, in CF the brush border enzyme activities are normal and there's enhanced active transport as has been shown regarding glucose and alanine. As a result, the gastrointestinal content in children affected by meconium ileus has lower acidity in the foregut and the accretion of mucins and proteins resulting in intestinal obstruction in the ileum but also in the colon. During development, the small intestinal mucosa does not function at maximal capacity. A better understanding of the CF gastrointestinal phenotype may contribute to improvement of the overall wellbeing of these newborn patients.

In recent years, the Na+-dependent amino acid transporter 'ATB(0)' which has been previously localised in the 19q13.3 region, did not appear to be associated with CF-MI disease: however, fine chromosomal mapping of other genetic factors and loci, in humans as well as in animal models should hopefully help to determine the association between CF and this intestinal phenotype. This will be a difficult task as more than 1,000 mutations have been identified in the CTFR gene and the final impact of these mutations on the genotype-phenotype correlation is unknown. In addition, the discordant phenotype observed in CF siblings suggests that genes other than CTFR modulate the CTFR phenotype. More recently, some author reported that the CTFR gene along with two or more modifier genes are the major determinants of intestinal obstruction in newborn CF patients, whereas intestinal obstruction in older CF patients is most probably caused by non-genetic factors.

42.5 Histopathology

In the meconium ileus, the intestine shows different aspects if we consider the proximal, the middle and the distal ileum. In the proximal ileum, the content has a semiliquid consistency and is not yet viscous. A marked and severe dilatation of the middle ileum is always seen: the intestine contains thick, dark green and putty-like meconium, firmly adherent to the walls. Iintestinal obstruction causing a hyperperistalsis is responsible for the congestion and hypertrophy of the walls. The distal ileum is full of concretions known as "rabbit-pellets", which are stained gray and typically have a beaded appearance. This small bowel condition is responsible for a narrow, empty and small colon, which is never used, and is termed a 'microcolon'. In complicated cases of meconium ileus, bowel wall perforation and secondary meconium peritonitis, and calcifications can occur. Spontaneous healing of the ileal perforation can lead to resorption of the involved portion of bowel and finally to an intestinal atresia. When the peristalsis is vigorous, twisting of the ileal tract full of dense meconium may result in a massive volvulus, with a high risk of perforation. Sometimes, when the bowel perforation is massive, an intense reaction to the meconial spillage may produce a giant meconial pseudocyst.

42.6 Clinical Pictures

Polyhydramnios is the most frequent feature observed in prenatal diagnosis of complicated forms of Meconium Ileus. The presence of fetal hyperechogenic bowel on the ultrasound, associated with dilated bowel and/or ascites could be indicative of an intestinal obstruction. A family history of **CF** is clearly evident in almost 25% of these patients. Meconium Ileus is uncommon in premature infants (5–12%), and associated congenital anomalies are rare.

Main symptoms include abdominal distension (96%) Fig. 42.1a, bilious vomiting (50%) usually the first sign of small bowel obstruction, and delayed passage of meconium (36%). In 45–55% of the newborns

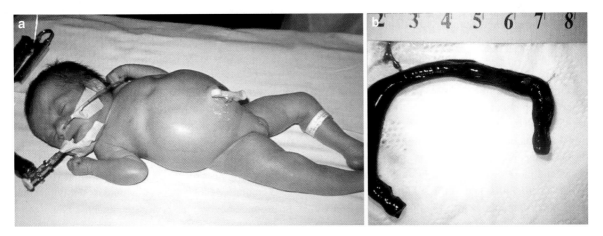

Fig. 42.1 a Newborn with intestinal obstruction and family history of cystic fibrosis. Gastrograffin enema failed and the baby needed laparotomy **b** Newborn with intestinal obstruction due to meconium plug syndrome passed a large meconium plug after digital examination

Table 42.1 Meconium Ileus: differential diagnosis in neonates

Diagnosis	Age	Incidence	Signs and findings	Treatment
Meconium ileus	Full term	1/2,500	Neonatal abdominal distention, cystic fibrosis	Enema, surgery
Meconium plugs	Premature	1/800	Meconium plugs	Enemas
Small left colons	Premature	Rare	Transition zone at splenic Flexure	Enemas, colostomy in selected cases
Hirschsprung's disease	Full term	1/3,800	Empty rectum, transition zone	Surgery
Anorectal malformation	Full term	1/6,000	Absent anus, flat perineum, fistula	Surgery
Neuronal intestinal dysplasia	Full term	Rare	Type A: mucosal flogosis	Medical, surgery
		Common	Type B: dilated colon	Medical, surgery in few cases
Maternal causes	drugs, $MgSO_4$			
Neonatal causes	hypothyroidism, >calcemia, <kalemia, sepsis, congestive hearth failure			

with *Meconium Ileus* the intestinal loops are undamaged and continuity is not interrupted.

From a clinical point of view, it is possible to recognize two different conditions: a simple, uncomplicated, and a complicated, severe type, with a mortality approaching 25% of all cases. In the first type (58%), sign and symptoms of a distal ileal obstruction are seen not later than 48h after birth: generalized abdominal distension with dilated and visible as well as palpable loops of bowel, bilious vomiting, no stools and narrowing of the anus and rectum, with only a dense and rubber-like gray meconium sticking to the anal wall. In the second type (42%), the neonate represent a surgical emergency, which must be treated within 24h after birth, when the signs of an hypovolemic shock or sepsis are not well established. Fetuses with complex Meconium Ileus are at increased risk for postnatal bowel obstruction and perforation. However, the Paediatric Surgeon have to decide in a series of intermediate cases when the most difficult management decision is whether the conservative management should precede or not the surgical time.

In this serious illness the progressive abdominal distension may culminate into a respiratory distress. If a perforation occurs, a pneumoperitoneum and sepsis are the unfavourable consequences. Fortunately, functional obstructions (Meconium Ileus, Hirschsprung's disease) should considered to be rare in preterm newborns and more often they are associated with necrotizing enterocolitis and only seldom correspond to idiopathic spontaneous intestinal perforation. Not frequently, meconium in the vagina or scrotum are evidence of a fetal perforation. Sometimes, the onset is directly with a meconium peritonitis, which could

involute in a giant meconial pseudocyst: when this happens, the abdominal skin edema and translucency are evident and associated with a palpable right lower mass (Table 42.1)

At present, whatever is the clinical presentation picture, the overall survival rate is at least 95%.

42.7 Prenatal Ultrasound and Radiologic Pattern

Meconium usually fill the small bowel during the 20th week of gestational age (GA), so that identification of *Meconium Ileus* before this period is rare. Prenatal ultrasound has led to confidence in the antenatal diagnosis of intestinal obstruction allowing counseling and birth planning. In this regard, the presence of fetal hyperechogenic bowel on the ultrasound, associated with dilated bowel and/or ascites could be indicative of an intestinal obstruction. The increased echogenicity of the intestinal loops is due to an higher density of the intraluminal content (hyperdense and dry meconium). However, is not easy to determine exactly if this feature is arising from intra- or from extraluminal structures and other different condition may present with similar ultrasound pattern, such as prenatal infections, neoplasm or chromosomal trisomy. In addition these findings may also represent transient normal variants.

When the Meconium Ileus evolute in a volvulus, the ultrasound shows enlarged hyperechogenic loops without peristalsis. Polyhydramnios is the most frequent feature observed in prenatal diagnosis of complicated forms of Meconium Ileus. Obviously, if the parents are found to be carriers for a **CF** mutation, the correlation between ultrasound findings and Meconium Ileus is done.

Plain radiographs shows distended and gas-filled intestinal loops. Sometimes, air–fluid levels are seen (one third of the cases), thus mimicking an ileal atresia. Where a sharp stop image is evident, this is the exact point of the obstruction. An usual image of fine, granular soap-bubble (the "Singleton's sign") or ground-glass appearance (the "Neuhauser's sign") is due to a dense meconium mixed with air, typical of the distal ileum: this picture is usually located in the mid-abdomen or in the right iliac fossa. Nevertheless, this image has also been observed in neonates with meconium plug syndrome, Hirschsprung disease, or small bowel atresia. The meconium hyperdensity may produce various images, depending from the length or from the localization of the obstructed bowel, but also from the filling (complete or partial) of the intestinal loops affected. When the Meconium Ileus is complicated, the abdominal radiograph may show calcification as a result of meconium peritonitis due to a fetal perforation of the intestine. A double-bubble image or air-fluid levels can be seen when a secondary ileal atresia (single or double) is the final bowel remodeling after a complete volvulus associated with a severe ischemic damage. If the intestinal perforation occur early in the antenatal period, the X-ray appearance of a round rim of calcification underlines a meconium pseudocyst. The colon is always a microcolon (unused colon), because the meconium never fills the large bowel during the fetal life. So, the length is normal but the caliber is small because of a little amount of feces (thick and dry meconium) passing through.

A water-soluble contrast enema is useful both for diagnostic and therapeutic purposes: the iso-osmolar agents facilitates evacuation of meconium without loss of large amounts of fluids and solutes.

42.8 Diagnostic Criteria and Differential Diagnosis

The sweat test provides a quantitative estimate of sodium and chloride on a collected sample of sweat usually from the forearm. A cholinergic drug act stimulating the sweat production with the help of a mild electrical current applied for 3–6 min (pilocarpine iontophoresis technique). Concentrations of these two cations above 60 mEq/L are diagnostic if at least 100 mg of sweat is collected. However, in the early neonatal age is really difficult to obtain a sufficient quantity of sweat to provide an accurate analysis and the collection must be done twice or three times before being satisfactory. In borderline cases, besides, results are not significant for **CF** and further analysis are needed. Another problem is represented by the high levels of sodium and chloride in neonates otherwise normals. In these situations we must wait and provide another series of results after an interval of at least 1 month from the first test. More recently, the DNA probe analysis test for the ΔF508 mutation and other common alleles allows for a precise diagnosis, which miss only a very little percentage of patients affected by **CF**. This method detects both affected children as well as heterozygote carriers. The serum immunoreactive trypsin levels (IRT), used as a screening test for **CF**, are not different in complicated as well as non-complicated form of this disease and this is why a single raised level of IRT in a neonate should prompt the analysis for the disease regardless of any surgical coexisting pathology.

Other causes of distal intestinal obstruction of the newborn may present with similar clinical patterns, including jejunoileal atresia, Hirschsprung's disease, meconium plug syndrome, Fig. 42.1b and neonatal small left colon syndrome. In particular, a congenital megacolon is suspected when the bowel contents are liquid and air–fluid levels are constantly seen in the dilated bowel.

Other conditions may mimic surgical obstruction, such as delayed peristalsis associated with prematurity (the so-called functional immaturity) and a dynamic ileus from sepsis. If a volvulus without malrotation or neonatal invagination are seen, these patients may underwent a sweat test to exclude **CF**. Although is unusual, Meconium Ileus exist as an isolated entity, not associated with **CF**. These patients accounts for 6–12% of the totality, and the course of the illness is more often benign and without complications.

42.9 Medical and Surgical Treatment

The first step of the treatment include a nasogastric tube decompression, an antibiotic prophylaxis with cephalosporin and aminogycosides, and correction of dehydration, electrolytes and hypothermia.

A contrast enema with water-soluble and hyper- or iso-osmolar contrast is the medical treatment of choice and mucosal safe, for uncomplicated *Meconium Ileus*. A recent study, which used various enema solutions, administered in a mice model showed that surfactant and Gastrographin (diatrizoate meglumine) were the most efficacious for the in vivo relief of constipation, in comparison with Perflubron, Tween-80, Golytely, DNase, *N*-Acetylcysteine and Viokase. Intestinal mucosal damage was absent and viscosity had been significantly reduced in vitro. Actually, the success rate using a Gastrographin enema varies from 20% to 50% as reported in Literature.

The enema evacuation should be obtained under fluoroscopic control, with a gentle and progressive increasing of the intraluminal pressure, thus avoiding unexpected rupture of the colon. A correct procedure prevents leakage of the contrast medium by taping buttocks as well as the catheter dislocation. If the contrast medium fails to progress into dilated small bowel loops, the presence of an acquired atresia is definite and the radiologist must stop the examination because of an high risk of perforation. Fifty percent of neonates submitted to this procedure benefits to enema alone over the next 48 h, without any additional treatment: in some cases, a second enema may be used with a complete evacuation of the meconium filling the ileal loops. Acetylcysteine administered by mouth is useful and helps to relieve the obstruction. Radiographs are taken at 3, 6, 12, 24 and 48 h intervals, with the aim of evaluating progression and possible complications. At this time feeding is begun. Hypovolemic shock and early perforation are round the corner, but an appropriate and meticoulous procedure can avoid these complications.

When the medical treatment is unsuccessful in spite of an uncomplicated Meconium Ileus, surgery is mandatory and an open evacuation, resection and ileostomy are the different options. In a simple Meconium Ileus surgeon should do the minimal procedure to obtain the lumen free from all kind of rubbish, such as pellets, sticky meconium and, sometimes, small calcifications. In this case, a limited enterotomy and repeated warm saline irrigations through a smooth catheter provide for the best result. In this evenience, meconium discharge may be manually supported, using the enterotomy placed in the dilated hypertrophic ileum. The catheter is two-way directed with care, clearing the small as well as the large bowel. At the time of the irrigation the surgeon also controls the enema progression and bowel may be inspected for

distension degree, mesenteric orientation, covered perforation, gangrenous tract and atretic single or multiple segments. The colon is inspected too, searching for possible perforation or microperforation. The T-tube ileostomy could be an additional effective and safe treatment, without any additional surgery in 90% of treated patients; the T-tube should be removed when full oral feeding is possible and regular bowel movements occur.

At the end of this treatment, discussion is about to resect or not, because some authors stress the risk of a leakage at the anastomotic-site: we must keep in mind that resection and termino-terminal anastomosis is possible, only if any sign of infection, or sepsis are absent.

Usually a resection is done with the aim to restore promptly the normal peristalsis: in these patients the intestinal resection is limited to a huge dilation, at risk for foci of regional infection. Actually, bowel resection with primary anastomosis has been proved to be as well effective and safe as stoma formation, but is associated with a reduced length of initial hospital stay.

Ileostomy can be performed in different fashion: the simplest one is a double-barreled ileostomy (Mikulicz), with the two loops brought out side-to-side; this solution is quick and avoids an intra-abdominal anastomosis (Fig. 42.2). However, neonates may loose a large amount of fluids and solute from this via and, in selected cases, in alternative to a peripheral line, a central venous catheter is scheduled, both for nutritional and medical purposes. Other alternatives have been described: distal ileostomy with end-to-side ileal anastomosis (Bishop-Koop), has been called as "distal chimney enterostomy" (Figs. 42.3 and 42.4.) The proximal chimney enterostomy

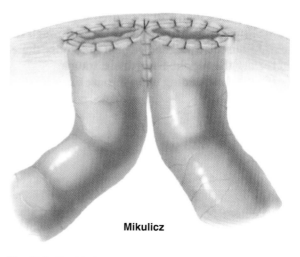

Mikulicz

Fig. 42.2 Double-barrell ileostomy according to Mikulicz

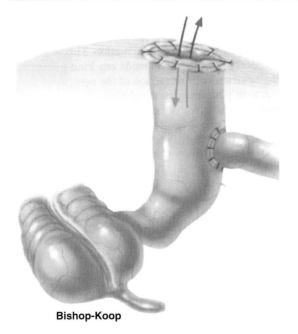

Bishop-Koop

Fig. 42.3 Distal ileostomy with end to side ileal anastomosis (Bishop-Koop)

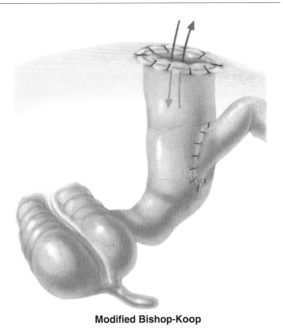

Modified Bishop-Koop

Fig. 42.4 Modified Bishop-Koop ileostomy

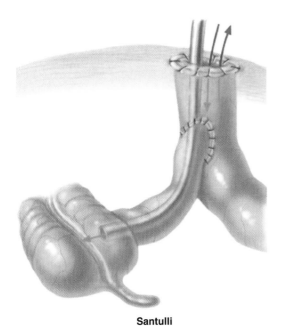

Santulli

Fig. 42.5 Proximal ileostomy with end to side ileal anastomosis (Santulli procedure)

is the Santulli procedure, with a proximal ileostomy with end-to-side ileal anastomosis (Fig. 42.5).

The enterostomy is closed between 7 and 12 days after surgery by an end-to-end anastomosis.

In a few selected cases, gastrostomy may be needed, but only when recovery of intestinal functions expected to be delayed.

Generally, the lowest the length of the intervention, the less extended the resection, the earliest the recovery of the peristalsis, and the less complicated and uneventful will be the postoperative care.

Complications include pulmonary infections, which is the most important one, with an incidence of at least 8–10%. Anastomotic leakage occurs for different reasons: a technical mistake, an insufficient blood supply, and a distal unrecognized obstruction. Delayed recovery of peristalsis is another frequently observed complication and is due to an abnormal stretching of the intestinal walls during the fetal life. Total Parenteral Nutrition is the support of choice and a central venous catheter is mandatory in these situations.

42.10 Prognosis

Meconium Ileus may be an early indication of a more severe phenotype of **CF**. This was suggested by the significantly lower pulmonary function found in children with a history of Meconium Ileus compared to age- and sex-matched children who did not have meconium ileus. However, an adequate initial nutritional and medical management allows to achieve a similar nutritional and pulmonary status compared with other early-diagnosed symptomatic CF patients and in this view, meconium Ileus did not represent an additional risk factor for the patient's life. The complicated form are susceptible to a higher number of long-term surgical complications, including small bowel obstructions and blind loop syndromes. Long-term complications in neonates affected by uncomplicated meconium Ileus who were nonoperatively treated are rarely seen, and only mild and transient complications had been observed in newborns treated with minor surgical procedures, such as enterotomies and irrigations.

Survival of neonates with Meconium Ileus has improved over the last two decades because of neo-natal intensive care, improved surgical technique and medical treatment. In general, an overall immediate survival of 90% is achieved using the modern protocols and nearly all deaths are pertinent to the adolescents. Long-term survival also in **CF** patients has improved significantly (83–90%), with many patients surviving into the fourth decade. Surgeons and Gastroenterologists should inform the parents that the future of Meconium Ileus is to be predisposed to late complications including fibrosing colonopathy and ongoing exocrine dysfunction. Pneumothorax in **CF** patients is an ominous predictor of mortality.

Only few children die because of liver and or septic complications. Deaths are mainly due to staphylococcal or Pseudomonas sepsis, primary or secondary to a pulmonary interstitial emphysema or to an aspiration pneumonia. In a large series reported, only one child died because of the *Meconium Ileus* itself. More recently, gene therapy vectors to the fetal intestinal tract should provide a novel means toward prevention of the early postnatal intestinal pathology of cystic fibrosis: obviously, prenatal treatment of genetic disease could avoid early-onset tissue damage and immune sensitization as well as the future surgical complications due to *Meconium Ileus* pre- and postnatal gut-perforation and fetal ascites sequelae.

Further Reading

Blackman SM, Deering-Brose R, McWilliams R et al (2006) Relative contribution of genetic and nongenetic modifiers to intestinal obstruction in cystic fibrosis. Gastroenterology 131(4):1030–1039

Burke MS, Ragi JM, Karamanoukian HL, et al (2002) New strategies in nonoperative management of meconium ileus. J Pediatr Surg 37:760–764

Escobar MA, Grosfeld JL, Burdick JJ et al (2005) Surgical considerations in cystic fibrosis: A 32-year evaluation of outcomes. Surgery 138(4):560–571

Fuchs JR, Langer JC (1998) Long-term outcome after neonatal meconium obstruction. Pediatrics 101:E7–E12

Munck A, Gerardin M, Alberti C, et al (2006) Clinical outcome of cystic fibrosis presenting with or without meconium ileus: A matched cohort study. J Pediatr Surg 41(9): 1556–1560

Rivosecchi M (2006) Meconium ileus. In P Puri, ME Höllwarth (eds) Pediatric Surgery. Springer, Surgery Atlas Series, Springer-Verlag Berlin Heidelberg, New York, pp 229–238

Duplications of the Alimentary Tract

43

Prem Puri and Alan Mortell

Contents

Duplications of the alimentary tract are rare spherical or tubular structures, which can occur anywhere in the tract from mouth to anus. Ladd, in 1937, introduced the term 'alimentary tract duplication' in the hope of clarifying the nomenclature which had previously included descriptive terms such as enteric or enterogenous cysts, giant diverticula; ileal, jejunal or colonic duplex, an unusual Meckel's diverticulum. Ladd proposed that the unifying term "alimentary tract duplications" be applied to congenital anomalies that involved the mesenteric side of the associated alimentary tract and shared a common blood supply with native bowel. Most duplications may indeed be called simply 'enterogenous cysts', since in only very few cases is there actual doubling of the alimentary tract and therefore deserving the name 'duplication'.

43.1 Embryology

Numerous theories have been developed to account for the multitude of gastrointestinal (GI) tract duplications. Recently, Stern and Warner outlined the most widely held theories regarding GI duplication.

Embryologically, duplications have been categorized into foregut, midgut, and hindgut (Fig. 43.1). Foregut duplications include the pharynx, respiratory tract, oesophagus, stomach, and the first portion and proximal half of the second portion of the duodenum. Midgut duplications include the distal half of the second part of the duodenum, the jejunum, ileum, cecum, appendix, the ascending colon, and the proximal two thirds of the transverse colon. The hindgut is composed of duplications of the distal third of transverse colon, the descending and sigmoid colon, the rectum, anus, and components of the urological system. In one series,

P. Puri and M. Höllwarth (eds.), *Pediatric Surgery: Diagnosis and Management,*
DOI: 10.1007/978-3-540-69560-8_43, © Springer-Verlag Berlin Heidelberg 2009

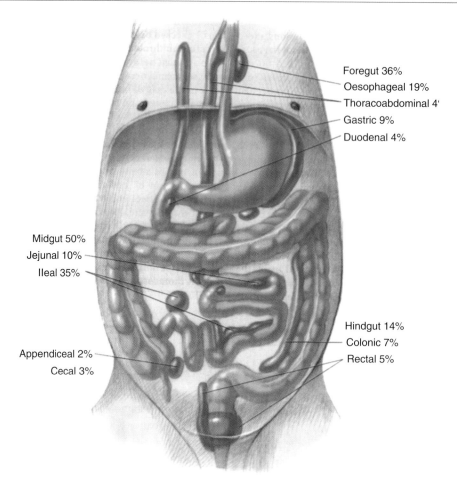

Foregut 36%
Oesophageal 19%
Thoracoabdominal 4'
Gastric 9%
Duodenal 4%

Midgut 50%
Jejunal 10%
Ileal 35%

Hindgut 14%
Colonic 7%
Rectal 5%

Appendiceal 2%
Cecal 3%

Fig. 43.1 Diagram demonstrating the common locations and incidence of gastrointestinal duplications

39% of duplication involved the foregut, whereas 61% represented duplications of both mid and hindgut.

43.1.1 Partial Twinning

Certain duplications appear to represent partial twinning, particularly the tubular duplications of the terminal ileum and colon. There is a wide spectrum of abnormalities, from complete twinning of the lower trunk and extremities to mere doubling of the lumen of hindgut structures. These lesions are often associated with duplication of the lower urinary tracts. Many rare examples of abortive cephalic twinning have also been described. When there is complete doubling of the colon, one or both lumens may open as a fistula into

the perineum or into the genitourinary tract, and may be associated with an imperforate anus. Doubling of the anus, vagina, and bladder all have been detailed and often can be associated with other severe deformities, such as double spines or two heads.

43.1.2 Split Notochord

The most satisfactory of several theories of the origin of GI duplications is that relating to the development of the neurenteric canal. Saunders, in 1943, noted that thoracic duplications are frequently associated with abnormalities of the cervical and thoracic vertebrae. These duplications may be attached to the vertebral bodies or connected to the spinal canal. These findings gave rise to the Bentley and Smith 'split notochord theory'. Initially the embryo has two layers, ectoderm and endoderm. Mesoderm forms between the two but for a short time these two layers remain adherent. A transient opening (the notochordal plate) appears, connecting the neural ectoderm with the intestinal endoderm. This notochordal plate normally migrates dorsally and becomes 'pinched' off from the endoderm by the ingrowth of mesodermal cells from each side. If the notochordal plate fails to migrate as a result of adhesions to the endodermal lining the spinal canal cannot close ventrally and a tract resembling a diverticulum is established with the primitive gut. This tract may remain open, leaving a fistula between the gut and the spinal canal, or closed leaving only a fibrous tract. However, in the majority of cases it disappears completely, leaving only the duplication of the GI tract. This theory explains the formation of thoracic and caudal duplications, which may be associated with vertebral anomalies. However the absence of spinal defects in many alimentary tract duplications makes this theory less tenable as a unifying model of origin.

43.1.3 Embryonic Diverticula and Recanalization Defects

Lewis and Thyng found in human embryos (4–23 mm), and in other animal embryos, tiny bands of intestinal epithelium protruding into the subepithelial connective tissue. The identification of numerous diverticula in the intestines of embryos, led to the proposal of extension of the diverticula into duplications. The frequent ileal position of these diverticula is congruous with the frequent ileal location of human GI duplications. Although this theory could explain duplications in the absence of spinal anomalies, it fails to account for the variability of the mucosal lining and specifically for the frequency of heterotopic gastric mucosa. Furthermore, the diverticula identified in this pathological series were located throughout the bowel circumference as opposed to the general locations of duplications on the mesenteric side of the intestine.

The occurrence of tubular duplications would also not be explained by this theory. Bremer believed that abnormal recanalization of the intestinal lumen after the solid stage of development of the primitive gut in the 6th–7th week resulted in duplications. Such duplications, however, would not be confined to the mesenteric side of the bowel. Also opposing this theory is the finding that the solid stage of development in the human does not usually extend beyond the duodenum.

In 1961, Mellish and Koop proposed environmental theory, which held that trauma or hypoxia could induce duplications and twinning in lower orders. Based on the work of Louw, they concluded that vascular insufficiency could lead to the recognized GI duplications seen in humans. Additionally, intrauterine vascular accidents are known precipitators of the other congenital anomalies, such as gastrointestinal atresias.

43.2 Pathology

Duplications are hollow structures that involve the mesenteric side of the associated GI tract. They tend to share a common muscular wall and blood supply with its mature bowel, although each has its own separate lining. They are usually isolated lesions and are more often cystic than tubular with a variable size. The lesions have a muscular coat in two layers and are usually lined with epithelium similar to that found in the associated portion of alimentary tract. The duplications, however, are occasionally lined with heterotopic epithelium; colonic mucosa has been described at the base of the tongue and sinuses lined with gastric mucosa have been found near the anus. Duplications containing gastric mucosa are at risk of peptic ulceration, perforation and haemorrhage. Patches of ectopic gastric mucosa along the GI tract may represent the mildest manifestation of duplication abnormalities. Ectopic pancreatic tissue has been reported in duplications of the stomach, ileum and colon. The contents of a duplication vary with the type of epithelial lining of the structure, the presence or absence of a communication with the proximate part of the GI tract and the absence or necrosis of the duplication wall. If an opening is present, the duplication contents will be similar to that of the adjacent intestinal tract. Communication between the two structures is rare and the cysts usually contain chyle or mucus. Multiple duplications can occur in the same patient. There is an increased incidence of other associated anomalies such as vertebral anomalies, myelomeningocele, imperforate anus, exomphalos, malrotation of bowel, genital anomalies, polysplenic syndrome and duodenal atresia. No genetic tendency has been demonstrated.

43.3 Incidence

Duplications of the alimentary tract are rare. Table 43.1 summarizes the larger published series of duplications. In many cases the numbers of patients reported represent up to 40 years' work in these centres. Only a small percentage of the total reported actually present in the neonatal period.

43.4 Oesophageal Duplication

The oesophagus is a relatively common site for foregut duplications (19%) with the majority being intramural, non-communicating cystic structures related to the right side of the oesophagus. Patients often present late in childhood as they cause relatively few symptoms, however cervical oesophageal duplications can cause significant respiratory distress requiring urgent surgery. Some lesions do not share a common wall with the oesophagus and can be easily removed through open or minimally invasive techniques. Plain radiographs may show an air or fluid-filled structure adjacent to the oesophagus although this is not usually enough to confirm the diagnosis. Contrast studies can provide useful information regarding the mass effect of the lesion and whether or not their lumens communicate. Ultrasound and computed tomography (CT) are useful for establishing a diagnosis and also for outruling multiple lesions, which can be present in 10–20% of cases. Technetium scans (^{99m}Tc) may reveal the presence of heterotopic gastric mucosa in the case of gastrointestinal bleeding.

43.5 Treatment

The surgical approach depends largely on the location of the cyst (Fig. 43.2). Cervical oesophageal duplications can be removed through a supraclavicular incision, with particular attention being paid to the vagus and phrenic nerves as well as the thoracic duct to avoid unnecessary damage. Intrathoracic duplications are resected through a standard postero-lateral thoracotomy or a thoracoscopic approach. A chest drain may be left in situ but is not always required.

43.6 Thoracoabdominal Duplication

Thoracoabdominal duplications are rare representing only 4% of all gastrointestinal duplications. They often lie separate from the oesophagus, more often on the

Table 43.1 Incidence and locations of duplications

Author	Total number	No. of neonates	Cervical	Mediastinal	Thoracoabd	Gastric	Duodenal	Jejunal/ileal	Colonic	Rectal
Carachi	21	10								
Gross	68	20	1	13	3	2	4	32	9	4
Sieber	25[a]	–	–	5	–	4	2	16	5	–
Grosfield et al.	20	–	–	4	–	1	–	9	4	–
Favara et al.	37[b]	–	3	4	2	3	4	20	4	–
Wren	22[c]	–	–	3	2	1	2	12	3	3
Lister & Vaos	32	24	–	3	–	1	–	20	5	3
Holcomb et al.	96[d]	36	1	20	3	8	2	47	20	–

[a]One patient had two, one had three and one had five duplications
[b]One patient had three duplications
[c]Two patients each had two duplications
[d]96 patients had 106 duplications

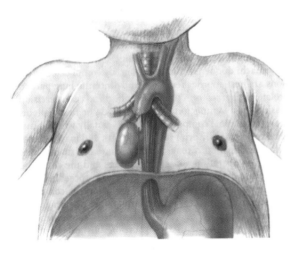

Fig. 43.2 Diagram demonstrating resection margin for simple cystic oesophageal duplication cyst

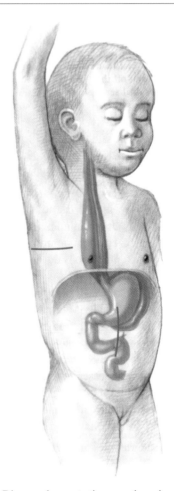

Fig. 43.3 Diagram demonstrating open thoracic and abdominal approaches to a thoracoabdominal duplication cyst

right than the left side, but may be attached to other important structures such as the aorta, azygous vein and tracheo-bronchial tree. They frequently lie in the posterior mediastinum and pass through the diaphragm to communicate with the stomach, duodenum or small bowel. The imaging studies employed are similar to those for oesophageal duplications, with special attention being paid to imaging of the vertebral column/spinal cord for a possible intra-spinal component. CT and/or magnetic resonance imaging (MRI) are particularly useful in this regard, especially if neurological symptoms of spinal cord compression or bony spinal abnormalities are present.

43.7 Treatment

These challenging duplications require resection of the thoracic and abdominal components through two different open procedures (Fig. 43.3) or alternatively they may be dealt with by a combined thoraco-laparoscopic approach. Although the abdominal portions are often asymptomatic the thoracic components can cause symptoms as a result of mass effect on the lungs and airway. The presence of gastric mucosa within the thoracic duplication cyst can lead to peptic ulceration and possible erosion into the lung parenchyma, presenting with haemoptysis. This complication may require a

lobectomy. Once the lesion is mobilised in the thorax, it is freed from the posterior aspect of the diaphragm prior to mobilisation and removal of the abdominal component.

43.8 Gastric Duplication

The stomach is one of the less common sites of duplications, accounting for only 9% of all GI duplications. Over 60% of cases are diagnosed during the first year of life, with a significant number (40%) appearing in the neonatal period by the finding of a palpable cystic mass in the upper abdomen accompanied by vomiting and weight loss. Rarely they undergo peptic ulceration and if the cyst communicates with the stomach, haematemesis

Table 43.2 Location of duplications of stomach in 87 reported cases

Location	No. of cases
Greater curvature	55
Lesser curvature	7
Anterior wall	9
Posterior wall	9
Others	7

and melaena may be the presenting feature. Rarely, a carcinoma may arise within a gastric duplication cyst. Gastric outlet obstruction mimicking hypertrophic pyloric stenosis also is a common presentation of this duplication. Gastric duplications occur twice as often in females as in males.

It is often difficult to make a preoperative diagnosis. Plain radiographs are usually negative. A barium meal may show compression of the stomach, usually along the greater curvature. Barium may demonstrate a connection between the stomach and duplication, but only in a small minority of cases. In these, barium may be retained in the duplication long after the remainder has passed from the GI tract. Ultrasonography has been shown to be useful in the diagnosis of gastric duplications. The vast majority of gastric duplications are located in the greater curvature (Table 43.2). Occasionally these are pedunculated, but most are closed spherical cysts or tubular structures.

Associated anomalies occur in 3% of gastric duplications. The most common is another cyst, usually of the oesophagus. Dual duplications of the stomach and pancreas have been reported. These are thought to arise from an error in rotation of the ventral pancreatic anlage.

43.9 Treatment

The management of gastric duplications is surgical because of the high incidence of complications due to obstruction, bleeding or peritonitis. As most duplications occur in the greater curvature, a wedge of stomach is excised together with the cyst and the gap closed with a single or double layer of horizontal inverting mattress sutures (Fig. 43.4). Partial gastrectomy should be avoided in children if possible, and if necessary only 25–30% of the stomach should be resected because of the associated long-term complications.

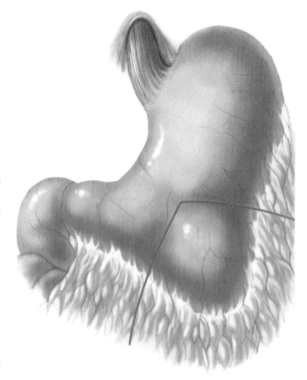

Fig. 43.4 Gastric duplication located at the greater curvature. A wedge of stomach is excised together with the cyst

When resection of the adjoining stomach is impractical, as in long tubular duplications of the greater curvature, the main part of the duplication is excised and the mucosa is stripped off. The remaining seromuscular cuff can be sutured over the denuded area after checking that the common wall between the stomach and duplication has not been perforated, by insufflating the stomach with air. The use of a linear stapling gun to divide the common wall along the length of the greater curvature has also been described.

43.10 Pyloric Duplications

True pyloric duplications are extremely rare, with very few being reported in the English literature and most of these presenting within the first week of life. They simulate the symptoms and signs of hypertrophic pyloric stenosis. Vomiting, weight loss and a palpable abdominal mass are the main findings. There are certain physical features which are consistent with duplication: the mass is usually large and smooth, in contrast to the smaller and often more mobile 'olive' mass in hypertrophic pyloric stenosis. Because of the non-specific physical examination, radiographic procedures are essential for diagnosis. Plain film radiography may show signs of gastric outlet or duodenal obstruction with a lack of distal bowel gas, or rarely calcification within a cyst wall. Ultrasonography may demonstrate an inner echogenic mucosal layer and outer hypoechoic muscular layer differentiating the duplication from a mesenteric cyst. Barium contrast studies may help differentiate the duplication from pyloric stenosis. If there is a clinical concern then preoperative endoscopic retrograde cholangiopancreatography (ERCP), percutaneous transhepatic cholangiography (PTC), or magnetic resonance cholangiography/pancreatography (MRCP) should be performed to evaluate the involvement of the biliary/pancreatic ducts.

43.11 Treatment

Of the cases of pyloric duplication reported, the majority underwent simple surgical excision after opening the pyloric canal longitudinally. The pylorus was then closed transversely with no complications. However, if there is a risk of damage to pancreatic or bile ducts an acceptable alternative is to drain the cyst into the duodenum or into a Roux limb of upper small bowel.

43.12 Duodenal Duplications

The duodenum is involved in only 4% of all duplications. They are often behind the duodenum and do not communicate with the bowel lumen. Vomiting secondary to partial or complete duodenal obstruction and an upper abdominal mass are present in the majority of cases. They may present with haematemesis, or perforation as gastric mucosa is present in 10–15% of cases. Alternatively, because of their location, they may present with biliary obstruction or pancreatitis. If the duplication is of sufficient size, it may appear in plain radiographs as a large opacity in the right side of the abdomen displacing the intestine. Barium studies will show the duodenum to be displaced upwards and a

'beak-like' projection due to compression of the duodenal lumen by the duplication. Contrast entering into the cyst confirms the presence of a luminal communication. Ultrasonography may show a cystic lesion below the liver and a classical "double-layered" appearance or "muscular rim sign".

43.13 Treatment

In view of the occasional occurrence of gastric mucosa in the duplication cyst, these lesions should, if possible, be dissected from the duodenum and excised, closing the resulting defect in the duodenum in two layers. Intraoperative cholangiography will help determine the relationship of the cyst to the bile and pancreatic ducts.

If the lesion is extensive, or if eversion of the cyst may compromise the biliary system, then cystoduodenostomy may be performed. The cyst may also be only partially excised, stripping off all the lining mucosa and leaving that part of the cyst which is adherent to the duodenum or pancreas.

43.14 Duplications of the Small Intestine

Small bowel duplications constitute 45% of all alimentary tract duplications. The vast majority of small bowel duplications are spherical cysts in the terminal ileum. Jejunal and ileal cysts are found on the mesenteric side of the bowel sharing a common muscularis with the adjacent bowel. They may cause obstruction by external pressure on the lumen, by acting as a lead point for intussusception or occasionally by causing a volvulus.

Tubular duplications have the same features as the cystic variety, but they communicate with the normal lumen of the intestine and they are more likely to contain gastric mucosa. Pancreatic mucosa has also been described in these duplications. Tubular duplications can range from a few millimetres to the whole length of the small bowel. The communication may be at the cephalad end which will cause the duplication to become grossly distended with intestinal contents, or if at the caudal end, will allow the duplication to drain freely. Communication at several different points may be present.

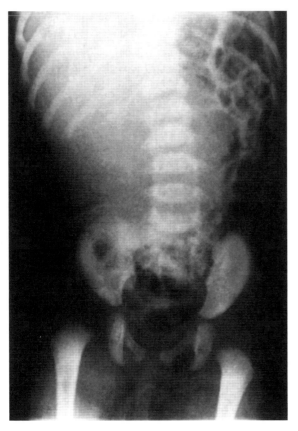

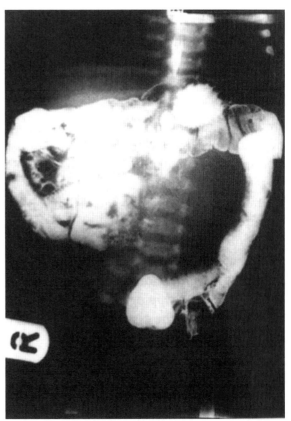

Fig. 43.5 Supine plain film of the abdomen in a 1-day-old baby showing a large soft tissue mass in the right upper and central abdomen displacing bowel loops to the left

Fig. 43.6 Contrast study in the same infant demonstrating a space-occupying lesion displacing bowel. At a large ileal duplication cyst was found

Haemorrhage occurs most often in tubular duplications, but perforation has been reported as well. Plain abdominal radiographs (Fig. 43.5) may show non-specific displacement of bowel gas shadows by the cyst or signs of intestinal obstruction or perforation. Ultrasonography can differentiate between a mesenteric and a duplication cyst. A barium meal will demonstrate displacement of the bowel (Fig. 43.6). Intraoperative ^{99m}Tc scanning may prove useful during this procedure to assure complete removal of all involved mucosa.

43.15 Treatment

Cystic duplications are relatively straightforward to deal with. Resection of the cyst with adjacent bowel (Fig. 43.7) is performed; the two ends of the bowel are

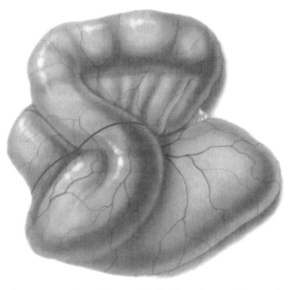

Fig. 43.7 Cystic small bowel duplication with resection margin incorporating duplication and adjacent normal bowel

anastomosed with one layer of horizontal inverting mattress sutures and the mesenteric defects closed.

Tubular duplications, if very short, can be resected as in a cystic lesion, but the majority involve a considerable length of small bowel and much ingenuity and patience may be required to meet the needs of any one particular case.

Wrenn suggested coring out the mucosal lining of a long tubular duplication through multiple seromuscular incisions in the wall of the duplication. The muscle and blood supply of the normal small bowel and duplication then need only be limited to the junction of the two.

Norris and colleagues employed a technique first described by Bianchi for bowel lengthening, to separate two leashes of blood vessels passing to each side of the small intestine. Using this method, the entire mucosa and almost the entire muscle wall can be excised. The remaining cuff of muscle wall can be oversewn, preserving the blood supply to the normal bowel.

Bishop and Koop described the techniques of anastomosing the distal end of the duplication to adjacent normal intestine, allowing free drainage of the contents. Malignant change in the mucosa has, however, been described as a late complication of this procedure. Whichever technique is utilised it is essential that the junction of normal and duplicated bowel is resected since heterotopic gastric mucosa is frequently present in tubular intestinal duplications.

43.16 Colonic Duplications

Colonic duplications are among the rarest reported. They are frequently diagnosed in infancy and some reports suggest a female predilection. McPherson and colleagues proposed a simple classification of colonic duplications: type I mesenteric cysts, type II diverticular and the more common type III tubular colonic duplication. A number of aetiological factors may be involved in the development of the 'double colon'. The most valid theory suggests division of the hindgut into two parts at a stage during which the anlage possessed a multi-organ developmental potential. The hindgut anlage normally forms the distal ileum, colon, rectum, bladder and urethra. Division of the anlage at the same initial stage could therefore be responsible for duplication of the lower urinary tract as well.

Simple cysts (type I) and diverticula (type II) occasionally result. They can be identified on plain radiographs or on barium studies. Barium enema may demonstrate a communication between the colon and duplication in types II and III. Associated genitourinary, and lumbosacral spine abnormalities can also be demonstrated on the appropriate radiographic studies, particularly when dealing with type III duplications. Isotope scans are rarely of benefit with colonic duplications, as they contain only colonic mucosa.

Complete duplication of the colon is usually asymptomatic in the neonatal period unless duplication of the anus or an abnormal orifice, in addition to the normal orifice in the perineum, is present. One or both orifices at the distal end of the colon may end as rectovaginal or recto-urethral fistulae.

43.17 Treatment

Surgery for colonic duplication is rarely indicated in the neonatal period unless there are complications, e.g. obstruction or an associated imperforate anus. All cystic and most tubular colonic duplications can be dealt with by simple resection and anastamosis utilising a single-layer extramucosal technique. With rare total colonic duplication (Fig. 43.8), the principal aim of management is to end up with two colons draining through one anal orifice. If one part of the colon has already reached the perineum, then the other colon is divided and anatomosed to its partner. This can be achieved by using a linear stapling device. If neither colon reaches the perineum, then a formal pull-through procedure will be required. Neonatal management in any of these situations is confined to fashioning a transverse defunctioning colostomy to drain both colons.

43.18 Rectal Duplications

Approximately 70 cases of rectal duplications have now been reported in the literature, comprising only 5% of all gastrointestinal duplications. More than 50% of these have been examples of hindgut twinning. Rectal duplications often present in the neonatal period with a fistula or perineal mucosal swelling extending to the perianal area (Fig. 43.9).

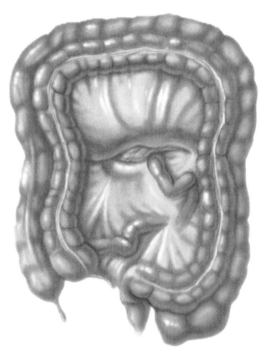

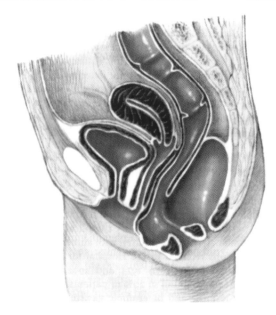

Fig. 43.10 Sagittal view of a rectal duplication cyst present in the retrorectal space

Fig. 43.8 Total colonic duplication from caecum to rectum lying lateral to normal bowel

ning', which occurs in the 10 mm embryo and is associated with complex hindgut anomalies.

Presentation of the cysts depends on (a) size and their mass effect, (b) fistulae, (c) infection, (d) ulceration if they contain gastric mucosa, and (e) malignancy. The duplication cyst usually forms in the retrorectal space (Fig. 43.10) and contains colourless mucous which can become infected. No cases of a fistula between the rectum and urinary tract have been described. Malignant degeneration has been reported in the rectal duplication from the fourth decade onwards.

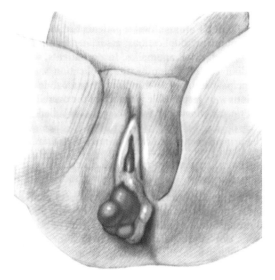

43.19 Treatment

Fig. 43.9 Rectal duplication presenting as a perianal mucosal swelling in the neonatal period

The embryogenesis of rectal duplication cysts is attributed to a 'pinching off' of a diverticulum in the 20–30 mm embryo, in contrast to the 'caudal twin-

The treatment of rectal duplication cyst is surgical excision or fenestration of the common wall. Depending on the anatomical variations, a transanal or transcoccygeal (Kraske) approach can be employed. For longer or more complicated cysts, a longer posterior sagittal incision will provide better exposure. As with other duplications, it is of prime importance to remove all mucosa in the duplication. The muscularis can be left in situ.

It is clear that duplications of the GI tract represent a diverse and complex group of anomalies. Small duplications in readily accessible areas (i.e. small intestine) may be excised with adjacent bowel. In other locations, where resection would endanger adjacent structures, simple anastomosis between the cyst and normal intestine can be performed, provided there is no gastric mucosa in the cyst. If bleeding has been a persisting complaint, one can assume the presence of gastric mucosa. If resection is contraindicated, the lining mucosa may be stripped from the cyst, leaving the muscle wall in situ.

Associated anomalies such as presacral tumours (16%) and anorectal malformations (21%) are frequently described in the literature. Management of these lesions may be difficult and often requires preoperative evaluation of both the GI and genitourinary tract. Continence of both systems is imperative, and, therefore treatment strategies must be individualized based on the findings of each patient.

Further Reading

Ladd WE (1937) Duplications of the alimentary tract. South Med J 30:363–371

MD Stringer (2006) Gastrointestinal Duplications. In P Puri, ME Höllwarth (eds) Pediatric Surgery, Springer Surgery Atlas Series. Springer-Verlag, Berlin, Heidelberg, New York, pp 239–256

Puri P (2003) Duplications of the alimentary tract. In P Puri (ed) Newborn Surgery, 2nd edn. Arnold, London, pp 479–488

Raffensperger JG (1990) Alimentary tract duplication. In JG Raffensperger (ed) Swenson's Pediatric Surgery, 5th edn. Appleton & Lange, Norwalk, CT, pp 579–585

Rothenberg SS (1999) Thoracoscopy in infants and children: Basic technique. In NMA Bax, KA Georgeson, AS Najmaldin et al (eds) Endoscopic Surgery in Children. Springer, Berlin, MA, pp 73–83

Stern LE, Warner BW (2000) Gastrointestinal duplications Semin Pediatr Surg 9(3):135–140

Stringer MD (1995) Duplications of the alimentary tract. In L Spitz, AG Coran (eds) Operative Surgery, 5th edn. Chapman & Hall, London, pp 383–395

Wrenn E (1992) Alimentary tract duplications. In T Holder, K Ashcraft (eds) Pediatric Surgery. W.B. Saunders, Philadelphia, PA, pp 455–456

Necrotizing Enterocolitis

44

Catherine J. Hunter, Henri R. Ford, and Victoria Camerini

Contents

44.1 Introduction Including Definition and Incidence

Necrotizing enterocolitis (NEC) is the most common life threatening surgical and medical emergency affecting the gastrointestinal tract encountered in the neonatal intensive care unit. NEC occurs in 2–5% of all preterm infants although the majority of cases develop in infants less than 36 weeks of gestational age. It has been noted that infants born at earlier gestational age, develop NEC at a later chronological age. The average age of onset of disease is 20.2 days for infants born less than 30 weeks of gestation whereas disease onset is reduced to 13.8 days for infants born at 31–33 weeks and 5.4 days for infants born after 34 weeks of gestation.

Epidemiological studies have identified multiple risk factors for NEC, although a history of hypoxia, asphyxia and the introduction of enteral feeding are characteristically associated with premature infants that develop NEC. Despite its predilection for premature infants, NEC has also been described in term infants particularly those with cyanotic heart disease. There is no clear evidence to suggest that geographical origin, ethnicity or gender alter the incidence of NEC.

NEC is characterized by intestinal inflammation accompanied by epithelial barrier disruption, bacterial overgrowth and submucosal invasion. In its most severe form, NEC is characterized by full-thickness destruction of the intestinal wall leading to intestinal perforation, peritonitis, sepsis and death. Although the overall mortality for patients with NEC ranges from 10% to 50%, it approaches 100% in infants with the most severe form of the disease, characteristically the smallest and most premature infants. Moreover, infants that recover from NEC may still require prolonged hospitalisation

P. Puri and M. Höllwarth (eds.), *Pediatric Surgery: Diagnosis and Management,*
DOI: 10.1007/978-3-540-69560-8_44, © Springer-Verlag Berlin Heidelberg 2009

due to complications from disease, such as intestinal obstruction due to scarring, short bowel syndrome and complete intestinal failure further impacting long-term survival, growth and development.

44.2 Etiology

Epidemiological studies have identified multiple perinatal factors that increase an infant's risk for the development of NEC, although prematurity and a history of hypoxia, asphyxia and the introduction of formula feeding are characteristic of infants that develop NEC. Three main factors are however required for the development of disease including immaturity, bacterial colonization, and enteral feeding. Figure 44.1 summarizes the pathogenic sequences and factors contributing to the development of NEC.

44.2.1 Immature Intestinal Barrier

The intestinal epithelium is a primary barrier between the inside of the body and the external environment. As such, the intrinsic function of this epithelial layer is to protect the host. The mucosal defence system can be divided into two categories: non-immunologic and immunologic defence mechanisms. Non-immunologic mechanisms include peristalsis, gastric acidity, prote-

olytic enzyme activity, mucin production and semi-permeable intestinal barrier function provided by tight junctions between the epithelial cells lining the gut. Peristalsis is the progressive wave of contraction and relaxation of the intestine. In full-term infants and adults, migrating motor complexes propagate these waves along the intestine. In humans migrating complexes are not present until approximately 34 weeks of gestation, which may contribute to intestinal stasis in premature infants, thereby altering the microbial ecosystem. Gastric acidity is thought to be a first line defence against bacterial passage into the proximal intestine. The premature human infant's gastric pH is initially high and then decreases towards mature levels with increasing age and ultimately reaching a pH < 4. Permeability is an important factor in the ability of bacteria to translocate, causing systemic infection, and the premature infant intestine is more permeable in the first 2 days of life. Mucus production provides a protective viscoelastic layer to the epithelial intestinal lining. In humans, mucus production and composition changes with age, and increases in response to bacterial challenge.

Immunologic defence mechanisms in the gut include both the innate and adaptive immune systems. Cells of the innate immune system include paneth cells, macrophages, polymorphonuclear leukocytes (PMN), dendritic cells, M cells (specialized epithelial cells overlying lymphoid aggregates called Peyer's patches) and epithelial cells. Paneth cells produce a variety of antibacterial substances including defensins, lysozymes, secretory phospholipase A2, and lectins. While PMN

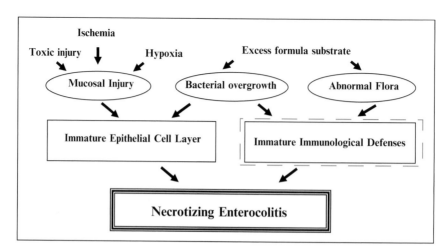

Fig. 44.1 Contributing factors in the development of NEC

are not regular inhabitants of the healthy intestine, PMN increase in number in response to intestinal injury and their production and function is known to be impaired in the newborn, contributing to the inadequate immature intestinal response. Dendritic cells and M cells function to capture and present antigens from the lumen of the bowel to T and B cells dispersed in the mucosal layer and in lymphoid aggregates along the length of the gut. Cells of the adaptive immune system include T and B lymphocytes and their differentiated effector cell subsets. T lymphocytes differentiate as cytotoxic T cells and are responsible for direct killing of damaged or infected epithelial cells and helper T cells are responsible for enhancing B cell differentiation and the production of plasma cells that secrete immunoglobulin in particular IgA. When compared to the adult, both the number and function of B and T cells is reduced in intestine contributing to defects in the intestinal epithelial barrier.

44.2.2 Role of Bacterial Pathogens and Other Microbes in NEC

NEC occurs in both sporadic and clustered distributions, causing speculation that specific infectious entities may be responsible. A variety of bacterial and viral pathogens have been implicated in the pathogenesis of NEC including *Enterobacteriaceae*, *Clostridia*, coagulase negative *Staphylococcus* and several viral species (Table 44.1).

Despite the fact that no single organism appears to be responsible for NEC the importance of bacteria in the pathogenesis of disease should not be discounted. It is known that NEC does not develop in animal models kept in sterile environments. At birth the intestine is devoid of bacterial flora, but is rapidly colonized by bacteria from the rectovaginal flora of the mother, and bacteria from the surrounding environment. Additionally, colonization by commensal bacteria is required for the normal development and maturation of the newborn intestine. Bacterial-host cross talk has been shown to modulate gut vascular development, and promote immune system development. Abnormal intestinal colonization patterns of neonates admitted to the neonatal intensive care unit may further increase susceptibility to NEC.

Table 44.1 Organisms implicated in necrotizing enterocolitis

Bacteria
- *Enterobacteriaceae* species
  - *Escherichia* species
  - *Salmonella* species
  - *Klebsiella* species
  - *Enterobacter* species
- *Clostridium* species
- *Staphylococcus* species

Viruses
- *Rotavirus*
- *Echovirus*
- *Coronavirus*
- *Torovirus*

Fungus
- ±*Candida* species

44.2.3 Role of Enteral Feeding

Rapid advancement of formula feeding has been associated with the development of NEC. Breast milk feeding is known to protect against NEC, and premature infants have a reduced incidence of infection when fed human breast milk rather than formula. A prospective multicenter study of preterm infants found almost a tenfold increase in the incidence of NEC in formula-fed infants as compared with those who were fed breast-milk. The positive effects of breast milk are likely due to a variety of potential anti-microbial products including immunoglobulins, oligosaccharides, lactoferrin and glycoproteins with anti-adhesive capacity for bacteria, and cytokines present in breast milk. Additionally breast milk promotes intestinal colonization by probiotic (beneficial) bacteria such as *Lactobacillus* species and *Bifidobacteria* species.

44.2.4 Inflammatory Mediators and NEC

A variety of inflammatory chemokines including tumor necrosis factor alpha (TNF-α), nitric oxide (NO), platelet activating factor (PAF), and several cytokines (IL-1, IL-6, IL-8 and IL-10) have been implicated in the pathogenesis of NEC. Elevated plasma levels of TNF-α have been found in infants with NEC, and local upregulation of IL-1, IL-8 and inducible NO synthase (iNOS) has been demonstrated in the intestine of infants with NEC. Nitric oxide plays a paradoxical role in the pathogenesis of NEC. Constitutive low-level production of NO enhances mucosal blood flow, and promotes local vascular health. However, sustained overproduction of NO due to upregulation of iNOS leads to intestinal damage. The pathologic effects of NO are postulated to be due to the strong oxidant effects of peroxynitrite (ONOO⁻) resulting in enterocyte cell death, and impaired mucosal healing. ONOO⁻ causes enterocyte cell death and impairs mucosal healing. The up-regulation of NO has been demonstrated in areas of intestinal epithelial injury in human infants with NEC. In infants who recover from NEC, iNOS, and NO return to baseline levels.

44.2.4.1 Maternal Factors

Several maternal risk factors increase an infant's risk of developing NEC, including placental insufficiency and maternal cocaine abuse. These factors may contribute to disease susceptibility by compromising placental blood flow and hence perfusion of vital organs in the foetus.

44.3 Pathology

Several pathological findings are associated with NEC. It is important to note however, that findings are highly variable. The terminal ileum is the most frequently involved site, however NEC may affect any part of the small or large intestine. Pan-necrosis is a highly morbid finding associated with fulminant disease (Fig. 44.2). Pneumatosis intestinalsis is a pathogneumonic finding in NEC characterized by the presence of air in the

intestinal wall (Fig. 44.3). The etiology of pneumatosis intestinalis is thought to be due to bacterial invasion, fermentation and hydrogen production in the intestinal wall.

Histologically, intestinal tissue may demonstrate epithelial layer sloughing, increased apoptotic bodies within epithelial cells, tissue oedema and submucosal air (Fig. 44.4). Evidence of the response of the immune

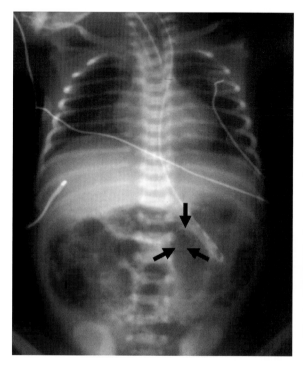

Fig. 44.3 Supine abdominal x-ray in a neonate showing diffuse pneumatosis intestinalis. Arrows indicate signet sign

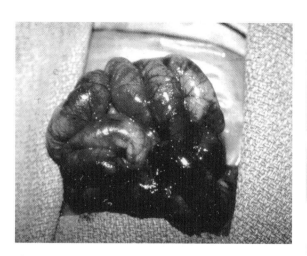

Fig. 44.2 Intraoperative image of pan intestinal necrosis, diagnosed at the time of laparotomy for NEC

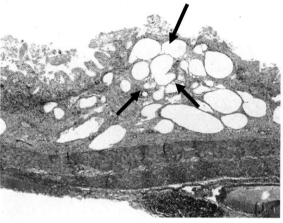

Fig. 44.4 Hematoxylin-eosin staining of intestinal tissue harvested from an infant with NEC. Arrows indicate epithelial destruction with submucosal gas collections

system is characterized by neutrophil infiltration and hypertrophy of intestinal lymphoid aggregates. However, ultimately the diagnosis of NEC is based on clinical findings.

44.4 Diagnosis

The assessment of an infant suspected of having NEC starts with a thorough history and physical examination. A typical presentation of NEC would be that of a premature infant advancing on enteral feedings who develops signs of feeding intolerance. These signs may be subtle and first noted by the nursing staff and include abdominal distension, high gastric residuals, and guaiac positive stool. In more advanced cases of disease, infants may present with progressive abdominal distention, evidence of peritonitis, frankly bloody stool and cardio-respiratory failure.

Although prompt diagnosis and intervention are desirable tenants of disease management, there is no clear evidence proving that early diagnosis and interventions alters patient outcome.

44.4.1 Clinical Features

In 1973 Bell et al proposed the NEC grading system, in an attempt to standardize diagnosis, disease severity scoring and, management. A slight modification of Bell's original criteria is in use today (Table 44.2). The presenting symptoms may vary and include feeding intolerance, abdominal distension, bloody stools, apnoea, lethargy, temperature instability and hypoperfusion. Classically, increased amounts of gastric residual and abdominal distension and visible loops of bowel are noted on physical exam. Occasionally discoloration of the abdomen wall may be present and the palpation of the abdomen may elicit tenderness with guarding. The progression of disease is variable; some infants have minor symptoms that resolve spontaneously over a period of days in response to bowel rest, while others progress over hours with respiratory failure requiring intubation, hypotension requiring fluid resuscitation and inotropic support and/or immediate surgical intervention.

Table 44.2 Modified Bell's stages of necrotizing enterocolitis

I. Suspected disease

IA.

Mild systemic signs (apnea, bradycardia, temperature instability)

Mild intestinal signs (abdominal distention, gastric residuals, occult blood in stool)

IB.

Mild systemic signs (apnea, bradycardia, temperature instability)

Mild intestinal signs (abdominal distention, gastric residuals, gross blood in stool)

Non-specific or normal radiological findings

II. Definite disease

IIA.

Mild systemic signs (apnea, bradycardia, temperature instability)

Additional intestinal signs (absent bowel sounds, abdominal tenderness)

Specific radiologic signs (pneumatosis intestinalis or portal venous air)

Laboratory changes (metabolic acidosis, thrombocytopenia)

IIB.

Moderate systemic signs (apnea, bradycardia, temperature instability, mild metabolic acidosis, mild thrombocytopenia)

Additional intestinal signs (absent bowel sounds, abdominal tenderness, abdominal mass)

III. Advanced disease

IIIA.

Severe systemic illness (same as IIB with additional hypotension and shock)

Intestinal signs (large abdominal distention, abdominal wall discoloration, peritonitis, intestine intact)

Severe radiologic signs (definite ascites)

Progressive laboratory derangements (metabolic acidosis, disseminated intravascular coagulopathy)

IIIB.

Severe systemic illness (same as IIIA)

Intestinal signs (large abdominal distention, abdominal wall discoloration, peritonitis, intestinal perforation)

Severe radiologic signs (definite ascites and pneumoperitoneum)

Worsening laboratory derangements (metabolic acidosis, disseminated intravascular coagulopathy)

44.4.2 Laboratory Findings

Common laboratory abnormalities include thrombocytopenia, leukocytosis, electrolytes imbalance, metabolic acidosis, hypoxia, or hypercapnia. Therefore a comprehensive laboratory analysis should be performed in infants with suspected NEC. A patient with NEC may present with an abnormal white blood cell count (WBC). Although it may be elevated, it is more commonly depressed, and a severely low white blood cell count ($<1.5 \times 10^9$/l) has been reported in 37% of cases. The granulocytopenia results from decreased production and increased utilization of leukocytes. Thrombocytopenia is also commonly seen in almost 90% of affected individuals. Serial C-reactive protein levels have been shown to be successful in differentiating benign abdominal etiologies such as ileus from NEC. Furthermore it has been suggested that persistently elevated CRP levels indicate the need for surgical intervention, although this is controversial. NEC is associated with bacteraemia in approximately one third of cases, and thus blood cultures should be obtained prior to administration of antibiotics.

44.4.3 Radiological Diagnosis

44.4.4 Abdominal Series X-rays

Serial plain films of the abdomen (anteroposterior radiograph and a left lateral decubitus or cross table lateral film) should be obtained at the first suspicion of disease. Several radiologic findings pathogneumonic of NEC can be identified on abdominal x-ray including intramural air (pneumatosis intestinalis), portal vein gas, the "fixed loop sign", "signet sign", and in advanced cases pneumoperitoneum.

Portal venous air is noted in approximately 30% of advanced cases, and occurs when intramural air is absorbed into the mesenteric venous circulation (Fig. 44.5). Portal venous air portends a worse prognosis. The finding of a fixed loop is referred to as a "signet sign" and results from a bowel loop that remains unchanged for 24–48h and is associated with transmural necrosis (Fig. 44.3). Despite some reports indicating an association between fixed loops and pan-necrosis, almost half of patients recover without surgical intervention. Free air can be seen in severe cases of NEC (Fig. 44.6). A large pneumoperitoneum can be seen as a central collection of air on the anteroposterior film, and is an indication for surgical intervention. Pneumoperitoneum in the absence of pneumotosis intestinalis may be more suggestive of focal intestinal perforation (FIP), rather than NEC.

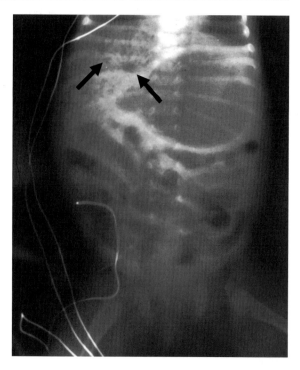

Fig. 44.5 Supine abdominal x-ray revealing an enlarged stomach bubble, stacking of bowel loops, and portal venous gas. Arrows indicate portal venous gas

Several common non-specific radiographic findings include a gasless abdomen, non-specific bowel gas patterns and ascites. Ascites has been reported to occur in approximately 10% of infants with NEC.

Computed tomography scans (CT) will reveal findings similar to those seen by X-ray, and is generally unnecessary and therefore not indicated.

44.4.5 Contrast Studies

The use of contrast enemas is contraindicated in the diagnosis of NEC. However, contrast studies may be indicated following recovery from acute disease. In patients with a history of NEC and new intestinal obstruction, contrast studies may localize a stricture secondary to scarring.

44.4.6 Ultrasound

Ultrasound can be useful in the diagnosis of NEC, allowing evaluation of intestinal wall edema, portal gas and free fluid. However ultrasound remains a

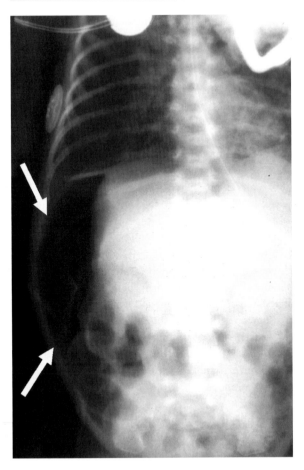

Fig. 44.6 Lateral decubitus abdominal x-ray of an infant with NEC, demonstrating intestinal free air

notoriously operator-dependent modality and may not be readily available in many centers.

44.5 Differential Diagnosis

The variability in the presentation and severity of NEC may mimic different conditions. Both sepsis and ileus can present with signs and symptoms of systemic infection and abdominal distension. Radiologic imaging may help in diagnosis, but often does not definitively rule in NEC unless pneumatosis intestinalis is present. Fortunately the therapy, to be discussed later, is the same for both early NEC and sepsis. Advanced cases of Hirschsprung's enterocolitis or severe gastroenteritis may present with intramural air. In advanced cases other aetiologies of intra-abdominal catastrophe

including volvulus, intussusception, inspissated meconium syndrome and intestinal vascular accident may be mistaken for fulminant NEC.

Focal intestinal perforation is important to consider in the differential of NEC. FIP is a distinct entity often characterized by the lack of signs and symptoms of sepsis. Despite the fact that FIP is typically seen in infants of smaller birth weight and more extreme prematurity, it has a higher survival rate. FIP is also associated with the use of pharmacologic agents including indomethacin and dexamethasone. Furthermore the most commonly associated organism of sepsis in FIP is *Candida* species, which is distinct from the agents associated with sepsis in NEC. It is important to note that infants with FIP who are culture-positive for *Candida* may be more severely ill, than those infants with FIP who are culture-negative.

44.6 Management

44.6.1 Medical Management

The majority of patients with NEC are treated non-operatively. Prompt resuscitative measures including evaluation of airway, breathing and circulation remain paramount in these patients. Many patients may require ventilator support, and tracheal intubation is preferred to prevent aerophagia and greater intestinal distension. Most patients with NEC will be hypovolemic and will require adequate fluid resuscitation, with intravenous crystalloids. If the patient is affected by coagulopathy then correction with platelets and/or fresh frozen plasma is indicated. States of acidosis should be corrected by optimal ventilation, fluid resuscitation, and if necessary, bicarbonate or Tris[hydroxymethyl]-aminomethane (THAM) administration. The use of inotropic support may be indicated in patients with refractory hypotension despite fluid administration. After blood cultures have been obtained broad-spectrum antibiotics should be started. Currently there is insufficient evidence regarding the choice of a specific antibiotic regimen or duration, although broad-spectrum antibiotics based on patterns of microbial resistance within individual neonatal intensive care units is recommended. The use of antifungal agents should also be considered in severely ill patients. Appropriate antibiotic therapy has been shown to improve the outcome and survival in infants with NEC.

All enteric feeds should be stopped and the stomach decompressed with an orogastric tube. Serial measurements of abdominal girth, frequent abdominal exams, and serial abdominal radiographs are obtained to monitor disease progression.

44.6.2 Probiotics

At birth, the intestine lacks bacterial flora, and with time becomes colonized with a variety of bacterial species. As previously mentioned, the microbial flora in the premature hospitalized patient is different from that of a healthy full-term infant. Typically, full-term infants have a predominance of favourable gram-positive organisms including *Lactobacilli* and *Bifidobacteria*, whereas premature infants are largely colonized by *Enterococcus* and gram negative organisms. The administration of exogenous probiotics may protect against NEC by altering the intestinal ecosystem from colonization by potentially harmful microflora to a more favourable or beneficial environment. Clinical trials investigating the potential benefit of probiotics have produced mixed results. A randomised prospective study by Bin-num et al found an absolute risk reduction of 12% in the incidence of NEC, and a decline in disease severity after daily feeding supplementation with probiotics. In a prospective study by Lin et al the overall patient mortality was lower after probiotic administration, with a lower incidence of NEC following probiotic therapy (1.1% vs. 5.3%). However, a similarly designed study revealed no benefit. Currently the role of probiotic therapy remains an area of investigation.

44.6.3 Surgical Management

Despite appropriate and timely medical management, over a third of patients with NEC require surgical intervention. In infants with a birth weight greater than 1,500 g laparotomy with resection of affected intestine is the preferred approach. In some cases the intestine is necrotic in only a single segment; while in others, the disease pattern is more complex involving multiple segments with intervening areas of questionable viability, or the entire extent of the small and large bowel (Fig. 44.2). The standard of care is to remove all necrotic areas, taking great care to preserve any bowel that appears viable. After resecting the necrotic regions, an area of viable intestine is used to create an ostomy with or without a mucus fistula. There are occasional reports of resection of isolated perforation with primary reanastomosis of the remaining intestine, however this is not a widely accepted approach. In patients who are found to have multiple areas of questionable intestinal viability, a "second-look" procedure may be planned to revaluate the bowel in 24–36 h prior to the formation of an enterostomy. In the past, if at the time of surgery many segments of intestine were found to be involved, the creation of multiple stomas was typically practiced. However, this strategy may result in the sacrifice of potentially viable intestine, hence some surgeons advocate the "patch, drain and wait" approach. In this case each perforation is sutured closed, penrose drains are placed and parenteral support is continued. In cases of pan-necrosis surgical therapy is often associated with extremely poor outcomes and intervention may be foregone.

In patients weighing less than 1,500 g the optimal choice of surgical intervention has been more controversial. Laparotomy with intestinal resection in very-low-birth weight infants is associated with a very high morbidity and mortality, and poor neurodevelopmental outcomes. Ein et al in 1977 reported a series of extremely low birth weight patients treated with a peritoneal-drainage procedure. They reported that three survived, two of which did not require a subsequent operation. It was postulated that peritoneal drainage allowed a release of intra-abdominal pressure, drainage of infection, and time for further medical optimisation and stabilisation. Despite remaining somewhat controversial, this approach was adopted for years by many surgeons as both a temporising measure and a definitive therapeutic approach to Bell stage III disease in extremely low birth weight patients. Moss et al. published a multi-institutional, randomised, controlled trial in 2006, comparing primary peritoneal drainage with laparotomy and bowel resection in infants less than 1,500 g. They found no statistical difference in survival, dependence on parenteral nutrition or length of hospital stay. Hence, while peritoneal drainage may have an important role in the surgical management of extremely low birth weight infants, careful individual assessment of each patient and consultation between medical and surgical personnel is required for determining an optimal treatment strategy.

In patients who improve after laparotomy with ostomy formation, re-establishing intestinal continuity within 6 weeks, assuming adequate bowel length, remains an optimal course of action.

44.7 Complications

44.7.1 Strictures

The most serious complications of acute NEC include intestinal necrosis and perforation, which may occur in up to one third of patients. However, some patients who initially appear to respond well to medical management develop gastric residuals associated with abdominal distension and bilious emesis upon resuming enteral feedings. This scenario is suggestive of the presence of intestinal strictures, which form in areas of partial intestinal necrosis or ischemia with healing, causing tissue contraction and scarring. The most commonly affected site is at the junction of the descending and sigmoid colon. Radiographic imaging may confirm bowel obstruction, with a transition zone and air-fluid levels. If a stricture is suspected a contrast enema (or an upper gastrointestinal study) should be performed to assess intestinal patency. If a stricture is demonstrated, surgical resection is indicated at this time. Intestinal strictures develop in approximately one third of patients with a history of NEC.

44.7.2 Short Bowel Syndrome

In addition to intestinal strictures, nearly 25% of patients with a history of NEC and surgical intervention develop short bowel syndrome. The intestine of a full-term neonate is approximately 250 cm, when a large segment or multiple segments of bowel is (are) resected, the amount of remaining intestine may not be sufficient to adequately absorb nutrients and fluids. The patient is then reliant upon intravenous nutrition, and is exposed to the risks of long-term parenteral support including line sepsis, cholestasis, cirrhosis and liver failure. Some success in survivors with short bowel syndrome has been reported after small bowel transplant.

44.7.3 Neurodevelopmental Delay

Neurodevelopmental delay continues to be a significant issue in survivors of NEC, as many as 50% of infants are affected. In a recent study, Blakely et al. found that patients with NEC who underwent laparotomy instead of peritoneal drainage had a lower risk of future developmental delay. Prior investigations suggested that neurodevelopmental delay was more related to prematurity and prolonged hospital stay, rather that NEC itself. However, Blakely et al controlled for the confounding factors of prematurity and severity of disease in their study. More investigation into this area is warranted.

Further Reading

Blakely ML, Tyson JE, Lally KP et al (2006) Laparotomy versus peritoneal drainage for necrotizing enterocolitis or isolated intestinal perforation in extremely low birth weight infants: Outcomes through 18 months adjusted age. Pediatr 117:e680–e687

Ford HR (2006) Mechanism of nitric oxide-mediated intestinal barrier failure: Insight into the pathogenesis of necrotizing enterocolitis. J Pediatr Surg 41:294–299

Hackam DJ, Upperman JS, Grishin A, Ford HR (2005) Disordered enterocyte signaling and intestinal barrier dysfunction in the pathogenesis of necrotizing enterocolitis. Semin Pediatr Surg 14:49–57

Lin P, Stoll B (2006) Necrotising enterocolitis. Lancet 368: 1271–1283

Moss RL, Dimmitt RA, Barnhart DC, et al (2006) Laparotomy versus peritoneal drainage for necrotizing enterocolitis and perforation. N Engl J Med 354:2225–2234

Puri P, Höllwarth M (2006) Pediatric Surgery. Springer, Berlin, Heidelberg

Strober W (2006) Immunology: Unraveling gut inflammation. Science 313:1052–1054

Constipation

45

Melanie C.C. Clarke, Bridget R. Southwell, and John M. Hutson

Contents

45.1 Introduction Including Definition and Incidence

Constipation is a common childhood condition that occurs in around 3% of children and accounts for 3–5% of visits to paediatricians and 10–15% of referrals to gastroenterologists. A positive family history can be found in 28–50% of constipated children and a higher incidence has been reported in monozygotic than dizygotic twins. The peak incidence of constipation occurs at the time of toilet training (between 2 and 4 years of age), with an increased prevalence in boys.

Constipation can be defined as being either organic or functional. Childhood Functional Constipation is further defined by the Rome III criteria (Table 45.1). Constipation can also be classified as being either acute or chronic. Chronic constipation, also referred to as chronic treatment-resistant constipation (CTRC), describes those children in whom there is no improvement in their symptoms after 2 years of medical therapy and/or behavioural modification.

45.2 Aetiology

Constipation may be caused by endocrine, metabolic, pharmacological, obstructive, systemic or central nervous system disorders (Table 45.2). Hirschsprung's disease, caused by aganglionosis of the bowel, must be excluded in children with severe idiopathic constipation especially if the constipation has been present since birth or has been associated with a delayed passage of meconium (beyond 24 h), failure to thrive or a positive family history.

P. Puri and M. Höllwarth (eds.), *Pediatric Surgery: Diagnosis and Management,*
DOI: 10.1007/978-3-540-69560-8_45, © Springer-Verlag Berlin Heidelberg 2009

Table 45.1 Diagnostic criteria for functional constipation (Rome III)

Must include two *or more* of the following in a child with a developmental age of *at least* 4 years
1. Two or fewer defecations in the toilet per week
2. At least one episode of faecal incontinence per week
3. History of retentive posturing or excessive volitional stool retention
4. History of painful or hard bowel movements
5. History of a large faecal mass in the rectum
6. History of large diameter stools that may obscure the toilet
Criteria must be fulfilled at least once per week for at least 2 months before diagnosis

45.3 Acute Constipation

Children with no obvious organic cause for their constipation should be managed by a combination of dietary changes, laxatives and/or stool softeners and/or bulking agents and behavioural modification and toilet training. Toilet posture education and pelvic floor muscle training by a physiotherapist should be considered. Seventy percent of children presenting with constipation will respond to this treatment strategy within 2 years.

45.4 Chronic Constipation

Despite aggressive medical management, constipation associated with faecal incontinence, recurrent faecal impaction and functional and emotional problems, persists in around 30% of patients. Chronic constipation, not associated with an obvious organic cause, was once thought to be entirely related to behavioural or psychological problems, however this is no longer the case. Instead, some of these children are now thought to have an organic cause for their constipation due to low motility of the colon known as slow transit constipation (STC). These children need to be distinguished from those with functional faecal retention (FFR) in whom there is a hold-up in the rectosigmoid colon but normal colonic transit. FFR is the most common cause of constipation and faecal incontinence in children and typically develops at the time of toilet training or when the child starts school. Children with FFR should respond to conventional medical and behavioural

Table 45.2 Causes of constipation

Congenital anatomic or structural defects
  Imperforate anus or anal stenosis
  Anteriorly displaced anus
  Meconium plug syndrome
  Hirschsprung's disease
  Pelvic mass
  Abnormal abdominal musculature—prune belly, gastroschisis, Down syndrome
Metabolic and endocrine disorders
  Diabetes insipidus
  Hypercalcaemia and hypokalaemia
  Renal tubular acidosis
  Hypothyroidism
  Dehydration
  Multiple endocrine neoplasia type 2B
Chronic intestinal pseudo-obstruction
Cystic fibrosis
Connective tissue disorders—scleroderma, SLE, Ehlers-Danlos syndrome
Coeliac disease
Neurologic causes
  Damage to the spinal cord—meningomyelocele, trauma, surgery, tumours, cauda equina syndrome and tethered cord
  Cerebral palsy
  Infectious polyneuritis
  Amyotonia congenita
  Muscular dystrophy
  degenerative disorders
  Neurofibromatosis
Cow milk intolerance or other food allergies
Other organic causes
  Colonic dysmotility (Slow Transit Constipation—STC)
  Outlet obstruction (Functional Faecal Retention—FFR)
Dietary
  Poor fibre intake
  Poor fluid intake
Medication
  Analgesics (Codeine preparations)
  Antacids
  Anticholinergics
  Anticonvulsants
  Tricyclic anti-depressants
  β-blockers
  Iron and calcium supplements
  Antispasmodics
  Diuretics
Behavioural causes
  Learned pattern of defecation (can be due to previous painful defecation)
  Adverse life event
  Defiant behaviour
  Intellectual disability

therapy, whereas those with STC may require more aggressive management.

45.5 The Pathology of Slow Transit Constipation

It is believed that in children with STC, the primary defect lies within the enteric nervous system.

The gastrointestinal tract contains its own nerve cell bodies that form an intrinsic network that is connected to the central nervous system via the vagal, coeliac and pelvic nerves. Enteric neurons have cell bodies within ganglia that lie in the myenteric or submucosal plexuses. The cell bodies have processes that penetrate the muscle layers where they release their neurotransmitters. Acetylcholine (Ach) and tachykinins (including substance P) cause gastrointestinal muscular contraction whilst relaxation is initiated by the release of vasoactive intestinal peptide (VIP), nitric oxide (NO) and ATP.

Interstitial cells of Cajal (ICC) are found in the tunica muscularis throughout the gastrointestinal tract and lie between enteric nerve terminals and smooth muscle. Although their precise role has remained undetermined for several decades, it is now thought that they act as a conduit for active transmission of electrical slow waves as well as serving as gastrointestinal pacemaker cells (Fig. 45.1).

STC has been associated with a decrease in substance P fibres and changes in NOS and VIP. A loss of ICC has been demonstrated in a range of motility disorders including STC.

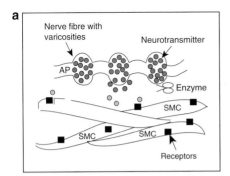

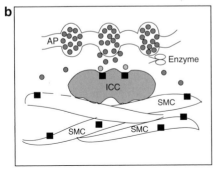

Fig. 45.1 Old and new models of neuromuscular transmission in the gastrointestinal tract. (**a**) Old two-cell model. Action potentials travelling along nerve fibres caused release of neurotransmitter from varicosities. Transmitter diffused across extracellular space and bound to receptors on muscle cells inducing contraction or relaxation. (**b**) New three-cell model. Interstitial cells of Cajal have receptors for transmitters and are connected to each other and to smooth muscle cells by gap junctions. ICC form a network among the smooth muscle cells. Transmitter released from nerve fibres binds to receptors on ICC, modifying excitation with changes conveyed to adjacent ICC and muscle cells by electrical conduction. ICC also act as pacemaker cells generating and conducting rhythmic electrical activity that produces slow waves. AP—action potential; ICC—interstitial cells of Cajal; SMC—smooth muscle cell; ●—transmitter; ■—receptor

45.6 Diagnosis

45.6.1 Clinical

Medical history and physical examination are essential when diagnosing constipation and a thorough ante-natal/birth/post-natal history should be obtained (Table 45.3). It is important to clarify what each individual family defines as "constipation" by determining the occurrence of specific symptoms and their frequency. Essential information includes an accurate gastrointestinal and general medical assessment as well as a developmental and psychosocial evaluation. Delayed first passage of meconium, frequent soiling, passage of large soft stools, abdominal distension and bloating are all common features associated with STC.

A thorough physical examination is essential in the initial assessment of a child with constipation (Table 45.4). This should include a general examination as well as an abdominal examination and external examination of the perineum and perianal area. A rectal

Table 45.3 Model of history taking in a child with constipation

Demographics
  Age
  Sex
Presenting symptoms
  Frequency of defecation
  Behaviour associated with defecation
  Consistency of stools
  Soiling
  Pain (abdominal, rectal or other)
  Rectal bleeding—associated with passage of stool, mixed or
    coating
  Appetite
  Vomiting
  Abdominal distension
  Weight loss/gain
  Toilet training
  Onset and duration of symptoms
Previous diagnoses and treatments
Current treatment
Peri-natal history
  Any ante-natal concerns/diagnoses
  Gestation
  Birth condition (need for ITU/special care)
  Time of passage of meconium
Developmental history
  Growth and attainment of developmental markers
Past medical history
  Hospital admissions (medical and surgical)
  Urinary symptoms
  Hypothyroidism associated symptoms (cold intolerance,
    coarse hair, dry skin etc…)
Dietary history
Medications
  Immunisations
  Allergies
Family history
  Gastrointestinal and other significant illnesses (including
    thyroid disease, cystic fibrosis, coeliac disease, neurologi-
    cal conditions, connective tissue disorders, diabetes)
Psychosocial history
  Age appropriate quality of life assessment

Table 45.4 Model of examination in a child with constipation

General appearance
  Failure to thrive
Routine observations
  Height and weight
  Pulse
  Blood pressure
General examination
  Including cardiovascular and respiratory examination
Abdominal examination
  Distension
  Hepatosplenomegaly
  Abdominal mass—including faecaloma
  Palpable bowel loops
Neurological and spinal examination
  Lower limb – tone, reflexes and power
  Sacral dimple/sacral hair tuft
  Obvious spinal deformity
  Muscle (especially buttock) wasting
Anal inspection
  Site
  Visible stool (skin and clothing)
  Skin condition
  Perianal skin tags
  Anal fissure
Rectal examination
  Anal wink
  Anal tone
  Pain
  Presence and consistency of stool
  Pelvic mass
  Explosive stool on finger withdrawal
  Bleeding

Blood samples should be obtained for coeliac disease screening, thyroid function testing and allergy testing (cows milk protein intolerance and high percentage of eosinophils in full blood count).

examination should be performed by an appropriately experienced practitioner.

In most cases, a comprehensive history and examination can determine whether or not an organic cause is responsible for the constipation. If the constipation is believed to be non-organic, although STC has some distinctive clinical features, sufficient information can rarely be obtained in order to distinguish STC from FFR.

45.6.2 Abdominal X-ray

Plain abdominal x-rays have debatable value in the assessment of constipation. If faecal impaction or loading is obvious on rectal or abdominal examination then little more information can be attained by means of a plain x-ray. Abdominal x-rays can be used to assess the presence and degree of abdominal loading, especially in obese subjects or in those in whom a rectal examination is refused or inappropriate, however interpretation can be subjective and x-ray timing in relation to defecation can be misleading.

45.6.3 Transit Studies

Colonic transit time takes between 1 and 3 days during which time there is extensive mixing of stool. The quantification of transit time demonstrates the presence of constipation and provides an objective evaluation of faecal clearance. Transit time has traditionally been measured using plastic, non-absorbable radio-opaque markers with transit time in different regions being determined by the ingestion of different shaped markers over 3–6 days. Studies measuring normal transit in children give the upper range of total colonic transit from 46 to 62 h. Transit rates in children less than 5 years old are faster, whilst children aged 6 years or more have a range of transit and frequency of defecation similar to adults. This mode of assessment of gastrointestinal transit time is widely available and until recently has been considered the gold standard. However, it has now been recognised that indigestible solid particles do not move with a meal, and may not be handled by the colon in the same manner as stool. Consequently, gastrointestinal transit is increasingly being investigated using scintigraphy (nuclear transit study). A tracer dose of technetium, or gallium, in 20 ml of milk is ingested and a first image obtained at 2 h to assess gastric emptying and a further image at 6 h to ascertain whether or not the tracer has reached the colon. Subsequently, images are obtained at 24, 30 and 48 h to document transit through the colon. The colonic transit index can be obtained based on the geometric mean of intestinal activity at 6, 24, 30 and 48 h post ingestion of tracer. By this means, patients with small bowel, right, left or pan-colonic (STC) or pan-intestinal transit deficits can be distinguished from those with normal gastrointestinal transit with FFR (Fig. 45.2).

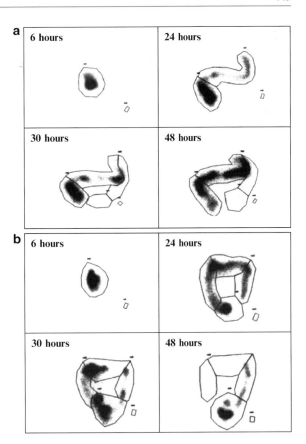

Fig. 45.2 Nuclear transit studies demonstrating (**a**) slow transit constipation (STC) and (**b**) functional faecal retention (FFR)

birth, a diagnosis of Hirschsprung's disease needs to be eliminated by performing a rectal biopsy. Biopsy specimens are obtained from approximately 3 cm above the anal verge and should be deep enough to include adequate submucosa. A diagnosis of Hirschsprung's disease is supported by an absence of ganglion cells, usually in the presence of hypertrophied nerve fibres, with a marked increase in acetylcholinesterase activity in the lamina propria and muscularis mucosa. A rectal biopsy is also useful in identifying those children with a food allergy, as recognised by increased eosinophils in the mucosa.

45.6.4 Rectal Biopsy

In cases of intractable constipation with a history of delayed passage of mecomium or symptoms since

45.6.5 Laparoscopic Colonic Biopsies

Recently, in those children with proximal colonic delay demonstrated by their transit study, laparoscopic seromuscular biopies are being performed in association with rectal biopsy, in some centres, in an attempt to identify any consistent histological anomalies. Biopsies are collected from the hepatic flexure, midtransverse colon, splenic flexure and sigmoid colon without the need for suturing the defect. Specimens are processed for immunofluorescence histochemistry and are stained for substance P, vasoactive intestinal peptide (VIP), nitric oxide synthase (NOS) or cKit (a marker for interstitial cells of Cajal (ICC)). It has been proposed that some children with STC have a form of intestinal neuronal dysplasia (IND), which represents an abnormality of intestinal innervation that is subtler than Hirschsprung's disease and can be diagnosed by abnormal immunohistochemistry.

45.6.6 Colonic Manometry

Colonic manometry involves the *in vivo* measurement of changes in intraluminal pressure within the colon. A multi-channel water-perfusion or solid-state pressure recording catheter is sited in the colon in either a retrograde manner, via colonoscopy, or an antegrade manner, via a pre-existing appendix stoma or via a naso-colic route (Fig. 45.3).

Colonic contractile activity produces changes in intraluminal pressure seen as a deviation from the baseline. Contractions can be non-propagating or propagating with propagating contractions being in either an antegrade or retrograde direction (Fig. 45.4). High amplitude contractions (>116 mmHg) are thought to represent mass movement within the colon. Standards for colonic manometry in children have been defined and parameters measured. Expected frequency of propagating sequences, ratio of antegrade to retrograde contractions, frequency of high amplitude propagating sequences, post-prandial response and diurnal variation have all been determined.

Although currently most studies are conducted under the auspices of research, manometric data are becoming increasingly valuable in demonstrating any underlying motility disorder. A correlation has been demonstrated that children with slow transit on nuclear transit studies have a lack of antegrade peristaltic sequences on colonic manometry (Fig. 45.4).

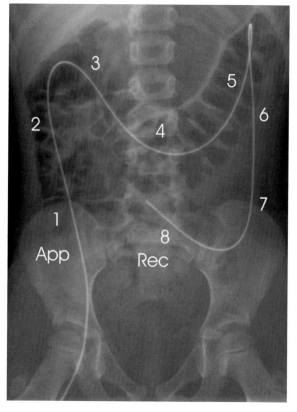

Fig. 45.3 Abdominal radiograph showing an antegradely inserted 8 channel manometry catheter passing from the appendix (App) to the rectum (Rec) with the position of the side holes shown

45.7 Treatment

45.7.1 Medical

For those children who have failed to improve with standard medical treatment (laxatives/stool softeners/ bulking agents, dietary changes, behavioural modification and toilet training) there still remain a few more aggressive medical therapeutic options. Polyethylene glycol, with or without electrolytes, acts as an osmotic laxative by increasing the amount of water retained in the faeces thus producing stools that are softer, bulkier and easier to pass. It is especially useful for overcoming impaction, although it can be used on a regular basis to manage chronic constipation. Alternatively, neurotrophin-3, a neurotrophic factor acting on the central nervous system, has been shown to increase stool frequency and enhance colonic transit.

a

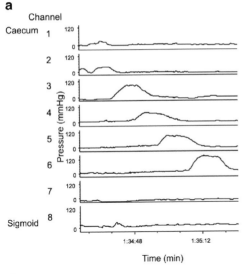

b

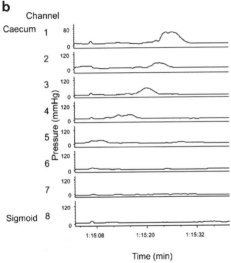

Fig. 45.4 Colonic manometry showing (**a**) an antegrade propagating sequence and (**b**) a retrograde propagating sequence

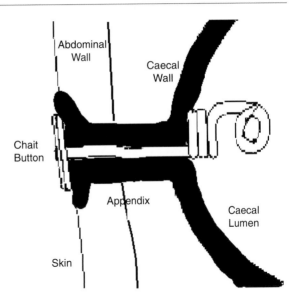

Fig. 45.5 Chait button in appendix stoma

tionally in either the right iliac fossa or at the umbilicus, and sutured to the skin to form an appendicostomy. Antegrade continence enemas (ACE) are then performed via the stoma to flush faeces from the caecum to the rectum. When the colon is intermittently (every 2–3 days) washed out in this manner it remains relatively empty and continence and soiling is improved. Washouts can be performed via intermittent stomal catheterisation or via a Chait caecostomy button (Fig. 45.5).

45.8 Complications

45.8.1 Disease Related

Ineffective treatment can lead to faecal impaction that may require either medical or surgical disimpaction. Constant soiling, if poorly managed, can result in perianal erythema and, in severe cases, excoriation.

45.7.2 Surgical

Until recently surgical management of chronic treatment resistant constipation consisted mostly of bowel resection with or without formation of a stoma. Now, however, a less invasive approach is regularly being taken with the formation of a continent appendix stoma as first described by Malone for the management of incontinence after correction of an anorectal malformation. The appendix is brought through the anterior abdominal wall, tradi-

45.8.2 Laxatives

There is widespread belief that chronic use of laxatives can lead to tolerance, habituation and even colonic damage and these misconceptions often lead to inappropriate prescribing practices. When used appropriately there are relatively few side effects to either bulk, osmotic or even stimulant laxatives.

45.8.3 Surgical

Intolerable stool leakage from an appendicostomy or stomal stenosis can both necessitate stomal revision.

45.8.4 Psychosocial

One of the biggest and least recognised complications of chronic constipation is the associated psychological insult. Chronic abdominal pain and constant faecal soiling can lead to disrupted peer relationships, undue family stress and social ostracism. Behavioural problems, which may be extreme, may be the cause in some patients, but more frequently are the result of years of living with constipation.

Further Reading

Constipation Guideline Committee of the North American Society for Pediatric Gastroenterology, Hepatology and Nutrition (2006) Evaluation and treatment of constipation in infants and children: Recommendations of the North American Society for Pediatric Gastroenterology, Hepatology and Nutrition. J Pediatr Gastroenterol Nutr 43(3):e1–13

Hutson JM, Catto-Smith T, Gibb S, Chase J, Shin YM, Stanton M, et al (2004) Chronic constipation: No longer stuck! Characterization of colonic dysmotility as a new disorder in children. J Pediatr Surg 39(6):795–799

Malone PS., Curry JI, Osborne A (1998) The antegrade continence enema procedure: Why, when and how? World J Urol 16(4):274–278

Southwell BR, King SK, Hutson JM (2005) Chronic constipation in children: Organic disorders are a major cause. J Paediatr Child Health 41:1–15

Puri P, Höllwarth ME (eds) (2006) Pediatric Surgery. Springer, Berlin, Heidelberg

Hirschsprung's Disease and Variants

46

Prem Puri

Contents

46.1 Introduction Including Definition and Incidence

Hirschsprung's disease (HD) is characterised by an absence of ganglion cells in the distal bowel and extending proximally for varying distances. The pathophysiology of Hirschsprung's disease is not fully understood. There is no clear explanation for the occurrence of spastic or tonically contracted aganglionic segment of bowel.

The aganglionosis is confined to rectosigmoid in 75% of patients, sigmoid, splenic flexure or transverse colon in 17% and total colon along with a short segment of terminal ileum in 8%. The incidence of HD is estimated to be 1 in 5,000 live births. The disease is more common in boys with a male-to-female ration of 4:1. The male preponderance is less evident in long-segment HD, where the male-to-female ratio is 1.5–2:1.

46.2 Etiology

In the human fetus, neural crest-derived neuroblasts first appear in the developing esophagus at 5 weeks, and then migrate down to the anal canal in a craniocaudal direction during the fifth to 12th weeks of gestation. The absence of ganglion cells in HD has been attributed to a failure of migration of neural crest cells. The earlier the arrest of migration, the longer the aganglionic segment.

Genetic factors have been implicated in the etiology of HD. HD is known to occur in families. The reported incidence of familial cases varied from 3.6% to 7.8% in different series. A familial incidence of 15–21% has been reported in total colonic aganglionosis and 50% in the rare total intestinal aganglionosis. Several genes and

P. Puri and M. Höllwarth (eds.), *Pediatric Surgery: Diagnosis and Management*,
DOI: 10.1007/978-3-540-69560-8_46, © Springer-Verlag Berlin Heidelberg 2009

signalling molecules have been identified which control morphogenesis and differentiation of the enteric nervous (ENS) system. These genes, when mutated or deleted, interfere with ENS development. One of these genes, RET with tyrosine kinase activity is involved in the development of enteric ganglia derived from vagal-neural crest cells. Mutations of RET gene account for 50% of familial and 15–20% of sporadic cases of HD.

The relationship with Down syndrome also tends to suggest a probable genetic component in the etiology of HD. Down syndrome is the most common chromosomal abnormality associated with aganglionosis and had been reported to occur in 4.5–16% of all cases of HD. Other chromosomal abnormalities that have been described in association with HD include: interstitial deletion of distal 13q, partial deletion of 2p and reciprocal translocation, and trisomy 18 mosiac. A number of unusual hereditary syndromes have been reported in patients with HD. These include: Waardenburg syndrome, Von Recklinghausen's syndrome, type D brachydactyly and Smith-Lemli-Optiz syndrome.

46.3 Pathology

The characteristic gross pathological feature in HD is dilation and hypertrophy of the proximal colon with abrupt or gradual transition to narrow distal bowel (Fig. 46.1). Although the degree of dilation and hypertrophy increases with age, the cone-shaped transitional zone from dilated to narrow bowel is usually evident in the newborn.

Histologically, HD is characterized by the absence of ganglionic cells in the myenteric and submucous plexuses and the presence of hypertrophied non-myelinated nerve trunks in the space normally occupied by the ganglionic cells. The aganglionic segment of bowel is followed proximally by a hypoganglionic segment of varying length. This hypoganglionic zone is characterized by a reduced number of ganglion cells and nerve fibers in myenteric and submucous plexuses.

46.4 Diagnosis

The diagnosis of HD is usually based on clinical history, radiological studies, anorectal manometry and in particular on histological examination of the rectal wall biopsy specimens.

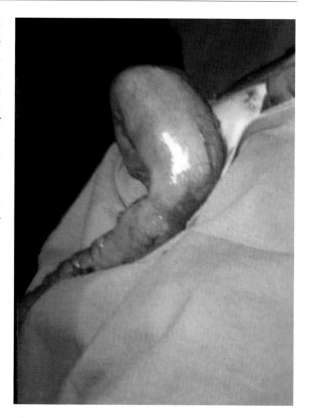

Fig. 46.1 Typical gross pathology in Hirschsprung's disease with transitional zone at rectosigmoid level

46.4.1 Clinical Features

Of all cases of HD, 80–90% produce clinical symptoms and are diagnosed during the neonatal period. Delayed passage of meconium is the cardinal symptom in neonates with HD. Over 90% of affected patients fail to pass meconium in the first 24 h of life. The usual presentation of HD in the neonatal period is with constipation, abdominal distension and vomiting during the first few days of life (Fig. 46.2). About one third of the babies with HD present with diarrhoea. Diarrhoea in HD is always a symptom of enterocolitis, which remains the commonest cause of death. Enterocolitis may resolve with adequate therapy or it may develop into a life-threatening condition, the toxic megacolon, characterised by the sudden onset of marked abdominal distension, bile stained vomiting, fever and signs of dehydration, sepsis and shock. Rectal examination or introduction of a rectal tube results in the explosive evacuation of gas and foul-smelling stools. In older children the main

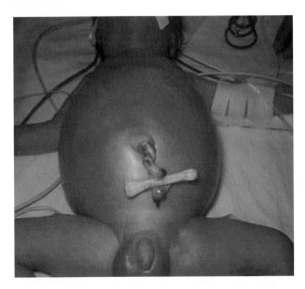

Fig. 46.2 A 2-day-old infant with abdominal distension and failure to pass meconium. Suction rectal biopsy confirmed Hirschsprung's disease

symptom is persistent constipation and chronic abdominal distension.

46.4.2 Radiological Diagnosis

Plain abdominal films in a neonate with HD will show dilated loops of bowel with fluid levels and airless pelvis. Occasionally, one may be able to see a small amount of air in the undistended rectum and dilated colon above it raising the suspicion of HD (Fig. 46.3). Plain abdominal radiographs obtained from patients with total colonic aganglionosis (TCA) may show characteristic signs of ileal obstruction with air fluid levels or simple gaseous distension of small intestinal loops.

In patients with enterocolitis complicating HD, plain abdominal radiography may show thickening of the bowel wall with mucosal irregularity or a grossly dilated colon loop, indicating toxic megacolon. Pneumoperitoneum may be found in those with perforation. Spontaneous perforation of the intestinal tract has been reported in 3% of patients with HD.

Barium enema performed by an experienced radiologist, using careful technique should achieve a high degree of reliability in diagnosing HD in the newborn. It is important that the infant should not have rectal washouts or even digital examinations prior to barium enema, as

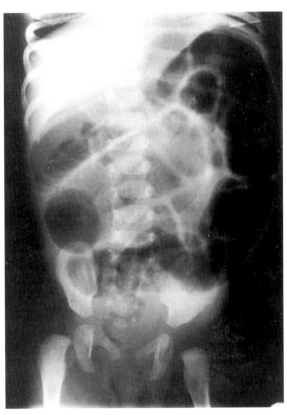

Fig. 46.3 Abdominal x-ray in a neonate showing marked dilatation of large and small bowel loops. Note gas in the undilated rectum. Rectal biopsy confirmed Hirschsprung's disease in this infant

such interference may distort the transitional zone appearance and give a false-negative diagnosis. A soft rubber catheter is inserted into the lower rectum and held in position with firm strapping across the buttocks. A balloon catheter should not be used due to the risk of perforation and the possibility of distorting a transitional zone by distension. The barium should be injected slowly in small amounts under fluoroscopic control with the baby in the lateral position. A typical case of HD will demonstrate flow of barium from the undilated rectum through a cone-shaped transitional zone into dilated colon (Fig. 46.4). Some cases may show an abrupt transition between the dilated proximal colon and the distal aganglionic segment, leaving the diagnosis in little doubt.

In some cases, the findings on the barium enema are uncertain and a delayed film at 24 h may confirm the diagnosis by demonstrating the retained barium and often accentuating the appearance of the transitional zone (Fig. 46.5).

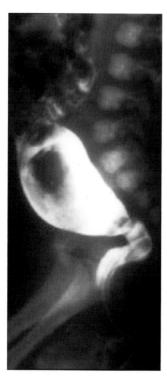

Fig. 46.4 Barium enema reveals Hirschsprung's disease with transitional zone at rectosigmoid

In total colonic aganglianosis (TCA), the contrast enema is not pathognomic and may not provide a definitive diagnosis. The colon in TCA is of normal calibre in 25–77% of cases.

46.4.3 Anorectal Manometry

In the normally innervated bowel, distension of the rectum produces relaxation of the internal sphincter rectosphincteric reflex. In normal persons, upon distending the rectal balloon with air, the rectum immediately responds with a transient rise in pressure lasting 15–20s; at the same time the internal sphincter rhythmic activity is depressed or abolished and its pressure falls by 15–20cm, the duration of relaxation coinciding with the rectal wave.

In patients with HD, the rectum often shows spontaneous waves of varying amplitude and frequency in the resting phase. The internal sphincter rhythmic activity is more pronounced. On rectal distension, with an increment of air, there is complete absence of internal sphincter relaxation (Fig. 46.6a, b). Failure to detect the rectosphincteric reflex in premature and term infants is believed to be due to technical difficulties and not to immaturity of ganglion cells. Light sedation particularly in infants and

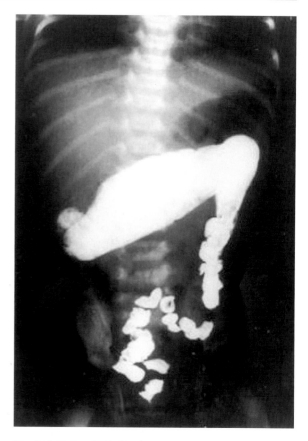

Fig. 46.5 Delayed 24h film showing barium retention with transition zone at splenic flexure in a 10-day-old infant

small children may overcome technical difficulties encountered in this age group.

46.4.4 Rectal Biopsy

The diagnosis of HD is confirmed on examination of rectal biopsy specimens. The introduction of histochemical staining technique for the detection of acetylcholinesterase (AChE) activity in suction rectal biopsy has resulted in a reliable and simple method for the diagnosis of HD. Full thickness rectal biopsy is rarely indicated for the diagnosis of HD except in total colonic aganglionosis. In normal persons, barely detectable acetylcholinesterase activity is observed within the lamina propria and muscularis mucosa, and submucosal ganglion cells stain strongly for acetylcholinesterase. In HD, there is a marked increase in acetylcholinesterase activity in lamina propria and muscularis which is evident as coarse, discrete cholinergic nerve fibers stained brown to black (Fig 46.7a, b).

In total, colonic aganglionosis (TCA), AChE activity in suction rectal biopsies presents an atypical pattern,

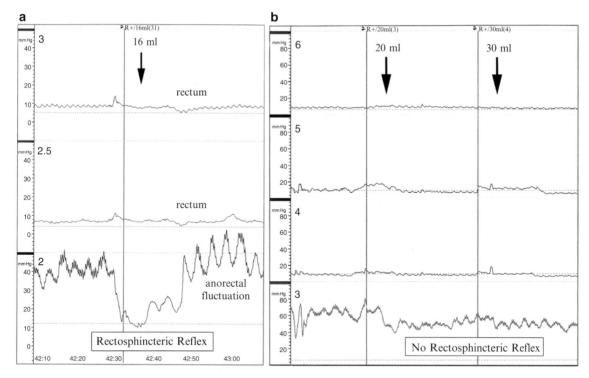

Fig. 46.6 Anorectal manometry (**a**) Normal rectosphincteric reflex on rectal balloon inflation. (**b**) Absence of rectosphincteric reflex and marked internal sphincter rhythmic activity in a patient with Hirschsprung's disease

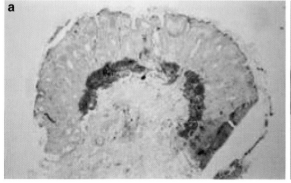
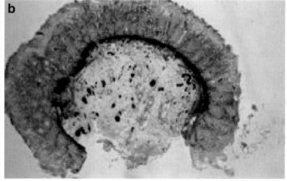

Fig. 46.7 Acetylcholinesterase (ache) staining of suction rectal biopsy. (**a**) Normal rectum showing minimal acetylcholinesterase staining of lamina propria and a ganglia in the submucosa.

(**b**) Hirschsprung's disease characterized by marked increase in acetylcholinesterase positive fibers in the lamina propria and hypertrophic nerve trunks in the submucosa

different from the classic one. Positive AChE fibers can be found in the lamina propria as well as the muscularis mucosae. However, cholinergic fibers present a lower density than in classical HD.

46.5 Differential Diagnosis

Several conditions must be considered where an infant is being evaluated for Hirschsprung's disease.

Table 46.1 gives the list of common differential diagnoses. Colonic atresia gives similar plain film findings to Hirschsprung's disease but is readily excluded with barium enema showing complete mechanical obstruction. Distal small bowel atresia shows gross distension of the bowel loop immediately proximal to the obstruction with the widest fluid level in it.

In meconium ileus the typical mottled thick meconium may be seen. Also clear, sharp fluid levels are not a feature in erect or lateral decubitus views. However,

Table 46.1 Differential diagnosis of Hirschsprung's disease

Neonatal bowel obstruction
Colonic atresia
Meconium ileus
Meconium plug syndrome
Small left colon syndrome
Malrotation
Low anorectal malformation
Intestinal motility disorders/pseudo-obstruction
Necrotizing enterocolitis
Medical causes: sepsis, electrolyte abnormalities, drugs, hypothyroidism, etc.

Chronic constipation
Functional megacolon
Intestinal motility disorders/pseudo-obstruction
Medical causes: electrolyte abnormalities, drugs, hypothyroidism, etc.

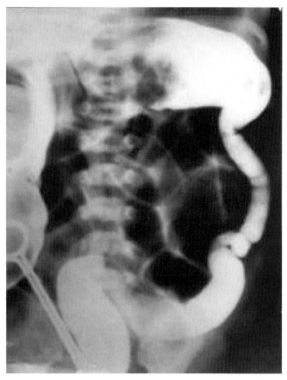

Fig. 46.8 The Small Left Colon Syndrome. The clinical and radiological features in this infant were indistinguishable from those in Hirshsprung's disease. Barium enema showed narrow descending colon with transition zone at splenic flexure. Suction rectal biopsy was ganglionic in this infant

Hirschsprung's disease can sometimes simulate meconium ileus in plain films and may give equivocal findings on Gastrografin or barium enema.

Meconium plugs obstructing the colon can present as Hirschsprung's disease with strongly suggestive history and plain films. Small left colon syndrome with marked distension proximal to narrowed descending colon also simulates Hirschsprung's disease at the left colonic flexure (Fig. 46.8). These two conditions usually resolve with Gastrografin enema but a minority of these cases will actually have Hirschsprung's which should be excluded clinically.

46.6 Management

Once the diagnosis of HD has been confirmed by rectal biopsy examination, the infant should be prepared for surgery. If the newborn has enterocolitis complicating HD, correction of dehydration and electrolyte imbalance by infusion of appropriate fluids will be required. It is essential to decompress the bowel as early as possible in these babies. Deflation of the intestine may be carried out by rectal irrigations but some babies may require colostomy.

In recent years, the vast majority of cases of HD are diagnosed in the neonatal period. Many centres are now performing one-stage pull-through operations in the newborn with minimal morbidity rates and encouraging results. The advantages of operating on the newborn are that the colonic dilation can be quickly controlled by washouts and at operation the calibre of the pull-through bowel is near normal, allowing for an accurate anastomosis that minimizes leakage and cuff infection. A number of different operations have been described for the treatment of HD. The four most commonly used operations are the rectosigmoidectomy developed by Swenson and Bill, the retrorectal approach developed by Duhamel, the endorectal procedure developed by Soave and deep anterior colorectal anastomosis developed by Rehbein. The basic principle in all these procedures is to bring the ganglionic bowel down to the anus. The long-term results of any of these operations are satisfactory if they are performed correctly. Recently, a number of investigators have described and advocated a variety of one-stage pull-through procedures in the newborn using minimally invasive laparoscopic techniques. More recently, a transanal endorectal pull-through operation performed without opening the abdomen has been used with excellent results in rectosigmoid HD.

46.7 Complications

Early postoperative complications which can occur after any type of pull-through operation include wound infections, anastomotic leak, anastomotic stricture, retraction or necrosis of the neorectum, intestinal adhesions, and ileus. Late complications include constipation, enterocolitis, incontinence, anastomotic problems, adhesive bowel obstruction and urogenital complications.

46.7.1 Anastomotic Leak

The most dangerous early post-operative complication following the definitive abdominoperineal pull-through procedure is leakage at the anastomotic suture line. Factors which are responsible for anastomotic leak include ischemia of the distal end of the colonic pull-through segment, tension on the anastomosis, incomplete anastomotic suture lines and inadvertent rectal manipulation. If a leak is recognized in a patient without a colostomy, it is imperative to perform a diverting colostomy promptly, to administer intravenous antibiotics and to irrigate the rectum with antibiotic solution a few times daily. Delay in establishing fecal diversion is likely to result in an extensive pelvic abscess which may require laparotomy and transabdominal drainage.

46.7.2 Retraction of Pullthrough

Retraction of a portion, or all of the colonic segment from the anastomosis can occur and is usually seen within 3 weeks of the operation. Evaluation under general anaesthesia is generally necessary. In occasional patients, resuturing the anastomosis may be feasible transanally. For those with separation of less than 50% of the anastomosis but with adequate vascularity of the colon, a diverting colostomy for approximately 3 months is necessary. For patients with wide separation at the anastomosis, early transabdominal reconstruction of the pull-through is recommended.

46.7.3 Perianal Excoriation

Perianal excoriation occurs in nearly half of the patients undergoing pull-through procedure, but generally resolves within 3 months with local therapy and resolution of diarrhoea. It is helpful to begin placing a barrier cream on the perianal skin promptly after the operation and to continue after each movement for the first few weeks. Resolution of diarrhoea will often hasten the clearance of perianal skin irration.

46.7.4 Enterocolitis

Hirschsprung's associated enterocolitis (HAEC) is a significant complication of HD both in the pre-and post-operative periods. HAEC can occur at any time from the neonatal period onwards to adulthood and can be independent of the medical management and surgical procedure performed. The incidence of enterocolitis ranges from 20% to 58%. Fortunately the mortality rate has declined over the last 30 years from 30% to 1%. This decrease in mortality is related to earlier diagnosis of HD and enterocolitis, rectal decompression, appropriate vigorous resuscitation and antibiotic therapy. It has been reported that routine post-operative rectal washouts decrease both the incidence and the severity of the episodes of enterocolitis following definitive surgery. In episodes of recurrent enterocolitis, which can develop in up to 56% of patients, anal dilatations have been recommended. However, prior to commencing a treatment regime, a contrast enema should be performed to rule out a mechanical obstruction. Patients with a normal rectal biopsy may require a sphincterotomy.

46.7.5 Constipation

Constipation is common after definitive repair of Hirschsprung's disease and can be due to residual aganglionosis and high anal tone. Repeated and forceful anal dilations or Botulin Toxin injection into the sphincter under general anaesthesia may resolve the problem. In some patients internal sphincter myectomy may be needed. In patients with scarring, stricture or intestinal neuronal dysplasia proximal to aganglionic segment, treatment consists of underlying cause.

46.7.6 Soiling

Soiling is fairly common after all types of pull-through operations, its precise incidence primarily dependent on how assiduously the investigator looks for it. The reported incidence of soiling ranges from 10% to 30%. The attainment of normal postoperative defaecation is clearly dependent on intensity of bowel training, social background and respective intelligence of the patients. Mental handicap, including Down's syndrome, is invariably associated with long-term incontinence. Those patients with preoperative enterocolitis would also seem to have a marginally higher long-term risk of incontinence. In some patients in whom soiling is intractable and a social problem, a Malone procedure may be needed to stay clean.

46.8 Variant Hirschsprung's Disease

Variant Hirschsprung's Disease includes conditions that clinically resemble HD despite the presence of ganglion cells on suction rectal biopsy results. These conditions can be diagnosed by providing an adequate biopsy and employing a variety of histological techniques. The motility disorders which comprise Variant Hirschsprung's Disease are intestinal neuronal dysplasia, hypoganglionosis, internal sphincter achalasia and smooth muscle disorders.

46.8.1 Intestinal Neuronal Dysplasia

Intestinal neuronal dysplasia (IND) is a clinical condition that resembles Hirschsprung's disease. IND has been described proximal to the aganglionic segment and less frequently as an isolated condition. IND is classified into two clinically and histologically distinct subtypes. Type A occurs in less than 5% of cases, is characterized by

congenital aplasia or hypoplasia of the sympathetic innervation, and presents acutely in the neonatal period with episodes of intestinal obstruction, diarrhoea and bloody stools. The clinical picture of Type B resembles HD and is characterized by malformation of the parasympathetic submucous and myenteric plexuses. IND occurring in association with HD is of Type B. The characteristic histologic features of IND Type B include hyperganglionosis of the submucous and myenteric plexuses, giant ganglia, ectopic ganglion cells and increased acetylcholinesterase (AChE) activity in the lamina propria and around submucosal blood vessels (Fig. 46.9).

Current treatment of IND Type B is in the first instance conservative, consisting of laxatives and enemas. In the majority of patients the clinical problem resolves or is manageable in this way. If bowel symptoms persist after at least 6 months of treatment, internal sphincter myectomy should be considered.

46.8.2 Hypoganglionosis

Hypoganglionosis as an isolated condition is rare. Failure to pass meconium may be the first symptom in the neonatal period, whereas infants and older children present with chronic constipation. The diagnosis of hypoganglionosis by means of suction rectal biopsy is difficult. Suction rectal biopsy in these patients demonstrates absence of submucosal ganglion cells with no or extremely low acetyl-cholinesterase activity in lamina propria or mucosal mucosae. Full thickness biopsy is usually required for the reliable diagnosis of hypoganglionosis. Characteristic histological features of hypoganglionosis include sparse and small myenteric ganglia, absence of or low AChE activity in the lamina propria and hypertrophy of muscularis mucosa and circular muscle.

The treatment of hypoganglionosis is similar to HD involving resection of the affected segment and pull-through operation.

46.8.3 Internal Sphincter Achalasia

Internal anal sphincter achalasia (IASA) is a clinical condition with presentation similar to Hirschsprung's disease but with the presence of ganglion cells on suction rectal biopsy. The diagnosis of IASA is made on anorectal

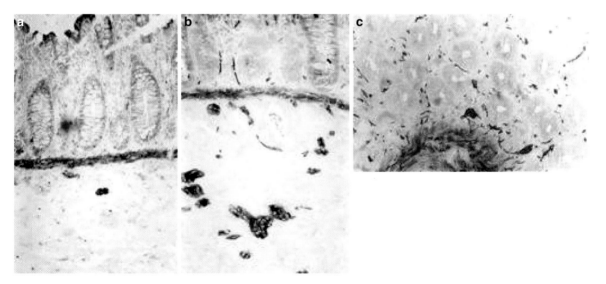

Fig. 46.9 Ache staining of suction rectal biopsy. (**a**) Normal biopsy showing a submucosal ganglion. (**b**) Biopsy from a patient with intestinal neuronal dysplasia shows hyperganglionosis and giant ganglia in the submucosa. (**c**) Ectopic ganglia in the lamina propria in a patient with IND

manometry, which shows the absence of rectosphincteric reflex on rectal balloon inflation. Previously, IASA has been referred to as ultrashort segment Hirschsprung's disease (HD). The ultrashort segment Hirschsprung's disease, which is a rare condition, is characterized by an aganglionic (AChE) activity in the lamina propria and increased AChE activity in the muscularis mucosae. Many patients who are considered to have ultrashort HD on abnormal anorectal mamometric findings show presence of ganglion cells and normal acetylcholinesterase (AChE) activity in suction rectal biopsies. Many investigators have therefore suggested that the term IASA is more suitable because it reflects more accurately failure of relaxation of the internal sphincter, which is the causative factor in this condition. The exact pathogenesis and pathophysiology of IASA is not understood fully. Altered intramuscular innervation has been reported in IASA and this is believed to be responsible for the motility dysfunction seen in these patients.

Posterior internal sphincter myectomy has been recommended as the treatment of choice for patients with internal sphincter achalasia. Recently, intraanal injection of botulinum toxin has been used to treat patients with IASA. This treatment modality has been found to be safe and effective but only as short-term treatment in these children.

46.8.4 Smooth Muscle Cell Disorders

These patients who show no apparent innervation abnormalities in the pathologic specimens demonstrate abnormalities of smooth muscle cells on electron-microscopy. The outcome of smooth muscle disorders is usually poor. There are two main types of smooth muscle cell abnormalities, perinuclear vacuolation and "central core" degeneration. Patients with Megacystis microcolon intestinal hypoperistalsis syndrome (MMIHS) usually have central core degeneration of smooth muscle cells. MMIHS is a rare and the most severe form of functional intestinal obstruction in the newborn. The major features of this congenital and usually lethal anomaly are abdominal distension, bile-stained vomiting and absent or decreased bowel peristalsis. Abdominal distension is a consequence of the distended, unobstructed urinary bladder with or without upper urinary tract dilation. Most patients with MMIHS are not able to void spontaneously. The outcome of smooth muscle disorders is generally fatal. The need for surgical intervention should be weighed carefully and individualized because most explorations have not been helpful and are probably not necessary.

Further Reading

Dasgupta R, Langer JC (2005) Transanal pullthrough for hirschsprung's disease. Semi Pediatr Surg 14:64–71

Puri P (2003) Newborn Surgery. Arnold, London

Puri P (2006) Hirschsprung's Disease. In P Puri, ME Höllwarth (eds) Pediatric Surgery, Springer-Verlag Berlin Heidelberg, New York, pp 275–288

Puri P, Shinkai T (2004) Pathogenesis of hirschsprung's disease and its variants: Recent progress. Semi Pediatr Surg 13:18–24

Anorectal Anomalies

47

Alberto Peña and Marc Levitt

Contents

The term "anorectal anomalies," encompasses a series of congenital defects that represent a wide spectrum. In the past, these malformations had been classified into two main categories, "high" and "low." Subsequently, some authors adopted a classification that included "high," "intermediate," and "low" categories. Those classifications were actually oversimplifications of a spectrum of defects. A more practical classification of these defects, with therapeutic and prognostic implications is presented here.

47.1 Classification

MALES (Figs. 47.1–47.5)

1. Rectobladder neck fistula
2. Rectourethral prostatic fistula
3. Rectourethral bulbar fistula
4. Imperforate anus with no fistula
5. Perineal fistula
6. Complex defects

FEMALES (Figs. 47.6–47.9)

1. Cloaca with a common channel longer than 3 cm
2. Cloaca with a common channel shorter than 3 cm
3. Rectovestibular fistula
4. Imperforate anus with no fistula
5. Perineal fistula
6. Complex malformations

Each one of the groups mentioned in this classification requires a specific type of treatment and has a well defined functional prognosis. The above classification is only an attempt to divide this wide spectrum of defects.

P. Puri and M. Höllwarth (eds.), *Pediatric Surgery: Diagnosis and Management,*
DOI: 10.1007/978-3-540-69560-8_47, © Springer-Verlag Berlin Heidelberg 2009

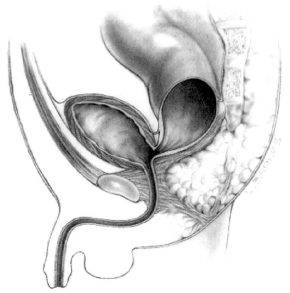

Fig. 47.1 Rectobladderneck fistula

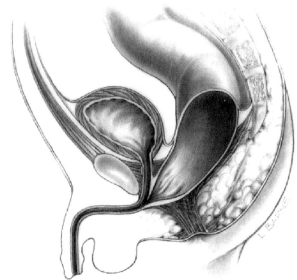

Fig. 47.3 Rectobulbar fistula

It is not unusual to see babies born with malformations that could be considered in between the categories mentioned above.

On the good side of the spectrum of anorectal anomalies, we find malformations with a very good functional post-operative prognosis, meaning that the majority of patients have normal bowel, urinary control, and sexual function. Unfortunately, on the bad side of the spectrum, we see malformations that we may be able to repair anatomically, but the patient will not have bowel control, sometimes he or she will not have urinary control, and sometimes they will also suffer from a significant degree of sexual dysfunction.

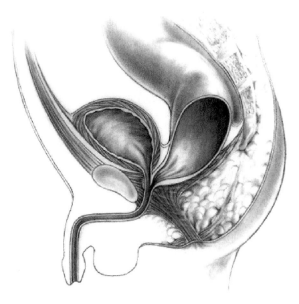

Fig. 47.2 Rectoprostatic fistula

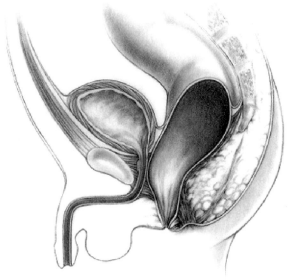

Fig. 47.4 Low malformation; rectoperineal fistula

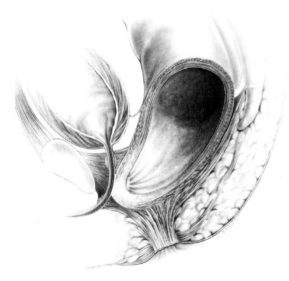

Fig. 47.5   Imperforate anus with no fistula

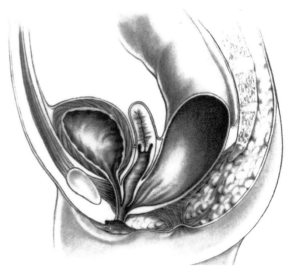

Fig. 47.7   Cloaca with common channel shorter than 3 cm

It is extremely important, therefore, to be sure that the patients born with what we call "benign defects," receive a technically correct operation to take advantage of their potential for bowel and urinary control.

47.2 Neonatal Approach

When we receive a call to see a newborn baby with an anorectal malformation, there are two important questions that must be answered:

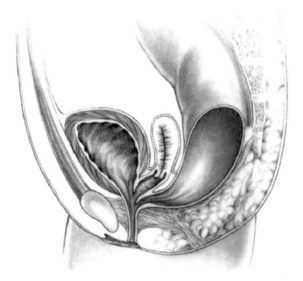

Fig. 47.6   Cloaca with common channel longer than 3 cm

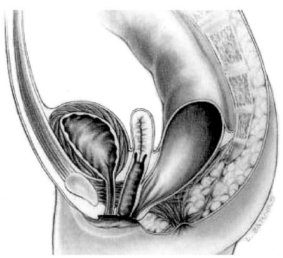

Fig. 47.8   Rectovestibular fistula

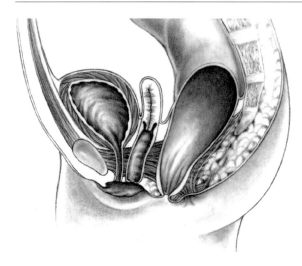

Fig. 47.9 Perineal fistula

(a) Does the baby have a serious associated defect that endangers his (her) life?
(b) Does the baby need a colostomy or should we perform a primary repair of the malformation?

These questions should be answered in the same order presented here. It is not unusual to see cases in which the surgeon deals first with the decision related to colostomy vs. primary repair and the baby had serious problems due to the fact that he suffered from an undi-

agnosed severe cardiac or urologic problem that put the baby's life at risk.

Newborns are not usually born with abdominal distention. Therefore, the first 24 h of life are relatively safe for observation and represent a window of opportunity to answer the first question. It is after 24 h that the second question should be addressed. (Figs. 47.10 and 47.11)

When trying to answer the first question, the surgeon must keep in mind the frequency of associated defects in cases of anorectal malformations:

1. Urologic defects (approximately 50%)
2. Spinal and sacral defects (approximately 30%)
3. Tethered cord and other cord abnormalities (approximately 25%)
4. Cardiovascular malformations (approximately 30%, but only 10% have important hemodynamic repercussions, requiring treatment)
5. Esophageal atresia (approximately 5–10%)

There are other defects, associated with anorectal malformations, but their diagnosis does not represent an emergency.

Based on the frequency of association of other defects mentioned above, newborns with anorectal malformations must have the following diagnostic tests during the first 24 h of life:

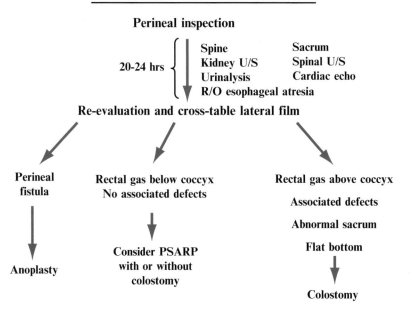

Fig. 47.10 Newborn male anorectal malformation algorithm

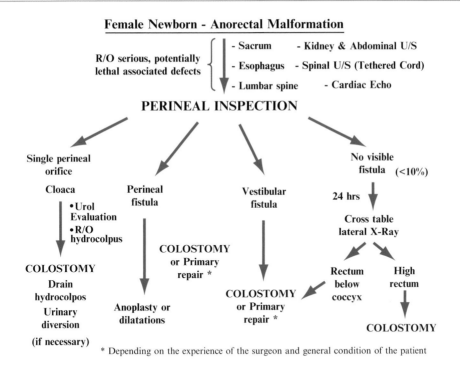

Fig. 47.11 Newborn female anorectal malformation algorithm

1. Ultrasound of the abdomen to rule out the presence of hydronephrosis and megaureter
2. Ultrasound of the pelvis in females, to rule out the presence of hydrocolpos
3. Ultrasound of the spine to rule out the presence of tethered cord
4. X-ray film of the lumbar spine and sacrum in AP and lateral positions to evaluate for hemivertebrae, assess the development of the sacrum, and look for a hemisacrum
5. Clinical evaluation for symptoms of cardiovascular disease and an echocardiogram if indicated
6. Clinical evaluation to rule out the possibility of esophageal atresia or other intestinal atresias, mainly duodenal

The above studies are mandatory, and must be performed in the first 24 h of life. More detailed and sophisticated diagnostic tests will be done, depending on the results of the basic screening tests mentioned above.

Babies with anorectal malformation should never be taken to the operating room without having ruled out the most important associated defects.

47.2.1 Second Question

47.2.1.1 Male

In order to answer the second question (colostomy or primary repair?) the surgeon should look at the perineum of the baby, looking for specific anatomic changes that are very important for the diagnosis.

In male newborns, the presence of a prominent midline groove, between both buttocks, in addition to an obvious anal dimple, is usually associated with a "benign type of defect" (perineal fistula, imperforate anus with no fistula, a rectourethral bulbar fistula). In such a case, the surgeon must look very meticulously for the presence of a small orifice in the perineum. That is called a perineal fistula. Usually, the meconium will come out through this orifice after 12 or 24 h of life, because it is a very narrow track and it takes a significant intrarectal pressure to force the meconium out.

The orifice of the perineal fistula is always located anterior to the center of the anal dimple, which represents the external sphincter mechanism (Fig. 47.12).

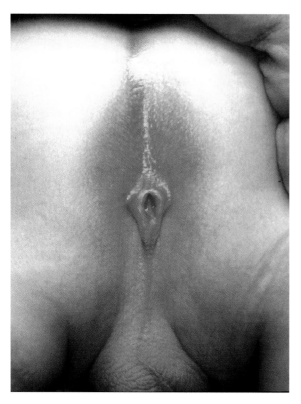

Fig. 47.12 Perineal fistula opening anterior to the sphincter mechanism

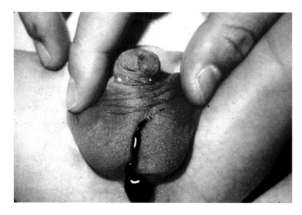

Fig. 47.13 Perineal fistula with subepithelial tract along scrotal raphe

Sometimes the orifice is located in the midline raphe of the scrotum or at the base of the penis following a subepithelial tract that can be filled with meconium or mucus (Fig. 47.13). If the baby has a "good looking perineum" (midline groove and anal dimple), but there is no perineal orifice, there is a possibility that the baby has a rectourethral bulbar fistula. In such a situation,

most likely the baby will pass meconium into the urine during the first 24 h of life. A urinalysis or a simple piece of gauze on the tip of the penis will reveal the presence of meconium in the urine.

If 24 h go by and there is no evidence of a perineal fistula and no meconium in the urine, there is a strong possibility that the baby has an imperforate anus with no fistula. If the baby suffers from Down's syndrome, then the possibilities are up to 90% that this is the correct diagnosis. If none of these findings are detected after 24 h, then the baby should have a crosstable lateral film, looking for the presence of gas in the rectum, to measure the distance from the rectum to the skin. It is very important to know that less than 5% of newborns need this x-ray. In other words, just by looking at the perineum in male babies, in the vast majority of cases, one can have a very good idea of the type of malformations that the baby was born with.

The "bad side" of the spectrum, includes malformations with poor functional prognosis. Those patients have different degrees of a "flat bottom," meaning that the midline intergluteal groove is less prominent and sometimes disappears, and there is no real anal dimple. A flat-bottom baby connotes a very high defect, either a rectourethral prostatic or a rectobladder neck fistula. In addition, the sacrum is frequently hypodeveloped. A "good or intact sacrum" is more frequently present in patients with benign malformations. An absent sacrum or a very abnormal short sacrum or hemisacrum is associated with higher defects. The presence of a bifid scrotum is usually related to higher malformations (Fig. 47.14)

47.2.1.2 Female

In female babies, the presence of a single perineal orifice makes the diagnosis of cloaca (Fig. 47.15). The length of the common channel can be evaluated endoscopically. If the baby has a single perineal orifice, a prominent midline groove, and an obvious anal dimple, most likely she has a cloaca with a common channel shorter than 3 cm, particularly if the sacrum is normal. On the other hand, if the baby has a single perineal orifice but also a flat bottom and an abnormal sacrum, most likely she has a cloaca with a common channel longer than 3 cm.

If the baby has an absent anus but one can see rather normal-looking female genitalia, including the presence of a urethra and vagina, most likely the baby has a

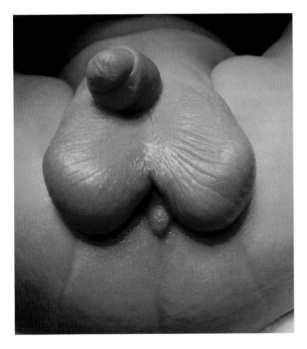

Fig. 47.14 Bifid scrotum

rectovestibular fistula which is the most common defect seen in females. In such a case, just in the vestibule of the genitalia outside the hymen, there is an orifice that we call recto- vestibular fistula (Fig. 47.16). Meconium may not pass in the first few hours of life, but most likely will start passing very soon after that. The diagnosis of a vestibular fistula requires a meticulous examination of the perineum of a female baby. A perineal fistula is a very obvious malformation and the diagnosis is made just by inspection of the perineum. These babies have an orifice located somewhere between the center of the anal dimple (sphincter) and the female genitalia. Usually, the orifice is abnormally narrow and is not surrounded by sphincter (Fig. 47.17).

If the female baby does not have a single perineal orifice, does not have a vestibular fistula, has no evidence of a perineal orifice, and does not pass meconium after 24 h, a crosstable lateral film is indicated. Again, this is necessary in female patients in less than 5% of the total number of cases. If the baby suffers from Down's syndrome, most likely the baby has imperforate anus with no fistula.

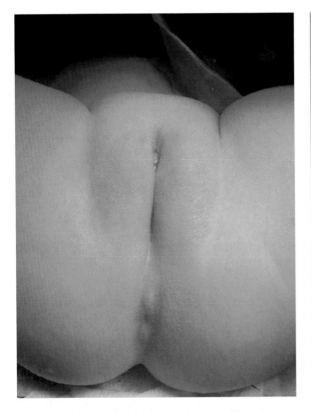

Fig. 47.15 Single perineal orifice, a cloacal malformation

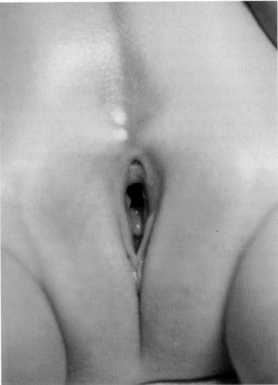

Fig. 47.16 Rectovestibular fistula

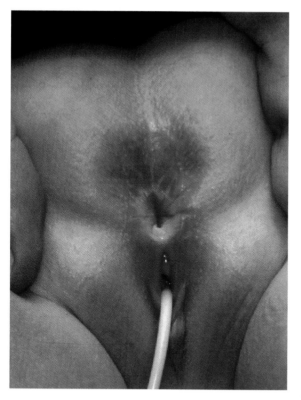

Fig. 47.17 Rectoperineal fistula

The analysis of the diagnostic tests already described, as well as the result of the examination of the baby's perineum, allow us to make an accurate diagnosis of the type of malformation and give us enough information to make a wise decision concerning the question of colostomy or primary repair.

The question of colostomy or primary repair does not have a dogmatic answer. We believe that the answer will depend on the specific circumstances of the surgeon, as well as the environment in which the baby is being treated. In other words, a surgeon with a significant experience in the management of anorectal malformation can repair primarily, without a colostomy, some of the patients born with anorectal malformations. Yet, the safest management for a baby is still the opening of a colostomy.

In general, newborns with rectobladder neck fistula, rectal prostatic fistula, and rectourethral bulbar fistula receive a colostomy and a secondary repair at several months of life. Females born with a cloaca receive a diverting colostomy. The question of colostomy in babies with vestibular fistula is still a matter of controversy. Experienced surgeons in the neonatal

management of this defect, frequently repair this malformation without a colostomy, without significant complications. Yet, we have seen many babies who underwent a previous failed attempted repair, without a colostomy, followed by catastrophic complications that changed the functional prognosis. If the surgeon does not have enough experience or the infrastructure of the institution where the baby is managed is not adequate, it is safer to open a colostomy.

Most surgeons in the world agree in repairing perineal fistulas without a protective colostomy.

Cases of imperforate anus with no fistula could be treated primarily, without a colostomy, provided the surgeon has experience with similar cases and evidence of the presence of rectal gas located below the coccyx and near the perineal skin.

47.3 Colostomy

Colostomy is an operation with a significant morbidity and therefore, it should be done with a delicate, efficient, and meticulous technique. We specifically recommend a descending colostomy

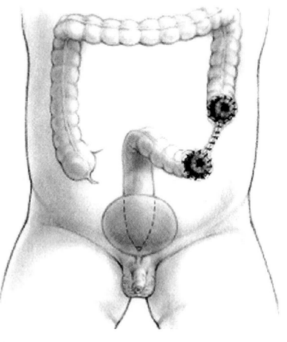

Fig. 47.18 Ideal colostomy for patients with an anorectal malformation

with separated stomas (Fig. 47.18) Loop colostomies, are not indicated in these patients because many of them will allow the passing of stool between the proximal and the distal limb. We must keep in mind that over 70% of patients with anorectal malformations have a connection (fistula) between the bowel and the urinary tract and therefore passing stool distally represents a direct fecal contamination of the urinary tract. We specifically recommend separating the stomas enough for the nurses and the parents to be able to accommodate a stoma bag over the proximal stoma without including the mucous fistula (distal stoma). The colostomy that we recommend is created in the first mobile portion of the descending colon at the junction of the descending colon with the sigmoid. We also recommend that the mucous fistula be made, very small, to avoid prolapse because it belongs to a mobile portion of the colon. It is only needed for irrigations and diagnostic tests. We recommend, when opening the colostomy, to make an oblique 6–8 cm incision running from the left flank to the midline in the lower abdomen. At the time of the colostomy opening, it is advisable to irrigate the distal limb of the colostomy to evacuate all the meconium and to have the distal bowel completely collapse.

47.4 Primary Repair (No Colostomy)

Most of the patients subjected to a primary repair are patients who have a perineal fistula. Fortunately, patients born with perineal fistula will enjoy bowel control with and without an operation. Usually, though, the perineal orifice is too narrow to have satisfactory evacuation of the stool. We prefer to perform a formal anoplasty consisting of making a small posterior sagittal incision the size of the extension of the sphincter mechanism as electrically demonstrated; the rectum is dissected and mobilized enough to be placed precisely within the limits of the sphincters. In females this ensures an adequate perineal body.

In male patients, the operation must be performed with a Foley catheter in place. Special care should be taken to avoid damage to the urethra during the separation of the rectum from its posterior aspect. Urethral injury is the most common and feared intraoperative complication in male babies subjected to attempted repairs of a perineal fistula. In female patients with perineal fistulas, it is very unusual to injure the vagina because in those cases there is a natural separation between the rectum and vagina.

Attempting a primary repair without a colostomy in malformations other than perineal fistula requires special expertise. One must be very careful in approaching newborn babies primarily without a colostomy. That approach is only justified if the surgeon has evidence that the rectum is located below the coccyx and near the skin. Surgical "explorations" of these babies usually end up with severe damage to the urinary tract or denervation of the urinary tract with serious secondary consequences.

47.5 High Pressure Distal Colostogram

By far, the most valuable diagnostic test in anorectal malformations is the high pressure distal colostogram. This study consists of the injection of hydrosoluble contrast material through the mucous fistula (distal stoma) under significant hydrostatic pressure, enough to overcome the tone of the striated muscle that surrounds the most distal part of the rectum, which will allow the distention of the distal rectum, as well as the passing of contrast material through the fistula into the genitourinary tract, showing the specific type of malformation that the patient was born with.

This study is performed by taking the baby to the fluoroscopy suite. It is usually performed 3–4 weeks after the colostomy has been done provided the baby recovered very well from that operation. A #8 Foley catheter is introduced into the mucous fistula. The catheter is introduced only 2 or 3 cm, and the balloon is inflated with 1 or 2 ml of water. Then, the radiologist or the surgeon must exert traction on the catheter. That way, the balloon will act as a plug in the mucous fistula and will allow injection of contrast material with significant pressure without leakage of the contrast material. The first films are taken while injecting contrast material under fluoroscopic control in the AP position. The first piece of information that we need from this study in the AP position is how much bowel is available from the mucous fistula down to the connection with the genitourinary tract (Fig. 47.19) Once we answer that question, the baby is then turned to the

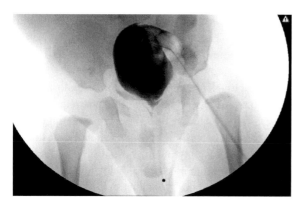

Fig. 47.19 AP view of colostogram showing length of the bowel available for the pull through

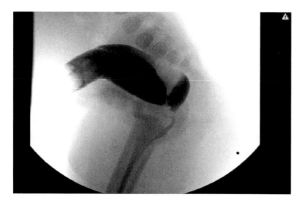

Fig. 47.20 Lateral view

lateral position. In the screen, we must see the entire sacrum, the tip of the coccyx, and an anal radiopaque marker located on the anal dimple. The injection must continue under hydrostatic pressure exerted with a syringe. The contrast material travels down and characteristically stops at the level of the pubococcygeal line creating a horizontal line (Fig. 47.20) When this happens, we know that that represents the effect of the muscle tone of the levator muscle. That should never be considered the end of the study. Many mistakes are made by assuming that the rectum is located very high and the misdiagnosis of "high anorectal malformation" is made. When the contrast material stops at the level of the PC line, all that means is that we have to inject with more pressure to overcome the muscle tone and very soon we see the contrast material going lower into the pelvis and ending in a characteristic peak, indicating that one is reaching the fistula site. The injection must continue, the contrast material passes through the fistula and usually goes up into the bladder. We inter-

pret this as manifestation of the muscle tone of the so called urinary external sphincter. The injection must continue until the bladder is full and even further until the baby starts voiding. During the voiding process, films must be taken that will show us an image of the bladder, posterior urethra, rectum, sacrum, coccyx, and anal dimple demonstrated by that marking (Fig. 47.21) That image is the one that we need in order to plan a satisfactory operation. The key question is the location of the distal rectum. It is with this study that we can classify the malformations in male patients into bladder neck (Fig. 47.22) rectoprostatic fistula (Fig. 47.23), and rectourethral bulbar fistula (Fig. 47.24).

A voiding cystourethrogram is not a good study to make a diagnosis of the fistula site.

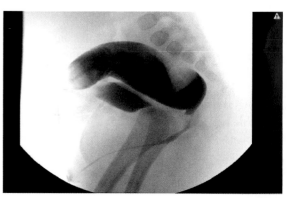

Fig. 47.21 Lateral view showing the rectourethral fistula

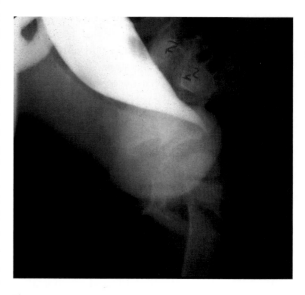

Fig. 47.22 Rectobladderneck fistula

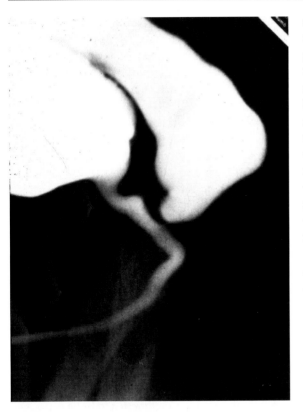

Fig. 47.23 Rectoprostatic fistula

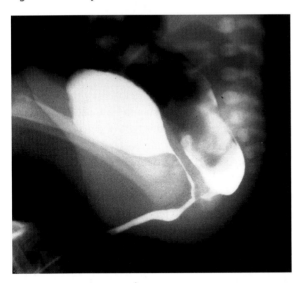

Fig. 47.24 Rectobulbar fistula

In a baby with perineal fistula we do not perform this kind of colostogram since we already have the diagnosis clinically.

In females, the distal colostogram is performed in order to try to make the diagnosis of the anatomic characteristics of the cloaca malformation. The injection is done in the way it was described for male patients, and the contrast material usually goes down to fill up one vagina or two hemivaginas (between 30% and 40% of the female babies with cloacas have two hemivaginas). It is very uncommon that the contrast material goes, in a female baby, into the urethra and the bladder. For that, it is necessary to pass a catheter through the single perineal orifice, which sometimes may go into the urethra and the bladder. Sometimes it will not and we will not be able to see the bladder during this type of study. The distal colostogram in patients with cloaca does not allow us to have an accurate diagnosis of the length of the common channel, which is something that we can only diagnosis with an endoscopy. 3-D fluoroscopy is improving the radiologic evaluation of cloacas.

We do not recommend doing a distal colostogram in a baby with a rectovestibular fistula because, it is not necessary as the diagnosis is made clinically, and second, one cannot distend the distal rectum because it is not possible to generate enough hydrostatic pressure, due to the fact that the contrast material leaks immediately through the vestibular fistula.

47.6 Definitive Repair

Most pediatric surgeons can be trained to repair the great majority of anorectal malformations. However, we believe that complex defects, cloacas with a common channel longer than 3 cm, covered exstrophies and cloacal exstrophies should be treated at centers with a special dedication to the repair of these malformations by surgeons with special training, not only in general pediatric surgery, but also in pediatric urology.

47.6.1 Males

Male patients born with rectobladder neck fistula are the only ones that require an abdominal approach in addition to the posterior sagittal approach, to be repaired. Therefore, those patients are ideal candidates for a laparoscopic assisted repair. The rectum opens in the bladder neck in a T-fashion and cannot be reached posterior sagittally. In fact, serious catastrophes occur when the surgeons enter posterior sagittally looking for a rectum that can never be reached this way. This usually happens in cases where the surgeon failed to perform a high pressure distal colostogram. The repair of an anorectal malformation should not be considered a surgical "exploration", but rather a well planned elective procedure, with a clear understanding of the patient's precise anatomy. The surgeon should know exactly what he or she is going to find based on a good anatomic diagnosis given by the high pressure distal colostogram. The abdomen should be entered either by laparotomy or by laparoscopy. The rectum is dissected near the peritoneal reflection with the dissection performed as close as possible to the rectal wall, until the rectum suddenly decreases in diameter, it becomes very narrow, and at that point, the rectum can be divided and the fistula ligated or sutured. The rectum then must be fully separated, dividing all the nonvascular attachments to the retroperitoneum and the blood supply of the rectosigmoid, namely the inferior mesenteric vessels and their branches should be visualized accurately. We have learned, in these very high defects, that one can divide the peripheral branches of the inferior mesentery vessels near the rectal wall. Provided the rectal wall is maintained intact, the intramural blood supply will be enough to maintain good perfusion of the most distal part of the rectum. One must be sure that some of the main, proximal branches of the inferior mesenteric vessels reach the rectum and that the rectal wall is intact if one wants to be able to pull the rectum down and still preserve a good blood supply. The center of the sphincter must be determined electrically, and the rectum can be pulled down under direct vision, using a small posterior sagittal incision. This can be done laparoscopically or by laparotomy depending on the training of the surgeon.

Rectourethral prostatic fistulas and rectourethral bulbar fistulas can be repaired in an expedited and efficient way. A posterior sagittal incision is performed, the rectum is meticulously separated from the urinary tract, the urethra fistula is repaired. Then the rectum must be subjected to a circumferential dissection, being sure to keep the bowel wall intact by burning and dividing all of the extrinsic blood supply while applying uniform traction to bring the rectum down to be placed within the limits of the sphincter.

It is a matter of debate as to whether or not some of the very high rectal prostatic fistulas (almost bladder neck fistulas) can or should be treated laparoscopically. We believe that this will depend very much on the experience of the operator. A surgeon who has a large experience in laparoscopy and not much experience in dealing with these very high prostatic fistulas, perhaps will do a better job laparoscopically.

We definitely believe that laparoscopy is not indicated in patients with rectourethral bulbar fistula. This malformation has an excellent functional prognosis and is easily treated with a posterior sagittal operation that takes approximately 2 h. The dissection performed in the rectum is minimal because the rectum is already located very low. A laparoscopic approach in this type of defect involves an unnecessary dissection of the entire rectum all the way from the peritoneum to the perineal skin and risks leaving behind the distal rectum as a diverticulum.

Anorectal malformation with no fistula should also be treated posterior sagittally. The fact that there is no fistula does not mean that the operation is necessarily easier, since it still requires the separation of the rectum from the posterior urethra that must be performed very meticulously.

47.6.2 Females

We believe that females with cloacas with a common channel longer than 3 cm should be treated in specialized centers. Fortunately, this type of defect occurs only in approximately 40% of the babies born with cloacas. The intraoperative, decision-making process, required for the repair of these malformations requires a large experience in the management of cloacas with the ability to perform vaginal replacement if necessary, as well as knowledge in pediatric urology. On the other hand, we believe cloacas with a common channel shorter than 3 cm can be treated by a pediatric surgeon who received good training in the management of these defects. These patients require a cystoscopy and vaginoscopy to measure the length of the common channel. For planning purposes it is recommended to do this during a separate anesthetic with a future plan for the definitive repair.

During the definitive reconstruction, the rectum is separated meticulously from the vagina, trying to respect both structures. The next step is a maneuver called "total urogenital mobilization", the vagina and urethra together, are dissected and mobilized, dividing the suspensory ligaments of urethra and vagina, which gains between 2 and 4 cm of length, enough to have a nice repair of the urethra and vagina with a good cosmetic and functional result. The limits of the sphincter are electrically determined and the perineum is repaired. The rectum is then placed within the limits of the sphincter and an anoplasty is performed.

A rectovestibular fistula is also repaired with a posterior sagittal operation. The incision is usually shorter than the one used for a cloaca. The rectum is identified and dissected meticulously. Special emphasis is placed in the separation of the rectum from the vagina, because they have a common wall without a plane of separation. Once the rectum is completely separated from the vagina and both structures are intact, the limits of the sphincter are electrically determined. The perineal body is reconstructed and the rectum is placed within the limits of the sphincters. An anoplasty is performed.

Perineal fistula in female babies is treated as previously described.

47.6.3 Results

Functional results also represent a spectrum. Males with rectobladder neck fistula have poor functional results (15% chance of voluntary bowel movements). Most of those babies have urinary control. The percentage of patients that have voluntary bowel movements by the age of three, in the authors' series are 60% for recto-prostatic fistulae, 85% for recto-bulbar, 90% for imperforate anus without fistula and (with no Down's syndrome), 80% for this same malformation with Down's syndrome, and 100% for perineal fistulae. All these results are in patients with a good sacrum. The overwhelming majority of male patients with a reasonable good sacrum will have urinary control, regardless of the type of anorectal malformation.

Occasional soiling may occur in about half of all those patients who have voluntary bowel movements; usually due to a poorly treated problem of constipation.

Constipation is by far, the most common postoperative sequela in anorectal malformations and should not be underestimated in its seriousness, because when constipation is not treated properly, babies tend to form a fecal impaction that produces overflow pseudoincontinence.

Patients operated on for a cloaca, frequently suffer from, an incapacity to empty their bladder; consequently, intermittent catheterization is indicated in 80% of those patients born with a common channel longer than 3 cm; and in 20% of those with a common channel shorter than 3 cm.

Depending on the quality of the sacrum, approximately 70% of the patients born with a cloaca will have voluntary bowel movements.

Patients with vestibular fistula with normal sacrum have a 95% chance of having voluntary bowel movements, but about half of them may soil depending on the degree of constipation that they suffer from.

All patients with perineal fistula have voluntary bowel movements with minimal soiling very occasionally, depending on the efficiency in the treatment for constipation.

For those patients that suffer from fecal incontinence, a bowel management program must be implemented. Such a program is 95% successful in keeping patients completely clean. This program consists of finding, by trial and error, the specific type of enema capable of cleaning the colon of a specific patient.

The overwhelming majority of patients born with an anorectal malformation, can remain completely clean in the underwear, either because they were born with a good-prognosis type of defect or because they are kept artificially clean due to the implementation of a good bowel management program.

When patients reach the age in which they are embarrassed to receive enemas, we offer them the creation of a continent appendicostomy, an operation that consists in connecting the tip of the appendix to the deepest portion of their umbilicus and plicating the cecum around the appendix to create a one-way-valve mechanism that allows the passing of a catheter to deliver an enema while sitting on the toilet. Those without an appendix can undergo a neoappendicostomy.

Further Reading

Levitt MA, Soffer SZ, Peña A (1997) Continent appendicostomy in the bowel management of fecal incontinent children. J Pediatr Surg 32:1630–1633

Peña A (1985) Posterior sagittal anorectoplasty as a secondary operation for the treatment of fecal incontinence. J Pediatr Surg 18:762–773

Peña A (1993) Management of anorectal malformations during the newborn period. World J Surg 17:385–392

Peña A (1997) Total urogenital mobilization – an easier way to repair cloacas. J Pediatr Surg 32:263–268

Peña A, DeVries PA (1982) Posterior sagittal anorectoplasty: important technical considerations and new applications. J Pediatr Surg 17:796–811

Peña A, Levitt MA (2006) Anorectal anomalies. In P Puri, ME Höllwarth (eds) Pediatric Surgery. Springer Surgery Atlas Series, Springer-Verlag Berlin, Heidelberg, New York, pp 289–312

Peña A, Guardino K, Torilla JM, Levitt MA, Rodriguez G, Torres R (1988) Bowel management for fecal incontinence in patients with anorectal malformations. J Pediatr Surg 33:133–137

Peña A, Levitt MA, Hong AR, Midulla P (2004) Surgical management of cloacal malformations: A review of 339 patients. J Pediatr Surg 39:470–479

Appendicitis

48

Jurgen Schleef and Prem Puri

Contents

48.1 Introduction

Acute appendicitis is the most common surgical emergency in childhood. Appendicitis may present at any age, although it is uncommon in preschool children. Approximately one-third of children with acute appendicitis have perforation by the time of operation. Despite improved fluid resuscitation and better antibiotics, appendicitis in children, especially in preschool children, is still associated with significant morbidity.

48.2 Epidemiology

The incidence of acute appendicitis has been reported to vary substantially by country, geographic region, race, sex and season, but the reasons for these variations are unknown. An epidemiological study of acute appendicitis in California revealed that the incidence of appendicitis in blacks and Asians was less than half that in whites. Epidemiological studies of acute appendicitis and perforation rates in California and New York have shown higher incidence rates of appendicitis among Hispanics than African Americans and Whites with Hispanics, Asians and African Americans having a higher risk of perforation than whites.

48.3 Etiology

The exact etiology and pathogenesis of appendicitis are poorly understood. While invasion of the appendiceal wall by micro-organisms is the ultimate pathological event, the primary initiating condition is not known.

P. Puri and M. Höllwarth (eds.), *Pediatric Surgery: Diagnosis and Management*,
DOI: 10.1007/978-3-540-69560-8_48, © Springer-Verlag Berlin Heidelberg 2009

Obstruction of the appendix lumen, from whatever cause, with resulting distension and disturbance of blood flow, is still considered the major factor in the pathogenesis of acute appendicitis. Other factors include low dietary fiber intake and bacterial and viral infections. Andersson et al. investigated temporospatial clustering and outbreaks (characteristics of infectious diseases) among appendicitis cases and found that appendicitis does occur in space-time clusters and outbreaks, thus supporting an infectious etiology theory. Recently, Gauderer et al. investigated the relationship between heredity and appendicitis and found that children with appendicitis are at least twice as likely to have a positive family history of appendicitis as compared with children with right lower quadrant pain without appendicitis or controls without abdominal pain.

48.4 Diagnosis

The diagnosis of acute appendicitis in childhood can sometimes be difficult. Definite diagnosis is made in only 43–72% of patients at the time of initial assessment. The rate of negative pediatric appendectomy is in the range 4–50% in various reports. The patient's history and clinical examination are the most important tools for the diagnosis of appendicitis. Periumbilical pain is often the first symptom, followed by vomiting and fever. When the inflammation progresses, the pain localizes to the right lower quadrant, and right lower quadrant tenderness develops. Appendices located in the retrocaecal position may cause pain, radiating to the back. Appendices in pelvic position may present with diarrhea. Clinical examination in a typical case with appendicitis reveals tenderness, guarding and rigidity in the right lower quadrant of abdomen.

Laboratory investigations and plain radiographs are neither sensitive nor specific in the diagnosis of appendicitis. Barium enema is an unreliable test because of its high false-positive and false-negative rates. In recent years, graded compression ultrasonography of the right lower quadrant has been shown to be a useful tool in the evaluation of patients with clinical findings that are suggestive but not diagnostic of appendicitis, with a sensitivity of 80–100%, a specificity of 78–98%, and an overall accuracy of 91%. Ultrasound is portable, fast, and free of irradiation exposure, of modest incremental cost and of use in

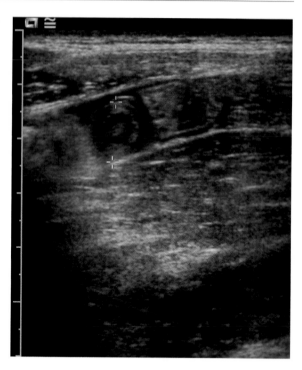

Fig. 48.1 Ultrasonography in a 12-year-old patient with acute appendicitis—enlarged and thickened (1.1 cm) appendix

delineating gynecologic disease. However, it is of limited use in obese adolescents and is highly user-dependent. The only sonographic sign that is specific for appendicitis is an enlarged, non-compressible appendix measuring greater than 6 mm in maximal diameter (Fig. 48.1). The appendix may not be visible following perforation. Recently, computed tomography (CT) has been used as an adjunct to the diagnosis of appendicitis and appeared to have an immediate impact, reducing negative appendectomy rates to 4.1% and perforation rates to 14.7%. The principal advantages of CT are its operator independency and enhanced delineation of disease extent in perforated appendicitis. Sensitivity, specificity and accuracy for unenhanced limited CT have approached 97%, 100% and 99%, respectively. However, with this improved diagnostic accuracy came a reduction in the degree of significance put on the initial clinical evaluation by the responsible surgical team. This management strategy must take into account the significant risk of exposure of the child to the CT dose of ionizing radiation. Recent studies have suggested that CT has not increased the accuracy of diagnosing appendicitis when compared to a careful history and physical examination performed by an experienced surgeon.

In patients with an uncertain diagnosis of acute abdominal pain, a policy of active observation in hospital is usually practiced. A repeated structured clinical examination is simple and noninvasive. However, the argument against this policy is that it may lead to a delay in specific management of these patients and may result in a high incidence of perforation. Bachoo et al. achieved a positive predictive value of 97.9% and a normal appendectomy rate of 2.6% with active observation alone and showed no correlation between post-operative morbidity and timing of surgery with this protocol. We have shown that the delay in appendectomy in children observed in a hospital setting does not increase the incidence of complicated appendicitis.

Table 48.1 Appendicitis

Most frequent differential diagnosis

- Abdominal pain of unknown origin
- Gastroenteritis
- Mesenteric lymphadenitis
- Intussusception
- Meckel's diverticulitis
- Primary peritonitis
- Inflammatory bowel disease
- Neoplasm (carcinoid, lymphoma)
- Urinary tract infection
- Testicular torsion
- Omental torsion
- Ruptured ovarian cyst
- Ovarian torsion
- Ectopic pregnancy
- Pelvic inflammatory disease

48.5 Differential Diagnosis

Several conditions must be considered where an infant is being evaluated for appendicitis. Table 48.1 gives the list of common differential diagnoses. Differential diagnoses are more frequent in small children (connatal malformations, intussusceptions) and adolescent girls (ovarian pathology, pelvic inflammatory disease).

48.6 Operative Techniques

Children with appendicitis are assessed for degree of sepsis and dehydration. Intravenous fluids are indicated preoperatively because most patients would have vomited and not eaten for over 24 h. Broad-spectrum antibiotics should be administered pre- and postoperatively in order to prevent infectious complications (Table 48.2).

Table 48.2 Appendicitis

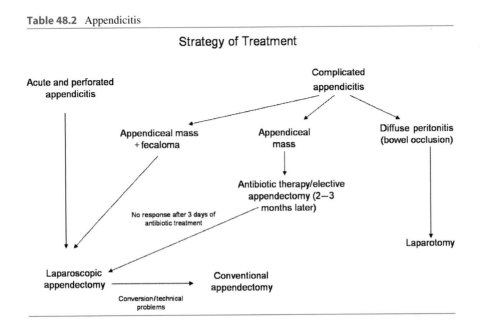

48.7 Open Appendectomy

A transverse right lower quadrant skin crease incision is recommended. The muscular layers are split in the direction of their fibers. The peritoneum is opened and fluid sent for culture. Recent studies have suggested it is unnecessary to send routine peritoneal fluid cultures. The mesoappendix is divided and the appendiceal base clamped and ligated. Stump inversion is optional. Engstrom and Fenyo found no difference as regards to wound infection and postoperative fever between one group in which the appendix was ligated and doubly invaginated and another group in which it was simply ligated. If pus is present, the abdomen should be irrigated with saline. The abdominal wall is closed in layers. The skin is usually closed by subcuticular absorbable sutures even in the case of perforation. Primary wound closure after perforated appendicitis is safe, economical and advantageous in pediatric practice.

48.8 Laparoscopic Appendectomy

An infraumbilical port is inserted using an open rather than percutaneous technique. Two 5 mm infraumbilical incisions are placed on either side of the midline. A third right lower quadrant incision is optional. After mobilization of the appendix, the mesoappendix is divided, the appendiceal stump is ligated with endoloops or an endoscopic stapler, and the appendix is removed.

In recent years, laparoscopic appendectomy has become an option as a safe alternative in the pediatric age group (Fig. 48.2). Although the rate at which laparoscopy is utilized in the treatment of appendicitis varies dramatically from center to center (range 0–95%), it is undoubtedly a reasonable surgical alternative to open appendectomy for the treatment of acute appendicitis in children. Recent studies have demonstrated that laparoscopic appendectomy is at least as safe and effective as open appendectomy. Despite the fact that laparoscopic appendectomy takes longer to perform at a marginally increased cost compared to open appendectomy, it has multiple advantages.

A large database study of adults and children in the United States showed laparoscopic appendectomy to be associated with a shorter median hospital stay and lower rates of wound infection, gastrointestinal complications and overall complications.

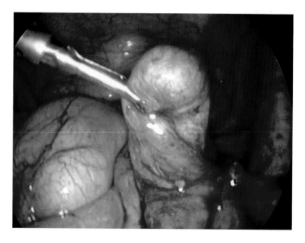

Fig. 48.2 A 14-year-old boy with phlegmon appendicitis during laparoscopy

The increased operative expense of laparoscopic appendectomy appear to be offset by an earlier return to normal daily activities.

48.9 Appendicitis in Preschool Children

Acute appendicitis in the preschool child accounts for a small fraction of all pediatric admissions with this diagnosis. In children under 2 years of age, it represents 1% of all cases of appendicitis in childhood. In a large series from Dublin, Puri et al. found that only 4.3% of their patients with appendicitis presented during the first 3 years of life. A recent 28-year review of appendicitis in children less than 3 years of age from Toronto showed that all children had perforated appendicitis at presentation. This resulted in very high morbidity (wound infection/abscess/dehiscence, pneumonia, small bowel obstruction, incisional hernia and enterocutaneous fistula) affecting 59% of these patients and although appendicitis is uncommon in this age group, it should be considered in the differential diagnosis of preschool children presenting with abdominal pain, tenderness or vomiting.

The diagnosis of appendicitis in preschool children can be difficult, resulting in delay and more severe disease. The young child's inability to communicate adequately with the parents, atypical disease presentation, and other associated illnesses may delay the diagnosis. Surana et al. reviewed 132 patients under 5 years of age treated for acute appendicitis in the two Dublin children's hospitals between 1987 and 1991, in order to identify factors that contribute to more serious disease in this age group. Of the 132 preschool children, 63 (48%) had perforated appendicitis and 29 (22%) had an appendix mass, 36 (27%) had uncomplicated appendicitis and 4 (3%) had a normal appendix. All the classic symptoms were present in the majority of patients. Atypical symptoms were found in many children and included diarrhea, cough/sore throat, dysuria, headache and earache. A diagnosis other than appendicitis was suspected in 53 (40%) patients, leading to a delay in management. Mean duration of symptoms before admission was as follows: acute appendicitis 39 hours, perforated appendicitis 53 h, and appendix mass 82 h. Postoperatively an intra-abdominal abscess occurred in 5% of the patients with perforated appendicitis and none with uncomplicated appendicitis: these patients were treated using antimicrobial agents, with complete resolution clinically and on ultrasound in all cases. One patient required laparotomy for adhesive intestinal obstruction. There were no deaths.

In view of the frequency of atypical presentation and the increased incidence of advanced appendicitis, a high index of suspicion is necessary in preschool children presenting with acute abdominal pain. Early diagnosis is the key to reducing morbidity from appendicitis in this age group.

48.10 Perforated Appendicitis

The reported incidence of perforated appendicitis in children is 18–40%. Two recent large series of appendicitis in children have reported 18% and 20% incidence respectively. The incidence is much higher in preschool children (see above).

Nowadays mortality is very rare. Several controversies have arisen over the years regarding the best approach to reduce the morbidity from appendicitis, especially infectious complications such as intra-abdominal abscess and wound infection. Many of the controversies relating to perforated appendicitis have been resolved. Several studies have confirmed the efficacy of antibiotics in reducing morbidity. Probably, the first preoperative dose of antibiotics is the most important. There is still some disagreement about the duration of antibiotic therapy and which drugs to use. Wound drainage is no longer thought to be beneficial,

and has been associated with an increased risk of infection. Current opinion overwhelmingly favors the approach of confining the use of drains to only those cases in which a clearly localized abscess cavity can be demonstrated. The placement of a peritoneal drain following perforated appendicitis has not been shown to improve outcome, with no reduction in the duration of hospitalization or nasogastric drainage time and is therefore not advocated. Intraoperative irrigation of the peritoneal cavity is a valuable procedure in perforated appendicitis. The majority of pediatric surgeons nowadays favor a protocol of irrigation, with or without antibiotics, until a clear effluent is returned. Subcuticular skin closure is safe after perforated appendicitis; wound infection rates are low and thus there is no compelling reason to opt for delayed closure of the appendectomy incision.

In Dublin, the protocol for the management of perforated appendicitis consists of preoperative administration of antibiotics that are continued for 5 days postoperatively. Intraoperative irrigation of the peritoneal cavity is carried out and the appendectomy wound is closed using subcuticular absorbable sutures. During a 5-year period (1987–1991), a total of 870 patients underwent emergency appendectomy for appendicitis at Our Lady's Hospital for Sick Children. One hundred and fifty-eight (18%) of the patients (98 boys) were found to have a perforated appendix. Their ages ranged from 18 months to 15 years (mean 7.8 years). Thirteen patients (8%) developed postoperative complications. Nine (5.6%) had a wound infection, which was managed by local drainage and antibiotics. Five children (3.2%), including one with a wound infection, developed an intra-abdominal abscess, which was confirmed by ultrasonography and resolved with antibiotic therapy (Fig. 48.3). Nine of the 13 patients with postoperative infective complications were readmitted to hospital; their mean hospital stay was 9.4 days (range 3–18). The mean duration of hospital stay in the 158 patients with perforated appendicitis, including those who were readmitted, was 6.8 days (range 3–47). There were no deaths.

An analysis of three recent studies of perforated appendicitis, using a protocol of preoperative antibiotics, intraoperative irrigation of the peritoneal cavity, primary subcuticular skin closure and a short course of postoperative antibiotics showed an intra-abdominal abscess rate of 1.3–3.2%, a wound infection rate of 1.3–5.7%, no deaths, and a mean hospital stay of

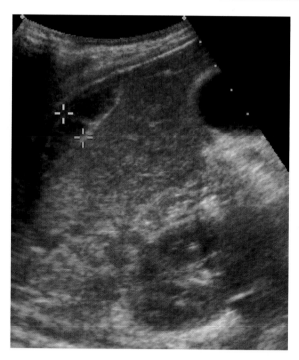

Fig. 48.3 Ultrasonography of a subdiaphragmatic abscess after complicated appendicitis (same patient as in Fig. 1)

6.8–11.4 days. These results set new standards in wound management, infectious complications and length of hospital stay in perforated appendicitis.

48.11 Appendix Mass

An appendix mass results from appendicitis that is localized by edematous, adherent omentum and loops of small bowel. In contrast, the appendiceal abscess is a localized suppurative process that may occur at any time in the course of appendicitis, or may complicate an appendiceal mass. Clinically, it is not possible in most cases to distinguish with certainty between the two conditions. An appendiceal mass at the time of presentation is discovered in about 10% of children with appendicitis. The incidence is higher during the first 3 years of life, when one-third of the patients with appendicitis have been reported to present with an appendiceal mass.

The management of an appendiceal mass in children is controversial. Many authors recommend non-operative management of an appendix mass, with

antibiotics followed by delayed appendectomy as the treatment of choice. Others favor immediate appendectomy in every case of appendicitis. Controversy around conservative management of appendiceal mass has arisen mainly from the belief that children, and particularly infants, have a poor ability to localize intraperitoneal inflammatory processes, and so children with an appendiceal mass should be managed operatively. The senior author has previously shown that a child's ability to localize appendiceal inflammation is well developed, even in infancy, and that one half of the patients developing appendicitis during the first 2 years of life, and one-third of those developing appendicitis during the first 3 years of life, have an appendiceal mass at the time of presentation.

Initial conservative management of appendiceal masses, followed by interval appendectomy, has been practiced at the author's institution for over 30 years. Gillick et al. recently reviewed the results of conservative management of patients with an appendix mass from Dublin. During the period 1982–2000, 427 children presented to one of Dublin's three pediatric hospitals with a diagnosis of appendix mass. There were 222 boys and 205 girls. Their ages ranged from 2 months to 18 years (mean 7.3 years). The duration of symptoms ranged from a few hours to 21 days, with 266 (62.3%) having had symptoms for longer than 3 days. The diagnosis was made clinically in 136 (31.9%) children, by ultrasonography in 61 (14.3%), by examination under anesthesia in 229 (53.6%) and by computed tomography in one child (0.2%). All were initially managed conservatively with intravenous antibiotics, nasogastric suction as required and intravenous fluids until oral fluids and diet were tolerated. In 346 (84.2%) of the 411 patients the mass resolved completely. The mean duration of hospital stay in this group was 6 days. Three hundred and thirty-one children had an elective appendectomy as planned, 4–6 weeks after discharge. Of these elective appendec-tomies, 15 (4.5%) were performed laparoscopically. The complication rate following elective appendectomy was 2.3% (five wound infections, two intra-abdominal abscesses and one hematoma). Histological assessment of the appendices removed electively demonstrates acute of subacute inflammation in 51% of the specimens. Two specimens had a carcinoid tumor. Sixty-five (16%) children with an appendix mass failed to respond to initial non-operative management: 17 required early appendectomy for ongoing symptoms and 27 developed an appendix abscess that required drainage and subsequent appendectomy. These data, as well as other studies, support the contention that initial nonoperative management of appendiceal mass, followed by an appendectomy, is a safe and effective policy.

We recommend interval appendectomy following resolution of the appendiceal mass. Some investigators have questioned the need for appendectomy after conservative management, on the assertion that the incidence of recurrent appendicitis is low and the complication rate with interval appendectomy is high. However, complications following interval appendectomy in children in our series were uncommon. Moreover, histological evidence of inflammation was present in almost 51% of these appendices. It is possible that the inflammation in some cases might have resolved spontaneously, but some patients develop recurrent appendicitis. Therefore, we recommend initial nonoperative management of appendiceal masses with antibiotics, followed by appendectomy 6–8 weeks later.

48.12 Mortality

In the United Kingdom, the number of deaths from acute appendicitis in children has decreased dramatically since the 1930s, largely as a result of the decline in incidence of appendicitis but also because of a marked reduction in the hospital case-fatality rate during the last 30 years. Three national audits between 1963 and 1997 covering all children dying of appendicitis in England and Wales showed an 85% decrease in the hospital case-fatality rate. This almost certainly reflects improvements in clinical care, which have occurred in parallel with expansion of specialist pediatric surgery and anesthesia. Delay in referral to hospital and/or diagnosis of acute appendicitis are the dominant factors responsible for the residual small number of avoidable deaths.

48.13 Long-Term Outcomes

The long-term outcome of the vast majority of patients who undergo appendectomy for childhood appendicitis is excellent. A small number of patients develop late adhesive intestinal obstruction. The belief that perforated appendicitis in girls is associated with reduced fertility rate in later life has been based on a few reports that do not stand up to critical analysis.

Further Reading

Esposito C, Borzi P, Valla JS et al (2007) Laparoscopic versus open appendectomy in children: A retrospective comparative study of 2,332 cases. World J Surg 31:750–755

Kosloske AM, Love CL, Rohrer JE, Goldthorn JF, Lacey SR (2004) The diagnosis of appendicitis in children: Outcomes of a strategy based on pediatric surgical evaluation. Pediatrics 113:29–34

Morrow SE, Newman KD (2007) Current management of appendicitis. Semin Pediatr Surg 16:34–40

Puri P, Mortell A (2007) Appendicitis. In MD Stringer, KT Oldham, PDE Mouriquand (eds) Paediatric Surgery and Urology: Long-term outcomes, 2nd edn. Cambridge University Press, New York, pp 374–384

Jasonni V (2006) Appendectomy. In P Puri, ME Höllwarth (eds) Pediatric Surgery, Springer Surgery Atlas Series. Springer-Verlag, Berlin, Heidelberg, New York, pp 321–326

Intussusception

49

Priya Ramachandran

Contents

49.1 Introduction

Intussusception is among the commonest emergencies in children requiring the attention of a pediatric surgeon. This condition in which one part of the bowel telescopes into another has been recognized since the 1600s and nonoperative measures of reducing the intussusception were the preferred mode of treatment till the early 1900s. Since then, surgical reduction became the treatment of choice and despite the high mortality associated with the operative method, it took almost 40 years to return to nonoperative methods of reduction. Today, these methods have been improved upon and are the standard of care for children with intussusception.

Intussusception occurs most commonly in infants between 15 and 19 months of age with only 10–25% of cases occurring after 2 years of age. Although 90% of intussusceptions occur in children between 3 months to 3 years of age, it has also been reported in utero, in neonates, and in adults.

49.2 Etiopathogenesis

In most cases there is no identifiable etiology for intussusception and hence is idiopathic. It is often preceded by a viral illness (respiratory or gastroenteritis). This may contribute to the hypertrophy of the Peyer's patches in the ileum, seen during surgery in most cases. Adenovirus and Rotavirus has been identified in 50% of children with gastroenteritis who develop intussusceptions. Ileocolic intussusceptions are more common than small bowel or colonic intussusceptions. In utero intussusception contributes to the development of

P. Puri and M. Höllwarth (eds.), *Pediatric Surgery: Diagnosis and Management,*
DOI: 10.1007/978-3-540-69560-8_49, © Springer-Verlag Berlin Heidelberg 2009

Table 49.1 Common pathological lead points

Meckel's diverticulum
Appendix
Polyps
Carcinoid tumour
Henoch-Schonlein purpura
Foreign body
Duplication of the bowel
Cystic fibrosis

intestinal atresia. Pathological lead points contribute to 2–10% of all intussusceptions (see Table 49.1). The incidence of lead points increases with age and in children over 4 years of age; 57% of intussusceptions have lead points.

The antegrade peristalsis of the bowel propels the segment of intestine with hypertrophic Peyer's patches or lead points into the adjacent distal bowel. As the proximal bowel (intussusceptum) invaginates into the distal bowel (intussuscipiens), the mesentery of the proximal bowel and its vessels are compressed between the layers of the bowel. This causes impaired venous return and edema of the bowel, which leads to congestion. Consequently there is bleeding and discharge of mucus, which has been described as red currant jelly stool. The proximal small bowel becomes dilated and in the absence of intervention gangrene occurs in the innermost layers of the bowel, which are the first to undergo vascular compromise and undergo perforation. The outer layers of the intussusception rarely lose their viability.

49.3 Clinical Presentation

The clinical presentation is more typical in infants and is characterized by episodes of abdominal colic associated with drawing up the legs and crying. These episodes occur in 15–30 min intervals. In between episodes the infant is quiet. Initially there may be vomiting of undigested food and streaks of blood in the stools.

Subsequently the child becomes lethargic between episodes, develops increasing abdominal distension, bilious vomiting, and passage of red currant jelly stools. Often these symptoms are preceded by an episode of diarrheal illness. Sometimes there is a history of change in diet with introduction of weaning foods. On examination the child may be febrile and dehydrated with signs of shock in case of bowel ischemia. A curved sausage-shaped

mass can be palpated anywhere in the abdomen when the infant is quiet. Rectal exam is positive for blood in 60–90% of cases. Rarely a cervix-shaped mass is seen protruding beyond the anal verge. The reported incidence of rectal prolapse of intussusception varies from 8–40% with the highest incidences being reported from the African and Indian subcontinent. Although this finding has been attributed to a delay in the presentation, increased intestinal peristalsis may lead to a rapid movement of the intussusception into the rectum. The classic triad of incessant cry due to abdominal colic, red currant jelly stools, and a palpable abdominal mass has been reported in 20–60% of cases.

In children over 2–3 years of age, the presentation of intussusception is subtler and the classic triad of symptoms may not be present. It is felt that since th diameter of the bowel is larger, the intussusceptions are looser and hence the symptoms and complications are less severe. In this group pathological lead points contribute to a majority of cases. Although the average incidence of intussusceptions caused by pathological lead points is about 8%, the incidence is much higher after the first year of life (20–40%). There may be symptoms associated with the primary disease that causes the intussusception, such as hemorrhagic patches in Henoch-Schonlien purpura (HSP) and joint swellings in coagulation disorders.

49.4 Diagnostic Studies

A plain film of the abdomen may be noncontributory early in the disease. A soft tissue shadow is seen in the right upper quadrant and there is paucity of gas in the right lower quadrant. The rectal gas shadow may be absent. Air fluid levels and dilated bowel loops are present in case of small bowel obstruction. The diagnostic accuracy of plain films is only 45% and is not indicated if there are facilities for ultrasonography.

Ultrasonography of the abdomen is often diagnostic for intussusception with a reported accuracy of up to 100% (Fig. 49.1). The characteristic "target sign" is described as two rings of low echogenicity with an intervening hyperechoic ring similar to a donut. The edematous walls of the intussusception appear as superimposed hyperechoic and hypoechoic layers described as the pseudo-kidney sign. Sonographic features of a thick hyperechoic rim of the intussusception, fluid

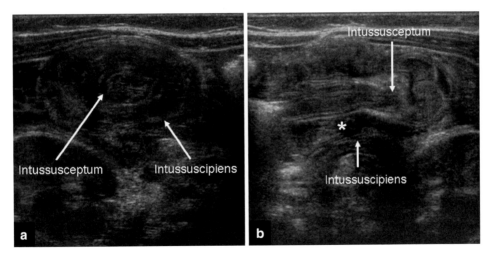

Fig. 49.1 Typical ultrasound finding of an intussusception

trapped in the layers of the intussusception, enlarged mesenteric lymph nodes dragged into the intussusception, free intraperitoneal fluid, pathologic lead points, and absence of blood flow in the intussusception have been evaluated to predict the reducibility of intussusception. However, none of the features are 100% accurate in predicting reducibility and hence are not contraindications for reduction by enema. The excellent diagnostic accuracy of ultrasonography and the advent of high-resolution machines have largely eliminated the need for radiologic contrast studies. Barium contrast enema was considered the gold standard for the diagnosis of intussusception with a diagnostic accuracy of 100%. It also becomes therapeutic when the barium is used to perform hydrostatic reduction.

Although the radiation exposure is small, it is significant that more than 50% of contrast enemas are negative when done to diagnose intussusception. Although computerized tomography and magnetic resonance imaging can be used for diagnosis, it is often not necessary given the diagnostic accuracy of ultrasonography.

49.5 Treatment

49.5.1 Resuscitation

The initial management of children with intussusception begins with fluid resuscitation in the emergency room. This can be assessed clinically and based on electrolyte values from blood samples drawn for complete hemogram and cross match at the time of placement of intravenous lines. The correction of dehydration is crucial before attempting reduction. Nasogastric decompression is instituted in all children in our institution although it may be argued that it is not indicated in children who do not present with vomiting. We do so because these children are irritable and prone to vomiting during attempts at reduction. Antibiotic prophylaxis including anaerobic coverage is started. The patient is then shifted to the radiology suite for attempts at reduction of the intussusception.

49.5.2 Nonoperative Reduction

The improvement in outcome of intussusception has been gratifying with negligible morbidity largely due to the success of nonsurgical modalities of treatment using pneumatic or hydrostatic reduction techniques.

49.5.2.1 Pneumoenema

Pneumoenema is a cheap, safe, and effective option for the treatment of intussusception. Various studies have quoted success rates of 80–92% in reducing the intussusception. When compared with barium the fluoroscopy screening times are shorter. Also, recurrences are less with air than barium and the morbidity is less should a perforation occur. Pneumoenema is easier to perform and teach to junior residents. Attempts have been made to establish predictors for outcome of pneumoenema in order to avoid excluding children from this procedure and also to avoid repeated attempts in children who fail the procedure. Several studies have considered long duration of symptoms, age less than 6 months, rectal bleeding, abdominal distension, prolapsing rectal mass, and a raised white cell count to be predictors of failure. However, the outcome of pneumoenema is excellent in most centers and it must be attempted in all children with intussusception except when there is peritonitis and bowel necrosis, which are the only contraindications to pneumoenema reduction. In our institution, pneumoenema reduction has been the treatment of choice for the last decade. The procedure is performed using a simple apparatus consisting of a three-way Foley and aneroid Sphygmomanometer with insufflation bulb (Fig. 49.2). The Foley is inserted into the rectum and the balloon is inflated. The buttocks are taped together. Two attempts are made of 5 min duration each using a maximum pressure of 120 mmHg with 10-min interval between each attempt. Reduction is considered complete when there is free flow of air into the terminal ileum. Following reduction the infant passes a large amount of flatus and falls asleep.

In children with rectal prolapse of intussusception, this technique is slightly modified. The balloon of the Foley is inflated partially outside the anal verge after manually pushing back the prolapse into the distal rectum. The intussusception is reduced back into the proximal rectum and the balloon is then repositioned within the rectum and the procedure is carried out as previously described. Using this technique, we have been able to reduce 57% of intussusceptions that presented with rectal prolapse. The disadvantage of pneumoenema reduction is that there is radiation exposure. Also, a tension pneumoperitoneum can develop if there is a perforation during the procedure. However, perforation rates reported are less than 1%. If a tension pneumoperitoneum develops, it must be immediately decompressed by inserting a needle into the peritoneal cavity.

49.5.2.2 Hydrostatic Reduction

Hydrostatic barium enema reduction under fluoroscopic guidance is also successful in children and is the preferred option in some centers. The barium defines the intussusception as it seeps between the layers and takes a concave shape around the head of the intussusception. This has been described as the crab claw sign. The column of barium is held at a height of 3 ft for 3–5 min and three attempts are made. At this height the pressure exerted by the mercury column on the intussusception is 120 mmHg. The reduction is considered complete when barium fills the distal ileum. The dissection of barium between the intussuceptum and the intussucepiens is considered to indicate irreducibility coupled with a prolonged history of 48 h and abdominal distension. This procedure is also cheap, safe, and effective. The disadvantages are that if perforation occurs, barium causes an intense inflammatory response in the peritoneal cavity. Hence, some centers use water-soluble contrast for hydrostatic reduction.

Ultrasound-guided reduction using water (diluted with water-soluble contrast at a ratio of 9:1) has also been reported to have a success rate of 90% in the reduction of intussusception. Reduction can be confirmed by a plain radiograph, which shows contrast in the terminal ileum. Although there is no radiation exposure in ultrasound-guided saline reduction and success rates are higher, expertise in sonography is required to perform the procedure. The technique is difficult to perform when there are multiple air fluid levels secondary to small bowel obstruction.

Following a successful reduction, it is customary to admit and observe the children in hospital for sometime. In children with small bowel obstruction, nasogastric decompression is continued until the aspirate

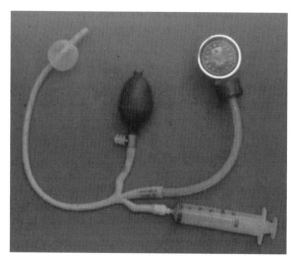

Fig. 49.2 Apparatus used for pneumoenema reduction

reduces and becomes nonbilious and the abdominal distension decreases. Intravenous fluids are discontinued when oral intake is established. In children with diarrhea, fluids are continued till the stools normalize. In the absence of a fever, antibiotics may be discontinued. The presence of a fever is an indication of ongoing bacteremia and antibiotics must be continued till the fever subsides. Experimental studies have shown that bacterial translocation occurs even in a viable intussusception with intact serosal surface. An ultrasonogram is recommended prior to discharge to confirm reduction and to identify pathologic lead points.

Sometimes significant edema of the ileocecal valve results in incomplete reduction. Spontaneous reduction may occur in such cases after the edema resolves. A delayed attempt can be made after 4–5 h if ultrasonography confirms persistent intussusception. Some surgeons would argue that these children require a laparotomy rather than a delayed attempt.

Spontaneous reduction of intussusception at laparotomy has been reported in 7–20% of children and this may be avoided by a delayed attempt at nonoperative reduction.

49.5.2.3 Recurrent Intussusception

Recurrent intussusception has been reported in 10% of children who undergo pneumatic or hydrostatic reduction. Although 30–60% of recurrences occur within 72 h, recurrences have been reported up to 36 months after reduction. The success rates of nonoperative reduction for recurrent intussusception are the same as with the first episode. There is no indication for a laparotomy in recurrent intussusception unless there is suspicion of a pathological lead point as is the case in children over 3 years of age and in children with multiple recurrences.

49.5.3 Operative Reduction

If the attempts at nonoperative reduction are unsuccessful, the patient is shifted to the operating room for a laparotomy and manual reduction of intussusception. This is done with the patient in the supine position through a small right lower quadrant incision. Although a midline incision grants better access to the peritoneal cavity, the caecum in infants is not a fixed structure and the intussusception can be easily delivered through the right lower quadrant incision. There is usually some serosanguinous fluid in the peritoneal cavity and this is suctioned out completely. The intussusception is then palpated and gently delivered through the wound. Most intussusceptions have an ileocecal component and ileoileal component. The intussusception is reduced by exerting gentle and persistent pressure at its distal end. The process is continued as long as there is gradual reduction despite serosal tears that may occur. After resection, the bowel is congested and edematous with hypertrophic Peyer's patches. The bowel may appear compromised and dusky. Usually the perfusion improves after warming the bowel with warm pads for 5–10 min. Any suspicious areas of the bowel must be resected.

The bowel is inspected for pathological lead points like Meckel's diverticulum or intestinal lymphomas, which are excised. The inflamed appendix can also act as a pathological lead point in which case appendicectomy is done. Some surgeons prefer to do an appendicectomy because the incision in the right lower quadrant may be assumed as an appendicectomy scar later and because the edema of the cecal mesentery is thought to cause vascular compromise of the appendix increasing the chance to develop appendicitis. The latter has not been proven in studies. If the intussusception remains immovable and large serosal tears develop attempt at reduction is abandoned in favor of resection. Resection of the entire irreducible mass includes the entire right colon and part of the transverse colon. Even if there is gangrene, the intussusception must be reduced as much as possible in order to avoid resecting a long length of colon. A primary anastamosis can be done in most instances unless the child is extremely unwell and the peritoneal cavity is soiled by fecal contamination.

In the case of infants who present with perforation or develop it during attempts at nonoperative reduction, the operative approach is the same. In such instances, the surgeon must compromise between worsening of the soiling due to tearing of the bowel if manual reduction is attempted and excising a longer length of bowel if it is not. When barium has been used for reduction there are longitudinal serosal tears plugged by barium. Also, barium admixed with stool cannot be removed and persists in the peritoneal cavity. Reports in the literature indicate that barium in the peritoneal cavity leads to longer operative time and prolonged postoperative morbidity in children.

Postoperatively feeds are resumed quickly if there has been no bowel resection. In children with bowel resection feeds are withheld for 5 days during which time the child is supported with intravenous fluids and antibiotics.

The complications of an open operation like infection are reduced with the usage of prophylactic antibiotics and intraoperative lavage of the peritoneal cavity. The incidence of small bowel obstruction is 5% and is the same as in a child who undergoes open appendicectomy. But the incidence increases considerably when there is resection of bowel for gangrene.

Laparoscopic reduction of intussusception has been described. Although there are no studies establishing clear advantages for this method, it has been shown that the duration of hospitalization is reduced and there is less pain than with open procedures. It must also be assumed that postoperative adhesions are less because of minimal bowel handing and consequently reduced scarring. However, in children requiring resection of the bowel and in children who have difficult intussusceptions the advantages of laparoscopy is not established.

49.6 Secondary Intussusception

Pathologic lead points contribute to 2–10% of intussusceptions and need to be differentiated from common ileocolic intussusception. They are commoner in children older than 3 years of age. The causes are listed in Table 49.1. Meckel's diverticulum is the commonest lead point.

Children with Henoch-Schonlien purpura (HSP) develop small bowel intussusception due to lymphoid hyperplasia. They present with severe abdominal pain and purpura. This occurs in about 3% of children with HSP. The initiation of steroid therapy may cause spontaneous reduction of intussusception by reducing the bowel wall edema. Nonoperative reduction is attempted in most cases in conjunction with steroid therapy.

Cystic fibrosis can present with intussusception commonly in children between 9–12 years of age and is caused by the thick, putty-like material in the mucosal lumen acting as a lead point. Sometimes the presentation is more chronic with longstanding symptoms. Nonoperative reduction is not often successful and most children require operative reduction.

Postoperative intussusceptions occur after major diaphragmatic or retroperitoneal surgery. It can occur up to 10 days after surgery and is usually exclusively in the small bowel. Operative reduction is often necessary.

Further Reading

Ashcraft KW, Holcomb III GW, Murphy JP (2005) Paediatric Surgery, 4th edn. Elsevier, Philadelphia

Bines JE, Ivanoff B (2002) Acute Intussusception in Infants and Children: Incidence, Clinical Presentation and Management: A Global Perspective, Vaccines and Biologicals. World Health Organisation, Geneva

Grosfeld JL, O'Neill Jr JA, Fonkalsrud EW, Coran AG (eds) (2006) Paediatric Surgery, 6th edn. Mosby, St. Louis, MO

Guo JZ, Ma XY, Zhou QH (1986) Results of air pressure enema reduction of intussusception: 6396 cases in 13 years. J Pediatr Surg 21:1201–1203

Hadidi AT, El Shal N (1999) Childhood intussusception: A comparative study of non surgical management. J Pediatr Surg 34:304–307

Heenan SD, Kyriou J, Fitzgerald N, Adam EJ (2000) Effective dose at pneumatic reduction of paediatric intussusception. Clin Radiol 55:811–816

Oldham KT, Colombani PM, Foglia RP, Skinner MA (eds) Principles and Practice of Paediatric Surgery. Lippincott, Williams & Wilkins, Philadelphia

Ramachandran P, Vincent P, Sridharan S (2006) Rectal prolapse of intussusception—A single institution's experience. Eur J Pediatr Surg 16:420–422

Sandler AD, Ein SH, Connolly B, Daneman A, Filler RM (1999) Unsuccessful air-enema reduction of intussusception: Is a second attempt worth while? Pediatr Surg Int 15:214–216

Talwar S, Agarwal S (1973) Intussusception in infants and children. Indian J Pediatr 40:403–409

Turner D, Rickwood AMK, Brereton J (1980) Intussusception in older children. Arch Dis Child 55:544–546

Wang K-L (2006) Intussusception. In P Puri, ME Höllwarth (eds) Pediatric Surgery, Springer Surgery Atlas Series. Springer-Verlag Berlin Heidelberg, New York, pp 313–320

Omphalomesenteric Duct Remnants

50

Dhanya Mullassery and Paul D. Losty

Contents

50.1 Introduction

The omphalomesenteric (or vitellointestinal) duct is an embryonic communication between the primitive yolk sac and the developing midgut. During normal development at the 6th week of embryogenesis, the midgut loop elongates and herniates into the umbilical cord. Within the 'physiological umbilical hernia', the midgut rotates 90° counter clockwise around the axis of the superior mesenteric artery. At the same time, as the midgut elongates the lumen of the omphalomesenteric duct begins a process of obliteration. By the 10th week of early fetal development, the midgut returns to the abdominal cavity and the omphalomesenteric duct becomes a thin fibrous band, which undergoes resorption. Persistence of the duct leads to a spectrum of anomalies that can present clinically in the newborn period, infancy or later childhood years.

50.1.1 Variant Pathology of Omphalomesenteric Duct Remnants

1. Meckel's diverticulum (Fig. 50.1) – the ileal remnant of the duct remains patent and usually contains heterotopic gastric mucosal tissue. The diverticulum is connected to the umbilicus by a fibrous band if the obliterated duct fails to be fully resorbed.
2. Umbilical fistula (Fig. 50.2) – a completely patent omphalomesenteric duct connects the ileal segment of small intestine to the anterior abdominal wall.
3. Omphalomesenteric cyst (Fig. 50.3) – develops when a segment in the midportion of the duct remains patent while each end portion of the tract obliterates.

P. Puri and M. Höllwarth (eds.), *Pediatric Surgery: Diagnosis and Management,*
DOI: 10.1007/978-3-540-69560-8_50, © Springer-Verlag Berlin Heidelberg 2009

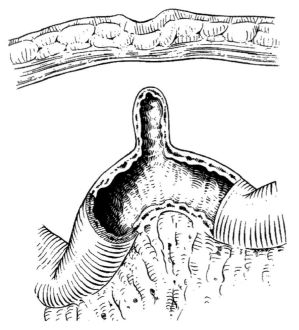

Fig. 50.1 Meckel's diverticulum

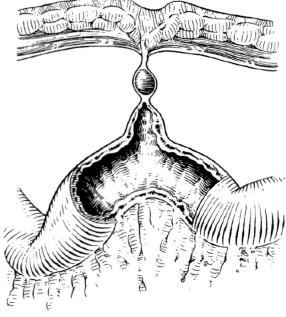

Fig. 50.3 Omphalomesenteric cyst

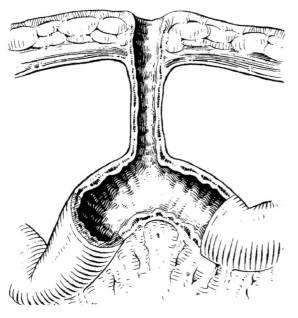

Fig. 50.2 Umbilical fistula

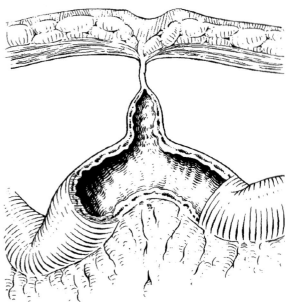

Fig. 50.4 Persistent fibrous cord

4. A persistent fibrous cord (Fig. 50.4) – connects the umbilicus to the small intestine where the duct obliterates but is not fully resorbed.

5. Umbilical polyp (Fig. 50.5) – a bright red nodule of sequestered ectopic gastrointestinal tissue resides in the umbilical dimple.

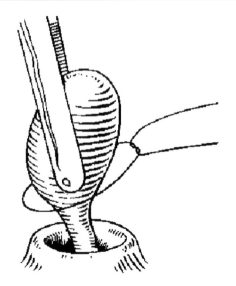

Fig. 50.5 Umbilical polyp

50.1.2 Meckel's Diverticulum

Meckel's diverticulum is the most common of the omphalomesenteric duct anomalies encountered in clinical practice. It results from a patency of the intestinal segment of the duct with a fibrous obliteration of the distal tract at the umbilicus. The lesion is usually located at the antimesenteric border of the ileum within 100 cm of the ileocaecal valve. The diverticulum is nourished by a rich blood supply from the vitellointestinal vessels that lie within a fold of the mesentery.

Originally described in 1809 by the German anatomist, Johann Friedrich Meckel (1781–1833), it is a true diverticulum, composed of all three layers of the intestinal tract. Frequently it contains heterotopic gastric, pancreatic and less commonly duodenal, colonic, or biliary mucosa.

50.1.2.1 Clinical Presentation

Clinical presentation usually results from complications arising from the presence of the diverticulum. These include lower gastrointestinal haemorrhage, abdominal pain secondary to diverticulitis and intestinal obstruction due to intussusception or volvulus. It was estimated in two large series that the lifetime probability of a MD becoming symptomatic is 4.2–6.4%. More than 75% of symptomatic MDs occur in children younger than 10 years of age.

Haemorrhage is the most frequent complication in the paediatric population secondary to active bleeding from peptic ulceration due to the ectopic gastric mucosa. The incidence of gastric mucosa is estimated at about 16–24% in asymptomatic and 50–80% in symptomatic Meckel's. The ulcer may be located in the diverticulum or adjacent ileum. Bleeding is usually profuse and painless manifesting as bright red bloody stools with clots and hypovolaemic shock. Rarely it may be occult in nature with a chronic anaemia.

Intestinal obstruction is the second commonest complication. It is more often encountered in older children. Symptoms include bile stained vomiting, abdominal distension and colicky pain. Findings at operation may reveal intussusception, volvulus or an internal hernia from persistent attachment of the diverticulum to the back of the umbilicus. Diverticulitis manifests as abdominal pain, fever, and vomiting. Presentation may be indistinguishable from that of acute appendicitis.

50.1.2.2 Investigations and Diagnosis

Imaging studies to aid definitive diagnosis should be tailored according to the varied clinical presentation. Haemorrhage is the major complication of a Meckel's diverticulum in the paediatric population. Technetium-99 m pertechnetate scintigraphy (Fig. 50.6)

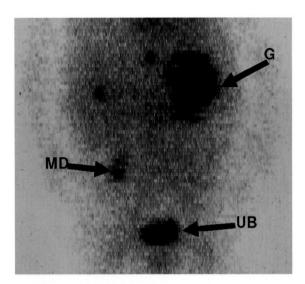

Fig. 50.6 Tc pertechnate isotope scan showing increased uptake in a Meckel's divertulum (M) bearing gastric mucosa. Note the normal uptake in gastric mucosa (G) and excretion through urinary bladder (UB)

is commonly employed to aid diagnosis. The gastric epithelial mucosa accumulates and secretes the pertechnetate isotope. After intravenous injection a focal area of increased isotope activity is apparent in the right lower quadrant within 30 min. However visualization may take up to 1 h if there are smaller amounts of heterotopic tissue. The sensitivity of Tc-99 m pertechnetate scintigraphy is approximately 85% with a specificity of 95%. This may decline with increasing age as seen in poorer yield of positive studies in the adult population. False-positive studies may occur when there is a gastric or small intestinal cystic or tubular duplication. False-negative reports are seen with Meckel's diverticula that do not contain adequate heterotopic gastric mucosa to sufficiently concentrate the Tc-99 m isotope.

Intestinal obstruction is readily diagnosed from plain film radiography. Ultrasonography may be of value in the further evaluation of children with a suspected Meckel diverticulum and a negative Tc-99 m pertechnetate scintigraphy scan. Diverticulae appear as a round or tubular, 'cyst like' structure. Echogenic foci in the lumen of the diverticulum may represent enteroliths or inflammatory debris. Colour Doppler may also demonstrate anomalous vessels. CT scanning has been used in some centres.

50.1.2.3 Differential Diagnosis

Differential diagnosis includes appendicitis, bleeding peptic ulcer, inflammatory bowel disorders or pelvic inflammatory disease in teenage girls.

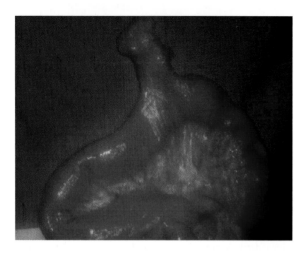

Fig. 50.7 Operative appearance of a Meckel's diverticulum

50.1.2.4 Management

The treatment for the symptomatic Meckel's diverticulum (Fig. 50.7) is open or laparoscopic surgical resection. This can be achieved either by diverticulectomy (Fig. 50.8a and b) or by a segmental limited small bowel resection and anastomosis (Fig. 50.9).

There has been ongoing debate about the merits of excision of a Meckel's diverticulum when found as an incidental finding at operation. During an operation, it is not always possible to determine by inspection or palpation whether an incidentally found Meckel's diverticulum is at increased risk of complications or not. Onen et al. recommended its removal in symptomatic as well as in asymptomatic cases in children younger than 8 years. Ueberrueck et al. proposed that in cases of gangrenous or perforated appendicitis, an incidentally discovered Meckel's diverticulum should be left alone, whereas in patients

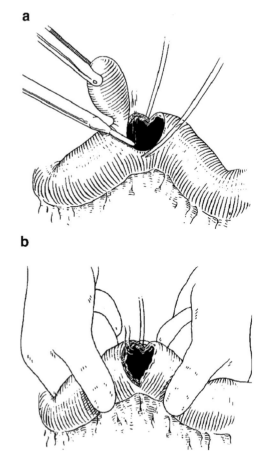

Fig. 50.8 A & B Diverticulectomy

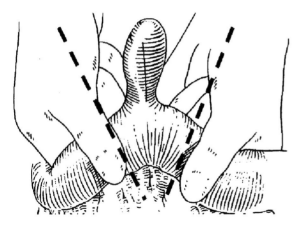

Fig. 50.9 Resection of a Meckel's diverticulum with adjacent small bowel segment

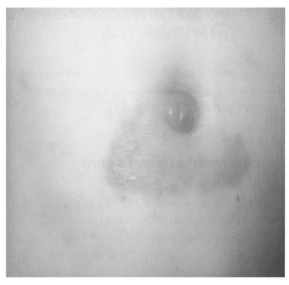

Fig. 50.10 Umbilical discharge from a patent vitellointestinal tract. Note the excoriation of the skin

with a mildly inflamed appendix removal is advisable. Soltero and Bill report a 4.2% lifetime complication risk for individuals harbouring a Meckel's diverticulum versus a 9% morbidity rate after routine incidental resection. These authors therefore do not favour incidental diverticulectomy. A recent systematic review does not support routine excision of asymptomatic Meckel's diverticuli.

50.1.2.5 Morbidity

Early postoperative complications (<10%) following resection include anastomotic leak, anastomotic stricture, adhesions, and post operative ileus. Intestinal obstruction from adhesions is a late event.

50.1.3 Umbilico-Ileal Fistula

A persistent fistula usually presents in the newborn period with discharge of intestinal content from the umbilicus with periumbilical excoriation (Fig. 50.10). Investigations (if indicated) may include a contrast fistulogram to confirm aberrant anatomy. Management includes resection via a cosmetic umbilical incision, identification of the fistula tract, intestinal resection and anastomosis.

Prolapse of a large patent vitellointestinal tract at the umbilicus presents as a characteristic 'double-horn' deformity with intestinal lumen clearly evident in the anomaly (Fig. 50.11).

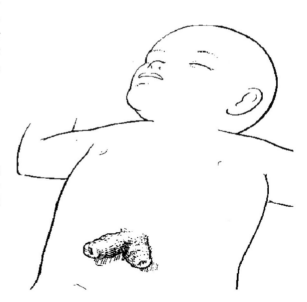

Fig. 50.11 Prolapse of a patent vitello-intestinal tract with the classic 'double-horn' anomaly

50.1.4 Umbilical Sinus

An umbilical sinus usually presents with a persistent serous or sero-sanguinous discharge from the navel area. When there is doubt about the nature of the discharge, often because of its intermittent nature, a sinogram may demonstrate the extent of the tract before formal resection.

50.1.5 Umbilical Cyst (Omphalomesenteric Cyst or Vitelline Cyst)

The cyst with the fibrous cord at either end can present with features of intestinal obstruction and is best managed by laparotomy and resection.

50.1.6 Persistent Fibrous Cord

Congenital fibrous bands are clinically significant because they may lead to intestinal obstruction or volvulus and need to be resected when symptomatic.

50.1.7 Umbilical Polyp

Polyps related to the presence of an OMD remnant can occasionally present as a nodular lesion in the umbilical dimple. They usually contain tiny fragments of intestinal or gastric mucosa. One should also consider the more common diagnosis of umbilical granuloma.

Further Reading

Cullen JJ (1994) Surgical management of Meckel's diverticula. An epidemiologic, population-based study. Ann Surg 220:564–568

Fa-Si-Oen PR, Roumen RM, Croiset van Uchelen FA (1999) Complications and management of Meckel's diverticulum: A review. Eur J Surg 165:674–678

Lloyd D (2006) Omphalomesenteric duct remnants. In P Puri, ME Höllwarth (eds) Pediatric Surgery, Springer Surgery Atlas Series. Springer-Verlag, Berlin, Heidelberg, New York, pp 327–332

Moore TC (1996) Omphalomesenteric duct malformations. Semin Pediatr Surg 5:116–123

Onen A, Cigdem MK, Ozturk H, Otcu S, Dokucu AI (2003) When to resect and when not to resect an asymptomatic Meckel's diverticulum? An ongoing challenge. Pediatr Surg Int 19:57–61

Park JJ, Wolff BG, Tollefson MK, Walsh EE, Larson DR (2005) Meckel's diverticulum: The Mayo Clinic experience with 1476 patients (1950–2002). Ann Surg 241(3):529–533

Soltero MJ, Bill AH (1976) The natural history of Meckel's diverticulum and its relation to incidental removal. A study of 202 cases of diseased Meckel's diverticulum found in King County, Washington, over a fifteen year period. Am J Surg 132:168–173

Zani A, Eaton S, Rees CM, Pierro A (2008) Meckel's diverticulum incidentally found: To resect or not to resect? Ann Surg 247(2):276–281

Hernias

51

Tomas Wester

Contents

51.1 Inguinal Hernia

51.1.1 Introduction

Inguinal hernias are among the most common surgical conditions in infants and children, with a peak incidence during the first 3 months of life. In children, inguinal hernias are almost always indirect hernias. Direct inguinal hernias are rare, particularly in neonates. The most important factor in the management of the neonate with a hernia is the high risk of incarceration. Hernias have been considered not to go away spontaneously, and should therefore always be repaired.

51.1.2 Aetiology

Congenital indirect inguinal hernia develops because the processus vaginalis remains patent after birth. The processus vaginalis is a potential hernia, which becomes an actual hernia when it contains some part of abdominal viscera. The processus vaginalis is an outpouching of the peritoneum that extends through the inguinal canal. The processus vaginalis is first seen during the 3rd month of intrauterine life. It follows the gubernaculum and testis through the inguinal canal and reaches the scrotum by the 7th month of gestation. In the female, the aetiology is less clear, although the processus vaginalis extends along the round ligament. Obliteration of the processus vaginalis starts soon after the descent of the testis is completed and continues after birth. Most infants have a patent processus vaginalis several months after birth. Patency has been reported to be 80–94% in the newborn period, approximately 60% in the 4–12 months age group and 20% in adulthood.

P. Puri and M. Höllwarth (eds.), *Pediatric Surgery: Diagnosis and Management*,
DOI: 10.1007/978-3-540-69560-8_51, © Springer-Verlag Berlin Heidelberg 2009

51.1.3 Epidemiology

The incidence of congenital indirect inguinal hernia in infants and children is 1–5%. The incidence of inguinal hernia in preterm infants is considerably higher and ranges from 9% to 11%. The incidence approaches 60% as birth weight decreases to 500–750 g. Inguinal hernia is more common in males than in females with a ratio ranging from 5:1 to 10:1. Approximately 60% of inguinal hernias occur on the right side, 30% are left-sided, and 10% are bilateral. Bilateral hernias are more common in premature infants and are reported to occur in 35–55% of the cases. There is a high familial incidence and inguinal hernia has been observed with increased frequency in twins and siblings of patients with inguinal hernia. There is no geographic or ethnic predominance reported in the literature.

51.1.4 Associated Conditions

There is an increased incidence of inguinal hernia in patients with various associated conditions (Table 51.1).

51.1.5 Diagnosis

51.1.5.1 Clinical Features

The presenting feature is a bulge in the groin, usually noticed by the parents, which increases in size with crying.

Table 51.1 Associated conditions showing an increased incidence of injuinal hernia

Urogenital conditions
Undescended testis
Bladder exstrophy
Increased amounts of peritoneal fluid
Ventriculoperitoneal shunts
Peritoneal dialysis
Increased intraabdominal pressure
Repair of gastroschisis or omphalocele
Meconium peritonitis
Chylous ascites
Necrotising enterocolitis
Chronic respiratory disorders
Cystic fibrosis
Connective tissue disorders
Ehler-Danlos syndrome
Marfan syndrome
Hurler-Hunter syndrome

The bulge may disappear spontaneously when the patient is quiet and relaxed. If the lump in the groin is reduced, it is usually possible to feel a thickening of the cord structures by the hernia sac. A reliable history along with palpation of a thickened cord is highly suggestive of inguinal hernia. Once the diagnosis of inguinal hernia is made, elective herniotomy should be done as soon as possible because of the high risk of incarceration particularly in the newborn infant. It is very important to examine the contralateral side.

51.1.5.2 Incarcerated Inguinal Hernia

Incarceration occurs when the contents of the sac cannot easily be reduced into the abdominal cavity. Strangulation refers to vascular compromise of the content of the sac because of constriction at the neck of the sac. If there is delay in the treatment, incarceration rapidly progresses to strangulation. The contents of the hernia sac may be small bowel, caecum, appendix, omentum or ovary and fallopian tube. The overall incidence of incarceration has been reported to be 6–18%. The incidence of incarceration in neonates and young infants is considerably higher and vary between 31% and 40%. Incarceration rate is much higher in premature infants compared with full-term infants. There have been several reports of testicular infarction, in association with an incarcerated inguinal hernia. In infants under the age of 3 months, gonadal infarction has been reported to occur in 30% of the cases. The incidence of testicular atrophy following incarceration of inguinal hernia has been reported to be between 10% and 15%. Most of the reports on testicular infarction or atrophy following incarcerated inguinal hernia, however, refer to infants who require emergency operation for the incarceration. One report showed that there was statistically significant difference in testicular volume between infants with incarcerated inguinal hernias, that first were reduced and then electively operated, and age-matched controls.

A newborn with incarcerated inguinal hernia usually presents with irritability, vomiting, moderately distended abdomen and a tender groin lump. Occasionally the infant may pass blood per rectum. Local examination reveals a tense, tender lump in the groin. The upper margin is not well defined. The testes may be normal or swollen and hard due to vascular compromise. Rectal examination usually is not necessary but, if done, contents of the hernia can be palpated at the internal ring.

The diagnosis of incarcerated inguinal hernia is usually made on clinical findings. Abdominal radiographs may occasionally show bowel gas within the lump in the groin and confirm the diagnosis. If intestinal obstruction is present, plain abdominal films will show dilated loops of bowel with fluid levels.

51.1.6 Differential Diagnosis

Clinical diagnosis of incarcerated inguinal hernia is usually easy, but it may sometimes be difficult to differentiate from a hydrocele, inguinal lymphadenitis and torsion of the testis. In hydrocele it is possible to get above the swelling, which is non-tender. Transillumination is not a reliable sign in infants, as bowel can be transilluminant because of its thin wall. Hydrocele of the cord is difficult to differentiate from incarcerated hernia. There is no previous history of reducible groin lump in these patients. Rectal examination may be useful in excluding incarcerated hernia. In lymphadenitis, examination of the area of drainage will reveal the source of infection. The cord and testis are normal. In scrotal testicular torsion it is possible to get above the swelling. Testis is tender and slightly higher than on the other side, while the torsion of the testis situated in the superficial inguinal pouch will be associated with an empty scrotum on the same side.

51.1.7 Management

The treatment of inguinal hernia is surgery. The ideal time for surgery is as soon as possible after the diagnosis has been made because of the risk of incarceration. In a recent survey of the members of the Surgical Section of the American Academy of Paediatrics, 79% responded that they repair asymptomatic reducible hernias in full-term boys electively. In full-term girl with reducible ovaries and no symptoms, 49% chose to repair electively. In former preterm babies the majority of surgeons would operate as soon as convenient, regardless of age. Others operate before discharge from the neonatal intensive care unit. In the survey of the members of the Surgical Section of the American Academy of Paediatrics, there is a trend towards earlier repair. Early repair is justified by the increased risk of incarceration during the waiting period. It has also been suggested that waiting can result in adhesions between the hernia sac and the spermatic cord increasing the risk of damage during the operation. Most of the inguinal hernia operations in older infants and children are done as day-case procedures, except in children with cardiac, respiratory, and other conditions that increase the risk for anaesthetic complications.

In patients presenting with incarceration, reduction is the preferred treatment as long as the patient is stable. The policy of non-operative reduction is based on the following facts: the likelihood of reducing strangulated bowel in infants is extremely high and the complication rate is higher with emergency operations for incarcerated hernia. The infant is placed in Trendelenburg position. This helps to relieve the oedema and allows mild traction on the contents of the hernia. Adequate sedation is given to the infant so as to relax abdominal muscles. If the hernia is not reduced within an hour with these measures, an attempt is made to reduce the hernia with gentle compression, where constant pressure is applied on the fundus of the sac in the direction of the cord. The vast majority of incarcerated hernias reduce with these non-operative measures. After the hernia is reduced, the infant is kept in the hospital and observed. Elective operation is carried out 24–48 h after the reduction when the oedema and swelling has subsided. Failure to reduce the hernia is an indication for emergency operation. These infants have to be stabilised before surgery. Nasogastric suction and correction of fluid end electrolyte balance are undertaken. Antibiotics are given.

51.1.7.1 Anaesthesia

General anaesthesia is required in the majority of infants and children with inguinal hernia. Endotracheal intubation is preferred in small infants. In older infants and children airway management with a mask or laryngeal mask are commonly used alternatives. Premature infants undergoing surgery have an increased risk of life-threatening postoperative apnoea. This risk correlates with postconceptual and gestational age. It has been reported that the risk of postoperative apnoea is less than 1% at a postconceptual age of 54 weeks. Except for age anemia is also an independent risk factor for postoperative apnoea. Regional anaesthesia is commonly used as a supplement to general anaesthesia and to give postoperative pain relief. It has also been shown that regional anaesthesia reduces the risk of postoperative respiratory complications. The most common forms are caudal block or regional nerve blocks, for instance ilioinguinal/iliohypogasric nerve block. Spinal anaesthesia can be an alternative to general anaesthesia in low birth-weight infants undergoing inguinal hernia repair, as it is associated with a lower incidence of postoperative apnoea.

51.1.7.2 Operation

Inguinal herniotomy is the procedure of choice. The operation consists of simple ligation of the hernia sac without opening the external ring. In older children the inguinal canal is longer and it is advisable to open the external oblique aponeurosis to make it possible to ligate the sac high enough. The child is placed in a supine position, infants on a heating blanket. A transverse inguinal skin crease incision is placed above and lateral to the pubic tubercle (Fig. 51.1). The subcutaneous tissue and the fascia of Scarpa are opened until the cord is seen emerging from the external ring (Figs. 51.2 and 51.3). The external spermatic fascia and cremaster are separated along the length of the cord by

blunt dissection. The hernia sac is identified and gently separated from the vas and vessels (Fig. 51.4). A haemostat is placed on the fundus of the sac. The sac is twisted so as to reduce any contents into the abdominal

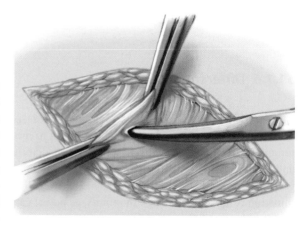

Fig. 51.2   The subcutaneous fat and fascia of Scarpa are opened

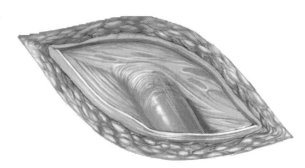

Fig. 51.3   The external inguinal ring is exposed

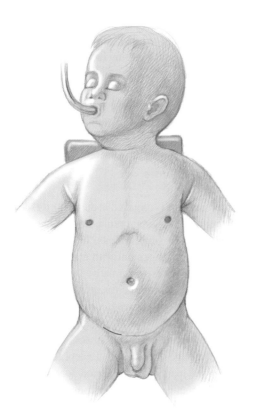

Fig. 51.1   A transverse inguinal skin crease incision is placed above and lateral to the pubic tubercle

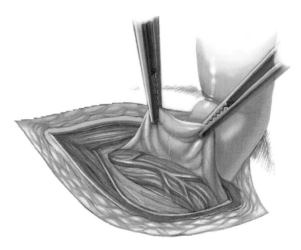

Fig. 51.4   The external spermatic fascia and cremaster are separated along the length of the cord by blunt dissection. The hernia sac is separated from the vas and vessels

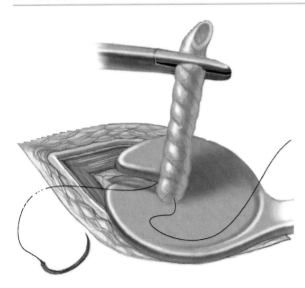

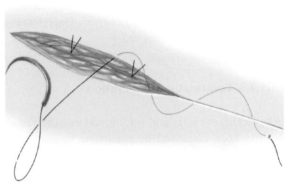

Fig. 51.7 The skin is closed with a continuous subcuticular suture

Fig. 51.5 The sac is transfixed at the level of the internal inguinal ring, which is marked by an extraperitoneal pad of fat

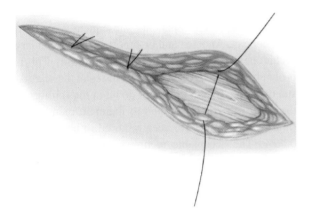

Fig. 51.6 The subcutaneous tissue is approximated with interrupted stitches

cavity. Some surgeons use a spoon to keep the vas and vessels away from the neck of the sac. The sac is transfixed with a 4-0 absorbable suture at the level of the internal ring, which is marked by an extraperitoneal pad of fat. The part of the sac beyond the stitch is excised (Fig. 51.5). 4-0 absorbable sutures, using 2 to 3 interrupted stitches approximate subcutaneous tissues (Fig. 51.6). The skin is closed with a 5-0 monofilament absorbable suture, using a continuous subcuticular stitch (Fig. 51.7). A small dressing is applied to the wound. At the end of the operation the testes must be pulled into the scrotum to avoid iatrogenic ascent of the testis.

Adequate postoperative analgesia is achieved by regional anaesthesia, caudal anaesthesia or ilioinguinal/iliohypogastric nerve block, which is administered either before or at the end of the operation. Feeding is resumed as soon as the child is awake. Most of the infants can be discharged the same day. Infants with a postconceptual age less than approximately 60 weeks are postoperatively monitored for 24 h for because of the risk of apnoeic episodes.

If the hernia is operated as an emergency procedure, the hernia often reduces spontaneously. The sac is then opened and the bowel inspected. If there is no evidence of intestinal ischemia a high ligation of the sac is done as in elective cases. If the are indications of ischemia, such as blood-stained fluid in the sac or if miscoloured bowel is seen through the opened sac, the bowel has to be examined through a laparotomy. If the bowel does not reduce spontaneously; no attempts are made to reduce the hernia when the patient is anesthetised. The sac is opened and the bowel examined. If the bowel is viable, it is reduced. The internal ring is split if this is difficult. On the other hand, if the viability of the bowel is questionable, it is delivered out and warm saline soaks are applied. The intestine is examined after about 5–10 min. If the colour of the intestine returns back to normal with adequate perfusion, peristalsis is visible and mesenteric arterial pulsations are seen, the intestine is returned to the abdomen and a herniotomy performed. If the bowel is non-viable, resection and anastomosis are performed either through the same incision or through a laparotomy. In a large series with 743 incarcerated hernias only two patients required a bowel resection, indicating that this is quite rare. Testes are put in the scrotum irrespective of whether they are normal or ischemic. Only frankly necrotic testes may be removed.

51.1.7.3 Contralateral Exploration

Whether the contralateral side should be explored or not has been discussed by paediatric surgeons for many years. Some surgeons perform a contralateral exploration in premature infants, because of the high incidence of bilateral hernias in this age-group. Others consider contralateral exploration unnecessary as only 5–31% of children will actually develop a metachronous hernia after ipsilateral repair. Except for prematurity, incarceration correlates with a higher risk for development of a contralateral hernia. In a recent survey of the current practice of 395 members of the Surgical Section of the American Academy of Paediatrics 44% reported that they routinely explore the contralateral side in boys less than 2 years of age. Forty-seven percent routinely explore the contralateral side in girls under the age of 4 years. It has been suggested that ultrasound is a good technique to show if there is a patent processus vaginalis on the contralateral side. The advantages are that the diagnostic accuracy is high and that ultrasound is non-invasive. Laparoscopy has also been shown to be a highly sensitive detecting a contralateral patent processus vaginalis. Although a patent processus vaginalis is shown, a majority of patients do not develop a metachronous hernia after ipsilateral repair. Contralateral exploration is therefore not considered to be justified.

51.1.7.4 Laparoscopic Repair of Inguinal Hernia

In recent years laparoscopic repair of inguinal hernias has become an option. Some reports have indicated a high recurrence rate, approximately 4%, which has not been confirmed by others, and longer operating time. One advantage may be the improved cosmetic result and less postoperative pain. Particularly in patients with recurrent hernia or incarcerated hernia laparoscopic repair may be advantageous as it lowers the risk of injury to the vas or testicular atrophy.

51.1.8 Complications

The overall complication rate with elective hernia repair is low, about 2%, while complications are much more frequent, 8–33%, for the incarcerated hernias requiring emergency operations. The most common complications are shown in Table 51.2. Haematomas can be avoided with meticulous attention to haemostasis. Rarely is it necessary to evacuate a haematoma. The wound infection rate is low at approximately 1–1.2% of the cases. Gonadal complications occur due to compression of the vessels. Although a large number of testes look non-viable in patients with incarcerated hernia, the actual incidence of testicular atrophy is low and has been reported to occur in 0.3% of the patients. Therefore, unless the testis is frankly necrotic, it should not be removed. Iatrogenic ascent of the testes is important as it may be avoidable. One investigator showed that at follow-up of 116 patients who had unilateral inguinal herniotomy performed before 6 months of age, three patients subsequently required orchidopexy. Another author reported that secondary orchidopexy was required in 0.5% of the cases. This is probably due to entrapment of the testes in the scar tissue or failure to pull the testes down in the scrotum at the end of the operation and to maintain them there. Injuries to the vas have been reported to be very low, 0.06%. The acceptable recurrence rate for inguinal hernia repair has been considered to be approximately 1%. Most of the recurrences occur within 5 years. The factors which predispose to recurrence are ventriculoperitoneal shunt, sliding hernia, incarceration, and connective tissue disorders. The recurrence may be indirect or direct. Indirect recurrences are due to either failure to ligate the sac at a high level enough, tearing of a friable sac, slipped ligature at the neck of the sac, or a wound infection. Direct hernia may be due to inherent muscle weakness or injury to the posterior wall of the inguinal canal. Today there should be

Table 51.2 Typical complications after hernia repair

Hematoma
Wound infection
Testicular atrophy
Vas injury
Iatrogenic ascent of the testis
Recurrence
Intestinal infarction

virtually no mortality as the result of an operation for inguinal hernia, which is confirmed by large series.

51.2 Congenital Hydrocele

Hydrocele is a common finding in newborn boys. Approximately 70% of the hydroceles are scrotal, 26% are hydroceles of the cord, and 4% are combined hydroceles. In females, an equivalent to hydrocele of the cord may occur as cysts of the canal of Nuck. Sixty percent of the hydroceles are right-sided, 33% are left-sided, and 7% are bilateral. There is consensus that asymptomatic scrotal hydroceles will usually spontaneously disappear during the first 1–2 years of life. Hydroceles that persist after 2 years of age are unlikely to resolve and requires operation. In the survey of North American paediatric surgeons' practice, 42% repair the hydrocele if it persists at 1 year of age. Some surgeons chose to operate communicating hydroceles earlier.

51.2.1 Management

A hydrocele should be operated with a high ligation of the processus vaginalis and emptying of the fluid. The procedure is identical to the operation for an inguinal hernia (Figs. 51.1–51.7).

51.3 Femoral Hernia

Femoral hernias are rarely seen in children. The aetiology is not clear. The diagnosis is based on the observation of a groin swelling located underneath the external inguinal orifice, although this location is easily missed because, unless the bulge is visible upon examination, parents and doctors will interpret its appearance as the expression of an inguinal hernia. This explains why 50% of these patients are mistakenly operated on for inguinal hernia and why, only when the sac is not found, exploration of the femoral area allows diagnosis and repair.

51.3.1 Management

The operative approach for femoral hernia is initially identical to the more commonly used approach for inguinal hernia. An inguinal skin crease incision is made and the subcutaneous layers and fascia of Scarpa are opened in order to expose the external oblique aponeurosis at the level of the external inguinal ring. The aponeurosis is incised longitudinally taking care to preserve the ilioinguinal nerve (Fig. 51.8). The inguinal canal is opened dorsally sectioning with cautery the conjoined tendon and the fascia transversalis. The spermatic cord is retracted in order to obtain access to the femoral region. The sac is identified and delivered into the wound avoiding damage to the femoral vein, which is in close contact with the sac laterally. It may be convenient to ligate and divide the inferior epigastric vessels in order to expose the femoral area from behind (Fig. 51.9). The sac is opened to ensure that it has no contents and it is subsequently suture-ligated with a fine stitch flush to the peritoneum. The femoral defect is then narrowed by approximating the internal insertions of the Cooper ligament and the inguinal ligament with two or three fine non-absorbable stitches taking care of

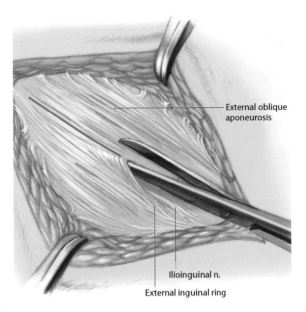

Fig. 51.8 The external oblique aponeurosis is opened laterally from the external ring

not compressing the femoral vessels. The inguinal canal is reconstructed and the superficial layers and the skin are closed as in inguinal hernias (Fig. 51.10). Femoral hernia repair can also be accomplished by an infra-inguinal approach.

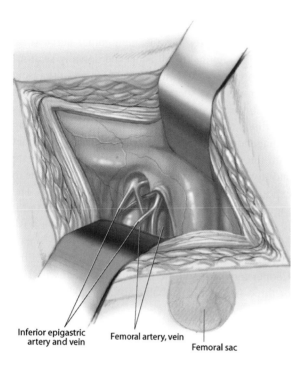

Inferior epigastric artery and vein　　Femoral artery, vein

Femoral sac

Fig. 51.9 The femoral hernia sac is identified medially to the femoral vein

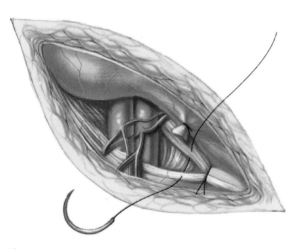

Fig. 51.10 The sac is suture-ligated close to the peritoneum and the inguinal canal is reconstructed

51.4 Umbilical Hernia

Umbilical hernia is the result of failure of closure of the umbilical ring. The hernia sac protrudes through the defect. Symptoms related to the hernia are rare. Most umbilical hernias have a tendency to resolve spontaneously. However hernias with a fascial defect greater than 1.5–2 cm have been considered less likely to close. Surgical intervention is limited to umbilical hernias persisting after 4 years of age. Occasionally incarceration of omentum occurs, which requires exploration

51.4.1 Management

Umbilical hernia repair is carried out under general anaesthesia. A semicircular incision is made in the skin crease immediately below the umbilicus (Fig. 51.11). The subcutaneous layers are dissected in order to expose the hernia sac. By blunt dissection, a plane is developed on both sides of the sac and the sac is encircled with a haemostat and is divided (Fig. 51.12). A clamp is placed on either side of the umbilicus defect for traction. The defect is closed by interrupted 2-0 absorbable sutures. A stitch is

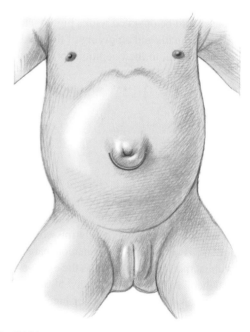

Fig. 51.11 A semicircular incision is made in the skin crease immediately below the umbilicus

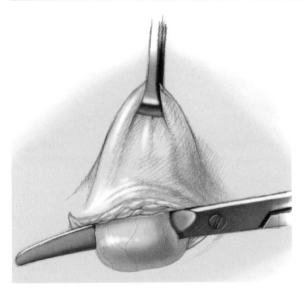

Fig. 51.12   The hernia sac is identified, mobilised, and divided

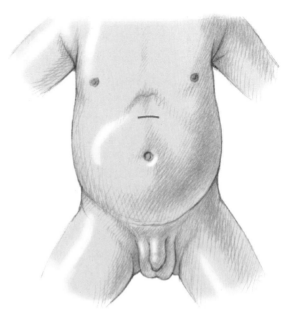

Fig. 51.14   A transverse incision is made over the marked hernia

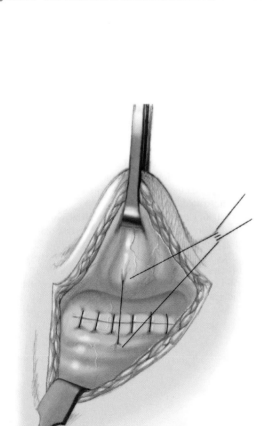

Fig. 51.13   The defect is closed and a stich fixes the umbilicus in the midline

used to invaginate the umbilical scar, tractioning it downwards and fixing it to the subcutaneous layer in the midline (Fig. 51.13). The wound is closed with several interrupted sutures placed in the sub-cuticular plane. A slightly compressive dressing is maintained for 24 h.

51.5 Epigastric Hernia

Epigastric hernia usually occurs in the midline of the anterior abdominal wall. It is usually small defects through which preperitoneal fat protrudes and may cause pain. Epigastric hernias do not resolve spontaneously.

51.5.1 Management

Epigastric hernias are repaired when they are prominent or when they are symptomatic. It is important to mark the location of the defect before anaesthesia, because in the recumbent position they are often impossible to palpate along the widened linea alba. A transverse incision is made directly over the previously marked location of the hernia (Fig. 51.14). The fat that

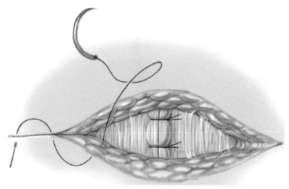

Fig. 51.16 The defect in closed layers

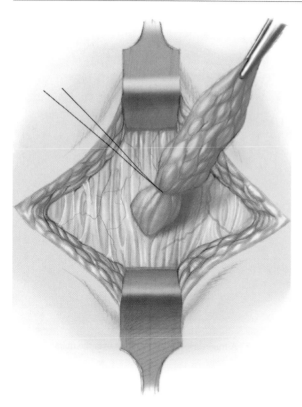

Fig. 51.15 The protruding fat is excised after a transfixation stich

protrudes through the linea alba defect is excised after a transfixation stitch (Fig. 51.15). The defect in the linea alba is closed with interrupted 3-0 absorbable sutures. The skin is approximated using subcuticular sutures (Fig. 51.16).

Further Reading

Antonoff MB, Kreyskes NS, Saltzman DA, et al. (2005) American Academy of Pediatrics Section on Surgery hernia survey revisited. J Pediatr Surg 40:1009–1014

Antonoff MB, Kreyskes NS, Saltzman DA (2005) American Academy of Pediatrics Section on Surgery hernia survey revisited. J Pediatr Surg 40:1009–1014

Ein SH, Njere I, Ein A (2006) Six thousand three hundred sixty-one pediatric inguinal hernias: A 35-year review. J Pediatr Surg 41:980–986

Fasching G, Höllwarth ME (1989) Risk of testicular lesions following incarcerated inguinal hernia in infants. Pediatr Surg Int 4:265–268

Lau ST, Lee Y-H, Caty MG (2007) Current management of hernias and hydroceles. Sem Pediatr Surg 16:50–57

Rintala RJ, Lloyd DA (1998) Inguinal hernia and hydrocele. In JA O'Neill, MI Rowe, JL Grosfeld et al (eds) Pediatric Surgery, 5th edn. Mosby, St. Louis, MO pp 1071–1086

Tovar JA (2003) Inguinal hernia. In P Puri (ed) Newborn Surgery. 2nd edn. Arnold, London, pp 561–568

Tovar JA (2006) Hernias – inguinal, umbilical, epigastric, femoral, and hydrocele. In P Puri, ME Höllwarth (eds) Pediatric Surgery. Springer, Berlin, Heidelberg, pp 139–152

Weber TR, Tracy TF, Keller MS (2005) Groin hernias and hydroceles. In KW Ashcraft, GW Holcomb III, JP Murphy (eds) Pediatric Surgery. 4th edn. Elsevier Saunders, Philadelphia, pp 697–705

Short Bowel Syndrome

52

Michael E. Höllwarth

Contents

52.1 Introduction

The term "*short bowel*" has been defined by Rickham in 1967 as a small intestinal remnant of 75 cm in the newborn, which equals 30% of normal small bowel length in that age group. In premature babies, the term also corresponds to 30% of the total calculated length for a given gestational age (Fig. 52.1). However, the antimesenteric measurement of intestinal length during surgical interventions yields highly variable results due to enormous contractibility of the bowel in length and diameter. Therefore, a more functional description is preferred by most authors defining a state of significant maldigestion and malabsorption due to an extensive loss of functional absorptive intestinal surface area as "*short bowel syndrome*" (SBS). Not included in this chapter are functional cases of SBS with an otherwise normal intestinal length.

In the past, extensive loss of small bowel in newborns and babies used to be a catastrophic event, which was nearly always followed by malnutrition and death. Significant progress was achieved by introducing sophisticated parenteral nutrition in the early 1970s when Wilmore reviewed 50 babies younger than 2 months with SBS. He found that survival was possible with 15 cm jejuno-ileum with ileocecal valve, or with 38 cm jejuno-ileum without ileocecal valve. It must be realized that little progress has been achieved since then: today, long-term survival on enteral nutrition is possible in infants with as little as 10 cm jejuno-ileum with ileocecal valve (5% of total), or with 25 cm jejuno-ileum without ileocecal valve (10% of total).

P. Puri and M. Höllwarth (eds.), *Pediatric Surgery: Diagnosis and Management,*
DOI: 10.1007/978-3-540-69560-8_52, © Springer-Verlag Berlin Heidelberg 2009

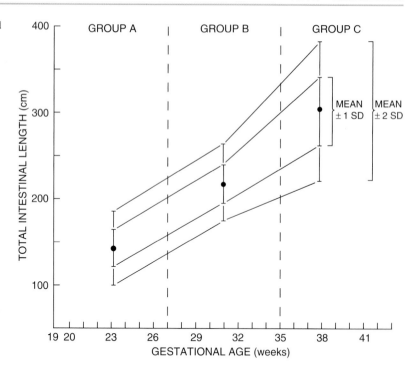

Fig. 52.1 Normal intestinal length and the ranges in premature babies (From Touloukian and Smith 1983. With permission)

52.2 Incidence and Aetiology

It has been estimated that severe SBS cases remaining dependent on long-term home parenteral nutritional support amount to two new patients per one million of population/year (including all age groups). The incidence of extreme SBS in the neonatal age group lies around 3–5/100,000 birth/year. The prevalence of SBS has been increasing over the last 2 decades, since enormous progress of intensive care medicine has significantly improved the initial prognosis of babies with severe intestinal disease and/or following major surgery.

In infancy, most cases of SBS occur in the neonatal age group. There are many different causes, which can be divided into three major groups. The first of these consists of neonates with prenatally acquired anomalies characterized by a vascular injury to the intestinal tract in utero, e.g. multiple intestinal atresias or gastroschisis with intrauterine volvulus of the prolapsed bowel. The second group comprises postnatally acquired diseases necessitating extensive intestinal resection, e.g. necrotizing enterocolitis or volvulus. A third group is defined by a genetically determined deficiency, e.g. in the embryological small bowel anlage causing a

Table 52.1 Causes of SBS in over 100 newborn babies collected from the literature

Necrotizing enterocolitis	36%
Volvulus	19%
Intestinal atresia	21%
Gastroschisis and atresia	10%
Hirschsprung's disease	7%
Trauma	1%
Others	6%

"true" congenital short bowel, or in its innervation, such as total intestinal aganglionosis (Table 52.1). Extensive intestinal resection leading to SBS is rarely required in older children. Indications may be severe Crohn's disease, traumatic avulsion of the intestinal tract and/or traumatic or iatrogenic mesenteric artery lesions.

52.3 Pathology

Following extensive loss of small bowel, the symptoms of an individual patient depend on the absorptive capacities as well as on inborn characteristics of the remaining bowel. In normal human individuals, most of the nutrients are digested and absorbed within the first part of the jejunum. After ingestion of food, luminal isotonicity is rapidly achieved in the upper jejunum either by water secretion (hypertonic meal) or water absorption (hypotonic meal). An isotonic aqueous medium is essential for proper digestion and absorption. However, the capacity of water and electrolyte absorption in SBS patients does not depend on the residual amount of small intestine alone, but also to a great extent on the presence or absence of colon as well.

Resection of the jejunum induces only a transient reduction of absorption of all nutrients due to an enormous adaptive capacity of the ileum, the intact enterohepatic circulation of bile salts and the preserved absorption of vitamin B_{12}. A minimum of ileum with at least 10–15 cm and the presence of the ileocecal valve are required that passage time allows at least partial absorption of bile salts, vitamins and nutrients. Therefore, despite different opinions in the literature, recent publications clearly show that the presence of an ileocecal valve has a beneficial effect on the outcome.

More serious consequences result from *resection of the ileum*. The ileum is responsible for absorbing all the water that has been secreted in the upper intestinal tract following a hypertonic meal. If the ileum is resected, this water spills over into the colon. Although the colon can increase water and solute absorption up to 400% of normal, there is a limit to the excess that may be reabsorbed. Another consequence of ileal resection is life-long malabsorption of vitamin B_{12} due to loss of site-specific receptors. Furthermore, the ileum is the major site of bile acid absorption. Nonabsorbed intestinal contents including bile acids spill over into the colon and may cause significant diarrhoea. Furthermore, loss of the ileum results in a depletion of the bile salt pool leading to a disturbed micelle formation, malabsorption of fat and fat soluble vitamins (A, E, D, and K). In consequence, hydrolyzed fatty acids and bile salts reach the colon. The former bind to calcium to form calcium stearate, preventing calcium absorption. Subsequently, oxalate—which is normally excreted with the faeces bound to intraluminal calcium—gets absorbed in increased amounts, leading to oxaluria and eventually kidney stone formation. Similarly due to the consumption of enteric calcium by undigested fatty acids, the deconjugated enteric bilirubin remains in solution resulting in a significant enterohepatic circulation of unconjugated bilirubin and increased secretion rates of bilirubin in the bile

responsible for biliary sludge formation and gallstone diseases in SBS patients.

Furthermore, resection of the ileum results in a loss of the 'ileal brake'. Consequently nutrients spend less time in the stomach and in the upper intestinal segments. Due to the shorter contact, digestion and absorption is reduced, and an unusual large fluid load imposed onto the distal remnants.

Intestinal adaptation is the term which characterizes the pathophysiology which follows intensive intestinal resection, and by which 90% of babies with SBS do finally reach a normal life on entirely oral nutrition. Adaptation is characterized by an early increase of blood flow to the intestinal remnants and by long-term stimulation of intestinal growth, which enormously enlarges the absorptive surface area. The latter includes an increase in villous height, crypt depth, intestinal length, thickness and diameter. Additionally, water and solute absorption is enhanced in the colon, colonic bacteria ferment undigested carbohydrates and proteins into short chain fatty acids, which act as important energy providers and apparently, as additional promoters of adaptation.

The precise mechanisms of adaptation are not clear, but intraluminal nutrients and endogenous intestinal secretions stimulate growth. In general, the higher the workload required for digestion and absorption, the more potent is the stimulus for adaptation.

In response of the nutrients and secretions a large number of trophic polypeptides and other mediators are secreted. Over the years, some of them have attracted attention regarding their possible clinical value in promoting adaptation in SBS patients. First, Gastrin was demonstrated to exhibit trophic effects on the small bowel. Later, enteroglucagon has been shown to stimulate the adaptive response on the intestinal tract in animal experiments and humans. Since monoclonal antibodies failed to block this trophic effect, recently precursors of enteroglucagon such as glucagon-like peptide 2 (GLP-2) are considered to be responsible for the intestinal effects. Limited studies have shown an increase in weight gain and energy absorption with GLP-2 administration after ileocecal resection in humans. Lately, human growth hormone (GH) in combination with epidermal growth factor, or with insulin-like growth factor-I (IGF-I) have been shown to regulate small intestinal growth and adaptation. IGF-I receptors have been identified in all segments of the gastrointestinal tract, and IGF-I stimulates

DNA and RNA synthesis and cellular amino acid uptake. The endogenous GH-IGF-I system is supposed to be an important regulator of small intestinal growth and adaptation. Among the amino acids, glutamine (GL) plays a key role in the maintenance of intestinal structure and function by providing the energy required by cells with a rapid turnover, such as macrophages and enterocytes. Patients after major trauma or in chronic catabolic states benefit from GL supplementation. It has been shown that human growth hormone increases glutamine uptake after intestinal resection, supporting the evidence that glutamine exerts trophic effects in the small intestine and colon of patients with SBS. More research however is needed, since other studies could not confirm a role for GL or GH as trophic agents for the intestinal tract. Thus, it remains controversial, whether or not GL alone or supplementation of GL and GH, or other trophic factors or hormones should be recommended for the treatment of SBS. There is a need for more controlled clinical trials in order to elaborate which agents have a lasting impact on intestinal adaptation and prove beneficial for the long-term.

Prostaglandin (Pg) E2 and polyamines have also been shown to stimulate cell proliferation in animal experiments by increasing blood flow and DNA synthesis. Experimental evidence exists that testosterone enhances adaptation after small bowel resection in cats.

52.4 Medical Therapy

The clinical course of SBS can be divided into three stages which require individual management: the acute phase, the adaptation phase, and the maintenance phase. The *acute phase*—the duration of which depends on the underlying disease—is characterized by insufficient absorption, dysmotility, diarrhoea, and gastric hypersecretion and hypergastremia. Therapeutic measures are guided by the underlying disease and the severity of illness of the patient. They are primarily aimed at restoring and maintaining fluid, electrolyte and acid-base equilibrium. The following *adaptation phase* is slower in humans compared to animals and often takes more than a year to reach its peak—unrelated to the absolute length of intestinal remnants. Treatment strategies during this phase include

parenteral nutrition and carefully balanced, stepwise increasing enteral feeding. Diligence and patience are necessary prerequisites to reach the maximum of what can be achieved in a given patient. Finally follows the *maintenance phase* in patients with a constant malabsorption rate of 30% or more, during which a surplus of enteral calories has to be consumed daily, supplemented by vitamins, trace elements and minerals, adapted to the individual demands.

Balanced fluid and electrolyte solutions must cover the basic demands and replace losses via a nasogastric tube, from an enterostomy, or due to excessive diarrhoea. Existing nutritional deficiencies should be restored by adequate supplementation of carbohydrates, protein, and fat. Calorie intake in children needs to be continuously advanced to accommodate the increasing demands of the growing organism. Growth in weight, height and head circumference are the basic parameters to ensure adequacy of parenteral nutritional solutions and enteral feeding. In newborns an infusion running continuously over 24 h is most appropriate. In contrast, when infants take at least 20% of their total calorie requirements by the enteral route, intermittent parenteral feeding can be attempted and the intervals increased as long as serum glucose levels are maintained. In the older age groups and in adults, a 12-h infusion time is usually well tolerated. Finally, parenteral nutrition can be restricted to the nocturnal period. The possibility of home parenteral nutrition considerably improves the quality of life for the patients and their families allowing a more normal lifestyle, and substantially reduces hospital costs.

Enteral feeding is usually introduced by continuous infusion via a gastric or jejunal tube as soon as the intestinal remnants resume normal motility. This technique avoids gastric distension and offers a constant load of carrier proteins to the microvilli. Elemental diets are started in a low concentration and are slowly increased to 0.67 kcal/ml in infants, and 1.0 kcal/ml in children and adults. High carbohydrate content represents a substantial osmotic load and may cause diarrhoea. A stool volume, which increases by >50% compared to baseline, is an indication to reduce the amount and/or concentration of enteral feedings. Stool samples positive for reducing substances also suggest that enteral feeding should not be advanced and carbohydrate uptake should be reduced. In infants with normal colon length, a decrease of stool pH below 5.5 signals carbohydrate malabsorption. Protein hydrolysate diets are beneficial due to their higher content of di- and tripeptides. In infants up to 6 months, protein containing diets might cause a protein sensitive enteritis/ allergy. Therefore, amino acid formulas are preferred. Medium chain triglycerides are water soluble and can be absorbed without the need for bile acid micelle formation, but their efficiency in enhancing the adaptation process is far lower in comparison to long-chain fatty acids. Therefore, elemental diets in paediatrics contain both medium and long-chain fatty acids, the mixture probably being the most efficacious for stimulation of adaptation. As soon as the neonate's condition improves, oral feeding of small amounts of breast milk three or four times daily should be attempted so that the child learns to suck, taste, chew and swallow properly with the aim of avoiding the problem of total refusal of any oral intake, not infrequently encountered after long-term total parenteral nutrition (TPN) and enteral tube feeding.

Blood levels of vitamins, trace elements and minerals must be checked regularly and any deficient substance has to be supplemented either orally or parenterally as appropriate. Dietary modifications are recommended depending on the individual situations. Patients suffering from SBS with the colon intact benefit from a high fibre intake because the colon is capable of fermenting carbohydrates. On the contrary, patients who have had the large bowel removed or excluded may fare better with a diet rich in fat providing a high energy concentration and a relatively low osmotic load. In animal experiments, triglycerides with highly unsaturated long-chain fatty acids such as menhaden oil have exerted more trophic effects on the intestinal remnants after resection than other long-chain fatty acid containing oils. In addition, recent studies in rats have shown that SCFA (w-3 fatty acids) supplementation of TPN enhances morphological and functional aspects of adaptation. From these results, one can speculate the further modifications of TPN formulas for humans might stimulate intestinal adaptation even before the introduction of enteral feeding.

Gastric hyperchlorhydria during the early phase after extensive loss of intestine can be suppressed successfully either with H2 receptor antagonists or with proton pump inhibitors, thereby improving absorption and reducing high output diarrhoea. Rapid intestinal transit can be slowed by opioid medication. In this group loperamide has proved effective and safe to use in the paediatric age group even over a long period of time. Octreotide acetate, a somatostatin analogue, which essentially inhibits all exocrine and endocrine gastrointestinal secretions, is apt to improve quality of life in patients with predominantly secretory losses, and has been judged beneficial in patients on long-term treatment. Unfortunately, it has more side effects in comparison to loperamide and is rather expensive. Interference with the adaptation process has been discussed, but recent work has not supported this fear. Cholestyramine binds bile acids and prevents choleretic diarrhoea induced by an excess of bile salts in the colon. While thus reducing diarrhoea, it may increase steaforrhoea. Ursodeoxycholic acid is known to counteract hepatic damage by restricting the absorption of potentially toxic bile acid metabolites from the colon. Of course, the latter considerations only apply if the colon is present. In patients with ileal resection but an intact colon, urinary oxalate levels should be monitored. Dietary oxalate restriction is to be recommended in patients with high levels of oxaluria. A surplus of calcium ingestion provides additional oxalate binding capacity. In order to avoid metabolic bone disease, calcium, vitamin D, and alkaline phosphatase levels in the serum should also be checked periodically, as well as other fat soluble vitamins, and vitamin B12 if the terminal ileum is lacking.

52.5 Surgical Therapy

A variety of surgical procedures to lengthen intestinal transit time have been invented and applied in humans. Reversed (antiperistaltic) intestinal segments (Fig. 52.2) have been used in over 40 patients, and in most of them a delay of chyme transport was achieved and increased absorption documented. However, all of these reports are anecdotal, and so far it remains uncertain whether these effects will be maintained. Intestinal valves and sphincters have been created in a few humans, mostly children, with doubtful results. A segment of colon can be interposed in the small bowel, more proximally in the isoperistaltic direction, or in an antiperistaltic manner distally (Fig. 52.3). Dilated intestinal loops with inefficient peristalsis and stagnant chyme are a common problem in patients with SBS, either as a consequence of the underlying pathology, e.g. remnants after multiple atresias, or following initially effective adaptive growth that finally overshoots to

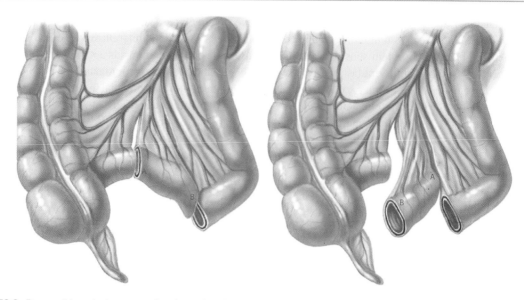

Fig. 52.2 Reversed intestinal segment aimed to reduce intestinal transit time. Appropriate length in newborn babies about 3 cm

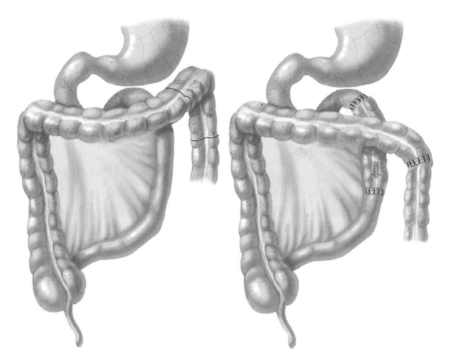

Fig. 52.3 Colon interposition can be used in an isoperistaltic manner to increase absorption and in the antiperistaltic manner the decrease transit time. The method has been used only in a few patients

result in large dilated bowel segments with insufficient and undirected motility. Bianchi introduced a very interesting procedure consisting of longitudinal division of the dilated part into two separate segments each comprising one half of the circumference. Both segments remain viable because the mesenteric vessels divide extramurally into branches supplying either side of the bowel separately. The two halves are then refashioned to tubes of normal intestinal diameter, which are lined up in the isoperistaltic direction and anastomosed one

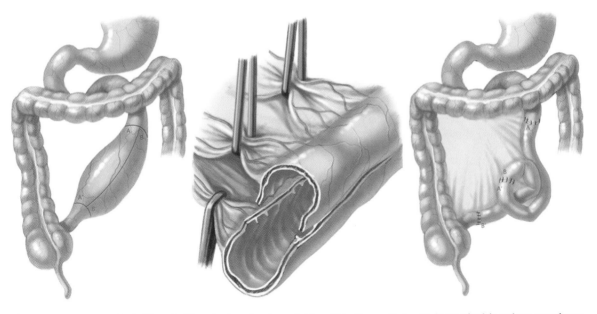

Fig. 52.4 Bianchi's method of intestinal lengthening aimed to refashion dilated loop with insufficient peristalsis and stagnant chyme

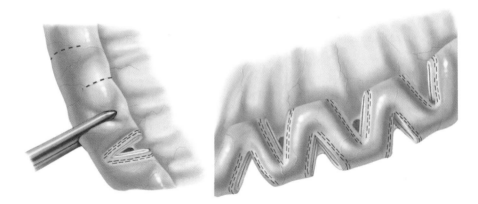

Fig. 52.5 The effects of serial transverse enteroplasty (STEP) is aimed to improve insufficient peristalsis and digestion

to the other yielding twice the length of the original part (Fig. 52.4). Although this technique has used in a larger number of patients, it has only proved successful when performed in a later stage of the disease, on so called "self-selected survivors", i.e. patients in stable general condition free of other severe complications such as liver insufficiency.

Serial transverse enteroplasty (STEP) (Fig. 52.5) is a new procedure that gained significant attention worldwide as a method to refashion dilated intestinal loops thereby improving peristalsis and motility. It is technically much easier when compared with the Bianchi method. First experiences show that the complication rate of the procedure is low and early outcome is encouraging. However, long-term results are still needed.

Intestinal refashioning can be achieved surgically by tailoring the antimesenteric side of a dilated loop, either by resection of abundant wall—provided that enough absorptive area remains available and stasis is the only problem—or by infolding the excessive part of the intestinal circumference in a longitudinal way (Fig. 52.6).

The most effective method to increase the absorptive area is intestinal transplantation (TPX) either

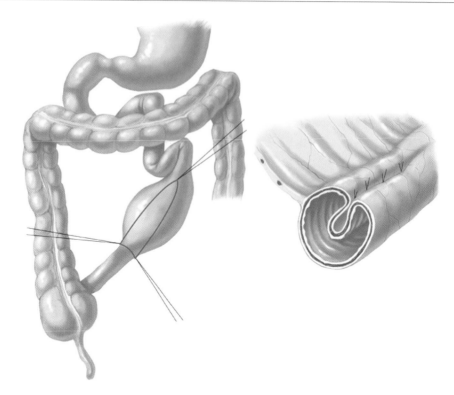

Fig. 52.6 Circumscript dilated instestinal loop can be refashioned by infolding the excessive part of the gut without losing absorptive area

with or without the liver. Indication for isolated intestinal TPX is given in infants with very little or no small bowel at all who are expected to always be dependent on TPN, and/or failure of venous access. Indication for combined TPX is intestinal failure together with progressive liver failure and recurrent sepsis. In the past, the results of intestinal TPX have been poor, mainly due to high rejection rate. Recently, significant progress has been achieved by introduction of new immunosuppressive agents (tacrolimus, evarolimus, OKT 3) and induction therapy (daclizumab, thymoglobulin), however 5-year survival rates of the grafts or the patients currently is still only 50%.

52.6 Complications

Despite the progress in intensive care medicine and long-term parenteral nutrition, many complications do occur in patients with SBS, some of which are life threatening. Among the most important ones are central venous catheter related problems, liver failure, and bacterial overgrowth and translocation.

Infections related to the central venous line have two major pathways, an external and an internal route. Today, bacterial contamination of the infusion solution has been virtually eliminated by developing detailed practice guidelines for aseptic care. However, bacteria may enter via the exit side and expand along the central venous line into the circulation. Colonisation of the catheter, especially by staphylococcus epidermidis, is highly resistant to antibiotic treatment as long as the foreign body is not removed. The incidence of this problem has been greatly reduced by using special ports, which are implanted subcutaneously for patients on home parenteral nutrition. In contrast, endogenous infections caused by continuous or intermittent bacteraemia from a distant focus, impose a significant problem and have gained increased attention. In this regard, bacterial translocation from the gut (BT) is being recognized as a major source of infection in a large variety of diseases including motility disorders and cholestasis. Over two thirds of systemic infections in neonates and infants on TPN are caused by germs which are normally encountered in the intestine. A variety of therapeutic options are available to reduce the incidence of endogenous catheter infection, either by medical or surgical improvement of gut motility or by intermittent decontamination of the gut with antibiotics and/or probiotic nutritional therapy.

Long-term parenteral nutrition is well known to cause liver steatosis in older children and adults. Steatosis may be directly related to the delivery of an inappropriate carbohydrate load and excess of calories. The course is usually uncomplicated with mild and often transient bilirubin and liver enzyme elevations, and recovery of hepatic function occurs once more than 50% of calorie intake is tolerated enterally. More *serious hepatic dysfunction* and cholestasis is mainly observed in infants. The severity of this complication is inversely related to the gestational age and birth weight and directly related to the number of septic episodes. The pathomechanism of cholestasis and biliary tract sludge—inspissated bile syndrome—in newborns and small infants with SBS may be related to enterohepatic cycling of bilirubin and high bilirubin concentration in bile. The problem is aggravated by TPN because direct toxic effects on the liver are attributed to the composition of parenteral solutions. Some damage to the liver may be caused by certain amino acids or lipids, whether administered parenterally or enterally (Glycin, Phytosterols). On the other side deficiency of specific amino acids such as taurin, serine or methionine may exert toxic effects on the hepatocytes. Bacterial driven bile salt deconjugation results in increased amounts of secondary bile salts such as desoxycholic or lithocholic acid, which are absorbed in the colon and impair bile flow. Ursodesoxycholic acid therapy replaces more harmful bile acids and reduces cholestasis according to experimental and clinical studies. Furthermore, it has been shown that all catheter infections are associated with a rise in bilirubin. Hepatic failure can be prevented experimentally by selective decontamination of the bowel and by binding endotoxin.

Stasis of nutrients and secretions due to insufficient propulsive peristalsis in dilated intestinal loops allows bacterial overgrowth despite an apparently short transit time. *Bacterial translocation* (BT) is the major harmful consequence of bacterial overgrowth. Intestinal motility, gastric acidity, the intact mucus layer, secretory IgA, and the ileocecal valve are supposed to be factors preventing bacterial overgrowth (Table 52.2). While under normal circumstances BT to mesenteric lymph nodes takes place at a rate of 5–8%, it increases up to 10-fold and systemic spread occurs if the mucosal

Table 52.2 Factors preventing bacterial translocation from the gut to the liver and circulation

1. Endogenous factors
Secretions: saliva
Gastric acidity
Pancreatic enzymes
Bile
Mucous
Intestinal motility
Ileocecal valve
Hormones
2. Immunologic factors
Secretory IgA
Other immunoglobulins
Mucosal mast cell system
3. Exogenous factors
Enteral nutrition
Breast milk factors (IgA, macrophages, lactoferrin, etc.)
Glutamine

barrier function is impaired and bacterial overgrowth prevails. If the predominant species are lactobacilli the resulting massive lactate production decreases intraluminal pH and causes L-lactic and D-lactic absorption. The latter is poorly metabolized and may be responsible for recurrent episodes of acidosis and coma. Elevated D-lactate in serum or urine can be used for diagnosis of lactobacilli overgrowth.

52.7 Prognosis

The mainstay of the treatment of a newborn or child with a SBS consists of a sophisticated enteral stimulation with an individually balanced nutritional equilibrium between carbohydrates, proteins and fatty acids. The enteral nutrition is the best stimulus for adaptation. The use of additional hormonal therapies has not yet been proved sufficiently by controlled studies. Patient age and adjusted length of intestinal remnant are considered to have the up-most impact on survival and disposition to complications (Table 52.3). Cholestasis ≥ 2.5 mg/dl has been identified as the complication with the strongest predictive value of mortality. One hundred percent of survival has been reported in children at or above 2 years of age while survival rates in newborn babies are around 75–83%. Approximately 20% of newborns with SBS will not reach infancy due to progressive liver failure, recurrent episodes of

Table 52.3 Factors which minimize the risk of complications

1. Control small bowel bacterial overgrowth
2. Pursue enteral feedings aggressively
3. Prevent catheter sepsis
4. Use appropriate nutrient mixture and amino acid solution at the correct dose
5. Cycle parenteral nutrition
6. Monitor for cholelithiasis

catheter sepsis, or from other causes. Some of them may benefit from intestinal TPX.

The length of the small bowel remnant—at least ≥10% of expected length—and the presence or absence of the ileocecal valve influences the time needed for weaning from parenteral nutrition. Crucial for a successful weaning is the presence of a good propulsive intestinal motility—with or without adjunct surgical measures. Approximately 10% of patients will benefit from surgical interventions, which are indicated only in some individual as a helpful adjunct therapy, either by prolongation of transit time or by remodelling parts of the intestine. However, even after successful weaning from parenteral nutrition some of these patients may suffer continuously from nutritional and digestive problems and may come after years to intestinal TPX due to insufficient absorption of nutrients.

Further Reading

Bianchi A (1997) Longitudinal intestinal lengthening and tailoring: Results in 20 children. JRSM 90:429–432

Goulet O, Baglin-gobet S, Talbotec C (2005) Outcome and long-term growth after extensive small bowel resection in the neonatal period: A survey of 87 children. Eur J Paediatr Surg 15:95–101

Hoellwarth ME (1999) Short bowel syndrome: Pathophysiology and clinical aspects. Pathophysiology 6:1–19

Höllwarth ME (2006) Short Bowel Syndrome. In P Puri, ME Höllwarth (eds) Pediatric Surgery. Springer Surgery Atlas Series, Springer-Verlag Berlin Heidelberg, New York, pp 257–274

Modi BP, Javid PJ, Jaksic T (2007) First report of the international serial transverse enteroplasty data registry: Indications, efficacy, and complications. Am Col Surg 204:365–371

Puri P, Höllwarth M (2006) Pediatric Surgery. Springer, Berlin, Heidelberg, pp. 257–274

SpencerAU, Neaga A, West B et al (2005) Pediatric short bowel syndrome. Redefining predictors of success. Ann Surg 242:403–409

Sudan D, Dibaise J, Torres C (2005) A multidisciplinary approach to the treatment of intestinal failure. Gastrointest Surg 9:165–176

Touloukian RJ, Smith GJ (1983) Normal intestinal length in preterm infants. J Paediatr Surg 18(6):720–723

Inflammatory Bowel Disease

53

Risto J. Rintala and Mikko P. Pakarinen

Contents

53.1 Ulcerative Colitis

53.1.1 Introduction

Ulcerative colitis (UC) is an inflammatory bowel disease of unknown etiology confined to rectum and colon. Males and females are equally affected. The incidence of UC (>10/100,000) is highest in the Nordic countries, in the British Isles and in the North America. About 5% of all cases of UC have their onset before the age of 10 years and about 20% before the age of 20 years. The incidence of paediatric cases has remained unchanged after 1980s.

53.1.2 Etiology

The etiology of UC is unknown and most likely multifactorial. Various potential contributing factors have been studied including environmental factors, infections, psychosocial factors, immunological factors and genetic factors. There is a clear inherited predilection for UC with 20% chance of UC in identical twins. No specific gene locus has been identified. It has been postulated that some inherited defect(s) in the immunoregulation may lead to clinical manifestation of the disease in certain environmental conditions including infective agents.

53.1.3 Pathology

UC is a chronic inflammatory disease of the rectum and colon affecting mucosa and submucosa of the bowel wall. The rectum is affected in more than 95%

P. Puri and M. Höllwarth (eds.), *Pediatric Surgery: Diagnosis and Management*,
DOI: 10.1007/978-3-540-69560-8_53, © Springer-Verlag Berlin Heidelberg 2009

of the cases and the inflammation extends contiguously to the more proximal large bowel. In children, UC is more aggressive and the entire colon is involved (pancolitis) more often than in adult patients. Ileal involvement strongly suggests Crohn's disease, although low grade unspecific inflammation of the ileal mucosa is often seen in patients with UC known as *backwash ileitis*.

The characteristic histological appearance of UC consists of diffuse superficial unspecific inflammation, neutrophilic epithelial invasion, crypt abscesses and crypt deformity. Progression of inflammation leads to mucosal ulceration and epithelial regeneration with pseudopolyp formation. Long-standing disease is associated with atrophic and dysplastic mucosa. The risk of colon cancer associated with UC is of special concern in paediatric patients and has been estimated as 1–3% 10 years after onset of the disease after which the risk is increased by 1–1.5% after every year.

53.1.4 Diagnosis

The diagnosis of UC is based on endoscopic findings and in particular histological examination of the colonic and ileal biopsy specimen.

53.1.4.1 Clinical Features

Bloody mucous diarrhoea is the cardinal symptom of UC. Other common presenting symptoms and signs include abdominal pain, tenesmus, fever, weight loss, poor appetite, growth retardation, malnutrition, delayed sexual maturation and iron deficiency anemia secondary to chronic intestinal bleeding. Other laboratory findings include increased blood sedimentation rate and fecal calprotectin concentration. Extraintestinal manifestations of UC may affect joints (arthralgias and arthritis), skin (erythema nodosum, pyoderma gangrenosum), skeleton (decreased bone density), eyes (uveitis) and hepatobiliary system (primary sclerosing cholangitis, autoimmune hepatitis).

53.1.4.2 Endoscopic Diagnosis

In addition to colonoscopy extending to the distal ileum, endoscopic work up should also include endoscopy

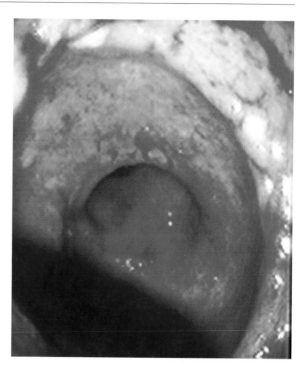

Fig. 53.1 Endoscopic view of fulminant acute ulcerative colitis

of the upper gastrointestinal tract in children. All the endoscopic examinations can be performed during the same anesthesia and multiple biopsies should be obtained. Characteristic macroscopic colonoscopy findings in UC include loss of vascular patterns, hyperemia, contact bleeding, exudates, ulcerations, denuation of the mucosa in some areas and pseudopolyps (Fig. 53.1). In chronic disease, normal colonic haustral folds disappear and mucosa becomes flat and featureless. Inflammation is typically diffuse and most severe in the distal colon and rectum. Pancolitis is common in children with UC. Mucosal granularity in the terminal ileum due to lymphonodular hyperplasia is normal finding in children and should not be confused with ileal inflammation. Excluding *backwash ileitis* any signs of extracolonic inflammation (ileum and/or upper gastrointestinal tract) should raise suspicion of Crohn's disease.

53.1.4.3 Microscopic Findings

Intestinal inflammation in UC is usually confined to mucosa and submucosa. Deeper layers may be affected in fulminant disease. Histology of the colonic biopsies in active UC shows mucosal neutrophil infiltration, goblet cell mucus depletion, crypt abscesses and crypt deformity. Although the mucosa may return to nearly normal in remission, cryptal deformity usually remains.

53.1.4.4 Differential Diagnosis

From a surgical point of view the major differential diagnosis of UC is Crohn's disease. Before any surgical therapy is undertaken Crohn's disease should be ruled out by every possible measure. These include small bowel follow through radiograph, capsule endoscopy of the small intestine and explorative laparoscopy in selected cases as well as advanced serologic investigations. It should be borne in mind that Crohn's disease may affect the entire gastrointestinal tract from mouth to anus. Clinical findings suggestive of Crohn's disease are weight loss, fever, lesions of the buccal mucosa and perianal disease. In colonoscopy segmental inflammation, stricture, fistulas and spared rectum also point to Crohn's disease. Focal inflammation extending beyond submucosa and granulomas are histological findings associated with Crohn's disease. Despite extensive investigations in up to 5–15% of children with UC the diagnosis is eventually changed to Crohn's disease. On the other hand, around 10–15% of all children with inflammatory bowel disease have colitis initially designated as *indeterminate colitis* because its shares features of both UC and Crohn's disease.

53.1.5 Medical Management

The main goals of the treatment are to alleviate symptoms, to provide normal growth and development and to avoid disease-related long-term complications. Children often present with widespread disease and pancolitis necessitating aggressive medical treatment. If patients are significantly malnourished or when there is growth retardation, intensive nutritional support is provided. Parenteral nutrition is very seldom indicated.

Corticosteroids are usually needed to control the initial disease. Remission is maintained with sulfasalazine and 5-aminosalisylic acid. However, a significant proportion of children with UC require high-dose systemic corticosteroids or, in selected cases other powerful immunomodulatory drugs (azathioprine, methotrexate, cyclosporine, tacrolimus, infliximab) to control the disease and prevent recurrences. The side-effects of these immunosuppressive preparations and high-dose systemic corticosteroid treatment on a growing and developing body are significant.

53.2 Surgical Management

Between 40% and 70% of children with UC undergo surgical treatment. In children UC is more aggressive than in adults. However, surgery should not be considered as a first-line treatment of UC. A significant proportion of patients achieves long-term symptom relief with conservative treatment and may remain in remission with minimal or no medication. Moreover, the functional outcome following restorative procto-colectomy is not comparable with normal bowel function.

53.2.1 Indications for Operative Treatment

The main indications for surgical treatment of UC are chronic persisting symptoms despite optimal medical therapy and corticosteroid dependency. The risk for colonic dysplasia and carcinoma may influence the decision to undergo colectomy.

53.2.2 Emergency Operation

As most patients can be stabilized by medical treatment, emergency operations for toxic megacolon and fulminant colitis as well as persistent colonic bleeding are rare today. In these cases the recommended operative approach is subtotal colectomy, closure of the rectal stump and end ileostomy. The restorative procto colectomy can be completed safely after few months when the patient has fully recovered and weaned of systemic immunosuppressive medication.

53.2.3 Restorative Proctocolectomy

Since the late 1970s restorative proctocolectomy with ileoanal anastomosis has gained worldwide acceptance as the standard operative procedure for adult and also pediatric patients with UC. Restorative proctocolectomy is a major operation with significant incidence of postoperative complications. Septic complications are the most common ones. In order to minimize the incidence of postoperative septic complications it is imperative that systemic corticosteroids are tapered preoperatively to as low as possible or, if possible, changed to locally acting budesonide with less systematic immunosuppressive effect. The nutritional status should also be optimized well before elective operation. This is usually possible by dietary measures, but parenteral nutritional support should be promptly used when indicated. Before the operation, the child and the parents should be openly informed about expected outcome and potential complications. The site of the covering loop ileostomy in the right lower abdominal quadrant should be marked preoperatively when the patient is sitting.

Restorative proctocolectomy consists of removal of the colon and rectum, ileal pull-through and ileoanal anastomosis. Most pediatric surgeons use an ileal reservoir; the most popular and the easiest to construct is the J-pouch (Fig. 53.2). The ileoanal anastomosis may be hand sewn necessitating mucosectomy. In this case the entire colonic mucosa is removed excluding about 5 mm of the anal transitional epithelium above the dentate line, which is saved for its critical function in anal sensation. Some surgeons prefer the use of circular stapler devices leaving several centimetres of rectal mucosa in situ. The latter practice is easier and faster to perform due to avoidance of mucosectomy and lesser anastomotic tension and it may be associated with less pelvic septic complications. Importantly, these children require life-long surveillance of the remaining rectal mucosa for dysplastic changes. The colectomy part of the operation may be performed laparoscopically.

In selected cases proctocolectomy with ileoanal anastomosis can be performed as a single procedure, although most pediatric surgeons employ a temporary covering ileostomy. A diverting ileostomy minimizes the risk of pouch leak and pelvic septic complications. The covering ileostomy may be closed after 2–4 months. Before the ileostomy closure a distal loopogram with pressure is performed to assess the integrity of the ileoanal anastomosis and the J-pouch. Recovery of patient's own cortisol production should also be confirmed before the ileostomy closure. Occasionally it is beneficial to perform the operation in three stages. In these cases the patient cannot be weaned from high-dose systemic corticosteroid treatment, the complications of long-term corticosteroid treatment have developed and there is a significant additional illness such as diabetes mellitus.

53.2.4 Postoperative Bowel Function

The immediate postoperative period is characterized by loose and frequent bowel movements up to 10–12 times per 24 h. Low residue lactose-free diet and dietary salt supplementation aid to decrease stomal output and increase stool consistency after closure of the ileostomy. Urinary sodium concentration should be kept above 20 mmol/l. Antipropulsive medication (loperamide) is also beneficial during adaptation period. Within following 3–6 months the frequency of bowel movements usually decreases to 2–7 per 24 h. The average long-term frequency of bowel movements is around four and five. A few patients will suffer from night-time soiling/staining that may require protective pads.

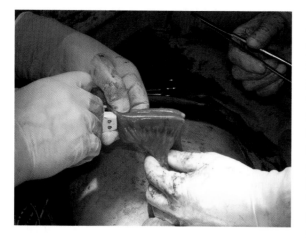

Fig. 53.2 Construction of a J-pouch by using a linear stapler

53.2.5 Complications

Early and late complications occur in 20–50% of the patients. Acute or chronic inflammation of the pouch (pouchitis) is an inherent complication of ileoanal pull-through operation for UC characterized by watery diarrhoea, fever and malaise. The etiology of pouchitis is unclear. Its incidence varies between 20% and 50% of the patients. Most acute episodes of pouchitis respond rapidly to a short course of oral antibiotics, for example metronidazole and ciprofloxacin. Chronic pouchitis is much less common and occurs in less than 10% of the patients. Its treatment consists of long courses of low-dose oral antibiotics and, in resistant cases locally acting corticosteroids.

Wound infection occurs in 5–15% of cases. Bowel obstructions are common and occur in up to 25% of the patients. Pelvic septic complications including anastomotic leakage and fistula formation occur in about 10% of the patients. Anastomotic stricture is uncommon. Only a few patients require temporary Hegar dilatations in order to ascertain anastomotic patency. The pelvic septic complications are especially important, because they are associated with worsened functional outcome. Overall about 15–45% of the patients require a repeat operation. A few patients eventually require pouch removal. In many of them the diagnosis is found to be Crohn's disease instead of UC.

53.3 Crohn's Disease

53.3.1 Introduction

Like in ulcerative colitis, Crohn's disease (CD) is a chronic inflammation of the bowel with unknown etiology. In children, CD is today usually reported to be more common than ulcerative colitis. Males and females are equally affected. Approximately 20–25% of patients with CD have the onset of the disease before 15 years of age. CD occurs more commonly in white population than in other ethnic groups. In many Western countries the incidence of CD has increased until last decades, in others the incidence continues to increase. There are some hereditary risk factors for Crohn's disease: 5–20% patients with CD have a first

degree relative who has inflammatory bowel disease and offspring of a CD patient have a 10% chance of developing CD.

53.3.2 Etiology

The etiology of Crohn's disease is unknown and is probably multifactorial. In addition to genetic factors immunological and microbiological factors as well as environmental factors are likely to play a significant role.

Extensive amount of testing of possible susceptibility genes for CD has occurred but no consensus concerning the genetic background of CD has been reached. One of the most studied genes is CARD15/NOD2 that is associated with bacterial recognition. This gene is associated with stricturising ileal CD.

53.3.3 Pathology

CD involves terminal ileum and colon in 60% of cases, small bowel only in 30% and colon only in 10% of cases. The involved bowel and also mesentery are thickened and fat often migrates towards the antimesenteric border of the bowel wall (creeping fat). Variable degree of stricturising is commonly seen in the segment of bowel that is mostly affected. Histologically, mucosa is often extensively ulcerated and the inflammation is usually transmural. The inflammation is often interspersed with almost normally appearing mucosal areas. The transmural inflammatory changes may develop to fistulas that erode to adjacent structures such as bowel, bladder, vagina, perineum and abdominal wall. Histological evidence of granulomas

Table 53.1 The Vienna classification of Crohn's disease

Age at diagnosis	A1, <40 years
	A2, >40 years
Location	L1, Terminal ileum
	L2, Colon
	L3, Ileocolon
	L4, Upper gastrointestinal
Behaviour	B1, Non-stricturing non-penetrating
	B2, Stricturing
	B3, Penetrating

that are the mainstay of histological diagnosis of CD occur in 40% of endoscopic biopsies taken from lesions in small bowel, in more than 60% of biopsies from gastric lesions and only 25% of biopsies from colonic lesions.

A simple classification of CD's location and behavior has been designed recently (Vienna classification, Table 53.1). This classification gives a reasonably solid basis for comparisons between different patient series. Moreover, the effectivity of various management modalities are more easy to assess in various forms of disease presentation when a commonly accepted classification exists.

53.3.4 Diagnosis

The diagnosis of CD is based on clinical history, endoscopic findings, imaging and to a limited extent on laboratory tests.

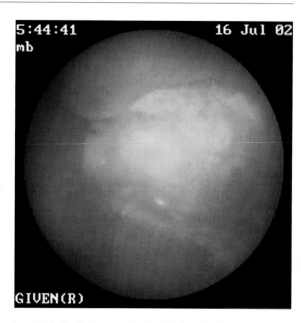

Fig. 53.3 Ileal ulcer associated with Crohn's disease at capsule endoscopy

53.3.4.1 Clinical Features

In children the onset of CD is most often after the age of 10 years. However, CD may occur almost at any age; about 5% of CD patients present before the age of 10 years. There is commonly a significant diagnostic delay, commonly longer than 1 year between the onset of symptoms and the definitive diagnosis. A typical early symptom of CD is non-specific abdominal pain. Other typical symptoms include diarrhea, weight loss and fever. Growth failure may be manifested by delayed onset of puberty. Patients with CD are commonly more ill than those with ulcerative colitis.

Perianal disease as a first presentation occur in up to 20% of CD patients. Typical findings are chronic anal fissures and skin tags, and chronic fistula-in-ano. In a preadolescent child any of these should alert the clinician to suspect CD.

Many children with CD have extraintestinal manifestations. Some of these may present years before the onset of bowel CD. Typical extraintestinal manifestations include arthritis, erythema nodosum and pyo-

derma gangrenosum as skin manifestations, and iritis and uveitis as eye symptoms.

Laboratory findings are not diagnostic but usually helpful. Many patients are anemic and most have elevated sedimentation rate. Serum albumin, prealbumin and transferrin are low in many CD patients reflecting their poor nutritional status. In CD increased serum ASCA (anti-*Saccharomyces cervisiae* antibody) has high specificity (>90%) but low sensitivity (<60%). The test is useful in differential diagnosis of CD, as it is always normal in ulcerative colitis.

Radiological imaging, especially small bowel follow-through, has been intensively used in CD to visualize the areas of bowel that cannot be reached by endoscopy. Today the whole length of small bowel can be observed by capsule endoscopy that has significantly decreased the need and number of radiographic small bowel imaging (Fig. 53.3).

53.3.5 Endoscopy

Endoscopic work-up for CD needs to include both upper and lower fiberoptic endoscopy. Granulomas that are diagnostic for CD may be found more easily from upper gastrointestinal biopsies than from biopsies from colon. Multiple biopsies should be obtained especially from macroscopic lesions. Typical findings in CD include segmental aphtous and linear ulcers, and stenotic areas that sometimes do not allow the passage of an endoscope. Typical for CD is that severely affected segment of bowel may rapidly change to an almost normal looking bowel. Sometimes, especially in colon, almost the whole length of the organ may be affected by the disease as in most cases of childhood ulcerative colitis. Even in cases of extensive colonic CD rectum may be completely or partially spared.

53.3.5.1 Differential Diagnosis

The major differential diagnostic problem in CD is ulcerative colitis. Usually it is easier to rule out ulcerative colitis in a patient with CD than CD in a child with ulcerative colitis. Indeterminate colitis occurs also in children but in less than 10% of the cases. From a surgical point of view ulcerative colitis should be definitively ruled out since today the golden standard for surgical management of ulcerative colitis is restorative proctocolectomy that is not a suitable surgical option for Crohn's disease. Typical clinical symptoms in CD and ulcerative colitis are summarized in Table 53.2.

53.3.6 Medical Management

The medical treatment of CD has evolved significantly during the last decade. The mainstay of medical management is immunomodulation. As medical management of ulcerative colitis is relatively straightforward and based on aminosalicylates and corticosteroids in different combinations depending on the activity of the disease, medical management of CD is much more complex. The modality of medical management is different in different localisations of the disease. Generally speaking, the more widespread and more distal in the bowel the disease activity is the more aggressive medical management is required. Predominantly ileal disease can be managed with corticosteroids, preferably with locally acting budesonide, and aminosalicylates. Colonic involvement requires often antibiotics such as metronidazole or ciprofloxacin in addition to the regimen used for ileal disease.

Elemental or semi-elemental enteral nutrition has also been used in pediatric CD with similar success rates as in those who have received corticosteroids. It appears that ileal and ileocolic disease responds better to enteral nutrition than isolated colonic disease.

Exacerbations, relapses or refractory CD require more effective medication; azathioprine, 6-mercaptopurine or cyclosporine is often helpful in inducing remission. Early use of these potent immunomodulators has also increased significantly in children because recent data from randomized controlled trials have shown significant decrease in relapse frequency.

Novel biological immunomodulatory drugs such as TNF-α antibodies (Infliximab) have been adopted for management of fistulizing and refractory CD. Internal and severe rectoperineal fistulas respond well to infliximab therapy and most patients resume a longer period of remission. Similar results have been reported in patients who have disease refractory to conventional medication. However, long term efficacy and safety of biological treatment of CD remains still unclear.

53.3.7 Surgical Management

There is no definitive curative treatment for Crohn's disease. As Crohn's disease is an affliction of the whole gastrointestinal tract surgery does not offer any permanent cure. Unlike in ulcerative colitis surgical treatment is palliative in nature and aimed to treat the complications of the disease. It is evident that the development of novel drug therapies has reduced the need for surgical therapy for Crohn's disease. The

Table 53.2 Incidence of different symptoms in Crohn's disease and ulcerative colitis

	UC (%)	CD (%)
Bloody stools	97	22
Diarrhoea	90	88
Abdominal pain	33	82
Weight loss	15	60
Fever	15	77
Growth failure	3	30

indications for surgery are limited to cases that are refractory to medical therapy or medical therapy is poorly tolerated. Acute indications include medically unmanageable toxic megacolon or acute bleeding, both of which are rare. Subacute or chronic conditions that may require surgery include refractory strictures, internal or external fistula and intra-abdominal abscesses.

The main principle in the surgical treatment of Crohn's disease is to save bowel length. Radical resections are not indicated; resection should be limited to the segment of bowel, which is causing symptoms. Isolated skip lesions are left alone if they do not cause obstruction. In adults strictureplasty has been shown to be an effective bowel saving surgical method for multiple fibrotic stenoses. The long-term outcome in terms of disease activity, risk of recurrence and quality of life has been very similar than following resectional surgery. There are only a few reports of strictureplasty for Crohn's disease in children but the preliminary results are similar as in adults. Although controversial, strictureplasty probably should be favoured also in children because it saves bowel length in patients who have early onset of the disease and are likely to be candidates for further surgery during their long life span.

Major bowel resections are sometimes required in association with severe and widespread colonic disease. In these cases rectum should be spared. Typical surgical solution for widespread colonic disease is colectomy and ileorectal anastomosis either in one or two stages. Either stages may be performed openly or laparoscopy-assisted. Ileoanal anastomosis with or without a pouch is not indicated for Crohn's disease; long-term outcome is very unpredictable and often poor, moreover, pouch complications are very common.

Perianal manifestations of Crohn's disease are common in children. These include skin tags, fissures and fistulas. In most cases perianal manifestations cause mild symptoms or are asymptomatic. Conservative approach is warranted and surgical treatment should be considered only in severely symptomatic high recto-perineal or rectovaginal fistulas that do not respond to increased immunomodulatory (infliximab, azathioprine) and antibiotic (metronidazole, ciprofloxacin) therapy. If surgery is required for a high perianal fistula resection

of the mostly diseased usually left colonic segment and temporary bowel diversion may increase the success rate of the fistula repair. In very severe perianal disease, especially if it is associated with severe rectal manifestation, proctectomy may be the only possibility to guarantee a reasonable quality of life.

53.3.8 Complications

Complications that occur after surgical management of CD are typical to all bowel resections. Anastomotic leaks may occur and strictureplasties may leak. A common procedure for widespread colonic disease is colectomy and ileorectal anastomosis. This is associated with an overall complication rate is 15–20% including septic complications and anastomotic leaks.

The main and typical complication of CD is disease recurrence. The rate of recurrence may be decreased by immunomodulatory medication, especially azathioprine, but recurrence still occurs in more than 50% of the patients within 5–10 years of time. Recurrences requiring surgery are less common but approach 25–35% in 5–10 years. Early recurrences appear to be more common if the disease is initially widespread. The risk of recurrence is not related to the indications or clinical presentation at primary surgery nor to age, sex and time from onset of the disease. The recurrence rate is highest in patients who have undergone surgery for perianal disease and lowest in those who have a permanent stoma. Permanent stoma for salvage is eventually used in a significant proportion (10–20%) of patients who have the onset of CD during childhood.

Further Reading

Baldassano RN, Han PD, Jeshion WC et al (2001) Pediatric Crohn's disease: Risk factors for postoperative recurrence. Am J Gastroenterol 96:2169–2176

Besnard M, Jaby O, Mougenot JF et al (1998) Postoperative outcome of Crohn's disease in 30 children. Gut 43:634–638

Caprilli R, Gassull M, Escher JC et al (2006) European evidence based consensus on the diagnosis and management of Crohn's disease: Special situation. Gut 55:36–58

Fonkalsrud EW (2006) Ulcerative colitis. In JL Grosfeld, JA O'Neill, EW Fonkalsrud, AG Coran (eds) Pediatric Surgery. Mosby, Philadelphia, pp 1462–1478

Griffiths AM, Buller HB (2000) Inflammatory bowel disease. In WA Walker, PR Durie, JR Hamilton, JA Walker-Smith, JB Watkins (eds) Pediatric Gastrointestinal Disease. B.C. Decker, Hamilton, pp 613–652

Patel HI, Leichtner AM, Colodny AH, Shamberger RC (1997) Surgery for Crohn's disease in infants and children. J Pediatr Surg 32:1063–1067

Rintala RJ (2006a) Crohn's disease. In P Puri, ME Höllwarth (eds) Pediatric Surgery, Springer Surgery Atlas Series. Springer-Verlag, Berlin, Heidelberg, New York, pp 347–354

Rintala RJ (2006b) Ulcerative colitis. In P Puri, ME Höllwarth (eds) Pediatric Surgery. Springer-Verlag, Berlin, MA, pp 333–346

Paediatric Small Bowel Transplantation

A.J.W. Millar, K. Sharif, and G.L. Gupte

54

Contents

54.1 Introduction

Intestinal transplantation (ITx) is now a well-established treatment for infants and children with intestinal failure (IF), who develop complications related to long-term parenteral nutrition (PN). Transplantation of other organs such as kidney, liver and heart developed during the 1960s but did not reach widespread clinical application until the cyclosporine era of immune suppression in the early 1980s. ITx lagged behind as the intestine was found to be an organ with special problems of its own immunogenicity, its interface with the enteric lumen colonized with bacteria and transfer of a heavy load of immune competent cells of the donor at the time of engraftment. In addition, organ preservation was more fragile and consequences of ischaemic reperfusion injury more severe. At the same time, treatment of intestinal failure with parenteral nutrition (PN) had developed to give children with IF a reasonable quality of life. Long-term PN, however, has its own complications including central venous catheter related sepsis, venous thrombosis and PN associated liver disease. PN therefore is not a lifetime treatment. Sporadic cases of ITx were reported in the 1970s but all recipients died of technical complications, sepsis or rejection. Optimism for success in the cyclosporine era was short-lived as most grafts were lost to rejection. A total of 15 cases were reported between 1985 and 1990 with one long term survivor. This child received a neonatal donor intestine and has survived 19 years post transplant. Introduction of more effective tacrolimus immune suppression by Starzl in 1990 allowed for reports of 60% 1 year graft survival by 1993. Currently 90% 1 year survival is reported from some centres.

Parenteral nutrition remains the current standard of care for infants and children with intestinal failure with a

P. Puri and M. Höllwarth (eds.), *Pediatric Surgery: Diagnosis and Management*,
DOI: 10.1007/978-3-540-69560-8_54, © Springer-Verlag Berlin Heidelberg 2009

Table 54.1 Causes of intestinal failure

Short bowel syndrome
  (a) Gastroschisis (atresia and dysmotility)
  (b) Necrotising enterocolitis
  (c) Intestinal atresia
  (d) Mid-gut volvulus
Older children
  Crohn's disease
  Mesenteric infarction
  Tumours
  Trauma
Dysmotility
  (a) Intestinal aganglionosis
  (b) Idiopathic intestinal pseudo-obstruction
  (c) Degenerative intestinal leiomyopathy
  (d) Megacystis microcolon hypoperistalsis syndrome
  (e) Hollow visceral myopathy
Congenital diarrhoeal disease
  (a) Microvillous inclusion disease
  (b) Tufting enteropathy
  (c) Autoimmune enteropathy

1 year survival of 90% and 5 year survival of 75%. The main causes of intestinal failure in the paediatric age group are short bowel syndrome, dysmotility syndromes and congenital diarrhoeal disease (Table 54.1).

54.2 Indications

Indications for transplant assessment in children with short gut and established IF are the potential lethal complications of PN namely loss of central venous access from thrombosis of central veins, life threatening recurrent line infections and PN induced cholestasis, which can rapidly progress to established irreversible liver disease. This is referred to as intestinal failure associated liver disease (IFALD). Common conditions resulting in short bowel syndrome and intestinal failure (IF) are summarised in Table 54.1.

There are few contraindications but complete loss of venous access, presence of other systemic malignant diseases, progressive neurological disorders and untreated immune deficiency syndromes because of the risk of unrestrained graft versus host disease (GVHD) are considered absolute. Relative contraindications would be the degree of other systemic co-morbidities. There is no lower age or size limit and a history of multiple previous laparotomies is not a contraindication but both may carry a waiting list mortality risk of nearly 50% in the <10 kg size recipients because of the shortage of size matched donors.

54.3 Pre-transplant Assessment

The pre-transplant workup for ITx is the same as other solid organ transplants with a focus on the assessment of central venous access patency, establishing the diagnosis of irreversible intestinal failure by assessing adequacy of function of the residual bowel and documentation of urinary tract anatomy in dysmotility syndromes because of the frequent association of bladder and ureteric dilatation in these patients.

It is important to assess the residual bowel for intestinal adaptation in children with short bowel syndrome. Patients with short bowel syndrome who have the potential to achieve independent enteral tolerance through intestinal adaptation and/or concomitant non-transplant surgery (closure of stomas, intestinal plication and lengthening procedures) should undergo procedures to optimise the residual bowel function before the development of end stage liver disease and portal hypertension.

Children with short bowel syndrome (SBS) who develop irreversible IFALD but show the potential for adaptation to autonomous enteral feeding should be considered for isolated liver transplant in the expectation that the adaptation process would be facilitated by replacement of a severely diseased liver with relief of portal hypertension.

The ideal donor would be that of a stable cadaver heart-beating donor (preferably CMV and EBV negative) 20% smaller than the recipient. However, because of the shortage of size match donors, techniques have been developed to accommodate larger sized donors by either increasing the size of the recipient abdomen (pre-transplant insertion of tissue expanders, use of prosthetic materials to close abdomen at the time of transplant, and staged abdominal closure) or reduce the size of the graft by back-table excision of part of donor liver and/or intestine in the case of multivisceral transplants.

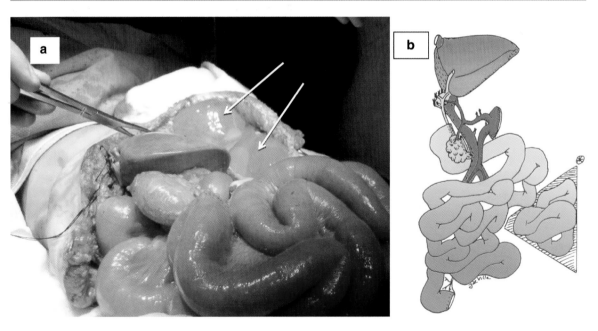

Fig. 54.1 A reduced size composite liver and small bowel transplant using segments 2 & 3 of the donor liver, small bowel from the duodenum with head of pancreas to the terminal ileum. Note the tissue expanders (white arrows in **a.**) used to assist in skin closure of a graft size too large for the recipient abdominal domain. A diagram representation of the graft is shown in **b.** The graft may be further reduced in size by excision of a segment of mid jejunum

54.4 Types of Transplant Procedures

Types of transplant depends on the severity of liver disease and portal hypertension

Different types of transplant are as follows:

1. **Isolated intestine** for minimal or mild liver disease and impaired venous access (Fig. 54.1)

    (a) Segmental or full length small intestine
    (b) Living related segmental small intestine
    (c) Small bowel and colon

2. **Liver and intestine** for moderate to severe liver disease with evidence of significant portal hypertension (Fig. 54.2)

    (a) 'Classical' separate liver and intestine
    (b) 'En bloc' liver, bile ducts, duodenum, head of pancreas and intestine in continuity as a composite graft whole or reduced

3. **Multi-visceral transplantation**, which includes liver, intestine and pancreas with an additional organ i.e. stomach and/or kidney (Fig. 54.2f).

54.4.1 Living Related Intestinal Transplantation

Living related intestinal transplantation is an option to address the deaths on the waiting list and expand the pool of donors. The proponents of the procedure claim the advantages of reduced cold ischemia time, the ability to select recipients in an optimal condition and the opportunity to plan a tolerance inducing immunosuppression protocol. However, the graft per se does not offer any immunological advantage, develops the same complications related to intestinal transplantation and all would still need to be maintained on life-long immunosuppression. Thus, living related ITx has not been widely adopted in major ITx centres.

54.5 Techniques of Transplantation

The procurement of organs is a complex procedure requiring a separate team of experienced transplant surgeons. The donor is given antibiotic and antifungal

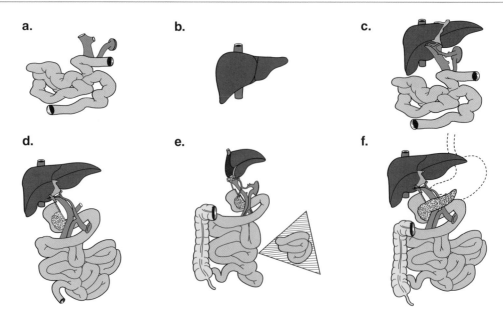

Fig. 54.2 Different types of grafts used for intestinal failure (a) isolated intestine (b) isolated liver for SBS (c) liver and intestine for IFALD (d) composite graft of liver and intestine with duodenum, bile ducts and head of pancreas (e) reduced size composite graft (f) multi-visceral graft, which could include the whole pancreas, stomach and right colon and even spleen

agents enterally by nasogastric tube as selective gut decontamination along with standard intravenous antibiotic prophylaxis. The graft must be handled with great care with in-situ cold flush and storage using the University of Wisconsin preservation solution. The donor organs are procured en bloc i.e. the hepatoduodenal-pancreas organ cluster is kept intact although the liver may be appropriately reduced in size as required. It is advisable to keep the cold ischaemic time to less than 8 h. Both stomach and colon may be included in the graft. The recipient operation may be challenging as there is frequently a history of multiple previous surgeries leading to dense vascularized adhesions from portal hypertension. Details of the procedures are well described but in principle the foregut portal circulation is decompressed with a porto-caval shunt. The diseased viscera are removed and the appropriate graft is then sutured in situ. It is acceptable for the venous drainage of the graft to be to the inferior vena cava in isolated intestinal transplants. In multivisceral transplants the 'clean sweep' operation may be performed whereby all the abdominal contents anterior to the main vessels are removed from the gastric body to the distal colon, including the duodenum, pancreas, spleen and rest of intestine.

A donor arterial conduit from the infra-renal aorta is anastomosed to an arterial patch including the orifices of both the coeliac axis and superior mesenteric artery.

The proximal bowel anastomosis may be a gastro-jejunostomy or jejuno-jejunostomy in continuity. The distal bowel continuity is restored by end to end anastomosis with a proximal venting stoma where distal colon has normal function. The stoma is used for biopsy access in the post transplant period or the distal end may be brought out as an end stoma. Stomas may be closed some time after the original engraftment when the graft has 'settled in' immunologically speaking. This is usually not considered until after the first year post transplant with a stable graft in the absence of rejection.

54.5.1 Immunosuppression in Small Bowel Transplantation

Tacrolimus, a powerful calcineurin 2 inhibitor along with steroids have been the mainstay of immune suppression protocols. Over the past decade, use of different agents like IL2 blockers (anti-CD25 monoclonal antibodies), Campath 1-H (anti CD52 monoclonal antibodies), Thymoglobulin (rabbit anti-thymocyte globulin) have been used in the induction regime, which has resulted in improved long-term outcome following ITx.

54.6 Medical Complications

Intestinal transplant is a complex and challenging procedure which requires a highly skilled multidisciplinary team to manage these patients. There are several reported complications associated with the procedure. Some of these are

54.6.1 Graft Rejection

Rejection usually occurs within the first few weeks after transplantation. Clinical features of rejection can be variable and include increased stomal output, fever, abdominal pain and malaise. Frequently it is difficult to distinguish rejection from viral enteritis. There are currently no reliable non-invasive markers of rejection. Serum citrulline, a marker of mucosal mass, has shown some promise, however the differentiation between rejection and infection can make the levels difficult to interpret. The diagnosis of rejection is made on histopatho-logical examination of graft tissue from stomal/endoscopic biopsies. Mild or moderate rejection is treated by optimising the immunosuppression and with pulse doses of intravenous methylprednisolone (10–20 mg/kg to a maximum of 400 mg/dose). Severe rejection is notoriously difficult to treat and is associated with a poor prognosis. Treatment strategies with OKT3, thymoglobulin and recently infliximab (anti TNF alpha monoclonal antibody) have been tried with variable success.

54.6.2 Infections

The intestinal transplant registry reports infections as cause in 60–70% of the deaths. There is a high incidence of infection in the post transplant period. The high incidence of bacterial infections is likely to be due to bacterial translocation from the gut lumen. Broad spectrum antibiotics are routinely administered during the early post-transplant period along with selective decontamination of the gut with oral antibiotics and antifungal agents. Infectious enteritis is reported in up to 40% of recipients with viruses (adenovirus, rotavirus and calcivirus) and protozoa (Giardia Lamblia, Cryptosporidium). As previously mentioned, prompt recognition of infectious enteritis can be difficult as the clinico-pathologic picture can mimic acute rejection. The treatments are diametrically opposite; one requires increased immune suppression (rejection) and the other reduced immune suppression (infection). Rotavirus and adenovirus enteritis can trigger episodes of acute moderate to severe rejection and can result in graft loss.

CMV (cytomegalovirus virus) and EBV (Epstein Barr virus) infection are seen more commonly in the paediatric intestinal transplant population because of a primary infection (seropositive donor to seronegative recipient). Different tests are used to make the diagnosis of CMV infection and can be effectively treated with intravenous gancyclovir. Post-transplant infectious enteritis, CMV and EBV infections can lead to significant morbidity and mortality.

54.6.3 Post-transplant Lymphoproliferative Disorder (PTLD)

PTLD is believed to be driven by EBV infection. The incidence of PTLD following intestinal transplantation, historically, was reported to be as high as 30–40%. Children presenting with recurrent infections, hypoalbuminemia, anaemia, thrombocytopenia and neutropenia should alert the physician to perform investigations to exclude PTLD. EBV viral load measured by polymerase chain reaction (PCR) is helpful to indicate ongoing EBV viraemia, but does not confirm the diagnosis of PTLD. Imaging of the abdomen and the chest with computed tomography (CT) or magnetic resonance imaging (MRI) for lymphadenopathy may be necessary to arrive at the diagnosis. Confirmation of EBV related PTLD needs histopathological examination of affected tissue. Endoscopic procedures along with EBER (EBV in situ hybridisation) staining of the gut biopsies may be necessary to confirm the diagnosis in children without lymphadenopathy. Pre-emptive reduction of immunosuppression in the context of EBV viraemia has been demonstrated to prevent the progression to PTLD. Occasionally anti CD 20 monoclonal antibody treatment (rituximab) and/or chemotherapy is required for control. The current cure rate with all modalities of treatment is around 70%.

54.6.4 Graft Versus Host Disease (GVHD)

Surprisingly, despite the high lymphocyte load within the intestine, the incidence of GVHD has been reported to be low, 8.5% from a large single centre experience. Optimisation of tacrolimus immunosuppression and steroid administration is the treatment of choice and usually leads to a favourable outcome.

54.7 Surgical Complications

Surgical complications have a significant impact on the morbidity and mortality following intestinal transplantation (ITx). Reported incidence of surgical complications following ITx is 40%.

54.7.1 Intestinal Perforation

Intestinal perforation (IP) is reported in 30–40% recipients following intestinal transplantation. This usually occurs within the first 2 weeks post-transplant and is sometimes difficult to manage. The use of steroids and viral infections are thought to be contributory factors in intestinal perforation but there is no definite evidence. The symptoms and signs of acute peritonitis can be masked as the children are heavily immunosuppressed and on high dose steroids thus needing a high index of suspicion. Abdominal imaging and contrast studies may be needed to confirm the diagnosis. Early second look operations to exclude IP in high-risk patients with minimal signs are frequently required. Surgical control of the perforation is achieved either by primary closure or by insertion of a T tube into the perforation to create a controlled enteric fistula.

54.7.2 Abdominal Compartment Syndrome (ACS)

ACS is relatively less recognised and an under-reported complication following ITx. There are several contributing factors including swelling of the graft in the first few days following ITx and reduced en-bloc liver small bowel transplant (LSBTx) in infants with small abdominal cavities and contracted scarred abdominal walls. These patients need skilled surgical management. Innovative surgical techniques have been developed which include insertion of tissue expanders pre-operatively; staged closure utilising a silastic pouch to contain the graft and shoelace sutures to the skin, which can be tightened daily to stretch the skin and achieve a degree of "skin creep". When it is apparent that the skin can be approximated without tension, the silastic patch is replaced by absorbable collagen protheses (Surgisis Gold® in infants & Permacol® in older children).

54.7.3 Pancreatic Complications

Shortage of size matched donors and high incidence of biliary complications following conventional liver and bowel transplants (LBTx) resulted in development of innovative techniques for LBTx. This included the use of reduced en-bloc liver small bowel transplant (LSBTx). Some of these children developed pancreatitis and pancreatic fluid collection presumably from the cut surface of the donor pancreas. These collections were usually treated conservatively with a percutaneous drainage tube however sometimes surgical intervention is required. Currently the whole pancreas is preferably included in the composite graft. This however results is bigger graft which in children with a small abdominal cavity increases the donor to recipient ratio and difficulties in abdominal closure

54.7.4 Vascular Complications

There is high incidence of vascular complication in some of the paediatric solid organ transplantation especially liver and kidney transplant. This complication has rarely been seen following ITx using current techniques as vascular reconstructions are with large arteries.

54.7.5 Other Complications

Other complications such as adhesive intestinal obstruction, development of biliary sludge with partial obstruction of donor common bile duct, wound dehiscence and stomal issues, e.g. prolapse are less frequent but can be successfully managed with appropriate interventions.

54.8 Nutritional Outcome and Quality of Life

More than 90% of the survivors can be established on full enteral nutrition in the early post-transplant period. The median time to establish children on an oral diet varies as it is dependent on the pre-transplant oral intake. Children with a diagnosis of pseudo-obstruction, who have not eaten normally prior to intestinal transplantation, find it extremely difficult to establish oral intake and may need psychological and speech therapy input. Few studies exist in the literature addressing long-term growth in intestinal transplantation but a normally functioning graft provides completely autonomous enteral nutrition.

With the recent advances and improved survival following intestinal transplantation, issues regarding the quality of life in long term survivors have come to the forefront.

54.9 Outcome

Data from the intestinal transplant registry presented at the IX small bowel transplant symposium in Brussels in 2005, reported a 1 year survival of 90% and 3 year survival of around 70–80% from some major centres in USA. In a univariate and multivariate analysis conducted within the registry the poor prognostic variables identified were: hospitalisation at the time of transplant; age under 2 years and centres performing less than 10 transplants in total.

At Birmingham Children's Hospital, 44 intestinal transplants have been done since 1993 and 21 are alive. The longest survivor at our hospital is 9 years post-transplant.

In conclusion, the advances in the surgical techniques and immunosuppressive strategies made in the last decade are reflected in the current era of improved outcomes following intestinal transplantation. ITx in the next 20 years will continue to evolve and has the potential to be considered as an alternative strategy to home PN in selected patients.

54.10 Key Points

- Early referral to a transplant centre before onset of IFALD so that children can be considered for isolated bowel transplantation, which may result in better utilisation of donor organs
- Children under 2 years of age needing a liver and small bowel transplant have a worse outcome due to scarcity of size matched donor organs and high waiting list mortality
- Innovative surgical techniques of graft size reduction, use of abdominal tissue expanders and staged abdominal closure have improved the chances of small children being considered for transplantation
- Improved immune suppression strategies using induction agents like IL2 blockers and anti-lymphocyte preparations have reduced the incidence of acute rejection
- Advances in both surgical strategies and medical management has resulted in a current 80% 3 year survival following intestinal transplantation.

Acknowledgments We thank Professor J. de Ville de Goyet for giving permission to publish his figures.

Further Reading

Grant D, Abu-Elmagd K, Reyes J et al (2005) 2003 Report of the intestine transplant registry: A new era has dawned. Ann Surg 241:607–613

Gupte GL, Beath SV, Kelly DA et al (2006) Current issues in the management of intestinal failure. Arch Dis Child 91:259–264

Kato T, Ruiz P, Thompson JF et al (2002) Intestinal and multivisceral transplantation. World J Surg 26:226–237

Kaufman SS, Atkinson JB, Bianchi A et al (2001) Indications for pediatric intestinal transplantation: A position paper of the American Society of Transplantation. Pediatr Transplant 5:80–87

Puri P, Höllwarth M (2006) Pediatric Surgery. Springer, Berlin, Heidelberg

Reyes J, Mazariegos GV, Bond GM et al (2002) Pediatric intestinal transplantation: Historical notes, principles and controversies. Pediatr Transplant 6:193–207

Sudan DL, Iyer KR, Deroover A et al (2001) A new technique for combined liver/small intestinal transplantation. Transplantation 72:1846–1488

Biliary Atresia

55

Mark Davenport

Contents

55.1 Introduction

Biliary atresia (BA) can be a devastating disease of infancy invariably leading, if untreated, to cirrhosis, liver failure and death. It is the commonest indication for pediatric liver transplantation throughout the developed world.

In common with North America and Western Europe, the incidence in the UK is about 1 in 16,000 live births. It is clearly higher in countries such as Japan, and probably China, at about 1 in 10,000. All large series have a slight female preponderance. Although usually an isolated abnormality found in otherwise normal term infants, there are a group of infants who should be distinguished by the presence of other abnormalities and a poorer prognosis. About 10% of infants in European and North American series (but only ~3% in Japanese series) will have a specific constellation of anomalies which we have termed the Biliary Atresia Splenic Malformation (BASM) syndrome. The possible associations include polysplenia, asplenia, situs inversus, preduodenal portal vein, absence of the inferior vena cava, malrotation and congenital heart abnormalities. Most infants with this syndromic form of BA are female.

55.2 Etiology

The cause of BA is not known and it may be that a number of factors may induce or cause the final common pathology of biliary inflammation, luminal obliteration and fibrosis (*etiological heterogeneity*). Nonetheless, of a number of hypotheses, two seem worthy of further consideration.

55.2.1 Congenital Embryopathy

Infants with BASM have a parallel range of anomalies which could only have arisen at key points in organ development within the embryonic phase of development (25–35 days gestation). A genetic etiology in these infants, although perhaps likely, has not been convincingly shown. Thus, there are certainly genes where there is obvious overlap between biliary and visceral (including acquisition of normal right-left determination) development (e.g. CFC-1, *INV*), but proof of linkage is lacking in clinical practice. There is also some evidence that such infants have been exposed to an abnormal intrauterine environment during the 1st trimester (e.g. maternal diabetes).

There is a remarkable similarity between the normal biliary appearance of the fetal porta hepatis at ~12 weeks gestation and what is seen pathologically in biliary atresia. There is a sieve-like appearance with multiple, microscopic biliary channels, some of which will be selected and conglomerate into the two macroscopic hepatic ducts with the remainder being deleted. The non-syndromic variant of BA may result if there is developmental arrest and failure of maturation at this stage.

55.2.2 Viral Exposure

There are a range of hepatotropic cholangiopathic viruses (e.g. Reovirus type 2, cytomegalovirus, rotavirus) which can cause biliary damage during the perinatal period. Such viruses are ubiquitous and a common source of gastrointestinal symptoms during infancy. Mouse models are available where perinatal viral exposure leads to biliary pathology reminiscent of BA, with a similar host immunopathological response. Serological evidence in humans is contradictory and although some studies using RT-PCR and PCR techniques have shown isolation of both viral RNA and DNA, others have not.

However given the prevalence of such viruses in the community it seems odd that BA remains such a rare disease, and it may be that there is some (possibly) genetic predisposition to develop biliary destruction given the virus as an initiating immune trigger.

55.3 Pathology

Both intra- and extra-hepatic parts of the biliary tree are affected and is characterised by cholangiole plugging and proliferation, moderate giant cell transformation, variable degrees of fibrosis, an inflammatory infiltrate in the liver and fibroinflammatory luminal obliteration within the extrahepatic bile ducts. In about 5% of cases, there is cyst formation within the biliary tree which may or may not contain bile (Figs. 55.1a and b).

The level at which the lumen is obliterated is the basis for the commonest classification in clinical use

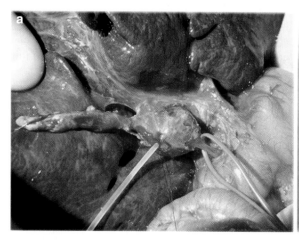
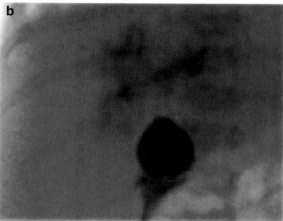

Fig. 55.1 Cystic biliary atresia, detected antenatally at 22 weeks gestation. Translucent obliterated distal common bile duct (yellow sling) and thick-walled mucus-containing cyst (**a**) The cholangiogram (**b**) showed typically abnormal intrahepatic biliary ductule "cloud" appearance. Cut surface of resected specimen appeared solid (i.e. Type 3)

Table 55.1   Classification of Biliary Atresia

Type	Incidence (%)	Description
1	~5%	**Level of obstruction within the common bile duct.**
		The gallbladder therefore contains bile.
		Typically these are cystic. The more proximal intrahepatic ducts are abnormal (scanty, irregular, and etiolated), sometimes with a hazy, cloud-like appearance rather than as actual ducts.
2	~3%	**Level of obstruction within the common hepatic duct.**
		The gallbladder will not contain bile but a transection of the proximal remnant should show two distinct bile-containing lumens
3	>90%	**Obstruction is within the porta hepatis with no visible bile-containing proximal lumen.**
		The gallbladder may look normal but if so will only contain clear mucus. A communication with the duodenum may be shown on cholangiography.

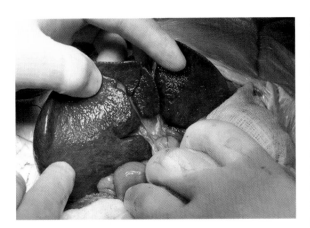

Fig. 55.2 Extra-abdominal mobilised liver with atrophic solid gallbladder just visible within its fossa

(Table 55.1). Type 3 is the usual manifestation of this with a level of obstruction within the porta hepatis combined with atrophic non-bile containing gallbladder and obliterated extrahepatic biliary tree (Fig. 55.2).

The nature of the inflammatory infiltrate and its molecular pathology has received a great deal of research attention recently and some aspects of its composition and relevance have still to be elucidated. It is still not known how specific the response is to biliary atresia, and some elements may be seen in other causes of neonatal cholestasis. In our study, the small cell infiltrate was largely composed of CD4+ T lymphocytes and CD56+ NK cells which exhibited markers for proliferation (CD71+) and activation (particularly LFA-1 + but also CD25+). Others have suggested a predominance of infiltrating CD8+ cells but which appear to be somewhat disabled and lack markers of activation such as perforin, granzyme B and Fas ligand. Macrophages/monocytes do seem to play an important role in the presentation of antigenic material (possibly derived from viruses) and in the initiation of later fibrosis, a hallmark of biliary atresia,

not seen in familial cholestatic syndromes. These may be resident as Kupffer cells or systemic and recruited and when activated and proliferating appears to be a key component in the prolongation of the inflammatory response. Certainly there is some evidence that the degree of macrophage infiltration and activation may have prognostic importance and worsen outcome.

Cell adhesion molecules are proteins involved in cell-cell binding and the initiation and maintenance of the inflammatory response. Intercellular adhesion molecule (ICAM-1) and vascular cell adhesion molecule (VCAM-1) are expressed on both hepatocytes and sinusoidal cell membranes and act to bind circulating leukocytes by interaction with cell-surface integrins leading to transendothelial migration. There is abnormal expression of the adhesion molecules, ICAM-1 and VCAM-1 but not E-selectin on the sinusoidal endothelium of virtually all infants with BA.

An abnormal parallel expression of soluble cellular adhesion molecules and a range of soluble cytokines can be found in the circulation of infants with BA. Thus there are elevated levels of soluble ICAM-1 and soluble VCAM-1 both at the time of portoenterostomy and for a considerable time after. Similarly, there appears to be a non-polarized soluble cytokine response characterized by often gross elevations of TNF-α, interferon-γ, IL-2, IL-4, IL-18, etc.

55.4 Clinical Features

The key clinical triad observable in virtually all infants with biliary atresia is a conjugated jaundice, pale acholic stools and dark urine (Fig. 55.3). There is an inability to excrete conjugated (i.e. water soluble) bilirubin into the gastrointestinal tract, which is then excreted into the urine darkening its colour. Some

Fig. 55.3 Schematic diagram illustrating modes of presentation of biliary atresia

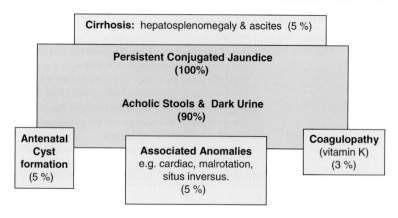

infants will have had an abnormal antenatal ultrasound scan (~5%), because of the cystic change in the biliary tree, and some infants present because of the other abnormalities associated with BASM (e.g. cardiac anomalies or malrotation). A small proportion of infants will present with features of Vitamin K dependent coagulopathy and bleeding, particularly in those communities where routine neonatal administration of parenteral Vitamin K is not usual practice. Clinical features of cirrhosis such as ascites, splenomegaly or a hard liver are unusual in infants presenting within 80 days of age.

55.5 Diagnosis

It is possible to make the correct diagnosis in >80% of cases before a laparotomy. The key diagnostic investigations in our centre are a detailed ultrasound of the liver and biliary tree followed by a percutaneous liver biopsy. Some centres, particularly in Japan, use duodenal intubation and measurement of intralumenal bile, rather than biopsy.

If there is still diagnostic doubt then other techniques such as ERCP (endoscopic retrograde cholangiopancreatography) or perhaps laparoscopy and percutaneous cholangiography can be performed, although both are difficult specialist tools. Currently MRCP (magnetic retrograde cholangiopancreaticography) does not appear to offer much advantage over standard ultrasonography simply because of the lack of detail required for a positive diagnosis. Similarly radioisotope hepatobiliary imaging lacks sufficient discrimination in borderline cases to be really useful.

55.6 Differential Diagnosis

This is long and needs perseverance to work out. The surgical causes other than biliary atresia, is uncommon but may include obstructed choledochal malformations, spontaneous perforation of the bile duct and the inspissated bile syndrome. Ultrasonography and MRCP will show a dilated common bile duct (usually >5 mm) or obvious cystic anomaly with a significant choledochal malformation. There should be some free peritoneal fluid and perhaps an echogenic mass at the porta hepatis in spontaneous biliary perforation with bile-staining of the skin in most. Infants with inspissated bile syndrome are usually premature and the ultrasound shows a dilated biliary tree with inspissated bile present. These infants usually require percutaneous cholangiography and occasionally surgery to clear the obstructed bile ducts.

Common medical causes include neonatal hepatitis, α1-antitrypsin deficiency, giant cell hepatitis, cytomegalovirus hepatitis and cystic fibrosis. Appropriate tests of exclusion include liver biopsy, viral serology, and a sweat test. Biliary hypoplasia may be a feature of Alagille's syndrome (abnormal "elfin" facies, butterfly vertebrae, pulmonary stenosis) and can cause diagnostic confusion.

55.7 Management

There are two possible strategies for infants with BA. Most infants are suitable for an attempt at restoration of bile flow and preservation of their native liver using a Kasai-type portoenterostomy. If this fails, or the child develops significant complications of chronic liver disease, then liver transplantation will be required if available. An alternative is simply to list all infants with BA for liver transplantation as a primary procedure. In our institution we consider the latter strategy only for infants where we feel an attempt at Kasai would be futile and these tend to be late-presenters (>100 days) who have already obvious features of cirrhosis such as ascites etc. In practice, this is <5% of all infants with BA.

55.7.1 Kasai Portoenterostomy

The aim of the surgery is to excise all extrahepatic biliary remnants allowing a wide portoenterostomy onto a portal plate, denuded of all tissue (Fig. 55.4). In the majority of cases, this will expose sufficient transected microscopic bile ductules which retain connections with the primitive intrahepatic bile ductule system to allow restoration of at least a degree of biliary drainage (Fig. 55.5). This should be the object not only in type 3, but also in those with types 1 and 2 BA.

Surgery consists of a liver mobilisation and eversion onto the abdominal wall (Fig. 55.1) to allow full exposure of the porta hepatis and a detailed meticulous dissection. The dissection itself must be wide and expose the origin of the umbilical vein from the left portal vein in the fossa of Rex, the extrahepatic bifurcation of the right portal pedicle and the caudate lobe behind the portal vein posteriorly. A portoenterostomy

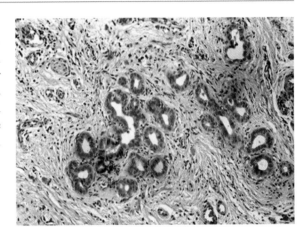

Fig. 55.5 H&E photomicrograph of transected proximal biliary remnants from Type 3 biliary atresia showing a predominantly fibro-inflammatory stroma within which are multiple biliary ductules (10–100 μm in diameter)

using a retrocolic Roux loop (~40 cm) completes the reconstruction.

Laparoscopic-assisted portoenterostomy has been described and is clearly possible although a true comparison with the open procedure as described above is yet to be performed.

55.8 Prognostic Factors

Biliary atresia remains a rare disease and one of the key prognostic factors is related to the experience of the surgeon and the centre where it is treated. The other main feature influencing outcome is the age at which the Kasai is carried out. Biliary atresia is a progressive disease which can only be halted by restoration of effective biliary drainage. This effect is actually difficult to quantify and almost certainly it is not a linear relationship. However, there probably is a finite time point beyond which the liver is irretrievable, so the worse outcomes are seen in the late Kasai's (arbitrarily > 100 days) with established cirrhosis. Whether those fortunate few who come to a Kasai at <40 days have a better prognosis is more difficult to define or quantify (Fig. 55.6).

Infants with BASM have poorer prognosis and reduced probability of clearance of jaundice although the degree of liver fibrosis at the time of the Kasai is comparable with age-matched non-syndromic infants.

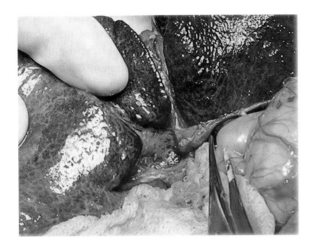

Fig. 55.4 Close-up of porta hepatis showing appropriate level of transection

Fig. 55.6 Graph showing relationship of age at time of Kasai portoenterostomy and outcome (resolution of bilirubin to ≤20 μmol/l). Solid lines are cumulative (from left to right) probability of clearance at defined time points for all cases of BA (*n* = 160, blue line), cases of syndromic BASM (*n* = 25, green line) and those with some cystic change within biliary remnant (*n* = 15). The cumulative age at Kasai (dotted line) for the whole cohort (1999–2005) is also illustrated (median age = 58 days)

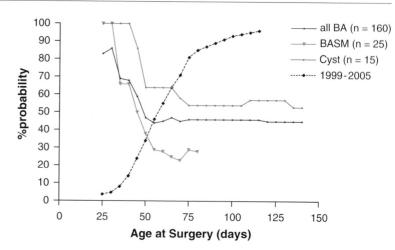

55.9 Complications

The main complication is simply that the procedure doesn't work. About 10–20% of all Kasais will have no effect on the course of the liver disease with persisting acholic stools and increasing jaundice. This is probably a function of the lack of exposed biliary ductules at the porta hepatis rather than the degree of established liver fibrosis and can only be treated by transplantation. Alternatively, restored bile flow in about 50% will be sufficient to allow their bilirubin levels to fall to normal with an excellent long-term prognosis. Nonetheless it is impossible to say that, even in these children, they are "cured" as if biopsied, the liver will show cirrhosis in over half. The remainder will have a degree of restoration of bile flow as evidenced by a fall in bilirubin and although some maintain reasonable biochemical liver function and absence of complications for long periods most tend to deteriorate over time.

55.9.1 Cholangitis

Re-establishment of bile drainage exposes the child to the risk of ascending cholangitis. This is seen in up to 40% of most series and is particularly prevalent in the first 2 years. The usual organisms are enteric in origin (e.g. *Escherichia coli*, *Pseudomonas*, *Klebsiella* spp.) and present with pyrexia and a worsening of jaundice and biochemical liver function.

The diagnosis can be difficult to establish beyond reasonable doubt but presumptive treatment should not wait for positive cultures (blood or liver) and should consist of intravenous broad-spectrum antibiotics. Most respond within 24 h and liver function is usually restored fairly quickly.

Recalcitrant cholangitis can be a problem in some children and should be initially treated by inserting a Hickman line and long-term administration of intravenous antibiotics, perhaps with cyclical oral antibiotics. Sometimes cholangitis can be associated with parenchymal cyst formation and some studies have advocated percutaneous aspiration or internal drainage to try and improve bile drainage. A brief course of high-dose steroids has also been advocated by some.

Occasionally cholangitis occurs as a late event in otherwise normal children or adolescents. A possible cause in these is a partial obstruction of their Roux loops, typically where it goes through the mesocolon, leading to bile stasis. A combination of radio-isotope scans and percutaneous cholangiography may aid the diagnostic process and subsequent Roux loop revision is usually straightforward and successful.

55.9.2 Portal Hypertension

Portal hypertension has been shown in virtually all infants at the time of the Kasai operation, however subsequent significant portal hypertension depends both on the degree of established fibrosis and, most importantly, the response to surgery. There is a relationship with biochemical liver function and variceal development. Thus, in those who fail and need early transplantation about 40% will have had a significant variceal bleed. In those who respond well to initial Kasai, but who perhaps have already established fibrosis then variceal development can be delayed. In these bleeding may be deferred until 2–4 years of age.

Infants and children with bleeding oesophageal varices need rapid access to a high quality paediatric facility with the resources and experience to manage them. Injection/banding is not a technique for the occasional endoscopist. Restoration of circulating blood volume and pharmacotherapy (e.g. octreotide) should precede endoscopy and achieve a measure of stabilisation. Sometimes a modified Sengstaken tube needs to be placed to achieve haemostasis. Invariably in children this can only be done under general anaesthesia but can be lifesaving. Older children are suited to endoscopic variceal banding, although injection sclerotherapy retains a role in treating varices in infants.

Liver transplantation needs to be actively considered as definitive treatment for portal hypertension where liver function is poor and the child is already significantly jaundiced. A few centres will consider portsystemic shunts for those where the varices become difficult to manage endoscopically but who have good liver function although this is not common.

Splenomegaly is invariably found with portal hypertension (at least in those with spleens!). This may cause hypersplenism (thrombocytopenia, anaemia and leucopenia) but of itself does not usually require specific intervention. Some centres in Japan advocate partial splenic embolization but the evidence for real benefit is sparse.

55.9.3 *Miscellaneous*

Less common complications include the development of the hepatopulmonary syndrome where there is chronic hypoxia secondary to the presence of abnormal pulmonary arteriovenous communications. This is related to established liver disease and is particularly prevalent in those with BASM. It can also be a cause of sudden death and if diagnosed active consideration for liver transplantation should be given.

Children with treated biliary atresia invariably have damaged abnormal livers, sub-normal bile flow and the potential for malabsorption and fat-soluble vitamin and perhaps trace element deficiencies. Vitamin levels should be checked at regular intervals and appropriate dietetic advice on calorie and protein supplementation sought if growth failure is suspected.

Further Reading

Davenport M (2005) Biliary atresia. Semin Pediatr Surg 14: 42–48

Davenport M, Kerkar N, Mieli-Vergani G, Mowat AP, Howard ER (1997) Biliary atresia: The King's College Hospital experience. J Pediatr Surg 32:479–485

Davenport M, Betalli P, D'Antiga L et al (2003) The spectrum of surgical jaundice in infancy. J Pediatr Surg 38: 1471–1479

Davenport M, Ville de Goyet J, Stringer MD et al (2004) Seamless management of biliary atresia in England & Wales 1999–2002. Lancet 363:1354–1357

Davenport M, Tizzard S, Underhill J, Mieli-Vergani G, Portmann B, Hadzic N (2006) The biliary atresia splenic malformation syndrome: A 28-year single-center retrospective study. J Pediatr 149:393–400

Ohi R, Nio M (2006) Biliary atresia. In P Puri, ME Höllwarth (eds) Pediatric Surgery. Springer Surgery Atlas Series, Springer-Verlag Berlin Heidelberg, New York, pp 357–370

Choledochal Cyst

56

Atsuyuki Yamataka and Yoshifumi Kato

Contents

56.1 Introduction

Choledochal cysts, or dilatation of the common bile duct, were first reported by Douglas in 1852. The condition is a relatively rare abnormality with an estimated incidence in Western populations of 1 in 13,000–15,000. However, this condition is far more common in the East, with rates as high as 1 per 1,000 having been described in Japan. The etiology remains unknown, but choledochal cysts are likely to be congenital in nature. The pathologic features of the condition frequently include an anomalous junction of the pancreatic and common bile ducts (pancreaticobiliary malunion: PBMU), intrahepatic bile duct dilatation with or without downstream stenosis, and various degrees of hepatic fibrosis.

Choledochal cysts are usually classified into three groups, based on anatomy. However, other forms and subgroups have been described, based on the cholangiographic findings of intrahepatic ducts or pancreaticobiliary malunion (PBMU), i.e., the so-called long common channel. Based on our experience, we prefer to classify choledochal cysts into groups associated with presence or absence of PBMU (Fig. 56.1). The majority of choledochal cysts are choledochal cysts with PBMU, and choledochal cysts without PBMU are extremely rare. Thus, the following comments are related primarily to cystic, fusiform, or forme fruste choledochal cysts (FFCC).

56.2 Etiology

A number of theories have been proposed for the etiology of the choledochal cyst. Congenital weakness of the bile duct wall, a primary abnormality of proliferation

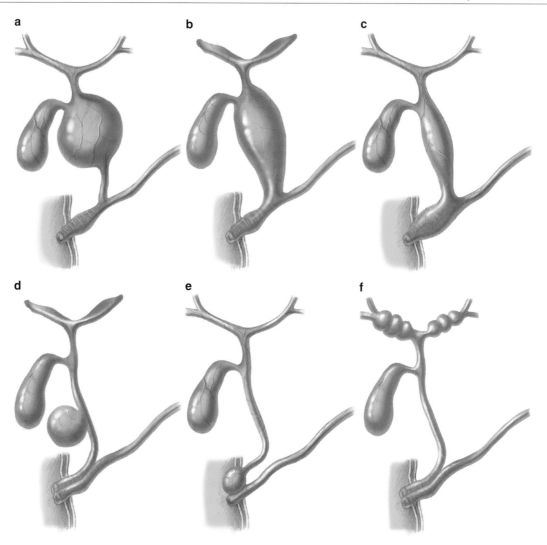

Fig. 56.1 Classification of choledochal cysts with PBMU. (**a**) Cystic dilatation of the extrahepatic bile duct. (**b**) Fusiform dilatation of the extrahepatic bile duct. (**c**) Forme fruste choledochal cyst. Without PBMU. (**d**) Cystic diverticulum of the common bile duct. (**e**) Choledochocele (diverticulum of the distal common bile duct). (**f**) Intrahepatic bile duct dilatation alone (Caroli's disease) (From Miyano et al., 2006, p373; Figure 34.1a–f)

during embryologic ductal development and congenital obstruction have been given as possible causes. Unequal proliferation of epithelial cells of primitive bile ducts when they are still solid is postulated as a hypothesis. If cellular proliferation is more active than that of distal portion of the duct, canalization will give rise to an abnormally dilated proximal end. An obstructive factor in the early developmental stage was stressed as a causative factor. It is based on an experimental study in which cystic dilatation of the common bile duct was produced by ligation of the distal end of the common bile duct in the neonatal lamb, but not in a later stage of development.

In 1969, the so called "long common channel theory" was proposed as a new concept. This explained that PBMU allows reflux of pancreatic enzymes into the common bile duct, and this leads to dissolution of the ductal wall. This theory is in vogue and supported by the high amylase content in the aspirated fluid from the choledochal cyst. In addition, it is stated that the common bile duct could become obstructed at the distal end of the cyst due to edema or eventually fibrosis caused by refluxed pancreatic fluid.

We support the "long common channel theory" based on our clinical experience since almost all choledochal cyst patients have PBMU, but we cannot agree with the hypothesis that the weakness of the choledochal wall due to the reflux of pancreatic fluid is the most basic causative factor of the cystic dilatation. However, with regard to the chemical reactions of the refluxed pancreatic fluid in the bile duct, we showed that this chemical reaction must be extremely mild, according to our animal experiments in puppies, in order to produce pancreatic fluid regurgitation into the bile duct. Also it is generally recognized that a number of patients who have PBMU and high amylase level in the gallbladder show no dilatation of the common bile duct. A diagnosis of choledochal cyst can be made antenatally as early as the 5th month of gestation, but at this time, fetal pancreas has not matured enough to produce functional enzymes, so the exact role of the pancreatic fluid is unclear. From research on human fetuses, it was demonstrated that the pancreaticobiliary ductal junction was outside the duodenal wall before the 8th week of gestation then moved inward toward the duodenal lumen, suggesting that PBMU may be caused by arrest of this migration.

Based on these studies, we believe that an anomalous pancreaticobiliary ductal junction (PBMU) combined with congenital stenosis are the basic causative factors of the choledochal cyst rather than weakness caused by reflux of the pancreatic fluid, at least in perinatal and young infants.

56.3 Pathology

56.3.1 Cystic Type or Fusiform Type Choledochal Cyst

The bile duct mucosa shows erosion, epithelial desquamation and papillary hyperplasia with regenerative atypia. Erosion, epithelial desquamation and dysplasia in the bile duct mucosa without carcinoma are frequently found in patients with choledochal cyst. Additionally, metaplastic changes, such as mucous cells, goblet cells and Paneth's cells, were observed. Such hyper plastic and metaplastic epithelia were apt to increase with age, and progress into dysplasia in adult cases, probably resulting in carcinogenic factors of the bile duct carcinoma.

The gallbladder mucosa in patients with PBMU shows cholecystitis, cholesterolosis, adenomyosis or adenomyomatosis, polyp including adenoma, and epithelial hyperplasia, which is particularly characteristic in PBMU.

56.3.2 Forme Fruste Choledochal Cyst (FFCC)

Bile duct mucosa with FFCC shows non-specific changes such as mucosal ulceration/sloughing, fibrosis, and inflammatory cell infiltration, indicating that children with FFCC may be at a high risk for carcinogenesis in the extrahepatic bile duct. These changes are the same ones as seen in cystic or fusiform type choledochal cysts.

The gallbladder mucosa showed diffuse epithelial hyperplasia characterized, with or without metaplasia of pyloric glands, goblet cells, and Paneth's cells.

56.4 Diagnosis

56.4.1 Clinical Features

Choledochal cysts can present at any age, but more than half of patients within the first decade of life. Clinical manifestations of choledochal cysts differ according to the age of onset.

In young infants, ranging neonates to 3 months old, the presence of obstructive jaundice, acholic stools and hepatomegaly, depending on the degree of obstruction, which resembles correctable biliary atresia, are the characteristic symptoms. These patients sometimes have advanced liver fibrosis. Notable difference from correctable biliary atresia is a patent communication to the duodenum and well-developed intra-hepatic bile ducts (IHBD) tree, as shown by surgical cholangiography. Another clinical presentation in young infants is a large upper abdominal mass without jaundice.

The presenting symptom of choledochal cysts in children after early infancy can be divided roughly into two groups: right upper quadrant mass with intermittent jaundice due to biliary obstruction, which is seen in patients with cystic choledochal cysts, and abdominal pain due to pancreatitis, which is characteristic in fusiform or forme fruste choledochal cysts.

Choledochal cysts in adolescence and adulthood appear to behave differently. Choledochal cysts undiagnosed for many years may ultimately lead to the development of cholelithiasis, liver cirrhosis, portal hypertension, hepatic abscess, and biliary carcinoma before cyst excision can be performed. Thus, surgery in this group is much more difficult than in children, and the incidence of postoperative complications is quite high even after primary cyst excision.

56.4.2 Ultrasonography

Currently abdominal ultrasonography is being used; this is probably the best screening method and should be applied first in patients who are suspected of having choledochal cyst. Furthermore, in recent years, the number of patients who are diagnosed by antenatal ultrasonography is increasing. This method also clearly demonstrates IHBD dilatation and the state of the liver parenchyma.

56.4.3 Radiological Diagnosis

For the diagnosis of choledochal cyst it is important to detect not only dilatation of the extrahepatic bile duct, but also PBMU. Endoscopic retrograde cholangiopancreatography (ERCP) can accurately visualize the configuration of the pancreaticobiliary ductal system in the detail and is unlikely to be replaced by other investigations, especially in cases where fine detail is required presurgically. However, it is invasive and therefore unsuitable for repeated use and is contraindicated during acute pancreatitis. Percutaneous transhepatic drainage followed by cholangiography via the drainage tube is also valuable, especially for choledochal cyst with IHBD dilatation and severe jaundice. Intraoperative cholangiography is unnecessary if the entire biliary system has been delineated before cyst excision using the previously mentioned radiological investigations; however, it should not be omitted if the pancreaticobiliary ductal system is not visualized entirely.

56.4.4 Magnetic Resonance Cholangiopancreatography (MRCP)

We have shown that MRCP can provide excellent visualization of the pancreaticobiliary ducts in patients with CBD and allow detection of narro-wing, dilatation, and filling defects with medium to high degrees of accuracy (Fig. 56.2). MRCP is noninvasive and can partially replace ERCP as a diagnostic tool for the evaluation of anatomic anomalies of the pancreaticobiliary tract. Another advantage of MRCP over ERCP is that the pancreatic duct can be visualized upstream to an obstruction of the area of stenosis. However, MRCP may not allow visualization of pancreaticobiliary ductal system in children aged less than 3 years because of their small caliber.

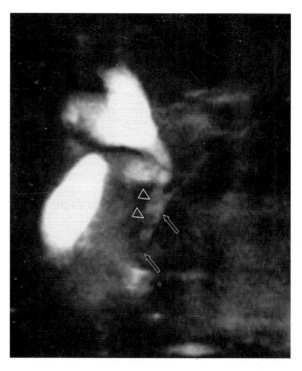

Fig. 56.2 Magnetic resonance cholangiopancreatography (MRCP) in a patient with a choledochal cyst showing fusiform dilatation of the extrahepatic bile duct, long common channel (between arrows), protein plugs (arrowheads), and pancreatic duct

56.5 Differential Diagnosis

In prenatal period, the differential diagnosis of CBD is intra-abdominal cystic lesions, such as Type I biliary atresia, ovarian cyst, giant cystic meconium peritonitis, duplication cyst and mesenteric cyst. After birth, CBD can be differentiated by combinations of the imaging studies.

56.6 Management

Cyst excision is the definitive treatment of choice for choledochal cyst because of the high morbidity and high risk of carcinoma after internal drainage, a commonly used treatment in the past. Recently, more attention has been paid to treatment of intrahepatic and intrapancreatic ductal diseases such as IHBD dilatation with downstream stenosis, debris in the IHBD, and protein plugs or stones in the common channel. The transection level of the common hepatic duct and excisional level of the intrapancreatic bile duct are also highly controversial.

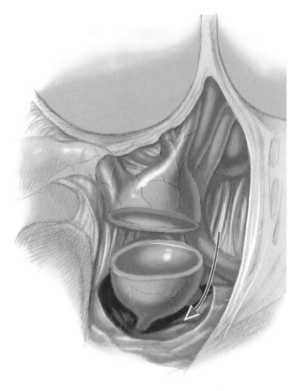

Fig. 56.3 Schema of transaction of choledochal cyst (From Miyano et al., 2006, p377; Figure 34.4)

56.6.1 Cyst Excision

There are usually more adhesions between a cystic type choledochal cyst and surrounding vital structures such as the portal vein and hepatic artery, especially in the older children, when compared with the fusiform type choledochal cyst. In the adolescent and adults, the adhesions are often very dense, and great care is required during cyst excision. Prior to dissection of the cyst, we always open the anterior wall of the choledochal cyst transversely (Fig. 56.3). By opening the anterior wall of the cyst, the posterior wall of the cyst is visible directly from the inside, and the choledochal cyst can be freed from surrounding tissues including the portal vein and hepatic artery more easily than by dissecting the cyst free without incising the anterior wall. If the cyst is extremely inflamed and adhesions are very dense, mucosectomy of the cyst (Figs. 56.4 and 56.5) should be performed rather than full-thickness dissection (Figs. 56.3 and 56.5) to minimize the risk of injuring the surrounding structures such as portal vein and hepatic artery.

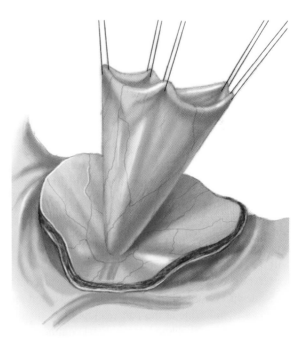

Fig. 56.4 Schema of mucosectomy of distal portion of choledochal cyst (From Miyano et al., 2006, p377; Figure 34.5)

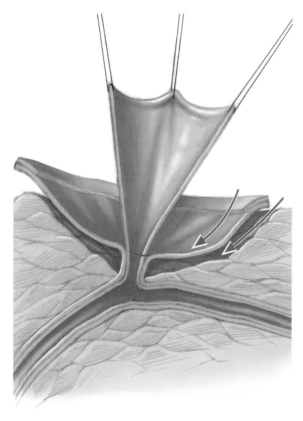

Fig. 56.5 Operative procedure for the excision of the distal portion of choledochal cyst (*arrows*; mucosectomy layer or full-thickness layer) (From Miyano et al., 2006, p377; Figure 34.6)

56.6.2 Excision of the Distal Common Bile Duct

In order to prevent postoperative pancreatitis and/or stone formation due to the formation of a residual cyst, the distal common bile duct should be resected as close as possible to pancreaticobiliary ductal junction. In the cystic type, the distal common bile duct is narrow, and sometimes so narrow that it looks blind-ended and cannot be identified specifically. Thus, in the cystic type choledochal cyst, it is unlikely that a residual cyst will develop within the pancreas. In contrast, in fusiform type choledochal cyst, excision of the distal common bile duct is more difficult since the distal common bile duct is still wide at the pancreaticobiliary ductal junction, and the likelihood of the distal common bile duct being left within the pancreas if not excised properly is high. If the distal common bile duct is resected

along the red line (Fig. 56.6), over time, a cyst will reform around the distal duct left within the pancreas, leading to recurrent pancreatitis, stone formation in the residual cyst, or malignant changes in the residual cyst (Fig. 56.7). In contrast, if the distal duct is resected along the blue line (Fig. 56.8), that is, just above the pancreaticobiliary ductal junction, cyst reformation due to residual duct within the pancreas is unlikely (Fig. 56.9).

Before the introduction of intraoperative endoscopy, it was difficult to excise the pancreatic portion of the fusiform type choledochal cyst completely and safely because of risk of injury to the pancreatic duct. Endoscopy now allows safe excision of most of the fusiform choledochal cyst wall in the pancreas without damaging the pancreatic duct, and we believe that this reduces the risk of postoperative complications such as recurrent pancreatitis, stone formation, and carcinoma.

56.6.3 Excision of the Common Hepatic Duct

The common hepatic duct is transected at the level of distinct caliber change. Because any remaining proximal cyst mucosa is prone to malignant changes, care must be taken to excise it completely, especially when there is a large anastomosis. (Fig. 56.10).

56.6.4 Dilatation of the IHBD

Dilatation of the peripheral portion of the IHBD in patients with choledochal cysts may be associated with late complications such as recurrent cholangitis, stone formation, and anastomotic stricture. Thus, dilatation of the IHBD can be managed by segmentectomy of the liver, intrahepatic cystoenterostomy, or balloon dilatation of the stenosis at the time of cyst excision. However, the incidence of the late complications appears to be low, especially in younger children, so such excessive surgical intervention may be unnecessary except in specific cases where there is massive dilatation of the peripheral IHBD with severe downstream stenosis. If IHBD dilatation persists even after definitive surgery, careful follow-up is mandatory.

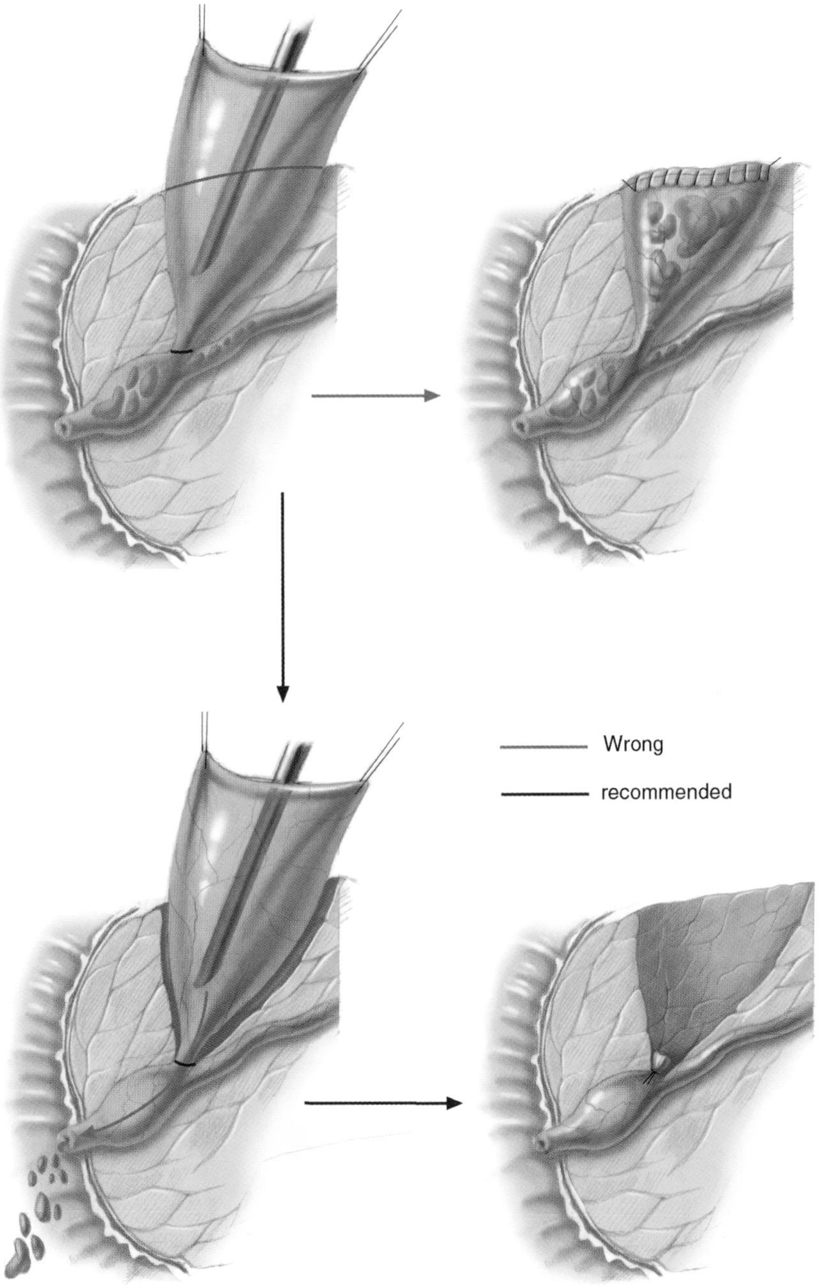

Figs. 56.6–56.9 Diagram of intraoperative endoscopy of the bile duct distal to a cyst with debris and protein plug. If the distal common bile duct is resected along the red line (Fig. 56.6), over time, a cyst will reform around the distal duct left within the pancreas, leading to recurrent pancreatitis, stone formation in the residual cyst, or malignant changes in the residual cyst (Fig. 56.7). In contrast, if the distal duct is resected along the blue line (Fig. 56.8), that is, just above the pancreaticobiliary ductal junction, cyst reformation due to residual duct within the pancreas is unlikely (Fig. 56.9) (From Miyano et al., 2006, p381; Figures 34.9–34.12)

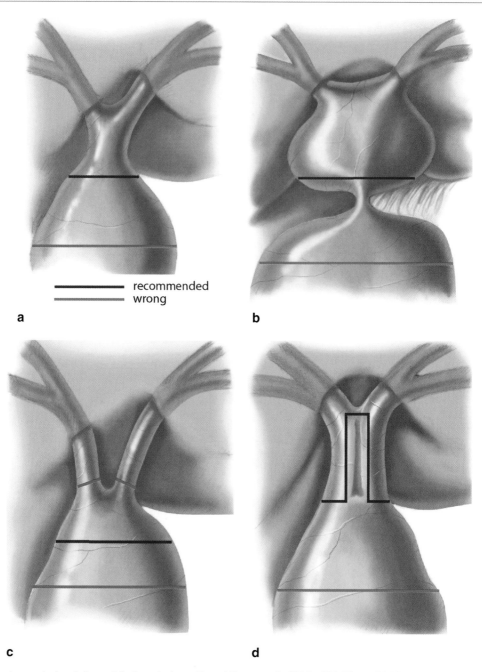

Fig. 56.10 Anatomical variations of the hepatic ducts (From Miyano et al., 2006, p383; Figure 34.14)

56.6.5 Intraoperative Endoscopy

Intraoperative endoscopy is also useful for examining for the presence of debris in the dilated IHBD (Fig. 56.11). Recently we found there was a high incidence of IHBD debris that was not usually detected by preoperative radiological investigations. In addition, some of IHBD debris was overlooked although the debris had been shown in the preoperative radiography by retrospective review. These facts indicate that intraoperative endoscopy is necessary at the time of cyst excision even if preoperative radiological investigations did not show the presence of IHBD debris. Another striking finding was that there could be debris even when the IHBD were not

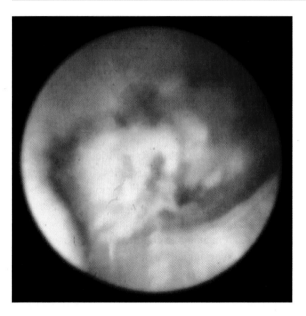

Fig. 56.11 Massive debris in the intrahepatic bile duct observed through the pediatric cystoscope

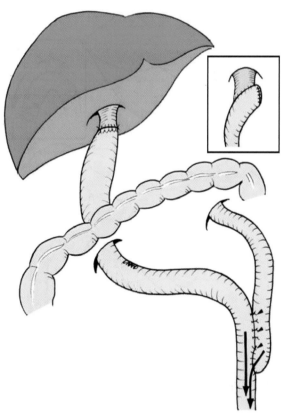

Fig. 56.12 Adequate Roux-en-Y (RY) hepatico-jejunostomy at the time of cyst excision. Arrowheads indicate approximated native jejunum and distal RY limb. Arrows indicate smooth flow without reflux of small bowel contents

dilated, although debris was more common when the IHBD were dilated. Thus, we believe, inspection even to non-dilated IHBD also should not be omitted.

56.6.6 Roux-en-Y Hepaticojejunostomy

End-to-end anastomosis during Roux-en-Y hepaticojejunostomy is recommended to prevent elongation of the blind pouch if the ratio between the diameters of the common hepatic duct and the proximal Roux-en-Y jejunum at the proposed site of anastomosis is less than or equal to 1 (common hepatic duct): 2.5 (jejunum) (Fig. 56.12). If end-to-side anastomosis is unavoidable, the common hepatic duct should be anastomosed as close as possible to the closed end of the blind pouch (Fig. 56.12, inset) so there will be no blind pouch at the hepaticojejunostomy anastomosis site; if an end-to-side anastomosis is performed far from the closed end of the blind pouch, elongation of the blind pouch will occur later in life as the child grows (Fig. 56.13). Elongation of the blind pouch can cause bile stasis in the blind pouch and IHBD (especially if they are dilated) leading to stone formation. We believe end-to-end hepaticojejunostomy anastomosis and our end-to-side anastomosis technique prevent stone formation in the blind pouch (or IHBD) and cholangitis.

Some surgeons predetermine the length of the Roux-en-Y jejunal limb, e.g. 30, 40, 50, or 60 cm without considering the size of the child, which causes the Roux-en-Y jejunal limb to be unnecessarily long especially in infants and the younger children. Redundancy of the Roux-en-Y limb is likely to occur later in life as the patient grows and may cause bile stasis in the Roux-en-Y limb itself as well as in the IHBD, leading to cholangitis or stone formation. Thus, the length of the Roux-en-Y limb should be individualized so the Roux-en-Y jejuno-jejunostomy fits naturally into the splenic flexure after the jejuno-jejunostomy is completed and returned to the peritoneal cavity (Fig. 56.12). In this situation, redundancy of the Roux-en-Y limb will not occur.

When a jejuno-jejunostomy and Roux-en-Y limb are used, we recommend that both the native jejunum and the Roux-en-Y jejunal limb proximal to the jejuno-jejunostomy be approximated for up to 8 cm from the jejuno-jejunostomy cranially to ensure both bile in the Roux-en-Y limb and the contents of the native jejunum flow smoothly

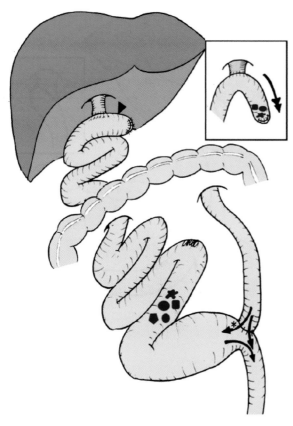

Fig. 56.13 Inadequate Roux-en-Y (RY) hepatico-jejunostomy (HJ) at the time of cyst excision HJ far from the closed end of the blind pouch (arrowhead). Double arrows in the inset indicate elongation of the blind pouch. Arrow with an asterisk indicates reflux of jejunal contents into the RY limb through a T-shaped RY jejuno-jejunostomy

down into the jejunum distal to the jejuno-jejunostomy (Fig. 56.12). Without performing this, the jejuno-jejunostomy tends to be T-shaped, and there may be reflux of jejunal contents into the Roux-en-Y limb, leading to the dilatation of the jejunal limb and biliary stasis in the Roux-en-Y limb, a situation we recently encountered in a patient who was operated on at another hospital (Fig. 56.13).

56.7 Complications

A satisfactory surgical outcome with low morbidity is expected in patients with choledochal cysts after cyst excision in the short to mid term. However, in the long term view, many complications are reported. So long term careful follow-up is mandatory.

In an American survey in 1981, 14 of 198 patients with choledochal cysts were reported to have died of biliary atresia, cholangitis with sepsis, hepatic failure, or carcinoma. The common late complications were cholangitis, obstructive jaundice, pancreatitis, stone formation, and portal hypertension. The survey showed that 36 patients were lost to follow-up, and 115 patients were alive without liver disease.

We reviewed 200 children who had cyst excision performed at the age of 15 years or less in 1997. The age of initial symptom development (various combinations of abdominal pain, abdominal mass, and jaundice) was 5 years or less in 175 children, and between 6 and 15 years in the remaining 25 children. The mean age when patients become initially symptomatic was 3.0 years. The mean age at cyst excision was 4.2 years. Primary cyst excision was performed in 176, five had cyst excision converted from internal drainage, and 19 had cyst excision converted from other biliary surgery such as percutaneous transhepatic cholangiodrainage, T-tube drainage, cholecystectomy, and so on. Intraoperative endoscopy was used in 70 children. The mean follow-up period was 10.9 years. Roux-en-Y hepaticojejunostomy was performed in 188 patients, 11 had standard hepaticoduodenostomy, and one had a jejunal interposition hepaticojejunostomy. There was no operative mortality. Eighteen (9.0%) children had 25 complications after cyst excision, including ascending cholangitis, intrapancreatic terminal choledochus calculi, pancreatitis, and bowel obstruction (Table 56.1). Fifteen of the 18 children required surgical interventions such as revision of the hepaticoenterostomy, percutaneous transhepatic cholangioscopic lithotomy, and excision of the residual intrapancreatic terminal choledochus, endoscopic sphincterotomy, pancreaticojejunostomy, or laparotomy for bowel obstruction. There was neither stone formation, anastomotic stricture, nor cholangitis in the 70 children who had intraoperative endoscopy. There was no occurrence of malignancy.

In patients who underwent cyst excision at the age of 5 years or less, there were no major complications such as the intrahepatic stone formation, or intrapancreatic terminal choledochus calculi, and anastomotic stricture of the hepaticoenterostomy. Thus, we believe early diagnosis followed by cyst excision and intraoperative endoscopy is extremely important to prevent postoperative complications.

Even after primary cyst excision, malignancy can arise from the intrapancreatic terminal choledochus,

Table 56.1 Complications after cyst excision in children versus adults

Incidence in 200 Children	Post-CEHE complications	Incidence in 40 adults
3	Ascending cholangitis	9
3	Intrahepatic bile duct stones	5
3[a]	Intrapancreatic terminal Choledochus calculi	1
1	Pancreatic duct calculus	1
1[a]	Stones in the blind pouch of the end-to-side Roux-en-Y hepaticojejunostomy	0
9[b]	Bowel obstruction	3[c]
0	Cholangiocarcinoma	2
0	Liver dysfunction	1
5	Pancreatitis	5
25 (18)	Total	27 (17)

The numbers in parenthesis indicate the no. of patients who had complications after cyst excision (18 children and 17 adults had 25 and 27 complications after cyst excision, respectively).

[a]One patient with intrapancreatic terminal choledochus calculi also had a stone in the blind pouch of the end-to-side hepaticojejunostomy.

[b]Adhesions in six and intussusception in three.

[c]Adhesions in all three.

the hepaticojejunostomy anastomosis site, and from the IHBD. Of the 40 adult patients in our series who had cyst excision at the age of 16 years or more, two died of cholangiocarcinoma. One of these patients had a primary cyst excision at the age of 25 years.

In a single institute for the past 18 years, we have performed a total of 92 Roux-en-Y hepaticojejunostomy (70 end-to-end anastomosis and 22 end-to-side anastomosis) using our cyst excision technique with intraoperative endoscopy, and our recommendations for the Roux-en-Y hepaticojejunostomy mentioned in the section of the treatment in this chapter, and all

patients are well after a mean follow-up period of 8.0 years (range 9 months–16 years) without any major complications.

Cyst excision and Roux-en-Y hepaticojejunostomy is the treatment of choice in both children and adults with choledochal cyst. Intraoperative endoscopy at the time of cyst excision is useful to prevent post-operative complications, especially those that develop in the over time. Roux-en-Y hepaticojejunostomy in children is different from that in adults, since the Roux-en-Y limb or blind pouch can grow and elongate as the child grows.

Further Reading

Miyano T (2005) Biliary tract disorders and portal hypertension. In K Ashcraft, G Holcomb III, J Murphy (eds) Pediatric Surgery, 4th edn. Elsevier Saunders, Philadelphia, pp 586–608

Miyano T (2006) Choledocal cyst. In M Stringer, K Oldham, P Mouriquand (eds) Pediatric Surgery and Urology Long-Term Outcomes, 2nd edn. Cambridge, Cambridge University Press, pp 465–479

Miyano T, Yamataka A (2003) Congenital biliary dilatation (choledocal cyst) In P Puri (ed) Newborn Surgery, 2nd edn. Arnold, London, pp 589–596

Miyano T, Urao M, Yamataka A (2006) Choledocal cyst. In P Puri, ME Höllwarth (eds) Pediatric Surgery. Springer Surgery Atlas Series, Springer-Verlag Berlin Heidelberg, New York, pp 371–386

O'Neill JA (1998) Pediatric Surgery, 5th edn. Mosby, St. Louis, MO, pp 1483–1493

Puri P, Höllwarth ME (2006) Pediatric Surgery. Springer, Berlin, Heidelberg

Shimotakahara A, Yamataka A, Yanai T et al (2005) Roux-en-Y hepaticojejunostomy or hepaticoduodenstomy for biliary reconstruction during the surgical treatment of choledochal cyst: Which is better? Pediatr Surg Int 21:5–7

Yamataka A, Kobayashi H, Shimotakahara A et al (2003) Recommen-dations for preventing complications related to Roux-en-Y hepatico-jejunostomy performed during excision of choledochal cyst. J Pediatr Surg 38:1830–1832

Hepatic Cysts and Abscesses

57

Priya Ramachandran

Contents

57.1 Introduction

Cystic lesions of the liver are seen in a multitude of conditions. Congenital simple cysts are asymptomatic in most cases except when associated with portal hypertension as in polycystic disease, portal fibrosis and Caroli's disease. Hydatid disease is the commonest cause of parasitic liver disease. Cystic neoplasms of the liver include hemangioendotheliomas, mesenchymal hamartomas and teratomas.

Liver abscesses are rarely asymptomatic and present with local and systemic signs of illness especially in pyogenic and amoebic abscesses. Fungal abscesses may not manifest with fever. Early diagnosis and prompt treatment has resulted in a dramatic reduction of the morbidity and mortality of this condition.

This chapter deals with the surgically relevant aspects of hepatic cysts and liver abscesses.

57.2 Hepatic Cysts

57.2.1 Congenital Liver Cysts

57.2.1.1 Simple Non Neoplastic Cyst

These cysts are uncommon in children and are often identified as incidental findings during imaging procedures. They are unilocular or mutilocular and contain clear or brownish liquid. They may be present entirely within the liver or as a pedunculated mass from the surface of the liver. The lining of the cyst wall is composed of an inner layer of epithelium (cuboidal, columnar or squamous) and an outer wall

P. Puri and M. Höllwarth (eds.), *Pediatric Surgery: Diagnosis and Management,*
DOI: 10.1007/978-3-540-69560-8_57, © Springer-Verlag Berlin Heidelberg 2009

which contains collagen and compressed liver tissue. When they enlarge they become symptomatic and present as a large abdominal mass. In such cases, deroofing of the cyst is preferable to cyst excision which may require resection of the adjacent lobe of the liver. In rare instances, if the cyst communicates with the biliary tract as confirmed by the presence of bile in the cyst and preoperative cholangiography, an internal drainage procedure into the small bowel is recommended.

57.2.1.2 Polycystic Disease

Liver cysts can occur in patients with Autosomal Dominant Polycystic kidney disease. In children, the kidney is more severely affected than the liver and although liver cysts have been reported, complications are rare. Surgical treatment is indicated only if the cysts cause pain and discomfort. Fenestration of the cyst is a better option than lobectomy.

In children with Autosomal Recessive Polycystic disease of the kidney, extremely dilated bile ducts are seen in the liver. However large cysts of the liver are rare. Most of these children have symptoms of portal hypertension because of portal fibrosis.

57.2.1.3 Congenital Hepatic Fibrosis

This condition occurs in various syndromes and presents with the clinical features of portal hypertension. The intrahepatic bile ducts are dilated and portal fibrosis is present. The outcome is good if the portal hypertension is well controlled.

57.2.1.4 Caroli's Disease

This condition is characterized by multiple strictures in the intra hepatic bile ducts. This leads to recurrent episodes of cholangitis and cholelithiasis. In children it is usually the larger intrahepatic bile ducts that are affected and they go on to develop portal hypertension. Segmental bile duct dilation is a variant of this disease. It affects only one part of the liver and is rare in children.

57.2.2 Parasitic Cysts

Hydatid disease of the liver is caused by two species, namely Echinococcus granulosus and Echinococcus multilocularis. This infection is endemic in the Middle-East, Australia and South Africa.

The parasite has a life cycle linked to the intermediate host and a definitive host. The worm lives in the intestine of animals like the dog (definitive hosts) and the ova are consumed by humans and animals like sheep and cattle who are the intermediary hosts. Humans are affected by contact with contaminated environments and infected animals.

In the intermediate host the ova that are not destroyed by the gastric juice reach the duodenum where the alkaline intestinal contents dissolve the membrane of the ovum thereby releasing the embryos. The embryos penetrate the bowel wall and reach the liver through the blood stream where they are filtered by the small capillaries of the liver. The embryos develop into cysts in the liver. These cysts have a pericyst layer composed of connective tissue, epithelial cells, giant cells and eosinophils. This layer is densely adherent to the liver tissue. Within the pericyst layer is the endocyst layer composed of an outer thick layer which allows permeation of nutrition into the cyst and an inner germinal layer which secretes hydatid fluid and produces scolices and daughter cysts. The hydatid fluid is very antigenic and spillage of this fluid can result in development of cysts in the peritoneal cavity.

The hydatid cysts in the liver are slow growing although in children they grow rapidly and may appear by 3 years of age. Small cysts remain uncomplicated while large cysts cause pressure on the adjacent liver tissue and this leads to obstructive jaundice and cholangitis. Large cysts also cause pain and may rupture into the peritoneal cavity or into the pleural space. Sometimes there can be secondary bacterial infection in the cyst.

Asymptomatic cysts may be incidental findings during ultrasound examinations. Especially in children from endemic areas, hydatid cysts must be considered in the differential diagnosis of hypoechoic lesions of the liver.

Ultrasound scans are accurate in the diagnosis of these cysts. CT scans show calcification of the cyst wall and the presence of daughter cysts. The reliability of the Casoni's skin test is less than the indirect hemagglutination tests and the enzyme linked immunosorbent assays (ELISA).

Mebendazole and Albendazole are the drugs of choice in the treatment of hydatid disease and must be continued for 1–2 months to prevent recurrence. Surgery is restricted to children with large cysts (<5 cm in diameter) or complicated cysts that have ruptured. During laparotomy, the large cysts are aspirated and carefully opened to avoid spillage. The endocyst wall is carefully removed by blunt dissection and the residual cavity is closed with mass sutures. Cyst perforation must be treated urgently and high dose steroids in the postoperative period reduce the effects of anaphylaxis. Recently percutaneous aspiration of the cyst with injection of hypertonic saline has been reported to be successful.

57.2.3 Cystic Neoplasms of the Liver

Hemangioendotheliomas present as hypoechoic lesions on ultrasound or CT scans and may be mistaken for abscesses. There may be small multifocal hypoechoic lesions scattered throughout the liver which are diagnostic of multifocal hemangioendotheliomas.

The histology shows orderly arrangement of endothelial vascular spaces and in the more aggressive variety the vascular spaces are complex with hyperchromatic and pleomorphic changes in the endothelial cells. Small tumors can be treated with corticosteroids and cyclophosphamide followed by embolisation of the feeding vessels. The tumor regresses slowly after embolisation which is successful in 60% of children. In infants, two or three attempts of embolisation are required because the vessels are small. Hepatic resections are restricted to lesions involving one lobe.

Mesenchymal Hamartomas present as cystic lesions because they arise from mesenchymal cells which give rise to blood vessels and bile ducts. Hence these structures are predominant in the cystic structure and are surrounded by connective tissue stroma. They may enlarge secondary to fluid accumulation and the children present with features of congestive heart failure. A large fluid filled cyst with fine septations is seen on ultrasound and CT scans. There is no role for aggressive surgical intervention since the lesion is essentially benign. Total resection is the treatment of choice whenever possible. Marsupialisation is advocated with large cysts which may recur with incomplete excision.

Cystic teratomas are rare and present with calcification in the margins of the cyst. Serum alpha fetoprotein is mildly elevated in some cases. Resection is the treatment of choice because of the potential for malignancy exists especially if there are immature elements.

57.3 Hepatic Abscesses

Bacterial infections are transmitted to the liver via the hepatic artery, bile ducts or portal veins. Most pyogenic abscesses in the western world are seen in children with immunodeficiencies and who are immunosupressed from chemotherapy and transplants. However in Asia and Africa, pyogenic abscesses are seen in neonates with omphalitis.

Pyogenic abscesses may arise in children who have recurrent cholangitis secondary to cholelithiasis and choledochal cysts, which causes inflammation and obstruction of the bile ducts. Following a portoenterostomy for biliary atresia, intrahepatic biliomas may develop into pyogenic abscesses in the presence of secondary infection. Infections of the gastrointestinal tract like acute appendicitis can lead to portal pyemia and liver abscesses. However, today such complications are rarely seen. Hematomas of the liver sustained from blunt abdominal trauma may develop into pyogenic abscesses. In generalized sepsis, bacterial seeding of the liver leads to pyogenic abscesses. Such abscesses have been reported in patients with pneumonia, osteomyelitis and endocarditis. Pyogenic abscesses develop in benign hepatic cysts following attempts at percutaneous drainage. Infection in these non neoplastic cysts may also occur in the absence of intervention. Infection leads to an increase in size of the cysts with thickening and inflammation of the cyst wall. The commonest pathogens found in hepatic abscesses are Staphylococcus aureus, Escherichia coli, Hemophilus influenza and Pseudomonas.

Clinical features include fever, abdominal pain, jaundice, shoulder pain and dyspnoea. The symptoms may be of long duration especially in chronic abscesses. These children also have weight loss and anemia. The liver is enlarged and tender and a pleural effusion may be present. Ultrasound and CT scans are the mainstay in the diagnosis of liver abscesses. A chest X-ray may show elevation of the right hemi diaphragm and a right sided pleural effusion. 70% of liver abscesses are multiple. Anemia, leucocytosis and a raised ESR are found in a majority of cases. Broad spectrum antibiotics and image guided percutaneous drainage is the treatment of choice especially in multiple abscesses. Percutaneous catheter placement can be facilitated by laparoscopy. Open drainage is advocated when there is associated intestinal pathology that needs intervention or when the diagnosis is in doubt.

Septicemia in children with liver abscesses is associated with a higher mortality. Large abscesses may rupture into the subphrenic space, the pleural cavity and the peritoneal cavity in which case these children require a drainage procedure and broad spectrum antibiotics.

57.3.1 Amoebic Liver Abscesses

Entamoeba histolytica infections are transmitted from person to person due to poor sanitation in overpopulated areas. It is endemic to Africa and Asia. Liver involvement is the commonest extra intestinal manifestation of amoebiasis. The trophozoites from the colon enter the liver via the portal vein and initiate abscess formation. The right lobe is more commonly affected. The clinical features include fever with rigor, weight loss and right upper quadrant pain. Dyspnoea is also seen in the presence of a right sided pleural effusion. The liver is enlarged and tender. Rapid increase in distension is an indication that rupture of the cyst is imminent.

Mild anemia, leucocytosis, raised ESR and mildly elevated liver enzymes may be present. The parasite is identified in the stool in only 30% of cases. Serological tests like indirect hemagglutination do not distinguish between old and new infections. Other investigations include a chest X-ray which may show an elevated diaphragm on the right side, pleural effusion and right lower lobe infiltration. An ultrasound scan will accurately identify the location and size of these abscesses and image aided percutaneous aspiration to identify amoeba on smear will confirm the diagnosis. CT scan offers no advantage over ultrasound.

Most cases of amoebic liver abscesses respond to Metronidazole. With intravenous Metronidazole in doses of 35–50 mg/kg, clinical remission is seen within 72 h in a majority of cases. Radiological remission takes longer. Closed aspiration is rarely necessary and is advocated in rapidly enlarging abscesses or when the diagnosis is in doubt and a pus culture is required. Intraperitoneal rupture causes peritonitis and shock. In such cases, urgent surgical exploration is necessary. Rarely the abscess ruptures into the pleural or pericardial cavity.

Rupture into the pleural cavity is marked by severe dyspnea and tachypnea with clinical signs of pleural effusion. Pleural collections can be drained by a tube thoracostomy. Rupture into the pericardial space is a serious complication leading to cardiac tamponade. The pericardial effusion requires urgent decompression. Percutaneous drainage of the liver abscesses will also drain the pericardial effusion since there is a communication between both cavities. Peritoneal rupture requires open surgical drainage and lavage.

Fortunately the mortality of the disease and the incidence of complications are on the decline due to early diagnosis and prompt treatment.

Further Reading

Andrews WS (2006) Gall Bladder disease and hepatic infection. In JA O'Neil, AG Coran, EW Fonkalsrud (eds) Pediatric Surgery. Mosby Elsevier, Philadelphia, pp 1635–1650

Cenk Buyukunal SW (2002) Hydatid disease. In ER Howard, MD Stringer, PM Colombani (eds) Surgery of the Liver, Bile Ducts and Pancreas in Children. Arnold, Hodder Headline Group, Euston, London, pp 355–362

Howard ER (2002) Cysts. In Howard ER, Stringer MD, Colombani PM (eds) Surgery of the Liver, Bile Ducts and Pancreas in Children. Arnold, Hodder Headline Group, Euston, London pp 239–246

Joseph VT (2002) Liver abscesses. In ER Howard, MD Stringer, PM Colombani (eds) Surgery of the Liver, Bile Ducts and Pancreas in Children. Arnold, Hodder Headline Group, Euston, London pp 355–362

Puri P, Höllwarth ME (eds) (2006) Pediatric Surgery. Springer, Berlin, Heidelberg

Portal Hypertension

58

Mark D. Stringer

Contents

58.1 Introduction

Portal hypertension (PHT) is a manifestation of a wide variety of conditions, each with a different natural history. It frequently presents with bleeding from esophageal varices which is the commonest cause of serious gastrointestinal bleeding in children. Precise diagnosis, a clear understanding of therapeutic options, and a multidisciplinary approach are essential for successful management.

58.2 Pathophysiology and Definition

The portal vein transports blood to the liver from the gastrointestinal tract and spleen (Fig. 58.1), contributing two-thirds of the liver's blood supply. The right and left portal veins undergo several divisions to supply each of the eight liver segments, where they terminate in the hepatic sinusoids.

Portal venous pressure is the product of blood flow and vascular resistance. Thus, PHT may develop as a result of increased vascular resistance (e.g. portal venous obstruction or hepatic fibrosis) or increased blood flow (e.g. arterioportal fistula). In cirrhosis of the liver, there is both an increase in splanchnic blood flow and an increased resistance to portal blood flow within the liver.

The normal portal venous pressure is 7–12 mmHg. A rise in portal pressure leads to splenomegaly and the development of varices at sites of portosystemic anastomoses: the distal oesophagus (esophageal varices); the anal canal (anorectal varices); the falciform ligament (umbilical varices); and in the abdominal wall and retroperitoneum. The junction between mucosal and submucosal varices in the distal 5 cm of the esophagus is the usual site of rupture causing

Fig. 58.1   The portomesenteric venous
system in portal hypertension

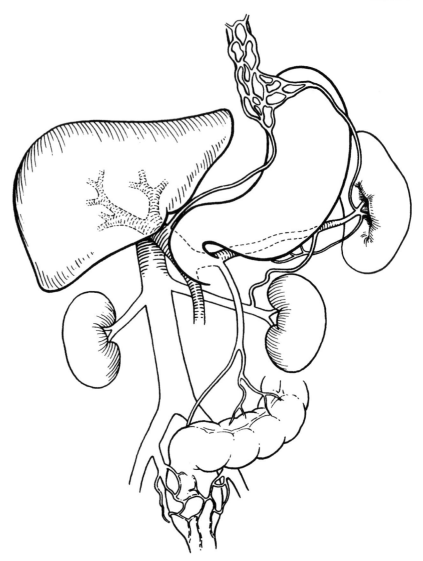

variceal bleeding. PHT is defined by an increased
hepatic venous pressure gradient of more than 5 mmHg,
i.e. the difference between the wedged hepatic venous
pressure (which reflects portal venous pressure) and
the free hepatic venous pressure. Esophageal varices
develop when the gradient exceeds 12 mmHg. The risk
of variceal bleeding is greatest in larger varices with a
higher internal pressure and wall tension.

58.3 Classification and Etiology

The vast majority of children with PHT have one of
the following underlying causes:

– Primary venous obstruction at a *prehepatic* (e.g.
  portal vein obstruction), *intrahepatic* (e.g. veno-
  occlusive disease) or *posthepatic* (e.g. Budd-Chiari
  syndrome) level (Table 58.1)
– Chronic liver disease (e.g. hepatic fibrosis or
  cirrhosis)

Chronic liver disease is the commonest overall cause
of PHT but portal vein occlusion (PVO) is the most
frequent cause of extrahepatic portal hypertension.
Occasionally, the picture is mixed as in the child with
cirrhosis complicated by portal vein thrombosis.

   Many etiologic factors have been implicated in the
cause of PVO which accounts for up to one-third of all
children with bleeding esophageal varices (Table 58.2).
Umbilical vein catheterization in the newborn, with or

Table 58.1   Etiology of portal hypertension in children

Primary venous obstruction	*Prehepatic*	Portal vein occlusion	Congenital
			Umbilical catheterization/sepsis in newborn
			Portal pyemia (e.g. appendicitis)
			Thrombophilic disorder
	Intrahepatic	Sinusoidal/venular occlusion	Veno-occlusive disease—toxic sinusoidal injury (e.g. chemotherapy, herbal toxins, bone marrow transplant)
			Schistosomiasis
			Hepatoportal sclerosis
	Posthepatic	Hepatic vein occlusion	Budd-Chiari syndrome
Chronic Liver disease		Liver fibrosis/cirrhosis	Biliary atresia, cystic fibrosis, chronic viral hepatitis, autoimmune hepatitis, alpha-1-antitrypsin deficiency, congenital hepatic fibrosis

Very rarely, PHT occurs without intrinsic obstruction of the portal/hepatic venous systems (e.g. chronic constrictive pericarditis or arterioportal venous fistula)

Table 58.2   Causes of portal vein occlusion

General factors

Developmental malformations

Septicaemia

Thrombophilia

Local factors

Umbilical sepsis/Umbilical catheterization ± infusion of irritant solutions in the newborn

Intra-abdominal sepsis and portal pyemia

Abdominal trauma (including surgical)

Structural lesions e.g. portal vein web

Cholangitis/choledochal cyst

Pancreatitis

Malignant disease/lymphadenopathy

Splenectomy

Post-transplant (local & general factors)

without infusion of irritant solutions, is a recognised cause of portal vein thrombosis although it is an uncommon complication of umbilical catheterization. Thrombophilic disorders such as deficiencies of protein C, S or antithrombin III or factor V Leiden gene mutations can predispose to portal vein thrombosis but are only rarely the cause. However, circulating levels of the natural anticoagulant proteins (C, S, and antithrombin III) are commonly decreased *as a result* of PVO.

In most children with isolated PVO the etiology is unknown. The portal vein is typically replaced by multiple venous collaterals, the so-called portal vein cavernoma. Occasionally, additional congenital anomalies such as congenital heart disease, intestinal malrotation, duodenal atresia and craniofacial dysostosis are present, suggesting that PVO may be a developmental malformation in these cases. The portal venous system

develops from paired vitelline and umbilical veins which drain the yolk sac and placenta, respectively. These veins intercommunicate around the embryonic duodenum and supply the developing hepatic sinusoids. Selective atrophy of these embryonic veins leaves the final arrangement of a single postduodenal portal vein. Aberrations in this process probably account for the majority of portal vein cavernomas.

58.4 Clinical Features

PHT typically presents with acute gastrointestinal haemorrhage and/or splenomegaly or as one of the manifestations of chronic liver disease. *Variceal bleeding* results in hematemesis and/or melena and may occur at any age. In some patients, bleeding is precipitated by an upper respiratory tract infection. Clinical examination usually reveals *splenomegaly*. Rarely, this is caused by isolated splenic vein obstruction rather than generalized portal hypertension. *Ascites* usually denotes the presence of chronic liver disease but may occur transiently after a major variceal bleed in those with extrahepatic portal hypertension. *Encephalopathy* can complicate an episode of bleeding in cirrhotics but is rare in children with PVO.

Portal hypertension may cause mucosal oedema in the small intestine leading to *malabsorption*, protein loss, and *failure to thrive*. In established portal hypertension dilated cutaneous collateral veins carry blood away from the umbilicus toward the tributaries of the vena cava (caput medusae). Rarely, *pulmonary hypertension* may coexist with portal hypertension, more often in children with cirrhosis than those with PVO. The development of varices at sites other than the esophagus or stomach (ectopic varices) poses small long-term risks, particularly in PVO. Ectopic varices may develop in the anorectum, at sites of previous intestinal anastomoses and around stomas. In long-standing PVO, varices around the common bile duct can cause obstructive jaundice.

Budd-Chiari syndrome due to hepatic vein thrombosis is rarely seen in children. In adolescent girls, onset may be precipitated by the oral contraceptive pill. Similar clinical features develop after hepatic vein occlusion from trauma, malignancy or surgery and with retrohepatic inferior vena caval obstruction. These include hepatomegaly, intractable ascites, symptoms and signs of portal hypertension, diarrhea, and progressive cachexia. Jaundice is variable. The caudate lobe is frequently spared and often hypertrophied because of its independent venous drainage directly into the inferior vena cava; compression of the vena cava may cause lower limb edema. Onset may be acute but is more often chronic.

58.5 Diagnosis and Investigation

- *Hematology*—A full blood count may show anaemia, leucopenia and thrombocytopenia from hypersplenism. The prothrombin time is often prolonged in patients with chronic liver disease. In patients with Budd-Chiari syndrome, an underlying myeloproliferative disorder or thrombophilia must be excluded.
- *Biochemical liver function*—In PVO, plasma albumin may be reduced after a variceal bleed but liver function tests are typically otherwise normal. Chronic liver disease causes abnormal liver function but routine biochemistry can be normal in well-compensated cirrhosis.
- *Abdominal ultrasound scan*—This confirms non-specific features of portal hypertension such as large collateral veins and splenomegaly. The hepatic echotexture is abnormal in chronic liver disease. In congenital PVO, the normal portal vein is replaced by a leash of collateral vessels. Color Doppler flow studies demonstrate the direction and velocity of flow in the portal vein, hepatic veins and vena cava.
- *Gastrointestinal endoscopy*—This can be used to evaluate gastro-esophageal and anorectal varices and mucosal features of portal hypertension. Esophageal varices are graded according to severity. Large varices may show 'red signs' of recent or impending variceal hemorrhage (Fig. 58.2a). Portal gastropathy is characterised by mucosal hyperaemia (Fig. 58.2b).
- *Computerised Tomography and Magnetic Resonance Imaging*—Both imaging modalities are useful in detecting focal liver lesions associated with portal hypertension. Magnetic resonance angiography provides detailed information about the patency

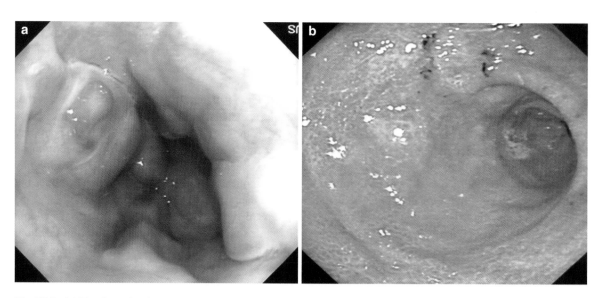

Fig. 58.2 (a) Esophageal varices with red signs. (b) Portal gastropathy in the gastric antrum (the pylorus is on the right)

and calibre of veins throughout the portomesenteric system (Fig. 58.3). This is essential when considering portosystemic shunt surgery and in the preoperative work-up of patients with an occluded portal vein before liver transplantation. Hepatic venography is useful in evaluating Budd-Chiari syndrome.

- *Percutaneous liver biopsy*—If there are no contraindications a percutaneous biopsy is usually undertaken to diagnose or exclude underlying liver

disease. In extrahepatic PVO, the liver architecture is essentially normal.

58.6 Treatment and Complications

If *acute* portal vein thrombosis is diagnosed promptly (e.g. after umbilical venous catheterization) thrombolytic therapy and/or anticoagulation can sometimes restore normal patency but this is an exceptionally uncommon scenario. More typically, the child presents with splenomegaly or variceal bleeding from chronic portal hypertension due to PVO or chronic liver disease. Initial treatment is focused on the emergency management of active variceal bleeding and the prevention of recurrent variceal bleeding. Subsequently, in those with good liver function (e.g. PVO or congenital hepatic fibrosis) control of portal hypertension remains the priority but in the child with cirrhosis, management is heavily influenced by the nature and severity of underlying liver disease. In children with known esophageal varices who have never bled, primary prophylaxis is worth considering.

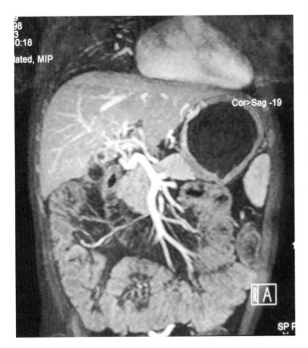

Fig. 58.3 Coronal magnetic resonance scan after gadolinium enhancement demonstrating a portal vein cavernoma in a child with extrahepatic portal hypertension. At the porta hepatis the main portal vein is replaced by a leash of collateral vessels rather than dividing into right and left branches

58.6.1 Emergency Management of Variceal Bleeding

Bleeding from esophageal varices is life-threatening. Resuscitation, investigation and initial treatment are outlined in Table 58.3. Octreotide, a long-acting analogue of somatostatin with a plasma half-life of more than 1 h, reduces splanchnic blood flow and portal pressure with minimal short-term side effects. Balloon

Table 58.3 Emergency management of bleeding esophageal varices (Modified from Stringer and Howard, 2004)

Resuscitation
- Airway (must be secure)
- Breathing (give oxygen if shocked)
- Circulation: insert two intravenous cannulae (22G or larger) and commence intravenous fluids (10 ml/kg crystalloid boluses)

Investigation
- Full blood count, clotting, urea, creatinine, electrolytes, liver function tests
- Blood cultures and cross-match (at least 2 units of packed red blood cells)
- Monitor and maintain blood glucose
- Accurate monitoring of (a) fluid balance and (b) cardiorespiratory status
- Watch for encephalopathy

(continued)

Table 58.3 (continued)

Treatment

- Transfuse packed red cells *slowly* aiming for Hb of 8–10 g/dl (avoid overtransfusion)
- Give vitamin K 300 μg/kg (maximum 10 mg) slowly i.v. and correct coagulopathy with fresh frozen plasma and platelets
- Start octreotide infusion: bolus dose of 1 μg/kg i.v. (maximum 50 μg) over 5 min followed by infusion @ 1–3 μg/kg/h (maximum 50 μg/h) via dedicated line. Continue infusion until 24 h after bleeding ceases and wean off slowly over 24 h
- Keep nil by mouth initially
- Give gastric protection: Ranitidine 1 mg/kg i.v. tds and oral Sucralfate
- Start i.v. antibiotics if any evidence of sepsis
- Ensure appropriate sized pediatric Sengstaken-type tube is available to provide balloon tamponade if necessary
- Consider prophylaxis against encephalopathy if poor liver function
- Urgent upper GI endoscopy within 24 h to confirm source of bleeding and to begin treatment of varices by banding or sclerotherapy, if appropriate

tamponade is rarely required to control active variceal bleeding. If necessary, A Sengstaken-type tube can be inserted after securing the airway by endotracheal intubation; only the gastric balloon is inflated and correct positioning must be verified radiographically. Moderate traction is applied by taping the tube to the side of the face; excessive traction may cause catastrophic balloon displacement. The balloon is deflated after 12–24 h at the time of endoscopy.

58.6.2 Endoscopic Treatment of Esophageal Varices

58.6.2.1 Injection Sclerotherapy

This is performed with a flexible fiberoptic gastroscope under general anesthesia with an endotracheal tube in place. A variety of injection techniques and sclerosants have been used. An intravariceal injection technique using 5% ethanolamine oleate is popular (Fig. 58.4a). Varices are initially injected every few weeks and then at monthly intervals until sclerosis is complete. Patients are often given oral Sucralfate and Omeprazole for 2 weeks after each injection session to reduce complications from ulceration. Endoscopic review is undertaken after 6 months and then annually; only large recurrent varices require further treatment.

Endoscopic injection sclerotherapy (EIS) is a highly effective treatment for esophageal varices. However, numerous complications have been reported. Transient retrosternal discomfort and fever are common after EIS and usually resolve within 48 h. Children with a pyrexia >38°C should be treated with intravenous antibiotics pending the results of blood cultures because they may have transient bacteremia. Antibiotic prophylaxis is given to patients at risk of bacterial endocarditis, those with cirrhosis and ascites, and the immunosuppressed. Major complications of sclerotherapy include esophageal stricturing (which responds to esophageal dilatation), recurrent esophageal varices, and intercurrent bleeding occurring between treatment episodes (due to a persistent varix or an injection ulcer). Some children experience intermittent dysphagia and heartburn secondary to oesophageal dysmotility and gastro-oesophageal reflux. Dissemination of the injected sclerosant causing distant complications has been rarely reported. Complication rates have fallen in recent years, probably as a result of injecting smaller volumes of sclerosant.

58.6.2.2 Variceal Ligation (Banding)

The varix is aspirated into a transparent cylinder fitted to the end of a flexible gastroscope and an elastic band released by a trip wire passing through the biopsy channel strangles the varix which thromboses and sloughs (Fig. 58.4b). Treatment begins with ligation of the most distal varix in the esophagus just above the cardia. Up to four bands are applied to the varices at each session; the treatment is repeated every few weeks and then monthly until the varices have been obliterated. Endoscopic variceal ligation (EVL) is now regarded as the optimum endoscopic method of treating active variceal bleeding and for preventing rebleeding from esophageal varices in children. Compared to EIS, EVL offers more rapid eradication with fewer treatment sessions and significantly lower complication rates.

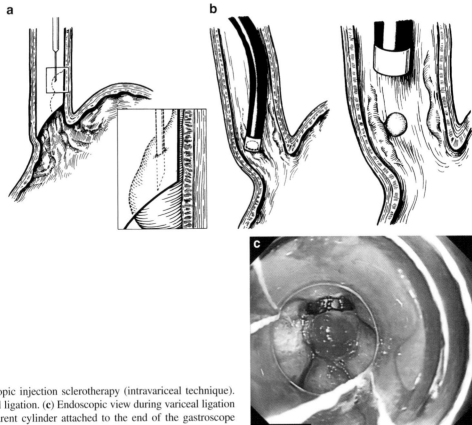

Fig. 58.4 (**a**) Endoscopic injection sclerotherapy (intravariceal technique). (**b**) Endoscopic variceal ligation. (**c**) Endoscopic view during variceal ligation (banding). The transparent cylinder attached to the end of the gastroscope holding the bands limits the view

Esophageal ulcers caused by banding are more superficial and resolve quicker than those induced by sclerotherapy. However, current EVL equipment is not suitable for infants.

Most gastric varices are fundal and directly contiguous with lower esophageal varices; these tend to be eradicated by treatment of the esophageal varices. Isolated gastric varices are less common and more difficult to treat using endoscopic techniques.

58.6.3 Primary Prophylaxis of Variceal Bleeding

Non-selective beta-blockers such as propanolol reduce portal pressure by causing splanchnic vasoconstriction and reducing cardiac output. These agents are effective in preventing variceal bleeding and rebleeding in adults with cirrhosis but there are no randomized controlled trials in children.

Prophylactic endoscopic therapy is controversial. Prophylactic EIS has not been shown to offer an overall survival advantage but EVS may be beneficial in preventing bleeding in children with large esophageal varices which have not bled.

58.6.4 Surgery for Portal Hypertension

Surgery and endoscopic therapy are complementary procedures in the management of portal hypertension. The indications for surgery have changed over the years as the relative merits of portosystemic shunt surgery, endoscopic therapy, and (most recently) mesoportal bypass have become clearer. Current indications for surgery are:

58.6.4.1 Primary Treatment of PVO

The mesenterico-left portal (Rex) bypass is becoming established as the optimum treatment of portal hypertension in children with extrahepatic portal hypertension secondary to PVO. In these patients, the liver is intrinsically healthy. The procedure is *contraindicated* in patients with chronic liver disease since the site of venous obstruction in these patients is intrahepatic. In the standard bypass, an internal jugular vein graft is interposed between the superior mesenteric vein and the intrahepatic left portal vein which is located in the Rex recess adjacent to the falciform ligament (Fig. 58.5). The portal vein occlusion is bypassed, hepatic portal blood flow is restored and portal hypertension is corrected. Ideally, the operation requires the presence of an adequate caliber, patent intrahepatic left portal vein and patent splenic and mesenteric veins; this is determined preoperatively using a combination of magnetic resonance angiography, ultrasound and/or retrograde hepatic venography. Both internal jugular veins should be patent on ultrasound. This shunt is an ideal

option for many children with PVO since it restores normal portal venous physiology. Alternative tributaries of the portomesenteric venous system (other than the superior mesenteric vein) can be used to provide inflow to the intrahepatic left portal vein. However, a mesenterico-portal bypass is not feasible in every child with PVO because the intrahepatic veins may be too abnormal.

58.6.4.2 Uncontrolled Bleeding from Esophageal Varices (Not Responding to At Least Two Treatment Sessions)

This is an unusual situation in PVO but if variceal bleeding cannot be controlled endoscopically and a Rex bypass is not feasible, a portosystemic shunt is an alternative option. A portosystemic shunt may also be used to control variceal bleeding in patients with chronic liver disease provided synthetic liver function is well preserved. However, this is often a palliative procedure in this circumstance and liver transplantation is often the definitive treatment. Many types of portosystemic shunt have been performed but mesocaval and spleno-renal shunts have been used most often in children (Fig. 58.6). The mesocaval shunt using an interposed segment of autologous jugular vein has been consistently reliable. The distal spleno-renal (Warren) shunt is considered to be a selective shunt in that it achieves gastrosplenic variceal decompression whilst maintaining portal perfusion.

58.6.4.3 Bleeding Gastric or Ectopic Varices That Cannot Be Controlled Endoscopically

Potential options include Rex bypass, portosystemic shunt, gastric devascularization, or liver transplantation, depending on the etiology of portal hypertension.

58.6.4.4 Massive Splenomegaly Causing Severe Hypersplenism or Abdominal Pain

A splenectomy or bypass/shunt procedure is sometimes indicated in these patients. There are a few reports of successful treatment with partial splenic embolization.

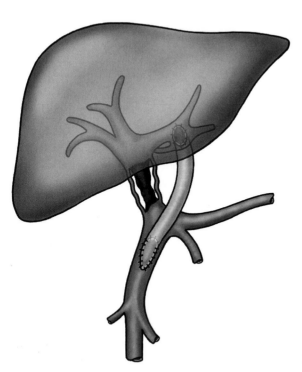

Fig. 58.5 Diagram illustrating the standard type of meso-Rex bypass. The bypass graft is typically autologous internal jugular vein

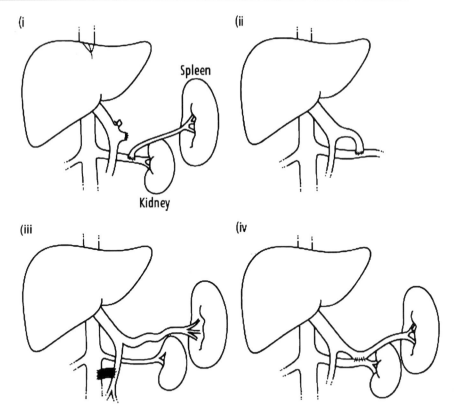

Fig. 58.6 Portosystemic shunt operations for portal hypertension. (**i**) Distal splenorenal, (**ii**) Proximal splenorenal, (**iii**) Mesocaval, and (**iv**) Side-to-side splenorenal shunt. (Modified from Stringer and Howard, 2004)

58.6.4.5 Lack of Access to Expert Endoscopy

This is now a rare indication for surgery in portal hypertension.

Patency of a Rex bypass or portosystemic shunt can be assessed *directly* by color Doppler ultrasound imaging (Fig. 58.7), magnetic resonance angiography, or conventional angiography. It may also be assessed *indirectly* by ultrasound from directional flow in portomesenteric and systemic veins and spleen size, and by endoscopic regression of varices. After successful bypass/shunt surgery, growth velocity and hypersplenism both improve (the latter reflected in an increased platelet count and a reduction in splenomegaly).

Thrombosis of a Rex bypass or portosystemic shunt is a major complication, likely to manifest as recurrent variceal bleeding. Patency rates after the standard Rex bypass using autologous jugular vein are typically greater than 90% between 1 and 5 years later. Failure rates have generally been slightly higher after portosystemic shunting. A shunt stenosis is another potential compli-

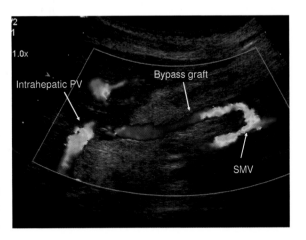

Fig. 58.7 Postoperative color Doppler ultrasound scan of Rex bypass graft confirming good patency and flow velocity. SMV = superior mesenteric vein, PV = portal vein

cation; this can usually be corrected by the interventional radiologist. Encephalopathy is a well recognised complication of portosystemic shunt surgery in cirrhotics but occurs only rarely in patients with PVO.

58.6.4.6 Liver Transplantation

Liver transplantation is the treatment of choice for most children with variceal bleeding complicating end-stage chronic liver disease. Previous portosystemic shunting does not compromise survival after liver transplantation although operative morbidity is less in those who have had a distal splenorenal or mesocaval shunt, both of which avoid surgery around the porta hepatis.

58.6.4.7 Surgery for Budd-Chiari Syndrome

Rarely, this has a radiologically or surgically treatable cause such as a caval web. Most children with hepatic vein thrombosis are successfully managed by medical therapy directed at controlling ascites and preventing progressive venous thrombosis. Portosystemic shunt surgery may be necessary for variceal bleeding, deteriorating liver function, and intractable ascites. Portosystemic shunting converts the portal vein into a venous outflow tract.

Transjugular intrahepatic portosystemic stent shunt (TIPS) is a less invasive but less durable alternative to portosystemic shunt surgery. This procedure is performed by the interventional radiologist and involves the percutaneous insertion of an expandable metal stent between the hepatic and portal veins in the liver. TIPS is also useful for treating refractory variceal bleeding in children with chronic liver disease awaiting liver transplantation.

58.7 Conclusions

Portal hypertension may be the predominant pathology in conditions such as congenital portal vein occlusion or it may be part of a spectrum of clinical features such as in chronic liver disease. The cause of portal hypertension must be precisely and fully elucidated in order to select the most appropriate therapy from the wide variety of available management options.

Further Reading

de Ville de Goyet J, Alberti D, Clapuyt P et al (1998) Direct bypassing of extrahepatic portal venous obstruction in children: A new technique for combined hepatic portal revascularization and treatment of extrahepatic portal hypertension. J Pediatr Surg 33:597–601

Howard ER, Stringer MD, Colombani PM (2002) Surgery of the Liver, Bile Ducts, and Pancreas in Children, 2nd edn. Arnold, London

Puri P, Höllwarth ME (eds) (2006) Pediatric Surgery. Springer, Berlin, Heidelberg

Stringer MD, Howard ER (2004) Surgical disorders of the liver and bile ducts and portal hypertension. In DA Kelly (ed) Diseases of the Liver and Biliary System in Children. Blackwell Publishing, Oxford, pp 345

Stringer MD, Oldham KT, Mouriquand PDE (2006) Pediatric Surgery and Urology: Long Term Outcomes, 2nd edn. Cambridge University Press, New York, pp 491–509

Gallbladder Disease

59

Shawn D. St. Peter and George W. Holcomb, III

Contents

59.1 Introduction

Gallbladder disease is being diagnosed more frequently in children, although it is not seen nearly as often as in adults. The disease processes contributing to gallbladder pathology are different in children compared with adults. There is a much higher incidence of black pigmented gallstones due to hemolytic disease in children. Moreover, acute and chronic cholecystitis with severe inflammation and/or scarring of the gallbladder and surrounding tissues are far less common in children. Aside from these fundamental differences, lessons gained from the vast published experience in adults can be useful in managing children with gallbladder disease.

59.2 Etiology

Gallbladder disease in children can arise from a range of underlying conditions. In most cases, gallbladder disease is related to the presence of stones. Gallstones develop for unknown reasons in many children. Gallstones in children are usually classified as being either hemolytic or non-hemolytic in etiology. Non-hemolytic disease includes a variety of causes for stone development or symptomatic gallbladder disease without stone formation. Stone formation is a complex interaction of several components centered around the lithogenic potential of a given individual. Hemolytic disease results in consumption of red blood cells leading to increased liver metabolism of bilirubin which precipitates stone formation.

P. Puri and M. Höllwarth (eds.), *Pediatric Surgery: Diagnosis and Management,*
DOI: 10.1007/978-3-540-69560-8_59, © Springer-Verlag Berlin Heidelberg 2009

59.2.1 Gallstone Formation

The major chemical components of bile which contribute to its lithogenic potential are bile salts, phospholipids, cholesterol, bilirubin, and electrolyte/water balance. The phospholipid component is mostly lethicin which, along with bile salts, serve as detergents in the bile. With polar and non-polar portions to these molecules, they form lecithin-bile acid-cholesterol micelles that keep the cholesterol soluble within the hydrophobic center of the micelle. An imbalance in the concentration of these substances is almost always due to an increase in cholesterol secretion, which results in cholesterol crystal precipitation. These crystals serve as the nidus for further precipitation resulting in macroscopically detectable gallstones. This pathway accounts for the majority of adult gallstones but is less common in children. In addition, cholesterol gallstones are extremely rare in prepubertal children. Obesity is a common risk factor for cholesterol stone formation. Within the pediatric population, obese children have been found to have an overall 2% incidence of gallstones.

The physiologic components contributing to stone formation include gallbladder emptying, bile duct emptying as well as the integrity and function of the biliary epithelium. Epithelial mucin production accelerates stone formation. Epithelial inflammation, which can result from cholesterol supersaturation, alters the electrolyte/water balance and leads to the epithelial release of procrystallizing proteins. Furthermore, bacterial colonization of biliary epithelium can cause deconjugation of bilirubin leading to stone formation as well.

59.2.1.1 Hemolytic Disease

Red blood cells are composed of a plasma membrane, the hemoglobin moiety, and a few cytoplasmic enzymes. These 3 basic components provide a functional outline for the major hereditary hemolytic diseases (Table 59.1). Their constant turnover requires the reticuloendothelial system to retrieve dying and dead red blood cells leading to the breakdown of the hemoglobin moiety to bilirubin. A nearly insoluble molecule, bilirubin requires conjugation by glucuronyl transferase to produce bilirubin diglucuronide, the

Table 59.1   The major hereditary hemolytic diseases

Membrane defects	Hemoglobin defects	Enzyme defects
Spherocytosis	Sickle cell disease	Glucose-6-phosphate deficiency
Eliptocytosis	α Thallasemia	Pyruvate kinase deficiency
Pyropoikilocytosis	β Thallasemia	
Hydrocytosis		
Xerocytosis		

molecule measured as "direct" bilirubin, which is more soluble. The enzymatic process of conjugation is saturable. Thus, the hemolytic states listed in Table 59.1 may cause an abnormal level of unconjugated (indirect) bilirubin in the bile. This results in calcium bilirubinate formation, which polymerizes with bilirubin to form black gallstones. This interaction is not linear but is affected by the physiologic function of the gallbladder, biliary system and the other variables of bile lithogenesis mentioned previously.

Fifty percent of patients with sickle cell anemia develop gallstones by 20 years of age. The incidence of cholelithiasis with hereditary spherocytosis is also around 50% and slightly more common in girls than boys. Previously, thalassemia patients were also at high risk for cholelithiasis. However, the incidence has decreased due to more aggressive transfusion management which prevents the production and release of native red cells with the defective hemoglobin.

59.2.1.2 Non-Hemolytic Disease

Conjugated bile salts are deconjugated by intestinal bacteria and resorbed, mostly in the terminal ileum. Through the portal circulation, they return to the hepatocytes for biliary excretion. Patients with short gut syndrome, ileal resection, or ileal disease (Crohn's disease) are at risk for stone development due to the decreased bile salt pool. Also, patients with bowel dysmotility or dysfunction may have altered bacterial flora which also affects the enterohepatic circulation.

The most common condition associated with the development of non-hemolytic cholelithiasis in neonates and infants is the use of total parenteral nutrition (TPN). Up to 40% of children receiving long-term TPN will develop gallstones. While many patients requiring long-term TPN have gastrointestinal disease, the complete picture of TPN associated cholestasis, liver disease, and gallstone formation is not completely understood. Decreased bile flow and gallbladder emptying from a lack of enteral stimulation has been postulated to be an important contribution to TPN associated gallstones. However, in one study, the use of cholecystikinin (CCK) to prevent stone development in TPN dependent children had no effect, implying that the role of CCK mediated bile flow may be less important than previously thought in gallstone formation for these patients. TPN has a primary lithogenic effect on bile causing increased bilirubin and calcium concentration. These effects have been shown to be prevented with glutamine supplementation suggesting there are intermediary steps that still need to be clarified. Septicemia, dehydration, and chronic furosemide therapy have also been implicated as contributing factors to lithogenesis in TPN dependent patients.

Cystic fibrosis, the phenotype of defective epithelial chloride channels, results in decreased transport of water and chloride which increases the viscosity of bile contributing to stone formation. Also, it can lead to obstruction of biliary ductules leading to liver failure.

Finally, cholelithiasis has been reported in children undergoing cardiac bypass, cardiac transplantation, and in patients who have previously undergone extracorporeal membrane oxygenation as a newborn.

59.2.2 Acalculous Gallbladder Disease

The gallbladder can be a source of symptoms in patients without gallstones. Acute inflammatory attacks of the gallbladder, called acute acalculous cholecystitis, occur more commonly in association with severe illness such as sepsis, burns, or trauma. This is much less common in children than adults, but can be seen in critically ill children.

Biliary dyskinesia, which is dysfunctional emptying of the gallbladder, is the most common gallbladder condition that does not involve stones. While the etiology of the symptoms is felt to be gallbladder distension secondary to poor emptying, bile stasis can promote sludge, microscopic bile crystallization and subsequent mucosal irritation. On pathologic examination, chronic cholecystitis is often documented on histologic examination of the gallbladder specimen. Overlapping with biliary dyskinesia is sphincter of Oddi hypertension as a cause of chronic acalculous symptomatic gallbladder disease. However, this condition is quite rare in children.

Hydrops is characterized by massive distention of the gallbladder in the absence of stones, infection, or congenital anomalies. It has been most frequently reported in association with Kawasaki's disease and is usually due to a transient obstruction of the cystic duct or to increased mucus secretion by the gallbladder resulting in poor emptying. With additional gallbladder distention, further angulation of the cystic duct may increase the obstruction.

Gallbladder polyps are unusual in children. Surgical recommendations have followed the adult literature that suggests that cholecystectomy should be performed if there are symptoms or if the polyp is ≥1 cm in size.

59.3 Diagnosis

59.3.1 Clinical Features

The diagnosis of gallstones in young children may be delayed due to vague and non-specific symptoms such as abdominal pain, nausea, emesis, and, occasionally, fever. Abdominal pain may vary from the typical right upper abdominal location due to poor localization of the pain by young children.

Older children and teenagers present with symptoms and physical findings similar to those in adults. Right subcostal pain with or without radiation to the subscapular area or central back is the most common complaint. The pain typically fluctuates with waves over a background level of pain due to gallbladder contractions against cystic duct obstruction. Nausea and vomiting commonly occur following the onset of pain. A precipitating fatty food can often be elicited.

Patients with symptomatic biliary colic will usually experience resolution of symptoms within 6h. These initial symptoms almost always resolve within a day. After the acute attack abates, patients will often describe a dull ache or soreness in the right upper quadrant for the next several days. These patients are sometimes tender to deep palpation, but not like the severe right upper quadrant tenderness seen in patients with cholecystitis. Murphy's sign, more indicative of acute cholecystitis, is the hesitation or inability to complete a deep inhalation when steady, gentle pressure is applied in a superior and posterior direction under the right costal margin. Patients with acute cholecystitis present similarly, but will usually appear more systemically ill. Moreover, they are more likely to have a fever and demonstrate leukocytosis. In these patients, the diagnosis is confirmed by inflammatory changes on imaging studies (see below).

59.3.2 Radiologic Diagnosis

Stones may be radio-opaque in up to 20% of patients with hemolytic disorders and in 15% of patients with cholesterol stones (Fig. 59.1a). Thus, abdominal radiographs are not usually a useful diagnostic or screening tool for gallstones. The anatomic appearance of the gallbladder and its contents is best evaluated by ultrasound (US) which is a very accurate (approximately 96%) imaging study for gallbladder disease (Fig. 59.1b). Also, it allows evaluation of hepatic and common bile duct stones or obstruction. Inflammatory changes as evidenced by gallbladder wall thickening, pericholecystic fluid, or tenderness elicited by probe placement directly over the gallbladder (sonographic

Murphy's sign) are indicative of acute cholecystitis. Stones without inflammatory changes must be associated with symptoms for the diagnosis of symptomatic cholelithiasis. Computed tomography (CT) scanning also defines the quality of the gallbladder and its contents, although delineation of the common bile duct is suboptimal with a routine abdominal CT. However, dedicated hepatobiliary CT scanning is extremely effective at evaluating the biliary tract. In children, an abdominal CT is often performed, instead of an ultrasound, prior to a surgical consult to exclude more common pediatric conditions.

Patients with typical symptoms but who do not have stones on US should be studied by cholescintigraphy, which is a nuclear medicine test referred to as hepatobiliary iminodiacetic acid scan (HIDA scan). ^{99m}Tc-labeled iminodiacitic acid (IDA) or an analogue is injected peripherally and is taken up by hepatocytes. The analogue is processed by the same mechanism as bilirubin and is excreted in bile. If the biliary tree is illuminated without filling the gallbladder, then the diagnosis of acute cholecystitis is confirmed. Occasional false positives occur in critically ill fasting patients for which intravenous morphine may be useful to enhance visualization of the gallbladder. The morphine constricts the sphincter of Oddi which can enhance filling of the gallbladder. When the gallbladder fills with

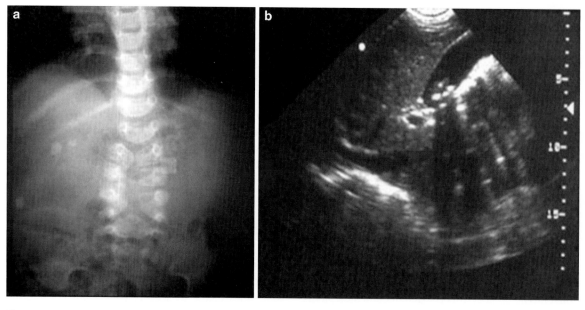

Fig. 59.1   In a small number of patients, gallstones may be radiopaque (**a**). Ultrasound is a very accurate imaging study for gallbladder disease (**b**). Note the acoustic shadowing that develops behind the gallstones on this study

radioactive substrate, emptying can then be quantified by calculating the ejection fraction of the gallbladder with cholecystikinin-assisted or lipomul challenge. The normal ejection fraction approximates 75%. Patients with an ejection fraction under 35% are considered to have biliary dyskinesia. Several series have shown that symptomatic patients diagnosed with biliary dyskinesia by cholescintigraphy have a high likelihood of symptomatic relief with cholecystectomy.

59.4 Management

The gallbladder is a functional reservoir to provide a bolus of bile for digestion, especially with large fatty meals. Because the need for a functioning gallbladder is marginal, it can be removed with few long-term consequences. Historically, gallstones have been treated with non-operative therapies including oral dissolution agents, direct instillation of dissolution agents, and extracorporeal shockwave lithotripsy. These measures have been abandoned due to failure, recurrence and high cost. Thus, once a patient presents with symptoms from their gallbladder disease, the risk of complications from the gallbladder disease is generally higher than the risks of laparoscopic cholecystectomy. Patients with symptomatic gallbladder disease who are older than 3 years should undergo laparoscopic cholecystectomy. The treatment of younger patients, particularly infants, should be individualized. Infant gallstones secondary to prolonged TPN have been reported to dissolve spontaneously. Therefore, in the absence of complications, these patients should be observed for 6–12 months following cessation of the TPN and the initiation of enteral alimentation.

When compared to the open operation, the laparoscopic approach provides less discomfort, reduces the length of postoperative hospitalization, improves cosmesis, and results in a much faster return to routine activities such as work, school, play, or participation in athletic activity.

Although most children can be discharged within 48 h, patients with sickle cell disease require special preoperative care to prevent postoperative complications. Several authors have reported favorable results with cholecystectomy in this patient population and have emphasized the need for preoperative transfusion.

The laparoscopic approach is not more hazardous for these patients and is therefore preferred. Because gallbladder sludge is frequently documented in patients with sickle cell anemia, elective cholecystectomy has been recommended when evidence suggests the presence of sludge, with or without stones. In one study of 35 patients with sickle cell disease and biliary sludge, 23 (65.7%) went on to develop gallstones.

Patients presenting with an acute episode of cholecystitis and signs of inflammation on laboratory or radiologic studies can be managed with either semi-urgent laparoscopic cholecystectomy or antibiotics followed by interval cholecystectomy. In adults, a recent prospective study found no difference in operative complications between early and delayed cholecystectomy, but found that delayed cholecystectomy was associated with more complications from the disease (relapse, choledocholithiasis, pancreatitis). Early intervention has also been shown to be much more cost-effective than interval cholecystectomy.

Because gallbladder polyps are an unusual finding in children, the natural history of these polyps is unknown. Due to the inability to assure life-long follow-up combined with the extremely poor prognosis when gallbladder cancer develops, we feel a laparoscopic cholecystectomy is a reasonable option for symptomatic children with gallbladder polyps or for patients with a polp ≥1 cm.

59.4.1 Concomitant Splenectomy

When patients are being evaluated for splenectomy due to hematologic disease, their gallbladder should also be evaluated by US. If gallstones are found, then cholecystectomy should be performed at the time of the splenectomy. A splenectomy should not be performed by the open approach except in extraordinary circumstances, and the cholecystectomy can be easily performed at the time of laparoscopic splenectomy. In the absence of stones, the splenectomy should decrease the possibility of future pigment stone development due to decreased hemolysis following splenectomy. In a series of 17 patients, none developed symptoms of cholelithiasis after splenectomy with a mean follow-up of 15 years. Thus, prophylactic cholecystectomy during splenectomy is not indicated in hemolytic patients without gallstones.

59.4.2 Choledocholithiasis

A variety of management strategies exist for patients who present with *suspected* common bile duct stones either clinically or on US. One strategy is to obtain a preoperative endoscopic retrograde cholangiopancreatography (ERCP) with sphincterotomy and stone extraction (if stones are found). A second option is to proceed with laparoscopic cholecystectomy with cholangiography and attempted transcystic extraction of the stones (if stones are seen on the cholangiography). If stones are found and cannot be extracted, then either laparoscopic or open choledochal exploration is performed or postoperative ERCP and sphincterotomy are attempted.

This decision is primarily influenced by the surgeon's experience with laparoscopic choledochal exploration, but also by the availability of an endoscopist experienced in ERCP in children. In many children's hospitals, an adult colleague from another hospital is called for consultation if an endoscopist experienced with ERCP and stone extraction is not available. For the majority of pediatric surgeons, the best option may be to perform a preoperative ERCP with sphincterotomy and stone extraction if stones are located. If successful, the surgeon can then proceed with laparoscopic cholecystectomy. However, if stones are found and cannot be extracted at ERCP and sphincterotomy, then the surgeon will know whether or not laparoscopic or open choledochal exploration is indicated at the time of the cholecystectomy. This latter approach is preferred at our institution (Fig. 59.2).

At operation, if common duct stones are found on cholangiography, flushing the common duct with saline through the cholangiocatheter may cause them to pass. This procedure can be augmented by the intravenous injection of 1 mg of glucagon to relax the sphincter of Oddi. This step can be repeated as needed. If glucagon is not available, naloxone and nitroglycerin have also been used successfully. Also, the cholangiocatheter can be gently passed into the common duct under fluoroscopy and used to push small stones through the sphincter of Oddi. Finally a choledochoscope can be passed through the cystic duct and into the common duct to push the stones through the sphincter. If unavailable, a standard ureteroscope is the same size (7 mm diameter) and is efficacious as well. If a stone is not amenable to any of these techniques, it is

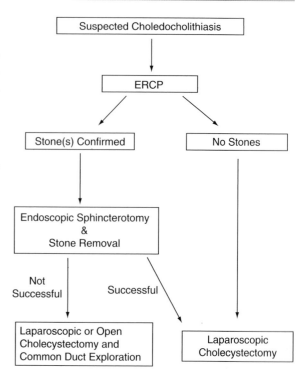

Fig. 59.2 This algorithm depicts our current management for suspected choledocholithiasis. Preoperative ERCP is preferred so that sphincterotomy and stone removal can be performed prior to the laparoscopic cholecystectomy. With this management strategy, the surgeon will know whether or not laparoscopic or open choledochal exploration will be required at the time of the laparoscopic cholecystectomy

likely to be stuck in the duct and will require basket retrieval. Currently, this is generally safer if approached by ERCP, which can be performed postoperatively. All of the aforementioned laparoscopic techniques can be performed through the cystic duct.

At the time of the laparoscopic cholecystectomy, surgeons have different opinions about the need for cholangiography. While there are advocates for routine intraoperative cholangiography, many surgeons do not support routinely increasing the operative time, cost and risk of the procedure for a large population of patients in whom it is not necessary. Contrary to individual, noncomparative series, review of complications leading to litigation has suggested that routine cholangiography does not reduce complications. Therefore, in children, cholangiography should be used selectively in patients in whom the anatomy is not clear or in whom there is the suspicion of choledocholithiasis.

59.4.3 Gallstone Pancreatitis

Patients who present with pancreatitis and who are found to have stones in the gallbladder or common duct are diagnosed with gallstone pancreatitis. In the majority of cases, considered simple or mild, the stone usually passes within 48 h without the need for pre-operative ERCP. In this scenario, the patient typically experiences a sudden and dramatic improvement in the epigastric pain when the stone passes after which the laboratory values usually resolve sharply over the next several days. Laparoscopic cholecystectomy can be safely performed when the pain is improved and the labs are on the decline without waiting until they normalize. These patients should undergo cholecystectomy prior to discharge due to the high rate of recurrence when these patients are scheduled for a later elective operation. In the unusual scenario where the pancreatitis becomes severe with systemic manifestations and pancreatic complications, then ERCP should be performed with sphincterotomy initially. Laparoscopic cholecystectomy can be performed later when the patient has recovered. In this situation, the cholecystectomy can be performed at the time of intervention for pseudocyst. We have had success with concomitant laparoscopic cyst-gastrostomy and cholecystectomy.

The most common etiology for pancreatitis in children is idiopathic. When idiopathic pancreatitis recurs a second time, these patients should be evaluated with an ERCP to evaluate an anatomic cause. If none is found, then these patients should be considered for sphincterotomy or cholecystectomy due to the high possibility of microlithiasis or biliary sludge as the underlying cause. Ursodeoxycholic acid therapy has also been reported to be successful in preventing recurrence by decreasing the viscosity of the bile, but this management strategy requires ongoing therapy and does not hold much promise for children. Therefore, children with a second episode of idiopathic pancreatitis are candidates for sphincterotomy or cholecystectomy.

59.4.4 Operative Considerations

While multiple variations are described and utilized, generally a 10 mm port in the umbilicus is the only large port necessary. A 5 mm subxiphoid port allows for the endoscopic clips to be applied to the cystic duct and cystic artery. In general, particularly in children, if a 5 mm clip is not of sufficient size for the cystic duct, then the anatomy should be re-examined starting from the gallbladder to assure this structure is the cystic duct. The other two ports placed on the right side of the abdomen are for retracting the fundus of the gallbladder cephalad and the infundibulum laterally. Port placement should be modified according to the patient's age. In thin or small children, the two right-sided sites are amenable to the "stab incision" technique for introducing instruments without a cannula (Fig. 59.3). This technique allows 3 or 5 mm instruments to be introduced through extremely small incisions in lean patients. Adequate cephalad retraction of the fundus and lateral retraction of the infundibulum along with reverse Trendelenberg positioning should allow good visualization of the triangle of Calot for dissection (Fig. 59.4). The dissection of the cystic duct should start at the level of the gallbladder to assure accurate identification of the cystic duct regardless of how short or anomalous its course. Likewise, the duct should be clipped and cut as distally as possible to avoid common bile duct injury (Fig. 59.5). Retained cystic duct stones or cystic duct complications have not been reported in children. Following ligation of the cystic artery and duct, the gallbladder is dissected from its liver bed with cautery and extracted through the umbilical incision. It can be placed into an endoscopic retrieval bag if necessary or desired.

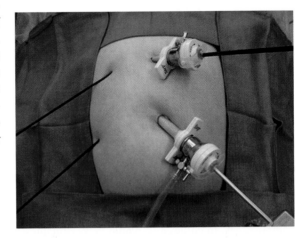

Fig. 59.3 This photograph shows placement of the ports for laparoscopic cholecystectomy in a 9-year-old girl with biliary dyskinesia. The two right-sided 3 mm instruments have been placed directly through the abdominal wall without the use of cannulas

Fig. 59.4 In order to create a 90° angle between the cystic duct and common duct, it is important to laterally retract the infundibulum. Lateral retraction of the infundibulum aids in accurate identification of the cystic duct (*solid arrow*) and common bile duct (*asterisk*). Note the cystic artery (*dotted arrow*) in this photograph

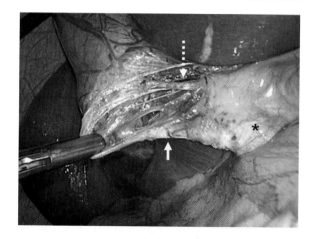

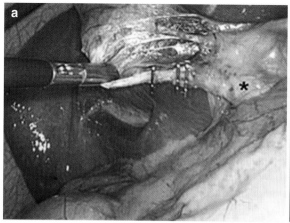
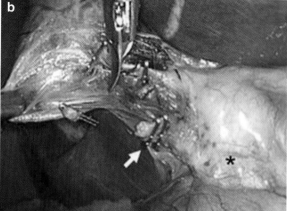

Fig. 59.5 The cystic duct is ligated so that two clips will remain on the cystic duct stump (**a**). In a similar fashion, the cystic artery is ligated and divided (**b**). Note the two clips (*arrow*) remaining on the cystic duct stump. The common bile duct is marked with an asterisk in both photographs

59.5 Complications

The most dreaded and severe complication from laparoscopic cholecystectomy is injury to the common bile duct. The rate of ductal injury after laparoscopic cholecystectomy is decreasing as experience continues to increase, but the number of patients who will require a ductal reconstructive operation remains about 1 per 1,000 undergoing a laparoscopic cholecystectomy. These numbers are derived from adult series as there are no published reports of ductal complications in children. It would be reasonable to expect that complications in children will remain less than adults given the high percentage of adult patients who require an operation due to severe inflammation obliterating the planes of dissection.

Very few pediatric patients present in this fashion. Regardless, any surgeon performing the operation should be aware of the complications that can occur and how to manage them.

When ductal injury is recognized at the time of the operation, conversion with open repair should be performed with a low threshold for performing a hepaticojejunostomy. Obstructive ductal injuries and delayed strictures detected after the operation can be temporized with percutaneous transhepatic drainage of the ductal system after which the patient should be referred to a center with a large experience reconstructing these injuries. In this setting, roux-en-Y hepaticojejunostomy has a 98% success rate.

Bile leaks after laparoscopic cholecystectomy are usually from the cystic duct stump or from the gallbladder fossa (ducts of Lushka). The sphincter of Oddi maintains a pressure gradient of about 10 mmHg in the biliary system. Thus, almost all post-operative leaks resolve promptly with sphincterotomy and/or stent placement which should be performed at the time of the ERCP that is useful for delineating the location of the leak.

Infectious complications are uncommon unless gallstones are spilled. Spilled stones should be removed to reduce these complications.

The most common complications following cholecystectomy in children occur with hemolytic disease, and are related to the manifestations of the underlying disease. In a report of 364 cases from a national sickle cell disease study group, the total complication rate was 39% with sickle cell events representing 19%; intraoperative or recovery room problems, 11%; transfusion complications, 10%; postoperative surgical events, 4%; and death in 1%. Acute chest syndrome can be seen in up to 20% of sickle cell patients undergoing abdominal surgery. In addition, the laparoscopic approach does not seem to decrease the incidence of this complication. Meticulous attention to perioperative management, transfusion guidelines, and pulmonary care should help reduce the incidence of these complications.

Further Reading

Agarwal N, Sharma BC, Garg S et al (2006) Endoscopic management of postoperative bile leaks. Hepatobiliary Pancreat Dis Int 5:273–277

Carney DE, Evan R, Kokoska ER et al (2004) Predictors of successful outcome after cholecystectomy for biliary dyskinesia. J Pediatr Surg 39:813–816

Kaechele V, Wabitsch M, Thiere D et al (2006) Prevalence of gallbladder stone disease in obese children and adolescents: Influence of the degree of obesity, sex, and pubertal development. J Pediatr Gastroenterol Nutr 42:66–70

Lillemoe KD (2006) Evaluation of suspected bile duct injuries. Surg Endosc 20:1638–1643

Lobe TE (2006) Cholecystectomy. In P Puri, ME Höllwarth (eds) Pediatric Surgery, Springer Surgery Atlas Series. Springer-Verlag, Berlin, Heidelberg, New York, pp 387–394

Mah D, Wales P, Njere I et al (2004) Management of suspected common bile duct stones in children: Role of selective intraoperative cholangiogram and endoscopic retrograde cholangiopancreatography. J Pediatr Surg 39:808–812

McLean TR (2006) Risk management observations from litigation involving laparoscopic cholecystectomy. Arch Surg 141:643–648

Schweizer P, Lenz MP, Kirschner HJ (2000) Pathogenesis and symptomatology of cholelithiasis in childhood. A prospective study. Dig Surg 17:459–467

Stringer MD, Ceylan H, Ward K et al (2003) Gallbladder polyps in children—Classification and management. J Pediatr Surg 38:1680–1684

Wu SC, Chen FC, Lo CJ (2005) Selective intraoperative cholangiography and single-stage management of common bile duct stone in laparoscopic cholecystectomy. World J Surg 29:1402–1408

Pancreatic Disorders

60

Paul R.V. Johnson

Contents

60.1 Introduction

Although most pancreatic disorders are rare in childhood, there are a number with which the paediatric surgeon must be familiar. These conditions may be congenital or acquired and may affect the exocrine or the endocrine components of the gland. In this chapter the most frequently encountered conditions are discussed including: structural pancreatic abnormalities, ectopic pancreatic tissue, acute and chronic pancreatitis, pancreatic trauma, hyperinsulinism, cystic fibrosis, pancreatic cysts and pseudo cysts, and pancreatic neoplasms.

60.2 Structural Abnormalities

A wide range of developmental structural abnormalities of the pancreas can occur. These include pancreas agenesis, aplasia and hypoplasia, hyperplasia and hypertrophy, and dysplasia. The commonest structural abnormalities are annular pancreas and pancreas divisum. Both these conditions result from abnormal pancreatic development and therefore an understanding of normal pancreatic development is important. The pancreas is formed from two endodermal buds

P. Puri and M. Höllwarth (eds.), *Pediatric Surgery: Diagnosis and Management*,
DOI: 10.1007/978-3-540-69560-8_60, © Springer-Verlag Berlin Heidelberg 2009

(a large dorsal bud and a smaller ventral bud) which both arise from the embryonic foregut during the 5th week of gestation. Each bud has its own duct and by the end of the 6th week the dorsal duct (duct of Santorini) drains into the foregut and slightly later the ventral one (duct of Wirsung) drains into the hepatic diverticulum. The dorsal bud develops faster than the ventral one and becomes larger overall. The rapid growth of the developing duodenum results in the ventral bud rotating behind the duodenum so that it comes to lie adjacent to the inferior and posterior aspects of the dorsal bud. During the 7th week, the two pancreatic buds fuse resulting in a single gland and a combined ductal system. The dorsal bud forms the body and tail of the definitive pancreas, whereas the ventral bud forms the head and uncinate process. The derivation of the definitive pancreatic ductal system is somewhat unexpected in that the minor accessory duct arises from the larger dorsal bud, whereas the main pancreatic duct arises distally from the dorsal bud and proximally including the ampulla from the ventral bud. Acinar cells and islet cells both appear to develop from the cells lining the pancreatic ducts. Whereas the acinar cells appear to remain non-secretory during foetal life, secretion from foetal islets seems to play an important part in foetal homeostasis.

60.3 Annular Pancreas

As its name implies, this condition results from normal pancreatic tissue encircling the duodenum. It is caused by abnormal rotation of the developing ventral pancreatic bud and the prevailing theory of pathogenesis is that the ventral bud splits into two with part rotating posteriorly and the remainder rotating anteriorly forming a complete or incomplete ring of pancreatic tissue.

60.3.1 Diagnosis

Whilst annular pancreas may be completely asymptomatic and be found incidentally at laparotomy or post mortem, the commonest presentation is that of partial or complete duodenal obstruction. The obstruction

either results from extrinsic compression of the duodenum by the encircling pancreas or can be due to an associated duodenal atresia (25% of duodenal atresias are associated with annular pancreas). The condition may be diagnosed antenatally by the presence of polyhydramnios and a dilated stomach and first part of duodenum on antenatal ultrasound. Postnatally, cases of complete duodenal obstruction classically present in the first few hours of life with the onset of vomiting. The vomit is usually bile-stained as the obstruction is most commonly in the second part of the duodenum distal to the ampulla of Vater. A plain abdominal x-ray demonstrates the typical 'double bubble' of duodenal atresia with absence of distal gas. Cases of incomplete obstruction often present more insidiously and diagnosis is often delayed. An upper gastrointestinal contrast study is useful in these cases.

60.3.2 Management

Once the diagnosis of duodenal obstruction has been confirmed, the stomach is decompressed with a nasogastric tube and fluid and electrolyte disturbances are corrected. After appropriate resuscitation and parental consent, the baby is taken to theatre. Once annular pancreas had been confirmed at laparotomy, the proximal and distal duodenum are carefully mobilised and a duodeno-duodenostomy is performed. The classically described 'diamond-shaped' anastamosis can be used, although a simple side-to side anastamosis is usually sufficient. The surgical procedure can be performed as an open or laparoscopic intervention.

60.4 Pancreas Divisum

Pancreas divisum is the commonest congenital abnormality of the pancreas and is found in up to 11% of patients at post mortem. It results from failure of the ventral and dorsal pancreatic ducts to unite during fusion of the ventral and dorsal pancreatic buds (see above). As a consequence, the duct of the dorsal bud (duct of Santorini) becomes the main pancreatic duct but drains into the duodenum through the minor papilla. A number of other anatomical variants of the ductal system are also encountered.

60.4.1 Diagnosis

Many individuals with pancreas divisum remain asymptomatic and as such it is often considered as a developmental variant rather than a pathological condition. Indeed this abnormal configuration of the pancreatic ducts is found in over 3% of patients under going endoscopic retrograde cholangiopancreatography (ERCP). However, the restricted drainage of the pancreatic secretions through the minor papilla can result in dilatation of the pancreatic duct and pancreatitis. In this group of patients, pancreas divisum can be confirmed by magnetic resonance cholangiopancreatography (MRCP) or ERCP. Although the latter is associated with a higher morbidity, it has the advantage that therapeutic intervention can be performed at the same time.

60.4.2 Management

The principal aim of treatment is to establish adequate drainage of the 'main' pancreatic duct in order to relieve symptoms and to prevent chronic pancreatitis and pancreas insufficiency from developing. Unfortunately, by the time of presentation chronic changes are often evident. Drainage of the pancreas can be achieved by sphincteroplasty or endoscopic sphincterotomy of the minor papilla. If chronic changes of duct dilatation have developed, a pancreatico-jejunostomy (Puestow procedure) may be indicated. Pancreatic resection may be required in severe forms of chronic pancreatitis (see below).

60.5 Ectopic Pancreatic Tissue

Ectopic pancreatic tissue is frequently found associated with foregut-derived structures. This is thought to be the result of transition of the embryonic epithelium. These pancreatic 'rests' are usually asymptomatic.

However, pancreatic tissue can be found at the base of a Meckel's diverticulum and can cause bleeding and inflammation.

60.6 Acute Pancreatitis

Acute pancreatitis is an inflammatory condition of the pancreas resulting from intrapancreatic activation, secretion and digestion of the pancreas by its own enzymes. It is rare in childhood but must always be considered in children presenting with abdominal pain. There are many different causes of acute pancreatitis and the principle ones are outlined in Table 60.1.

60.6.1 Diagnosis

The diagnosis of acute pancreatitis is based on a careful history and physical examination, and confirmed by the results of both laboratory and radiological investigations. A careful history is essential both for the diagnosis to be made and for determining the underlying cause. Acute pancreatitis classically presents with

Table 60.1 Principle causes of acute pancreatitis

Idiopathic	
Hereditary	
Systemic infections	– Mumps
	– Coxsackie B
	– Rubella
Trauma	
Iatrogenic injury	
Developmental anomalies of pancreatico-biliary system	
	– Pancreas divisum
	– Pancreatcobiliary malunion
	– Choledochal cyst
Gallstones	
Drugs	– Azathiorpine
	– Steroids
	– Valproic acid
	– Tetracycline
	– L-Aspariginase
	– Immunosuppressants
Metabolic Abnormalities	– Hypercalcaemia
	– Hyperglyceridaemia
	– Cystic fibrosis
Miscellaneous	

epigastric pain radiating through to the back and left upper quadrant. However, the pain may be less well localised and particularly in younger children, nausea and vomiting is often the predominant feature. In determining the underlying cause, it is important to elucidate a history of abdominal trauma, gallstones, recent mumps, familial pancreatitis, or pancreatitis-associated medication. Physical examination may elicit a range of signs including low-grade pyrexia, epigastric tenderness, generalised peritonitis, and in severe forms of pancreatitis the child may present with the signs of hypovolaemic shock. In cases of necrotising or haemorrhagic pancreatitis, pathognomonic patterns of bruising may be present on the abdominal wall either around the umbilicus (Cullen's sign) or in the flanks (Grey-Turner sign). Grossly elevated serum amylase levels are usually diagnostic of acute pancreatitis but normal levels do not exclude the diagnosis, and mildly elevated levels can be present in a number of other conditions including salivary inflammation, intestinal perforation, and renal failure. Elevated urinary amylase levels occur only if the serum amylase is greatly elevated. As a result of these discrepancies with amylase, some centres measure serum lipase levels instead, as lipase is specific to the pancreas.

A plain abdominal x-ray is important to exclude perforation. Other features that may be seen include gallstones, a dilated loop of small bowel (sentinel loop), and a dilated ascending colon with 'cut off' of air in the transverse colon. A chest x-ray may demonstrate pulmonary oedema or a left sided pleural effusion. Abdominal ultrasound can be useful for identifying pancreatic oedema and can be helpful in identifying pancreatic anatomy. However, overlying dilated bowel loops frequently obscure the visibility of the pancreas. Computed tomography (CT) with double contrast is therefore often indicated and provides a more accurate picture of the degree of pancreatic damage and better visualisation of the ductal anatomy (Fig. 60.1). Apart from its therapeutic use following pancreatic trauma, ERCP is rarely indicated in the acute phase of pancreatitis. Indeed, non-interventional ERCP is itself associated with a 10% incidence of acute pancreatitis. If duct anatomy needs to be further elucidated, a MRCP is useful.

Other laboratory tests are performed to determine the severity of the disease including a full blood count, liver function tests, serum calcium, blood glucose, and an arterial blood gas (see below).

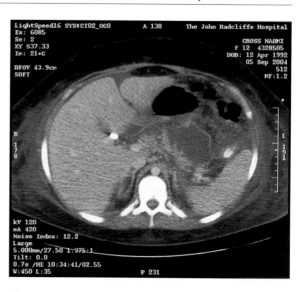

Fig. 60.1 An abdominal CT scan of a 12 year old girl presenting with acute necrotizing pancreatitis secondary to gallstones. The scan demonstrates a diffusely swollen pancreas with 75% necrosis

60.6.2 Management

There are three main aims of management of these patients, namely to support the child during the acute phase of the disease, to help prevent the sequelae of the disease, and to identify and treat any underlying causes.

Children with acute pancreatitis require very close monitoring throughout their admission. Early signs of multi-organ failure must be treated aggressively as the child can deteriorate rapidly. This is often best achieved by the child being located in a high dependency unit or an intensive care unit.

Active resuscitation is essential from the onset in all patients. Oxygen is administered and breathing carefully assessed. Children with severe pancreatitis may require ventilation. Acute pancreatitis is associated with large volume fluid loss and therefore aggressive fluid replacement and close monitoring of urine output are vital. A nasogastric tube is inserted to decompress and 'rest' the bowel. Analgesia is administered as soon as the child has been assessed, but opiates are used selectively due to their spasmodic effects on the sphincter of Oddi and hence their indirect effects on intra-pancreatic pressure. Broad-spectrum antibiotics are often administered and indeed it is the author's preference to do so. However, there is no conclusive evidence-base for this approach. A number of different regimes have been attempted in order to reduce pancreatic enzymatic activation in the acute phase but it is unclear which have a clear advantage. There does seem to be moderate evidence that somatostatin analogues are beneficial. In addition, many clinicians start the child on H$_2$ antagonists or proton pump inhibitors in order to prevent gastric ulceration and also potentially prevent gastric acid from triggering pancreatic secretions within the duodenum. Total parenteral nutrition is commenced early in the treatment regime not only because prolonged bowel rest is the norm, but also because a positive nitrogen balance has been shown to be associated with a more favourable outcome. Surgical intervention is rarely required in the acute phase of the disease. Peritoneal lavage has been used widely in the past but is rarely indicated in children. Necrotising pancreatitis may require necrosectomy or pancreatic debridement and this may sometimes need to be done repeatedly. The complications of acute pancreatitis such as pancreatic abscess and pancreatic pseudocyst may also require surgical treatment (see below).

Once the child has been stabilised, the underlying cause of the acute pancreatitis should also be addressed and treated appropriately. This includes correcting conditions such as hyperlipidaemia and hypercalcaemia and also planning surgical treatment for gallstones and correction of any underlying pancreatico-biliary malformations.

60.6.3 Prognosis

A number of different systems for predicting patient outcome have been devised. These include the Ranson and Imrie Criteria, and Apache II. However, none of these systems have been worked out on children and they also tend to make a presumption that all the parameters being measured rise and fall at similar stages in the disease.

The majority of children with acute pancreatitis make a good recovery.

60.6.4 Complications

The main complications of acute pancreatitis are pancreatic abscess, pancreatic pseudocyst, pancreatic fistula, and relapsing pancreatitis.

Pancreatic abscesses require open drainage having first been confirmed by CT-guided aspiration. There is some evidence that delaying abscess drainage beyond the first 2 weeks of the onset of the disease is associated with a better outcome.

A pancreatic pseudocyst results from accumulation of leaked pancreatic enzymes enclosed within an inflammatory non-epithelial lining. They commonly appear 10–14 days after the onset of acute pancreatitis and should be suspected if elevated amylase levels reappear after having settled. About half of acute pancreatic pseudocysts settle spontaneously. If they persist, maturation of the pseudocyst wall is essential before definitive treatment is performed. It is conventional to allow 6–8 weeks for this process to occur. Treatment usually consists of internal drainage of the pseudocyst either by open gastro-cystostomy or by minimally invasive procedures such as endoscopic insertion of gastro-cystic stent or percutaneous drainage. Occasionally if the pseudocyst is confined to the tail of the pancreas, excision can be considered. Complications of pancreatic pseudocysts include bleeding, infection, and rupture.

A pancreatic fistula is usually a post-operative complication and can be associated with a low or high output. Most low output fistulae close spontaneously. Treatment is therefore directed at maintaining adequate nutrition of the child, attempting to reduce secretions with pharmacological agents such as somatostatin analogues, and ensuring that the fistula tract does not become prematurely obstructed. Persistent fistulae may require surgical intervention.

Although the majority of cases of acute pancreatitis are single episodes and self-resolving, some children may develop acute relapsing pancreatitis and others may develop irreversible damage of the pancreas leading to chronic pancreatitis.

60.7 Chronic Pancreatitis

Chronic pancreatitis occurs when the pancreas has been permanently damaged by inflammation. Several classifications exist for this disease and the simplest is an anatomical one sub-dividing the condition into either being calcifying or obstructive. The former is more common and is associated with dense fibrosis and intrapancreatic stone formation. The commonest aetiology in children is hereditary or familial pancreatitis (Fig. 60.2). Obstructive chronic pancreatitis on the other hand is associated with less aggressive scar formation

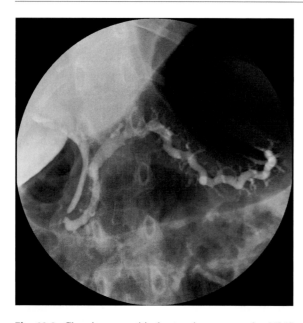

Fig. 60.2 Chronic pancreatitis due to missense mutation N34S (SPINK 1 gene). The pancreatic duct is dilated up to 1 cm. After a Puestow procedure (long side-to-side pancreatic jejunostomy) the further time course was uneventful (by courtesy of M. E. Höllwarth)

and most commonly arises as a result of congenital structural abnormalities such as pancreas divisum.

60.7.1 Diagnosis

High amylase or lipase levels are less of a feature in chronic pancreatitis. CT scans are helpful in determining the extent of damage to the pancreas, to look for calcification, and to determine the anatomy of the ductal system. An ERCP is useful if intervention to the ducts is required in the form of stenting or sphincterotomy at the same time as elucidating ductal anatomy. MRCP is the investigation of choice if a detailed view of the pancreatic ducts is required without intervention.

The main presenting features are chronic intractable pain and weight loss, but the child's first presentation may be with one or more of the complications described below. Although up to 15% of patients with chronic pancreatitis are relatively pain free, for the remainder chronic pain in the epigastrium and back dominates their lives.

This pain can be exacerbated by food or alcohol. The aetiology of the severe pain is unclear, but theories include the effects of pancreatic obstruction and distension, and also the exposure of peri-pancreatic nerves as a result of pancreatic damage.

The cause of weight loss in these patients is multifactorial in that it can be simply due to the reduced food intake of many of these patients due to the associated exacerbation of pain, but can also be due to malabsorption, as well as the fact that many of the adult patients with this disease have a chronic alcohol problem.

60.7.2 Management

The intractable pain associated with chronic pancreatitis is often difficult to control. Whilst patients can get some relief from simple measures such as leaning forward while sitting, the main stay of treatment is strong analgesia. As a result, patients with this condition frequently become opiate-dependent. Pharmacological and surgical nerve blocks can help with pain control. Some surgeons advocate partial or total pancreatectomy for pain control earlier in the disease process than others, but careful patient selection is always critical. If total pancreatectomy is performed and the individual is shown pre-operatively to have maintained endocrine function, there is a strong case for stating that the patient should also be offered a simultaneous islet autotransplant. Whilst this procedure may enable the patient to remain insulin-independent, even if it does not, it should enable the patient to avoid the particularly brittle form of diabetes that often follows pancreatectomy. Drainage procedures may be indicated if ductal dilatation is present. Longitudinal pancreaticojejunostomy (Puestow procedure) works well if the obstruction of the pancreatic duct is distal to the pancreatic neck. However, frequently the head and neck of the pancreas are also fibrosed.

Exocrine insufficiency is treated with long-term oral pancreatic enzyme replacement. The number of enzyme capsules required is titrated by the patient against the appearance of the stool.

When endocrine insufficiency has fully developed, it requires insulin treatment. As stated above, the brittle form of the disease associated with chronic pancreatitis is often difficult to control and needs close input from the diabetes team.

Obstruction of the structures adjacent to the pancreas often requires radiological or surgical intervention in the form of stents or bypass surgery.

60.7.3 Complications

The complications of chronic pancreatitis may present late in the disease process or particularly if the disease has been preceded by acute relapsing pancreatitis, may be one of the presenting features. The principle complications are exocrine insufficiency, endocrine insufficiency, and damage to adjacent structures.

Exocrine insufficiency is usually a late feature and presents with steatorrhea. Stools are bulky with a particularly offensive smell, and are difficult to flush away in the toilet. This can be exacerbated by a high lipid diet.

Despite the islets of Langerhans accounting for only 2% of the pancreatic tissue, the endocrine component of the pancreas is often surprisingly spared until the later stages of the disease. Before frank diabetes develops however, abnormal patterns of glucose-tolerance tests can often be detected.

The pancreas is associated with a number of other structures including the common bile duct, the duodenum, and the splenic vessels. All these structures can become partially or completely obstructed as a result of chronic fibrosis. Colonic obstruction can also occur if the inflammation is extensive.

The precise link between chronic pancreatitis and pancreatic cancer is unclear, but several studies have suggested a direct correlation.

60.8 Pancreatic Trauma

Although pancreatic injury occurs in less than 3% of adults who have suffered blunt or penetrating abdominal trauma, the anatomical position of the pancreas traversing the upper lumbar vertebrae means that this organ is vulnerable to transection and this injury is greatly increased in young children due to their thin abdominal walls. Whilst pancreatic trauma often presents with all the features of acute pancreatitis described above, it has some unique treatment dilemmas that warrant separate discussion.

60.8.1 Diagnosis

A history of blunt abdominal trauma to the epigastric region is frequently given. This may be in the context of a motor vehicle accident or is frequently due to an object such as a bicycle handle being caught in the upper abdomen. Examination may reveal traumatic bruising within the epigastric region. Penetrating abdominal injury is rare in children in the UK.

Non-accidental injury (NAI) must be considered especially if the history is inconsistent, the history is at odds with the clinical findings, or if any other stigmata of NAI are present.

Pancreatic injury may not be an isolated injury and associated injuries to the duodenum, small bowel, and spleen are common. The child may therefore, present with profound shock or signs of peritonitis.

Sometimes the initial pancreatic injury can go unnoticed and instead the child presents later on with a complication of pancreatic injury such as a pseudocyst.

Some degree of hyperamylaseaemia or hyperlipaseaemia is usually present, but this does depend on the severity of injury and the timing of presentation.

Abdominal ultrasound can be useful in cases of minor pancreatic trauma. However, this modality is poor for assessing injuries of the pancreatic duct and therefore CT scan with double contrast is required in most patients (Fig. 60.3). This also enables a full assessment of adjacent structures including the duodenum. MRCP can also be useful for further delineation of the duct.

Based on CT findings pancreatic trauma is classified into 4 grades of severity (see Table 60.2).

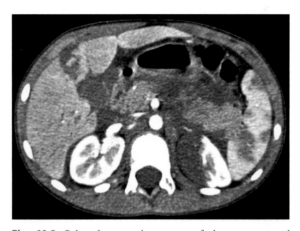

Fig. 60.3 Subtotal traumatic rupture of the pancreas and infarction of the dorsal part of the kidney after an abdominal trauma (by courtesy of the Dept. of Paediatric Radiology, Medical University of Graz)

Table 60.2 Classification of Pancreatic Injury (American Association for the Surgery of Trauma)

Grade I	Minor contusion or superficial laceration without ductal injury
Grade II	Major contusion or laceration without ductal injury or tissue loss
Grade III	Distal transection or parenchymal injury with ductal injury
Grade IV	Proximal transection (to the right of the superior mesenteric vein) or parenchymal injury involving the ampulla
Grade V	Massive disruption of pancreatic head

60.8.2 Management

As with all cases of major trauma in children, the systematic approach of advanced paediatric life support is essential. The child is carefully assessed and resuscitation started. The pancreatic injury may be an isolated injury or multiple injuries may be present and treatment is tailored accordingly.

As far as the pancreatic injury is concerned, the majority of grade I and II injuries can be treated conservatively. Close observation of the child must be continued throughout to detect clinical deterioration and repeated serum amylase or lipase levels taken and repeat imaging performed to determine whether complications such as pseudocyst have developed.

If transection of the distal pancreas has occurred, early distal pancreatectomy with splenic preservation (if possible) is advocated and is associated with good recovery in most patients. However, in cases of delayed presentation, this procedure can be difficult, and a more conservative approach is often preferable in the first instance. Treatment is then targeted at the sequelae of the acute injury such as pancreatic pseudocyst. Major injuries to the pancreatic head provide the greatest challenge. In the acute phase, major bleeding sometimes requires immediate packing and abdominal closure. If the child is haemodynamically stable and the injury to the pancreatic head is major and involves the duodenum, a pancreaticduodenectomy is indicated. Major ductal injuries with preservation of pancreatic tissue can either be managed by endoscopic stenting or by pancreaticojejunostomy (Fig. 60.4).

60.8.3 Complications

The commonest complication of pancreatic trauma is a persistent ductal leak, which can manifest itself as a

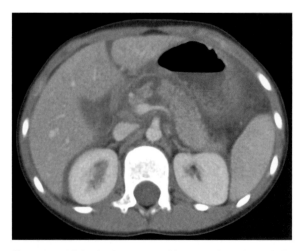

Fig. 60.4 Abdominal trauma with total disruption of the pancreatic head from the corpus. In this case the proximal part of the pancreas was closed with sutures and the distal part was anastomosed to a Roux-en-Y jejunal loop (by courtesy of the Dept. of Paediatric Radiology, Medical University of Graz)

pancreatic pseudocyst or pancreatic fistula (Fig. 60.5a,b). A pseudocyst is managed as for acute pancreatitis but surgery may be required if the ductal leak persists (see above). Surgery for pancreatic fistulae is only indicated after several months of conservative treatment have been attempted.

60.9 Persistent Hyperinsulinaemic Hypoglycaemia of Infancy (PHHI)

Hyperinsulism in neonates is relatively common but is usually transient. Persistent hyperinsulinism is a rare condition affecting 1 in 50,000 live European births but can affect up to 1 in 2,800 in familial cases. A number of different terms have been used for this condition including pancreatic endocrine dysregulation syndrome (PEDS) and the more extensively used term nesidioblastosis. However, whilst the latter term was favoured by surgeons it was a pathological definition and did not take into account different forms of the disease, and as a result a few years ago the more general term PHHI was introduced. PHHI is characterised by persistent non-ketotic hypoglycaemia and the baby can present with fits and early brain damage. It is therefore imperative that all neonates are checked for hypoglycaemia immediately after birth.

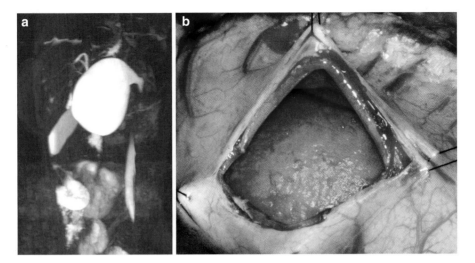

Fig. 60.5 a The patient of figure 60.3 developed a pancreatic pseudocyst (by courtesy of the Dept. of Paediatric Radiology, Medical University of Graz) **b** The pseudocyst was treated by a cystogastrostomy. The photograph shows the bulging of the dorsal gastric wall by the pseudocyst (by courtesy of M.E. Höllwarth)

Detailed research over recent years has helped elucidate the pathogenesis of the disease at a molecular level and also identified two subtypes of the disease namely diffuse PHHI and focal PHHI. The former is characterised by abnormal islets with large pleomorphic, hyperchromatic nuclei being present throughout the pancreas (see Fig. 60.2). Focal PHHI on the other hand, involves nodules of adenomatous islet cell hyperplasia with normal islets surrounding these areas. Familial and sporadic forms of PHHI have also been identified. The genetic defect for certain forms of this condition has been located to the gene encoding the sulphonylurea receptor on the short arm of chromosome 11.

60.9.1 Diagnosis

Diagnosis is based on the confirmation of persistent non-ketotic hypoglycaemia in the presence of hyperinsulinism, with a glucose requirement of >12.5 mg/kg/min and a hyperglycaemic response to glucagon. A number of different diagnostic tests have been advocated for imaging the PHHI pancreas and determining whether the disease is diffuse or focal. These have included serial venous sampling of insulin and more recently laparoscopic pancreatic biopsy. However, the current 'gold standard' is positive emission tomography (PET), which seems to locate the lesions with greatest accuracy.

60.9.2 Management

Glucose infusions are commenced immediately. The mainstay treatment for these babies is medical with drugs such as diazoxide which acts on the potassium-ATP channels within beta cells, and somatostatin analogues. Both these reduce insulin secretion and may be required for many years. Surgery is indicated for diffuse PHHI that fails to respond to medical management, in which case a 95% pancreatectomy is required, and for focal disease in which limited pancreatic resection can be curative. Surgery can be performed as an open procedure or laparoscopically.

60.9.3 Complications

The complications of delayed diagnosis of hypoglycaemia can be catastrophic. For this reason early diagnosis is vital. Prolonged treatment with diazoxide is associated with profound facial hirsutism, which can be particularly problematic for older children on long-term treatment. For those infants undergoing surgery, incomplete resection of focal disease can result in unresolved hyperinsulinism. Further resection of the remaining 'cuff' of pancreatic tissue is required. Persistent symptoms in babies who have undergone surgery, is either a result of incomplete excision of the focal area or multi-focal disease. More accurate pre-operative localisation with PET scanning will potentially minimise this problem. Even in the most experienced hands, pancreatic resection involving the proximal pancreas in neonates is associated with not inconsiderable morbidity of surrounding structures including bile duct and superior mesenteric vein. The majority of patients who have undergone 95% pancreatectomy for PHHI are insulin-dependent by the age of 20. Pancreatic insufficiency is also common.

60.10 Pancreatic Cysts

Pancreatic cysts can be congenital or acquired. Congenital cysts are either single or multiple and can be also be part of gastro-intestinal duplication (Fig. 60.6).

Single congenital cysts are most commonly present in the tail and body of the pancreas and usually do not communicate with the pancreatic duct. There is a female predominance. These developmental cysts can present at any age but the majority are diagnosed before 2 years of age. Multiple congenital cysts can be confined to the pancreas or be part of a polycystic systemic disorder such as von Hippel-Landau syndrome.

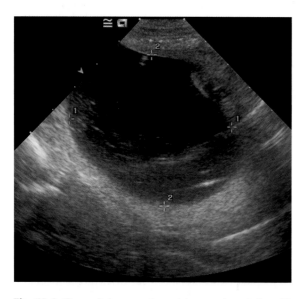

Fig. 60.6 Congenital pancreatic cyst in a newborn baby with sedimentation phenomenon on the dorsal part of the cyst. The cyst was anastomosed to a Roux-en-Y loop (by courtesy of M. E. Höllwarth)

A number of different types of acquired pancreatic cysts occur. The most frequent is a pancreatic pseudocyst (discussed above). Retention cysts secondary to pancreatic duct obstruction and tropical cysts usually associated with hydatid disease also occur.

60.10.1 Diagnosis

Clinically, such cysts may be incidental findings during physical examination or ultrasound or may present with a palpable abdominal mass. In addition, they may present with symptoms resulting from the effects of pressure on surrounding structures such as nausea and vomiting, epigastric pain, and jaundice. Abdominal ultrasound is helpful in confirming the diagnosis and CT or MRI scan help to further delineate the nature of the cyst and its anatomical relations.

60.10.2 Management

The treatment of pancreatic cysts is dependent on the exact nature of the cyst. Single congenital cysts are excised if they occur in the body or tail of the pancreas and internally drained if they are located in the pancreatic head. Small incidental, asymptomatic congenital cysts can be left and observed if neoplasia has been excluded. Symptomatic multiple congenital cysts may require extensive pancreatic resection. The treatment of pancreatic pseudocysts has already been discussed. Duplication cysts are often amenable to resection whereas the priority for hydatid cysts is to treat the underlying cause. Hydatid cysts sometime resolve spontaneously and there are also a range of surgical options including marsupilization, cystectomy, and partial pancreatectomy.

60.11 Pancreatic Tumours

Pancreatic tumours are rare in childhood but a large number of different types of pancreatic tumour can occur. These can be primary or secondary, cystic or solid, involve the exocrine or endocrine component of the gland, and can be secretory or non-secretory. An extensive discussion of pancreatic tumours is beyond the scope of this chapter but a brief overview of primary tumours of the exocrine and endocrine pancreas will be given.

60.11.1 Tumours of the Exocrine Pancreas

Benign tumours of the exocrine pancreas include serous adenomas (microcystic and oligocystic), mucinous cystadenomas, and mature cystic teratomas. Serous adenomas do not require excision unless symptomatic but mucinous cystadenomas should undergo wide excision because they belong to the same spectrum of tumours that include mucinous cystadenocarcinoma and have definite malignant potential. This malignant tumour spreads locally in the same manner as ductal adenocarcinoma. However, if complete excision is achieved, prognosis is excellent. Ductal adenocarcinoma is rarely encountered in the paediatric age group but has been reported in teenagers. Prognosis for this condition is poor. Acinar adenocarcinoma is also rare but has a slightly better prognosis than ductal adenocarcinoma. The commonest pancreatic neoplasm in children is a pancreatoblastoma. This tumour can present at any age but the mean age for presentation is 4 years of age. The tumour is more common in males (2:1) and is associated with Beckwith-Widemann syndrome. Tumours tend to be large and solitary, and can be located in any region of the pancreas. The tumour has a mixed histology and although a malignant tumour, the presence of a capsule means that it behaves in less aggressive manner than acinar adenocarcinoma. Treatment is by radical surgical excision and metastatic disease often responds favourably to chemotherapy. Radiotherapy is used for local recurrence. Overall 30% of patients with this tumour are tumour-free 5 years after initial treatment.

Papillary-cystic tumour (also termed a Frantz tumour) is classified as being 'low-grade' malignant. Occurring predominantly in young women, these tumours present as large, round, solitary masses and can arise from any region of the pancreas. Tumours may be found incidentally or may present with abdominal discomfort. Complete excision is associated with a 95% cure rate.

60.11.2 Tumours of the Endocrine Pancreas

Both benign and malignant tumours of the endocrine pancreas can be secretory (functioning) or non-secretory. Insulinoma is the commonest functioning pancreatic endocrine tumour. Over 90% of these are benign although malignant forms do exist. Most are solitary but multiple lesions have been reported. Clinical presentation usually consists of intermittent episodes of profound hypoglycaemia. Treatment is by surgical enucleation or excision. The commonest malignant pancreatic endocrine tumour of childhood is a gastrinoma. These may occur in the pancreas itself or in extrapancreatic sites. It is associated with the Zollinger-Ellison syndrome and is also a feature of multiple endocrine neoplasia 1 syndrome (MEN 1). These are well-circumscribed, non-encapsulated lesions. Treatment is by aggressive resection which may require pancreaticoduodenectomy if the tumour is in the pancreatic head. Other endocrine pancreatic tumours encountered in children include VIPomas and islet cell carcinomas.

60.12 Conclusions

Pancreatic disorders present a number of different challenges to the paediatric surgeon. As these cases are infrequent and often complex, there is a strong case for these children to be managed in a small number of specialist centres where the facilities and expertise for investigating and treating the full range of pancreatic disorders is available.

Further Reading

Bax KN, van der Zee DC (2007) The laparoscopic approach toward hyperinsulinism in children. Semin Pediatr Surg 16(4):245–251

Hines OJ, Reber HA (2000) Acute pancreatitis. In PJ Morris, WC Wood (eds) Oxford Textbook of Surgery, 2nd edn. Oxford University Press, Oxford, pp 1765–1777

Johnson PRV, Spitz L (2000) Cysts and tumors of the pancreas. Semin Paediatr Surg 9(4):209–215

Miyano T (1998) The pancreas. In JA O'Neill et al (eds) Paediatric Surgery, 5th edn. Mosby-Year Book, Philadelphia, pp 1527–1544

Spitz L (2006) Surgery for persistent hyperinsulinaemic hypoglycaemia of infancy. In P Puri, ME Höllwarth (eds) Pediatric Surgery, Springer-Verlag, Berlin, Heidelberg, New York, pp 395–402

Splenic Disorder

61

Thom E. Lobe

Contents

61.1 Introduction

The spleen is the largest organ or component of the reticuloendothelial system. Its primary functions include hematopoiesis and immune protection. As part of the reticuloendothelial system, the spleen acts as a filter for abnormally shaped blood cells and some metabolic products. It has the ability to store blood and contract in response to acute changes in blood volume such as in the case of trauma and it becomes the focus of surgical attention in a variety of circumstances that we will discuss in detail in this chapter.

61.2 Anatomy and Physiology

The spleen serves as a hemopoietic organ during the hepatosplenothymic phase (beginning in the 2nd month). The spleen mainly produces cells of the erythroid lineage in the fetus and lymphocytes in the newborn. Thymic and B-lymphocytes migrate to the spleen and populate the white pulp associated with the trabeculae. (The sinuses contain erythroblastic tissue, or red pulp.) The spleen contains phagocytes that remove "exhausted" erythrocytes and foreign bodies from the blood and it is a major reservoir for blood. Absence of the spleen predisposes to certain infections.

The organ is located in the upper left part of the abdomen, behind the stomach and just below the diaphragm. In normal adult individuals this organ measures about $125 \times 75 \times 50$ mm ($5 \times 3 \times 2$ in.) in size, with an average weight of 150 g. It consists of masses of lymphoid tissue of granular appearance located around fine terminal branches of veins and arteries.

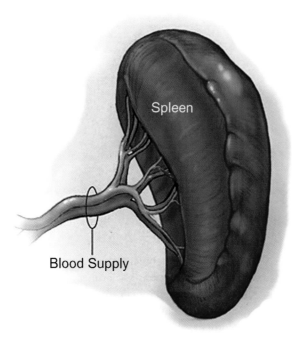

Fig. 61.1 Splenic vascular anatomy

These vessels are connected by modified capillaries called splenic sinuses.

The splenic artery the largest branch of the celiac artery, is remarkable for the tortuosity of its course as it passes horizontally to the left side, behind the stomach and the omental bursa of the peritoneum, and along the upper border of the pancreas. Some surgeons identify and ligate the splenic vessel in this location before splenectomy to minimize the risk of hemorrhage. Pre-operative embolization of the splenic artery also has been described. The artery is accompanied by the splenic vein, which lies below it; the artery crosses in front of the upper part of the left kidney, and, on arriving near the spleen, divides into branches, some of which enter the splenic hilum between the two layers of the phrenicosplenic ligament to be distributed to the tissues of the spleen; some are given to the pancreas, while others pass to the greater curvature of the stomach between the layers of the gastrosplenic ligament (Fig. 61.1).

The short gastric arteries consist of five to seven small branches, which arise from the end of the splenic artery, and from its terminal divisions. They pass from left to right, between the layers of the gastrosplenic ligament, and are distributed to the greater curvature of the stomach, anastomosing with branches of the left gastric and left gastroepiploic arteries.

Approximately 10% of people have one or more accessory spleens. They may form near the hilum of the main spleen, the junction at which the splenic vessels enter and leave the organ.

There are several peritoneal ligaments that support the spleen: the gastrosplenic ligament connects the stomach to spleen; the splenorenal ligament connects spleen to kidney and the phrenicocolic ligament connects left colic flexure to the thoracic diaphragm – the middle of it connects to the spleen.

The splenic red pulp is composed of: "sinuses" (or "sinusoids") which are filled with blood; "splenic cords" of reticular fibers and "marginal zone" bordering on white pulp. Its function is mechanical filtration. Removes unwanted materials from the blood, including senescent red blood cells.

White Pulp, on the other hand, is composed of nodules, called Malpighian corpuscles. These are composed of: "lymphoid follicles" (or "follicles"), rich in B-lymphocytes and "periarteriolar lymphoid sheaths", rich in T-lymphocytes. It's function is to help fight infections.

Other functions of the spleen are less prominent including: the production of opsonins, properdin, and tuftsin.

Creation of red blood cells occurs in the spleen up until the 5th month of gestation, the spleen has important hematopoietic functions. After birth, no significant hematopoietic function is left in the spleen except in some hematologic disorders: e.g. myelodysplastic syndrome and hemoglobinopathies.

61.3 Pathology

The spleen is the largest collection of lymphoid tissue in the body. It is normally palpable in preterm infants, in 30% of normal, full-term neonates, and in 5–10% of infants and toddlers. A spleen easily palpable below the costal margin in any child over the age of 3–4 years should be considered abnormal until proven otherwise.

Splenomegaly can result from antigenic stimulation (e.g., infection), obstruction of blood flow (e.g., portal vein obstruction), underlying functional abnormality (e.g., hemolytic anemia), or infiltration (e.g., leukemia

Table 61.1 Diseases or conditions for which splenectomy is indicated

Traumatic injury to spleen

Hematologic diseases including hereditary spherocytosis; thalassemia major; certain forms of immune thrombocytopenic purpura (ITP) unresponsive to medical management; myeloproliferative disorders; thrombotic thrombocytopenic purpura (TTP)

Hydatid cysts

Hodgkin's disease (clinical stage I-A or II-A)

Intraoperative splenic injury

Splenic abscesses

Non-parasitic cysts that are symptomatic and greater than 5 cm

Sinistral portal hypertension secondary to isolated splenic vein thrombosis or obstruction

Splenic mass presumed to be a primary or undiagnosed neoplasm, malignancy in an adjacent organ

Metabolic storage diseases such as Gaucher's disease

Infarcted wandering spleen

or storage disease, such as Gaucher's disease). The most common cause of acute splenomegaly in children is viral infection, which is transient and usually moderate. Basic work-up for acute splenomegaly includes a complete blood count with differential, platelet count, and reticulocyte and atypical lymphocyte counts to exclude hemolytic anemia and leukemia. Assessment of IgM antibodies to viral capsid antigen (a rising titer) is indicated to confirm Epstein-Barr virus or cytomegalovirus. Other infections should be excluded if these tests are negative.

Conditions for which splenectomy is indicated are listed in Table 61.1.

61.4 Splenic Trauma

A direct blow to the abdomen may bruise, tear or shatter the spleen. Trauma to the spleen can cause varying degrees of damage, the major problem associated with internal bleeding. Mild splenic subcapsular hematomas are injuries in which bleeding is limited to small areas on and immediately around the spleen. Splenic contusions refer to bruising and bleeding on and around larger areas of the spleen. Lacerations are the most common splenic trauma injuries. Tears tend to occur on the areas between the three main blood vessels of the spleen. Because of the abundant blood supply, splenic trauma may

cause serious internal bleeding. Most injuries to the spleen in children heal spontaneously. Severe trauma can cause the spleen or its blood vessels to rupture or fragment.

61.4.1 Causes and Symptoms

The most common cause of injury to the spleen is blunt abdominal trauma. Blunt trauma is often caused by a direct blow to the belly, car and motorcycle accidents, falls, sports mishaps, and fights. The spleen is the most commonly injured organ in blunt abdominal trauma; splenic injury occurs in nearly 25% of injuries of this type. Penetrating injuries such as those from stabbing, gunshot wounds, and accidental impaling also account for cases of splenic trauma, although far less frequently than blunt trauma.

A spleen that has become enlarged and fragile from disease is sometimes ruptured by a doctor or medical student in the course of palpating (feeling) the patient's abdomen, or damaged by a surgeon in the course of an operation on other abdominal organs.

Damage to the spleen may cause localized or general abdominal pain, tenderness, and swelling. Fractured ribs may be present. Splenic trauma may cause mild or severe internal bleeding, leading to shock and for which symptoms include rapid heartbeat, shortness of breath, thirst, pale or clammy skin, weak pulse, low blood pressure, dizziness, fainting, sweating. Vomiting blood, blood in the stools or urine, deterioration of vital signs, and loss of consciousness are other symptoms.

61.4.2 Diagnosis

The goal of diagnosis of all abdominal traumas is to detect and treat life-threatening injuries as quickly as possible. Ultrasonography – particularly focused abdominal sonographic technique (FAST) – has now become a standard bedside technique in many hospitals to check for bleeding in the abdomen. Imaging tests allow doctors to determine the necessity and type of surgery required. The CT scan has been shown to be the most available and accurate test for abdominal trauma. MRI tests are accurate but costly and less available in some hospitals, while radionuclide scanning requires more time and patient stability. Peritoneal lavage is another diagnostic technique in which the abdominal cavity is entered and flushed to check for bleeding. When patients exhibit shock, infection, or prolonged internal bleeding, exploratory laparoscopy may be warranted.

61.4.3 Treatment

Improved techniques of diagnosis and monitoring (particularly the introduction of CT scans), as well as understanding that removal of the spleen creates future risk of a lowered capacity to fight infection has modified treatment approaches. Research over the past two decades has shown that the spleen has high healing potential, and confirmed that children are more susceptible to infection after splenectomy (post splenectomy sepsis, PSS). PSS has a mortality rate of over 50% and standard procedure now avoids splenectomy as much as possible.

61.4.4 Nonoperative Treatment

In nonoperative therapy, splenic trauma patients are monitored closely, often in intensive care units for several days. Fluid and blood levels are observed and maintained by intravenous fluid and possible blood transfusions. Follow-up scans may be used to observe the healing process, but in the asymptomatic patient these are of little benefit. Today non-operative treatment of a blunt splenic injury is the rule and splenectomy is rarely needed.

61.4.5 Prognosis

The ample blood supply to the spleen can promote rapid healing. Studies have shown that intra-abdominal bleeding associated with splenic trauma stops without surgical intervention in up to two out of three cases in children. When trauma patients stabilize during non-operative therapy, chances are high that surgery will be avoided and that spleen injuries will heal themselves. Splenic trauma patients undergoing diagnostic tests

such as CT and MRI scans have improved chances of avoiding splenectomy and retaining whole or partial spleen.

61.5 Hematologic Diseases

Indications for splenectomy should be determined with the close cooperation of a hematologist/oncologist. Common indications include hereditary spherocytosis, thalassemia major, and certain forms of immune thrombocytopenic purpura (ITP) unresponsive to medical management. Myeloproliferative disorders may lead to massive splenomegaly and can cause symptoms that are best relieved by splenectomy, primarily for symptomatic relief.

61.6 Hodgkin's Disease

Selected patients with clinical Stage I-A or II-A Hodgkin's disease may be candidates for a staging laparotomy or laparoscopy. In the absence of obvious liver or intra-abdominal nodal disease, splenectomy is an integral part of the staging procedure to exclude splenic involvement, which would alter the method of treatment.

61.7 Iatrogenic (Intraoperative) Splenic Injury

The spleen may be injured inadvertently during the performance of intraperitoneal procedures, especially those involving the distal esophagus, stomach, distal pancreas, or splenic flexure of the colon. These injuries may occur directly from operative retractors or, more often, secondary to inadvertently avulsed capsular adhesions that can lead to persistent bleeding. Hemostasis should be attempted using suture plication, topical hemostatic agents (including absorbable mesh), electrocautery, or argon beam coagulation so that splenectomy is not required. However, if rapid hemostasis is not possible, hemorrhage severe enough to require blood transfusion is better managed by formal splenectomy than by repeated attempts at splenic salvage.

61.8 Other Indications for Splenectomy

Less common indications for splenectomy include splenic abscesses, cysts, sinistral portal hypertension secondary to isolated splenic vein thrombosis or obstruction, or splenic mass presumed to be a primary or undiagnosed neoplasm. Splenectomy is occasionally included in en bloc resection for malignancy in an adjacent organ, such as the stomach, colon, adrenal gland, or pancreas. Distal pancreatectomy may include splenectomy if preservation of the splenic artery and vein is either contraindicated (malignancy) or technically impossible.

61.9 Prophylaxis Against Post-splenectomy Sepsis

The absence of a spleen predisposes to some septicemia infections. Vaccination and antibiotic measures are discussed under asplenia. Some people congenitally completely lack a spleen, although this is rare.

The absence of the spleen is best confirmed with a technetium-99m radionuclide scan. This agent is taken up by the reticuloendothelial cells and enables better assessment of splenic function.

Sickle-cell disease can cause a functional asplenia (or autosplenectomy) by causing infarctions of the spleen during repeated sickle-cell crises.

Medical care involves four key components: antibiotic prophylaxis, appropriate immunization, aggressive management of suspected infection, and parent education.

61.9.1 Antibiotic Prophylaxis

Antibiotic prophylaxis should be initiated immediately upon the diagnosis of asplenia because these patients are at significant risk of pneumococcal infections. For children younger than 2 years, oral penicillin V may be given twice a day. Amoxicillin has also been recommended as an appropriate prophylactic antibiotic. Erythromycin is an alternate choice in patients who are allergic to penicillin.

In general, antimicrobial prophylaxis should be considered for all children with asplenia or splenic dysfunction until 5 years of age and for at least 1 year after surgical splenectomy. Some experts recommend continuing prophylaxis into adulthood, particularly for high-risk patients. The need for long-term prophylaxis for children who have splenectomy after trauma has not been agreed upon.

61.9.2 Immunization

All patients should receive all standard childhood and adolescent immunizations at the recommended age. Most importantly, vaccinations against encapsulated organisms, including pneumococcal conjugate and/or polysaccharide, H influenzae type b conjugate, and meningococcal conjugate and/or polysaccharide vaccines, should be administered on the standard schedule.

Approximately 80% of the pediatric pneumococcal bacteremias in the United States are caused by the seven serotypes covered in the vaccine: 4, 6B, 9V, 14, 18C, 19F, and 23F. The conjugated vaccine has been effective in dramatically reducing the occurrence of invasive pneumococcal disease. In children younger than 2 years, the incidence of all invasive pneumococcal infections has decreased by 80% after conjugated vaccine was recommended in the routine childhood immunization schedule. Infections caused by vaccine and vaccine-related serotypes have decreased by 90% in older children and adults.

The immunization schedule for pneumococcal conjugate vaccine (PCV7) consists of a primary series of four doses (0.5 ml each) at age 2, 4, 6, and 12–15 months. Catch-up immunization schedules are published regarding appropriate dosing schedules for children aged 5 years or younger. Administration of a single dose of PCV7 to children of any age is not contraindicated, especially for patients with asplenia or splenic dysfunction who are at high risk for invasive pneumococcal disease.

The pneumococcal polysaccharide vaccine against 23 serotypes (PPV23) should be given after age 24 months for supplemental protection. PCV7 should be administered first, with administration of PPV23 at least 8 weeks after the last dose of PCV7. A booster dose 3–5 years after the first dose of PPV23 is appropriate.

Patients should also receive quadrivalent meningococcal vaccine. Two licensed meningococcal vaccines are available in the United States against serotypes A, C, Y, and W-135. Meningococcal conjugate vaccine (MCV4) was licensed in 2005 for people aged 11–55 years. Meningococcal polysaccharide vaccine (MPSV4) is licensed for children aged 2 years and older. Immunization with MPSV4 is recommended for children aged 2–10 years and older who have functional or anatomic asplenia. MCV4 should be used if the patient is aged 11 years or older. Because of its ability to induce a T-cell response, MCV4 is expected to confer immunity for approximately 10 years, as opposed to about 4 years of immunity from MPSV4. Immunization with MCV4 should be considered in adolescents aged 3–5 years after receiving MPSV4. Revaccination schedules with MCV4 are ongoing.

The recommended vaccination schedule for H influenzae type b is a primary series of three doses given at age 2, 4, and 6 months or two doses given at age 2 and 4 months, depending on the particular conjugate vaccine product administered. A booster dose at age 12 months is recommended for all vaccine products. Children who are undergoing scheduled splenectomy after completion of their primary series and booster dose, may benefit from an additional dose of conjugate vaccine at least 7–10 days before surgery. Catch-up immunization schedules regarding H influenzae type b vaccine are published.

Yearly influenza vaccine is also recommended to minimize the likelihood of secondary bacterial infections.

61.9.3 Management of Suspected Infection

The risk of serious bacterial infection is ever present in these patients. Many patients have trivial symptoms yet rapidly develop fulminant sepsis and death within hours.

All patients with impaired splenic function with suspected infection must be urgently and promptly evaluated. Obtain blood; urine; and, if indicated, cerebrospinal fluid (CSF) cultures. Initiate broad-spectrum intravenous antibiotics effective against S pneumoniae, H influenzae type b, and N meningitidis. Second- or third-generation cephalosporins may be the initial choices. If multiple-drug resistance is a concern, vancomycin should be added to the regimen. In addition, many patients require supportive care with intravenous fluids, volume expanders, and pressor support.

Because of the potential rapid progression of a serious bacterial infection, some experts recommend that asplenic patients have access to "stand-by" antibiotics, which can be initiated at the first sign of infection (fever, chills, or malaise). That the initiation of "stand-by" antibiotics is not a substitute for seeking immediate medical attention at the onset of an illness cannot be overemphasized.

Patients with asplenia are at an increased risk of sepsis, shock, and meningitis secondary to Capnocytophaga canimorsus resulting from dog, cat, or rodent bites. The diagnosis may be made by means of Gram staining of the buffy coat, blood, and CSF cultures. Early treatment with penicillin is the therapy of choice, but cephalosporins, clindamycin, and erythromycin may also be used.

61.10 Wandering Spleen

Congenital wandering spleen is a rare, randomly distributed birth defect characterized by the absence or weakness of one or more of the ligaments that hold the spleen in its normal position in the upper left abdomen. The disorder is not genetic in origin. Instead of ligaments, the spleen is attached by a stalk-like tissue supplied with blood vessels (vascular pedicle). If the pedicle is twisted in the course of the movement of the spleen, the blood supply may be interrupted or blocked (ischemia) to the point of severe damage to the blood vessels (infarction). Because there is little or nothing to hold it in place the spleen "wanders" in the lower abdomen or pelvis where it may be mistaken for an unidentified abdominal mass.

Symptoms of wandering spleen are typically those associated with an abnormally large size of the spleen (splenomegaly) or the unusual position of the spleen in the abdomen. Enlargement is most often the result of twisting (torsion) of the splenic arteries and veins or, in some cases, the formation of a blood clot (infarct) in the spleen. Thrombocytosis is the hallmark of an infarcted or recently removed spleen.

61.11 Surgical Approaches

The technical aspects of removing the spleen depend on the specific indication and the experience of the surgeon. There appears to be no data to support the routine use of prophylactic antibiotics in the perioperative period.

The traditional approach is an open one. In cases of traumatic injury to the spleen and in cases of massive splenomegaly, a midline incision may be preferred. Uncontrolled hemorrhage from traumatic splenic injury will immediately focus the surgeon's attention on the left upper quadrant of the open abdomen. Coagulated blood is quickly removed to faciliate visualization and the surgeon (standing on the patient's right side with the patient supine), cups the left hand on the spleen as the splenoreno and splenophreno ligaments are quickly divided either with scissors or bluntly with the surgeon's right hand so that the spleen can be delivered from the surgical wound for inspection.

At that point, the surgeon will assess whether the spleen can be repaired. Pre-operative images may suggest the degree of injury so that the surgeon can anticipate the findings, however, direct inspection will be required to make a final determination.

If the spleen is amenable to repair, this can be done using any of a variety of techniques. These include: using topical agents to promote coagulation, direct suturing, enveloping the fractured spleen in surgical mesh and other techniques. Ischemic segments can be discarded. The important point is to control ongoing hemorrhage. If hemorrhage cannot be controlled, then removal is justified.

All forms of splenectomy incorporate similar surgical steps: the spleen must be mobilized from its ligamentous (peritoneal) attachments; the short-gastric vessels must be divided; the colon must be dissected free of the tail of the pancreas and lower pole of the spleen; the splenic arteries and veins must be divided; the pancreas should be preserved and left intact; any accessory spleen should be searched for and removed and in the case of hematological diseases, the spleen must be removed and hemostasis assessed.

In the case of trauma, all this happens rather quickly so as to prevent further hemorrhage.

When an open midline approach is used for massive splenomegaly, the incision should be extended sufficiently to allow the surgeon easy access to all these maneuvers and to prevent accidental rupture of the

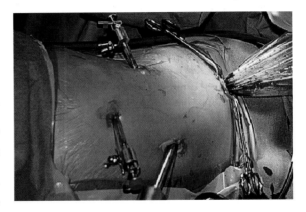

Fig. 61.2 Trocar sites with patient in lateral position. Spleen in sac with neck exteriorized from umbilicus

spleen. The surgeon should not have to struggle to perform the operation.

A lateral open approach is used by many for elective splenectomy, primarily for hematological or storage diseases. The difference in the case is principally the type of incision. The patient in this instance is positioned in a lateral decubitus position with the left side up. A roll is usually placed under the patient's right flank to accentuate elevation of the left side and to flex the patient to help get the lower ribs out of the way.

A transverse incision then is made through the layers of the abdominal wall just below or off the tip of the 12th rib. This puts the incision directly over the spleen which can be elevated into the wound to complete the operation. This incision is not ideal for cases of hematological diseases that require concomitant cholecystectomy for cholelithiasis as the gallbladder is rather inaccessible from this approach.

When cholecystectomy is required at the time of a planned open procedure, a midline or upper transverse incision is preferred to the lateral flank incision.

More recently, surgeons have adopted the laparoscopic approach to the spleen. Except in the instance of traumatic injury accompanied by ongoing hemorrhage and in the hemodynamically unstable patient, most splenic surgery can be performed safely and effectively using the laparoscopic approach.

Trocar positions and number will vary depending on the surgical goal and the surgeon's preference. Laparoscopic splenectomy can be performed using as few as three strategically placed trocars, one for the telescope (usually placed in the umbilicus), and two for instrumentation. One or more additional trocars may facilitate retraction and dissection and can be placed at the surgeon's discretion (Fig. 61.2).

The patient's position is also a matter of preference and depends somewhat on the planned procedure.

For simple splenectomy, this author prefers to operate between the legs (the so-called "French Style") and aims the telescope and instruments toward the upper abdomen. The patient then is supine and in a reversed Trendelenburg position, perhaps with the table rotated to elevate the left side. This position allows for maximal access and permits the intestines to gravitate toward the pelvis and away from the left side so as to best visualize the spleen. This approach also allows easy access to the gallbladder for its removal when indicated. And, for surgeons who prefer to use a surgical robot, little has to change to accommodate the robot.

Other surgeons prefer to position the patient in a lateral position, or to start supine and move the patient after the initial trocars have been placed. This author has tried every position and found that approaching the upper abdomen as described above is the simplest and most reliable in his hands.

The steps to the operation are essentially as described earlier: We divide the short gastric vessels first as cephalad as is feasible without risking hemorrhage. We then divide the lateral attachments and carry this dissection cephalad and medial. We often leave a small attachment to the diaphragm intact so the spleen when freed will stay in place when trying to place it in a bag. We then divide the splenic vessels at the hilum. This can be done individually or en masse and can be done with an energy device, with sutures or with an endoscopic stapler, depending on the size of the patient and on the expertise of the surgeon (Fig. 61.3).

We then use an endoscopic pouch or bag inserted through one of the trocar sites to snare the freed spleen. If we have left a small peritoneal attachment to the diaphragm, we divide it after the spleen is in the pouch (Fig. 61.4). We then withdraw the open end of the pouch through the trocar site and fracture or morcellate the spleen so that it can be removed in segments without spilling its contents in the abdomen (Fig. 61.5). Depending on the surgeon's preference, this can be accomplished with a finger, a sponge forceps or other similar device. The important point is not to rupture the bag and spill its contents.

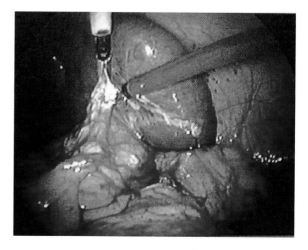

Fig. 61.3   Laparoscopic view of splenic hilar dissection

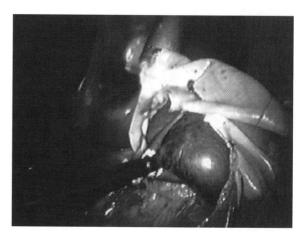

Fig. 61.4   Spleen in sac for laparoscopic extraction

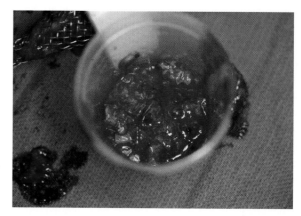

Fig. 61.5   Morcellated spleen

After the spleen is removed, the left upper abdomen is inspected for hemostasis. If the gallbladder is to be removed, we usually do this after the spleen has been removed successfully. Careful trocar placement can obviate the need to insert additional trocars for the cholecystectomy.

Some pediatric hematologists advocate partial splenectomy for certain conditions such as hereditary spherocytosis. This can be accomplished easily using conventional laparoscopic techniques. One aid to accomplishing this is to take a piece of umbilical tape, tie it around the diameter of the spleen that is to remain intact and to use this as a handle to grasp when manipulating the spleen. We then divide segmental vessels as they are encountered and after the segment to be removed is devascularized, we use an energy device such as a Ligasure (Tyco, USA) or similar device to hemostatically divide the parenchyma at the line of ischemia.

Splenic autotransplantation with a free-graft for maintenance of specific splenic immunity is still experimental and of unproven efficacy.

In the case of the wandering spleen, a peritoneal pocket can be created into which the spleen can be placed. Or, a pouch can be made from surgical mesh into which the spleen can be placed. The pouch is then sutured to the abdominal wall to keep the spleen from wandering.

The laparoscopic approach has also proved beneficial in the management of congenital and acquired splenic cysts. Splenic cysts may be a form of cystic hygroma within the splenic parenchyma or may be the result of a traumatic injury. These can be identified laparoscopically and their wall can be excised. Simple fenestration is possible but often results in recurrance.

Echinococcal or hydatid cysts are rare and also can be treated laparoscopically. Their diagnosis should be made preoperatively by laboratory and imaging characteristics that are diagnostic. Under laparoscopic view, these cysts can be aspirated and refilled with hypertonic saline.

All patients with hydatid disease should be considered for percutaneous or surgical treatment because of the risk of life-threatening complications of untreated disease. More complicated cysts are better managed by open surgery. Treatment of hydatid cysts is associated with two technical problems: risk of anaphylaxis from spillage of cyst fluid containing eggs and larvae into the peritoneal cavity and recurrence caused by residual eggs in incompletely removed germinal membranes. To prevent these problems, most surgeons use a technique in which the cyst contents are aspirated and replaced with a hypertonic saline solution to kill residual daughter cysts in the germinal membrane before unroofing and pericystectomy. The goal of the latter procedure is to excise the germinal membrane, leaving the inflammatory and fibrous components of the cyst wall *in situ*.

We no longer leave a nasogastric tube in children undergoing splenectomy unless we are worried about the integrity of the stomach where the short-gastric vessels were divided. Similarly, we do not leave a urinary bladder catheter in place after surgery.

Instead, we encourage patients to ambulate immediately and we advance their diet as tolerated from the immediate post-operative period (Fig. 61.6).

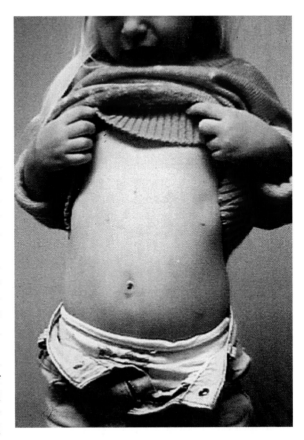

Fig. 61.6 Post-op appearance of abdomen

61.12 Complications and Adverse Effects

The risk of postsplenectomy infections depends on the etiology of the disease. The majority of infections occur within 2 years after splenectomy and are fatal in almost 50% of cases. The incidence is low in patients with spherocytosis, ITP and splenic trauma and higher in Hodgkin's disease (8%).

Splenoportal thrombosis following splenectomy is a rare complication. The true rate of thrombotic complications after splenectomy is not defined, but early diagnosis and prompt initiation of anticoagulant therapy is mandatory. Port site splenosis has been reported after laparoscopic splenectomy and has to be considered in the differential diagnosis of port site pain and a palpable nodule. Leaks along the pancreatic tail can also rarely occur after splenectomy.

Other post-operative complications of splenectomy depend somewhat on the procedure.

Wound complications may be seen after an open splenectomy, though the frequency of these appear to be independent of the procedure and are more closely related with surgical technique. Trocar site infection, hemorrhage and herniation can occur but these are rare and can be related more to trocar technique than to splenectomy.

Patients undergoing open procedures may be more prone to pulmonary complications, though we have seen one case of pneumonia after a laparoscopic splenectomy in a teenage girl with hematological disease who was poorly motivated to ambulate after surgery. In general, atelectasis and pneumonia are more closely correlated with open incisions.

Intraabdominal infections and left upper quadrant abscess is another potential complication, but we have not seen this in laparoscopic surgery. When this occurs, it is probably related to inadequately controlled hemorrhage in the surgical bed.

And finally, high grade injuries to the spleen are at risk for delayed presentation of splenic artery aneurysms. We recommend examination for abdominal bruit and follow-up abdominal ultrasounds in all high grade (III and IV), injuries.

In general, the laparoscopic approach tends to be associated with fewer adhesions and thus fewer postoperative bowl obstructions when compared to open procedures. This seems to hold true for laparoscopic splenectomy.

The results of laparoscopic splenectomy in children are excellent. We routinely use the da Vinci robotic system to remove the spleen from children. The result of this approach are equivalent to the more conventional laparoscopic technique.

Further Reading

Borzi P (2006) Splenectomy. In P Puri, ME Höllwarth (eds) Pediatric Surgery, Springer Surgery Atlas Series. Springer-Verlag, Berlin, Heidelberg, New York, pp 403–410

Hansen MB, Moller AC (2004) Splenic cysts. Surg Laparosc Endosc Percutan Tech 4:316–322

Kappers-Klunne MC, Wijermans P, Fijnheer R et al (2005) Splenectomy in the treatment of thrombotic thrombocytopenic purpura. Br J Haematol 130:768–776

Shatz DV (2005) Vaccination considerations in the asplenic patient. Expert Rev Vaccines. 4:27–34

Silecchia G, Paparelli L, Casella G, Basso N (2005) Laparoscopic splenectomy for non-traumatic diseases. Minerva Chir 60:363–374

Thompson SR, Holland AJ (2006) Evolution of non-operative management for blunt splenic trauma in children. J Paediatr Child Health 42:231–234

Paediatric Liver Transplantation

62

K. Sharif and A.J.W. Millar

Contents

62.1 Introduction

Liver transplantation is accepted as a life saving treatment for children with end stage liver disease. Until recently, treatment options for the debilitating effects of liver disease in children were limited to supportive therapy, anti-viral agents and immunosuppressive agents. With surgical conditions such as biliary atresia, some success has been achieved with timely diagnosis and early surgical intervention. However, in many cases even with expert management there was inevitable progression of liver disease. Liver transplantation offers the only chance of a cure for these unfortunate children. Although the first attempted human transplant was performed in 1963, it was not until 5 years later that long-term success was achieved. Advances in surgical technique, anaesthetic management, pre- and post-operative care and refinements in immunosuppression over the last 4 decades have resulted in a much improved outcome and wide acceptance of liver transplantation among paediatricians with an ever-increasing list of indications being identified.

The full story of liver transplantation for children is yet to be told but the current expected 5-year survival is now greater than 85% in major paediatric transplant centres. Excellent quality of life is the rule rather than the exception. The longest survivor is well more than 35 years after transplantation. Current anxieties are over organ donor scarcity, long-term side effects of the immunosuppressive therapy and some ethical issues. The focus of attention has now shifted from an initial target of early post-transplant survival to quality of life in the long-term. The transformation of a miserable jaundiced invalid into an active healthy child remains a powerful stimulant for paediatricians and transplant surgeons alike.

P. Puri and M. Höllwarth (eds.), *Pediatric Surgery: Diagnosis and Management,*
DOI: 10.1007/978-3-540-69560-8_62, © Springer-Verlag Berlin Heidelberg 2009

62.2 Indications

Liver disease has generally been underestimated as a cause of death in children. In general, liver transplantation should be considered as a therapeutic option in all cases of acute and chronic liver disease before the end stage liver disease is reached. The most common indications for paediatric liver transplantation are biliary atresia (43%), metabolic diseases (13%) and acute liver failure (11%) A list of conditions for which liver transplant has been performed is summarized in Table 62.1. For approximately 75% of children with acute hepatic failure, the cause is unknown. Among the worldwide accepted indications for liver transplantation, inherited metabolic disorders constitute a major portion. In some paediatric

Table 62.1 Indications for which liver transplantation has been performed in children

I Metabolic (inborn errors of metabolism).
   (a) Alpha-1 antitrypsin
   (b) Tyrosinaemia
   (c) Glycogen storage disease type III and IV
   (d) Wilson's disease
   (e) Neonatal haemochromatosis
   (f) Hypercholesterolaemia
   (g) Cystic fibrosis
   (h) Hyperoxaluria (+ renal transplant)
   (i) Haemophilia A + B
   (j) Protein C deficiency
   (k) Crigler-Najjar syndrome
II Acute and chronic hepatitis
   (a) Fulminant hepatic failure (viral, toxin or drug induced)
   (b) Chronic hepatitis (B, C, etc. toxin, autoimmune, idiopathic)
III Intrahepatic cholestasis:
   (a) Neonatal hepatitis
   (b) Alagille syndrome
   (c) Biliary hypoplasia
   (d) Familial cholestasis
IV Obstructive biliary tract disease
   (a) Biliary atresia
   (b) Choledochal cyst with cirrhosis
V Neoplasia
   (a) Hepatoblastoma
   (b) Hepatocellular carcinoma
   (c) Sarcoma
   (d) Haemangioendothelioma
VI Miscellaneous
   (a) Cryptogenic cirrhosis
   (b) Congenital hepatic fibrosis
   (c) Caroli's disease
   (d) Budd-Chiari syndrome
   (e) Cirrhosis from prolonged parenteral nutrition

centres this indication runs second after extrahepatic biliary atresia. The aim of liver transplantation in inherited metabolic disorders is twofold: the first is to save a patient's life by addressing the immediate consequences of the pathologic defect and the second is to accomplish phenotypic and functional cure of disease. In some metabolic diseases, the manifestations are widespread and affect other organs as well. Examples are heamochromatosis, tyrosinemia, Wilson's disease, glycogen storage diseases and hyperoxaluria. With experience, certain disorders have moved from the list of contraindications to acceptable indication. One such example is hepatic respiratory chain disorders, although it is essential to exclude extra-hepatic disease before transplantation.

In recent years the outcome of the operation is so improved that indications for early transplant would be evidence of impaired synthetic function, including prolonged prothrombin time, reduced serum cholesterol levels and low serum albumin. Clinical indicators include presence of ascites, bleeding from oesophageal varices not controlled by endoscopic banding or sclerotherapy and poor response to nutritional resuscitation. Those with acute hepatic failure who develop encephalopathy, hypoglycaemia, a prothrombin time of greater than 50 s and a Factor V level of less than 20% should be considered for transplant, as almost all of these children die without transplantation. Timing of liver transplantation not only affects survival rate, but may also influence neurodevelopmental outcome.

62.2.1 Contraindications

There are few reasons for refusal for transplantation. These include disorders as listed in Table 62.2. Until recently, hypoxemia (hepato-pulmonary syndrome) was considered as a relative contraindication for liver transplantation.

Table 62.2 Contra-indications

1. Absolute:
   Uncontrolled systemic infection
   Malignancy outside the liver
   Disease in other organs incompatible with quality survival
2. Relative:
   Cyanotic pulmonary arteriovenous shunting with pulmonary hypertension
   Hepatitis B, eAg positive, HIV positive
   Psychosocial factors
   Inadequate vascular supply

However it has been shown that liver transplantation can be successfully achieved in severely hypoxemic children and that postoperative correction of the right to left shunt is then obtained. HIV/AIDS as well as other major cardio-respiratory, neurological or renal disease, which would be incompatible with quality of life and long-term survival, are also considered as contraindications.

62.2.2 Assessment

Liver transplant assessment includes thorough evaluation of the child and family. This process allows detailed disease assessment and time for discussion of treatment options, to prepare for the transplant procedure and afterwards. This also provides opportunity to assess the family's commitment to sustain long-term compliance after transplantation and to put in place supportive strategies to ensure adherence to treatment regimens, which need to be lifelong. However, detailed assessment is not possible in children presenting with acute liver failure or those with acute deterioration of chronic liver disease. The pre-transplant assessment protocol from our center is summarized in Table 62.3.

(A) **Child assessment**: All children require initial confirmation of the diagnosis, intensive medical investigation and nutritional resuscitation to treat the complications of the liver disease, portal hypertension and nutritional deprivation. Disease assessment includes identification of contraindications.

Table 62.3 Pre-transplant assessment

Anthropometry:
- Height and Weight
- Head circumference—under 2 years of age (OFC)
- Mid-xyphisternal umbilical circumference (girth)
- Mid-arm circumference (MAC) & Triceps skin fold (TSF)

Routine Bloods:
- Blood group
- FBC
- PT,PTT, Fibrinogen
- AST, ALT, αGT, Alk. Phos, Cholesterol
- Total protein, Albumin
- Na, K, Urea, Creatinine, Calcium, Potassium, Magnesium Phosphate
- Vitamin A/E

N.B. Additional bloods may be required if Metabolic Liver Disease is suspected

Serology:
- EBV (IgG)
- CMV (IgG)
- Measles
- Varicella
- Hepatitis A (IgG)
- Hepatitis B (Hepatitis B sAg + Hep B core antibody – hepatitis B s antibody if previously vaccinated)
- Hepatitis C antibody
- HIV 1 and 2

Microbiology
- MRSA
- VRE – Pseudomonas—B cepacia screen if chronic patient or CF
- Blood C&S if indwelling catheter

Urine
- MC + S
- Protein/creatinine ratio
- Tubular re-absorption of phosphate

Assessment of severity of liver disease:
- Upper Gastrointestinal Endoscopy (if required)
- Liver biopsy (if indicated, otherwise obtain previous biopsy result)
- Paediatric hepatology scores (PHS and PELD)

Radiology:
- Chest X-ray
- Bone age for rickets or metabolic bone disease
- Abdominal ultrasound and Doppler study to evaluate diameter of portal vein and direction of flow, size of spleen, ascites, vascular anatomy, resistivity index if biliary atresia or reverse flow in portal vein
- MRI and/or angiography if vascular anatomy uncertain

Cardiology:
- ECG
- ECHO
- Cardiology opinion if needed
- Blood Pressure

Neurology:
- EEG
- Developmental Assessment

Renal Function:
- Chromium EDTA
- Calculated GFR (Schwartz index)
- Urine tubular phosphate re-absorption (TRP)
- Urine protein/creatinine ratio

Respiratory:
- Oxygen saturations (resting and on exercise)
- For children with cystic fibrosis:
- Pulmonary function tests
- Cough swab sputum for MC + S
- Lung perfusion study only if cyanosed

Immunisations:
Arrange pre-transplant immunisation as needed–Suspend from list for 2 weeks if live vaccine given.
- Check hand held record for routine DPT, polio, HIB, MenC and MMR
- Ensure live vaccines are given if time permits i.e. VZ, MMR (if over 6 months) plus advice on completing other vaccinations such as Prevenar®, Pneumovax II®, Hepatitis A and B, influenza.

(B) **Family assessment**: Transplant candidacy inevitably results in enormous emotional stress for parents while waiting for the appropriate donor. Family life may become disrupted especially for those who live afar. Compliance is more difficult to predict in children with acute hepatic failure, as time from presentation to decision to transplant is much shorter. Living related transplant includes extensive evaluation of the potential donors including both physical and psychological assessment.

62.3 Surgical Technique

(A) **Donor operation**: Age limits for suitable donors are being extended due to shortage of organs. Paediatric donors can be accepted from 1 month of age while livers procured from older children and even young adults can be transplanted into small children after ex-vivo reduction of the size of the graft. However, stable cadaver donors from patients with a short intensive care unit stay (less than 3 days), little requirement for inotropic support and normal or near normal liver function are preferred, with an expected < 5% incidence of impaired function after transplant. Liver biopsy is useful if steatosis is suspected. Viral screening of the donors is essential. This would include Hepatitis A, B & C, CMV, EBV and HIV screening. Core HBV antibody and HCV positive donors would only be considered in selected viral infected recipients.

Surgical techniques used for donor retrieval and recipient liver removal and engraftment have evolved over the last 30 years. The majority of donor livers are removed as part of a multi-organ procurement procedure, which would include various combinations of kidneys, liver, heart or heart and lungs, small bowel and pancreas. University of Wisconsin solution is widely used as the preservation solution of choice.

The two procurement techniques used are a careful dissection and excision technique or the so-called 'rapid' technique described by Starzl. A mid-line incision is made from the supra-sternal notch to the pubis and the sternum is opened. The abdominal part of the operation includes quick assessment of all the abdominal organs. Control of the aorta is achieved above the coeliac axis by incision of the right crus of the diaphragm. The inferior vena cava and aorta are identified, dissected and encircled with tapes below the renal vessels. After a careful search for any vascular abnormalities, the liver is mobilised by division of the left coronary ligament. An appropriate sized cannula is placed in the inferior mesenteric or superior mesenteric vein so that the tip lies at the junction with the splenic vein. A large bore cannula is placed in the aorta with the tip approximately opposite the renal arteries, the distal common iliac vessels are tied off and the donor is given a heparin (3 gm/kg). A large bore cannula may be placed in the inferior vena cava, which is connected to an away suction. Procurement commences with infusion of preservation solution through both the portal vein and aorta after cross clamping the aorta at the level of the diaphragm and incising the supra-hepatic vena cava within the pericardium. The porta hepatis is divided distal to the gastro duodenal artery, which is ligated and the portal vein is divided at the junction with the splenic vein. The proximal part of the superior mesenteric artery is defined and is dissected down to the aorta.

The liver is now removed with a patch of aorta including the base of the superior mesenteric and the celiac axis. The resected liver includes a cuff of diaphragm around the bare area along with the retrohepatic cava and part of the right adrenal gland, which is cut through. The infrahepatic inferior vena cava is divided above the renal veins. Once the organs have been removed, they are placed in a plastic bag and the liver is further perfused with 500 ml of preservation solution via the portal vein, hepatic artery and through the bile ducts. The liver then is placed in a further two plastic bags and packed in ice for transportation.

A major constraint has been the shortage of donor organs of appropriate size. The use of reduced size adult organs has partially alleviated this problem but the previous technique employed was limited to a donor to recipient body-weight disparity of not greater than 3:1. Innovative techniques have been described that allow safe transplantation with a donor to recipient weight ratio of greater than 15:1.using further of a left lateral segment graft to a monosegment, usually segment 3. Splitting the donor liver into two functioning units for two recipients is now routine in good donors.

(B) **The recipient operation**: The recipient operation commences with an upper abdominal transverse or curved subcostal laparotomy incision, which may be extended in the midline to the xiphoid process for extra exposure. The porta hepatis is dissected first and in children with biliary atresia, this requires the portoenterostomy to be taken down. The portal vein is dissected and isolated. The rest of the liver is carefully mobilised. This includes the gastrohepatic ligament, the falciform and triangular ligaments together with the right retroperitoneal reflexion. Mobilisation of the liver off the inferior vena cava which is frequently preserved to facilitate reduced size transplantation or piggy-back engraftment should be done and is assisted by carefully dividing the vena cava ligament and ligating the right adrenal vein. The suprahepatic and infrahepatic vena cava are dissected and encircled with tape. Haemostasis of the retroperitoneum must be ensured with a combination of suture ligation and cautery. If the recipient inferior vena cava is to be preserved, this is simply done by carefully incising the diseased liver clear of the cava and when the liver has been removed, individually suturing all small areas of leakage from divided direct caudate lobe hepatic veins. The IVC is prepared for the donor liver by dividing the bridges between the separate hepatic veins. This creates a wide orifice for the hepatic vein to cava anastomosis. The inferior vena cava should be incised distally for approximately 1–2 cm to make a triangular orifice for the 'piggy-back' graft. Engraftment should begin with the upper caval anastomosis, which is usually performed with continuous posterior sutures of polypropolene and interrupted anterior sutures if a conventional transplant is being done. Prior to completion of the anastomosis, the liver is flushed clear of potassium rich preservation solution via the portal vein with either normal saline or a colloid solution. The lower cava anastomosis is then performed if required being sure not to cause any stricture or kinking, a growth factor of about a third of the diameter of the vessel is usually sufficient to prevent this occurring. The recipient portal vein is usually used for the anastomosis and in reduced size transplants where the donor liver is of large diameter, the bifurcation of the recipient portal vein is opened to create a trumpeted end for anastomosis. If the portal vein is hypoplastic, then the anastomosis is done at the level of the confluence of the splenic vein after careful dissection under the head of the pancreas. Another technique is to place a graft of donor iliac vein onto this area first during the anhepatic phase. The portal vein anastomosis is carefully performed using continuous posterior and interrupted anterior sutures or the use of a generous growth factor. In reduced size grafts, plenty of portal vein length should be left to avoid having any tension on the vein, which may result in stretching thus compromising flow. The donor hepatic artery is flushed with heparin saline to remove air and blood clots and an anastomosis is done to the recipient common hepatic artery. End to end microvascular techniques are preferred while others have used donor

iliac artery vascular grafts to the infra-renal aorta or from the supra celiac aorta with success. The donor liver is usually revascularised with removal of the suprahepatic clamp followed by the infrahepatic clamp, portal vein and artery. After careful haemostasis of bleeding areas, either from the free edge of a reduced size liver or from any of the other major bleeding points, the operation is completed, by performing the biliary reconstruction. The bile duct is trimmed back such that good bleeding from the edges is obtained and the end is spatulated. In biliary atresia patients and those with a reduced size graft, a Roux-en-Y choledochojejunostomy is performed with fine absorbable sutures. Occasionally in paediatric cases, a duct-to-duct anastomosis may be performed with a whole liver graft in a recipient with a normal extrahepatic biliary system. Stents or T tubes are optional with some evidence of increased biliary complications associated with their use. The only real advantage is access to the biliary system during the postoperative period. Finally haemostasis is obtained and the wound closed with drainage to the suprahepatic and infrahepatic spaces. If there is any tension at sheath closure due to bowel oedema or graft size, it is wise to insert a temporary patch of gortex or other non-adherent material as a 'tight' abdominal closure is associated with an increased incidence of vascular thrombosis and graft dysfunction. It is usually possible to obtain skin closure over the patch without too much tension. The patch can be removed 5–10 days later (Fig. 62.1).

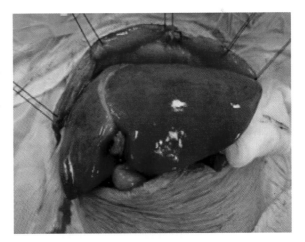

Fig. 62.1 This shows a reduced size liver (segments 2, 3 and part of 4) after transplantation before abdominal closure. In this case a silastic patch would be required to accommodate the large liver without any compression

62.4 Living Related Donors

Living related donation of the left lateral segment, first successfully performed by Strong, has become widely accepted as a method of acquiring a liver graft in the face of severe donor shortages, particularly in countries with cultural or religious reticence to accept brain death in a ventilated heart-beating donor. There are clear advantages in the planned nature of the procedure preferably before end stage liver disease in the recipient, the excellent quality of the graft and short ischaemic time. The use of a living donor also increases the availability of donor organs in general for other patients on the waiting list. The only advantage to the donor is a psychological one and there is a current morbidity of around 10% (wound sepsis, hernia, bile leak and adhesive bowel obstruction). There is also a reported mortality of around 0.2% although in Japan more than a 1,000 of these operations were done without donor mortality. There are ethical concerns, which appear justified, as with more widespread transplant activity increasing mortality and morbidity has been recorded. The donor should first undergo a thorough screening, both clinical and psychological without coercion and be given an option to withdraw from the procedure at any time before the transplant. It is important to recognize limitation of living related liver transplantation as the major source of organs for children. Parents usually approach living related liver transplantation with enthusiasm. They should be advised of the high chance of unsuitability, including the finding of significant pathology and complications, including death.

62.4.1 Split Liver Transplantation

The donor pool for children has been extended by the use of cut-down, split, living-related and, recently, non-heart-beating donor and isolated hepatocyte transplantation. In the split technique, the liver of the donor is divided into two functional units thus making maximum use of this very scarce resource. The procedure may be performed in-situ, which has been associated with less post-reperfusion bleeding from the cut surfaces and improved graft function. However, this technique is time-consuming and may not be feasible in many cases. Early results with ex-situ dissection on the back table were poor and this was in part due to a technical learning curve, prolonged preservation times and the use of grafts, for only those recipients in the worst condition. Recent results are much improved. Clearly the infrastructure must be in place to either perform two transplants simultaneously or alternatively one hemi-liver graft is exported to another centre. The in-situ technique is similar to a living related transplant. Cholangiography is essential as there is considerable variety in the intrahepatic biliary anatomy. Angiography is desirable but not essential. Some centres leave the hepatic artery with the right lobe making it more acceptable as an 'export'. The left lateral segment graft remaining is then used locally. Segment 4 should be used with the left graft if size is compatible; otherwise it is better to resect it prior to transplant as the segment 4 duct usually drains into the left hepatic duct. Likewise arterial anatomy is carefully examined and apportioned to each hemi-liver. There is usually a sufficient periductular vascular network to ensure adequate blood supply to the relevant duct systems so long as the main hepatic artery branch to each hemi-liver is preserved. Accessory arteries can be ligated if there is adequate 'back bleeding' after reperfusion.

62.5 Medical Management

62.5.1 Postoperative Care

Patients are monitored intensively postoperatively and usually require ventilation for a period of 24–48 h. Post-transplant protocol from our centre is summarised in Table 62.4.

1. Liver ultrasound with colour flow doppler is performed for the first 5 days and later as clinically indicated to confirm vascular patency and the absence of biliary dilatation.
2. Hypertension is almost universal in paediatric transplantation and can be initially managed with nifedipine sublingually in conjunction with diuretic agents. Subsequently calcium channel blockers may be given in appropriate dosage.
3. Aspirin 3 mg/kg given on alternate days is used as prophylaxis against arterial thrombosis and a proton pump inhibitor is given for gastric mucosal protection.
4. Nutritional and vitamin supplementation should

Table 62.4 Post-transplant management

Immediate management on arrival to ITU:
- Baseline measurements of FBC, U & E, Astrup, Ca, PT, PTT, chest X-ray, lactate.
- HB must be kept between 8 and 10 g/dl (or PCR < 0.35)
- Measurements of fluid, urine and drain output

Frequency of monitoring and investigations:
- **Hourly:**
  - BP, HR by ECG monitor, CVP, core/peripheral temperature difference, cutaneous oxygen saturation, fluid balance including colloid, wound drainage, urine output and drug volumes.
- **4 hourly for 24 h if required:**
  - Arterial blood gases, serum Na, K, Ca, blood glucose and lactate.
  - Gastric pH is recorded 6 hourly by nasogastric aspiration (aim to keep pH > 5).
- **Daily:**
  - Chest X-ray if indicated
  - FBC and clotting (PT, PTT)
  - Cyclosporin/Tacrolimus level
  - Urea, creatinine, calcium, phosphate, magnesium, total proteins, albumin, CRP
  - Full LFTs (bilirubin total & unconjugated, ALP, ALT, AST, GGT)

Culture: Wound swabs

Drain fluid

ETT aspirates if indicated

(i) Anti-microbials
1. Cefuroxime 25 mg/kg/dose tds for 48 h (max 750 mgs tds)
2. Amoxicillin 25 mg/kg/dose tds for 48 h (max 500 mgs tds)
3. Metronidazole 8 mg/kg/dose (maximum 500 mg) tds over 1 h (can give over 30 min) for 48 h
4. Cotrimoxazole: Up to 5 years 240 mgs od orally

Over 5 years 480 mgs od orally

Over 5 years 480 mgs od orally

(ii) Anti-virals

If the donor status for EBV and CMV is known, all transplanted children are to be started on antiviral prophylaxis.

If donor is EBV NEGATIVE

Recipient Status	Donor Status	Treatment
CMV –ve	CMV –ve Stop	Aciclovir
CMV +ve	CMV –ve	Stop Aciclovir
CMV +ve	CMV +ve	Continue Aciclovir
CMV –ve	CMV + ve	Continue Aciclovir

If donor is EBV POSITIVE

All to continue on aciclovir irrespective of recipient EBV/CMV status

(iii) Anti-fungals

Nystatin 100,000 units (= 1 ml) orally qds if > 10 kg

50,000 units (= 0.5 ml) orally qds if < 10 kg

Ambisome 3 mg/kg for 7–10 days

(iv) Gastric acidity prophylaxis

Ranitidine 3 mg/kg/dose (I/V) tds, if pH still < 5 use sucralfate PO/NGT 250–500 mg QDS and consider using

omeprazole 0.5 mg/kg/bd iv or orally.

(v) Immunosuppression

Standard immunosuppression (i.e. first graft, no renal failure) begins post-operatively.

(a) **Daclizumab (3 doses)** 1 mg/kg in 50 ml of sodium chloride 0.9% over 15 min (in fluid restriction or in smaller patients dilute to 1 mg/ml).

Intra-operatively, Day 4 post transplant and Day 18 post transplant

(b) **Tacrolimus (Prograf)**

First dose 0.2 mg/kg/dose orally given within 6 h of transplant.

Then 0.1 mg/kg/dose bd orally to maintain levels of 10–15 nanogram/ml in first 2 weeks.

Subsequently adjust dosage to achieve:

7–11 ng/ml in 3rd/4th weeks

4–7 ng/ml in 2nd/3rd month

2–4 ng/ml thereafter

(c) **Steroids**

From Day 0: **Hydrocortisone IV OD (First dose to be given as child reaches ITU):**

Weight kg	Dose
<20	50 mg bd
>20	100 mg bd

When oral diet is tolerated please commence oral steroids (maximum daily dose 40 mg):

(vi) Anti—platelet treatment

(a) **Aspirin (if platelet > 75,000)** 3 mg/kg/day OD orally/NGT

(maximum dose 75 mg)

(b) **Dipyridamole (if platelets > 50,000)**

If patient weighs < 10 kg 25 mg tds orally, if weighs > 10 kg 50 mg tds orally

(vii) Heparin infusion

For vascular anastomosis at risk (complex vascular reconstruction or small diameter arteries or portal vein)

(viii) Analgesia and sedation

Analgesia is achieved with morphine in the routine transplant patient with reasonable graft function and is titrated against pain level

be commenced within 72 h of surgery and may be supplemented by nasogastric feeding or parenteral nutrition in the early phase if there is a delay in restoration of bowel function. Phosphate and magnesium deficiency is common and requires replacement therapy in nearly all patients.

62.5.2 Immunosuppression

There is considerable variation in the selection of immunosuppressive agents. Most protocols currently employ triple therapy with Tacrolimus, methylprednisolone and a monoclonal interleukin-2 inhibitor (CD 25) antibody. Some centres use steroid free immunosuppression. In addition, there are a number of other strategies in place to reduce the amount of nephrotoxicity, which is a toxic side effect to both calcineurin inhibitors. Thus, mycophenolate mofetil, an inosine monophosphate dehydrogenase inhibitor may be used instead from early on in what is called "nephron sparing immunosuppression". Rapamycin, a drug structurally similar to tacrolimus, which prevents proliferation of T cells but acts at a different stage of T cell activation than either cyclosporin or tacrolimus, has the advantage that it is not nephrotoxic and does not interfere with transcription and production of interleukin 2, rather it antagonises the action of interleukin 2 on its receptor. It has no adverse effects on liver function and may be synergistic with cyclosporin.

The methylprednisolone dosage is reduced over the 1st week to about 1 mg/kg/day for the first month and then reduced to a level of 0.3 mg/kg/day to 0.2 mg/kg as maintenance. This can be later reduced in some patients to alternate day therapy or even withdrawn completely. Both mycophenolate mofetil and rapamycin can be used as renal sparing should nephrotoxicity become evident. Use of humanised anti-CD25 monoclonal antibodies given before and during the 1st week of the transplant have reduced the incidence of acute rejection in the first 3 months by around 30% but long term graft survival is essentially the same as when these agents have not been used. The other polyclonal anti-lymphocyte immunoglobulins are rarely used.

62.5.3 Anti-Infection Agents

Immunosuppression naturally leads to susceptibility to bacterial, fungal and viral infections. Fungal infection (FI) is a major and potentially fatal complication in liver transplantation (LT). Fungal prophylaxis is given before the transplant as mycostatin orally to reduce Candida colonisation of the gut and after transplant as amphotericin and continued for a period of several months. From two to 3 weeks after the transplant, for at least the 1st year, trimethoprim-sulphamethoxazole is given at a dose of 6 mg/kg/day in two divided doses 3 days a week for prevention of pneumocystis carinii infection. Intravenous ganciclovir 5 mg/kg/dose 12 hourly is used as prophylaxis against cytomegalovirus (CMV) and Epstein Barr virus (EBV) infection, initially for 2 weeks and this may be extended for up to 3 months in high risk patients who have not previously been exposed to CMV or EBV but have received a donor graft with previous exposure. This considerably reduces the incidence of both cytomegalovirus disease and post transplantation lymphoproliferative disorder. Either hyper-immune cytomegalovirus globulin or immunoglobulin is also given to assist viral prophylaxis. Leucocyte filtered blood products are used throughout to reduce CMV load. Prophylactic antibiotics are given with induction of anaesthesia and continued for 3–5 days. These are changed according to cultures taken of blood, secretions, sputum and urine. Anti-tuberculosis prophylaxis is given only if the reason for transplant is a reaction to anti-tuberculosis drugs with fulminant hepatic failure, where evidence of tuberculosis is found before surgery and if a close family contact has tuberculosis. Ofloxacin, rifampicin and ethambutol or ethionamide may be used in addition to isoniacid but very careful monitoring of liver function tests is required because all of these drugs may be hepatotoxic and particularly rifampicin may result in a decrease in cyclosporin or tacrolimus levels due to enzyme P450 induction with increased drug metabolism.

62.6 Surgical Complications

Surgical complications may be reduced to an absolute minimum with meticulous technique. These may present early and late as summarised in Table 62.5. Most common surgical complications are as follows.

(A) **Biliary complications** continue to be a significant problem with an overall incidence of between 10–20%, particularly in living related left lateral segment grafts. These complications include bile leak, anastomotic strictures, and non-anastomotic strictures of the donor bile duct with sludge formation. Most biliary complications (72%) occur

Table 62.5 Summary of common postoperative problems

1. **Biliary tract**
   (a) Stenosis or stricture
   (b) Anastomotic leak—often associated with hepatic artery thrombosis
   (c) Infection
2. **Rejection**
   (a) Acute
   (b) Chronic (vanishing bile duct syndrome)
3. **Infection**—bacterial, viral, (CMV, EBV, Herpes Zoster, hepatitis B). fungal (Candida, Aspergillus), parasitic (pneumocystis)
   (a) Abdominal (peri or intra-hepatic abscess)
   (b) Biliary tree
   (c) Pulmonary
   (d) Re-activated virus
   (e) Gastro-intestinal tract
   (f) Catheter associated (intravenous, urinary tract)
4. **Graft vascular injury (thrombosis, stenosis)**
   (a) Hepatic artery
   (b) Portal vein
   (c) Inferior vena cava (supra and infrahepatic)
   (d) Hepatic vein (left lateral segment grafts), Budd-Chiari recurrence
5. **Renal dysfunction**
   (a) Tacrolimus/Cyclosporin or other drug induced injury
   (b) Tubular necrosis due to hypoperfusion
   (c) Pre-existing disease (hepato-renal syndrome)
   (d) Hypertension
6. **Miscellaneous**
   (a) Encephalopathy (cyclosporin, tacrolimus, hypertensive, metabolic)
   (b) Bowel perforation (steroid, diathermy)
   (c) Diaphragm paresis/paralysis
   (d) Gastrointestinal haemorrhage (peptic ulceration, variceal)
   (e) Obesity (steroids)
   (f) Other drug side effects

in the first 2 weeks following transplantation. Ultrasound and cholangiography are the principle imaging modalities used for detection of these complications. Ultrasound is important in the post-operative surveillance of paediatric liver transplants, with cholangiography having a complementary role. It is imperative with all suspected biliary complications to ensure that the hepatic artery is patent using doppler ultrasound or angiography as hepatic artery thrombosis will cause ischaemia and necrosis of the biliary tree. Simple bile leaks are diagnosed in the early postoperative period by the presence of bile in drainage fluid or in per-cutaneous aspirate of fluid collections around the liver. Early biliary complications are best treated by immediate surgery and re-anastomosis if required. Late stricture formation may be satisfactorily dealt with by endoscopic or percutaneous balloon dilatation or stenting.

(B) **Graft ischaemia** either from hepatic artery thrombosis or portal vein thrombosis can be a devastating complication. Hepatic artery thrombosis (HAT) represents a significant cause of graft loss and mortality after pediatric orthotopic liver transplantation (OLT). The reported incidence of this complication is 7.8%. The incidence is much less frequent with the use of reduced size liver transplants and microsurgical techniques for living donor transplants. Most centres recommend routine Doppler ultrasound in the early post-operative period ranging from 3–7 days to confirm the patency of these vessels. Consequences of vascular thrombosis are graft necrosis, intrahepatic abscess, biliary necrosis and bile leakage. A massive rise in enzyme activity, particularly in the first few days after transplant, may be the first signs. Immediate intervention with thrombectomy and re-anastomosis may be successful if the diagnosis and treatment is carried out as soon as the complication is diagnosed. If thrombectomy fails, urgent re-transplant is required. Late thrombosis may be asymptomatic and if so can be ignored. Although technical factors usually account for most cases, it is advisable to maintain the haematocrit at around 30 to improve microvascular flow and most centres use aspirin and dipyrimidole as long term prophylaxis.

(C) **Portal vein thrombosis** usually presents with a degree of liver dysfunction with prolonged clotting and portal hypertension, which may be heralded by an oesophageal varicoele bleed. Immediate thrombectomy may be successful. Where graft thrombosis is established, a meso-portal (Rex) shunt, with a vein graft taken from the internal jugular vein of the patient or donor veins from vascular bank (if available) and interposed between the superior mesenteric vein and the left branch of the portal vein, may be curative. Significant risk factors for portal vein thrombosis are young age and weight at the time of LT, small portal vein, and emergency LT. Overall risk of portal vein thrombosis (PVT) is 2.2% in teams using aspirin with or without dipyridamole compared with 7.8% when no antiaggregative agents are given.

(D) **Bowel perforation** is a well-recognized complication following orthotopic liver transplantation (6.7%). Contributory factors include previous operation, steroid therapy and viral infection. The incidence is higher in children who underwent transplantation for biliary atresia after a previous Kasai portoenterostomy. Diagnosis may be difficult and a high index of suspicion is needed.

(E) **Post-operative fluid collections** arising from the cut surface of the liver has the reported incidence of 39% and 44% of which nearly 50% required intervention. These collections can be due to biliary anastomosis leaks or bowel perforation however the overall incidence of fluid collections are not increased by the use of reduced-size liver transplants. Late presentations may be less acute and typically present with gram-negative sepsis, liver abscess or biliary complications.

(F) **Inferior vena cava thrombosis** is now rare Thrombosis in the IVC may develop either in the immediate postoperative period presenting with ascites and lower body oedema or later on due to regeneration of the graft and twisting of the caval anastomosis. Thrombolytic therapy may be successful in late thromboses but should be avoided in early thromboses as uncontrollable bleeding may occur from raw surfaces particularly if a reduced/split liver was transplanted.

(G) **Hepatic venous outflow obstruction** is a more frequent complication. This can be due to redundancy of hepatic vein (when the graft hepatic vein is kept long) in reconstruction of a partial graft. The correction of the redundancy is made by pulling the graft caudally and to the left or right side of the abdominal cavity as determined by Doppler ultrasonography. It can also be suspected if there is persistence of ascites in the early post transplant period. This is usually confirmed either by angiography or by liver biopsy findings of congestion and red cell extravasation around central veins.

(H) **Diaphragmatic paresis and hernia** are rare complications of liver transplantation. The possible role of several contributing factors include cross clamping of the IVC at the level of the diaphragmatic hiatus, trauma at operation (dissection and diathermy) and diaphragm thinness related to low weight and malnutrition.

62.7 Late Medical Complications

Most patients can be discharged from the intensive care unit within the 1st week after transplantation. Complications of transplantation include bacterial, viral, fungal and opportunistic infections, renal function impairment, hypertension, rejection and particular concern is the post-transplant lymphoproliferative syndrome.

(A) **Infections:** The reported incidence of infection in the liver transplant population is 1.36 infection/patient. The most common sites of infection are bloodstream (36.5%) and abdomen (30%). Gram-positive bacteria (78%) predominated over gram-negative bacteria (22%). Detailed analysis of risk factors shows that age < 1 year, body weight < 10 kg, extrahepatic biliary atresia, intraoperative transfusion > 160 ml × kg(−1), mechanical ventilation > 8 days and PICU stay > 19 days are associated with higher risk of infection.

(B) **Acute rejection:** Despite the availability of potent immunosuppressive drugs, rejection after organ transplantation in children remains a serious concern, and may lead to significant morbidity, graft loss, and death of the patient. Diagnosis of rejection can be made on the basis of clinical, biochemical and histologic changes and usually presents in the first few weeks after transplant with fever, malaise, a tender graft and loose stools. Diagnosis is confirmed by liver biopsies performed using the Menghini technique (Hypafix needle (Braun), diameter 1.4 mm), unless biliary dilatation is observed on ultrasonography. Biopsies are also routinely assayed for viral and bacterial activity. The grade of rejection is assessed according to established histological criteria on a scale of 0–4. Some centres are trying to evaluate non-invasive tools to diagnose acute rejection such as radiologic findings on post-transplant Doppler ultrasound. Others are using Interleukin 5 (IL-5), it is produced in the liver and is a T cell-derived cytokine that acts as a potent and specific eosinophil differentiation factor in humans. During liver allograft rejection, intragraft IL-5 mRNA and eosinophilia have been observed. It may be a useful as a specific marker of allograft rejection. However once diagnosed acute rejection is treated with three doses of methyl prednisolone 10 mg/kg on successive days with adjusted baseline immunosuppression. Some patients experience corticosteroid resistant acute rejection, the management of which is not standardized. Various agents used include the addition of mycophenolate mofetil or sirolimus. The use of antithymocyte globulins (ATG) or monoclonal anti-CD3 antibodies, muromonab CD3 (OKT3) is hampered by numerous adverse effects, including a significant risk of over-immunosuppression. These therapies are nowadays indicated in only few selected cases. Other treatments such as plasmapheresis and high dose immunoglobulins may be useful in difficult cases. In patients with refractory rejection despite therapeutic escalation, the risks of over-immunosuppression, including opportunistic infections and malignancies (especially the Epstein-Barr virus related post-transplant lymphoproliferative disease) have to be balanced with the consequences of graft loss due to rejection.

(C) **Late acute cellular rejection**: Although acute rejection is mostly encountered during the first 3 months after liver transplant, it may occur later on. Late cellular rejection in children is usually due to low or decreased immunosuppression and is associated with long-term complications. Prompt intervention to correct inadequate immunosuppression and careful follow-up to identify other treatable conditions is essential.

(D) **Chronic rejection** is an irreversible phenomenon which is chiefly intrahepatic and ductular rather than a vascular phenomenon in contrast to other organ transplants. This is usually manifested by disruption of bile duct radicals with development of the vanishing bile duct syndrome. The incidence seems less frequent with tacrolimus based immunosuppressive regimens as opposed to cyclosporin where an incidence of up to 10% has been recorded. Late chronic rejection may also be associated with a vasculopathy affecting larger arteries.

(E) **Chronic graft hepatitis** occurs in 20–30% children after liver transplantation but the prevalence and causes are not known. Serum liver associated autoantibodies are often positive. It is most frequently seen in children transplanted for cryptogenic cirrhosis (71%). However neither hepatitis C nor hepatitis G infection was associated. Management is with re-introduction or increase in steroid dose.

(F) **Cytomegalovirus (CMV) infection**: Cytomegalovirus (CMV) infection (seroconversion or virus isolation) and CMV disease (infection plus clinical signs and symptoms) have a reported incidence of 37% and 11.5% respectively with significant morbidity and mortality. The high prevalence of CMV infections supports the view that clinical signs alone are inadequate to direct investigations for CMV. Cytomegalovirus (CMV) infection is best monitored with PP65 antigen and polymerase chain reaction (PCR) measurement of the virus. Ganciclovir remains an important therapeutic option for the prevention and treatment of CMV disease in transplant recipients. Prophylactic treatment with ganciclovir appears the best strategy to implement in high risk patients. A rare association with cytomegalovirus (CMV) reactivation is Haemophagocytic syndrome (HPS). It is a rare event, which is often fatal. These patients are treated with a combination of antiviral agents, immunomodulatory and supportive therapy.

(G) **Epstein-Barr virus (EBV) and post-transplant lymphoproliferative disease (PTLD)**. EBV infection is the main cause of PTLD. Since many infants are EBV seronegative at the time of transplantation, PTLD is a major concern for these patients. Post transplantation lymphoproliferative disorder (PTLPD) presents from the first few weeks after transplant to several years later with a mean time of onset around 9 months. First manifestations of PTLD are adenoidal and/or tonsillar involvement. A typical presentation is usually with acute membranous tonsillitis and associated cervical lymphadenopathy, which is resistant to antibiotic therapy. It is important to remember that tonsillar enlargement in paediatric liver transplant patients does not necessarily imply a diagnosis of PTLD. Furthermore, the presence of increased numbers of EBV infected cells in tonsils from liver transplant recipients by itself does not indicate an increased risk of developing PTLD. However, the disease may be widespread and gastrointestinal and central nervous system involvement is common. Currently there are no tests to accurately identify paediatric liver transplant patients at risk for post-transplant lymphoproliferative disorder (PTLD). Attempts have been made to use cytokine polymorphisms and real-time quantitative polymerase chain reaction (qPCR) Epstein-Barr virus (EBV) viral load to identify patients at risk for PTLD development. Use of cytokine genotyping in conjunction with qPCR for EBV viral load can significantly improve the predictive value of diagnostic tests for identification of patients at high risk for

PTLD. Management strategies include reduction of immunosuppression, which may require complete withdrawal along with standard anti-lymphoma chemotherapy, particularly with the monoclonal type. Mortality varies from 20% to 70% or more. Prophylactic intravenous ganciclovir given for a prolonged period may be effective in preventing EBV activation which is the promoter of PTLD in most cases. Rituximab, an anti-CD 20 monoclonal antibody has been used with good effect. As B cells are largely ablated, replacement immunoglobulin therapy is required until B cell recovery has occurred.

(H) **Renal impairment**: A degree of renal impairment is almost inevitable in those patients suffering from chronic liver disease and with the additional burden of the use of nephrotoxic immunosuppressive drugs such as cyclosporin and tacrolimus with other neprotoxic antibiotics and antifungal agents may result in significant renal impairment of function in the long term. The importance of renal sparing strategies in immunosuppression is becoming increasingly evident as long-term survivors present with drug induced renal failure.

62.7.1 Re-Transplantation

Ten percent to 15% of patients may suffer graft failure at some time and need re-transplantation. Early indications may be primary non-function, early hepatic arterial thrombosis, severe drug resistant acute rejection and established chronic rejection. Early re-transplantation is technically a much less traumatic procedure than the original transplant, although the patient may be in a poorer condition. Outcome largely depends on the indication for re-transplantation and is quite good for technical causes but less satisfactory for rejection and infection. An increasingly poorer outcome can be expected after third and fourth re-transplants and the efficacy and ethics of these interventions are in question.

62.7.2 Longterm Survival and Quality of Life

One year survival of > 95% is being achieved in the best centres with predicted 10 year survivals of around 80–85%. Patients grafted for acute liver failure have done less well with a higher early death rate usually associated with cerebral complications and multi-organ failure. Excellent quality of life can be achieved and most children are fully rehabilitated. It is however increasingly evident that prolonged cholestatic jaundice and malnutrition in infancy may have late effects and despite good physical rehabilitation evidence of significant cognitive deficits, which present during early schooling as learning difficulties and attention deficit disorder, are common. Quality of life may not reach perfection, and depends also on the way society accepts these imperfections. As with any immunosuppressed patient, the incidence of neoplasia in a lifetime is greatly increased.

62.8 Conclusion

Careful planning, extensive preparation of personnel and a broad base of skills along with good teamwork between health professionals are required for the development of a successful paediatric transplant programme. Surgical technique, anaesthetic skills, and medical care of the highest order are essential. A patient with a liver transplant is a patient for life and requires complete commitment from the transplant medical and surgical team, which cannot be abrogated after discharge from hospital. Endemic viral and bacterial infections particularly HBV, CMV, EBV and PTLD, impact negatively on any programme. Extended hospital stay may be required and this, along with long-term therapy may be extremely expensive.

The need for paediatric liver transplants has been assessed at approximately 1–2 children per million per year. Thus transplant activity should be concentrated in specific centres preferably doing more than 12 transplants a year. The shortage of donor organs will continue and future efforts must be focused on maximum use of cadaver donors and increasing living related donation. Transplant activity is rapidly increasing throughout the developing world. This endeavour should be strongly supported as poor socio-economic status is not a contraindication to transplantation and we have frequently been impressed by how parents with relatively few material resources have been able to diligently care for their children. No child with end stage liver disease should be denied the opportunity of receiving appropriate treatment. As with any new development, knowledge and experience improve, costs decline and success is ensured. These challenges must be met to offer any infant or child requiring liver replacement a chance of a life. The ultimate aim is to restore the child to normal health such that he/she can grow up into a productive healthy adult who can make his/her contribution to society and develop all of his/her human potential.

Further Reading

Baker A, Dhawan A, Heaton N (1998) Who needs a liver transplant? (new disease specific indications). Arch Dis Child 79(5):460–464

Cox KL, Berquist WE, Castillo RO (1999) Paediatric liver transplantation: indications, timing and medical complications. J Gastroenterol Hepatol 14(Suppl):S61–S66

de Ville de Goyet, J et al (1995) Standardized quick en bloc technique for procurement of cadaveric liver grafts for pediatric liver transplantation. Transpl Int 8(4):280–285

Muiesan P, Vergani D, Mieli-Vergani G (2007) Liver transplantation in children. J Hepatol 46(2):340–348

Otte JB (2004) Paediatric liver transplantation–a review based on 20 years of personal experience. Transpl Int 17(10):562–573

Otte JB (2002) History of pediatric liver transplantation. Where are we coming from? Where do we stand? Pediatr Transpl 6(5):378–387

Puri P, Höllwarth M (2006) Pediatric Surgery. Springer, Berlin, Heidelberg

Shepherd RW (1998) The treatment of end-stage liver disease in childhood. Aust Paediatr J 24(4):213–216

Shneider BL (2002) Pediatric liver transplantation in metabolic disease: clinical decision making. Pediatr Transplant 6(1):25–29

Vilca-Melendez H, Heaton ND (2004) Paediatric liver transplantation: the surgical view. Postgrad Med J 80(948):571–576

Omphalocele and Gastroschisis

63

Duane S. Duke and Marshall Z. Schwartz

Contents

63.1 Introduction

Gastroschisis and omphalocele represent two distinct congenital abnormalities of the anterior abdominal wall. Dudrick's development of total parenteral nutrition in the late 1960s and Schuster's successful application of an extra-abdominal housing (silo) for eviscerated bowel in 1967, provided surgeons with much needed tools to enhance the treatment for and improve the survival of infants with gastroschisis and omphalocele. Advancements in prenatal ultrasonography, neonatal monitoring and ventilator management continue to improve outcomes for critically ill infants with abdominal wall defects.

63.2 Types of Anterior Abdominal Wall Defects

Congenital abdominal wall defects include gastroschisis, omphalocele, hernia of the umbilical cord, cloacal exstrophy (infraumbilical omphalocele, exstrophy of the bladder, imperforate anus), and Cantrell's Pentalogy (supraumbilical omphalocele, sternal cleft, intracardiac anomaly, diaphragmatic hernia, and pericardial defect). This chapter will specifically address gastroschisis and omphalocele (Table 63.1).

63.3 Gastroschisis

Gastroschisis (Gr. *gaster*-, belly + -schisis, fissure) is a congenital defect of the anterior abdominal wall most often to the right of the umbilicus. The abdominal wall

Table 63.1   Clinical features: Gastroschisis and omphalocele contrasted

	Gastroschisis	Omphalocele
Location	To the right of intact Umbilical cord	Umbilical ring
Defect size	Small: 2–4 cm	Large: 2–10 cm
Covering sac	Absent	Present
Intestinal rotation	Nonrotation	Nonrotation
GI motility	Adynamic ileus	Normal
Associated anomalies	Intestinal atresia (10–15%)	Common and often major
Associated syndromes	None	Beckwith-Wiedemann
		Trisomy 13–15, 16–18, 21
		Lower Midline Syndrome
		Cantrell's Pentalogy
Survival	90%	30–70% largely dependent on associated anomalies

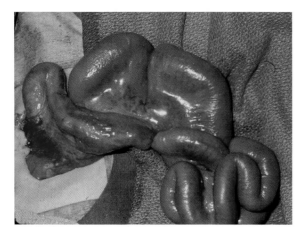

Fig. 63.1   Gastroschisis defect with eviscerated bowel

defect ranges in size from 2–4 cm: notably smaller than the defect encountered with omphalocele. All patients with gastroschisis have intestinal nonrotation. The stomach, small and large intestines and occasionally the gonads can be found outside of the abdominal wall (Figs. 63.1 and 63.2). The liver is almost never eviscerated. There is no peritoneal sac over the herniated contents. Therefore, the bowel is subjected to amniotic fluid (pH 7.0), which later in pregnancy becomes irritating and results in a thick fibrotic inflammatory peel over the eviscerated bowel. Another proposed cause of the thickened, inflamed bowel is the constriction of the abdominal wall defect late in gestation leading to venous congestion. Although the etiology is unclear, patients with gastroschisis sustain intrauterine growth retardation. The typical birth weight for these infants is between 2,000–2,500 g. Associated anomalies are uncommon; intestinal atresia can complicate gastroschisis in 10–15% of cases. With modern neonatal intensive care, nutritional supplementation, and appropriate surgical care, overall survival is excellent and surpasses 90%.

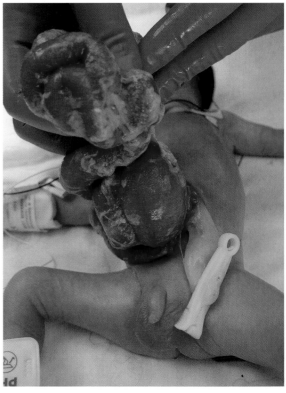

Fig. 63.2   The eviscerated bowel typically shows evidence of a fibrin "peel", bowel wall thickening, bowel dilatation, and mesenteric foreshortening

63.3.1   Etiology and Incidence

The abdominal wall forms from infolding of the cranial, caudal, and two lateral embryonic folds. The rapid growth of the intestine at this time causes it to migrate external to the forming abdominal wall. By the 10–12th gestational week the abdominal wall is well formed and the intestinal tract has returned to its intraperitoneal location with normal rotation and fixation.

The etiology of gastroschisis has not been fully elicited. One hypothesis suggests that the abdominal wall defect results from an ischemic event during the formation of the abdominal wall. The right paraumbilical area is vulnerable because it is supplied by the right umbilical vein and right omphalomesenteric artery until they involute. If their development and/or involution is disturbed it can result in the right paraumbilical abdominal wall having its blood supply interrupted and lead to an abdominal wall defect. An alternative hypothesis suggests that gastroschisis results from an intrauterine rupture of an omphalocele with subsequent resorption of the omphalocele sac. This hypothesis is less likely because of the other clear differences between these two abdominal wall defects such as the marked increase in associated anomalies in infants with omphalocele.

The incidence of gastroschisis worldwide is increasing. Presently, gastroschisis occurs in roughly 0.4–3 per 10,000 live births. Gastroschisis is commonly seen in young mothers with 25% of cases involving teenage mothers. Maternal exposure to cigarette smoking, illicit drugs, vasoactive over the counter drugs (pseudoephedrine, aspirin, acetaminophen), and environmental toxins have been linked to gastroschisis.

63.3.2 Associated Anomalies

Associated anomalies are uncommon with gastroschisis. Intestinal atresia/stenosis is present in 10–15% of cases. The areas of atresia/stenosis are attributed to intrauterine volvulus, intussusception, or secondary to the bowel's blood supply being impeded by a narrow abdominal wall defect. Bowel perforation occurs in 5% of patients. Other less common anomalies include: undescended testes, hypoplastic gallbladder, hydronephrosis, Meckel's diverticulum, and intestinal duplications. The incidence of chromosomal abnormalities is not higher than the normal population.

63.3.3 Prenatal Diagnosis

Abdominal wall defects can be detected with abdominal ultrasonography as early as the 10–12th week of gestation. This modality is limited by the timing and objective of the ultrasonography, fetal position, and the experience of the sonographer. Ultrasound diagnosis has a specificity of 95% and a sensitivity of 60–75% for identifying abdominal wall defects. The prenatal differential diagnosis based on ultrasound includes bladder exstrophy, cystic cord lesion, urachal cysts, as well as omphalocele and gastroschisis. Ultrasonography cannot reliably detect whether gastroschisis is complicated by areas of intestinal atresia. However, serial ultrasonography especially in the third trimester can detect increasing bowel diameter and thickening suggestive of vascular obstruction. These findings have been used as an indication for urgent delivery to avoid midgut infarction, a devastating complication in gastroschisis patients.

Maternal serum levels of alpha fetoprotein (AFP) can be elevated up to nine times the mean in gastroschisis. Elevation of AFP is less dramatic in omphalocele and is only 3–4 times the mean.

When diagnosed prenatally, gastroschisis patients should be referred to a high-risk obstetric unit with neonatal intensive care and pediatric surgery capability. Serial ultrasonography should be performed looking for changes in the size and thickness of the bowel as well as the diameter of the abdominal wall defect. Significant bowel wall thickening and bowel dilatation accompanied by a decrease in defect diameter may be indications for earlier delivery to avoid bowel infarction. When compared to normal vaginal delivery, preterm elective delivery, and term cesarean section delivery have not been shown to improve outcomes. Vaginal delivery is an acceptable birth route for gastroschisis patients. The benefit of preterm fetal amniotic fluid exchange is currently under investigation.

63.3.4 Perinatal Care

As a result of the absence of a hernia sac and exposure of the eviscerated contents to fluid and evaporative heat loss, infants with gastroschisis will have profound fluid and temperature regulation difficulties upon delivery. After addressing any airway, breathing or circulation issues, immediate placement of the lower half of the infant into a sterile bowel bag will ameliorate the fluid and heat losses. The bowel bag should extend from the axilla to the feet and must include the herniated viscera. A nasogastric tube should be placed to facilitate decompression of the gastrointestinal tract.

Empiric parenteral antibiotics with broad spectrum coverage are administered. Ampicillin 100 mg/kg/day and gentamicin 7.5 mg/kg/day in combination are commonly used. Maintenance of normothermia is critical to facilitate an optimum outcome.

Fluid resuscitation should be guided by hemodynamic status, urine output, tissue perfusion, and correction of metabolic acidosis (if present). An initial fluid bolus of 20 ml/kg with 10% dextrose in lactated Ringer's solution should be administered followed with 125–150% maintenance intravenous fluid.

Once adequate urine output is obtained and any acidosis corrected, the newborn can undergo either primary closure of the abdominal defect or temporary silo placement as described below.

63.3.5 Operative Management

Primary closure should be attempted whenever feasible. The abdominal wall defect can be enlarged 1–2 cm cephalad to facilitate reduction. Caudal extension of the abdominal wall defect is not recommended due to the risk of injuring the bladder. Peak inspiratory pressures greater than 25 mmHg, increases in central venous pressure of 4 mmHg or more, and elevated bladder pressures greater than 20 mmHg upon fascial apposition should steer the surgeon away from performing primary closure. The consequences of creating an abdominal compartment syndrome with an ambitious primary closure maybe catastrophic and there should be a low threshold to convert to silo placement with delayed closure.

The temptation to debride the fibrotic membranous peel or to search for areas of intestinal atresia should be avoided. These maneuvers only serve to prolong the procedure and further the likelihood of iatrogenic bowel injury. Additionally, some pediatric surgeons have employed abdominal wall stretching and efforts to manually decompress the luminal contents from the thickened, dilated intestine in an effort to accomplish primary closure. It is the view of the authors that these maneuvers are not safe and the risks outweigh the benefits.

The abdominal silo can be constructed from rectangular shaped Dacron reinforced Silastic sheeting. The silastic pieces are attached to each side of the abdominal wall fascia with interrupted mattress suture of 3.0 or 2.0 silk (Figs. 63.3a and b. The top can be narrowed at each side thus creating a trapezoid with a wide base. This modification will protect the bowel from potential strangulation from a narrow silo base during reduction. The apex of the silo is usually closed with a running monofilament suture but other techniques have been employed (Fig. 63.4). The goal is to progressively reduce the eviscerated bowel over no more than 5–7 days. Daily reductions of the silo is usually possible until it is flush with the abdominal wall.

A pre-formed spring loaded silo is also available for use (Figs. 63.5–63.7). This device has been successful

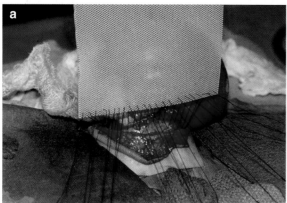
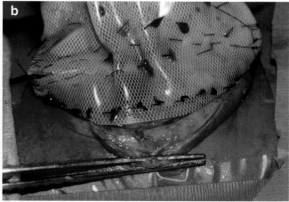

Fig. 63.3 (a) In infants who cannot undergo complete reduction of herniated intestinal contents, an abdominal wall silo is created by suturing a Dacron reinforced Silastic sheet to the fascial edges using horizontal mattress, 2-0 silk sutures placed through the fascia to anchor the Silastic mesh. (b) Close up view of Silastic mesh anchored to the fascia and also showing several suture lines in the mesh indicating serial reductions of the herniated contents

in accomplishing the reduction of the herniated contents and can be placed in the NICU without anesthesia. Once the bowel has been completely reduced into the peritoneal cavity, the fascial edges are approximated enough to allow the removal of the silo, and a primary fascial and skin closure is performed (Figs. 63.8a and b).

Gastric decompression and parenteral nutrition should be continued until return of bowel function. If an ileus persists beyond 3–4 weeks, contrast studies of the gastrointestinal tract should be considered to rule out mechanical obstruction due to atresia, stenosis, or adhesive bands.

63.3.6 Complications

All gastroschisis patients will have some degree of postoperative ileus. While awaiting return of bowel function, gastroschisis patients will require parenteral nutrition via a central venous access thus subjecting them to risks like catheter sepsis. Ten percent of patients with gastroschisis will have persistent bowel hypoperistalsis and some infants will require long term parenteral nutrition. Gastroschisis, complicated by intestinal atresia or perforation, can result in short bowel syndrome. Other postoperative complications include surgical site infection, sepsis, aspiration pneumonia, necrotizing enterocolitis, and complications related to increased abdominal pressure (gastroesophageal reflux and inguinal hernia).

Most postnatal deaths are attributed to prematurity, overwhelming sepsis and complications of short bowel syndrome such as liver failure secondary to parenteral nutrition induced cholestasis and hepatic fibrosis.

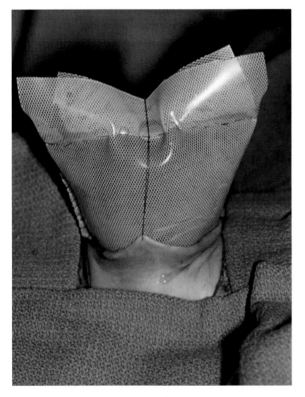

Fig. 63.4 A completed abdominal wall "silo". The single monofilament suture is used to prevent the skin from retracting

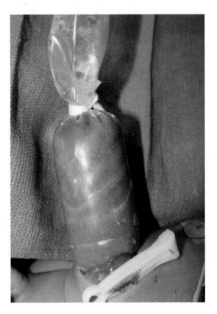

Fig. 63.6 The viscera are progressively reduced using gentle pressure from the apex of the silo. Gradual reduction can be carried out in the NICU with minimal to no anesthesia

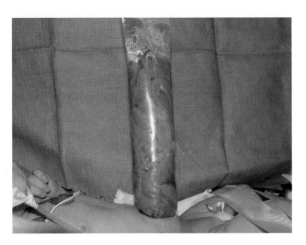

Fig. 63.5 A preformed spring loaded silo bag in place in an infant with gastroschisis

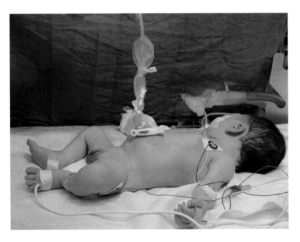

Fig. 63.7 Once the bowel has been completely reduced into the peritoneal cavity, the infant is returned to the OR where the silo is removed and the fascia and skin are closed primarily

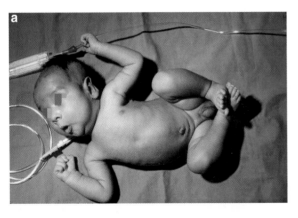

Fig. 63.8 (**a**) An infant status post gastroschisis closure

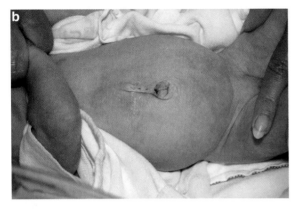

Fig. 63.8 (**b**) Close up of a recent primary closure of a gastroschisis

63.4 Omphalocele

Omphalocele (Gr. *omphalos* – umbilicus + Gr. *kele* – swelling; hernia; syn. Exomphalos) is a congenital anterior abdominal defect present at the umbilical ring. It represents a wide spectrum of pathology ranging from an uncomplicated hernia of the umbilical cord to a large defect with extrusion of all abdominal viscera (giant omphalocele) and life threatening associated anomalies (Figs. 63.9a and b). The abdominal wall defect can range in size from 2–10 cm. Virtually all intraabdominal structures can be eviscerated including the liver. The omphalocele is covered by an outer layer of amnion, a middle layer of Wharton's jelly, and an inner layer of peritoneum. This robust covering protects the gastrointestinal tract during intrauterine life and bowel function is usually normal at birth. Associated anomalies can involve the cardiovascular, alimentary, genitourinary, musculoskeletal and nervous systems. The presence of such significant associated anomalies suggests that the omphalocele defect is simply one element of a global intrauterine developmental disruption. The severity of the associated anomalies ultimately determines the morbidity and mortality of infants with omphalocele.

63.4.1 Etiology and Incidence

The etiology of omphalocele is not fully understood. It is believed that an omphalocele results from failure in the fusion of the three embryonic folds. The infolding process is a delicate balance of cell proliferation and cell apoptosis. When the cranial embryonic fold has unsuccessful infolding, epigastric omphalocele results and can be accompanied by diaphragmatic hernias, sternal clefts, pericardial defects, and intracardiac defects as in the Pentalogy of Cantrell (Figs. 63.10a and b). When the caudal embryonic fold has unsuccessful infolding, a hypogastric omphalocele results and can be accompanied by exstrophy of the bladder or cloaca, vesicointestinal fissure, colon atresia, imperforate anus, sacral vertebral defects, or meningomyelocele as in the Lower Midline Syndrome. The classic central omphalocele is thought to result from an infolding error of the lateral embryonic folds.

Omphalocele is less common than gastroschisis with an incidence of 1–2 per 10,000 live births. Males are more

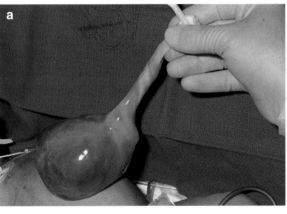
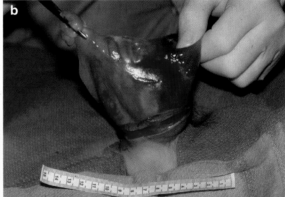

Fig. 63.9 (a) A typical omphalocele protruding through a large central defect of the umbilical ring. The omphalocele contains the liver (seen) and small intestine. (b) An omphalocele sac containing several loops of intestine. An incision has been made at the junction of the omphalocele sac and skin

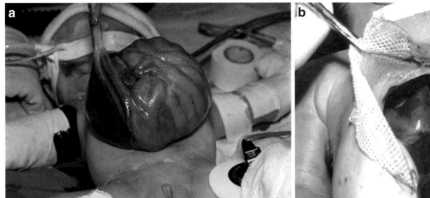
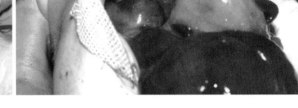

Fig. 63.10 (a) A giant omphalocele with ectopia cordis (see Fig. 63.10b) (b) Omphalocele with accompanying diaphragmatic hernia. The heart is visible in the cephalad part of the defect through large diaphragmatic and pericardial defects

affected than females. Whereas gastroschisis is seen in young mothers, omphalocele is more frequently associated with maternal age over 30 years old. No teratogens have been linked to the formation of an omphalocele.

63.4.2 Associated Anomalies

The survival of an infant with an omphalocele depends more on the severity of its associated anomalies than the abdominal wall defect itself. Multiple anomalies are seen in 40–70% of infants with omphaloceles. Cardiac anomalies are present in 50% of cases (septal defects, tetralogy of Fallot, ectopia cordis). Gastrointestinal anomalies can occur (e.g. duodenal atresia, etc.). Malignant tumors

such as Wilms' tumor, neuroblastoma, and adrenocortical tumors have an increased incidence with omphalocele. Ambiguous genitalia can also accompany omphalocele providing the additional clinical hurdle of sex determination.

Chromosomal anomalies are seen in 30–40% of omphalocele cases (trisomy 13–15, 16–18, 21, Turner's syndrome, Klinefelter's syndrome, and triploidy). Omphalocele is a part of the Beckwith-Wiedemann chromosomal syndrome (umbilical defect, gigantism, macroglossia, visceromegaly, and pancreatic islet cell hyperplasia). Chromosomal anomalies are seen more frequently when there is a small defect and no liver is present in the omphalocele hernia. There is a reported higher incidence of Wilms' tumor associated with Beckwith-Weidmann Syndrome.

63.4.3 Prenatal Diagnosis

Abdominal viscera in the base of the umbilical cord can be visualized with ultrasonography as early as the 10th gestational week. Ultrasound can also determine if the liver has herniated outside the abdominal wall. Maternal alpha fetoprotein is elevated 3–4 times the normal mean in omphalocele. If omphalocele is detected, amniocentesis with chromosomal analysis should be offered to screen for lethal anomalies.

For small omphaloceles without lethal associated anomalies, serial ultrasonography should be continued and term vaginal delivery pursued. There are no absolute indications for cesarean section; however, for large omphaloceles with eviscerated liver most centers will recommend term cesarean section to avoid liver injury with hemorrhage upon parturition.

The main advantage of prenatal ultrasonography and chromosomal analysis is that it allows for more informed prenatal counseling. If severe or lethal anomalies are detected, the option of terminating the pregnancy can be discussed with the parents.

63.4.4 Perinatal Care

After addressing any airway, breathing or circulation issues, assessment of the neonate with omphalocele should include a complete physical examination, chest radiograph, and an echocardiogram of the heart and ultrasonography of the kidneys to identify associated anomalies. Baseline laboratory values should be obtained with attention to immediate serum glucose analysis; omphalocele complicated by Beckwith-Wiedemann syndrome can present with profound hypoglycemia resulting in brain injury and mental retardation if not rapidly corrected. If not already established, karyotype analysis also should be performed. A nasogastric tube should be inserted to decompress the gastrointestinal tract. Empirical broad spectrum antibiotics should be initiated as with gastroschisis. Intravenous fluids using 10% dextrose and 0.25–0.50% normal saline solution run at a 125% maintenance rate. A non-adherent plastic sheet may be placed over the omphalocele sac to protect the sac from inadvertent tear during patient transport. The neonate should be maintained in a thermoneutral environment while in transport or awaiting further care.

A rupture of the hernia sac occurs in 10% of infants with omphalocele. If the sac has a minor tear it may be carefully sutured closed at the bedside. Fluid resuscitation for a neonate with a ruptured omphalocele sac should be approached as described above for gastroschisis.

63.4.5 Operative Management

The operative strategy for the repair of omphalocele depends on the size of the defect, the extent of visceroabdominal disproportion (VAD), and the severity of the associated anomalies.

Primary closure of the omphalocele can be accomplished 60–70% of the time (generally 2–5 cm in diameter). In large omphaloceles with the liver herniated, care must be taken in the reduction of the liver to avoid torsion of the hepatic veins, obstruction of portal vein inflow, obstruction of the inferior vena cava, or injury to the hepatic capsule. Resection of the hernia sac prior to reduction of the hernia is not necessary but in small defects is recommended. In very large defects that require staged reduction, failure of this approach allows the hernia sac to still be present. Regardless, if a portion of the sac overlying the liver is densely adherent it should be left in place, as attempts at debridement can cause difficulty to control liver hemorrhage.

When there is significant VAD and loss of abdominal domain the reduction of the hernia can be approached via a staged silo technique as described for gastroschisis (Fig. 63.11). The abdominal wall can

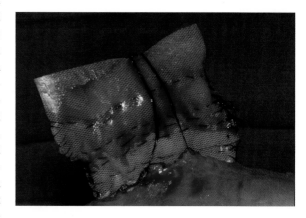

Fig. 63.11 Appearance of the silastic silo after complete reduction of the herniated contents. Note the six horizontal suture lines indicating the number of sequential reductions. This sac has been 'painted' with Betadine antiseptic ointment

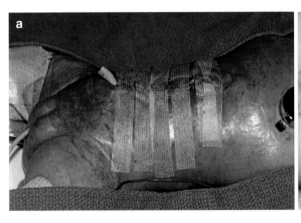
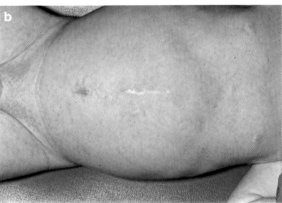
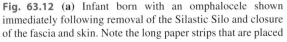

Fig. 63.12 (**a**) Infant born with an omphalocele shown immediately following removal of the Silastic Silo and closure of the fascia and skin. Note the long paper strips that are placed to distribute the tension over a wide distance (**b**) A well healed omphalocele repair

then be closed in layers resulting in an intact abdominal wall (Figs. 63.12a and b). Alternatively, the surgeon can create an intentional ventral hernia by elevating skin flaps or inserting a prosthetic mesh. This planned hernia can be repaired at 1 year of age.

For neonates with giant omphaloceles (>8 cm), significant pulmonary or cardiac abnormalities, or significant chromosomal abnormalities, a non-operative approach can be employed by induction epithelialization of the hernia sac. Topical eschar forming agents are painted on the hernia sac twice a day. Silver sulfadiazine is presently the most commonly used eschar forming agent in the United States. When using this agent, sodium levels should be monitored because this compound is hypotonic and can cause sodium loss through the sac. Mercurochrome was a popular topical agent in the past but is not generally used now.

63.4.6 Complications

Early post repair complications include surgical site infection, sepsis, dehiscence, ventral hernia, bowel obstruction, bowel perforation, necrotizing enterocolitis, fistulas, renal failure and respiratory distress. Iatrogenic injury to the eviscerated liver can result in hepatic hematoma and hepatic infarction.

A significant increase in intraabdominal pressure following abdominal wall closure can induce respiratory distress and require long-term ventilatory support. The increase in intra-abdominal pressure can also lead to inguinal hernias and gastroesophageal reflux.

Antenatal mortality ranges from 30–60% and largely depends on the severity of associated anomalies.

Further Reading

Ledbetter DJ (2006) Gastroschisis and omphalocele. Surg Clin N Am 86:249–260

Puri P, Höllwarth ME (eds) (2006) Pediatric Surgery. Springer, Berlin, Heidelberg

Schuster SR (1967) A new method for the staged repair of large omphaloceles. Surg Gynecol Obstet 125:837–850

Weber TR, Au-Fliegner M, Downward CD, Fishman SJ (2002) Abdominal wall defects. Curr Opin Pediatr 14:491–497

Wilson DR, Johnson MP (2004) Congenital abdominal wall defects: An update. Fetal Diag Ther 19:385–398

Yokomori K, Olikura M, Kitano Y, Hori T, Nakajo T (1992) Advantages and pitfalls of amnion inversion repair for the treatment of large unruptured omphalocele: Results of 22 cases. J Pediatr Surg 27:882

Bladder Exstrophy

64

Amanda C. North and John P. Gearhart

Contents

64.1 Introduction Including Definition and Incidence

Bladder exstrophy is part of a spectrum of genito-urinary tract anomalies ranging from epispadias to cloacal exstrophy. It involves defects in the abdominal wall, bladder, genitalia, pelvic bones, rectum, and anus. There is a triangular fascial defect which is occupied by the exstrophied bladder and posterior urethra. This defect extends from the umbilicus, which is situated below the horizontal line of the iliac crest, to the intra-symphyseal band. Indirect inguinal hernias are frequently present.

It is characterized by the absence of a portion of the lower abdominal wall and the anterior vesical wall, with eversion of the posterior vesical wall through the deficit.

The bladder mucosa may be normal at birth or there may be hamartomatous polyps, or more rarely ectopic bowel mucosa, or an isolated bowel loop on the surface. The ureters follow an abnormal course due to the enlarged and deep pouch of Douglas. This forces the ureters to be inferiorly and laterally displaced. With bladder closure vesico-ureteral reflux occurs in 100% of cases.

Patients with classic bladder exstrophy have widening of the pubic symphysis, external rotation of the posterior aspect of the pelvis, retroversion of the acetabulum, external rotation of the anterior pelvis, and a 30% shortening of the pubic bones.

The incidence of bladder exstrophy is estimated to be between 1 in 10,000 and 1 in 50,000 live births. There is a male preponderance with a male to female ratio of 5:1 to 6:1.

P. Puri and M. Höllwarth (eds.), *Pediatric Surgery: Diagnosis and Management,*
DOI: 10.1007/978-3-540-69560-8_64, © Springer-Verlag Berlin Heidelberg 2009

64.2 Etiology

There are several theories as to the cause of the exstrophy-epispadias complex. One idea is that exstrophy is caused by the failure of the cloacal membrane to be reinforced by ingrowth of mesoderm. The cloacal membrane is a bilaminar layer at the caudal end of the germinal disc. Mesenchymal ingrowth between the ectodermal and endodermal layers of this membrane leads to the formation of the lower abdominal muscles and pelvic bones. This mesenchymal ingrowth is followed by downward growth of the urorectal septum which divides the cloaca into the bladder anteriorly and rectum posteriorly. The paired genital tubercles then migrate medially and fuse in the midline. Premature rupture of the cloacal membrane leads to either bladder exstrophy, cloacal exstrophy, or epispadias depending on the timing of the rupture.

Another theory, held by Marshall and Muecke, is that abnormal overdevelopment of the cloacal membrane prevents medial migration of the mesenchymal tissue. Again, the timing of the rupture of the cloacal membrane determines the extent of the defect. Other theories include the concept that an abnormal caudal development of the genital hillocks with fusion in the midline below rather than above the cloacal membrane. Another suggests an abnormal caudal insertion of the body stalk with failure of interposition of the mesenchymal tissue in the midline which prevents translocation of the cloaca into the depths of the abdominal cavity. The superficial position of the cloacal membrane predisposes to disintegration. This last theory is somewhat controversial.

There appears to be a genetic component to exstrophy-epispadias complex. The incidence of bladder exstrophy in offsprings of a parent with exstrophy has been reported at 1 in 70 live births. Other studies have found a lower incidence. Twin studies have found examples where only one twin was affected and where both twins were affected. No cases have been reported where both nonidentical twins were affected. There have been five sets of male identical twins with both twins affected; one set of identical male twins with one twin affected; and three sets of female identical twins with only one twin affected. The risk of recurrence in a given family has been reported at about 1 in 100. One review study found that increased incidence of bladder exstrophy occurred in infants of younger mothers and mothers with high parity.

64.3 Pathology

Bladder exstrophy involves the urinary tract, genitalia, musculoskeletal system, and sometimes the gastrointestinal tract.

64.3.1 Musculoskeletal Defects

The characteristic finding in bladder exstrophy is widening of the pubic symphysis caused by malrotation of the innominate bones. There is outward rotation of the pubic rami at their junction with the iliac bones, external rotation of the posterior aspect of the pelvis, retroversion of the acetabulum, external rotation of the anterior pelvis, and shortening of the pubic rami by 30%. The sacroiliac joint angle is 10% larger in the exstrophy pelvis. The bony pelvis has 14.7% more inferior rotation than normal. Finally, the sacrum has a 42.6% larger volume and 23.5% more surface area in exstrophy.

64.3.2 Abdominal Wall Defects

There is a triangular defect caused by the premature rupture of the cloacal membrane. This is occupied by the exstrophied bladder and posterior urethra. The fascial defect is limited inferiorly by the intrasymphyseal band and superiorly by the umbilicus. The distance between the umbilicus and anus is foreshortened. Although an umbilical hernia is usually present, omphaloceles are rarely seen in bladder exstrophy but are frequently associated with cloacal exstrophy. Inguinal hernias are present in 81.8% of boys and 10.5% of girls with bladder exstrophy.

64.3.3 Anorectal Defects

Bladder exstrophy patients have a short and broad perineum. The anus is displaced anteriorly, directly behind the urogenital diaphragm. The levator ani and puborectalis muscles are divergent and the majority are displaced behind the rectum. Rectal prolapse rarely occurs after bladder closure.

64.3.4 Male Genital Defects

Anterior corporal length is 50% shorter and 30% wider than normal controls. Autonomic nerves are displaced laterally. There is prominent dorsal chordee and a shortened urethral groove. The vas deferens, seminal vesicles, and ejaculatory ducts are normal. The urethra is located anterior to the prostate. Testes are frequently undescended but appear to be otherwise normal (Fig. 64.1).

64.3.5 Female Genital Defects

The vagina is shorter than normal but normal caliber. The orifice is frequently stenotic and anteriorly displaced. The clitoris is bifid and the labia, mons pubis, and clitoris are divergent. The cervix is located in the anterior wall of the vagina. The defective pelvic floor predisposes even nulliparous females to pelvic prolapse (Fig. 64.2).

64.3.6 Urinary Defects

The bladder mucosa may appear normal at birth or may have a hamartomatous polyp present. The mucosa

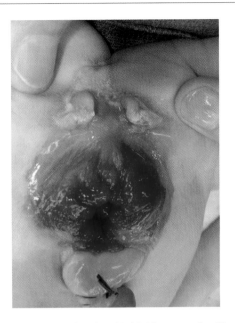

Fig. 64.2 Newborn female with bladder exstrophy. Note the bifid clitoris

needs to be frequently irrigated with saline and protected from surface trauma to prevent cystic or metaplastic changes. The exstrophy bladder has an increase in the collagen to smooth muscle ratio compared to controls with an increase in type III collagen. Additionally, there is a decrease in the average number of myelinated nerve fibers in the newborn exstrophy bladder which appears to be due to a lack of small fibers. There is variability in the size, distensibility, and neuromuscular function of the exstrophy bladder which may alter the decision to attempt closure.

64.4 Diagnosis

Bladder exstrophy can be diagnosed prenatally. Diagnosis is made by: an absence of bladder filling, a low-set umbilicus, widening of the pubic ramus, diminutive genitalia, and a lower abdominal mass that increases in size as the pregnancy progressed.

64.5 Management

The umbilical cord should be tied with 2-0 silk so the umbilical clamp does not cause trauma to the bladder. The bladder should be covered with nonadherent film

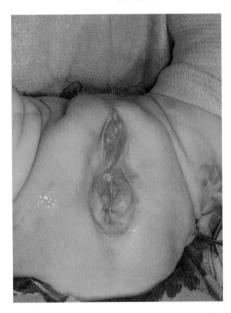

Fig. 64.1 Infant male with bladder exstrophy prior to closure. Traction suture is in the glans of the epispadiac penis. This bladder was too small to close at birth

of plastic wrap to prevent the mucosa from sticking to clothing or diapers. With each diaper change the plastic wrap is removed, the bladder is irrigated with saline, and new plastic wrap is placed.

The bladder needs to be evaluated to determine the suitability for closure. A small, fibrotic bladder patch without elasticity or contractility may be unsuitable for newborn primary closure. Primary closure should not be undertaken is patients with penoscrotal duplication, ectopic bowel within the exstrophied bladder, a hypoplastic bladder, or significant bilateral hydronephrosis. The alternatives to primary closure include waiting and allowing the bladder template to grow, excision of the bladder and a nonrefluxing colon conduit or ureterosigmoidostomy, urinary diversion with a colon conduit while preserving the small bladder inside to be used for the posterior urethra in an Arap-type procedure, or bladder augmentation.

For bladders that are suitable for primary closure there are multiple approaches which have been used. One involves complete primary closure with bladder closure and epispadias repair in a single stage and later bladder neck reconstruction in over 70% of patients. The second involves the modern staged closure with early closure of the bladder, posterior urethra, and abdominal wall, usually with pelvic osteotomy; epispadias repair around 6 months to 1 year of age; reconstruction of the bladder neck with ureteral reimplantation around age 4–5 years. Other repairs such as the Kelly repair have been done but no long term outcome data exists.

Pelvic osteotomies should be considered when bladder closure is performed after 72 h of age, if the pelvis is not malleable, or if the diastasis is greater than 4 cm. Bilateral transverse innominate and vertical iliac osteotomies allow easy reapproximation of the symphysis, decrease tension on the abdominal wall closure, eliminate the need for fascial flaps, help place the urethra deep within the pelvic ring which increases bladder outlet resistance, and bring the pelvic floor muscles near the midline where they can support the bladder neck and aid in later continence. Other types of osteotomy have been used including: simple bilateral anterior innominate osteotomies, pubic ramotomy, or posterior iliac osteotomy. However, the latest series and experience has been with the combined approach.

64.6 Complications

Following initial closure of bladder exstrophy, the main complications are bladder prolapse, complete wound dehiscence, and posterior urethral outlet obstruction. Bladder or renal calculi are a potential secondary complication.

64.6.1 Complications of Initial Closure

To minimize potential complications related to infection, the bladder should be protected with plastic film to prevent denuding of the mucosa. It should be washed with sterile saline. Preoperative antibiotics should be given, usually in the form of ampicillin and gentamicin, and continued for 7–10 days postoperatively.

The pubic bones need to be brought into apposition to minimize wound tension. If the initial closure is performed within the first 72 h of life and the pubis is mobile, osteotomy may be avoided. Otherwise, bilateral pelvic osteotomy will help protect the closure.

Fixation and immobilization of the wound and pelvis are critical to healing. The coapted pubic bones are fixed by a nylon horizontal mattress suture. External fixation of the closed pelvic ring is necessary. In newborns closed without pelvic osteotomy, modified Bryant's traction for 4 weeks is used. In patients who undergo osteotomy, modified Buck's traction and fixation is used. Furthermore, any muscular activity by the child must be controlled to prevent wound mobility. A combination of continuous caudal epidural catheters, analgesics, antispasmodics, and tranquilizers are used to maintain a calm postoperative course.

Dehiscence may be precipitated by incomplete mobilization of the pelvic diaphragm, inadequate pelvic immobilization postoperatively, wound infection, abdominal distention, or urinary tube malfunction. It necessitates a 6 month recovery period prior to attempted re-closure. When repeat closure is undertaken, tension-free closure with osteotomy and postoperative immobilization are important. Bladder prolapse also necessitate reclosure/revision. In patients who undergo a second closure, we perform epispadias repair at the time of reclosure. The patient receives testosterone enanthate intramuscularly 5 weeks and 2 weeks prior to surgery and undergoes an osteotomy at the time of surgery. For a patient who undergoes a second closure, the chance of obtaining a bladder capacity adequate for bladder neck reconstruction is only 60% and the chance of continence is 30%. This decreases with subsequent closures.

64.6.2 Complications of Osteotomy

Although osteomyelitis used to be seen in patients when pins were used to suspend the legs, this is rare with broad-spectrum antibiotic coverage. Pin sites should be cleaned 3–4 times a day with full strength peroxide on a cotton swab and then bacitracin ointment is applied.

Transient femoral nerve palsy and temporary abductor weakness has been reported in one patient. Blood loss from osteotomy is more common in patients with previous failed closure and blood transfusion may be necessary. Recurrent pubic diastasis has been seen in some patients, especially in infants.

64.6.3 Bladder Outlet Obstruction

A urinary tract infection (UTI), early hydronephrosis on ultrasound, or dry diapers early on after closure suggest bladder outlet obstruction. A bladder ultrasound along with cystoscopy is immediately indicated. Paraexstrophy skin flaps, although used rarely, can be a cause along with erosion of the intrapubic stitch into the posterior urethra. Strictures associated with paraexstrophy skin flaps, if found early, usually respond to simple dilation or internal urethrotomy. If stitch erosion is found, it is removed through a simple suprapubic incision.

64.6.4 Other Complications

Penile lengthening procedures may be complicated by bleeding or damage to the corporal bodies. Severe corporal body damage has occurred and is permanent. Damage has been especially associated with the penile disassembly technique.

Hypertension and oliguria following closure can be avoided by ureteral intubation at the time of closure. The ureteral catheters may need to be irrigated at regular intervals to maintain patency. Bladder drainage is accomplished by a suprapubic catheter.

64.6.5 Complications of Epispadias Repair

The most common complication of epispadias repair is urethrocutaneous fistula which occurs in about 10–15% of cases. The fistula may close spontaneously in about 25% of patients. A secondary procedure will be required in the rest. The most common location for fistula is at the base of the penis where the urethra comes up between the corporal bodies.

The second most common complication is urethral stricture. Prior failed epispadias repair seems to be the biggest risk factor for stricture formation. Another complication is loss of penile skin. This is a rare complication with a Cantwell-Ransley repair.

Persistent chordee may occur, especially when the patients reach the age of sexual maturity. In older children it may be necessary to incise the corpora and use a dermal graft to achieve straightness and obtain more penile length at puberty.

64.6.6 Complications of Bladder Neck Reconstruction

The complications following bladder neck reconstruction include difficulty urinating, persistent incontinence, hydronephrosis, and bladder stones. If the patient is unable to void following the 3rd week healing period, they may be managed by continuos suprapubic drainage, gentle urethral dilation, indwelling urethral catheterization, or clean intermittent catheterization. Initially, an 8-Fr foley is placed under anesthesia and left for 3–5 days. After removal of this catheter, another voiding trial is given.

Urinary continence may take as long as 1–2 years to achieve. In patients who have had a successful primary closure, urinary continence may be achieved in up to 81%. If stress incontinence or dribbling is present in the early post-operative period, the patient is unlikely to gain continence without further intervention. In patients with incontinence following bladder neck reconstruction, there are several options available. Patients may undergo bladder augmentation and placement of an artificial urinary sphincter. A re-do bladder neck repair with augmentation cystoplasty can be performed, with or without a continent stoma. Finally a continent stoma can be placed with bladder neck transaction and augmentation or bladder replacement.

Hydronephrosis may persist after bladder neck reconstruction. Careful follow-up is necessary. Patients with persistent hydronephrosis may require augmenta-tion. Stones may also develop in patients following bladder neck reconstruction.

Further Reading

Frionberger D, Gearhart JP (2006) Bladdes Exstrophy and Epispadis. In P Puri, ME Höllwarth (eds) Pediatric Surgery, Springer Surgery Atlas Series. Springer-Verlag Berlin Heidelberg, New York, pp 589–606

Gearhart JP (2001) Pediatric Urology. W.B. Saunders, Philadelphia

Gearhart JP (2002) Operative Pediatric Urology. Harcourt, London

Gearhart JP, Lakshmanan Y (2001) Complications of Urologic Surgery. W.B. Saunders, Philadelphia

Cloacal Exstrophy

65

Moritz M. Ziegler

Contents

65.1 Introduction

Cloacal exstrophy is a rare and complex malformation that affects between 1 in 200,000 and 1 in 400,000 live births. Despite its complexity, survival is expected; and instead, management is focused on patient outcomes and the achievement of an optimal quality of life. This has been born out in the last 3 decades where the shift for improving the quality of life has included appropriate gender assignment, independence from stoma appliances, and improved physical and social independence and mobility.

65.2 History

Cloacal exstrophy, also known as vesicointestinal fissure, ileovesical fistula, or extrophia splanchnica, was first described by Littre in 1709 and again by Meckel in 1812. The era of operative correction began with Rickham's 1960 report of a three-stage procedure performed over 8 months. Although only 17 of 34 patients survived correction during the years 1968–1976, survival of 13 of 15 patients at a single institution was reported in the early 1980s; and since that time, survival has ranged from 90% to 100% in a variety of reported series.

Today, survival from cloacal exstrophy is nearly universal, the mortality being a product of associated renal or cardiac disease. Rather, the focus has shifted to urinary, gastrointestinal, and genital reconstruction, designed to render the patient appliance-free and of appropriate psychologic and physiologic gender (Groner and Ziegler, 1995; Schober et al., 2002).

P. Puri and M. Höllwarth (eds.), *Pediatric Surgery: Diagnosis and Management,*
DOI: 10.1007/978-3-540-69560-8_65, © Springer-Verlag Berlin Heidelberg 2009

65.3 Embryogenesis

The classic description of cloacal exstrophy is that it results from incomplete coverage of the infra-umbilical wall by the secondary mesoderm of the primitive streak, resulting in a 'rupture' of the midline structures during the 5th embryonic week (Gray and Skandalakis, 2004). Were this developmental defect to occur after fusion of the genital tubercles in the 7th week, bladder exstrophy would result. If, however, the rupture occurs before the 5th week, the genital tubercles will have not fused and the urorectal septum will have not descended to separate the future bladder from the future large bowel. The result is a large midline defect with exposure of both bowel and bladder elements and duplication of the genitalia. Furthermore, the absence of the urorectal septum may cause a marked retardation in the development of the colon, resulting in the blind-ending, foreshortened distal gut typically seen in these patients.

However, challenge to this classic explanation has occurred from three fronts: studies in twins, the diagnosis of cloacal exstrophy in the fetus, and the development of a chick model that simulates this anomaly. Twin studies include reports in which cloacal exstrophy was present in one of two monozygotic twins, while the twin sibling was normal. This same finding has occurred in a set of conjoined twins. In two additional reports of the fetal diagnosis of cloacal exstrophy, rupture of the cloacal membrane occurred as late as 18–24 weeks and 22–26 weeks, a contrasting observation that may account for the broad scope of anatomic variations seen in this anomaly. The chick studies suggest a role for space occupation by the swollen dorsal aorta that produces a widening of pelvic structures and a secondary stretching or thinning of the infraumbilical abdominal wall before eventual rupture (Manner and Kluth, 2005).

65.4 Anatomy

Cloacal exstrophy is the most severe form of a ventral abdominal wall defect (Fig. 65.1). An omphalocele of variable size is always present. Inferior to the omphalocele, a complex midline lesion with exposed mucosal surfaces is readily apparent. The two lateral mucosal "plates" represent the right and left hemibladder, and typically a ureteral orifice is present in the lower portion of each. The central mucosal plate is

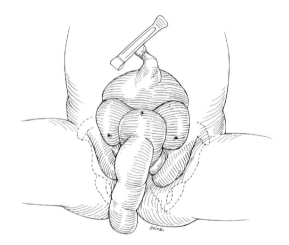

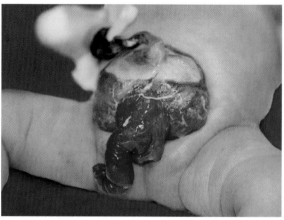

Fig. 65.1 A patient with cloacal exstrophy and a diagram depicting the component parts of the deformity: a prolapsing terminal ileum (elephant trunk deformity); a cephalad membrane covered omphalocele; two separated bladder halves; orifices depict an appendiceal lumen and two ureteral orifices; and it can be observed that the pubic rami are separated and along their superior margin can be seen bifid corporal bodies

composed of intestinal epithelium and represents the ileo-cecum. Up to five orifices may be present on this surface. The most superior orifice belongs to the terminal ileum, which may be prolapsed as an "elephant trunk" deformity. In the middle of the bowel plate is one or two orifices, representing the single or duplicated appendix. Finally, the most inferior orifice, which may also be single or duplicated, represents the distal colon, and it is almost always of shortened length and ends blindly.

Genital abnormalities are universally present. For male infants, testes are typically undescended and located intraabdominally, the penis is bifid and laterally positioned on the separated pubic rami, the urethra is epispadiac, and the vas deferens may be normal, absent or duplicated. In the female, the clitoris is bifid and separated or it may be absent, the vagina is typically duplex, though it too could be exstrophied or even absent, and the uterus is bicornuate in type.

65.5 Preoperative Management

65.5.1 Associated Anomalies

Anomalies of organ systems remote from the basic cloacal exstrophy defect are common, occurring in as many as 85% of cases. Interestingly, survivors of cloacal exstrophy are generally of normal intelligence. Abnormalities include the upper urinary tract (42–60%): hydronephrosis, hydroureter, ureteral atresia, ureteral duplication, pelvic kidney, renal agenesis, multicystic kidney, and crossed fused renal ectopia. Vertebral anomalies occur in 48–75% of cases, with myelodysplasia syndromes present in 29–46%. The tethered cord anomaly must also be excluded. Associated gastrointestinal anomalies include malrotation, duodenal atresia, Meckel's diverticulum, and intestinal duplications. What is more inconsistent as well as controversial is the association of short bowel syndrome. Therefore, ileal as well as colon preservation becomes a very important strategy for long-term intestinal rehabilitation. Associated orthopedic anomalies (26–30%) include club-foot, congenital dislocation of the hips and other potentially severe deformities.

Prune belly syndrome features may be associated with the omphalocele of cloacal exstrophy, such babies also demonstrating myelodysplasia.

In postpubertal girls with cloacal exstrophy, a recent association of ovarian cysts, severe pelvic pain and urinary obstruction has been reported.

65.5.2 Diagnosis and Preoperative Evaluation

Prenatal ultrasound has become commonplace for the diagnosis of cloacal exstrophy, and major diagnostic criteria include the following: non-visualization of the bladder, a large midline infraumbilical anterior abdominal wall defect or cystic abdominal wall structure, the protruding proboscus, an omphalocele, or myelomeningocele. Less frequently defined minor criteria include lower extremity defects, renal anomalies, ascites, widened pubic arches, a narrow thorax, hydrocephalus, and a single umbilical artery. This diagnostic prepartum information allows appropriate education of the parents, planning for the pregnancy, timing and location of the delivery, as well as optimal newborn management, preferably in a center experienced in the care of this complex anomaly.

At birth, immediate management is stabilization of the baby, protection of the exposed omphalocele, bladder and bowel, and if present, protection of the myelomeningocele. After a screening physical examination and baseline laboratory studies that include an evaluation of renal function and serum electrolytes, an ultrasound of the genitourinary tract along with chest/abdominal radiographs is done to complete the initial screening for associated anomalies. Cardiac evaluation should be individualized. Normal body temperature is maintained either by covering the exposed mucosa and membranes with warmed sterile saline followed by a plastic wrap, or by enclosing the lower half of the torso in a warm saline-filled plastic bag. A prenatal or postnatal chromosome study would be useful in determining the genetic sex of the baby.

At this time it is imperative to assemble the team of pediatric surgeon and urologist, and if other organ system involvement has been identified, e.g. myelomeningocele, the appropriate additional consultants. It is also prudent to add to the evaluative team an endocrinologist as well as a psychiatrist/psychologist versed in gender assignment issues. At that time a team meeting with the family, if not done prenatally, must be arranged, and the magnitude of the problems and their potential solutions discussed. It is then important to prioritize and define a step-wise management plan that defines all of the issues including gender. All parties should be in agreement with the plan.

This complex anomaly requires the combined efforts of both pediatric surgeon and pediatric urologist. The team leader must also coordinate input from a variety of ancillary personnel including a stoma therapist, physical therapist, social worker, psychiatrist or psychologist, and endocrinologist. A neurosurgeon or orthopedic surgeon may also need to be involved if indicated.

65.6 Operative Management

65.6.1 The Sequence

The successful therapy of this complex anomaly requires an orderly approach of both sequential and simultaneous steps. (Lee, Grady and Joyner et al., 2006) We would propose a modification of the original management phases recommended by Ricketts (Table 65.1). If a myelomeningocele is present it must first be covered, and attention to a possible tethered cord can be delayed. The next focus is a multi-step procedure that includes coverage/closure of the omphalocele, take-down of the exposed ileal plate and exstrophied hemibladders, establishment of gastrointestinal continuity by tubularizing the bowel plate and salvaging all of the small and large bowel length including the appendices, and creation of a colostomy that should exit the left upper abdomen. The hemibladders are connected in the posterior midline, and if possible tubularized into a reservoir. The sepa-

rated pubic rami are approximated in the midline, a maneuver that facilitates both omphalocele closure as well as bladder closure. The gonads and external genitalia are addressed as the final step of this initial procedure. In light of recent data, though still controversial, a decision for gender conversion and /or reassignment is best deferred at this time. A genetic female is likely best managed by delayed clitoroplasty or vaginoplasty in the neonatal period, and any reconstruction for bifid or duplicated internal genitalia can be deferred. A genetic male with an adequate but bifid phallus can have approximation of the corporal bodies in the midline as the pubis is closed, but the repair of the epispadius/exstrophy complex is best deferred. Attention to the undescended and typically intraabdominal testes can also be delayed until a time of further reconstruction. The subsequent phases of therapy are individualized and planned in a discussion with the family led by the care team.

In cases with a huge omphalocele, it is practical to consider leaving the intact membrane in place as a barrier for a potential staged closure. However, since in dissecting out the exstrophied bladder and bowel the peritoneal cavity will be entered, the usual approach is to open the abdomen extending the incision vertically with removal of the omphalocele membrane. This will permit eventual primary fascial closure of the omphalocele, aided by approximation of the pubic rami. This same exposure is optimal for staged closure techniques including the application of a prosthetic silo. Newer approaches to abdominal wall coverage and closure include application of an expanded thoraco-epigastric myo-cutaneous flap or application of an absorbable matrix on which to lay a mobilized skin flap.

The central bowel plate is then separated from the two lateral hemibladders. Intestinal reconstruction including the blind-ending colon segment should emphasize bowel conservation. The exstrophied ileocecal junction should be tubularized to restore continuity of the ileocolonic lumen. Appendices, single or duplicated, should always be considered as potential catheterizable conduits for achieving urinary dryness and thus should not be sacrificed. Similarly, duplicated colon segments, even though blind ending, can be used as interposed pro-peristaltic and anti-peristaltic colon conduits to potentially slow intestinal transit time. This is especially beneficial in the usual circumstance of a foreshortened colonic length or in the unusual circumstance of a concomitant limited small bowel length. An extra colon may also prove to be useful in urinary

Table 65.1 Step-wise management plan for cloacal exstrophy

Management phase	Patient age	Therapeutic procedures
Phase 1	Newborn	Meningocele coverage
		Closure/coverage of omphalocele
		Separation of bowel/bladder plates
		Ileal reconstruction
		End colostomy
		Hemibladder approximation/ closure
		Pubic bone approximation
Phase 2	1–6 months	Feeding access
		Manage short bowel syndrome
Phase 3	6 months –2 years	Bladder closure if not done Phase 1
		Iliac osteotomy
		First stage genital reconstruction/ gender decision
		Tethered cord release
		Midline sagittal anorectoplasty
Phase 4	2–8 years	Bladder augmentation
		Construction catheterizable urinary reservoir
		Second stage genital reconstruction/gender decision
Phase 5	8–18 years	Completion genital reconstruction
		Exogenous hormone therapy

conduit reconstruction later in the child's life, and for these reasons it should never be sacrificed. After mobilizing the blind-ending colon, the tubularized bowel must then be exited as an end colostomy. The placement of this fecal stream stoma will optimally be exited more lateral and more cephalad than is usual, especially if a prosthetic pouch is used to close the omphalocele.

The free hemibladders are then re-approximated into a single midline posterior bladder wall plate by suture technique, taking care to identify and protect the ureteral orifices. If sufficient bladder surface exists from which to construct an adequate capacity reservoir, then the bladder is also closed anteriorly, forming a urine-collecting chamber. The tubularized bladder is then positioned behind the approximated pubic rami, and the bladder neck drains inferiorly onto the perineum. Practically, most patients will have only the bladder halves approximated posteriorly, which will drain as a cutaneous vesicostomy onto the perineum. Other urinary diversion techniques include end or loop ureterostomies, or cutaneous pyelostomies.

Primary abdominal closure is possible in most patients. Such primary closure can be done most easily in the first 48 hours of life, with the benefit of circulating "relaxin" and permanent high-tensile strength suture material placed into either end of the separated pubis.

For genetic XY babies with a microphallus or a bifid phallus, gender conversion would previously have been accomplished at the neonatal procedure by assigning a female phenotype. However, current practice would not proceed to that decision until exploration of the options had occurred with a team that would include a urologist, endocrinologist, psychologist, and the baby's parents. The discussion would include the role of prenatal as well as pubertal genetic male imprinting as well as the options for phallic reconstruction that even might include total replacement phalloplasty. Corporal and glanular tissue should always be preserved for eventual reconstruction, and the separated hemiscrota should be preserved and reapproximated in the midline. Completion orchidopexy should be delayed until a definitive gender decision is made. Vaginal reconstruction should be deferred to a later age for genetic XX babies to permit full evaluation and correction of double systems, potential vaginal atresia, or potential vaginal exstrophy, the latter located caudal to the exstrophied bladder mucosa. This will also allow an informed decision to be made about which tissue might best be used to augment any deficiency in vaginal tissue (Hughes, Houk and Ahmed, 2006).

65.7 Post-operative Care

Postoperatively, the patient should receive fluid and electrolyte management which takes into account a potentially diminished renal reserve. A circumferential wrap should encircle the lower extremities from ankles to mid-abdomen to "strap" together the upper thighs, minimizing pelvic tension and possible distraction of the closed pubic rami. Suspension in a modified Bryant's traction can also be done. Staged closure of the omphalocele should follow in those cases with an applied prosthetic silo. The fecal and urinary stream should be isolated, either by temporary bladder or ureteral catheters or by permitting free drainage of urine onto the bladder exstrophied plate, an appliance covering the colostomy.

After completion of the newborn repair, the associated anomalies should be prioritized and addressed. The myelodysplasia occurring in almost 50% of such patients should be covered and selected use of shunts to treat hydrocephalus should follow. Orthopedic assessment of extremity, pelvis and spinal deformities is necessary, and a long-range treatment plan should be outlined. If the pelvis was not primarily reapproximated, eventual plan for pelvic osteotomy can be made so that at the time of reoperation, pelvic closure becomes a reality.

65.8 Long-Term Management

65.8.1 Gender Assignment/Genital Reconstruction

Although there is a genetic male predominance in cloacal exstrophy, the commonly found inadequate corporal structures associated with a bifid penis make adequate penile reconstruction difficult. Historically, therefore, most such patients underwent a female gender assignment. Despite their genetic sex, they were reared as a girl, and an eventual reconstructive operation was designed to develop phenotypic female anatomy complimented by female hormonal replacement. However, in recent years there has been a call to re-examine genotypically congruent sex assignment, even in those newborns with an inadequate phallus, both because of a high frequency of sexual dysfunction in gender converted children and adolescents as well as a realization of the potential for penile reconstruction. Certainly genetic males with adequate bilateral or even unilateral phallic structures should receive a male gender assignment. In any case where gender reassignment or conversion is considered, there is a considerable need for parental counseling, endocrinology input, and input on a longitudinal basis from a trained psychiatrist/psychologist for both the parents and child. All corporal and scrotal/labial tissue needs to be preserved. The corporal tissue, typically bifid, becomes critical whether reconstructing a penile shaft or a clitoris. In the phenotypic male, penile reconstruction and orchidopexy will be the two steps of significance, and they can be delayed beyond the neonatal period. In genotypic males with cloacal exstrophy, the testes are typically located intra-abdominally. If a genotypic congruent sex assignment is maintained, orchidopexy will be needed. Fortunately as a group, the testes, despite their location, retain near-normal histology. In contrast, when gender conversion to the female phenotype is considered, eventual orchiectomy will be required. Penile reconstruction will likely need to be deferred to an older age if the bifid phalli are inadequate for simple re-approximation.

In genetic females, the bifid clitoris and labia are initially preserved but left alone. As the child grows, staged operations are used to create an adequate appearance. Failure of midline fusion, a key characteristic of cloacal exstrophy, is frequently manifested in the female reproductive system by duplication of the vagina, uterus, and fallopian tubes. Atresia and exstrophy of the vagina are also possible. The latter is difficult to distinguish in the newborn period, due to the large exstrophic bladder above or anterior to the exposed vaginal tissue. However, diagnosis of this entity is important in planning the eventual staged vaginal reconstruction. An atretic vagina will require reconstruction with a combination of perineal skin flaps and a small or large bowel pull-through. An intact vagina may contain a septum or be duplicated, and it is most prudent to resect the more rudimentary of the two, attaching the remaining uterus to the vaginal vault. Other than the propensity for cyst formation, the ovaries should be normal.

65.8.2 Continence and Stomas

The goal for most children with cloacal exstrophy is a stoma-free existence. At a delayed interval, we prefer to use pelvic magnetic resonance imaging or computer tomographic imaging, coupled with electrical stimulation of the perineum, to define the presence of an anorectal pelvic muscle complex. If such muscle is present, a midline sagittal anorectoplasty is feasible in selected patients who also have an adequate small and large bowel length for establishing a continent anorectum. Others have advocated for a primary rectal pull-through procedure done in the newborn period following the anterior approach used for abdominal wall reconstruction. Though anorectal reconstruction is an attractive and preferred outcome, those children amenable to this plan who also have a good outcome are few. As a result, either a permanent colostomy or a colostomy or pull-through aided by an antegrade continent enterostomy (ACE Procedure) may be preferred.

Urinary "dryness" is frequently accomplished utilizing the principle of a catheterizable stoma into a reservoir. Using a "continent nipple valve" of the Mitrofanoff principle with an appendix or a tubularized portion of small bowel: a catheterizable conduit is attached to the reservoir. The reservoir itself could be bowel or bladder augmented with stomach, small or large bowel. These procedures are typically deferred until the child has grown out of infancy.

65.9 Patient Outcomes

With the progressively improving survival of cloacal exstrophy, attention has shifted to optimizing bowel, bladder and sexual function. Historically these children were at best committed to a chronic bowel as well as a chronic urinary stoma, and when that was coupled with a degree of genital ambiguity, short-bowel syndrome, or spinal dysraphism, the quality of life was best described as unfortunate. What has now been realized is that the majority of such children has a preserved intellect, and also has an anatomy that lends itself to imaginative but real "continent" outcomes.

A bowel pull-through procedure is feasible in selected patients, and only in the face of an absent gluteal cleft, poor response of muscle to perineal stimulation, severe sacral deformity, a lipomeningocele, or a "rocker-bottom" should a permanent bowel stoma be considered. The remainder of the patients can undergo a pull-through procedure, and if a degree of incontinence exists, a bowel management program or application of the ACE procedure will be an adjunct (Koyle and Malone, 2006). The most challenging of the group are those children who also have a short small bowel, and in that circumstance various nutritional, pharmacological, and operative manipulations may be in order. In one series of 26 patients with cloacal exstrophy, four had colon duplication, one a duodenal web and one had malrotation. Of six patients with short bowel syndrome, five were eventually weaned from parenteral nutrition. Interestingly, two of four patients who underwent abdominal-perineal colon pull through were continent of stool. In another series of 22 patients, ten had an ileostomy, seven a colostomy, three were stoma free, and two had died. In this series an association of spinal dysraphism increased intestinal morbidity, and the presence of an ileostomy increased dependence on parenteral nutrition and its inherent morbidity. In a third series of 50 patients, 25 had a colon pull-through, and of these, 4 were failures, 2 were continent, and 19 were managed by a colon washout regimen.

The reconstructed urinary reservoir is typically of small volume and it is non-dynamic. Bladder augmentation has been a process in evolution and includes the use of stomach, large bowel and small bowel, or a potential combination thereof. Ileal urinary conduits can also be used. To enhance bladder continence mechanisms, the bladder neck can be tightened, a bowel nipple valve can be added, Teflon can be injected, and these changes coupled with intermittent catheterization can render the majority of patients dry. A catheterizable conduit attached to the urinary reservoir has also been proven to be effective. Spontaneous voluntarily controlled perineal voiding is currently an unrealistic outcome expectation. The magnitude of urinary reconstruction is indicated in one series of fifty patients where 21 had narrowing of the bladder neck, 7 had a bowel nipple constructed, 12 a Mitranoff procedure, 4 a ureterostomy, and 35 had a bladder augmentation. Dryness was achieved 75% of the time.

The outcomes from genital reconstruction in females are satisfactory, but the ability of a bifid uterus and reconstructed vagina to permit fertility has, as of yet, not been reported. The greater controversy arises in a genetic male who has a penile reconstruction. Since the testes, even if located intra-abdominally, appear to be histologically normal, fertility may be preserved; however, to date, a fertile male has also not been reported. More than 30% of males have a diminutive or absent penis. If an inadequate phallus is the result of a series of failed operative reconstructions, reported emotional disasters are common. More controversial yet are those genetic males who have undergone reassignment to the female phenotype. Acting-out male behavior imprinted genetically or hormonally has been witnessed. At adolescence, such "phenotypically-assigned-females" have declared their "maleness" and have emotionally struggled with their sexual identity (Reiner and Gearhart, 2004). Whether early removal of the testes will diminish such a testosterone imprinting affect or whether such imprinting is prenatal is currently unknown. In one assessment of quality of life, child behavior and social cognition, no difference was reported for the gender ambiguous children who underwent a gender reassignment when they were compared to the control exstrophied group who had no gender issue. However, in another series of 29 genetic males with cloacal exstrophy reassigned to the female phenotype, all patients in adolescence had declared themselves male.

Though staged management has the inherent difficulty of multiple operative procedures, the expectations for an excellent outcome should remain high. The vast majority of these children can be rehabilitated to have a meaningful and functional quality of life through a careful, individualized, staged reconstruction accomplished by a team experienced in the care of this complex anomaly (Baker Towell and Towell, 2003).

Further Reading

Baker Towell DM, Towell AD (2003) A preliminary investigation into quality of life, psychological distress and social competence in children with cloacal exstrophy. J Urol 169: 1850–1853

Gray SW, Skandalakis JE (2004) The bladder and urethra. In Embryology for Surgeons. W.B. Saunders, Philadelphia, pp 519–552

Groner JI, Ziegler MM (1995) Cloacal exstrophy. In P Puri (ed) Newborn Surgery, 2nd edn. Arnold, London, pp 629–636 (2003 new edition)

Hughes IA, Houk C, Ahmed PA (2006) Consensus statement on the management of intersex disorders. J Ped Urol 2:148–162

Koyle MA, Malone PSJ (2006) The Malone antegrade continence enema revisited. Dialogues in Pediatr Urol 28:1–11

Lee RS, Grady R, Joyner B et al (2006) Can a complete primary repair approach be applied to cloacal exstrophy? J Urol 176:2643–2648

Manner J, Kluth D (2005) The morphogenesis of the exstrophy-epispadias complex: A new concept based on observations made in early embryonic cases of cloacal exstrophy. Anat Embryol 210:51–57

Puri P, Höllwarth M (2006) Pediatric Surgery. Springer, Berlin, Heidelberg

Reiner WG, Gearhart JP (2004) Discordant sexual identity in some genetic males with cloacal exstrophy assigned to female sex at birth. N Engl J Med 350:333–341

Rickham PO (1960) Vesico-intestinal fissure. Arch Dis Child 35:97–102

Wilcox D, Shenoy M (2006) Cloacal Exstrophy. In P Puri, ME Höllwarth (eds) Pediatric Surgery. Springer Surgery Atlas Series, Springer-Verlag Berlin Heidelberg, New York, pp 607–612

Schober JM, Carmichael PA, Hines M, Ransley PG (2002) The ultimate challenge of cloacal exstrophy. J Urol 167: 300–304

Prune Belly Syndrome

66

Thambipillai Sri Paran and Prem Puri

Contents

66.1 Introduction

Prune belly syndrome is characterized by three abnormalities: an absence or deficiency of abdominal wall musculature, bilateral cryptorchidism and a dilated dysmorphic urinary tract. The incidence of this syndrome is estimated to be 1 in 29,000 to 1 in 50,000 live births. It is mostly seen in males with only 3–5% of cases seen in females. In females, it is obvious that the bilateral cryptorchidism is not applicable. Hence the term 'pseudo prune belly syndrome' has been used to describe the children in whom one or two of the characteristics from the classical triad are absent.

66.2 Aetiology

The aetiology of prune belly syndrome remains controversial. Several theories including genetic inheritance, foetal urinary outlet obstruction, and an embryological aberration of mesenchymal development have been proposed by various authors in an attempt to explain this complex of abnormalities. However, none appears to completely explain all the observations made within this group of children. It is suffice to say, that the theory of mesodermal arrest, as proposed by Stephens and Gupta, appears to explain the triad of abnormalities best. Nevertheless this theory does not explain the male predominance of this syndrome, or the myriad of other associated congenital anomalies seen amongst these children.

P. Puri and M. Höllwarth (eds.), *Pediatric Surgery: Diagnosis and Management*,
DOI: 10.1007/978-3-540-69560-8_66, © Springer-Verlag Berlin Heidelberg 2009

66.3 Pathology

Prune belly syndrome represents a spectrum of disease severity, ranging from those that die within the first few days of life to those that survive with relatively stable renal function into adulthood. The most obvious defect in newborns is the shrivelled prune belly-like appearance of the abdominal wall due to a deficiency in the abdominal wall musculature (Fig. 66.1). Biopsies from the abdominal wall have shown that functioning musculature exists in the lateral and upper quadrants of the abdomen, while none is seen in the lower central portions. This lack of abdominal muscle strength contributes to the symptoms of constipation, respiratory infection and postoperative pulmonary complications. It also means that these children cannot sit up from a lying down position without using their arms for support.

The cryptorchids could be found anywhere from just inferior to the lower pole of the kidney to near the ureterovesical junction. The maldescent of the testes may be part due to the absence of the abdominal muscles and part due to the absence of gubernaculums seen in these children. Atypical germ cells have also been reported in testicular biopsies from these children, and follow-up is advised regarding future risk of germ cell neoplasia.

The renal tract abnormalities could range in severity from those that result in severe renal insufficiency and death within few days of life, as mentioned earlier, to near normal renal function. The commonest abnormality seen is that of dilated tortuous ureters. These ureters show poor ineffective peristalsis over their entire length. Vesicoureteric reflux is seen in up to 85% of patients.

The microscopic analysis of the ureteric wall reveals a higher ratio of collagen to smooth muscle and also marked decrease in the number of nerve plexuses and non-myelinated Schwann fibres. This in turn contributes to the poor ureteral peristalsis even after corrective surgery. The bladder is thick walled and grossly enlarged. Presence of urachal remnant gives the bladder an hourglass configuration. The trigone is surprisingly large, and the ureteric orifices are located laterally, contributing to the vesicoureteric reflux. The bladder neck is often wide and ill defined.

The bladder in prune belly syndrome has efficient low-pressure storage and good compliance. Though

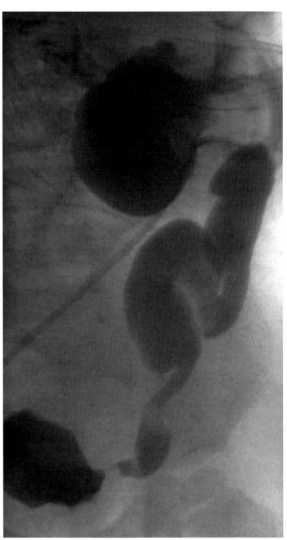

Fig. 66.2 MCUG showing left grade V vesicoureteric reflux into a dilated tortuous ureter. In this 4-week-old boy, no right kidney was identified on a subsequent CT scan

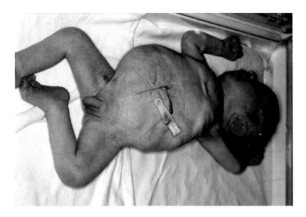

Fig. 66.1 Shrivelled prune–belly like appearance of the abdominal wall in a patient with prune–belly syndrome

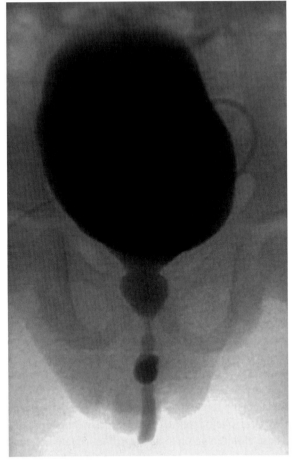

Fig. 66.3 Irregular bladder appearance with ill-defined bladder neck and enlarged prostatic urethra. No urethral obstruction was demonstrated in this 2-week-old infant

the voiding pattern may be different, it does not correlate with residual urine volume. The main compromise to voiding is usually secondary to the vesicoureteric reflux and poor bladder contractility. Changes in voiding efficiency are not unusual and mandate the need for regular urodynamic assessment. Surgical intervention or intermittent self-catheterization may be necessary to avoid further complications.

Urethral abnormalities such as wide prostatic urethra, narrow urogenital diaphragm, large prostatic utricle and prostatic hypoplasia may all cause a 'functional obstruction' to bladder outflow. The membranous and anterior urethra are sometimes atretic or extremely hypoplastic. Penile abnormalities include hypospadias, ventral and dorsal chordee and hypoplastic or absent corpora cavernosa. Ejaculation is possible, but often is retrograde due to the open bladder neck. In females, genital anomalies include bicornuate uterus, vaginal atresia, urogenital sinus and ambiguous genitalia.

66.4 Associated Anomalies

Anomalies other than the classical triad described above are seen in as many as 75% of children with prune belly syndrome. Severe pulmonary hypoplasia, with associated oligohydramnios and renal dysplasia, is incompatible with life, and is seen in as many as 20% of newborns. Pneumothorax, pneumomediastinum, chest wall deformities and chronic bronchitis are some of the other problems associated with these children.

Cardiac anomalies such as patent ductus arteriosus, atrial and ventricular septal defects, tetralogy of Fallot are seen in up to 10% of children with prune belly syndrome. Gastrointestinal anomalies are seen in up to 30% of these children and include malrotation, atresia, stenosis, anorectal malformations, exomphalus, gastroschisis and persistence of the embryonic wide mesentery with absent fixation to the posterior abdominal wall. Chronic constipation, secondary to poor abdominal wall pressure, needs constant attention in these children.

Orthopaedic problems are also very common and include congenital dislocation of the hips, lower limb problems secondary to oligohydramnios, talipes equinovarus, polydactyly, syndactyly and torticollis. Pectus carinatum, pectus excavatum and scoliosis are also commonly seen.

66.5 Antenatal Diagnosis

With improved quality of antenatal scans, major renal tract abnormalities are being diagnosed as early as in 11 weeks of gestation. However, differentiating between posterior urethral valve and prune belly syndrome could be difficult. Foetal vesicoamniotic shunts have been used in the hope of preventing renal parenchymal damage in children with enlarged bladder and upper renal tract dilatation in the past. However, studies have failed to document a beneficial effect of foetal intervention on subsequent renal function or pulmonary development.

66.6 Newborn Assessment and Investigations

The prune belly appearance of the abdominal wall together with bilateral undescended testes allows easy diagnosis of this condition in a newborn. When antenatal oligohydramnios is evident, pulmonary complications should be anticipated, and an immediate chest X-ray to exclude Pneumothorax and pneumomediastinum is necessary.

Initial creatinine measurements reflect maternal renal function and repetitive sampling is necessary. A serum creatinine >1.0 mg/dl in a term infant or >1.5 mg/dl in a preterm infant after 72 h indicates poor renal function, and poor overall outcome. On the other hand, if initial creatinine is < 0.7 mg/dl, then subsequent renal failure is unlikely. Urine should be checked for any infection and antibiotic prophylaxis to prevent urinary tract infection started. Renal ultrasound will provide information regarding kidneys, cortical thickness, renal tract dilatations, and bladder volume and post micturition residue. A micturating cystourethrogram (MCUG) will provide information regarding vesicoureteric reflux, and rare presence of posterior urethral valve. However, contrast medium should be sparingly used in the presence of poor renal function and impaired glomerular filtration rates to avoid rapid rise in serum osmolality and subsequent intraventricular haemorrhage. Mercaptoacetyltriglycine (MAG3) and Dimercaptosuccinic acid (DMSA) studies are requested as indicated to assess the differential renal filtration and drainage.

66.7 Management

Based on the severity of renal disease, patients with prune belly syndrome could be classified into three groups: Group 1 is characterized by oligohydramnios, pulmonary hypoplasia, possible urethral obstruction or patent urachus. These children also have very poor renal function and will usually die in the immediate postnatal period due to pulmonary complications. Aggressive surgical approach in these children should be avoided. Group 2 children have mild impairment of renal function and may progress to renal failure. During early infancy a cutaneous vesicostomy may improve drainage of urine and allow time for definitive reconstructive surgery later. Definitive surgery is better postponed till 1 year of age.

Group 3 consists of the majority of children with prune belly syndrome that has normal renal function and dilated renal tracts. Surgical intervention is not necessary, as long as the renal function is maintained and no infection is seen. When problems are encountered, an urodynamic study is needed to evaluate bladder emptying and unbalanced voiding. When deterioration is noted, these children should be managed as the children in group 2, with early vesicostomy.

Definitive surgery includes abdominoplasty, bilateral orchidopexies and suitable antireflux procedure around 1 year of age. The surgical management strategy should be tailored to suit individual cases. Surgical options include internal urethrotomy (when obstruction to outflow is evident on urodynamics study), ureteral tailoring and ureteric reimplantations, reduction cystoplasty with concomitant excision of a dilated urachal diverticulum, and or intermittent catheterisation. Approximately 30% of the long-term survivors will develop renal failure as a result of renal dysplasia, recurrent pyelonephritis or obstructive nephropathy. These children go on to have renal transplantation and reported to have a graft survival rate of 66.7% at 5 years. However, good bladder emptying must be achieved prior to transplantation to avoid significant risk of infection in the presence of immunosuppressant therapy.

Further Reading

Becker A, Baum M, Obstructive Uropathy, Early Human Development (2006)82:15–22.

Fusaro F, et al., Renal transplantation in prune-belly syndrome, Transpl Int (2004)17:549–552.

Hudson RG, Skoog SJ, Prune belly syndrome. In Canning DA, Khoury AE (Eds) Clinical Pediatric Urology, Informa Healthcare, London (2007), pp. 1081–1110.

Puri P, Miyakita H, Prune belly syndrome. In Puri P (Eds) Newborn Surgery, Arnold, London (2003), pp. 637–640.

Puri P, Höllwarth M (2006) Pediatric Surgery. Springer: Berlin, Heidelberg.

Conjoined Twins

67

Juan A. Tovar

Contents

67.1 Introduction

Conjoined twinning is an uncommon condition (1:100,000 live births) in which two genetically identical individuals are joined by a part of their anatomy and eventually share one or more organs. When confronted with one of these sets, pediatric surgeons face one of the most challenging situations in their specialty. This form of twinning raises many interesting issues that we shall try to address in order: history, embryonal mechanisms, anatomical varieties, imaging definition of the anatomy, ethical issues, technical aspects and results.

67.2 History

Since it is an obvious condition that often poses obstetric problems, it has been known from ancient times. Probably two-faced deities (Jano) or multiple-headed creatures (Hydra) were introduced into mythology after observation of such twins. There are pictures and carvings depicting conjoined twins in all cultures from the European, Asiatic, African and American continents. Some cases represented moral dilemmas and prompted risky definitions (for instance, how many souls they have) by religious authorities. One of the first descriptions of esophageal atresia was based on the autopsy of a set of conjoined twins. This condition became popular because the twins were often exhibited as freaks or circus attractions. This was the case of Chang and Eng Bunker, the original siamese twins, who were taken for this purpose from Siam to the US, where they eventually settled and lived for more that 50 years. Many examples have been publicized ever since and they are often reported particularly in the current media era.

P. Puri and M. Höllwarth (eds.), *Pediatric Surgery: Diagnosis and Management*,
DOI: 10.1007/978-3-540-69560-8_67, © Springer-Verlag Berlin Heidelberg 2009

Due to the complexity of the technical problems involved it is understandable for the first separations to be relatively recent (seventeenth century). However, many unsuccessful separations are never reported and the high mortality of this condition is still hidden in part.

67.3 Mechanisms

The only apparently possible mechanism for conjoined twinning is an early failure of the division of a primitive embryonal disk destined to produce identical, monozygotic, monochorionic, isosexual twins that share the same genome and the same fingerprints. The causes for this incomplete division are unknown but it is interesting that three quarters of these twins are females. It has been pointed out appropriately by R. Spencer, who produced a very complete monography on this subject, that the twins are always joined by central parts of their anatomies and never by their periphery. This author also pointed out that the twins are always homologous in the sense that they never have the head or the lower limbs on opposite sides. This suggests that the original mechanism is the missed cleavage of the primitive embryonal plate along the longitudinal axis.

Some ancient experiments in amphibians and a few modern molecular genetic observations suggest that fusion of two originally separated embryos may be the explanation for some rare cases in which there is genetic sex discordance and some asymmetric heteropagus that have to be otherwise interpreted as resulting form a partial atrophy of one of two originally symmetric joined individuals.

67.4 Classification

There are multiple classifications based on various criteria. Spencer proposed to divide them into ventrally and dorsally joined and to subdivide them within the groups according to the level of fusion. We preferred to adhere to a wider classification, which takes into

Table 67.1 Classification of conjoined twins

Asymmetric
fetus in feto
Acardius acephalus
Heteropagus
Symmetric
Craniopagus
Thoracopagus
Omphalopagus
Parapagus
Rachiopagus
Ischiopagus
Pygopagus

account their asymmetric or symmetric nature and the level of the fusion. This is in each case defined by the suffix *pagus* (Table 67.1).

Among the asymmetric twins we include the organoid teratomas and "**fetus in fetu**", the **acardius acephalus** and the **heteropagus** parasitic twins. The first ones are hardly ascribable to the family of conjoined twins and, except for some very "organoid" ones in which a more or less rudimentary spine is present; they are rather considered as teratomas. **Acardius acephalus** are connected by marginal placental vessels that allow the healthy twin (the *autositus*) to maintain circulation and feeding to the incomplete parasitic one, characteristically devoid of heart and head. When they come to term, only the *autositus* survives after umbilical cord division. However, prenatal diagnosis is possible nowadays and intrauterine coagulation of the umbilical vessels of the *parasitus* is an alternative to postnatal demise. **Heteropagus** twins (Fig. 67.1) are in general attached to the umbilical region of an anatomically normal *autositus* twin, without or with exomphalus, as organoid parasitic masses containing various organs and limbs unable to sustain independent circulation by them and therefore unviable if separated.

Symmetric conjoined twins may be joined by the head (**craniopagus**), the thorax (**thoracopagus**), the abdomen (**omphalopagus**), the spine (**rachiopagus**) or by the caudal pole (**ischiopagus** and **pygopagus**). Occasionally they are laterally fused along the body axis (**parapagus**) (Table 67.1).

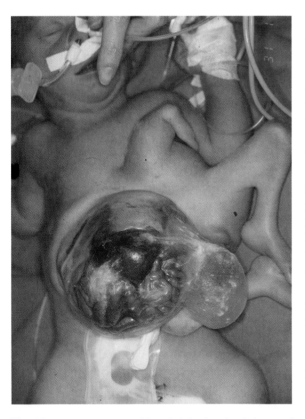

Fig. 67.1 Heteropagus parasitic twin joined to the abdomen of the autositus. Exomphalos is frequent in this particular form of conjoined twinning

67.5 Ethical Issues

Conjoined twinning is a unique situation in terms of ethical dilemmas. The usual principles that regulate our profession are particularly difficult to respect in these cases:

The principle of **autonomy** (we shall respect the decisions of the patient), that in pediatric surgical patients is usually exerted by proxy by the parents and only very rarely by others, may generate conflicts among parents, doctors or even the courts when unanimity regarding decisions is not reached. When unseparated twins come into adolescent or adult age, they may be involved in the conflict themselves (for instance, if only one would accept separation).

The principle of **justice** (similar chances for both patients) is obviously at risk when it comes to separation that may involve mutilation or sharing of organs.

The principles of **beneficiency** and **non-maleficiency** (we shall act on the benefit of our patients and we shall not harm them), that are considered as the ethical backbone of medical decision-making are also difficult to apply if separation is necessary for the survival of only one twin, if distribution of organs is uneven and if separation involves, as it is usually the case, loss of some functions that might be preserved without separation.

All these considerations are not philosophical but rather very down-to-earth. When separation of conjoined twins is considered, the patients are usually too young for deciding by themselves, the parents are heavily influenced by information delivered by doctors and the team involved is usually so large and often ethically discordant that keeping a unified line of decision becomes difficult. Acknowledgement of a strong moral leadership after open discussion of every issue is required before passing on to the parents information regarding the chances and the consequences of separation. In case of serious discrepancies among all participants in the process of decision, the courts might be involved.

Furthermore, the ethical difficulties may be seriously aggravated by broadcasting the information in the media (and this is rarely avoidable nowadays due to the large number of people involved in these cases). The twins and their family should be protected from the media and, if possible, the entire process of decision-making and even the separation should be kept in the shade. However, as we said, this is rarely, if ever, possible nowadays.

67.6 Imaging

Modern imaging considerably facilitates the understanding of the often unusual anatomy of these twins, which is necessary for planning separation strategies when possible, or to rule them out when unviable. Standard radiology, including plain X-rays, g.i. tract or urogenital contrast studies may depict the points of junction and other features of the corresponding organs but due to the atypical anatomy, they rarely produce a totally accurate picture of its details. Ultrasonography is used advantageously at every diagnostic stage. Angiography that was the only way of detecting the nature of the blood influx and outflow of the shared organs has been largely replaced in the last few years by MR angiography. MRI is the best way to depict the anatomy of the fused neural and meningeal tissues in the heads or spines of craniopagus, rachiopagus, ischiopagus, pygopagus or parapagus. It is also crucial for understanding the anatomy of conjoined hearts. Helical CT reconstruction of the bony junctions may be crucial for preparing surgical strategies. Nuclear imaging may help to define the functional anatomy of the liver, kidney or other organs.

However, the team facing separation of one of these sets must be prepared for unexpected anatomical surprises that may change the order or the nature of the participation of the different specialists involved. In most cases, the expected anatomy does not totally correspond with the surgical findings and a lot of ingenuity is often required for improvising solutions.

67.7 Technical Issues of Separation

When separation has been decided, it is very useful to schedule one or more meetings with scrub nurses, nurses, anesthesiologists and surgeons that may involve several specialties (general pediatric, orthopedic, plastic, urologic, neurologic and cardiovascular surgery). All technical aspects should be discussed and eventually rehearsed. Installing comfortably the set of twins on the table, skin prep and draping, moving one twin with the corresponding anesthetic equipment to another table for reconstruction after separation are problems to be solved according to a previously established pattern. The expected order and extent of the participation of each specialist team in the separation should be scheduled as well. The surgeon in charge of the direction of the operation acts as an orchestral conductor and his/her coordinating activity extends well beyond the end of the separation itself.

Anesthesia for separation is already a great challenge not only because of the obvious anatomical difficulties for intubation, insertion of lines and invasive monitoring but mainly because both twins are to a variable extent in a situation of cross-circulation in which they share more or less directly one single internal environment. The drugs administered to one pass on into the other one and biochemical and gas monitoring

may be confusing. It is a good policy to take the patients to the anesthetic or ICU area the day before surgery in order to perform these tasks that may last hours, without interfering with the already tightly scheduled surgical time.

Asymmetrical conjoined twins do not represent in general surgical challenges beyond those that are usual in our specialty and we are not going to address these in the present chapter.

The separation of **Craniopagus** is usually a difficult task given the complexity of the neural, arterial and venous connections involved. Modern imaging is particularly useful in these cases. Separation may be extremely difficult or even impossible. The final results depend to a great extent on the amount and nature of the brain tissue and the vascular network shared by the twins.

Separation of **Omphalopagus** twins involves variable difficulties depending on the extent of organ sharing (Fig. 67.2). These twins have more often fused livers and g.i. tracts. A small liver bridge without major vascular connections is relatively easy to take down but a large mass of anatomically atypical liver with wide arterial, venous and biliary connections may be a serious undertaking. Perioperative ultrasonography and parenchyme dividing devices used for liver resection are very useful for this purpose. The most common form of g.i. tract connection involves fusion of the small bowel from the upper jejunum down and divergence near the distal ileum. Separation consists in most cases of allocating half the available gut to each twin. Additional problems may be found when atresia of one of the tracts or a common cystic dilatation of the mid bowel are present.

Thoracopagus twins are rarely separable because sharing cardiac tissue makes the operation impossible in most cases (Fig. 67.3). Only when small atrial bridges exist, the operation can be realistically faced with all the facilities for cardiopulmonary bypass available. In addition, most of these twins have malformations of the connected hearts and the great vessels that may further complicate or preclude the separation. The aorta and the pulmonary arteries may be hypoplastic and the infradiaphragmatic aortas are often largely connected by thick trunks that compensate for other circulatory deficits. Only a few survivors after separation of thoracopagus with common cardiac tissue have been reported and most involve survival of only one of the twins. Of those who cannot be separated, most die

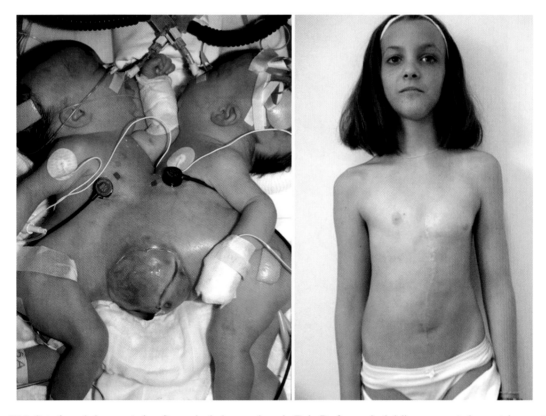

Fig. 67.2 Set of omphalopagus twins. Severe brain haemorrhage in Twin B after vaginal delivery prompted neonatal separation. Twin A survived

of the associated heart dysfunctions in the 1st months or years of life.

Rachiopagus, **Ischiopagus**, **Pygopagus** and **Parapagus** twins share to different extent parts of the spine, central nervous system, g.i. and g.u tracts and they may represent major challenges (Figs. 67.4 and 67.5). The separation of the bony parts requires highly skilled orthopedic surgeons. In some cases the reconstruction of the pelvic rim requires bilateral iliac osteotomies and pubic fixation. In some cases, even refashioning a bony pelvis is impossible and the subsequent prosthetic treatment is difficult. The spine has often some malformations at other levels, and scoliosis has to be taken into account during follow-up.

Neurosurgical separation may involve dividing a common spinal cord with reconstruction of the dural sacs on each side. Since fusion of neural tissue is usually distal, the motor and sensitive effects tend to be limited.

The distribution of a common lower g.i. tract between both twins entails the loss of continence for one or both of them. In frontally-united twins there is usually ileal confluence near the ileocecal valve and a single colon. The functional reconstruction of the pelvic organs is therefore rarely possible. Seldom the rectal function can be preserved in one twin but more often this is impossible and ostomies have to be fashioned at some stage. All refinements of advanced bowel management are necessary to obtain subsequent adaptation of these patients to a more or less normal life.

The same can be said about distributing the urogenital tract structures between the twins. Keeping a bladder and urethra for one twin is rarely possible in most frontally- united sets. Again all refinements of reconstructive urology, bladder augmentation, clean intermittent catheterization and continent urinary diversion may help to readapt these patients. The native genital tract can be reconstructed if duplicated but sometimes vaginal replacement is necessary.

One of the major technical problems posed by separation of conjoined twins is the coverage of the huge parietal defects left. When only one of the component

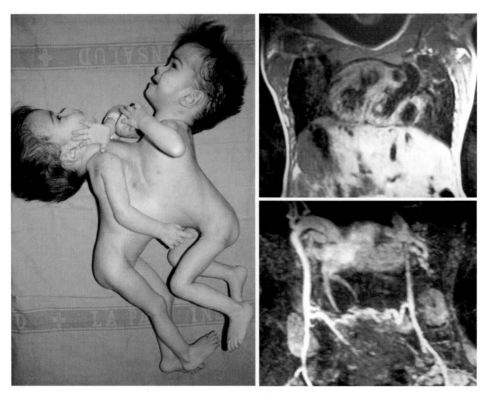

Fig. 67.3 Thoracopagus twins. They shared ventricular muscle as depicted in MRI. Angio MRI showed that, in addition, they had pulmonary stenoses, aortic stenosis (twin B) and a thick inf- radiaphragmatic arterial trunk connecting both aortas at that level. Separation was considered impossible

of the set survives, part of the wall of the other one can be used to bridge the defects but in other cases, all sorts of plastic procedures have to be put into practice. The skin can be expanded with subcutaneous expanders prior to separation. The use of synthetic patches may help but often they have to be inserted in contaminated operative fields that increase the risk of bacterial colonization and infection. Occasionally, vascularized musculo-cutaneous material from an extra limb can be used for coverage and this is very convenient.

67.8 Results

Mortality in conjoined twins is high. When diagnosis is firm in early pregnancy, interruption of gestation is common practice in developed countries particularly for the forms with bad prognosis. Fetal mortality or stillbirth is also frequent. Obstetric mortality or severe birth trauma remain a real risk when prenatal diagnosis has not been made and this happens more often in less sophisticated health environments in which pregnancies are not monitored. A considerable proportion of twins have multiple malformations that cause demise in the first hours or days of life. When separation is deemed possible, it must be reminded that neonatal operations involve higher mortality not only because they are better performed later when most anatomical and functional features of the set have been ascertained, but also because neonatal separation in the newborn period has often to be undertaken for life-threatening reasons (for instance, one twin may be very ill or develop intestinal obstruction).

Thoracopagus twins rarely survive because most have severe malformations in addition to the common heart. There are only a few reports of survival of one of the twins after separation and practically none of survival of both.

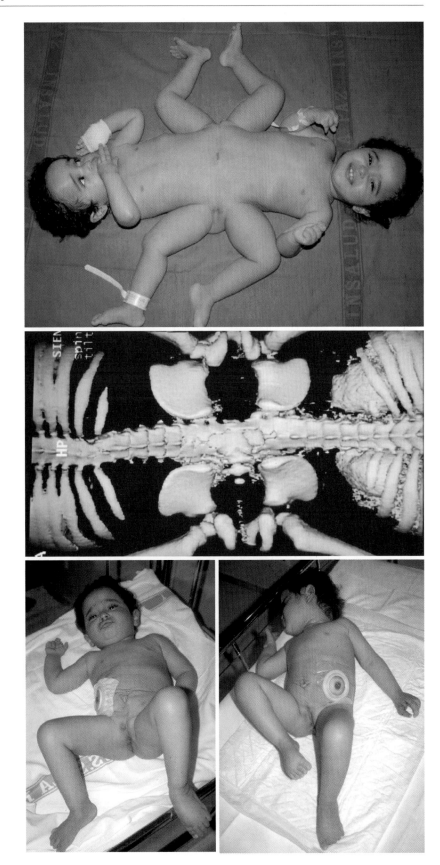

Fig. 67.4 Ischiopagus tetrapus (four legs) twins. The spines and the spinal cords were joined at the caudal end as shown by helicoidal CT reconstruction. During separation, the spines were divided, the meningeal sacs were reconstructed, a quadruple iliac osteotomy was performed for joining both pubic bones in each twin, the urogenital system was reconstructed and colostomies were fashioned. Both patients deambulate normally and enjoy relatively normal lives

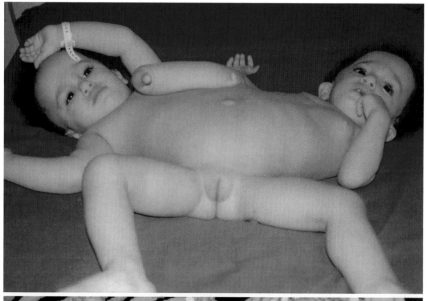

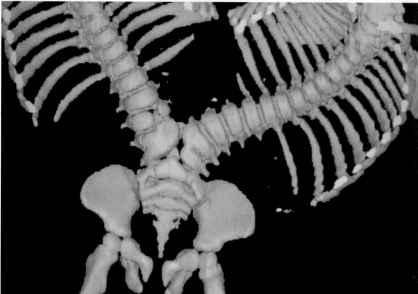

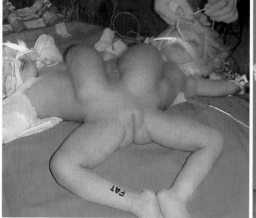

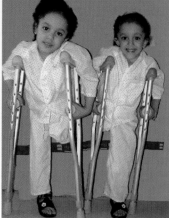

Fig. 67.5 Caudal parapagus twins with an extra thoracic limb irrigated from the abdominal aorta of twin A. Separation involved two surgical steps. First, the spinal cords and meningeal sacs were separated and subcutaneous expanders were inserted. Secondly, the sacrum, the g.i. and g.u. tracts were divided and the parietal defects were closed. In twin A the skin and muscle of the additional limb were used as a vascularized flap. In twin B a synthesis mesh was used for this purpose. Colostomies were fashioned. Both twins are able to deambulate with braces

Most omphalopagus twins can survive if no obstetric trauma or severe associated malformation are present. All other forms of conjoined twinning may allow survival of both twins but usually with more or less extensive deficits that require follow-up for life and often additional operations. Fecal and urinary continence problems become dominant with the passage of time and orthopedic and motor deficits may require prosthetic appliances.

It is particularly discouraging that the sophisticated medical and social environments in which these children have the better chances of maintaining good quality of life produce the minority of these cases probably because such pregnancies are terminated. In contrast, patients that come to separation are often from less privileged countries where they lack facilities for long term follow-up and all additional support including complementary operations, rehabilitation and social integration.

Separation of conjoined twins is a major test for the quality of pediatric surgical care. Only institutions in which the higher level of sophistication for all pediatric surgical subspecialties are available can undertake these operations with any chance of overall success.

Further Reading

Al Rabeeah A (2006) Conjoined twins—Past, present, and future. J Pediatr Surg 41:1000–1004

Annas GJ (2001) Conjoined twins—The limits of law at the limits of life. N Engl J Med 344:1104–1108

Cywes S, Millar AJ, Rode H, Brown RA (1997) Conjoined twins—The Cape Town experience. Pediatr Surg Int 12:234–248

Fieggen AG, Dunn RN, Pitcher RD, Millar AJ, Rode H, Peter JC (2004) Ischiopagus and pygopagus conjoined twins: Neurosurgical considerations. Childs Nerv Syst 20:640–651

Martinez L, Fernandez J, Pastor I, Garcia-Guereta L, Lassaletta L, Tovar JA (2003) The contribution of modern imaging to planning separation strategies in conjoined twins. Eur J Pediatr Surg 13:120–124

McHugh K, Kiely EM, Spitz L (2006) Imaging of conjoined twins. Pediatr Radiol 36:899–910

Pearn J (2001) Bioethical issues in caring for conjoined twins and their parents. Lancet 357:1968–1971

Puri P, Höllwarth ME (eds) (2006) Pediatric Surgery. Springer, Berlin, Heidelberg

Spitz L, Kiely E (2000) Success rate for surgery of conjoined twins. Lancet 356:1765

Vascular Anomalies

68

Emily Christison-Lagay and Steven J. Fishman

Contents

68.1 Introduction

Most vascular anomalies involve the skin, the largest, most visible organ of the body, and therefore are noted at birth. For centuries, vascular birthmarks were referred to by vernacular names derived from folk beliefs that a mother's emotions or patterns of ingestion could indelibly imprint her unborn fetus. The present day use of such terms as "cherry," "port wine stain," and "strawberry" can be referenced to this false doctrine of maternal impressions.[1] Virchow may be credited with the first effort to categorize vascular anomalies on the basis of histologic features, breaking them down into three principal categories: *angioma simplex*, *angioma cavernosum*, or *angioma racemosum*.[2] While these more formal terms attempted a more microanatomic-based classification of vascular lesions, the lack of specificity or identifying features perpetuated the confusion over vascular anomalies well into the late twentieth century. Today, vascular anomalies may be separated into two major categories: tumors and malformations. While this distinction is clinically and heuristically useful, there are some anomalies that appear to span both categories. Progress in understanding the biology and pathogenesis of these lesions will facilitate a more comprehensive molecular classification of this diverse collection in the future.

68.2 Hemangiomas and Other Vascular Tumors

68.2.1 Incidence

Hemangiomas represent the most common tumor of any type seen in infancy with a documented perinatal

P. Puri and M. Höllwarth (eds.), *Pediatric Surgery: Diagnosis and Management,*
DOI: 10.1007/978-3-540-69560-8_68, © Springer-Verlag Berlin Heidelberg 2009

incidence of 1.0–2.6% but increasing in incidence over the first year of life. They are speculated to affect 4–12% of Caucasian children. The incidence appears to be lower in Asian infants and is very low in children of African descent. Preterm infants with low birth weight (<1,000 g) have an increased incidence of hemangioma, possibly as high as 30%. A female to male ratio of 3:1 to 5:1 has been observed. There is no clear genetic tendency toward hemangioma formation. A family history can be elicited in approximately 10% of infants, and although studies have demonstrated no difference in the frequency of co-expression in monozygotic and dizygotic twins, a subset of patients with hemangiomas have been identified as having a missense mutation in the genes encoding vascular endothelial growth factor receptor-2 (VEGFR2) or tumor endothelial marker-8 (TEM8).

68.2.2 History and Physical Examination

Hemangiomas typically appear in the neonatal period, generally around the 1st or 2nd week of life. Approximately one third of hemangiomas are nascent at birth, presenting as a premonitory pink macular stain, pale spot, telangiectasia, or purplish ecchymotic patch. The typical cutaneous hemangioma permeates the dermis so that the skin becomes raised, bosselated, and vivid crimson in color. (Fig. 68.1) This knobby, scarlet appearance of the superficial hemangioma historically provided inspiration for its common name of "strawberry hemangioma." Deeper hemangiomas located in the lower dermis, subcutis, or muscle may present as raised bluish lesions with indistinct borders manifesting at 2–3 months of life or later.

In addition to the typical postnatal ("infantile") hemangioma, tumors, frequently referred to as *congenital hemangiomas*, evolve in utero and present fully-grown at birth. The hemangiomas can vary in appearance but are most commonly present as raised dome-like purple masses, often surrounded by a pale halo. Occasionally, a congenital hemangioma exhibits an area of central necrosis.

Hemangiomas are most commonly located in the head and neck region (60%), followed in frequency by the trunk (25%) and extremities (15%). Approximately 80% of hemangiomas are isolated to a single location,

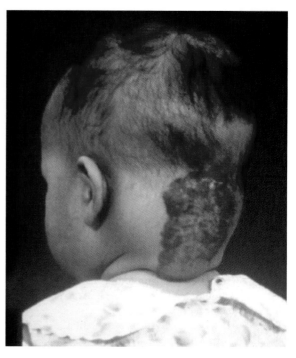

Fig. 68.1 Occipital hemangioma in a year old child. The center of the lesion has begun to involute into fibro-fatty tissue, while the borders are more indicative of proliferating endothelium

but nearly one fifth proliferate in multiple sites. Infants with multiple skin lesions may also have visceral organ involvement. Gastrointestinal hemangiomas may present with anemia or rectal bleeding. While most hepatic hemangiomas are probably clinically silent, a subset becomes symptomatic, manifesting as cardiac failure secondary to high volume shunting, hypothyroidism secondary to overproduction of type III iodothyronine deiodinase, fulminant hepatic failure, and/or abdominal compartment syndrome.

68.2.3 Clinical Course

Hemangiomas exhibit unique biologic behavior: they grow rapidly during the first 6–12 months of life (the *proliferative phase*), enter a second stage of growth proportionate with that of the child, and finally enter a phase of slow regression (*involuting phase*) lasting 1–7 years during which the endothelial matrix of hemangiomas is replaced by loose fibrous or fibro-fatty tissue.

Regression is complete in half of the children by age 5, in 70% of children by 7 years, and in the remainder by age 10–12 years. In the involuted phase, nearly normal skin is restored in approximately 50% of children. Otherwise, the involved skin is damaged with telangiectasias, crepe-like laxity, and yellowish discoloration or scarred patches. In rare cases, a large facial tumor can be associated with cartilaginous or bony overgrowth (presumably secondary to a local environment of increased blood flow) or produce a mass effect on the local facial skeleton.

Congenital hemangiomas, defined as a tumor present at birth, occur in two forms. The rapidly involuting congenital hemangioma (RICH) begins to regress during early infancy and is fully involuted by age 12–14 months. The noninvoluting congenital hemangioma (NICH) demonstrates proportional growth to that of the child and never undergoes regression. These tumors may be distinguished from the more common infantile hemangiomas by a variety of molecular and histopathologic markers.

68.2.4 Pathogenesis

Despite its overwhelming incidence, little is known about the pathogenesis of infantile hemangioma. Evidence supports the development of hemangiomas from clonal expansion of endothelial cells subject to either abnormal local cellular signals or an initial somatic mutation favoring rapid expansion. However, even the tissue of origin of these endothelial progenitors remains elusive. Some studies suggest that a population of resident angioblasts, arrested in an early stage of vascular development, give rise to these endothelial cells. A second theory suggests that these endothelial cells are derived from a distant population of endothelial precursors carried by existing vascular pathways to a receptive environment. One such possibility is the bone marrow; another suggested alternative is the placenta. A small embolic nidus of placental endothelial cells could reach fetal tissues through the permissive right to left shunt of fetal circulation. This could, in part, explain the threefold increased risk of hemangiomas observed in infants subjected in utero to chorionic villus sampling, as local placental injury might predispose the shedding of cells into the fetal circula-

tion. Moreover, at least five markers of hemangiomas are uniquely co-expressed in the placenta: GLUT1, merosin, Lewis Y antigen, Fcγ-RIIb, and type III iodothyronine deiodinase (DIO3). Recently, a comparison of the transcriptomes of human placenta and infantile hemangioma supported a placental origin of the tumor. This evidence would also support a common precursor cell of the placental and hemangioma endothelium. Recently, an animal model of hemangiomas has been developed using a population of hemangioma "stem cells". This model shares immunophenotypic characteristics with human hemangiomas and shows in vivo proliferation and involution. A placental stem cell with the same properties has yet to be identified and it remains possible that hemangioma and placenta share a common transcriptional profile but not a common ontogeny.

68.2.5 Associated Malformative Anomalies

Historical association of hemangiomas with a wide variety of syndromes is most likely secondary to miscategorization of another vascular lesion. However, certain true hemangiomas do occasionally occur in association with other malformations. A large cervicofacial hemangioma can be accompanied by ocular abnormalities (e.g. microphthalmia, congenital cataract, or optic nerve hypoplasia), sternal clefting, supraumbilical raphe, persistent intracranial and extracranial embryonic arteries, absence of ipsilateral carotid or vertebral vessels, coarctation of a right sided aortic arch, and Dandy-Walker cystic malformation or other posterior fossa malformations (PHACES syndrome). Lumbosacral hemangioma is one of several ectodermal lesions, such as hypertrichosis, capillary malformation (port-wine stain), achordoma, and sacral dimple that are known to signal underlying occult spinal dysraphism (e.g. lipomeningocele, tethered spinal cord). In patients with sacral hemangioma, ultrasound can be used to screen infants less than 4 months of age for occult spinal dysraphism, whereas MRI is usually necessary to identify spinal cord abnormalities in older children. Additionally there are rare reported incidences in which pelvic and perineal hemangioma is associated with urogenital and anorectal anomalies.

68.2.6 Differential Diagnosis

68.2.6.1 Kasabach-Merritt Phenomenon

In 1940, radiologist Kasabach and pediatrician Merritt reported a child with profound thrombocytopenia, petechiae, and bleeding in the presence of a "giant hemangioma." Only recently has it become known that persistent, profound thrombocytopenia is never associated with common hemangioma of infancy. Common infantile hemangioma markers Glut1 and Lewis Antigen Y are absent in the vascular tumors associated with Kasabach-Merritt phenomenon. Instead, the so-called Kasabach-Merritt phenomenon occurs with more invasive types of infantile vascular tumor like *kaposiform hemangioendothelioma* (KHE) or *tufted angioma* (TA). Both types of tumor are typically present at birth. Unlike infantile hemangioma, KHE and TA affect both genders equally, are unifocal, and generally involve the trunk, shoulder, thigh, or retroperitoneum. The overlying skin is deep red-purple in color, tense, and shiny (Fig. 68.2). Ecchymosis appears over and around the tumor in association with generalized petechiae and may falsely raise concern for child abuse. Thrombocytopenia unresponsive to platelet transfusion can be profound (<10,000 mm³), but coagulation values (partial thromboplastin time and prothrombin time) are normal to mildly elevated. The child with Kasabach-Merritt thrombocytopenia is at risk for intracranial, pleural-pulmonic, intraperitoneal, or gastrointestinal hemorrhage with an associated mortality of 20–30%. Diagnosis can be aided, if necessary, by MRI, which demonstrates enhanced signal on T2-weighted images and dilated feeding/drain vessels like other vascular tumors but, specific to KHE, demonstrates a poorly defined tumor margin with extension across tissues, prominent subcutaneous stranding and small vessels relative to tumor size. Histopathologic examination differs according to underlying cause. KHE demonstrates an aggressive cellular pattern of infiltrating sheets or nodules of slender epithelial cells, slit-like vascular spaces filled with hemosiderin and fragments of red blood cells, and coexistent dilated lymphatic spaces. TA, while macroscopically similar to KHE, is histologically composed of small tufts of capillaries (cannonballs) in the middle to lower dermis with lymphatics present at the periphery.

Several dermatologic entities of early infancy are sometimes confused with an infantile hemangioma. The *nevus flammeus neonatorum,* known by lay terms as "angel's kiss," "stork bite," or "salmon patch," is a non-evolving macular stain typically vanishing by the first year of life. A deep hemangioma can be confused with either a localized lymphatic or venous malformation causing the overlying skin to assume a bluish tinge with a few telangiectasias or draining veins. Diagnosis may be aided by palpation of the lesion: just as with a superficial hemangioma, those of the deeper tissues are rubbery in consistency. Venous and lymphatic malformations are usually quite soft and compressible unless intralesional bleeding or thrombosis has occurred. Hemangiomas can also imitate port-wine stains (capillary malformations) and the blush of silent arteriovenous malformations (AVMs).

Hemangiomas can be confused with another common cutaneous vascular tumor known as a *pyogenic granuloma*. These are small lesions rarely appearing before 6 months of age (average age 6.7 years). There is an association of pyogenic granulomas with port wine stains. The lesions grow rapidly, erupting through the skin on a stalk or pedicle. Epidermal breakdown with crusting is the norm associated with recurrent, often copious, bleeding. The best treatment is curettage or excision.

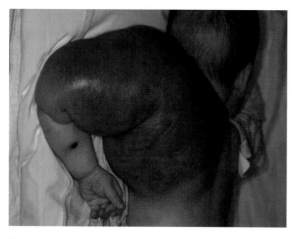

Fig. 68.2   An infant with kaposiform hemangioendothelioma involving the right arm, shoulder, and trunk. The overlying skin is crimson-purple and shiny with significant associated edema. A separate lesion lower in the forearm is not uncommon

68.2.7 Treatment

Most hemangiomas are small, regressing without need for cosmetic or therapeutic intervention. They should be allowed to undergo proliferation and involution under the careful observation by a pediatrician with gentle and sympathetic parental education and reassurance. Referral to a specialty center should occur in the event of equivocal diagnosis, dangerous location, large size, rapidity of growth, or potential for other complications.

Spontaneous epithelial breakdown, crusting, ulceration, and necrosis occur in 5% of cutaneous hemangiomas, and are most common in mucosal hemangiomas of the lips or anogenital region. Initial treatment should be the application of a petroleum based antibiotic salve along with viscous lidocaine to assist with pain control. If there is an eschar on the surface of the tumor, sharp debridement and wet-to-dry dressing changes are used to stimulate granulation tissue. Ulceration of larger than several millimeters is an indication for referral. Pharmacologic treatment with corticosteroid can accelerate healing and minimize recurrence. Flashlamp pulsed-dye laser is also reported to aid healing and alleviate pain. Total resection of an ulcerated hemangioma is often the most expedient treatment and should be considered if the resultant scar would be the same as if the regressing tumor were removed later in childhood.

Punctate bleeding can occasionally complicate a bosselated, protuberant hemangioma. Parents should be instructed to apply a full ten minutes of pressure to the area with a clean pad. In very rare instances, a suture is required for control of a local bleeding site.

68.2.7.1 Endangering Complications

The incidence of fatal or significantly morbid complications caused by hemangioma has been estimated at 10%. Such complications are most commonly localized to the cervicofacial region and may cause destruction, distortion, or obstruction. A large hemangioma can cause a mass effect and expansion of tissue. A periorbital hemangioma can block the visual axis and cause deprivation amblyopia or extend into the retrobulbar space causing ocular proptosis. Similarly, a hemangioma of the upper eyelid can distort the growing cornea, producing astigmatic amblyopia. Such cases should be referred for immediate evaluation by a pediatric ophthalmologist.

Even a small hemangioma can obstruct the subglottis; hence any cervical hemangioma should be treated with a high index of suspicion. Symptoms include hoarseness and, later, typically around 6–8 weeks of age, biphasic stridor and may be confused with croup. Approximately one half of these infants have cutaneous cervical hemangioma, often in the "beard distribution."

Other rare (approximately 1%) complications include high-output congestive heart failure in association with a hepatic hemangioma and gastrointestinal bleeding from mucosal hemangiomas of the bowel. Many GI hemangiomas may be symptomatically controlled with pharmacologic treatment, endoscopy, or surgery; however, large diffusely infiltrating hemangiomas may be unamenable to surgical resection and should be managed by transfusion, parenteral nutrition, and pharmacologic therapy to hasten involution. Hepatic hemangiomas may rarely present with high-output cardiac failure or massive hepatomegaly and abdominal compartment syndrome. Certain hepatic hemangiomas may also cause profound hypothyroidism due to the expression of a deiodinase that inactivates thyroid hormones. Infants with symptomatic hepatic hemangiomas should be referred to specialty centers. Pharmacologic therapy should be used to accelerate hemangioma regression, embolization may be employed to correct high-output arteriovenous or portohepatic shunting, and aggressive thyroid replacement therapy should be instituted in those infants with documented hypothyroidism. In rare cases, liver transplantation may be indicated.

68.2.7.2 Pharmacologic Therapy

Small, well-localized cutaneous or mucosal hemangiomas in critical locations may be considered for intralesional injection of corticosteroid. Systemic therapy using oral prednisolone (2–3 mg/kg/day) is favored as a first line of treatment of large, problematic, or life-threatening hemangiomas. For an acute situation, such as an upper airway constriction, an equivalent dose of intravenous corticosteroid may result in a rapid involution of a sensitive tumor. Most hemangiomas demonstrate accelerated regression in response to corticosteroids, some have stabilized growth, and few demonstrate no response at all. Signs of responsiveness occur within several days to 1 week after initiation of the treatment and include a diminished rate of growth, fading color, and softening of the tumor.

Until recently, recombinant interferon alpha (IFNα-2a or 2b) had been considered a second-line agent for endangering or life-threatening hemangiomas after failure of or contraindication to corticosteroid treatment. However, toxicity has significantly curtailed its use. Complications and side effects include a low-grade fever, reversible elevation in hepatic transaminases, transient neutropenia, and anemia. The most concerning toxicity with the use of interferon is the idiopathic occurrence of spastic diplegia, with an incidence estimated at 5–15%. Children should be followed closely with neurologic examinations and IFN discontinued if the long-tract signs appear. Spastic diplegia generally improves after discontinuation of the drug.

Vincristine has been effective in some children unresponsive to interferon and is now chosen by some practitioners as the second line agent after corticosteroids for both hemangioma and kaposiform hemangioendothelioma (KHE). In managing thrombocytopenia associated with KHE, platelet transfusion should be avoided unless there is active bleeding or a planned surgical procedure and heparin should not be administered because it can stimulate tumor growth and aggravate platelet trapping.

68.2.7.3 Laser Therapy

Although there is widespread interest in the application of laser technology to the treatment of hemangiomas, true indications for its use are relatively few. Flashlamp pulsed dye laser only penetrates 0.75–1.2 mm into the dermis, typically affecting only a superficial portion of a hemangioma. This does result in lighting of its surface color, but does not affect its subsequent proliferation. Small, flat lesions can be successfully treated, but these very same lesions would regress naturally to leave little or no scar. Moreover, overzealous use of the laser can result in ulceration, partial-thickness, skin loss and consequent scarring. Two well-accepted indications for laser use are the obliteration of telangiectasias, which persist into the involuting/involuted phase of hemangioma growth and reduction of a unilateral subglottic hemangioma with a continuous-wave carbon dioxide laser.

68.2.7.4 Surgical Therapy

Surgical excision of a hemangioma may be indicated in any stage of its life cycle. A well-localized, pedunculated hemangioma, particularly one demonstrating ulceration or subject to recurrent episodes of bleeding, may be removed early in infancy during the tumor's proliferative phase. Similarly, problematic hemangiomas of the upper eyelid which do not respond to corticosteroid therapy should be considered for surgical excision to prevent the attendant changes in vision. Focal or multifocal GI hemangiomas which persist in bleeding despite pharmacotherapy may be considered for removal, although one cannot always assume that an endoscopically visualized lesion is the only source for bleeding.

As children progress through their preschool years and develop a sense of physical awareness, consideration should be given to staged or total excision of a large or protuberant involuting phase hemangioma, if the lesion risks significantly compromising the child's body image. Most commonly, it is preferred to wait until late childhood to remove the hemangiomatous residuum of the involuted phase. Protrusive hemangiomas frequently leave in their wake unsightly expanded skin and fibrofatty tissue. Staged resection is often indicated to minimize distortion and recreate a cosmetically acceptable outcome.

68.3   Vascular Malformations

Vascular malformations are localized or diffused errors of embryonic development which may affect any segment of the vascular tree including arterial, venous, capillary, and lymphatic vessels. It is useful to subcategorize vascular malformations on the predominant type of channel abnormality and flow characteristics. According to this distinction, two major categories exist: (1) slow-flow anomalies (capillary malformations, lymphatic malformations, and venous malformations) and (2) fast-flow anomalies (arterial malformations [e.g. aneurysm, coarctation, ectasia, and stenosis], AVMs, and arteriovenous fistulas). Complex, combined vascular malformations also exist including slow-flow (capillary-lymphatic [CLM], capillary-lymphaticovenous [CLVM], and lymphaticovenous [LVM]) malformations and fast-slow (capillary-lymphatic AVMs [CLAVMs] and capillary-lymphatic AVFs [CLAVFs]).

Congenital vascular malformations are present in approximately 1.2–1.5%, making them a relatively common defect in embryogenesis. Most vascular malformations are sporadic (i.e. nonfamilial), but some exhibit classic Mendelian inheritance. While much of the pathogenesis of vascular malformations remains unelucidated, recent strides have been made in understanding the development of the blood vascular and lymphatic systems opening the door for greater insight into observed aberrancies.

68.3.1 Capillary Malformation

Still commonly referred to as port-wine or claret stains, capillary malformations (CMs) are dermal vascular anomalies that are reported to occur in 0.3% of newborns with an even gender distribution (Fig. 68.3). They can be localized or extensive, occurring anywhere on the body but are rarely multiple. CM must be differentiated from the fading macular stain *nevus flammeus neonatorum*, the most common vascular birthmark. These latter represent a minor transient dilation of dermal vessels and must be relabeled if they persist into childhood. CMs are composed of dilated,

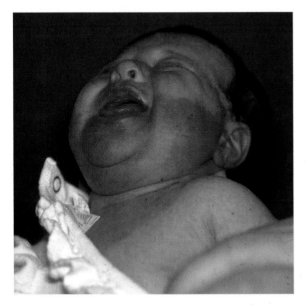

Fig. 68.3 Capillary malformation on a young infant. Facial lesions can darken with age and the skin can become thickened and cobblestoned

ectatic capillary-to-venule sized vessels in the superficial dermis. Immunohistochemical studies demonstrate normal endothelial and smooth muscle cell morphology and mitotic index, but a paucity of surrounding normal nerve fibers. With age, the vessels gradually dilate, probably accounting for the darkening color and tendency to nodular ectasias. Although CMs are usually sporadic, a familial pattern of autosomal dominant inheritance with incomplete penetration has been reported.

CMs are often associated with hypertrophy of the soft tissue and underlying skeleton. They can also signal underlying structural abnormality. A midline occipital CM can overlie an encephalocele or ectopic meninges. A CM over the cervical or lumbosacral spine can be a clue to occult spinal dysraphism. A child with a CM of the first or first-second trigeminal nerve distribution should be evaluated for Sturge-Weber syndrome, an associated vascular anomaly of the ipsilateral choroid and leptomeninges with clinical manifestations of seizures, contralateral hemiplegia, and variable developmental motor and cognitive delay. Choroid involvement leads to increased risk for retinal detachment, glaucoma, and blindness. Fundoscopic examination and tonometry are essential and should be performed twice annually for 2 years and yearly thereafter for life. Early diagnosis can be suggested by MRI demonstrating pial vascular enhancement. Angiographic findings include parenchymal blush and apparent cortical venous occlusions and collaterals. Other syndromes associated with capillary malformation include Klippel-Trenaunay syndrome, a combined slow-flow CLVM with axial elongation and overgrowth in girth involving one or more extremities, and Parkes Weber syndrome, a fast-flow vascular anomaly comprised of a capillary stain with AVM or AVFs of a limb. While the cause of most CMs remains idiopathic, a mutation in the gene RA5AI is associated with hereditary CMs, sometimes in combination with arteriovenous malformations.

Flashlamp pulsed dye laser is currently the treatment of choice for selective photothermolysis of CM. The optimal timing is controversial. In general, significant lightening is observed in approximately 70% of patients with better outcomes observed on the face than on the trunk and limbs. Soft tissue and skeletal hypertrophy require surgical strategies. Children with Sturge-Weber syndrome and seizures refractory to pharmacologic treatment may require neurosurgical resection of the involved brain.

68.3.2 Telangiectasias

Tiny acquired capillary vascular marks, commonly known as spider nevus or spider telangiectasis typically appear on children in the preschool and school-aged years. Epidemiological studies suggest they may be present in nearly half of all children with an equal gender distribution. Spontaneous disappearance is possible, but pulsed dye laser successfully removes the lesion.

Cutaneous marbling of the skin of Caucasian infants placed at a low temperature, so-called, *cutis marmorata* or *livido reticularis* is an accentuated pattern of normal cutaneous vascularity which improves with age as the skin thickens. In one rare congenital pathologic disorder, the newborn has a distinctive deep purple, serpiginous, and reticulated vascular staining pattern, called *cutis marmorata telangiectatica congenital*. This vascular birthmark occurs in a localized, segmental distribution, usually involving the trunk and extremities. Neonatal ulceration of the depressed purple areas can occur; sometimes there is hypoplasia of the affected limb and subcutaneous tissues. Almost all infants with cutis marmorata telangiectatica congenital demonstrate steady improvement during the first year of life. In time, venous dilation becomes more prominent and persists into adulthood, together with residual cutaneous atrophy and staining.

Hereditary hemorrhagic telangiectasia (HHT; Rendu-Osler-Weber syndrome) is an autosomal dominant disorder with high penetrance and an age-dependent phenotype estimated to occur at a frequency of 1–2 per 100,000 Caucasian populations. Patients with HHT have mucocutaneous telangiectasias, cerebral and pulmonary AVMs, and hepatic vascular anomalies. Two causative genes (HHT1 and ACLVRL1) have been identified; both are associated with loss of function of TGF-β.

Ataxia-telangiectasia (Louis-Bar syndrome) is an autosomal recessive neurovascular disorder that appears at 3–6 years of life. Bright-red telangiectasias are first noted on the nasal and temporal area of the bulbar conjunctiva and subsequently manifest on the face, neck, upper chest, and flexor surfaces of the forearms. Cerebellar ataxia begins nearly synchronously followed by progressive motor neuron dysfunction. Endocrine

and immunologic deficiencies become manifest and death usually occurs in the second decade from recurrent sinopulmonary infections or from lymphoreticular malignancy. The defective gene (ATM) is believed to cause abnormalities in DNA repair, as its primary function is to detect double-stranded breaks.

68.3.3 Lymphatic Malformation

Historically termed *lymphangioma* or *cystic hygroma*, slow-flow vascular anomalies of the lymphatic system consist of localized or diffuse malformations of lymphatic channels best characterized as *microcystic, macrocystic* or both. Lymphatic malformations (LMs) most commonly appear as ballotable masses with normal overlying skin, although a blue hue may result if large underlying cysts are present (Fig. 68.4). Less common dermal involvement is manifest as puckering or deep cutaneous dimpling. LMs in the subcutis or submucosa manifest as tiny vesicles. Intravesicular bleeding is evidenced by tiny, dark-red dome-shaped nodules.

Prenatal ultrasound can detect macrocystic LM in the late first trimester. Those LMs not diagnosed prenatally are generally evident at birth or before 2 years of age; however, occasionally they can manifest suddenly in older children and adults. Radiologic documentation is best performed by MRI, although ultrasound is a useful auxiliary agent to confirm the presence of macrocystic LM. Although conventional

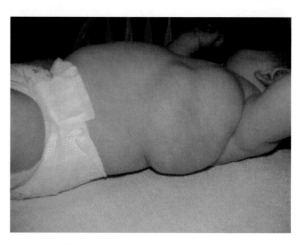

Fig. 68.4 Truncal lymphatic mutation on an infant. In this instance the overlying skin is unaffected and the malformation presents as a soft, ballotable mass

contrast lymphangiography is rarely performed, it may be useful for determining the precise location of lymphatic or chylous leaks in a patient with a diffuse thoracic lymphatic anomaly.

LMs are most commonly located in the axilla/chest, cervicofacial region (70–80%), mediastinum, retroperitoneum, buttock, and anogenital areas. Facial LM is the most common basis for macrocheilia, macroglossia, macrotia, and macromala. Cervicofacial LM is associated with the overgrowth of the mandibular body, causing an open bite and underbite. LMs in the floor of the mouth and tongue are characterized by vesicles, intermittent swelling, bleeding, and the possibility of oropharyngeal obstruction. Cervical LMs involve the supraglottic airway and tracheostomy may be necessary early in infancy. Diffuse thoracic lymphatic anomalies or rare abnormalities of the thoracic duct or cisterna chylii can manifest as recurrent pleural and pericardial chylous effusion or chylous ascites. Anomalous lymphatics in the GI tract can cause hypoalbuminemia as the result of chronic protein-losing enteropathy. LMs in an extremity cause diffuse or localized swelling or gigantism with both soft tissue and skeletal overgrowth. Progressive osteolysis, caused by diffuse soft tissue and skeletal LM, is called *Gorham-Stout syndrome* and is known also as "disappearing bone disease" or "phantom bone disease."

Lymphedema should also be included as a type of LM. Type I hereditary lymphedema (*Milroy disease*) is an autosomal dominant disorder presenting early in life with localized areas of edema. The initial superficial lymphatics of these areas are thought to be hypoplastic or absent, although superficial lymphatics are observed in non-edematous areas. Type II hereditary lymphedema (*Meige disease*) is a late-onset autosomal dominant disorder with variable penetrance and phenotype. Associated features include distichiasis (a double row of eyelashes), ptosis, cleft palate, yellow nails and congenital heart disease. The disorder is thought to arise from an impairment of lymphatic drainage and lymphoscintigraphy demonstrates numerous dilated lymphatic vessels.

68.3.3.1 Treatment

The two main complications of LMs are intralesional bleeding and infection. Bleeding, spontaneous or the result of local trauma, causes rapid, painful enlargement of an LM. The LM becomes firm and ecchymotic. Analgesia, rest and time are generally sufficient. Hemorrhage and infection can transform a macrocystic lesion into a microcystic and scarred lesion.

LMs often swell in the event of a viral or bacterial infection. Most often this is a harmless event likely related to change in lymphatic flow. Bacterial cellulitis, however, is a more dangerous condition. Prolonged intravenous antibiotic therapy is frequently indicated, with choice of antibiotic agents based upon the presumptive pathogens of the affected area.

The two strategies for treating lymphatic anomalies are sclerotherapy and surgical resection. Sclerotherapy works through obliteration of the lymphatic lumen by endothelial destruction with subsequent sclerosis/fibrosis. Success depends upon the sclerotic agent selected and the damage inflicted upon the endothelial and deeper muscular and connective tissue layers. Macrocystic LM is more likely than microcystic tissue to shrink after an injection of sclerosant. Ethanol is widely considered to be the most effective sclerosing agent for low flow malformations. Injection is quite painful, often requiring general anesthesia and subsequent pharmacologic pain relief. Edema following sclerosant injection is associated with prolonged recovery and increased therapeutic effect. Side effects include local necrosis and blistering as well as local neuropathy. Systemic absorption of ethanol may lead to cardiac arrest, pulmonary vasoconstriction, or systemic hypotension. Other sclerosant agents include doxycycline, sodium tetradecyl sulfate and OK-432.

Resection is the only way to potentially "cure" LM. Often staged excision is necessary and total excision is often possible. In each resection a surgeon should focus on a defined anatomic region, attempt to limit blood loss, perform as thorough a dissection as possible and to be prepared to operate as long as necessary. Even with such an intensive approach to resection, the "recurrence" rate is reported to be 40% after an incomplete excision and 17% after a macroscopically complete excision.

68.3.4 *Venous Malformation*

Venous malformations are the most common of all vascular anomalies and are frequently misdiagnosed as hemangiomas or mislabeled "cavernous hemangiomas." While present at birth, they are not always immediately evident. The typical description of a VM is of a blue, soft, and compressible mass (Fig. 68.5). VM can vary greatly in size, shape, and degree of associated deformation. Venous malformations demonstrate proportional growth with the growth of the child. Histologically, VMs are composed of thin-walled, dilated, sponge-like abnormal channels. The normal architecture of vascular smooth muscle is distorted into clumps. This mural muscular abnormality is likely responsible for the tendency of VMs toward gradual expansion. Microscopy often reveals evidence of clot formation, fibrovascular ingrowth and phleboliths. Phlebothrombosis is common and can be painful.

Most VMs are solitary, but multiple cutaneous or visceral lesions can occur. There are well-documented pedigrees of familial, usually multifocal, VMs. *Blue-rubber bleb nevus syndrome* is a rare, sporadic disorder composed of cutaneous and gastrointestinal VMs. It is the most common vascular anomaly causing chronic gastrointestinal bleeding. Cutaneous lesions can occur anywhere on the body, but there is a predilection for the trunk, palms, and soles of the feet. The lesions increase in size and become more apparent with age. Gastrointestinal lesions are located throughout the GI tract but are most frequently located in the small bowel (Fig. 68.6). In addition to bleeding, these lesions can provide a lead point for intussusception or volvulus.

Complications of venous malformations depend upon their location. VMs of the head and neck can cause progressive distortion of facial features, exophthalmia, dental malalignment, and obstructive sleep apnea. VMs of the extremities can cause limb length discrepancies, painful hemarthrosis, and degenerative arthritis. Intraosseous VMs can cause structural weakening of the bone shaft and pathologic fracture. VMs of the gastrointestinal

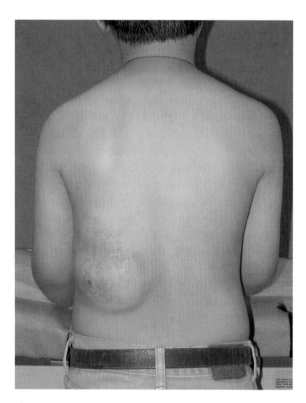

Fig. 68.5 Characteristic venous malformation on the back of a school age boy. Dilated venous channels contribute to a pale blue appearance. The lesion itself is soft and compressible

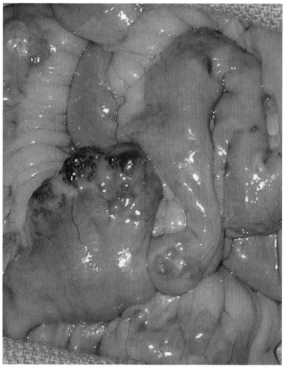

Fig. 68.6 Intraoperative findings in a patient with blue-rubber bleb nevus syndrome. Hundreds of millimeter to multi-centimeter sized lesions throughout the small and large bowel and mesentery can be responsible for gastrointestinal hemorrhage. Treatment is surgical resection of all lesions which, though laborious, typically eliminates the need for subsequent blood transfusion

tract can manifest with chronic bleeding and anemia. While VMs may be localized throughout the length of the bowel, they are most commonly found encompassing the entire left colon and rectum and surrounding pelvic and retroperitoneal structures. Lesions that involve the foregut can be associated with central mesenteric and portal venous anomalies.

Like other vascular malformations, venous malformations are best imaged by MRI which demonstrates T2 enhancement and differ from lymphatic slow flow lesions by the presence of contrast enhancement of the vascular spaces.

68.3.4.1 Treatment

As with lymphatic malformations, the mainstay of therapy for venous malformations is sclerotherapy and surgical resection. For small cutaneous or oromucosal VMs, injection with 1–3% sodium tetradecyl sulfate is often successful. Ethanol is also used as described for lymphatic malformations. Venous anomalies have a propensity for recanalization and recurrence. Excision of a VM is usually successful for small, well localized lesions. In some locations, staged subtotal surgical removal can be accomplished without preoperative sclerotherapy. However, sclerotherapy may be used as a first line approach to attempt to shrink the VM prior to surgical resection. Complete resection of large, focal GI VMs is often necessary because of chronic bleeding, anemia, and transfusion dependence. Multifocal GI lesions are best treated by multiple excisions (sometimes numbering in the hundreds). Bowel resections should be minimized and used only in segments in which there is a high density of VMs.

Diffuse VMs of the colo-rectum and surrounding pelvic structures can be left alone if bleeding does not necessitate blood transfusions. When bleeding is more severe, control may occasionally be established with sclerotherapy. The definitive surgical alternatives are to divert the fecal stream by colostomy, or, preferably, to perform a colectomy with endorectal mucosectomy and coloanal endorectal pull-through. This procedure entails a risk of pulmonary embolism because of the manipulation of abnormal pelvic veins.

Elastic support stockings are indispensable in the treatment of venous malformation of the extremity. Additionally, low dose aspirin (81 mg/day or every other day) helps to minimize phlebothromboses.

68.3.5 Arteriovenous Malformations

Most often arteriovenous malformations are latent during infancy and childhood and expand during adolescence manifesting as a warm, pink patch in the skin and an underlying thrill or bruit. Later, cutaneous consequences may include ischemic changes, ulceration, pain and intermittent bleeding (Fig. 68.7). The hormonal changes of puberty or local trauma seem to trigger expansion. Nonetheless, there are rare examples of an AVM or AVF presenting at birth with life-threatening high-output heart failure. The natural history of AVMs can be documented by a clinical staging system introduced by Schobinger (Table 68.1). Like other vas-

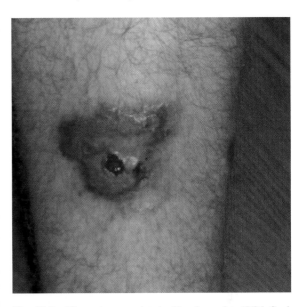

Fig. 68.7 Ulceration associated with a lower leg AVM. Such lesions can be quite painful and, due to their high flow, present with difficult to control bleeding

Table 68.1 Schobinger clinical staging system for AVMs

Stage	Description
I (Quiescence)	Pink-bluish stain, warmth and arteriovascular shunting by continuous Doppler scanning or 20 MHz color Doppler Scanning
II (Expansion)	Same as stage I plus enlargement, pulsations, thrill, bruit, and tortuous/tense veins
III (Destruction)	Same as stage II plus either dystrophic skin changes, ulceration, bleeding, persistent pain, or tissue necrosis
IV (Decompensation)	Same as stage III plus cardiac failure

cular malformations, AVMs are best imaged by MRI and MRA.

68.3.5.1 Treatment

Prompt embolization may be necessary in the uncommon occurrence of postnatal congestive heart failure caused by an AVF or AVM. Treatment is rarely indicated during infancy or early childhood for a quiescent (stage I) AVM, however the child should be re-examined annually for signs of expansion. Conventional dogma dictates that intervention should be delayed until there are symptoms or endangering signs (e.g. recurrent ulceration refractory to treatment, pain, bleeding, increased cardiac output or Schobinger stage III-IV). Ligation or proximal embolization of feeding vessels should never be attempted as it causes the rapid recruitment of flow from nearby arteries to supply the malformation. Rather, the usual strategy is arterial embolization for the temporary occlusion of the nidus 24–72 h prior to surgical resection. If the arteries are tortuous or if the feeding arteries have been ligated, sclerotherapy may play a role in conjunction with local arterial and venous occlusion. Whenever possible, the lesion should be resected completely. Extensive preoperative planning is often necessary to determine the exact extent of resection necessary. Intraoperative frozen sectioning of the resection margins can be helpful, but the most accurate way to determine whether resection is complete is by observation of the pattern of bleeding from the wound edges. Unfortunately, many AVMs are not localized and may permeate throughout the deep craniofacial structures or the soft and/or skeletal tissues of an extremity. In these instances, embolization is usually palliative and surgical resection is rarely indicated.

68.3.6 Combined (Eponymous) Vascular Malformations

Combined (or complex) vascular malformations are associated with the overgrowth of soft tissue and the skeleton. Many are named after the physicians who are credited with the most memorable description of the condition.

68.3.6.1 Slow-Flow Anomalies

Klippel-Trenaunay syndrome is a well described combined CLVM associated with soft tissue and skeletal hypertrophy of a limb or trunk. Bilaterality is not uncommon. The capillary malformations are multiple and typically arranged in a geographic pattern over the lateral side of the extremity, buttock, and/or thorax (Fig. 68.8). The CM component is macular in the newborn but becomes studded with lymphatic vesicles as the child ages. Anomalous lateral veins become prominent because of incompetent valves and deep venous abnormalities. Lymphatic hypoplasia is present in more than 50% of patients with associated lymphedema or isolated lymphatic microcysts. Thrombophlebitis occurs in 20–45% of patients and pulmonary embolism can occur. Management is fundamentally conservative.

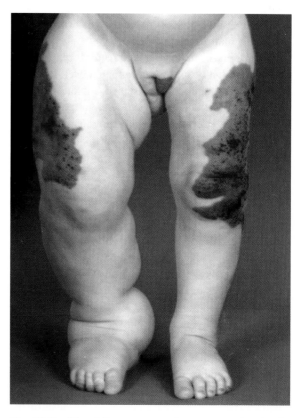

Fig. 68.8 Klippel-Trenaunay syndrome presenting in the bilateral lower extremities of a young child. Note the lateral CMs with vesicular studding. Medially the bluish hues of the venolymphatic component are apparent. Lymphedema is present bilaterally, but is more marked in the right lower extremity and associated with foot deformity

Children should be seen annually and limb length followed by serial radiographs. If a limb length discrepancy of greater than 1.5 cm develops, a shoe-lift is prescribed to prevent limping and secondary scoliosis. Elastic compression stockings are recommended. Grotesque enlargement of the foot requires selective ablative procedures (i.e. ray, midfoot, or Syme amputation) to allow the child to wear proper footwear. In selected patients, sclerotherapy can be used to obliterate incompetent superficial veins and to shrink focal VMs or lymphatic cysts. Debulking procedures can be very effective in selected patients. Laser photocoagulation or injection with 1% sodium tetradecyl sulfate can provide temporary control over intermittent lymphatic oozing or bleeding from the lymphatic vesicles.

Proteus syndrome is a sporadic vascular, skeletal, and soft tissue disorder of asymmetric overgrowth and gigantism. Its salient clinical features include verrucous nevus, lipomas and lipomatosis, macrocephaly, asymmetric limbs with partial gigantism of the hands and feet or both, and cerebriform plantar thickening ("moccasin" feet). It has been suggested that Joseph Merrick, the unfortunately entitled "Elephant Man" suffered from Proteus syndrome.

Maffucci syndrome, a variant of *Ollier's disease*, is a low flow malformation of exophytic vascular anomalies associated with multiple enchondromas and bony exostoses. The children appear normal at birth with osseous lesions becoming manifest as small nodules on a finger or toe during childhood and the vascular lesions appearing later. The vascular anomalies are predominantly venous and occur in the subcutaneous tissue and bones of the extremities. Early recognition is important as greater than half of these patients develop spindle cell tumors with potential for malignant transformation into chondrosarcoma.

68.3.6.2 Fast-Flow Anomalies

The *Parkes Weber syndrome* shares many similarities with Klippel-Trenaunay syndrome, but should be distinguished by a component of an additional capillary-arteriovenous malformation/fistula. The lesions are obvious at birth and the involved, asymmetrically enlarged limb is covered by a geographic pink, warm, macular stain with an underlying bruit or thrill. There may be associated lymphatic abnormalities. Large lesions may be associated with high output cardiac failure. MRI/MRA complemented by angiography is important for diagnosis and anatomic delineation.

68.4 Conclusions

The last two decades have witnessed remarkable forays into understanding the pathogenesis of vascular anomalies. Improved definitions based upon this genetic-anatomic-histologic classification have allowed the development of multidisciplinary approaches toward disease treatment and management. As our appreciation of the embryonic and developmental contributions to disease increases, so does our ability to develop novel strategies for management of previously insurmountably complex lesions. Molecular and pharmacologic manipulation of vascular anomalies holds great promise.

Further Reading

Boon LM, Enjolras O, Mulliken JB (1996) Congenital hemangioma: Evidence of accelerated involution. J Pediatr 128:329–335

Christison-Lagay ER, Burrows PE, Alomari A et al (2007) Hepatic Hemangiomas: Subtype classification and development of a clinical practice algorithm and registry. J Pediatr Surg 42:62–68

Dadras SS, North PE et al (2004) Infantile Hemangiomas: Are arrested in the early development vascular differentiation state. Mod Pathol 17:1068–1079

Finn MC, Glowacki J, Mulliken JB (1983) Congenital vascular lesions: Clinical application of a new classification. J Pediatr Surg 18:894–900

Fishman SJ, Burrows PE, Leichtner AM, Mulliken JB (1998) Gastrointestinal manifestations of vascular anomalies in childhood. J Pediatr Surg 33:1163–1167

Fishman SJ, Burrows PE, Upton J, Hendren H (2001) Life-threatening anomalies of the thoracic duct: Anatomic delineation dictates management. J Pediatr Surg 36(8): 1269–1272

Fishman SJ, Smithers CJ Folkman J et al (2005) Blue rubber bleb nevua syndrome: Surgical eradication of gastrointestinal bleeding. Ann Surg 241(3):523–528

Mulliken JB, Young AE (1988) Vascular Birthmarks: Hemangiomas and Malformations. W.B. Saunders, Philadelphia

Puig S, Casati B et al (2005) Vascular low-flow malformations in children: Current concepts for classification, diagnosis and therapy. Eur J Radiol 53:35–45

Puri P, Höllwarth M (2006) Pediatric Surgery. Springer, Berlin, Heidelberg

Van der Horst CMAM, Koster PHL et al (1998) Effect of the timing of treatment of port-wine stains with the flash lamp pulsed dye laser. New Engl J Med 338:1028–1033

Congenital Nevi

69

Alexander Margulis, Julia F. Corcoran and Bruce S. Bauer

Contents

69.1 Introduction

Congenital melanocytic nevi (CMN) are composed of clusters of nevo-melanocytes that are generally present at birth but occasionally arise as late as several years. These lesions arise from melanocytic stem cells that migrate from the neural crest to the embryonic dermis and upward into the epidermis. They may also migrate into the leptomeninges.

Although the bulk of these lesions are small and benign, some cover large portions of the body or can be in conspicuous locations, presenting challenging reconstructive problems. Furthermore, their potential for malignant degeneration causes anxiety for the parent, primary care physician and surgeon alike. Although small pigmented nevi are present in one out of 100 births, large nevi are present in only 1 in 20,000 births, and the giant lesions are even less common. As a result, most surgeons have little experience with them and little opportunity to develop a rational protocol for their treatment.

The goal of this chapter is to classify the more common cutaneous lesions, review the pathophysiology and natural history, summarize the risk of malignant degeneration and provide a rational approach to treatment.

69.2 Congenital Nevi

Congenital nevi are those cutaneous lesions apparent at birth or that become apparent prior to 1 year of age. The word nevus is a 'generic' term best defined as a hamartoma that is an overgrowth of mature cells normally present in the affected part, but with disorganization

P. Puri and M. Höllwarth (eds.), *Pediatric Surgery: Diagnosis and Management*,
DOI: 10.1007/978-3-540-69560-8_69, © Springer-Verlag Berlin Heidelberg 2009

and often with one element predominating. This broad definition applies to a variety of cutaneous lesions that can be congenital or acquired.

The majority of congenital lesions are melanocytic in nature, including common congenital melanocytic nevi, nevi of Ota, nevi of Ito, nevus spilus, café au lait spots and Mongolian spots. Other non-melanotic lesions such as sebaceous nevi (of Jadassohn), neural nevi and epidermal nevi can be evident at birth. Several other nevi have a propensity to appear in childhood and will be discussed here, including intradermal nevi, blue nevi and Spitz nevi.

69.2.1 Congenital Melanocytic Nevi (CMN)

It is important to have a frame of reference in discussing the treatment of CMN. Multiple definitions have been used, and without some uniformity it is difficult to compare different studies. The authors believe that the following definitions are becoming accepted and used in most studies: small nevi are those measuring 1.5 cm or less, medium nevi measure from 1.5 to 19.9 cm, and large nevi are 20 cm or greater. Giant nevi are a subset of large nevi that measure 50 cm or greater. Another definition of large and giant nevi classifies them as those that cover 2% or more of total body surface (Fig. 69.1).

Congenital melanocytic nevi are composed of nevus cells of melanocytic origin, which vary in the amount of pigment they carry. At birth, these lesions can be quite faint. During the first 6 months of life, some nevi can appear to "grow" significantly as tardive pigment becomes more visible. Some satellite nevi may become visible for the first time over the first 2–3 years (tardive CMN). After the first 6 months, the lesions grow proportionally to the particular area of the body involved. The diameter of the lesion grows by a factor of 1.7 times in the head, 3.3 in thigh and leg, and 2.8 in the torso, arms, hands and feet. The

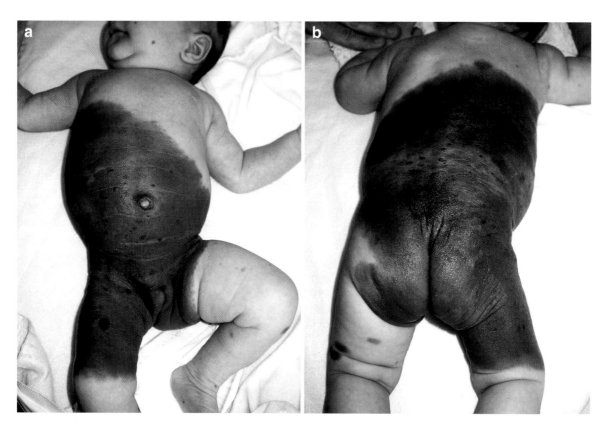

Fig. 69.1 a, b This infant female was born with a giant congenital melanocytic nevus covering large portions of her trunk with extension to lower extremities. This patient should be worked up for potential meningeal and cerebral melanosis

large nevi are at least 6 cm in diameter on the infant's body and 9 cm on its head.

Embryologically, these lesions are ectopic rests of nevus cells. Melanoblasts, the precursors to melanocytes, migrate from the neural crest to the skin, mucus membranes, eyes, mesentery, chromaffin system and meninges, where they differentiate into dendritic melanocytes. When a disturbance of this migration and differentiation occurs, the result is an ectopic population of nevus cells. Nevus cells are melanocytes that differ from ordinary melanocytes histologically by being arranged in nests or clusters, having a rounded rather than dendritic shape and tending to keep their pigment in their cytoplasm rather then transferring it to surrounding keratinocytes.

Histologically, efforts have been made to identify characteristics specific to CMN in contrast to nevi acquired later in life. A reliable microscopic differentiation between the two could help determine the true rate of melanoma in association with these lesions. Nevus cells when found within the eccrine ducts or glands, follicular epithelium, and blood vessels are specific for congenital melanocytic nevus but not all CMN will demonstrate these findings. In large congenital melanocytic nevi, nevus cells have been found in underlying subcutaneous fat, fascia and musculature.

69.2.2 Small Congenital Melanocytic Nevi

Most congenital pigmented nevi are small and are excised easily in a single procedure. The life-time risk for melanoma in these patients has been quoted to occur in 4.9 out of 100 people when the patient provides the history that the lesion is congenital, and in 0.8–2.6 out of 100 people when determined by histological criteria of findings consistent with CMN in melanoma specimens. Practically speaking, however, the risk of melanoma before puberty is nil, being quoted as 1 in 200,000 individuals. For this reason, many pediatricians, pediatric dermatologists and pediatric surgeons defer the removal of these lesions to an age when excision can be performed under local anesthesia in the office, eliminating the risks associated with general anesthesia. Clearly, some lesions lie in cosmetically sensitive areas and for the psychological benefit of the child should be

removed earlier, even if general anesthesia is required. From a practical point of view, these procedures are best done either before the child starts toddling or just prior to school entrance. The stage in between these two ages is fraught with falls, scrapes, fear and lack of patient cooperation. The experience is better for the patient, parent and surgeon alike by avoiding elective nevus removal in the toddler. There is little benefit to delaying surgery in those lesions, which because of their location, will likely require general anesthesia at any age.

69.2.3 Large Congenital Melanocytic Nevi

Two immediate concerns face the family of a child with a large or giant nevus. The first is the risk of the child- developing melanoma, and the second is the stigma of this very visible lesion and how it will affect the child's psychological development. Early consultation with a pediatric surgeon or pediatric dermatologist can help educate the family and decrease the stress of the situation by providing concise information about the nature of the nevus, its natural history and the options for its management.

In the literature, the estimated risk of developing melanoma ranges from 2% to 31%. The different populations and numbers in these studies explain the wide variance. In a retrospective study, Quaba and Wallace examined patients with CMN covering more than 2% of total body surface and found the melanoma risk to be 8.5% during the first 15 years of life. Sandsmark et al. have quoted a risk of 6.7% in childhood. Marghoob et al. have quoted a lifetime risk of 4.5–9% for melanoma arising in large and giant CMN. Approximately 50% of the malignancies that develop in large CMN do so in the first 3 years of life, 60% by childhood, and 70% by puberty. Another important point is that less than 0.5% of melanomas appear in preadolescent children, but 33% of those are thought to arise from CMN.

There is an ongoing controversy regarding the risk of melanoma transformation. In the Swedish prospective trial, the risk of malignant transformation was reported as 0.2%. Other studies reported only extracutaneous melanoma in patients with CMN. No studies convincingly show that excision of large CMN effectively reduce the rate of malignant transformation to melanoma. We have treated a patient who developed a metastatic malignant melanoma 20 years after a complete excision of a large CMN of the face.

Another factor that needs to be considered and discussed with families is the issue of neurocutaneous melanosis (NCM). Recent reports have demonstrated the association of nevus cells in the leptomeninges in a percentage of children with large nevi in an axial orientation or those with an extensive number of satellite nevi (Fig. 69.1). Although symptomatic NCM is characterized by mental retardation, hydrocephalus and seizures, many children are asymptomatic. These children can be identified by T1 shortening in MR imaging. It has been reported that 23% of at-risk patients had evidence of central nervous system involvement (melanotic rests within the brain and meninges) on MR imaging. Marghoob and Dusza have seen this finding in only 3% of children in the Nevus Outreach Registry of over 600 patients. The latter figure coincides with the authors' experience. Although the presence of a lesion on MRI does not typically alter the decision to treat or not treat a child with a large or giant nevus, the approach may be altered in cases of symptomatic NCM.

The rationale for early treatment of large and giant nevi has four components. These are (1) the presence of the greatest risk for malignancy in the first 3 years, (2) the elasticity and healing capacity of the skin in the early years (3) the greater parent tolerance of surgery in this time and (4) the psychological benefit on the child. Taking all this into account, and assuming that the child is otherwise healthy, the authors begin treatment of the large and giant nevus by 6 months of age in most cases, provided that they have seen the child from early infancy. Although many of the tissue-expansion procedures used in treatment of giant nevi can be applied to older children and selected adults, the intolerance for repeated procedures and the decreased elasticity of the skin may make the excision of extensive lesions impractical in older patients.

Patches of darker color and raised areas often exist within large CMN. The areas can represent neuroid nevus, which is a form of nevus with melanocytes that appear to be histologically like Schwann cells and with nerve organelles such as Meissner's and Pacinan corpuscles. The patches also can represent areas of local proliferation but do not necessarily behave in an aggressive manner. Histological findings of low mitotic rate, lack of necrosis, evidence of maturation in the cell population and lack of high grade nuclear atypia are clues to a benign course. Sometimes, the best description of these areas, however, is melanocytic tumor of uncertain potential. Unusual areas such as these should be addressed earlier in the course of reconstruction.

69.2.4 Other Congenital Nevi

69.2.4.1 Café Au Lait Macules

Café au lait macules are sharply demarcated areas of light tan to brown pigmentation which present in normal individuals or can be associated, when multiple, with syndromes such as neurofibromatosis. Histologically, there is increased pigment in macromelanosomes within keratinocytes in the basal layer. These lesions are benign. If they are in cosmetically sensitive areas, LASER ablation can be considered. Recurrence after LASER therapy is commonly reported, but successful ablation has also been reported.

69.2.4.2 Nevus Spilus

Nevus spilus, also called speckled lentiginous nevus, also has light tan to brown macules with areas of speckling within it. The presence of the "speckles" or freckles within it separates it clinically from the café au lait macule. Histologically, there is both increased pigment within the keratinocytes of the basal layer and an increased number of melanocytes as well. The speckles can be areas of freckling, congenital melanocytic nevi or blue nevi. Any suspicious areas within the lesion can be excised for biopsy as a nevocellular portion of the lesion may still carry a malignant potential. If the entire defect is in a cosmetically sensitive area, it can be removed surgically.

69.2.4.3 Blue Nevus

Blue nevi are smooth, almost blue-black lesions, which can be present at birth but are more likely to appear during childhood and puberty. Frequently they are found on the extremities or the head. Females are affected more than males. Two variants exist: common and cellular. The common blue nevus is a relatively small, <1 cm, sharply demarcated and dome shaped. In this benign lesion, the melanocytes are dendritic in nature, within the dermis and possibly into the subcutaneous tissue, but the epidermis is normal. The cellular blue nevus tends to be larger, 1–3 cm, has less regular borders and is found frequently in the lumbosacrum. Melanocytes can be spindle-shaped and found in aggregates admixed with dendritic melanocytes. The lesions tend to be wider at the surface than at the base. There are reported cases of malignant degeneration within cellular blue nevi. For this reason, removal of blue nevi is recommended.

69.2.4.4 Spitz Nevi

Although not usually congenital, Spitz nevi occur frequently in young children. They are pink, raised, firm lesions that often are confused with pyogenic granulomas because of the appearance and history of rapid growth and onset. On occasion, they are pigmented as well. The original name for these lesions was "benign juvenile melanoma" and under the microscope the rather bizarre histology can be confusing, if the patient's age and history are not supplied to the pathologist. These lesions are not malignant, but do grow rapidly and tend to recur aggressively if not completely excised. A generous border of normal tissue (i.e. 3–4 mm) should be excised along with the lesion to decrease the chances of recurrence.

69.2.4.5 Mongolian Spots

Mongolian spots commonly appear as blue-gray macular discoloration resembling a bruise over the lumbosacral area of newborn infants, especially in darker skinned individuals. On occasion they can appear in atypical locations such as the upper thorax or extremities. Usually these benign lesions regress spontaneously by the age of 3–4 years, but can persist in unusual cases. Histologically, widely scattered dendritic melanocytes lie in the lower two thirds of the dermis. No specific therapy is necessary, however LASER treatments can obliterate persistent lesions.

69.2.4.6 Nevus of Ota/Nevus of ITO

The nevus of Ota and the nevus of Ito are macular, blue-gray field defects in the area of the first and second branches of the trigeminal nerve or in the scapular, del-toid and supraclavicular area, respectively. The mucosae of the nose and mouth and the sclera, retina and conjunctiva can also be involved in the nevus of Ota. These lesions are field defects of dermal melanocytosis, like Mongolian spots. Unlike Mongolian spots, these lesions do not spontaneously regress and can become hyperpigmented during puberty. Usually these lesions are present at birth, but may become apparent around puberty, only rarely appearing during childhood. They are more common in females and more frequent in darker skinned individuals, being reported most frequently in Indian and Asian populations. In 10% of the cases, the nevus of Ota is bilateral, and these cases are associated with extensive Mongolian spots. Histologically, the dermis contains elongated, dendritic melanocytes scattered among the collagen bundles, mostly located in the upper third of the reticular dermis; they can have raised areas within them that are indistinguishable from a blue nevus beneath the microscope. These lesions are considered to be benign; however reports of malignant changes exist in a few cases, with the tumors having the histologic appearance of a malignant or cellular blue nevus.

Good results in treatment of these nevi have been obtained with the Q-switched ruby laser, the Q-switched Alexandrite laser and the Q-switched Nd:YAG laser. Multiple treatments are required with each of these modalities.

69.2.4.7 Sebaceous Nevi

The sebaceous nevus was described by Jadassohn at the turn of the century. It presents as a waxy, hairless, yellow-orange plague, usually on the scalp, head or neck (Fig. 69.2). It is a hamartoma of sebaceous glands. The lesions tend to become more verrucous, itchy and excoriated during puberty. Sebaceous nevus syndrome is the combination of large sebaceous nevi of the scalp and face associated with developmental delay, seizures, and ophthalmologic and bony abnormalities. Removal is recommended for these lesions because of a documented risk of malignant degeneration, usually basal cell carcinoma. For extensive lesions involving cosmetically sensitive areas, some centers reported using CO2 laser ablation with good results. Complete surgical excision, however, remains the gold standard for treatment of these challenging nevi.

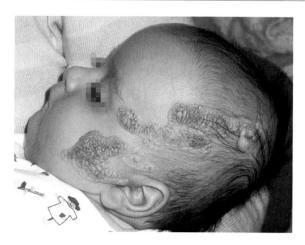

Fig. 69.2 A newborn boy with a large sebaceous nevus covering portion of the left scalp, lateral forehead, lateral temporal area and the cheek. Clinically, these lesions are significant for a chance of development of a basal cell carcinoma later in life

69.3   Treatment of Congenital Nevi

The treatment of large and giant nevi is controversial. Many feel that the risk of degeneration is too low to warrant the unsightly scars or grafts that may follow treatment. Others feel that, in the presence of NCM, the greatest risk lies within the central nervous system, so the excision of the cutaneous lesion can only have limited benefits. However, the appearance of these lesions clearly produces a stigma with significant psychological implications. Removal on this basis is often warranted. The challenge for the surgeon involved in treating these often complex lesions is to develop treatment modalities that do not only accomplish the excision of all or most of the nevus but also lead to an optimal aesthetic and functional outcome.

Treatment choices include observation, dermabrasion or curettage, and staged excision and reconstruction. Some giant nevi are so extensive as to have no available "donor" tissue for reconstruction. In other cases, the family situation or lack of available resources may speak for a less "aggressive" approach. The treating surgeon should be well versed in the available treatment options, honest about the potential risks and outcomes of the various surgical modalities of treatment, and able to present these to the family.

69.4   Dermabrasion, Curettage, and Laser Treatment

Dermabrasion and curettage are both techniques that have been applied in the neonatal period in an effort to remove the more concentrated population of nevus cells near the lesion's surface. The technique can be effective in reducing the overall nevus "cell load" but cannot fully remove the nevus, because of the well-known depth of nevus cells in CMN. Although this treatment may result in significant lightening of the color of the lesion, it is quite common to see later "bleed-through" of the deeper nevus, with gradual darkening and reappearance of the lesion. This result may present a difficult treatment problem in visible areas like the face, where other techniques for excision may then be less tolerated.

The same issues arise in consideration of the LASER as a means of treating nevi. Many patients request information about the use of the LASER to manage these lesions, hoping for removal without scarring. Selective photodermolysis is appropriate in macular dermal melanocytosis such as nevus of Ota or nevus of Ito, non-regressing Mongolian spots, nevus spilus and café au lait macules in cosmetically sensitive locations. These particular lesions have minimal thickness, are not located in the epidermis and are unlikely to be malignant, which makes them ideally suited for management with lasers. Treatment hinges on the surgeon picking a LASER of correct wavelength and pulse-width to allow selective destruction of the melanocytes without damaging the overlying epidermis and underlying adnexal structures. Serial treatments are required. Inappropriate selection of the wavelength or dosimetry can lead to secondary scarring with LASER treatments. Temporary hyperpigmentation and hypopigmentation can occur as well.

Increasing number of centers are treating extensive facial sebaceous nevi with carbon dioxide laser, with greatly improved cosmetic appearance. Unfortunately, there is no data in the literature regarding the prevention of cancerous transformation of these lesions with this treatment modality.

Because large and giant congenital melanocytic nevi have nevus cells in all layers of the epidermis, dermis, subcutaneous tissue and sometimes fascia and muscle, it is unrealistic to think that any laser would be capable of eliminating the nevus without damaging, i.e. burning and scarring the tissue. Furthermore, because the lesion is vaporized there is no surgical specimen for histologic confirmation of the benign or malignant nature of the lesion. While it may prove to be of use for reducing pigmentation in sensitive facial areas (e.g. on the eyelids) it would be expected to be of limited benefit and likely to require repeated treatment over time. Whether or not the radiant energy required for laser treatment has a negative impact on the nevus cells within the remaining lesion has yet to be determined, and may not be apparent for many years into the future.

69.5 Methods of Excision of Small and Intermediate Nevi

Smaller nevi can be excised with elliptical, wedge, circular or serial excision.

69.5.1 Elliptical Excision

Simple elliptical excision is the most commonly used technique. Elliptical excision of inadequate length may yield "dog-ears", which consist of excess skin and subcutaneous fat at the end of the closure. To prevent "dog-ears", the length of the ellipse should be at least three times the width. "Dog-ears" do not disappear on their own.

69.5.2 Wedge Excision

Lesions located at or adjacent to free margins can be excised by wedge excision. This applies to lesions located on the helical rim, eyelids and lips.

69.5.3 Circular Excision

When preservation of skin is desired or the length of the scar must be kept to a minimum, circular excision might be desirable. Circular defects can be closed with full thickness skin graft, local flap or with a purse-string suture. A purse-string suture causes significant bunching of the skin. This is allowed to mature for many months and may result in a shorter (but often a wider) scar.

69.5.4 Serial Excision

Serial excision is the excision of a lesion in more than one stage. Serial excision is frequently employed for treatment of congenital nevi. The inherent viscoelastic properties of skin are used, allowing the skin to stretch over time. These techniques enable wound closure to be accomplished with a shorter scar than if the original lesion was elliptically excised in a single stage.

69.6 Overview of Current Surgical Treatment of Large and Giant Pigmented Nevi

As previously mentioned, the challenge in surgical treatment of large and giant nevi is to select a treatment program that will allow complete excision and reconstruction at an early stage, minimize scarring, and minimize the need for later treatment. Surgical planning must satisfy these requirements in order to provide an optimal functional and esthetic outcome. The optimal choice of treatment varies by body region, and the remainder of this chapter summarizes the authors' thoughts on these different treatment modalities.

69.6.1 Scalp

Tissue expansion is a treatment modality of choice for excision and reconstruction of large and giant nevi of the scalp. As surgical experience increases and planning improves, larger defects can be reconstructed with fewer procedures and better restoration of normal hair patterns. Rectangular expanders with soft bottoms and remote injection ports are used, with the expanders in place for an average of 10 weeks. Expanders are typically injected weekly (increased to every 4–5 days in some cases). The typical scalp expanders range from 250 to 500 cc in size. Treatment starts with patients as early as 8 months, with some cranial molding expected

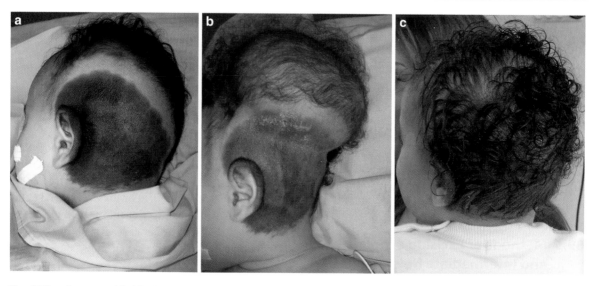

Fig. 69.3 a One year old girl with congenital large pigmented nevus of the left parietal-occipital scalp, with extension into the auricle. **b** Expander in place in the parietal-occipital scalp above the nevus. **c** Nevus excision was followed by reconstruction with expanded transposition flap. Postoperative view demonstrates accurate hairline and hair growth directions

by the time the expanders are removed, but with no instance of long-term cranial deformity noted (remodeling usually occurs over 3–4 months) (Fig. 69.3).

Application of transposition flaps to the scalp has dramatically improved our ability to cover larger defects with more aesthetically acceptable restoration of a normal hair pattern and the frontotemporal hairline. The benefit of this modification is most apparent with the use of the expanded occipital transposition flap for covering the entire parietal scalp and reconstruction of the temporal hairline and sideburns. The nevus or the scar must never be resected until the extent of flap transposition is determined. If a complete excision cannot be accomplished, the remaining nevus or scar is reconstructed after additional expansion.

69.6.2 Face

Large and giant nevi of the face present some of the greatest challenges in treatment of these lesions. These are the most visible nevi with which the patient and family must deal and the ones that are most likely to be associated with significant psychological sequelae. They also represent the area where unsightly scarring is most readily visible; consequently, the planning and execution of the reconstructive plan must be very

detailed. A description of all the nuances of treatment of facial nevi is beyond the scope of this chapter. What follows is the summary of the highlights.

Tissue expansion of the hemiforehead for unilateral lesions or the bilateral or lateral forehead for central lesions can very effectively treat even extensive lesions. Because many of these nevi involve the adjacent scalp, the combined "attack" on both of these regions often facilitates the excision and lessens the number of stages required. The planning of expansion and reconstruction for nevi of the forehead must be directed at minimizing any possibility of distorting the eyebrow and the normal distance from brow to hairline (Fig. 69.4).

Nevi of the cheek are best reconstructed with expanded or non-expanded postauricular flaps (the cheek and neck can be considered as a single anatomic unit sharing similar hair-bearing characteristics and relatively thin skin). Reconstruction of the entire aesthetic unit of the cheek may require two or even three expansions. The use of a transposition flap significantly reduces the risk of downward traction and distortion of the lower eyelid, which are seen as common sequelae of direct advancement of expanded flaps from below the mandible to the cheek (Fig. 69.4).

Expanded or non-expanded full-thickness skin grafts have been used effectively for excision and reconstruction of nevi of the periorbital and eyelid areas and occasionally the nasal dorsum. A single, large, expanded

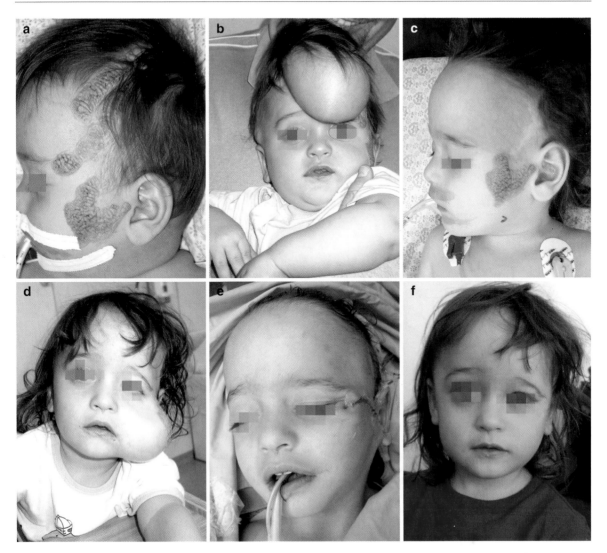

Fig. 69.4 a Patient with an extensive sebaceous nevus covering portion of the left scalp, lateral forehead, lateral temporal area and the left cheek. His reconstruction was performed in two stages. **b** Tissue expander in place. Note that both the hair bearing scalp and the non-hair bearing forehead are expanded. **c** Partial excision of the nevus is followed by reconstruction with expanded flap, advanced laterally. Postoperative view demon-strates accurate hairline and hair growth directions and excellent contour of the forehead without distortion of the eyebrow. **d** In the second stage tissue expander was placed in the medial cheek. **e** Resurfacing of the cheek with medially based expanded flap, transposed to reconstruct the cheek aesthetic unit. **f** Postoperative view

full-thickness graft from the supraclavicular area can reconstruct eyelids, canthus and the region between eyelid and brow, without the multiple "seams" that follow use of multiple smaller grafts (Fig. 69.5).

Extensive nevi of the central face (nose, lips, chin) are some of the most challenging that we have to deal with, and their treatment requires both ingenuity and a solid grasp of plastic surgery reconstructive techniques.

69.6.3 Neck

The posterior and the posterolateral neck are commonly involved with large nevi. Posterior and posterolateral neck defects can be successfully reconstructed with expanded flaps from the upper back and the shoulders. The tissue expanders are placed adjacent to the lesion to be excised. The flaps are designed in such a way that they can be wrapped around the neck, eliminating the

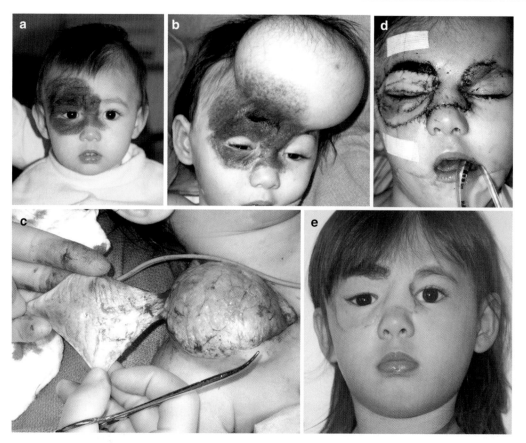

Fig. 69.5 a Patient with a congenital melanocytic nevus involving eyelids with extensions to the eyebrow and the forehead, the cheek and the nose bilaterally (areas involved 1-8). **b, c** Tissue expanders were placed in the contra-lateral forehead and the ipsi-lateral supraclavicular areas. An expanded full thickness skin graft was harvested from the supraclavicular area. **d** Immediate postoperative view. The forehead and the nasal dorsum and sidewalls were reconstructed with an expanded flap transposed from the contralateral forehead. The eyelids were resurfaced with a single unit expanded full thickness skin graft split at the aperture. A small portion of the nevus was left to mimic the eyebrow. **e** Postoperative views after one year. Note the thin rims of the nevus left deliberately at the margins. These rims are excised in a second procedure, combined with scar revisions

"webbing" created by pure upward advanced flaps. With this design the reconstructed neck has a better contour and more favorable scar location (Fig. 69.6).

69.6.4 Trunk

Some of the most significant strides have been made in better understanding and applying tissue expansion to the treatment of giant nevi of the trunk. Better expanded flap design and, when regional expansion is not possible, using expanded distant flaps with microvascular transfer, has resulted in both functional and esthetic outcomes where previously large grafted areas diminished the outcome in both these aspects.

The most common location of giant nevi was found to be over the posterior trunk, often extending anteriorly in a dermatome distribution.

Tissue expansion can be very effective on the anterior trunk, provided that the lesion is confined either to the lower abdomen or central abdomen and that there is sufficient uninvolved skin above or above and below the nevus to expand. Expansion must be avoided in or around the area of the breast bud in females, and lesions of the breast should be left until after breast development, regardless of the psychological implications of delaying the treatment till that age.

The use of expanded transposition flaps has enabled excision of nevi of the upper back and buttock/perineal region, where previously it was thought that only skin

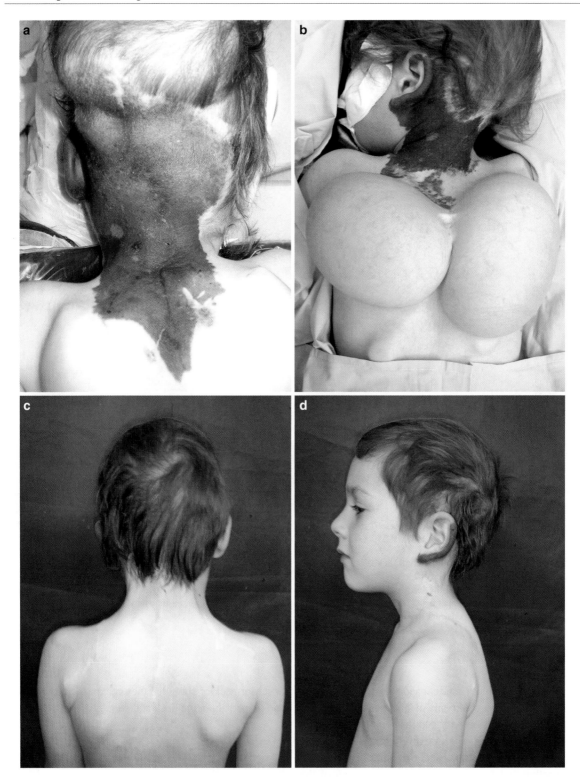

Fig. 69.6 a Two years old boy with a large congenital melanocytic nevus of the posterior neck, extending to the upper back and the occipital scalp. **b** Expanders in place after 3 months of serial expansion. **c, d** Postoperative views. Excellent contour of the neck was achieved with expanded flaps transposed upwards and wrapped around the neck

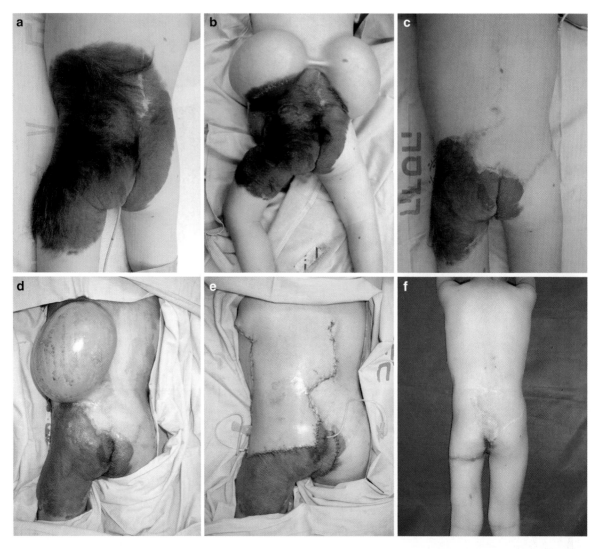

Fig. 69.7 a Patient with a bathing trunk nevus starting at the junction of the middle and lower of the back and covering the entire buttocks, perineum and the left thigh circumferentially. **b, c** After expansion of the upper back, two large medially based flaps are transposed to reconstruct the lower trunk. **d, e** These flaps can be re-expanded to allow for further nevus excision. **f** View after four rounds of tissue expansion and near total nevus excision (a small rim of nevus was left around the anus to prevent scarring in this area that may lead to incontinence of the sphincter)

grafting was possible. Tissue expanders in the 500–750 cc range are used most commonly in infants and young children. Serial expansion with careful planning has made possible the excision of progressively larger nevi of the back and buttocks with excellent outcomes (Fig. 69.7).

Another tool for reconstruction of giant nevi of the upper back, shoulders and neck has been the expanded free transverse rectus abdominis myocutaneous (TRAM) flap, which can be positioned in the upper back and

posterior neck or shoulder, then reexpanded, contoured, and draped about the neck and shoulders.

69.6.5 Extremities

Large and giant nevi of the extremities present a challenge that is still not fully met. Tissue expansion has been of some help in the treating smaller lesions, where tissue is available both proximal and distal to the lesion and the lesion is confined to a fairly small segment of the limb. The geometry of the extremity, as well as the limited flexibility of the skin (particularly in the lower extremity) makes regional expansion of limited use.

In the past decade, the authors have begun to find a way around these limitations, using large expanded transposition flaps from the scapular region to cover the upper arm and shoulder and expanded pedicle flaps from the flank and abdomen for circumferential nevi from the elbow to the wrist (Fig. 69.8). Expanded full thickness skin grafts have been used effectively for the dorsum of the hand with excellent aesthetic outcome.

Although pedicled flaps are not readily available for coverage of more extensive lesions of the arm, thigh, or leg, the authors have had some success with expanded free flaps from the abdomen and scapular region. These

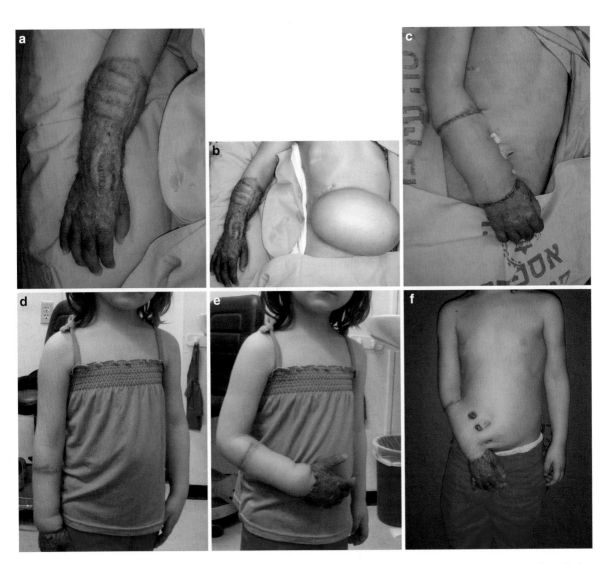

Fig. 69.8 a 3½ year old girl with a giant nevus extending circumferentially around the forearm from elbow to the hand and the fingers. **b, c** The arm is positioned against the flank and abdomen after expansion of the site. The forearm nevus is excised to the fascia level and the forearm is placed within the expanded pedicle flap. **d** The arm is placed for 3 weeks within the expanded "tunnel", and the pedicle is gradually tightened with through and through bolster sutures, gradually reducing the blood flow through the pedicle. **e, f** Postoperative views after division of the pedicle. Clearly noted are the excellent contour and quality of the skin of the forearm gained with this approach. Residual nevus is still present at the hand and will be excised and reconstructed later with expanded full thickness skin graft

procedures have been used only in very carefully selected cases, and the optimum timing of these complex reconstructive procedures is still under consideration.

69.7 Satellite Nevi

Satellite nevi may appear anywhere over the course of the first few years of life, and their number seems to correlate directly with the likelihood of NCM. They may vary in size from small to medium lesions. To date, no case of melanoma has been reported arising in a satellite nevus. With this in mind, it is generally agreed that the primary reason for excision of satellite nevi is an aesthetic one. The authors generally excise some of the larger lesions early, often with serial excision, and leave the smaller lesions until the child expresses specific concerns about them. A significant benefit may also result from excising multiple satellite nevi on the face before the child enters his or her school years.

69.8 Summary

Although the exact risk of malignant degeneration may never be determined, there is still evidence that large and giant congenital nevi carry this potential. Excision and reconstruction are warranted, provided that they can be accomplished with an optimal aesthetic and functional outcome. The ability to present organized discussion of current views of malignant change to parents, patients (when old enough) and other allied health care workers is critical. Experience with a large population of children with large and giant CMN has demonstrated that thoughtful application of the full spectrum of

reconstructive options, heavily weighed toward the use of tissue expansion (as well as expanded pedicled and free flaps) can result in total or near total excision of many of these extensive nevi with predictably good outcomes.

Further Reading

Bauer BS, Byun MY, Han H, Vicari FA (1997) A new look into the treatment of congenital giant pigmented nevi in infancy and childhood: a follow-up study and review of 200 patients. Plast Surg Forum 20:76

Bauer BS, Few JW, Chavez CD, Galiano RD (2001) The role of tissue expansion in the management of large congenital pigmented nevi of the forehead in the pediatric patient. Plast Reconstr Surg 107:668–75

Bauer BS, Margulis A (2004) The expanded transposition flap: shifting paradigms based on experience gained from two decades of pediatric tissue expansion. Plast Reconstr Surg 114:98–106

Berg P, Lindelof B (2002) Congenital nevocytic nevi: follow-up of a Swedish birth register sample regarding etiologic factors, discomfort, and removal rate. Pediatr Dermatol 19(4):293–297

Bruce SB, Julia C (2005) Treatment of large and giant nevi. Clin Plastic Surg 32:11–18

Foster RD, Williams ML, Barkovich AJ, et al. (2001) Giant congenital melanocytic nevi: the significance of neurocutaneous melanosis in neurologically asymptomatic children. Plast Reconstr Surg 107:933–41

Marghoob AA, Dusza SW, Oliveria SO, Halpren AC (2004) Number of satellite nevi as a correlate for neurocutaneous melanocytosis in patients with large congenital melanocytic nevi. Arch Derm 140:171–5

Margulis A, Bauer BS, Fine NA (2004) Large and giant congenital pigmented nevi of the upper extremity: an algorithm to surgical management. Ann Plast Surg 521:158–67

Puri P, Höllwarth M (2006) Pediaric Surgery, Springer: Berlin, Heidelberg

Watt AJ, Kotsis SV, Chung KC (2004) Risk of melanoma arising in large melanocytic nevi: a systematic review. Plast Reconstr Surg 113:1968–74

Lymphatic Malformations

70

Mohammed Zamakhshary and Jacob C. Langer

Contents

70.1 Introduction

The term "lymphatic malformation" refers to a group of benign vascular anomalies which result from embryologic abnormalities in the development of the lymphatic system. Lymphatic malformations occur in about 1:1700 live births, with an incidence that has remained relatively stable. Lymphatic malformations are generally divided into three major groups: Cystic (by far the most common), lymphangiectasia, and lymphedema. This chapter will focus on the clinical diagnosis and treatment of cystic lymphatic malformations.

70.2 Nomenclature and Classification

Historically there has been significant confusion regarding the nomenclature of vascular malformations in general and lymphatic malformations in particular. In 1996, the Society for the Study of Vascular Anomalies adopted a classification system aimed at minimising such confusion (Table 70.1). "Cystic hygroma" and "lymphangiomas" are commonly used to describe lymphatic malformations. These terms should be abandoned and the term lymphatic malformation should be used instead. Morphologically, cystic lymphatic malformations can be classified as microcystic, macrocystic or combined.

70.3 Pathology and Embryology

The lymphatic system develops from five primitive sacs: two in the neck, one in the retroperitoneum and two sacs posterior to the sciatic veins. Later on it was

P. Puri and M. Höllwarth (eds.), *Pediatric Surgery: Diagnosis and Management*,
DOI: 10.1007/978-3-540-69560-8_70, © Springer-Verlag Berlin Heidelberg 2009

Table 70.1 Classification of Vascular Malformations including: Lymphatic malformations

Vascular tumors	Slow-flow VM	Fast-flow VM	Combined VM
Hemangioma	Capillary Malformations	Arteriovenous Fistula (AVF)	Klippel-Trenaunay syndrome (CLVM)
Kaposiform Hemangioendothelioma (KHE)	Venous Malformation	Arteriovenous malformation (AVM)	Parkers-Weber syndrome (CAVM)
Tufted Angioma	Lymphatic Malformation		

suggested that lymphatic malformations actually result from failure of the lymphatic spaces to join the venous system. Whether the cause of lymphatic malformation is related to sequestration of lymphatic sac, failure of fusion with the venous system or obstruction of lymph drainage remains unknown.

Lymphatic malformations consist of cystic cavities filled with clear or straw coloured fluid, which is usually eosinophilic and protein rich. Occasionally haemorrhage into the cyst can be seen. These lesions usually have an infiltrative pattern of growth, a factor that may complicate planning for operative treatment.

Due to the close development of the lymphatic system with that of the venous system, the cysts are usually lined with a single layer of endothelial cells. The relationship between the developing lymphatic system and the cardiovascular system have led to a number of theories to explain the pathogenesis of lymphatic malformations, including abnormalities in the development of extracellular matrix and neural crest migration. The wall of a lymphatic malformation usually also contains abnormal muscle cells of both the smooth and striated variety. Histologically these malformations can be composed of one or more of the following architectural patterns: capillary, cavernous and cystic. Whether growth of these lesions is due to neo-tissue formation or thrombosis with ongoing re-organization within the malformation remains a subject of debate. It is important to note that the microcystic, macrocystic or combined micro and macrocystic classification is based on morphology. The exact aetiology remains unclear.

70.4 Epidemiology and Prenatal Diagnosis

Lymphatic malformations are often diagnosed prenatally. The natural history ranges from progression to hydrops, to complete resolution, a possibility that has been well documented.

Prenatally diagnosed lymphatic malformation may be a marker of aneuploidy (>50%), syndromicity and other congenital structural anomalies. This subgroup is usually diagnosed early in pregnancy, is predominantly nuchal, and is associated with diffuse lymphatic abnormalities (Fig. 70.1). Isolated lymphatic malformations presenting early in pregnancy often resolve spontaneously. This is in sharp contrast to isolated lymphatic malformation diagnosed late in pregnancy, which are similar to those presenting to pediatric surgeons postnatally. This "late" group is rarely associated with aneuploidy (<1%), affects a variety of sites, and almost never resolves.

The incidence of lymphatic malformation is variable. In a population-based study from Wessex region the incidence was estimated at 1 in 1,750 live births. It is important to note that the incidence in spontaneous abortions is much higher, estimated at 1 in 200. The rate of aneuploidy seen in association with prenatal diagnosis of lymphatic malformation is estimated at 50–60%. Of the multiple syndromes associated with

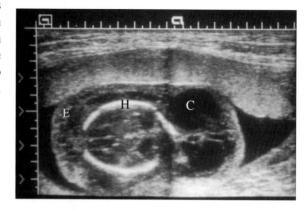

Fig. 70.1 Prenatal ultrasound of a fetus with Turner syndrome and a large posterior cervical cystic hygroma. Note the diffuse subcutaneous edema (E), which is indicative of hydrops fetalis. H = fetal head, C = cystic hygroma

Table 70.2 Syndromes commonly associated with prenatally diagnosed LM

Non-aneuploidies	Aneuploidies
Noonan's	Turner
Multiple pterygium	Down
Achondrogenesis type-1	Edward
Short-rib-polydactyly syndrome	Patau
Fryn's	
Robert's	
Fetal alcohol	

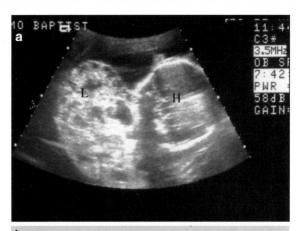

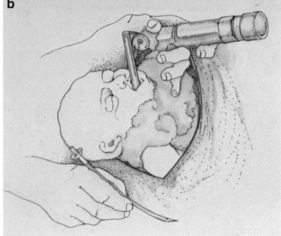

Fig. 70.2 (a) Prenatal sonogram showing a large pretracheal lymphatic malformation. H = fetal head, T = lymphatic malformation. (b) The EXIT procedure, in which intubation is accomplished prior to delivery while still on placental support

the prenatal diagnosis of lymphatic malformation, Turner's syndrome and Noonan's syndrome are probably the most common (Table 70.2).

In a key study, Howarth et al. reported population based estimates of prevalence and natural history of lymphatic malformation in the United Kingdom. The database included more than 175,000 live births over a 3-year period, of which 99 patients with lymphatic malformation were identified, (yielding a prevalence of 1 in 1,775 live births). Karyotyping was performed in 88% of pregnancies, of which 61% were abnormal. Moreover, structural abnormalities were seen in 21 patients. Cardiac anomalies were the most prevalent, especially A-V canal defects. This could not be explained only by aneuploidy, since almost 40% of these defects were seen in euploid fetuses. Other structural anomalies seen included: exomphalos, renal, skeletal and central nervous system anomalies. Of the 99 pregnancies identified with an associated lymphatic malformation, 19 suffered spontaneous fetal demise, and 64 underwent pregnancy termination. The other 16 went on to live birth. Of these, only 6 were completely normal postnatally. One required surgery for the lymphatic malformation but was otherwise normal, four died, and the remaining patients had significant chromosomal anomalies and neurological impairment. This "hidden mortality" of lymphatic malformation has been well documented by others.

Because of the high risk of associated syndromes, parental counseling should take place in a specialized center, where complete fetal investigation, including karyotype analysis and detailed ultrasound examination, can be undertaken.

Prenatal diagnosis of a large cervical mass should raise suspicion for potential airway obstruction that may impact planning for delivery. The treating team should include a surgeon, and should be prepared to perform life-saving procedures such as ex-utero intrapartum treatment (EXIT), endoscopy and a surgical airway (Fig. 70.2).

70.5 Clinical Features

Most lymphatic malformations are diagnosed postnatally. More than half are evident at birth and more than 80% are diagnosed by the age of 5 years; rarely lymphatic malformations may present later in the first 2 decades of life. These lesions vary widely in size. The most common anatomic location is the head and neck (Figs. 70.3 and 70.4); Table 70.3). Other areas commonly affected are: axilla, mediastinum, groin and retroperitoneum (Fig. 70.5). The predilection to these sites is thought to be related to the rich lymphatics in these areas.

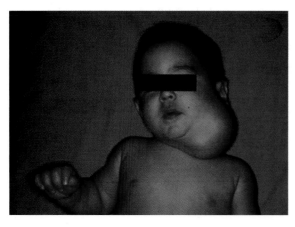

Fig. 70.3 Five month old child with moderate-sized lymphatic malformation, which was relatively asymptomatic

Table 70.3 Lymphatic malformations of the head and neck at The Hospital for Sick Children (1988–2000)

Sites of Involvement (130 Patients)

Site	Number of cases
Neck[a]	97
Posterior	40
Anterior	38
Submandibular	37
Face and Oropharynx[b]	46
Tongue	14
Floor of mouth	14
Cheek	17
Parotid	14
Larynx	5
Mediastinum and chest wall	14

[a] Neck Only–69, Entire Neck (all three sites)–17
[b] Face and Oropharynx Only–19

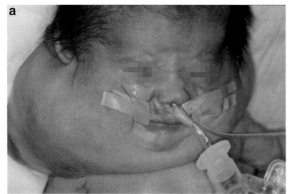

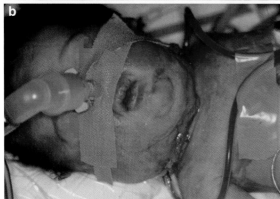

Fig. 70.4 Newborn with large cystic hygroma and airway obstruction. (a) Preoperatively, (b) Postoperatively

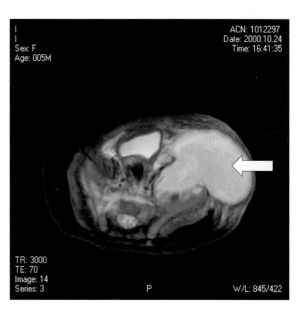

Fig. 70.5 MRI image of a retroperitoneal cystic hygroma presenting as an asymptomatic abdominal mass in a newborn (arrow)

Microcystic lymphatic malformations usually present as clear small vesicles infiltrating underlying tissues and are commonly found above the level of the mylohyoid muscle. Macrocystic lesions on the other hand are usually large, compressible masses under normal or bluish skin and are commonly below the level of the mylohyoid in the anterior or posterior triangles of the neck. Lymphatic malformations of the extremities are relatively uncommon but can be quite disfiguring.

Symptoms caused by lymphatic malformations are related to anatomical site, size and the presence or absence of complications such as bleeding or infection. However, most lymphatic malformations are asymptomatic and their effect on cosmesis is related to their site and size. Complications of lymphatic

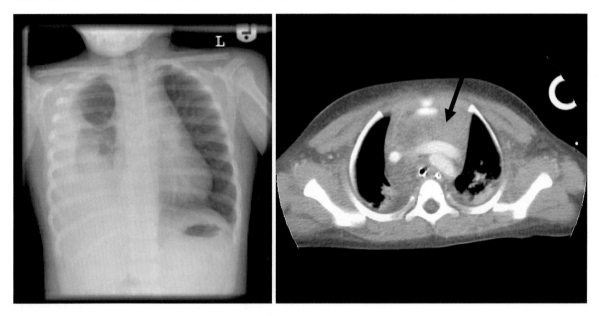

Fig. 70.6   Chest X-ray and CT from a child with persistent chylothorax due to a mediastinal lymphatic malformation (arrow)

malformations include *infections* which may be caused by bacteria contaminating cutaneous vesicles related to the malformation, or which travel to the malformation from distant sites through lymphatic channels. Such infections must be treated expeditiously and aggressively, since they can progress to life-threatening sepsis.

Hemorrhage into the cyst is also a well-described complication and may be spontaneous or related to minor trauma. Both infection and/or trauma may account for sudden rapid increase in the size of the malformation and may be the first presenting symptom. Less commonly, large malformations may cause airway obstruction. Such complex lesions require prompt treatment by an expert multi-disciplinary team. Rarely, *chylothorax*, *chylopericardium*, or *chylous ascites* may complicate lymphatic malformations (Fig. 70.6).

70.6 Investigations

No laboratory tests are necessary to diagnose a lymphatic malformation. If oncological diagnoses such as teratoma or lymphoma are being considered, measuring tumor markers specific to the tumor in question would be appropriate.

Ultrasound is usually the first imaging study to be performed. In some cases, no further testing is necessary, since ultrasound often provides adequate information regarding the consistency and location of the mass. However, it is often necessary to further delineate surrounding anatomy and relationships of the lesion to nearby vital structures, and for these cases *computerized tomography (CT)* and *magnetic resonance imaging (MRI)* are superior to ultrasound. Of these two imaging studies, most authors believe that MRI provides superior information, particularly with respect to the relationship of the lymphatic malformation to nearby neurovascular structures (Fig. 70.7).

70.7 Treatment

70.7.1 Non-operative Treatment

70.7.1.1 Expectant Treatment

The risk of complications associated with sclerotherapy and surgery must always be weighed against the risk of infection and bleeding, and the cosmetic implications of the lymphatic malformation. There is no risk for malignant transformation of these lesions. For

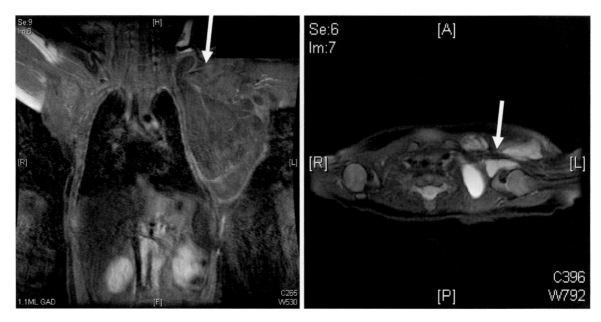

Fig. 70.7 Child with a large lymphatic malformation of the chest wall, extending into the axilla. The MRI demonstrates clearly the relationship of the lesion with the axillary neurovascular structures (arrows)

some asymptomatic lesions, or for lymphatic malformations that are located in a sensitive anatomic location that creates significant risk, some authorities would recommend expectant treatment.

70.7.1.2 Sclerotherapy

The increasing interest in sclerotherapy in recent years is a response to the relatively high complication rate reported after surgical resection, including recurrence, injury to vital structures, and large scars. The risk for neurovascular injury is higher in remedial surgery; hence, use of sclerosing agents has been recommended both as primary and adjuvant therapy. Multiple agents have been used with varying degrees of success, including: OK 432, Bleomycin, Ethibloc, dextrose solutions and fibrin glue. Injecting sclerosing agents is best performed under ultrasound guidance. The cyst is usually emptied prior to injecting the sclerosant.

OK432

OK432 is a compound derived by incubating a lyophilized group A streptococcus pyogenes in benzyl peni-

cillin. This agent was initially developed in Japan, and is still not approved for use in the United States. Advocates of this sclerosing agent note the relatively safe profile of the drug, particularly in contrast to bleomycin which may be associated with pulmonary fibrosis. Likewise, ethanol and sotradecol may produce life-threatening complications if injected in the blood stream. It remains unclear how OK432 produces its sclerosing effect. Although the agent produces an intense inflammatory reaction, no necrosis is seen on pathologic examination. This suggests that OK 432 causes cytokine-induced permeability of the endothelial lining of the malformation. The proposed increase in plasmin induced by OK 432 might allow for diffusion of OK 432 throughout the lesion, explaining its surprising effectiveness on microcytic lesions.

There are some well known complications of OK 432.

Anaphylaxis can be life threatening and is a result of the penicillin component in OK 432.

Swelling compressing vital structures: Swelling can result in significant airway compromise and it is advised that patients with lesions in the head and neck be admitted to hospital for observation post injection. Significant swelling is observed in up to 50% of patients. *Fever* is almost a universal finding in patients injected with OK 432. Fever is usually more than 38 degrees and persists on average for a day or two. There have been reports of fever lasting up to 10 days post injection.

No long-term studies are available yet to examine recurrence after treatment with OK 432. However in a recent report from Italy, recurrence was seen in a third of patients treated with this agent. Re-treatment with OK 432 is reasonable.

The use of OK 432 for the treatment of lymphatic malformations was first reported by Ogita et al. in 1987 with a subsequent report from the same group in 1994. However, very few studies have reported similar results outside Japan in part due to the relative difficulty of obtaining the material elsewhere. In a recent review from Sweden, Claesson et al. reported their experience with OK 432 in 32 patients, 28 of whom were children. In this series the authors excluded patients with an allergy to penicillin and those with significant medical problems. The mean age at the time of treatment with OK 432 was 3 years and 9 months (2 months to 11 years). In this cohort the injection treatment was used as primary treatment in 93% of patients (26 children). The authors rated the results of their treatment visually based on the response of the lesion to injection treatment. Results were said to be excellent when no residual disease was seen, fair when a > 50% reduction was observed and poor if such reduction was less than 50%. Fifteen patients had large cysts that were not previously treated; an excellent response was recorded after a mean of 2.6 injections (range 1–7). Another four children had microcystic disease and an excellent result was seen in two. A third developed a recurrence after 6 months, the results however were still considered fair. In the group of patients who had combined malformations (n = 8), all received OK 432 primarily. 87.5% (7 patients) had excellent results; the eighth patient had a large malformation for which he received a tracheostomy at birth. The neck part of the malformation responded well to OK 432, but due to the persistence of the mediastinal part of the malformation operative treatment was performed with excellent results. The authors note that there was no increased difficulty observed secondary to the use of the sclerosing agent. Claesson et al. concluded that the OK 432 is an excellent alternative to surgery in the treatment of lymphatic malformations.

A more recent case series on the use of OK 432 from New Zealand in 2004 reported 7 children under the age of 5 years who were treated with OK 432. In this series the surgeons used ultrasound guidance to aspirate the malformations and inject a maximum of 0.1 mg per session. Two lesions were in the neck, four in the axilla and one in the floor of the mouth extending to the anterior neck. Of note the injection therapy was performed as day surgery. The authors report "excellent" results in macrocystic lesion and "disappointing" results in their microcystic counterparts.

The most recent review is a case series by Luzzatto et al. In this study the authors report two separate cohorts. The first cohort comprised 29 children with lymphatic malformations who underwent treatment with OK 432 over a period of 4 years from 1999 to 2003. The second cohort described long term follow up of a previously reported series of 15 patients who underwent the same treatment in an earlier time period. In the recent group of 29 patients 12 had complete resolution with OK 432 treatment. Eight patients had more than 50% reduction and seven had no change in their lesions. The remaining two patients were lost to follow up. When the lesions were stratified by type the authors noted that about a half of the patients had no response in the microcystic and combined groups. As for long term results, the authors also reported an overall 30% recurrence rate in the cohort that was treated in earlier years. Two important lessons are learned from this report: the authors noticed ongoing regression beyond 6 weeks, and have become less aggressive in terms of repeat injections so long as the lesion continues to involute on ongoing clinical and ultrasound follow up. The second lesson is that persisting with injections beyond two sessions was worthwhile in early "non-responders", once the lesion did not respond to the third injection then further persistence was not indicated.

Bleomycin

The advantages of bleomycin are low cost and ready availability. Bleomycin as a chemotherapeutic agent works by DNA inhibition. It is postulated however, that it produces the sclerosing effect by inducing non-specific inflammation of the endothelial cells. The most feared complication of Bleomycin is the development of pulmonary fibrosis. The association of pulmonary complications and bleomycin are well documented in the oncology population. Even when the drug is not injected directly in the blood stream—as seen when using it for pleurodesis—there is significant systemic absorption. Currently in most North American centers the use of this agent has been abandoned.

In a recent review from India seven patients with lymphatic malformations were treated with Bleomycin with technique described above. All the lesions were confined to the neck. All malformations were macrocystic. All patients showed an initial response, with three patients having complete resolution of their lesions. The rest of the patients had a greater than 50% initial response, but subsequent recurrence in three patients necessitated surgical excision. Sanlalip reported similar results.

were mainly micro-cystic where only 23% had excellent results.

Analogous to most other sclerosing agents, patients experienced post injection pyrexia that lasted on average 1–2 days. Interestingly five patients required surgery post injection: two for scar revision, two for persistent drainage and one for a salivary fistula. Contrary to most surgeons' expectations, the authors claimed that the surgical resection was not more difficult due to scar formation from the previous sclerotherapy.

A common complication of Ethiblock injection is extravasation from the lesion post-injection. In the Montreal study, 80% of the patients experienced this problem. Although a cause for parental concern, the authors consider such extravasation a "good" sign, indicating the sclerosing effect of the agent is underway.

Ethiblock (Alcohol Solution of Zein)

Ethiblock is a mixture consisting of ethanol, contrast agents, and amino acids, which has been used as a sclerosing agent for vascular malformations as well as other applications

Ethiblock is both biodegradable and thrombogenic. The mechanism by which it produces its sclerosing effect is not completely understood.

Ethiblock has been used in Europe since the early 1990s. The agent has yet to be approved by the FDA in the US. In a recent review from Montreal, 63 patients underwent treatment with this agent for 67 lymphatic malformations. Most lesions (67%) were in the head and neck region. Median follow up time in this report was 3.5 years. Purely microcystic lesions were excluded.

The majority of the patients underwent sclerosing therapy as primary treatment. Only six patients had had previous resection. The average treatment sessions per patient were 1.5 session /patient (range 1–6). The results were classified in a similar fashion to the aforementioned studies. Cosmetic results were generally encouraging. 49% of patients in the predominantly macrocystic lesions had excellent results. This is in sharp contrast to lesions which

70.7.2 Surgical Management

Most lymphatic malformations remain readily amenable to surgical resection. With recent advances in surgical technique, anesthesia and critical care, postoperative mortality has significantly decreased.

When attempting surgical resection of a lymphatic malformation certain surgical principals must be remembered and adhered to. *First*, these malformations are benign lesions and hence, radical resection sacrificing vital structures is contraindicated. In all cases, slow careful dissection must be used, and all neurovascular structures must be identified (Fig. 70.8). *Second*, wide exposure with meticulous haemostatic dissection should be always carried out. Such dissection can be aided by the use of microbipolar techniques. *Thirdly*, intra-operative identification and individual ligation of lymphatic channels feeding into the lesion should be performed wherever possible. This is thought to decrease the likelihood of clinically significant post-operative lymphatic leak. *Finally*, closed suction drains should be left at the operative site to prevent accumulation of lymphatic fluid which could compress underlying structures.

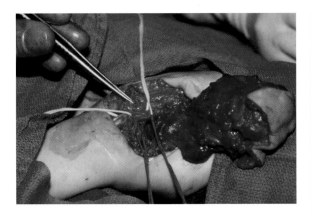

Fig. 70.8 Exposure of an axillary lymphatic malformation. Neurovascular structures must be identified and preserved, even if it means leaving some of the lesion behind.

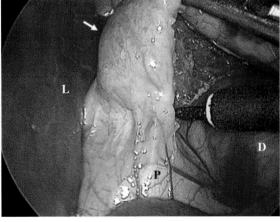

Fig. 70.10 Thoracoscopic resection of a mediastinal lymphatic malformation (arrow). P = pericardium, D = diaphragm, L = collapsed lung

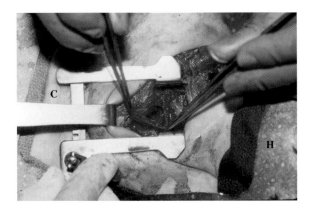

Fig. 70.9 Use of a "hockey stick" incision for a large cervico-mediastinal lymphatic malformation. C = chest, H = head

70.7.3 Surgical Resection Versus Sclerotherapy

Very few studies have compared surgical versus sclerosing treatment for lymphatic malformations. In a recent review from Japan, Okazaki et al. compared 78 patients who underwent surgical resection for lymphatic malformations with a group of 50 patients who were treated with OK 432 over a 26-year period. Similar to other reports, the most common location was head and neck (53.9%). The authors noted a significant increase in the utilization of primary OK 432 over the study period. Surgical treatment was effective for eradication of the malformation in 88.5% of patients compared to 64% in the OK 432 group. This difference was statistically significant. Eighteen patients failed initial OK 432 treatment and subsequently underwent surgical resection with good results. As observed in other series, the authors noted that surgical resection was not difficult after OK 432 injection. Although surgical treatment was more effective, it was associated with a higher rate of complications. In particular, 27% of surgical patients suffered lymphatic leaks, a complication that was not seen in the OK 432 group. The authors concluded that because OK 432 treatment was not as effective as reported in the literature, surgical treatment, especially in an area where there is little risk of damage to vital structures, is probably the initial treatment of choice.

The surgical approach should be individualized according to the anatomical position of the malformation. In the neck most surgeons would approach such lesions with a transverse incision. Lesions extending into the mediastinum could be approached by extending the neck incision into a median sternotomy (a "hockey stick" incision) as described by Grosfeld et al. (Fig. 70.9). Lesions in the chest and abdomen can be approached using laparoscopic or thoracoscopic techniques, as long as the aforementioned principals are adhered to (Fig. 70.10).

70.8 Complications

70.8.1 Treatment of Recurrence

Little has been written about the indications and techniques for treatment of recurrent lymphatic malformations, or the morbidity associated with it. In the aforementioned study, 52.9% of patients had recurrent disease. Factors predisposing to recurrence include microcystic disease and/or incomplete initial resection. Location of the malformation—particularly lesions in the floor of the mouth and tongue—influences the rate of recurrence. The choice of treatment for recurrent lymphatic malformation should be individualized, based on the degree of symptomatology, the risk of injury to vital structures, and the cosmetic implications of further surgery.

70.8.2 Other Complications

Complications of sclerosing agents have been discussed previously. In the modern era, the mortality associated with surgical resection of a lymphatic malformation should approach zero. In a large series of 263 procedures performed for lymphatic malformations, 31.3% of the cohort experienced a complication over the 10-year period of the study. Local complications, mainly seromas and hematomas, occurred in 50% of

Table 70.4 Perioperative complications–120 cases

Complication	Number
Infection	6
Bleeding[a]	5
Cranial neuropathy	12
Marginal mandibular branch VII [b]	10
Cranial nerve XI	1
Cranial nerve XII	1
Horner's syndrome	1
Seroma	4
Salivary fistula	1
Wound dehiscence	3
Tongue edema	3

[a]Requiring blood transfusion
[b]Paresis resolved completely

patients. Neurological complications were seen in 17% of patients. These results are similar to our own experience, outlined in (Table 70.4).

70.9 Conclusion

Lymphatic malformations are rare, challenging lesions that require significant expertise. A multidisciplinary approach is optimal for providing excellent care and maximizing the chances for a favorable outcome. With the current increasing interest in non-operative treatment, a standardized well-organized comparative study is needed to help define the role of these agents as primary treatments for lymphatic malformations.

Further Reading

Elluru RG, Azizkhan RG (2006) Cervicofacial vascular anomalies. II. Vascular malformations. Semin Pediat Surg 15:133–139

Emran MA, Dubois J, Laberge L et al (2006) Alcoholic solution of zein (Ethibloc) sclerotherapy for treatment of lymphangiomas in children. J Pediatr Surg 41:975–979

Howarth ES, Draper ES, Budd JLS et al (2005) Population based study of the outcome following the prenatal diagnosis of cystic hygroma. Prenat Diagn 25:286–291

Langer JC, Fitzgerald PG, Desa D et al (1990) Cervical cystic hygroma in the fetus: Clinical spectrum and outcome. J Pediatr Surg 25:58–62

Luzzatto C, Piccolo RL, Fascetti F et al (2005) Further experience with OK-432 for lymphangiomas. Pediatr Surg Int. 21:969–972

Mathur NN, Rana I, Bothra R et al (2005) Bleomycin sclerotherapy in congenital lymphatic and vascular malformations of head and neck. Intl J Pediatr Otorhinolaryngol 69:75–80

Ogita S, Tsuto T, Nakamura K et al (1996) OK-432 therapy for lymphangioma in children: Why and how does it work? J Pediatr Surg 31:477–480

Okazaki T, Iwatani S, Yanai T et al (2007) Treatment of lymphangiomas in children: Our experience of 128 cases. J Pediatr Surg 42:386–389

Ozen O, Moralioglu S, Karabulut R (2005) Surgical treatment of cervicofacial cystic hygromas in children. ORL 67:331–334

Smith BM, Albanese CT (2006) Cystic hygroma. In P Puri, ME Höllwarth (eds) Pediatric Surgery. Springer, Berlin, Heidelberg pp 13–18

Sacrococcygeal Teratoma

71

Thambipillai Sri Paran and Prem Puri

Contents

71.1 Introduction

Teratomas are uncommon tumours comprised of mixed dermal elements derived from the three germ cell layers. They attract attention because of their bizarre histology and gross appearance. Sacrococcygeal teratoma is the commonest teratoma seen in children, with an incidence of 1 in 40,000 live births. They are congenital and arise from the coccygeal region and can grow into the pelvis or externally into the caudal region or into both these regions. Though the majority are benign, malignancy is reported in some resected specimens. However, the overall prognosis is excellent, dependent on ease of surgical resection, timing of diagnosis, and malignant potential of the tumour.

71.2 Embryology and Pathology

The commonly accepted Embryonic (Blastomeric) Cell Theory suggests that these teratomas arise from pluripotent cells from Hensen's node, which have eluded the influence of the primary organizer during early embryonic development. Willis defined a teratoma as a 'true tumour or neoplasm composed of multiple tissues of kinds foreign to the part in which it arises'. Extragonadal teratomas tend to occur in midline structures such as the anterior mediastinum, retroperitoneum, sacrococcygeal region, and pineal gland. They are composed of mixed dermal elements derived from the three germ cell layers, and are known to contain virtually any tissue type including skin, teeth, endocrine structures, central nervous tissue, respiratory mucosa and alimentary mucosa. The tumour may comprise of cells that are totally benign

P. Puri and M. Höllwarth (eds.), *Pediatric Surgery: Diagnosis and Management,*
DOI: 10.1007/978-3-540-69560-8_71, © Springer-Verlag Berlin Heidelberg 2009

(mature teratoma) to that are frankly malignant. A third group of cells that appear malignant (usually described as 'immature') can confuse the diagnosis. For this reason, the diagnosis of malignant sacrococcygeal teratoma can only be made if there are distant metastases at the time of diagnosis.

71.3 Altman's Classification

Altman et al. have classified sacrococcygeal teratomas into four groups in 1974 (Fig. 71.1). Type I tumours are almost exclusively exterior with a minimal pelvic component; type II tumours have a significant pelvic component ('hour-glass pattern'); type III tumours have a larger proportion of intra-abdominal and intrapelvic component than the external component; type IV tumours are exclusively presacral with no external component. Furthermore, Altman et al. also reported that type I tumours were rarely malignant (0% in the

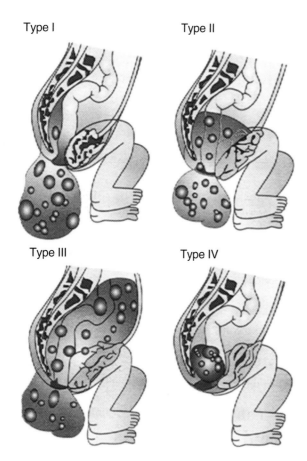

Fig. 71.1 Altman's Classification

71.4 Antenatal Diagnosis

In contrast to the overall prognosis of a newborn with Sacrococcygeal teratoma, a foetus remains at high risk for perinatal complications and death. Neonatal death may result from the maternal obstetric complications of tumour rupture during labour, preterm labour from polyhydramnios, dystocia or high-output cardiac failure due to the tumour size. Foetal hydrops is usually the result of a vascular steal syndrome leading to the shunting of blood away from the placenta and causing high-output cardiac failure, the earliest signs of which are polyhydramnios and placental thickening leading inexorably to preterm labour. Foetal hydrops and placentomegaly also have grave complications for maternal health. This is known as maternal "mirror" syndrome, because the mother suffers the same symptoms as the sick foetus. She will become ill and have signs of preeclampsia: water retention, high blood pressure and proteinuria.

Hedrick et al. reported their experience with 30 antenatally diagnosed Sacrococcygeal teratoma, which included 4 terminations, 5 foetal demises, 7 neonatal deaths and 14 survivors. In three of the five intrauterine foetal deaths, high-output cardiac failure and hydrops was evident. One child died for partial tumour rupture with pericardial and pleural effusions, while the cause of death is unknown in the fifth foetus. The seven neonatal deaths were at a mean of 28.6 weeks of gestational age due to tumour rupture during labour in three, intraoperative bleeding in two, severe oligohydramnios and pulmonary hypoplasia in one, and due to cardiac complications following open foetal surgery in one. Fourteen survivors were all born by caesarean section at a mean of 36 weeks gestational age, and were operated on 1st or 2nd day of life.

Makin et al. followed up 41 foetuses in their series of antenatally diagnosed sacrococcygeal teratoma, with 6 elective terminations, 12 elective foetal interventions with 50% survival and 17 non-interventions with 94% survival. Foetal intervention for hydrops resulted in 86% mortality.

American Academy of Pediatric Surgical Section Survey), while 6% of type II and 20% of type III and 8% of type IV tumours were malignant. It is also well documented that most tumours that are benign at birth can become malignant after about 2 months.

71.5 Neonatal Diagnosis

The most common neonatal presentation is large sacral mass that is obvious at birth (Fig. 71.2). The mass may be in the midline or paramedian. The overlying skin is usually normal, but there may be evidence of a haemangioma or necrosis with ulceration. When there is intrapelvic extension of tumour, the anus and vagina are pushed anteriorly. Intrapelvic tumours are often not diagnosed until later in life when they may present with symptoms due to pressure on the rectum or bladder. Associated congenital anomalies are found in 20% of cases and include vertebral, renal, cardiac and gastrointestinal anomalies. Infants presenting with malignant tumours usually present with a rapidly growing buttock mass. In such cases distant metastases are usually present at diagnosis. Even in these children with malignant sacrococcygeal teratoma, recent advances in multimodal therapy have resulted in survival rates as high as 80%.

Major differential diagnosis of a large sacral mass in a neonate is an anterior meningocoele. While most sacrococcygeal teratomas are solid, meningocoele are

cystic with a sacral defect. Dillarad et al. reported that during rectal examination of a meningocoele, the anterior fontanelle is seen to bulge. Lemire et al. have produced a list of 20 different lesions that can possibly enter into the differential diagnosis including a sacrococcygeal chordoma.

71.6 Investigations

Plain X-ray of the pelvis and spine may show calcification or structures such as teeth and bones or there may be a bony defect as in neural tube defect.

Abdominal ultrasonography is useful to determine the size and consistency of any pelvic or abdominal component. Computed tomography (CT) scan and Magnetic resonance imaging (MRI) both will provide more details regarding tumour size, extension and even vascular anatomy, but will need sedation or even general anaesthesia in these newborns (Fig. 71.3). If oil is instilled into the rectum during the MRI examination while T1-wieghted images are gathered, then the oil can act as contrast medium. MRI should clearly distinguish between sacrococcygeal teratoma and anterior meningocoele,

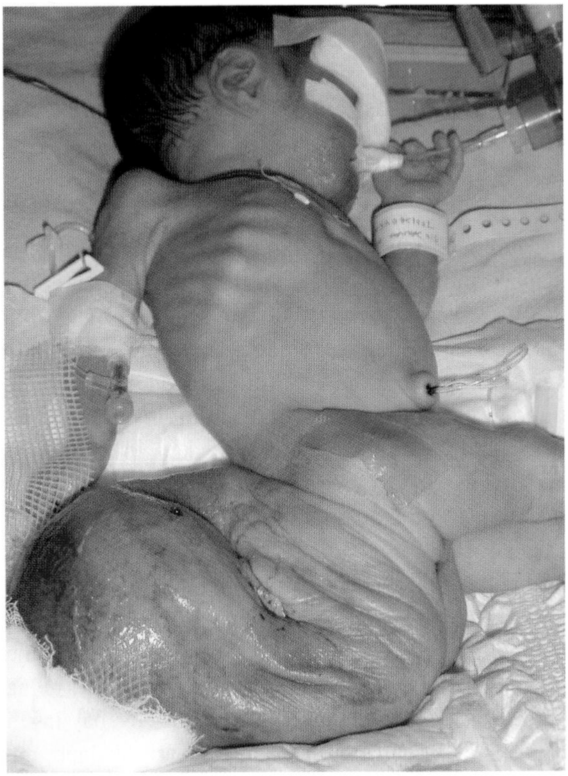

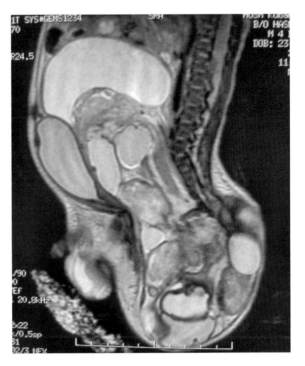

Fig. 71.2 Newborn with a large Sacrococcygeal Teratoma

Fig. 71.3 MRI scan showing large Type II tumour

and may be able to detect the occasional extension of the tumour through the sacral hiatus into the spinal canal.

Alpha-Fetoprotein is elevated when there is a malignant component to the tumour and is a useful serum marker in detecting postoperative malignant recurrence.

71.7 Preoperative Management

Blood should be cross-matched, and adequate venous access and arterial access for blood pressure monitoring should be established. If the tumour is ruptured, a pressure bandage may be necessary to stop the blood loss, while emergency surgery is being planned.

If the surgery is being carried out within the first 2 days of life, then bowel preparation is not necessary. However, when surgery is delayed beyond this period for various reasons, proper bowel prep must be carried out. In our institution we give Amoxycillin, Gentamicin and Metronidazole antibiotic prophylaxis preoperatively in all children, and continue this for 48 h postoperatively.

71.8 Surgery

Following general anaesthesia and catheterisation of the bladder, the patient is placed in prone position with rolls across the anterior superior iliac spines and the shoulders (Fig. 71.4).

A chevron incision with its apex over the lower sacrum is made with preservation of as much of the normal skin as possible (Fig. 71.5). The incision is deepened down to the fascia, with ligation of large subcutaneous veins.

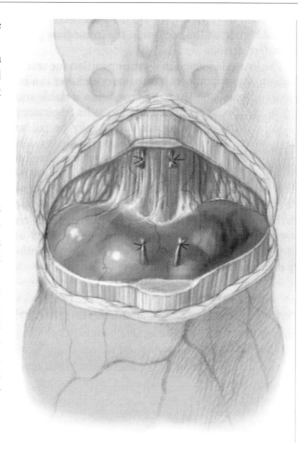

Fig. 71.5 Chevron incision above the coccyx

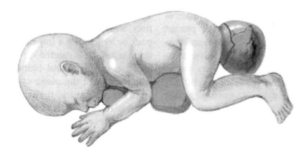

Fig. 71.4 Positioning of the child for surgery

The incision is deepened down to the coccyx or even the lower sacrum in the midline, and the edges of the sacrum are defined. A clamp is passed across the sacrum at this level, keeping the tips of the forceps against the ventral surface of the bone to ensure that the forceps pass between the sacrum and the underlying middle sacral vessels, which are usually substantial vessels, supplying the bulk of the blood supply to the tumour. Following this the sacrum is divided and the middle sacral vessels are ligated in continuity and divided.

Following this, the tumour is dissected outside the capsule from thinned out levator and gluteus muscle. The pelvic component is displaced anteriorly until its upper extent is reached. The tumour is dissected out from the pelvis and rolled inferiorly. At this point the upper end of the rectum could be identified by Vaseline gauze pack (placed preoperatively) or by passing a Hagar dilator. Once the rectum is clearly defined, the tumour is dissected off the rectum, anal canal and the inferior skin flap. Following meticulous haemostasis, the pelvic floor is reconstructed by suturing the central portion of levator sling to the perichondrium of the sacrum and muscle and facial reconstruction along the midline. These initial fascial sutures should determine the sitting of the anus. A drain may be placed within the presacral space and brought out through the subcutaneous tissue of the buttock. Excess skin is trimmed and the skin is closed in two layers when possible with absorbable sutures or in a single layer with nylon sutures. Vaseline pack is left within the anus.

Abdominal exploration is indicated when there is a large abdominal component of tumour or when there is significant bleeding either due to tumour rupture or vascular injury during the perineal approach. A transverse infra-umbilical incision will allow access to aorta below the origin of inferior mesenteric artery. The middle sacral vessels could be ligated via the abdominal approach, and the abdominal component of the tumour mobilised safely. The abdominal wound is temporarily closed with running 3/0 nylon suture, and patient repositioned for tumour resection as described above. At the end of tumour removal, the abdominal wound is closed in layers with absorbable sutures.

71.9 Postoperative Management

The infant is nursed in prone position until the wound is healed. Vaseline pack is removed after 24 h, if it is not passed spontaneously. Infant could be fed the same day, as long as there is no damage to the rectum during the tumour resection, once fully recovered from anaesthesia. Urinary catheter is removed as soon as baby's condition is stable. The wound drain can also be removed after 48 h.

Alpha-Fetoprotein levels are measured soon after surgery before discharge. The infant is then followed up with three monthly checks of Alpha-Fetoprotein and PR examinations for 1 year to detect any recurrence.

71.10 Long-Term Follow-Up

Though a 5-year follow-up was recommended in the past, latest reports by Derikx et al. and Gabra et al. highlight the need to monitor these children into their teenage years. Derikx et al. reported malignant recurrence in 4 out of 148 children with age at recurrence ranging from 10 months to 10.6 years. When alpha-Fetoprotein is raised or when clinical suspicion is raised, the CT or MRI scan must be used to detect and localize recurrent disease.

Long-term bowel and bladder dysfunction in children following sacrococcygeal tumour resection is also well recognised. Bowel dysfunction varied from constipation (17%), soiling (13%) to involuntary bowel movements (9%) in the report by Drikx et al. They also reported a 31% urinary incontinence within their group of children. Gabra et al. have also reported such high incidence of bowel and bladder dysfunction. Whether these complications are a result of tumour mass compressing the pelvic nerves or a secondary result of surgical damage to the pelvic nerves is unknown. Renal ultrasound is necessary to assess the kidneys when symptoms suggestive of neuropathic bladder are encountered. In fact, routine ultrasound monitoring of the renal tracts annually is recommended by some authors. Urodynamics, anorectal manometry, and sphincter-mapping stimulation studies must be performed as dictated by clinical symptoms.

71.11 Prognosis

In the absence of distant metastases and when the tumour is resected completely with the coccyx, the life expectancy is normal. When distant metastases are present, the prognosis must be guarded. However, with present multimodal treatment > 90% survival could be expected in children with distant metastases.

Bowel and bladder dysfunction are common following sacrococcygeal teratoma resection. Clean intermittent catheterisation for neuropathic bladder and bowel management programs for faecal incontinence can improve the quality of life for these children. As for the cosmetic results after reconstruction of buttock region following resection of large tumours (>500 cm³), further referral to plastic reconstructive surgeons may be necessary.

Further Reading

Derikx JPM et al (2007) Long-term functional sequelae of Sacro-coccygeal teratoma: A national study in the Netherlands. J Pediatr Surg 42(6):1122–1126

Docimo SG (2007) Clinical Pediatric Urology, Informa Healthcare, Oxon

Gabra HO et al (2006) Sacrococcygeal teratoma – A 25-year experience in a UK regional center. J Pediatr Surg 41(9):1513–1516

Hedrick HL et al (2004) Sacrococcygeal teratoma: Prenatal assessment, fetal intervention and outcome. J Pediatr Surg 39(3):319–323

Makin EC et al (2006) Outcome of antenatally diagnosed Sacrococcygeal teratomas: Single – center experience (1993–2004). J Pediatr Surg 41(2):388–393

Pringle KC (2006) Sacrococcygeal Teratoma. In P Puri, ME Höllwarth (eds) Pediatric Surgery. Springer Surgery Atlas Series, Springer-Verlag Berlin Heidelberg, New York, pp 435–442.

Puri P (2003) Newborn Surgery. Arnold, London

Puri P, Höllwarth ME (2006) Paediatric Surgery. Springer, Berlin, Heidelberg, pp 435–442

Stringer MD, Oldham KT, Mouriquand PDE (2006) Pediatric Surgery and Urology. Cambridge University Press, Cambridge

Neuroblastoma

72

Edward Kiely

Contents

72.1 Introduction

Neuroblastoma arises in primitive cells of the sympathetic nervous system. Consequently it is found at sites where collections of sympathetic cells are encountered – adrenal medulla and sympathetic ganglia. A wide spectrum of tumour activity is seen ranging from spontaneous regression to rapid growth and widespread dissemination. In between these extremes are children whose tumours behave in an indolent fashion with long periods of static size and absent growth.

In addition a number of tumours mature to a less malignant phenotype.

72.2 Incidence

About 1 in 100,000 children is diagnosed with neuroblastoma in childhood. It is the commonest extra-cranial solid tumour in children and comprises about 10% of all childhood cancer.

About 30% of tumours occur in infancy; a further 50% between the ages of 1 and 4 years and the remainder are in older children and adolescents. There is a slight male preponderance.

72.3 Pathology

The macroscopic appearance of these tumours varies from firm pale grey discreet masses to friable haemorrhagic ill-defined tumours.

Histologically firmer tumours are composed of mature ganglion cells with abundant pink cytoplasm

P. Puri and M. Höllwarth (eds.), *Pediatric Surgery: Diagnosis and Management*,
DOI: 10.1007/978-3-540-69560-8_72, © Springer-Verlag Berlin Heidelberg 2009

and well-defined nucleoli. In between the ganglion cells is mature schwannian stroma. These ganglioneuromas are generally associated with a benign clinical course.

At the opposite end of the histological spectrum are tumours comprised of sheets of immature small round blue cells. These sometimes show rosette formation – a circular arrangement of cells with central neurofibrillary material (Fig. 72.1). On occasion, dystrophic calcification is seen. Those tumours composed predominantly of neuroblasts, exhibit more aggressive behaviour.

When there is a substantial infiltration of immature neuroblasts in an otherwise mature tumour, the lesion is termed a ganglioneuroblastoma.

Although many of these tumours may be diagnosed on standard haematoxylin and eosin staining, a battery of immuno-histochemical stains is routinely used to confirm the diagnosis. Rapidly evolving laboratory techniques allow more detailed genome and proteome analysis and will further define risk group and likely tumour behaviour.

Various pathological grading systems have been used to predict tumour behaviour and to direct therapy. The most widely used is the Shimada classification, which has formed the basis of the International Neuroblastoma Pathology Classification. Use of these classifications has produced favourable and unfavourable histological groups and has allowed a reduction in therapy for the former and more intensive therapy for the latter group.

72.4 Sites of Disease

The adrenal medulla is the commonest site of primary neuroblastoma – about 50% of the total. Other abdominal sites – sympathetic chains or pre-aorta locations – are involved in about 20%. The posterior mediastinum is the site of primary tumour in perhaps 10% and the pelvis in about 7% of the total.

In the majority, metastatic spread has already occurred at the time of diagnosis – up to 70%. Metastatic spread is predominantly to lymph nodes, bone and bone marrow. The disease is localised in perhaps 25% and about 10% of the total have the special infant form of the disease – stage 4S disease.

72.5 Markers of Disease Behaviour

72.5.1 Biochemical Markers

Biochemical markers are widely used to help predict likely tumour behaviour. The three commonly used markers are lactate dehydrogenase (LDH), ferritin and neuron specific enolase (NSE). Elevated levels of these markers are associated with a worse clinical outcome (LDH > 1,500 IU per ml, feritin > 142 nanograms per ml, NSE > 15 nanograms per ml). In general elevated levels of these markers are associated with advanced clinical stage and a worse outcome.

72.5.2 Molecular Markers

Increasing numbers of genetic markers of disease activity have been defined. The sheer number of these markers is sometimes considered a hindrance to understanding disease behaviour and in planning clinical care. At the present time MYCN status, 1p deletion, 11q deletion, 17q gain and DNA ploidy are frequently assessed at diagnosis. The information gained from different combinations of these markers, combined with clinical stage, age and pathological classification, is used to define high as against lower risk groups. More intensive therapy is then given to the high-risk group.

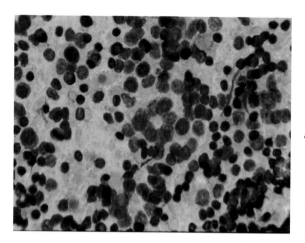

Fig. 72.1 Histology from the tumor surface: round cells with rosette formation. (by courtesy from Michael Höllwarth)

The MYCN proto-oncogene is located on chromosome 2 and amplification, especially more than ten copies, is associated with more aggressive clinical behaviour independent of age and disease stage. About 20% of neuroblastoma patients show MYCN amplification and this increases to 50% in those presenting with locally advanced or metastatic disease.

Loss of genetic material from the short arm of chromosome 1—1p deletion—is usually associated with MYCN amplification and with worse clinical outcome. 1p deletion is found in about 25% of all neuroblastomas.

11q deletion is found in about one third of all neuroblastomas and is not associated with MYCN amplification. This abnormality is independently associated with reduced survival.

17q gain is in the form of an unbalanced translocation. It is found in almost 60% of all neuroblastomas and again, is associated with a worse outcome.

DNA ploidy also affects tumour behaviour. Polyploidy—greater than diploid DNA content—is associated with improved survival. Tumours with diploid DNA content have a significantly worse outcome.

At the present time, the manner in which these genetic markers result in altered tumour behaviour is not clear. Obviously chromosomal deletions may involve tumour suppressor genes. However, the exact mechanism of altered cell survival and behaviour is not understood at present.

72.6 Staging

The International Neuroblastoma Staging System (INSS) is widely applied. The clinical stage is the main factor directing therapy. At the present time, different oncology groups use other markers of disease activity to define high-risk and low-risk groups and to direct intensified therapy towards those in high-risk groups (Table 72.1).

In the near future it is likely that a new risk classification will be applied – the International Neuroblastoma Risk Group Staging System (INRGSS). This system will combine clinical stage, histological tumour differentiation, ploidy, MYCN amplification and 11q deletion to define the risk groups. These will be low, intermediate, high and ultra high-risk groups and different treatment strategies will be used for each group.

Table 72.1 INSS staging criteria

Stage	Definition
1.	Localised tumour with complete gross excision, with or without microscopic residual disease; representative ipsilateral lymph nodes negative for tumour microscopically (nodes attached to and removed with the primary tumour may Be positive).
2A.	localised tumour with incomplete gross excision; representative ipsilateral nonadherent lymph nodes negative for tumour microscopically.
2B.	Localised tumour with or without complete gross excision, with ipsilateral nonadherent lymph nodes positive for tumour. Enlarged contralateral lymph nodes must be negative microscopically.
3.	Unresectable unilateral tumour infiltrating across the midline, with or without regional lymph node involvement; or localised unilateral tumour with Contralateral regional lymph node involvement; or midline tumour with bilateral extension by infiltration (unresectable) or by lymph node involvement.
4.	Any primary tumour with dissemination to distant lymph nodes, bone, bone marrow, liver, skin and/or other organs (except as defined for stage 4S).
4S.	Localised primary tumour (as defined for stage 1, 2A or 2B), with dissemination limited to skin, liver and/or bone marrow (limited to infants < 1 year of age).

In most case series, patients with stage 1 or 2 disease make up about 25% of the total. 60–70% of patients have stage 3 or 4 disease and the remaining 10% have stage 4S disease.

The midline is defined as the vertebral column. Tumours originating on one side and crossing the midline must infiltrate to or beyond the opposite side of the vertebral column.

Marrow involvement in stage 4S should be minimal, i.e. <10% of total nucleated cells identified as malignant on bone marrow biopsy or on marrow aspirate. More extensive marrow involvement would be considered to be stage 4. The MIBG scan (if performed) should be negative in the marrow.

72.7 Presentation

A small number—about 3%—of neuroblastomas are detected antenatally. The infants usually have low stage disease with good biology.

A second group of infants with Stage 4S disease present with skin nodules and/or hepatomegaly (Fig. 72.2a and 72.2b).

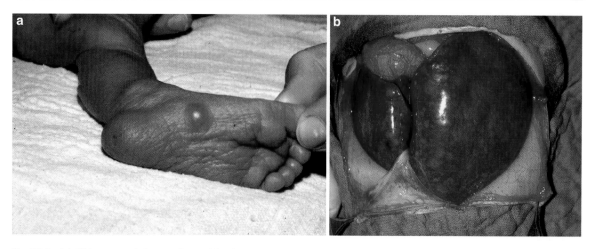

Fig. 72.2 (**a**). Skin metastasis in a newborn with a Stage IV S neuroblastoma (by courtesy from Michael Höllwarth) (**b**). Multiple liver metastases in a newborn with Stage IV S neuroblastoma (by courtesy from Michael Höllwarth)

The majority of patients however, present with symptoms from either the mass or the metastases. An abdominal mass may be palpated during clinical examination for non-specific symptoms. Bone pain, arthralgia or periorbital bruising are a consequence of bony metastases. Increased sweating is occasionally reported and hypertension from renal artery compression is not unusual. Generally the children with metastases have a period of general malaise and ill health preceding diagnosis.

Thoracic tumours are usually detected on a chest X-ray taken for presumed chest infection. Pelvic tumours interfere with bowel or bladder function and are found during investigation for these problems.

Uncommon presentations include paraplegia from spinal cord compression, diarrhoea as a consequence of vaso-active intestinal polypeptide secretion. Finally, a small group presents with opsomyoclonus (dancing eye syndrome).

Physical examination may reveal a fixed, hard, irregular abdominal mass. A pelvic mass may be detected on rectal examination but otherwise, in the absence of periorbital bruising or skin nodules, there is little to find on clinical examination.

72.8 Diagnosis

A diagnosis may be suspected on the basis of the history and the physical findings. The diagnosis is confirmed by detecting raised levels of urinary catecholamine metabolites – vanillyl mandelic acid (VMA) or homovanillic acid (HVA). Raised levels of these metabolites are found in about 85% of neuroblastomas.

Tissue diagnosis is nowadays considered mandatory. As assessment of tumour biology is essential before planning treatment, tissue from the tumour or from the metastases is needed. Sufficient tissue may be obtained by needle core biopsies for all relevant investigations.

Plain X-rays of chest or abdomen will frequently give useful information. Over half the tumours showed dystrophic calcification.

Ultrasound is used to assess the nature and extent of the tumour as well as to define the size of the tumour. The echo pattern is heterogeneous and unlike other childhood cancers. Ganglioneuromas present a more uniform appearance than undifferentiated neuroblastomas and an experienced radiologist will often suspect the diagnosis from the ultrasound appearance.

Cross sectional imaging in the form of MRI or contrast enhanced CT is also mandatory. These images provide precise anatomical information but usually underestimate the full extent of the tumour (Fig. 72.3).

Isotope scanning is essential for staging purposes. Metaiodobenzylguanidine (MIBG) scanning is widely available and is considered the optimal form of imaging for these tumours. Technetium bone scanning is also used.

Finally, bone marrow aspirates and trephines are essential to fully define the clinical stage.

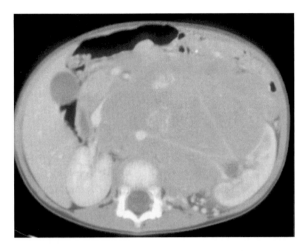

Fig. 72.3 Significant elongation of the renal artery due to a giant abdominal neuroblastoma involving most of the major intestinal vessels. Calcifications can be seen. (by courtesy from Michael Höllwarth)

72.9 Management

Available treatment modalities include chemotherapy, surgery and radiotherapy. In most centres care is coordinated by paediatric oncologists and the various steps in treatment are in accordance with agreed national and international protocols.

A large team is needed to look after these children. The surgeon's role includes provision of tissue for diagnosis; provision of vascular access and of course tumour resection.

The timing of surgical intervention is also protocol driven and should take place after discussion with oncologists and radiologists. Decisions about surgery can only be taken by surgeons who alone can evaluate what is or is not possible.

In general, low stage localised tumours are amenable to excision, often without the need for any other form of treatment.

Locally advanced or metastatic tumours are best managed by use of preoperative chemotherapy followed by delayed tumour excision. This allows for a less hazardous and potentially more complete operation.

Many infants with stage 4S disease need no specific treatment. In some, the tumour matures and eventually disappears without treatment. If hepatomegaly is progressive, then chemotherapy may be too slow to inter-

rupt the process. Should ventilation be required then progressive multi organ failure may result unless the liver growth can be interrupted.

Under these circumstances, hepatic artery embolisation may be life saving.

72.10 Chemotherapy

Combination chemotherapy has been responsible for the improved survival in the past 30 years. Oncology groups worldwide use a combination of alkylating agents (cyclophosphamide, platinum agents), topoisomerase inhibitors (topotecan, etoposide), vinca alkaloids (vincristin) and anthracyclines (doxorubicin). Dose intensity and length of treatment are increased for those with advanced or histologically unfavourable tumours.

72.11 Surgery

Neuroblastomas frequently surround and are in close proximity to major blood vessels. These include the aorta and its branches as well as the inferior vena cava and its branches. The aim of surgery is to remove the tumour whilst preserving essential blood vessels.

For paediatric surgeons this poses an unusual problem. The usual dissection techniques may be inadequate or unduly hazardous.

However, these tumours rarely invade the tunica media of major blood vessels and therefore the dissection may take place in the subadventitial plane. This is most easily accomplished using knife dissection.

Complete resection is not always possible. The surgical failure rate is 10%. The incidence of nephrectomy to achieve more complete excision is about 15%.

72.12 Radiotherapy

This is used either in the form of targeted therapy to improve local control or in the form of total body irradiation as part of conditioning for bone marrow transplantation.

72.13 Outcome

In one generation, the survival of patients with neuroblastoma has quadrupled – from 15 to 60%.

The outlook for those with localised stage 1 or 2 disease is a survival rate in excess of 90%.

For those with stage 3 disease the outlook has greatly improved and is now well over 70%.

Little change in survival has been seen in children presenting with stage 4 disease. About 30% of this group now survive long term and this figure has not changed in the past 15 years. For those with stage 4 disease and poor biology, survival rates may be less than 20%.

For infants with stage 4S disease, reported survival varies from 50–80%. Progressive hepatomegaly producing respiratory compromise has been associated with multi organ failure and death. The majority of these tumours have a favourable biological profile but some do not and may progress to stage 4 disease.

An age of 18 months or less at presentation is associated with markedly improved survival, independent of disease stage. The older the age of presentation, the worse the outcome.

As noted above, elevated levels of LDH, ferritin and NSE at diagnosis are associated with worse clinical outcome.

MYCN amplification, diploid DNA content, 1p deletion, 11q deletion and 17q gain all confirm a worse outlook.

Surgical resection is curative in those with localised stage 1 and 2 disease. Complete surgical resection more than doubles the survival rate for those with stage 3 disease.

The literature is contradictory in regard to the effect of surgery in those with stage 4 disease. Although some report improved survival for these children after complete surgical resection, our own figures do not suggest that complete resection necessarily confers an advantage.

72.14 Conclusion

The outlook for children with this tumour has improved. Research has yielded insights into the biology of the tumour but recent reports do not show progressively improving survival for those with advanced disease. Improved outcome for this group of children and for those with poor biology tumours awaits either novel chemotherapeutic agents or an entirely different form of treatment.

Further Reading

Brodeur GM, Maris JM (2006) Neuroblastoma. In PA Pizzo, DG Poplack (eds) Principles and Practice of Pediatric Oncology, 5th edn. JB Lippincott, Philadelphia, pp 933–970

Gutierrez JC et al (2007) Markedly improving survival of neuroblastoma: A 30-year analysis for 1,646 patients. Pediatr Surg Int 23:637–646

Kiely E (2006) Neuroblastoma. In P Puri, ME Hollwarth (eds) Pediatric Surgery. Springer Surgery Atlas Series, Springer-Verlag Berlin, Heidelberg, New York, pp 443–450

Kiely E (2007) A technique for excision of abdominal and pelvic neuroblastomas. Ann Roy Coll Surg Engl 89:342–348

Maris JM, Hoganty MD, Bagatell R et al (2007) Neuroblastoma. Lancet 369:2106–2120

Puri P, Höllwarth M (2006) Pediatric Surgery. Springer, Berlin, Heidelberg

Shilyansky J (2006) Neuroblastoma In Stringer M, Oldham K, Mouriquand P (eds) Pediatric Surgery and Urology: Long-term outcomes, 2nd edn. Cambridge University Press, Cambridge pp 745–758

Wilms' Tumor

73

Michael E. Höllwarth

Contents

73.1 Introduction

The Wilms' tumor (WT) is an embryonal tumor of renal origin, but extrarenal localization may rarely occur. The first description of a kidney tumor as myoma sarcomatodes is from Eberth in 1872. In 1898, Birch-Hirschfeld classified a similar kidney tumor as embryonal adenosarcoma. In 1899, Wilms reviewed the literature and added seven more cases with the clinical picture of the tumor that now bears his name, or nephroblastoma. It is the most common kidney tumor, the second common solid tumor after neuroblastoma, and represents 6–10% of all childhood cancer cases. The incidence varies between 1 per 50.000 to 1 per 200.000 neonates. It is more common in the US with 10.9 per million than in China with 2.5 per million. Most cases are diagnosed around the age of 3 years (range 1–5 years). Males and females are affected equally. Ninety-two to ninety-five percent of the WT occur in only one kidney and are unilateral. Anomalies associated with WT are the WAGR syndrome (aniridia, genitourinary anomalies, mental retardation), the Denis-Drash syndrome (intersex, nephropathy), the Beckwith-Wiedemann syndrome (exomphalos, macroglossia, viscero-megaly), and hemihypertrophy. Patients with bilateral tumor or other associated anomalies are diagnosed significantly earlier. About 2% of patients have a positive family history with one relative who also suffered from a WT. The association with other anomalies as well as the occurrence in families suggest that altered genes are involved in the tumor pathogenesis. Several genetic loci are involved. The two more important genes are the WT 1 and WT 2 suppressor gene on chromosome 11, but additional loci have been described on several other chromosomes, so far.

P. Puri and M. Höllwarth (eds.), *Pediatric Surgery: Diagnosis and Management*,
DOI: 10.1007/978-3-540-69560-8_73, © Springer-Verlag Berlin Heidelberg 2009

73.2 Pathology

The tumor compromises most parts of the kidney and may invade the urinary collecting system, the renal vein, or the surrounding tissues. The section shows partly solid, partly cystic regions with hemorrhagic areas (Fig. 73.1). If the WT occupies only one pole there exists a clear demarcation line to the normal kidney. The origin of the tumor is the metanephrogenic blastema; thus the histology mimics the development of a normal kidney, showing the three tissue components: blastema, tubules, and stroma (favorable histology) (Fig. 73.2). The proportions of these cell elements may be different from one tumor to the other. However, each component can exhibit focal or diffuse anaplastic cell elements (unfavorable histology), which are indicators for a poor outcome (Fig. 73.3). In 25–40% of WT patients, additional abnormal cell clusters can be found within normal parts of the kidney, the so-called *nephrogenic rests* (NR). They consist of foci of persisting blastemic cells, which are situated either intralobar or perilobar (Fig. 73.4). NR are common in neonatal kidneys and are either transformed into normal kidney tissue or into WT cell elements. Rarely both kidneys consist of diffuse nephrogenic rests—a pathology that is called *nephroblastomatosis.*

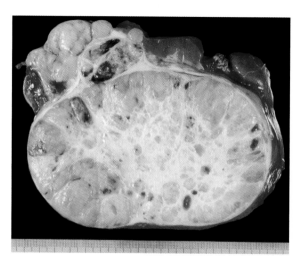

Fig. 73.1 Typical appearance of the tumor consisting of solid and cystic parts as well as hemorrhagic regions

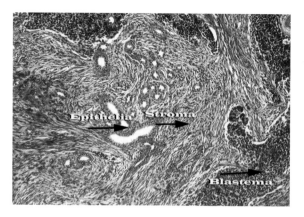

Fig. 73.2 Medium-power microscopic view of a typical Wilms Tumor with elements of tubules, blastema, and spindel cells

73.3 Clinical Presentation and Diagnosis

Most children present with an asymptomatic but rapidly growing abdominal mass. About 30% of patients suffer from abdominal pain, malaise, and weight loss.

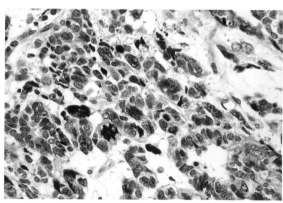

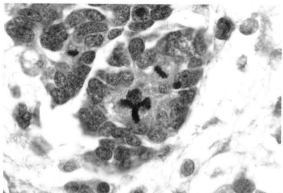

Fig. 73.3 High-power microscopic view of an anaplastic part of a Wilms Tumor with polymorphic cell nuclei and atypical cell mitosis

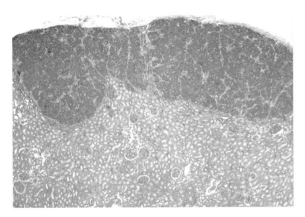

Fig. 73.4 Medium-power microscopic view of perilobar nephrogenic rest consisting of mesonephric blastema cells within normal kidney tissue

Some patients may show additionally a leftsided varicocele (occlusion of the renal vein by tumor invasion) or a symptomatic hydrocele. Ten percent of patients suffer from hematuria, mostly microscopic, when the tumor invades the urinary collecting system.

The availability of ultrasound in the private practice of GP and pediatricians today allows early diagnosis of WT and referral to the pediatric centre. The ultrasound study documents the position, size and volume of the tumor, the intravascular extension, metastatic involvement of regional lymph nodes and the liver, and the examination of the contralateral kidney. Furthermore, regular ultrasound investigations during preoperative chemotherapy allow weekly measurement of tumor volume, thereby indicating whether the tumor responds immediately to the therapy or not. The abundant availability of ultrasound today allows regular screening in patients with associated anomalies and increased risk for WT. Recommended screening intervals are two times a year.

The abdominal CT scan with contrast administration shows in detail the location of the tumor in the kidney, whether it extends into the surrounding tissues and the metastatic involvement of regional or distant lymph nodes. A chest X-ray is obtained to evaluate for the presence of pulmonary metastases. When the chest X- ray is negative, we order an additional CT scan for more precise evaluation of small pulmonary metastases, which has a significant impact on the tumor staging. To perform an MRI is optional, but it may provide additional information to confirm the diagnosis by imaging methods alone, thereby excluding different kidney pathologies. Differential diagnosis includes benign diseases such as hydronephrosis or a cystic kidney disease and malignancies such as clear cell sarcoma or rhabdoid tumor of the kidney.

73.4 Therapy

The mainstay of therapy is the radical surgical excision of the tumor and additional metastases. The international protocols include detailed recommendations for diagnosis, controls, and chemotherapeutic regimen in WT patients.

The basis of the therapy is the clinical Staging in regard to the tumor extent and the histological Grading (favorable or unfavorable histology). The National Wilm's Tumor Study Group (NWTS) and the International Society for Paediatric Oncology (SIOP-Societé Internationale pour Oncolgie Paediatrique) use a similar staging system:

Stage I: Tumor limited to the kidney and completely resected. No tumor rupture.

Stage II: Tumor extends beyond the kidney but is completely resected; regional extension of the tumor, vessel infiltration, tumor biopsy, or local spillage.

The SIOP protocol differentiates between Stage IIa—no lymph nodes involved—and Stage IIb—regional (hilar) lymph nodes involved.

Stage III: Residual nonhematogenous tumor, involvement of paraaortic or paracaval lymph nodes, diffuse spillage, peritoneal implants, local infiltration of vital structures.

Stage IV: Distant metastases.

Stage V: Bilateral tumor.

The study protocols of the NWTS and the SIOP are significantly different in that regard that SIOP includes preoperative chemotherapy—biopsy is only optional—and the NWTS protocol recommends primary surgery and biopsy if primary resection is not feasible or recommended (Table 73.1). The benefit of primary chemotherapy consists of a significant shrinkage of the tumor, evidenced by weekly ultrasound controls, and as a result a reduced incidence of intraoperative rupture

Table 73.1 Differences between the SIOP protocol and the protocol of the NWTS-Group

NWTS	SIOP
• Tumor nephrectomy or biopsy	• Chemotherapy, biopsy optional
• Postoperative chemo-(radio-)therapy	• Secondary tumor nephrectomy
	• Postoperative chemo-(radio-)therapy
Disadvantages	
• Tumor rupture and spillage	
• More complications	• Diagnostic error
• Extensive resection	• Downstaging
• Increased mortality	• Downgrading

Table 73. 2 Advantages and disadvantages of the protocols of SIOP and NWTS

- Downstaging
  - Less stage III (less radiation)
  - More stage I and II
  - More relapses in stage II
  - Therefore adriamycin is included in all stage II (late heart failure)
- Complications → 9.8% vs. 6.8%
- Tumor rupture and spillage 15.3% vs. 2,2%
  - Stage III → more radiation therapy
  - Less relapse-free survival but same overall survival

with diffuse spilling. The preoperative chemotherapy results in a downstaging of the tumor. This effect after chemotherapy may raise doubts in regard to Stage II, because it might have been in reality a stage III. Therefore, within the SIOP protocol, Stage II patients receive additionally antracyclin to adjust for this problem. The WT trial in the UK recommends preoperative chemotherapy also, but includes percutaneous biopsy to obtain histological confirmation. This procedure has the risk of tumor leakage along the needle tract leading to recurrences within the biopsy tract.

Radiotherapy of the tumor region is recommended for Stage III; therefore, tumor spillage during surgery should be avoided at all costs. Lung radiation can be omitted if pulmonary metastases disappear under chemotherapy or when they have been resected successfully. However, pulmonary radiation is inevitable if additional pulmonary metastases reappear.

One of the criticisms in regard to the SIOP protocol was the uncertainty of diagnosis without a preoperative biopsy. The SIOP arguments are that imaging methods today are so excellent that misdiagnosis is extremely rare. In SIOP-9, only 2% of patients received preoperative chemotherapy inappropriately for non-malignant processes and 3% had other malignant diseases. However, neither dactinomycin nor vincristine is associated with much short-term toxicity, and no long-term complications have been identified so far. Furthermore, biopsy is recommended if the tumor does not significantly respond to chemotherapy with a shrinking volume within 1 or 2 weeks. The disadvantage of the NWTS protocol is caused by the fact that the surgical procedure for the usually very large tumor is more difficult. Thus, surgical complication rates are

higher (9.8% vs. 6.8%) although not significant, but tumor rupture occurs significantly more often (15.3% vs. 2.2%). As a consequence, the number of Stage III patients with the additional need for local radiation is significantly higher (30.4% vs. 14.2) (Table 73.2).

The surgical procedure consists of a transabdominal tumornephrectomy via a large transverse incision. Whether or not the contralateral kidney must be explored during surgery is a matter of debate. We think that today's preoperative imaging methods are so excellent that this extension of the procedure is rarely necessary.

The hilum of the kidney is approached first and the vessels are ligated in order to avoid intraoperative spread of malignant cell elements through the renal vein. However, this part of the procedure is often not feasible due to the huge size of the tumor and the close connection to the vena cava or aorta. The adrenal gland may be left in place if it is not abutting the tumor. The ureter is ligated and divided as low as possible. Careful sampling of regional and distant lymph nodes is essential for correct staging. Metastatic lesions in the liver or lungs must be excised surgically if they are present after appropriate chemotherapy.

73.5 Special Problems

Tumor extension into the renal vein and vena cava presents a particular problem. The preoperative imaging examinations show the extension of the invasion accurately. Preoperative chemotherapy often reduces not only the size but also the intravascular extension of

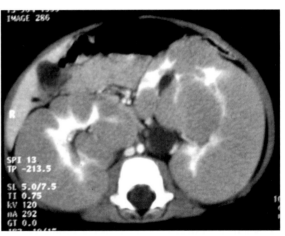

Fig. 73.6 Diffuse bilateral microscopic nephroblastomatosis. This kidney responded well to chemotherapy, but the patient developed a unilateral Wilms Tumor 2 years later, which was resected by nephron-sparing surgery

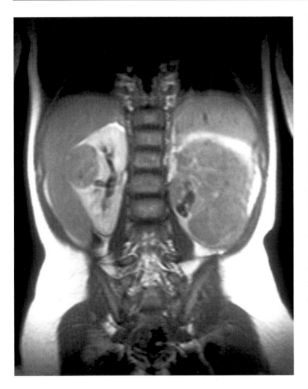

Fig. 73.5 Bilateral Wilms Tumor. In this case tumor enucleation on the right side is not a violence of the protocol

the tumor. If the tumor thrombus is located within the infradiaphragmatic vena cava it can be removed through a horizontal cavatomy after occlusion of the vein above the liver or within the pericardium. If the tumor extends beyond the diaphragm into the right atrium cardiopulmonary bypass is recommended.

The protocols agree that primary chemotherapy is necessary if a *bilateral WT* is present. Four to 6 weeks of chemotherapy result in a significant reduction of tumor size and volume and kidney-sparing surgery can be performed (Fig. 73.5). The surgical procedure should always start at the more difficult side; if a kidney-sparing surgical procedure on this side is not possible and tumornephrectomy is inevitable, the surgeon should do the best to save as much normal kidney tissue as possible on the other side, even by tumor enucleation. Some authors recommend a bench dissection of the tumor with autotransplantation of the kidneys for these difficult cases. Results in bilateral tumors are excellent and exceed 80% after 2 years. *Metachronous tumors* occur in about 1% after therapy of unilateral WT. Partial nephrectomy is recommended after preoperative chemotherapy.

WT in horseshoe kidneys is approximately two times more common than in the general population. We recommend preoperative chemotherapy to reduce the tumor size and to allow an easier resection of the involved side.

Nephroblastomatosis is a diffuse mostly bilateral, microscopic, or macroscopic presence of NR in the kidneys, usually in children under 2 years of age. Microscopic nephroblastomatosis is common in children with bilateral WT, or in children younger than 1 year, or in patients with associated syndromes. Macroscopic nephroblastomatosis is characterized by significantly enlarged and lobulated kidneys (Fig. 73.6). Therapeutic regimen includes biopsy and reduced chemotherapy until the kidneys achieve the normal appearance. However, long-term regular controls are mandatory, because a unilateral or bilateral synchronous or metachronous Wilms' tumor may occur months or years later.

73.6 Nephron-Sparing Surgery

Nephron-sparing surgery is a well-established method in adult patients with unilateral renal cell carcinoma—a comparable tumor with good overall results. In contrast, renal salvage procedures in unilateral WT remain a controversial issue and tumor nephrectomy is recommended as the standard surgical procedure. On the basis of today's excellent survival rate of more than 90% of patients, the question whether in some carefully selected cases of unilateral WT a kidney-sparing surgery could represent a valid option preserving a maximum of healthy renal tissue for the patient must be asked.

Any reduction of kidney tissue causes structural and functional hypertrophy of the remaining nephrons. While the overall function is normal, the glomerular filtration rate rises in the remaining kidney by 70%, the creatinine clearance is reduced to 75% of normal, and the systolic blood pressure increases. In young children, the minimal amount of renal tissue is about 25% of total in order to keep the glomerular filtration rate at a level greater than $50 \, mL/m/1.73 \, m^2$. In adolescence, about 40% of the total is needed to avoid renal insufficiency. The risk of end-stage renal insufficiency after nephrectomy in otherwise normal patients is considered to be as low as 0.2% and 0.6%. In bilateral WT, the incidence of end-stage renal disease 20 years after treatment is between 5.4% and 12% in the literature. Unilateral nephrectomy bears the additional long-term risk of focal glomerulosclerosis caused by hyperfiltration of the remaining kidney tissue. Microalbuminuria, proteinuria, and a decreased glomerular filtration rate can be observed in adults as a long-term sequel of renal agenesis or unilateral nephrectomy. The cumulative incidence of end-stage renal disease is significantly higher in patients with Denish-Drash syndrome, Wilm's tumor aniridia syndrome, hypospadias or cryptorchidism, or other genito-urinary anomalies (Table 73.3). However, this group of patients represents only 0.75% of overall WT population.

A further argument for renal salvage procedures in unilateral WT lies in the advantage of renal tissue preservation in cases of secondary contralateral nephrectomy, i.e., due to metachronous WT or trauma. The main argument for a partial nephrectomy, however, comes from findings during the surgical procedure,

when a comparable small WT is located on one pol of the kidney and a heminephrectomy could easily be performed. This finding is more often encountered when patients are treated according to the SIOP protocol with a 4-week course of chemotherapy before surgery. Significant reduction in volume, measured weekly by ultrasound reflects a favorable histology. A reduction in tumor volume to at least 50% after chemotherapy, the location of the tumor on the upper or lower pole of the kidney, Stage I (or local Stage I in a Stage VI patient), and salvage of at least half of the normal kidney are the prerequisites for a nephron-sparing strategy (Table 73.4; Fig. 73.7). These criteria have been included in the recent SIOP protocol as an option for centers that can provide the necessary surgical experience. Only occasionally a lesion will be small enough to allow partial nephrectomy without preoperative chemotherapy.

The tumor heminephrectomy needs a 10–15 min occlusion of the renal vessels. Thereafter, careful coagulation of the bleeding vessels on the cut surface and closure of the urinary collecting system by single or continuous sutures is necessary. In most cases with a small WT on one pol of the kidney, tumor resection can be easily performed including a rim of healthy renal tissue. It is important to emphasise that when the resection through normal renal tissue seems to be doubtful an intraoperative ultrasound examination is necessary to define the appropriate resection line. If this option is not available, tumor nephrectomy should be better preferred. Inadvertent opening of the tumor must be avoided strictly, since it changes the stage from I to III, which then needs additional local radiation therapy.

The preoperative imaging studies provide only a vague hint whether renal salvage will be possible. It is our experience that only the intraoperative situs is decisive for the definite surgical approach. Moreover, some WTs that have responded well to primary

Table 73.3 Significant decreased risk of renal failure after unilateral nephrectomy in syndromic patients

	n	Renal failure—%
DDS	22	62.4
WAGR syndrome	46	38.3
Male GU anomalies	153	10.9
Bilateral disease	397	5.5
Unilateral disease	5358	1.0

Table 73.4 Nephron-sparing surgery may be performed if these criteria are fulfilled

- Local Stage I (IV)
- Tumor involving one pole
- No invasion of renal vein
- At least 50% of normal kidney tissue remaining
- Resection must be possible with tumor-free margins
- Surgeon and oncologist agree about the decision

Fig. 73.7 Significant reduction of tumor volume and tumor localization on one pole of the kidney. Heminephrectomy including the tumor is easily possible and saves the other normal half of the kidney

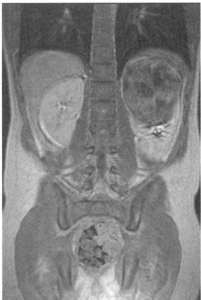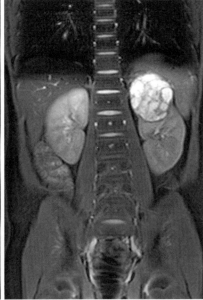

chemotherapy but remain a large mass preoperatively and are therefore determined for tumor nephrectomy. However, during surgery they can turn out as a resectable tumor with the possibility of preservation of at least 50% of the healthy renal tissue. Thus, the final decision should be felt during the surgical procedure and in accordance with the present oncologist. In regard to the discussion in the literature about the risks or the advantages of nephron-sparing surgery in WT patients, we should consider a statement of Beckwith "…the proven efficacy of modern chemotherapy for Wilm's tumor, coupled with the power of imaging technology, provides a basis for considering more conservative management of problems that formerly would have required destruction of most or all renal function."

Table 73.5 5-year survival results according to the SIOP-Study 93-01

Relapse free after 4 years:	
Stage I	97%
Stage II and III	86%
Stage IV	60% (80%)
Stage V	82%
Survival with a local relapse	50%
Survival with systemic relapse	40%

Furthermore, the preliminary results of partial nephrectomy in the SIOP 93-01 study show that the relapse-free survival was not different to total nephrectomy. We conclude that modern techniques of diagnosis and treatment allow less aggressive strategies with lower morbidity and excellent cure rates.

73.7 Prognosis

Current result in the treatment of WT is one of the most impressive success stories in pediatric oncology. While in the fifties of the last century about 50% of all patients with WT died despite the introduction of radiation, survival rates reach more than 90% now with a multimodal therapy including tumor nephrectomy in unilateral WT. Despite the differences in protocols between the NWTS and the SIOP, the overall long-term results are similar. The recent results of the SIOP study are presented in Table 73.5.

Further Reading

Beckwith JB, Kiviat NB, Bonadio JF (1990) Nephrogenic rests, nephroblastomatosis, and the pathogenesis of Wilms' tumor. Pediatr Pathol 10:1–36

Carachi R (2006) Wilms Tumour. In P Puri, ME Höllwarth (eds) Pediatric Surgery, Springer Surgery Atlas Series. Springer-Verlag Berlin Heidelberg, New York, pp 451–458

Cozzi F, Schiavetti A, Morini F et al (2005) Renal function adaptation in children with unilateral renal tumor treated with nephron sparing surgery or nephrectomy. J Urol 174: 1404–1408

Grosfeld JL, O'Neill JA Jr, Fonkalsrud EW, Coran AG (2006) Pediatric Surgery. Mosby–Elsevier, Philadelphia

Hall G, Grant R, Weitzman S et al (2006) Predictors of surgical outcome in Wilms' tumor: A single institution comparative experience. J Pediatr Surg 41:966–971

Linni K, Urban C, Lackner H, Höllwarth ME (2003) Nephronsparing procedures in 11 patients with Wilms' tumor. Pediatr Surg Int 19:457–462

Mitchell Ch, Pritchard-Jones K, Shannon R, et al (2006) Immediate nephrectomy versus preoperative chemotherapy in the management of non-metastatic Wilms' tumor: Results of a randomized trial (UKW3) by the UK children's cancer study group. Eur J Cancer 42:2554–2562

Wu H-Y, Snyder HM, D'Angio GJ (2005) Wilms' tumor management. Curr Opin Urol 15:273–276

Soft Tissue Sarcoma

74

Robert Carachi

Contents

74.1 Introduction Including Definition and Incidence

74.1.1 Definition

The term sarcoma etymologically means a tumour of the flesh. Any malignancy arising from the muscle layer of the body integument is technically a sarcoma. The common term used, soft tissue sarcoma, is a misnomer as the tumour is rarely soft and it is a descriptive term with no scientific basis. The word sarcoma encompasses a wide variety of tumours of the integument, not just those arising from muscle but all structures that make up this mesoderm layer. In addition certain organs in the body have sarcomatous elements, e.g. the genitourinary system, the biliary tree, the gastrointestinal tract as well as the kidney can develop malignancies that are sarcomatous.

74.1.2 Incidence

Soft tissue sarcomas account for about 5–6% of all childhood malignancies. There is an increased incidence in males compared to females. They are divided into two groups. The rhabdomyosarcoma group (RMS), which originate from striated muscle and are by far the commoner and the second group are a heterogeneous collection of sarcomas referred to as non-rhabdomyosarcoma soft tissue sarcomas (NRSTS). These tumours behave in a very different biological manner from those tumours arising from blastemal elements.

P. Puri and M. Höllwarth (eds.), *Pediatric Surgery: Diagnosis and Management,*
DOI: 10.1007/978-3-540-69560-8_74, © Springer-Verlag Berlin Heidelberg 2009

74.2 Age of Presentation and Epidemiology

This is usually bimodal occurring early on between the ages of 2 and 5 years and a secondary peak occurring in the teenage years. However all ages are susceptible to develop these tumours and some may present in the neonatal period which makes them very difficult to treat (Fig. 74.1).

The clinical evaluation of the patients includes a careful history and a physical examination because by their very nature rhabdomyosarcomas may occur anywhere in the body. A family history may be significant since soft tissue sarcomas may occur in cancer families as a component of the Li-fraumeni syndrome as well as the Beckwith-Wiedemann syndrome. The genetics of these two syndromes are associated with soft tissue sarcomas.

The Beckwith-Wiedemann syndrome has a complex genetic makeup. It is often associated with several 11p15 chromosomal changes. It is an overgrowth syndrome often associated with hypoglycaemia. Other tumours associated are Wilms' tumour and liver tumours.

The Li-fraumeni syndrome is an autosomal dominant disorder where soft tissue sarcoma occurs at an early age in a cancer family. Other tumours associated are brain lesions, breast cancer and leukaemia.

Rhabdomyosarcoma has also been associated with neurofibrosarcoma.

74.3 Symptoms and Signs

Over 80% of the patients have localised disease at the time of presentation. The symptoms at presentation often depend on the primary site. In general there are three main areas that can be affected. These are the head and neck, the trunk and limbs and the genitourinary system.

74.3.1 Clinical Presentation of Rms in the Head and Neck

These tumours often present early with a swelling or bleeding from an orifice, which might be the ear or the nose or even proptosis of the eye. Such tumours may mimic parotitis or even cause neurological dysfunction secondary to extension of parameningeal lesions affecting the central nervous system. These tumours may be confused with commoner lesions initially but gradually the progression of tumour growth is relentless and it soon becomes obvious that this is not an infective condition when they do not respond to standard regimes of antibiotic chemotherapy. These tumours are aggressive and gradually erode bony margins and can infiltrate from one space in the head and neck to another. Regional lymph nodes are often involved and can initially present as an enlarged lymph node in the neck region (Fig. 74.2).

Head and neck tumours may arise in the orbit at parameningeal or nonparameningeal sites. Orbital rhabdomyosarcomas may present with proptosis, chemosis or a conjunctival mass. This may lead to blindness and ophthalmoplegia later on. Tumours that arise from parameningeal sites are associated with erosion of the cranial

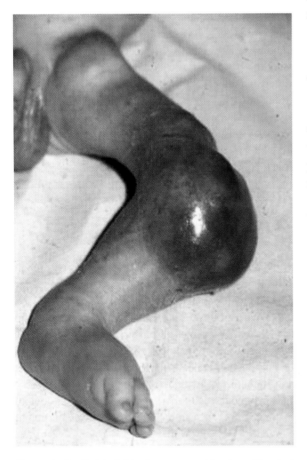

Fig. 74.1 RMS of the left leg in a neonate with enlarged inguinal lymph nodes

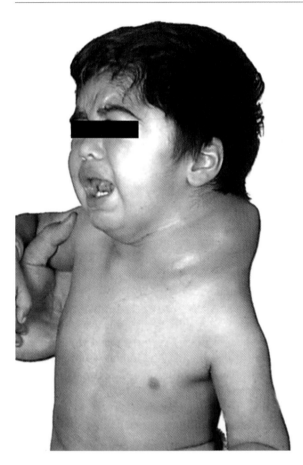

Fig. 74.2 RMS of the neck presenting as a lump

bones, which can present with meningeal symptoms and cranial nerve manifestations. A tumour arising in the nasopharynx may cause airway obstruction and bleeding. Those arising in the paranasal sinus present with pain and nasal discharge. A tumour in the middle ear or mastoid region may present as a polypoidal tumour with obvious facial nerve palsy. The commonest histology in this group of tumours is embryonal. Thus a clinical presentation may at first present to the general practitioner, to the ear, nose and throat surgeon or even to the ophthalmologist.

74.3.2 Clinical Presentation of RMS of the Trunk and Limbs

Truncal RMS can present as a nodule or a mass occasionally going into the chest wall causing respiratory symptoms or neurological ones if cord compression results from a paraspinal tumour.

Rhabdomyosarcomas of the extremities are more common in the lower limbs and occur in the older age group. There is a higher incidence of nodal involvement in these cases. There is often a delay in presentation and occasionally may present with a metastasis in a groin node. Rhabdomyosarcomas of the trunk and the limbs usually present with a localised swelling, which can be confused with a haematoma following a minor injury. The lesion may be associated with bruising and may have an inflammatory component to it, which can be very confusing for the diagnostician. The tumour grows relentlessly and does not behave like a simple haematoma and metastise early to the regional glands. Another potential confusion is a sudden change in a congenital haemangioma/lymphangioma. If it suddenly changes in characteristics and becomes hard, it can be confused with the development of a rhabdomyosarcoma. Occasionally clinical presentation may be with metastatic disease to other parts of the body and especially to the lungs from a small primary in the periphery.

74.3.3 Clinical Presentation of RMS of the Genitourinary System

The sites that are generally affected include the bladder, prostate and paratesticular region in the male and the bladder, vagina, uterus and vulva in the female. The histopathology of this tumour is very often of the embryonal variety and carries a good prognosis. The poor sites include the rhabdomyosarcomas that arise in the base of the bladder and the prostate. Rhabdomyosarcoma of the genitourinary system can manifest with urinary frequency or retention or the presence of sarcoma botryoides, which are fleshy polyps that protrude from the vaginal orifice and may be found in the nappy of a child (Fig. 74.3a and b). Rhabdomyosarcoma of the genitourinary system usually present earlier because of the confined space within the pelvis causing an obstructive uropathy. During the examination of the child a full examination of the pelvic region and a digital rectal examination is mandatory in order to pick this up and avoid confusion with what maybe mistakenly diagnosed as a constipated child. In the genitourinary tract some of these masses may be very large and present as an abdominal mass. This can be a true tumour or can be due to an obstructed bladder, which may enhance the

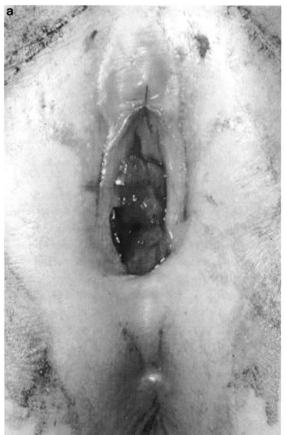

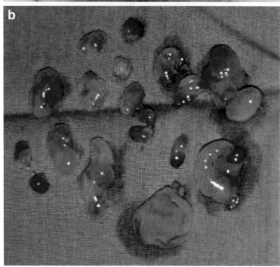

Fig. 74.3 (**a**) Sarcoma botryiodes protruding from the vagina, (**b**) Botryoid fleshy masses in nappy of the same patient

size of the mass. Paratesticular tumours are usually hard, painless scrotal swellings that can present with signs and symptoms secondary to a larger intraperito-

neal mass and have a characteristic spindle cell on histology.

74.4 Imaging at Presentation

The commonest imaging used is a plain X-ray, which may demonstrate a soft tissue mass with calcification if haemorrhage has occurred into the tumour. In a tumour of the head and neck the bony structures may be eroded especially in orbital meningeal/parameningeal tumours. In a tumour arising from the neck, the mediastinum may be shifted and the trachea may be pushed away from its central position. In truncal lesions there may be bony erosions, metastases in the lung or pleural effusions.

Ultrasound is another modality that can be very helpful initially to define a solid from a cystic lesion. It is most helpful in genitourinary rhabdomyosarcomas to identify the origin of the tumour and detect any obstructive lesion causing an obstructive uropathy i.e. a large bladder and hydronephrosis (Fig. 74.4).

Computerised tomography (CT) and magnetic resonance imaging (MRI) are essential in the evaluation of the primary site and to detect any extension of the tumour and its relationship to other surrounding structures (Fig. 74.5). CT scans are very useful to confirm metastatic lung lesions in rhabdomyosarcoma. Similarly assessment of retroperitoneal lymphadenopathy in tumours that arise in the testis have replaced extensive retroperitoneal surgery to identify these lesions.

MRI scans are particularly useful in extremities, pelvic, head and neck regions and give very clear definition and differentiation between the different tissues and planes. There is still however a lot of doubt and debate whether MRI scans are able to differentiate between malignant soft tissue tumour from a benign condition.

74.5 Staging and Surgical Biopsy for Diagnosis

There is no place for needling a tumour, which could be a sarcoma whether it is to take a percutaneous biopsy or aspiration cytology. This approach compromises the care of the patient because it inevitably will seed tumour along the track and spread it resulting in upstaging of this type

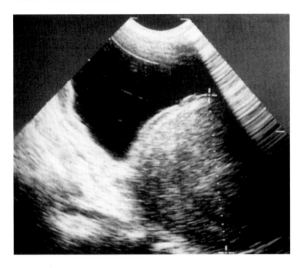

Fig. 74.4 Ultrasound of bladder with RMS of the base of the bladder

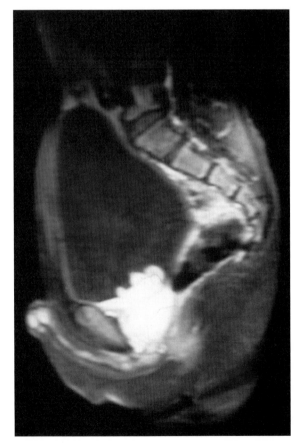

Fig. 74.5 CT scan of a extensive bladder neck RMS with outlet obstruction

of tumour. The role of the surgeon is to ensure that under a general anaesthetic an adequate open incision is made over the site of the tumour and a careful incision is made through the capsule of the tumour if there is one. This is in order to obtain a proper representation of the tumour. An adequate sample of the tumour will give an accurate diagnosis and allow proper staging as well as histological typing for the appropriate chemotherapy. The tumour must be sent fresh to the pathology department because of the variety of biological and histochemical tests that need to be carried out on this type of tissue. It is important that the pathologist is aware that this type of tumour surgery is being performed and can provide advice as to whether adequate amount of tissue has been obtained to be able to provide a diagnosis. The site where the incision is made has to be carefully planned so that this area is included in the eventual total resection of the tumour after chemotherapy has been instituted. All attempts at removal of the tumour en bloc at initial presentation should be resisted. The tumours are often gross at presentation and there is a real risk of compromising adjacent tissues, which may have been invaded by this tumour. Extirpative surgery and extensive surgery in these types of tumours should no longer be carried out at initial presentation. Trunk and extremity biopsies should be performed along the long axis of the tumour so that subsequent excisions are not compromised.

A clinical staging system has been developed to determine prognosis (Table 74.1). It has been demonstrated that the site of origin of the tumour, the size, the invasiveness as well as whether regional lymph nodes involvement is affected have a significant impact on the survival for non-metastatic rhabdomyosarcoma patients.

The diagnosis of Rhabdomyosarcoma depends on open surgical biopsies. These need to be open biopsies which should be generous so that full investigation of the tissue can take place which should include a chromosome analysis, surface markers and a whole range of histochemical testing and special stains which are available for these tumours. The detection of metastatic disease is very often included during the scanning of the chest by CT scans and MRI scans of the whole body. Regional lymph nodes should be sampled at the time of surgery for patients with lymph primaries. However the role of retroperitoneal lymph node sampling in patients with paratesticular tumours is still very controversial.

74.6 Histopathology

The histopathology of rhabdomyosarcoma falls into the small round blue cell tumours of childhood, which

Table 74.1   Pretreatment clinical staging[a] for rhabdomyosarcoma in IRS

Stage	Site	Size	Nodes	Distant mets
1	Favorable	$\leq$ or > 5 cm	N_0 or N_1	None
2	Unfavorable	≤ 5 cm	N_0	None
3	Unfavorable	> 5 cm	N_0	None
4	Unfavorable	$\leq$ or > 5 cm	N_1	None
	Either	$\leq$ or > 5 cm	N_0 or N_1	Yes

Primary sites

Favorable	**Unfavorable**
Orbit	Parameningeal head and neck
Superficial head and neck	Bladder prostate
Paratesticular, vagina, uterus	Extremities
	Other

[a] Based on *clinical* evaluation *before* surgery, chemotherapy and/or radiation therapy begins.
IRS: Intergroup Rhabdomyosarcoma Study.

Table 74.2   Histologic variants of childhood rhabdomyosarcoma: International Rhabdomyo-sarcoma Pathologic Classification

I	Favourable prognosis
	(a) Botryoid
	(b) Spindle-cell
II	Intermediate prognosis
	(a) Embryonal
	(b) Pleomorphic (rare)
III	Poor prognosis
	(a) Alveolar
	(b) Undifferentiated

also include neuroblastoma, Ewing's sarcoma, small cell osteogenic sarcoma and lymphomas. It is possible for the histopathologist to differentiate between the different tumour types by a combination of microscopic appearance and immunohistochemical staining as well as the molecular genetic characteristics of these different types of tumours (Tables 74.2 and 74.3). The presence of rhabdomyoblasts or skeletal muscle and muscle-specific proteins can be identified by immunohistochemical staining. The commonest type of tumour encountered is the embryonal type of rhabdomyosarcoma, which consists of spindle shape rhabdomyoblasts and small round cells and longitudinal cytoplasmic striae. It is the commonest type of tumour in the younger age group and 80% of urinary tract tumours are made of the embryonal type whereas 60% of the head and neck tumours are embryonal and only half of the extremity ones fall into this category. The sarcoma botryoid a variant of the embryonal sarcoma can occur in the vagina, uterus, bladder. These are small round cells with a very mixed stroma and they are typical of this type of tumour. The prognosis in this age group is excellent. The alveolar type of tumour, which is second in frequency following the embryonal, most commonly occurs in the extremity and trunk.

The pleomorphic type of rhabdomyosarcoma is the least common in children and has large pleomorphic cells with large giant cells also present. This is seen in the extremity and trunk and carries a very poor prognosis. Thus the prognostic and therapeutic implications of biologic, immunologic and cytologic techniques makes it essential for the surgeon to obtain adequate quality and quantity of tissue to ensure proper transfer of the specimens to the laboratory while they are fresh. It has to be noted that the site where the open biopsy is carried out must be included in the planning for future so that when the final resection is carried out this site of biopsy is also included in the area of excision. The common sites for metastatic spread include the lungs, bones, bone marrow and these need to be evaluated by scans as well as bone marrow aspiration. In general patients with an alveolar histopathology have a poorer prognosis both for stage and site of disease. Histological grading in soft tissue sarcoma is dependent on the number of mitoses, the presence or absence of necrosis of tumour cells and the differentiation of the tumours. They are graded from I to III according to the scoring system. Table 74.4.

74.6.1 Cytogenetics

Specific chromosomal translocation is useful where light microscopy may be insufficient for a diagnosis,

Table 74.3 Examples of antibodies useful in pediatric tumor diagnosis

Antibody	Antisera/cell lineage marked	Tumor
CD45 Leukocyte common antigen	Leukocytes	Lymphomas
CD20 (L26)	B lymphocytes	Lymphomas
CD45RO (UCHL-1)	T lymphocytes	Lymphomas
CD30 (Ber H-2)	Activated lymphocytes/macrophages/ Anaplastic large cell lymphoma	Hodgkin's disease/Reed-Sternberg cells
CD15 (LeuM1)	Reed-Sternberg cells	Hodgkin's disease
CD68 (KP1)	Macrophages	Histocytic neoplasms
Kappa/Lambda proliferation	Ig light chains	Lymphoid clonal
Neuron-specific enolase (NSE)	Neuroectoderm	Neuroblastoma
S100	Glial/Schwann cells/others	Neurofibroma, etc. Langerhan's cells
b2-microglobulin	b2-microglobulin	PNET
Synaptophysin	Neuroectoderm/neuroendocrine	Ewing's/PNET
MIC-2 (CD99)	MIC-2 gene product (glycoprotein P30/32)	Ewing's/PNET
Vimentin	Intermediate filaments/mesenchyme	Ewing's/soft tissue Sarcoma
Actin (common, smooth muscle, sarcomeric)	Muscle filaments	Rhabdomyosarcoma
Desmin	Muscle (smooth/striated)	Rhabdomyosarcoma
Myoglobin	Striated muscle	Rhabdomyosarcoma
Myo D-1	Skeletal muscle	Rhabdomyosarcoma
Cytokeratins (AE1-AE3, CAM 5.2, etc.)		Epithelial
	Synovial sarcoma	
CD1a	Langerhan's cells	Langerhan's cell histiocytosis

Table 74.4 Histological grading in soft tissue sarcoma

Feature		Score
Mitoses	0–9 (per 10 high power fields)	1
	10–19 (per 10 high power fields)	2
	>20 (per 10 high power fields)	3
Necrosis	None	1
	<50% of the tumor	2
	>50% of the tumor	3
Differentiation	Very highly differentiated	1
	Moderately differentiated but cell type easily recognizable	2
	Poorly differentiated or cell type uncertain	3
Grade is determined by aggregate score for all these features, i.e.		
Grade I	Score 3–4	
Grade II	Score 5–6	
Grade III	Score 7–9	

e.g. t(2:13) (q35:q14) in alveolar RMS and t(x:18) (p11.2:q11.2) in synovial sarcoma.

74.7 Management

In general once the diagnosis has been made the patient has a double lumen central line inserted and a regime of chemotherapy commenced.

74.7.1 Chemotherapy

The standard drugs used over the years has been a triple regimen of Vincristine, Actinomycin-D and Cyclophosphamide (VAC). Overall survival rate is above 70%. The site of origin as well as size of tumour and tumour spread determine the 5-year survival rate. It is best for localised lesions who can get a 95% rate. The patients with embryonal histology do well and need less aggressive treatment than those with pleomorphic or alveolar histology who even with early stage disease and aggressive therapy do badly. Other drugs active in this disease include Doxorubicin, ifosphamide, etoposide, cisplatin, carboplatin, melphelan, topotecan, methotrexate, mitoycin C. In the majority of cases the chemotherapy is successful in shrinking tumours to allow surgical resection to take place.

74.7.2 Radiotherapy

Radiation therapy is used to mop up residual microscopic disease to achieve local control or gross residual disease that surgical removal was unable to excise because of dangers to the patient's life. It is very effective in reducing the mutilating surgery seen in days gone past. It may be delivered in the form of intracavitary brachytherapy in RMS of the vagina and uterus.

74.7.3 Surgery

The goal of the surgeon is to attempt a complete resection of the primary tumour with surrounding margins which are uninvolved but this must also be done to preserve organs and be cosmetically acceptable. There is no place for debulking operations in this type of tumour. Regional lymph nodes are often removed for pathological examination and evaluation at the time. If residual disease is present it is important to re-excise the area until there is microscopic clearance of the edges of the excised region. This may require raising of flaps to cover the area of the wound eventually. Second look surgery for patients who have had an incomplete response to therapy is important to determine how responsive the tumour was to the chemotherapy regime used and to have a second attempt at total excision of the tumour.

The resection margin in children is variable whereas in adults a 2 cm margin is usually adequate, in children this is at times not possible. This is especially so when one approaches a neurovascular bundle and at the risk of damaging this one may have to compromise on the amount of clear margin at the tumour edge. Another common pitfall in tumour surgery with these types of tumours – especially the synovial sarcoma – is that they

develop a pseudocapsule which is thought to be the boundary of the tumour whereas the capsule itself is part of the tumour and may be left behind thus leaving behind residual disease. In these situations recurrence rates are extremely high and in high-grade tumours a need to adopt a more aggressive approach to extirpative surgery.

Lymph node dissection is not done routinely for the disease and one often depends on imaging techniques to decide if there is lymph node involvement. This of course is not always accurate since one knows that a large lymph node may be due to inflammation whereas a normal size lymph node may still contain metastatic tumour cells. Some centres still advocate the biopsy of the sentinel lymph node for a variety of these tumours and lymph node resection can be performed.

Patients who have a tumour close to organs i.e. the eye and the genitourinary system benefit from primary chemotherapy followed by radiation therapy. This may alter excision of a tumour as a result of shrinkage by chemotherapy with or without radiotherapy. Taking regional lymph node biopsies, especially sentinel lymph node biopsies has improved the outcome in some situation.

Solitary lesions may be amenable to surgical resection and can produce long-term survival. This has been attempted by minimaly invasive surgery e.g. thoracoscopic approach for solitary lung lesion. However occurrence very often carries a poorer prognosis and these may relapse within the 1st years after treatment.

74.8 Genital Urinary Rhabdomyosarcoma

Patients with bladder and prostatic tumours may undergo radiation therapy and have a slightly higher survival rate and less recurrence. Attempts at intracavital or brachytherapy for tumours of the bladder and the prostate have been successfully treated with these conservative managements, however not without a price and in some instances tumour recurs and also complications of the radiation may result in necrosis and fistula formation. However with the increase in survival and with bladder preservation, which has been the main aim in recent years, it is certainly possible with tumours arising from the dome of the bladder where partial cystectomy can be performed. Prostatectomy with preservation and urethra reconstruction is possible in some patients with bladder and prostatic rhabdo who do not respond to treatment. However, in some cases a total cystectomy is required in these patients and a urinary diversion would be necessary. Vulva, vaginal and uterine rhabdomyosarcoma carries a good prognosis with chemotherapy. It is possible to treat the majority of these tumours by conservative surgery.

74.9 Nonrhabdomyosarcoma Soft Tissue Sarcoma (NRSTS)

Although initially reported as an adult disease, more and more cases are reported in children and this group now form less than half of all the soft tissue sarcomas found in the paediatric age group. They may occur in association with neurofibromatosis. They occur most commonly in the lower limbs then the trunk followed by the chest and head and neck. Synovial cell sarcoma is the commonest of this group of tumours followed by the malignant fibrous histocytomas and fibrosarcoma.

This group of sarcomas is slightly less than half of the total number of sarcomas encountered in childhood and occasionally occur in older children and young adults. The clinical presentation is very often that of a localised mass and again presenting following a minor trauma and regional lymph nodes may be palpable in some instances. There is a slight preponderance of males and the most common type of tumour encountered in childhood is the synovial cell sarcoma which can be very misleading thinking it is a benign lesion. There are a whole variety of these tumours with their own histopathological pattern.

Imaging usually consists of CT scanning with contrast and MRI scans.

Synovial carcinomas are high-grade malignant neoplasms that account for the majority of the non-rhabdomyosarcoma soft tissue cell sarcoma. They occur in the teenage group and can present with metastases in the lung. Many of these tumours have got a pseudocapsule which gives a false impression during the time of surgery that the tumour has totally been excised. Many of these cases need to undergo re-excision for microscopic disease that might have been left behind at the time of the initial surgery. Chemotherapy is not of much value in this type of tumour, however

Table 74.5 Intergroup RMS Study Group Surgicopathological Staging System and Clinical Outcome According to Clinical Group

Group	Description	5-Year event-free survival %	5-Year survival %
I	Localised disease, completely resected	72–83	84–90
II	Microscopic residual, completely resected with nodes, nodes Involved with microscopic residual	65–72	84–88
III	Incomplete resection	—	35–54
IV	Distant metastases	15 (2 years)	34 (2 years)

radiation therapy may have some benefit (Table 74.5). Another type of tumour is infantile fibrosarcoma. Fibrosarcoma is one of the commonest NRSTS that occur in the paediatric population. It is histologically similar to the malignant adult counterpart. This tumour in infants is very often of a benign nature and does not metastasise although local recurrence may occur. Local excision of this tumour is adequate. The principles that have been learned from the past large studies from the United States indicated the following:

1. Patients with localised completely resected disease have the best prognosis. Patients with metastasis at diagnosis have the worst prognosis thus in an attempt to remove all the visible tumour without excessive morbidity is an important consideration in these patients.
2. When a lesion has been incompletely resected, re-resection is important and any doubt about margin status should have a resection of that area.
3. It is desirable to preserve organ function and space structures such as the paraorbital region and the genitourinary system. These patients generally have a good prognosis.

The principles of management include adequate tissue biopsy, regional lymph node evaluation followed by chemotherapy. Eventually only radical surgery offers a cure.

Radiation therapy is particularly useful specially in limb involvement. The role of chemotherapy is unclear in NRSTS.

Further Reading

Pediatric Surgery – Sixth Edition – Volume 1, Chapters 32–33, P524–553, Mosby. Jay L Grosfeld, James A. O'Neill Jr., Eric W. Fonkalsrud and Arnold G. Cowan

Puri P, Höllwarth M (2006) Pediatric Surgery. Springer, Berlin, Heidelberg

The Surgery of Childhood Tumors, 2nd Edition, Springer. Robert Carachi, Jay L. Grosfeld and Amir Azmy

Hepatic Tumors in Childhood

75

Thambipillai Sri Paran and Michael P. La Quaglia

Contents

75.1 Introduction

Primary neoplasms of the liver are rare in childhood and constitute 0.3–2% of all pediatric tumors. Malignant neoplasms account for 1% of all pediatric malignancies and are the third most common intra-abdominal neoplasm after neuroblastoma and nephroblastoma. The two primary malignant neoplasms of the liver are hepatoblastoma and hepatocellular carcinoma. For both these malignant tumors, complete resection of the tumor is necessary to achieve a cure. Detailed description of hepatic segmental anatomy has enabled surgeons to resect larger tumors in the recent years. This appreciation of the anatomy and the regenerative capability of the liver, which allows up to 85% of the liver to be safely removed in small infants, have greatly increased the scope for cure.

The incidence of benign liver tumors in children is less than their malignant counterpart, and in a large series of pediatric liver tumors, benign tumors accounted for less than 35%. The benign tumors include hemangiomas or vascular malformations, hepatocellular adenomas, focal nodular hyperplasia, mesenchymal hamartomas, and various types of cysts and cystic disease. With widespread use of ultrasonography, fortuitous discoveries of benign tumors are being made in a large number of children, and this raises the question of optimal surgical management for the surgeon.

75.2 History

A first glimpse of the hepatic anatomy was presented by Herophilus and Erasistratus between 310 BC and 280 BC. The first attempt at hepatic resection did not take place till the late 1880s. Though Martin et al.

reported that hepatoblastomas could be treated by hepatic lobectomy in 1969, real progress in hepatic surgery was mostly seen following the detailed description of hepatic segmental anatomy by Couinaud. This knowledge allowed surgeons to get good vascular control before attempting to divide the liver parenchyma, and thereby avoid catastrophic bleeding.

Holton et al. showed that hepatoblastoma was sensitive to systemic chemotherapy in 1975. Following this, various authors have shown that neoadjuvant chemotherapy is useful in reducing the tumor size in hepatoblastoma and thereby enabling complete surgical resection of previously unresectable tumors. Presently, the standard of practice is to administer neoadjuvant systemic chemotherapy to patients with hepatoblastoma unless the tumor is clearly resectable at diagnosis.

The first application of hepatic transplantation to a childhood liver tumor was reported by Heimann et al. in 1987. Tagge et al. reported the first series of pediatric liver tumor patients treated by hepatic transplantation in 1992. Total hepatectomy with liver transplantation now has become a recognized treatment for unresectable hepatoblastoma confined to the liver and this treatment modality is part of the SIOPEL 3 protocol.

75.3 Surgical Anatomy

The liver has two main lobes, a large right and a smaller left and conventional description places their line of fusion on the upper surface of the liver along the attachment of the falciform ligament. However, knowledge of the detailed internal functional anatomy of the liver is essential for planning surgical resections. The anatomical description of the liver by Couinaud is the most complete and exact and also the most useful for the operating surgeon (Fig. 75.1). Essentially the three main hepatic veins within the scissurae divide the liver into four sectors each of which receives a portal pedicle with alternation between the hepatic veins and portal pedicles. The main portal scissura contains the middle hepatic vein and progresses from the middle of the gallbladder bed anteriorly to the left of the vena cava posteriorly. The right and left liver, demarcated by the main portal scissura, are independent in terms of portal and arterial vascularization and of biliary drainage. The distribution of the portal pedicles and hepatic veins delimits the hepatic segments, each of which has a unique portal

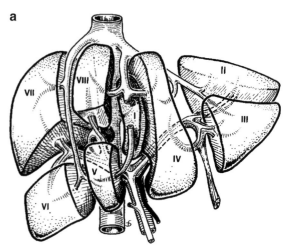

a

As seen in patient

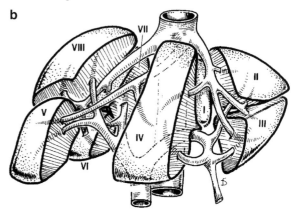

b

Ex-vivo

Fig. 75.1 Couinaud's description of liver into eight functional divisions. (**a**) As seen in patient (**b**) Ex-vivo. Each segment receives a branch of the portal vein, hepatic artery and is drained by a branch of either the right or left hepatic duct. The three main hepatic veins demarcate the liver into its four portal sectors (Blumgart 2000)

vein, a branch of hepatic artery and bile duct. Knowledge of this anatomy allows control of the vascular structures before division of the hepatic parenchyma, thereby making major hepatic resections feasible.

75.4 Evaluation of a Child with a Hepatic Mass

Most hepatic tumors present as an asymptomatic abdominal mass. Patients presenting with a suspected hepatic mass are first evaluated by history and physical examination. Blood should be drawn for the following tests: complete blood count, liver function tests, coagulation studies, and measurement of tumor markers such as serum α-fetoprotein and β-human chorionic gonadotropin.

Usually the initial radiological evaluation is with ultrasonography. Ultrasonography will determine whether the hepatic mass is solid or cystic and the extent of the mass. A Doppler ultrasonography is useful in determining the patency of hepatic vasculature. This is followed with either a CT scan or magnetic resonance imaging (MRI). In our experience, MRI provides the greatest amount of information concerning both the lesion and surrounding veins and bile ducts. If a malignant liver tumor is suspected following the initial scans, then a thoracic CT scan is necessary for the purpose of tumor staging.

A tissue diagnosis is necessary to confirm malignancy. Percutaneous needle core biopsy is useful for the diagnosis of hepatoblastomas but may not be definitive in the case of hepatocellular carcinoma. When larger samples are needed, an open or laparoscopic liver biopsy is necessary. Once a diagnosis of malignancy is made it is advisable for the pediatric surgeon to include an oncologist and an experienced hepatobiliary surgeon in the planning of definitive surgery.

75.5 Malignant Liver Tumors

The most common malignant hepatic tumors are hepatoblastoma, hepatocellular carcinoma (hepatoma) and sarcomas. It is estimated that about 57.8% of these are hepatoblastoma, 33.4% are hepatocellular carcinoma and 8.8% are sarcomas.

75.5.1 Hepatoblastoma

75.5.1.1 Incidence and Etiology

Hepatoblastomas are the most common primary hepatic tumors in children, accounting for up to 64% of hepatic malignant tumors. Hepatoblastoma affects one child in one million per year under 15 years of age. This translates into approximately 50–70 new cases per year in the United States with a male to female ratio of 1.7:1.0. Over 75% of these tumors occur in children less than 2 years of age. The median age at diagnosis of hepatoblastoma is 18 months. Though congenital hepatoblastomas and adult onset hepatoblastomas have been described in literature, these are rare. Blair et al. noted a borderline, but significant increase in the incidence of hepatoblastoma in 1994. However, Stiller et al. found no such increase in the incidence of hepatoblastoma between 1978 and 1997.

Hepatoblastoma may occur in siblings and there is an increased incidence in first degree relatives of the patients with familial polyposis coli. Other conditions associated with hepatoblastoma include Gardner's syndrome and the Beckwith-Wiedemann syndrome. Beckwith-Wiedemann Syndrome is also associated with several abdominal tumors, of which the majority are Wilms' tumors.

There is a significant association between hepatoblastoma and low birth weight. It is unknown as to whether developmental abnormalities associated with prematurity or interventions, such as early total parenteral nutrition, are the cause of the increased incidence of hepatoblastoma in these children. The increased survival of these children may somewhat explain the increased overall incidence of hepatoblastoma noted by some authors.

75.5.1.2 Histopathological Subtypes

There are five histological subtypes of hepatoblastoma reported based on the light microscopic findings. These subtypes are fetal (cells grow in trabeculae and resemble fetal hepatic cells), embryonal (cells grow in noncohesive sheets), mixed mesenchymal (contain mesenchymal tissue along with the epithelial component), macrotrabecular, and anaplastic or small cell. The histological subtyping of hepatoblastoma is important as there is an association between prognostic risk and the various subtypes as illustrated in Fig. 75.2. Some authors have indicated that the fetal histological subtype has a better prognosis compared to others. However, a review of 105 cases at the Armed Forces Institute of Pathology failed to confirm this finding. The histological subtype anaplastic or small-cell variant is a rare subtype, but is particularly virulent with a strong metastatic potential.

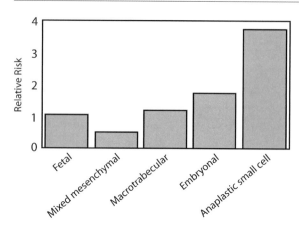

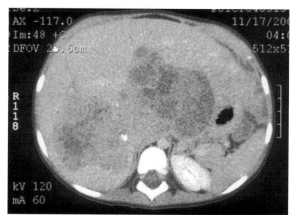

Fig. 75.2 Relative risk of death associated with histopathological subtypes of hepatoblastoma (La Quaglia 2000). The small cell undifferentiated or anaplastic variant has a very poor risk in comparison to the other three histopathological subtypes.

75.5.1.3 Clinical Findings

As mentioned above, the most common presenting sign of a hepatoblastoma is an asymptomatic abdominal mass. The child is often in good health and the tumor mass is discovered incidentally when an attentive parent, grandparent, or clinician discovers the mass on a routine examination or while bathing the child. A small minority may have other symptoms such as pain, irritability, minor gastrointestinal disturbances, fever, pallor, failure to thrive and even tumor rupture. Patients with the anaplastic variant of hepatoblastoma who often have distant metastases at diagnoses are more frequently symptomatic. A mild anemia associated with a markedly elevated platelet count is observed in the majority of patients at diagnosis. The platelet count can range into the millions and the etiology is probably secondary to an abnormal cytokine release.

Measurement of the serum α-fetoprotein is well established as an initial tumor marker in the diagnosis of hepatoblastoma and a means of monitoring the therapeutic response. When interpreting the α-fetoprotein level it is important to realize that normal α-fetoprotein levels are very high at birth and decrease over the first 6 months of life. Usually by 6 months of age, the levels should be below 100 ng/mL, though in some children this may take up to 1 year of age. It is estimated that the α-fetoprotein will be markedly elevated in 84–91% of patients with hepatoblastoma. Low initial

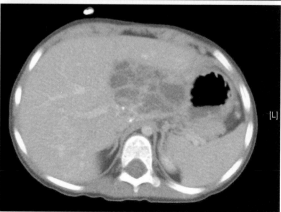

Fig. 75.3 Typical response of hepatoblastoma to neoadjuvant chemotherapy. CT findings at diagnosis in a child with hepatoblastoma. The tumor involves both right and left hepatic lobes and is inoperable. CT scan in the same child following four cycles of chemotherapy. The tumor is confined to left lobe and is eminently resectable.

α-fetoprotein levels have been associated with poor survival outcome.

75.5.1.4 Imaging

As mentioned earlier, the first imaging study is usually an abdominal ultrasound and, if duplex technique is employed, tumor vascularity can be gauged and the hepatic veins assessed. This is usually followed by computerized axial tomography or magnetic resonance imaging. A computerized axial tomography with oral contrast is useful in identifying any pulmonary metastases, and in determining the hepatic involvement and resectability (Fig. 75.3).

75.5.1.5 Staging

Most studies to date have used the clinical grouping defined by the Children's Cancer Group and the Pediatric Oncology Group as listed in Table 75.1. This classification is based on the postoperative extent of disease. Although this classification is useful in

Table 75.1   Post-surgical clinical group staging

Stage I	No metastases, tumor completely resected
Stage II	No metastases, tumor grossly resected with microscopic residual disease (positive margins or tumor rupture/spill at the time of surgery)
Stage III	No distant metastases, tumor unresectable or resected with gross residual tumor or positive lymph nodes
Stage IV	Distant metastases regardless of the extent of liver involvement

predicting postoperative prognosis, it does not provide preoperative information. To assess tumor response and resectability before and after neoadjuvant chemotherapy, the International Society of Pediatric Oncology (SIOP) developed the PRETEXT (pretreatment extent of disease) staging system (Fig. 75.4). The PRETEXT system is based on the radiological findings and describes both the number and the location of involved liver sectors and takes into account the invasion of the hepatic and portal veins as well as extrahepatic and metastatic disease. More recently, the TNM classification has been used (Table 75.2).

75.5.1.6 Treatment and Prognosis

Following initial assessment, the first decision regarding treatment is whether to initiate neo-adjuvant chemotherapy

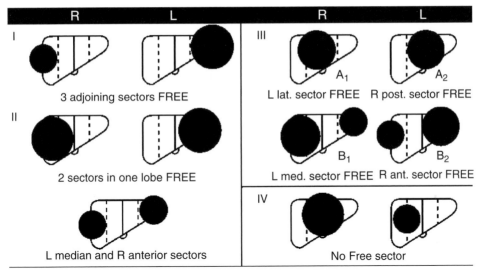

Liver is divided into four sectors, based on its surgical anatomy.

- PRETEXT I- three adjoining sectors are free of tumor
- PRETEXT II- two adjoining sectors are free of tumor
- PRETEXT III- one non Sector or two non-adjoining sectors are free of tumor
- PRETEXT IV- no tumor free sectors

In addition, extrahepatic tumor is expressed as follows:

V - tumor involving hepatic vein
P - tumor involving pertal vein
E - extrahepatic direct spread, limited to enlargement of the hilar lymph nodes
M - presence of distant metastases

Fig. 75.4   International Society of Paediatric Oncology PRETEXT staging (Brown, Perilongo et al. 2000)

Table 75.2 TNM staging of hepatic tumors

Stage I	T1, N0, M0
Stage II	T2, N0, M0
Stage III	T1, N1, M0
	T2, N1, M0
	T3, N0, M0
Stage IVA	T4, any N, M0
Stage IVB	Any T, any N, M1

T0 = no tumor

T1 = solitary tumor $\leq$ 2 cm

T2 = solitary tumor $\leq$ 2 cm with vascular invasion or multiple tumors limited to one lobe without vascular invasion

T3 = solitary tumor $\geq$ 2 cm with vascular invasion or multiple tumors limited to one lobe with vascular invasion

T4 = multiple tumors in more than one lobe or involvement of a major branch of the portal or hepatic vein

N0 = no nodal disease

N1 = nodes involved

M0 = no distant metastases

M1 = distant metastases

or proceed with resection. About 46% of hepatic malignancies are resectable at diagnosis. Resection at diagnosis will avoid or lessen the need for chemotherapy and its associated morbidity. However, when resection at presentation is not feasible, neo-adjuvant chemotherapy can shrink the tumor size extensively and enable safer and complete resection at a later stage. This requires good clinical judgment and good communication between the pediatric surgeon, oncologist, radiologist, and if necessary, an experienced hepatobiliary surgeon.

For unresectable tumors at diagnosis, the initial surgical procedure should include a diagnostic biopsy and placement of a vascular access device for neo-adjuvant chemotherapy. At present, the recommendation for initial treatment of hepatoblastomas is with Cisplatin, 5-fluorouracil, and vincristine. Single agent doxorubicin is sometimes used in very young infants who undergo complete resection. This regimen consists of just three doses and may be associated with less long- and short-term toxicity than multi-agent regimens. Definitive resection of tumor is undertaken after four cycles of chemotherapy, if complete resection is feasible. With complete resection of the primary tumor, overall survival of 60–70% is achievable with non-stage IV hepatoblastoma except in the very small group of children with aggressive anaplastic variant.

It is estimated that approximately 20% of children will have stage IV disease at the time of diagnosis. The overall survival rates are lower in this group of children, but in our experience a rate of 50% is achievable as long as complete resection at the primary site is accomplished. Some patients with microscopic residual at the primary site are curable with continued chemotherapy and may benefit from external beam radiotherapy to this primary hepatic site. Most pulmonary metastases will resolve fully with chemotherapy while resection is reserved for larger or persistent metastatic lesions.

Hepatic transplantation for unresectable primary lesions can be effective for tumors confined to the liver. Cases with extensive extrahepatic extension or vascular invasion have had poor outcomes with total hepatectomy and hepatic transplantation. Chemoembolization shows promise and involves arteriographic injection of occluding thrombogenic materials (Angiostat collagen) or stainless steel coils combined with chemotherapeutic agents like Cisplatin or doxorubicin, into the arterial circulation to the tumor. Using this technique the concentration of chemotherapeutic agents can be increased 50- to 100-fold in the embolized tumor. Others have treated pulmonary metastases with external beam radiotherapy in an approach similar to that used for Wilms' tumors but with 18–20 Gy administered. Pulmonary radiation may be associated with significant pulmonary toxicity.

75.5.2 Hepatocellular Carcinoma (or Hepatoma)

75.5.2.1 Incidence and Epidemiology

Hepatocellular carcinoma accounts for 23% of pediatric liver tumors and affects about 0.5 children in one million per year under the age of 15. The incidence is bimodal with an early peak before the age of 5 years, and a second peak between 13 and 15 years of age. It is rare in infancy, though historical series without pathological review may report a higher rate of infantile hepatocellular carcinoma due to misdiagnosis of some early hepatoblastomas. The Liver Cancer Study Group of Japan reported no cases below the age of 4 years in a series of 2,286 patients (Japan 1987). There is a male predominance that ranges from 1.3 to 3.2:1 for hepatocellular carcinoma. In areas endemic for hepatitis B the male to female ratio may be reversed at 0.2:1.

The relative risk for the development of hepatocellular carcinoma is 250 for patients with chronic active hepatitis compared to those without hepatitis surface antigen positivity. This knowledge has enabled the health workers in Taiwan to reduce their incidence of hepatocellular carcinoma in children from 0.70 per 100,000 children to 0.36 per 100,000 in 5 years following the introduction of a universal vaccination program against hepatitis B. Other conditions associated with the development of hepatocellular carcinoma include cirrhosis, alpha-1-antitrypsin deficiency, tyrosinemia, aflatoxin ingestion, hemochromatosis, hepatic venous obstruction, androgen and estrogen exposure, the Alagille syndrome (arteriohepatic dysplasia), and thorotrast administration.

75.5.2.2 Clinical Findings

Unlike children with hepatoblastoma, children with hepatocellular carcinoma are usually symptomatic at diagnosis. Pain is common (38%) and may even occur in the absence of an obvious mass. But most of these symptoms are nonspecific and include anorexia, fatigue, nausea, and vomiting and weight loss. The α-fetoprotein is elevated in approximately 85% of patients with most levels more than 1,000 ng/mL. Though elevated, these levels are usually lower than those measured in hepatoblastoma patients. Up to 10% may present with tumor rupture with signs and symptoms of a hemoperitoneum. The tumors that rupture are not necessarily large and long-term survival with complete resection has been reported.

75.5.2.3 Staging

The staging schemes listed for hepatoblastoma are also used for hepatocellular carcinoma in childhood.

75.5.2.4 Treatment and Outcome

Again, complete resection of the primary tumor is essential for long-term survival. However, this is usually difficult at presentation due to the multifocal nature of the tumor with its extrahepatic involvement of regional lymph nodes and distant metastases. Infiltration with thrombosis of portal and hepatic venous branches is common and even the vena cava may be involved. Chen et al. reported a 18.2% complete resection rate in their series of 55 children. Combination chemotherapy with doxorubicin, cyclophosphamide, vincristine and 5-fluorouracil has not been found effective in reducing tumor size in hepatocellular carcinoma. All this translates into an overall survival rate of zero for children with hepatocellular carcinoma that is not fully resectable at presentation.

Liver transplantation has shown to be useful in selected patients with unresectable tumor. However, positive hepatitis B viral serology, non-fibrolamellar histological type and high frequency of local or metastatic spread make most patients unsuitable for liver transplantation.

75.5.3 Rhabdomyosarcoma of the Extrahepatic Bile Ducts

This form of rhabdomyosarcoma is a very rare tumor with 40% of patients presenting with distant metastases. But mortality is most often due to the effects of local invasion. Rhabdomyosarcoma of the liver, not involving the bile ducts, has also been reported, but is extremely rare. The patients' ages range from 1 to 9 years at presentation. The typical symptoms include intermittent jaundice and sometimes loss of appetite and episodes of cholangitis (Charcot's triad). Hepatomegaly or a palpable abdominal mass is usual, and the diagnosis may be confused with hepatitis or a choledochal cyst.

As with hepatoblastoma and hepatocellular carcinoma, tissue diagnosis is necessary. Neo-adjuvant chemotherapy will reduce the tumor size and allow a cleaner resection at second-look surgery. During the initial biopsy, hilar and left gastric lymph node sampling is performed to determine whether these nodal echelons require added radiotherapy. Resection appears to improve survival. Whether these patients may be treated by chemotherapy alone after establishment of the diagnosis and simply observed if a complete radiologic response is documented remains to be confirmed with future studies.

75.5.4 Primary Hepatic Non-Hodgkin's Lymphoma

Primary non-Hodgkin's lymphoma of the liver occurs in childhood and may account for up to 5% of primary hepatic malignancies. These tumors respond well to chemotherapy, and surgery is not necessary.

75.5.5 Metastatic Hepatic Tumors

Several tumors, including non-Hodgkin's lymphoma, neuroblastoma, rhabdomyosarcoma, rhabdoid tumors, Wilms' tumor, the desmoplastic small round cell tumor, adrenal cortical carcinoma, and osteogenic sarcomas are known to metastasize to the liver in children. There is little data to determine the correct surgical approach to these lesions. Criteria for surgical removal of hepatic metastases include control of the primary site, a solitary or limited number of metastases, good performance status, and a reasonable expectation of prolonged survival or cure.

Hepatic metastases from neuroblastoma are seen in newborns and infants with Stage 4S disease, and are a distinct characteristic of this disease. These lesions usually resolve with time. Wilms' tumor metastasizes to the liver in about 12% of cases and this is usually associated with unfavorable histology. In selected patients, resection of these lesions may have a survival benefit. Most of the other tumors metastasize to the liver in the late stages of disease, and surgical resection does not appear to provide any survival advantage.

75.5.6 Benign Hepatic Tumors

Benign tumors of the liver that occur in childhood include hemangiomas or vascular tumors, hepatocytic adenomas, focal nodular hyperplasia, mesenchymal hamartomas, and various types of cysts or cystic disease. Vascular tumors are the most common and compose greater than 50% of these benign hepatic tumors.

75.5.6.1 Vascular Tumors

Hemangioma: Hemangiomas are lesions characterized by endothelial-lined vascular spaces that can vary in size and extent. They are sometimes classified as hamartomas. The overall incidence of endothelial lined vascular tumors of the liver in childhood is probably unknown since many are asymptomatic. Vascular lesions taken together represent 13–18% of symptomatic hepatic tumors in childhood. Hepatic hemangiomas are twice as common in females as in males.

Diagnosis can be fortuitous on a routine ultrasonography or when presented with an abdominal mass. Multiple hemispherical cutaneous hemangiomas may be present and warn the physician of possible visceral lesions. MRI study is all that is needed to confirm diagnosis and asymptomatic lesions are best left alone, as they tend to regress after the 1st year of life. Large lesions may cause congestive heart failure; if medical treatment is not successful, either hepatic artery embolization or direct surgical ligation may be necessary.

Hemangioendothelioma: These are highly proliferative cellular lesions of variable malignant potential. In one report of 16 infants and children, 15 presented with hepatomegaly, 7 with congestive heart failure, and 4 had associated cutaneous lesions. The Kasabach-Merritt syndrome, a platelet-trapping coagulopathy, has also been observed. These lesions may appear very cellular but do not metastasize. If a primary lesion produces symptoms, resection is indicated for relief.

Hemangioblastoma: Hemangioblastoma of the liver is usually associated with Lindau-von Hippel disease. In infancy and childhood these lesions appear very cellular but distant metastases are uncommon. Complete resection should be performed and is usually curative.

75.5.6.2 Mesenchymal Hamartoma

Mesenchymal hamartomas account for six percent of primary liver tumors in childhood and there is a male predominance. Two-thirds of these tumors are diagnosed at less than 1 year of age. These are usually multicystic and the cysts are lined with flattened biliary epithelium, or endothelium. It is postulated that mesenchymal hamartomas arise in areas of focal intrahepatic biliary atresia. This results in distal bile duct obstruction and hepatocellular necrosis.

The majority of mesenchymal hamartomas present as an enlarging abdominal mass or hepatomegaly, and are usually not symptomatic. They can grow to great sizes causing respiratory distress or evidence of caval obstruction. Often an open biopsy is necessary to make the diagnosis. Anatomical resection is the recommended treatment for large lesions. Because of the mesenchymal component, these lesions have a definite capsule that facilitates enucleation of large central mesenchymal hamartomas that are not amenable to lobectomy. Prognosis is good and in one study of 18 patients, 13 who were available for follow-up were alive and well 1 month to 24 years after treatment (mean = 5 years).

75.5.6.3 Focal Nodular Hyperplasia and Hepatocellular Adenoma

These are benign hepatocellular proliferations that are rare in children. Less than 2% of hepatic tumors in childhood are focal nodular hyperplasia or hepatocellular adenomas. The presence of fibrous septa containing bile ducts and inflammatory infiltrate distinguishes focal nodular hyperplasia from hepatocellular adenoma. These fibrous septa are seen as a distinct central scar in the ultrasound and computerized axial tomogram images. Most patients are less than 5 years of age at presentation and there is a female predominance. There is an association with contraceptive use in adults but no such association is reported in childhood and adolescence.

It is best to remove adenomas because of the difficulty in histologically differentiating them from low-grade hepatocellular carcinomas, and because of the uncertainty surrounding future malignant degeneration. Resection may also result in symptomatic relief in some children. In general anatomic resection is preferred for focal nodular hyperplasia and most do well after the hepatic resection. However, asymptomatic lesions can be observed using serial abdominal ultrasonography.

75.5.6.4 Cysts and Cystic Disease

There are multiple case reports of solitary, congenital, non-parasitic liver cysts in childhood. They are extremely rare but have been increasingly noted as incidental findings on ultrasounds or computerized axial tomograms performed for other reasons. These usually are simple cysts and are asymptomatic. To the best of our knowledge, there has been no report indicating any malignant degeneration of these cysts.

If there are associated symptoms, such as pain or jaundice, then aspiration followed by ethanol injection (sclerotherapy) may be of benefit. If this is not successful, surgical intervention including resection, marsupialization or cyst wall excision may be considered.

Further Reading

Abbasoglu L, Gun F et al (2004) Hepatoblastoma in children. Acta Chir Belg 104(3):318–321

Czauderna P, Mackinlay G et al (2002) Hepatocellular carcinoma in children: Results of the first prospective study of the International Society of Pediatric Oncology group. J Clin Oncol 20(12):2798–2804

Fuchs J, Rydzynski J et al (2002) Pretreatment prognostic factors and treatment results in children with hepatoblastoma: A report from the German Cooperative Pediatric Liver Tumor Study HB 94. Cancer 95(1):172–182

La Quaglia MP (2000) Hepatic tumors in childhood. In L Blumgart, Y Fong (eds), Surgery of the Liver and Biliary Tract, 2nd vol. W.B. Saunders, London, pp 1451–1473

Pimpalwar AP, Sharif K et al (2002) Strategy for hepatoblastoma management: Transplant versus nontransplant surgery. J Pediatr Surg 37(2):240–245

Stiller CA, Pritchard J et al (2006) Liver cancer in European children: Incidence and survival, 1978–1997. Report from the Automated Childhood Cancer Information System project. Eur J Cancer 42(13):2115–2123

Su WT, La Quaglia MP (2006) Liver Tumours. In P Puri, ME Höllwarth (eds) Pediatric Surgery, Springer Surgery Atlas Series. Springer-Verlag, Berlin, Heidelberg, New York, pp 459–476

von Schweinitz D (2006) Management of liver tumors in childhood. Semin Pediatr Surg 15(1):17–24

Xuewu J, Jianhong L et al (2006) Combined treatment of hepatoblastoma with transcatheter arterial chemoembolization and surgery. Pediatr Hematol Oncol 23(1):1–9

Lymphomas

76

Christian Urban

Contents

76.1 Principle Considerations

The role of surgery in the treatment of children with lymphomas (Hodgkin lymphoma (HL) and non-Hodgkin lymphoma (NHL)) is limited to diagnostic biopsies and treatment complications. There are no indications for performing major tumour resections or debulking procedures, since chemotherapy is so effective and major surgery delays may complicate chemotherapy. Only in children with ileocecal intus-susceptions due to Burkitt's lymphoma complete resection of the involved bowel segment is advised. Second-look surgery is also generally not recommended. Particularly, children with NHL may have rapidly growing tumors that can cause life-threatening complications requiring prompt intervention and treatment. Thus, a rapid diagnosis with the least invasive procedure should be done. In case of suspected lymphoma other options to establish the diagnosis before surgery should be considered like examination of blood and bone marrow and in case of pleural effusion/ascites puncture with cytologic and immunophenotypic examination. If the diagnosis with these simple measures cannot be established the most peripheral suspected lesion should be biopsied, e.g. in case of mediastinal tumor the nearest extrathoracic lymph node. The optimal way is that the surgeon, the pediatric oncologist and the pathologist cooperate in planning the biopsy, so that the biopsy material can be taken over by the pathologist already in the operation room for further appropriate processing.

P. Puri and M. Höllwarth (eds.), *Pediatric Surgery: Diagnosis and Management,*
DOI: 10.1007/978-3-540-69560-8_76, © Springer-Verlag Berlin Heidelberg 2009

76.2 Non-Hodgkin Lymphoma (NHL)

76.2.1 Classification and Pathology

Early classification systems in use have been confusing for clinicians and also led to disagreement even between expert pathologists, since non-Hodgkin lymphoma (NHL) is a heterogenous collection of diseases and their description was solely on cytomorphologic features. Immunophenotyping, cytogenetic and molecular studies now allow for a more precise classification according to the lineage of the malignant cells (WHO and REAL classification).

In contrast to the wide diversity of adulthood NHL, childhood NHL can mainly be divided among four major subgroups: Burkitt and Burkitt-like-lymphomas, diffuse large B-cell-lymphomas, anaplastic large cell lymphomas and lymphoblastic precursor T- and B-cell-lymphomas. The malignant cells in childhood NHLs appear to arise from different lymphocyte precursors at various stages of maturation or from mature lymphocytes. Approximately 40–50% of childhood NHL are either from T-cell lineage or from mature B-cells expressing surface immunoglobulin, whereas fewer than 10% are of early B-cell origin lacking surface immunoglobulin (Table 76.1).

Table 76.1 Correlation of histopathology, immunophenotype, clinical features, cytogenetic and molecular features in childhood non-Hodgkin lymphoma*

Histology	Immunology	Clinical features	Cytogenetics	Genes involved
Burkitt and Burkitt-like	B cell (sIg$^+$)	Abdominal masses, gastrointestinal tract tumors, involvement of Waldeyer's ring	t(8;14)(q24;q32) t(2;8)(p11;q24) t(8;22)(q24;q11)	IgH-cMYC Igκ-cMYC Igλ-cMYC
Diffuse large B-cell (DLBCL)	B cells of germinal center or post germinal center	Abdominal masses, gastrointestinal tract tumors, involvement of Waldeyer's ring	t(8;14)(q24;q32) t(2;17)(p23;q23)	IgH-cMYC CLTC-ALK
Mediastinal large B-cell	B cells of medullary thymus	Mediastinum		
Anaplastic large cell (ALCL)	T cell (mostly), null cell or NK cell (CD30$^+$)	Skin, nodes, bone	t(2;5)(p23;q35) t(1;2)(q21;p23) t(2;3)(p23;q21) t(2,17)(p23;q23) t(X;2)(q11–12;p23) inv 2 (p23;q35)	NPM-ALK TPM3-ALK TFG-ALK CLTC-ALK MSN-ALK ATIC-ALK
Precursor T lymphoblastic (pT-LBL)	T cell (thymocyte phenotype)	Anterior mediastinal mass with upper torso adenopathy	t(1;14)(p32;q11) t(11;14)(p13;q11) t(11;14)(p15;q11) t(10;14)(q24;q11) t(7;19)(q35;p13) t(8;14)(q24;q11) t(1;7)(p34;q34)	TCRαδ-TAL1 TCRαδ- RHOMB2 TCRαδ- RHOMB1 TCRαδ-HOX11 TCRβ-LYL1 TCRαδ-MYC TCRαδ-MYC TCRβ-LCK
Precursor B lymphoblastic (pB-LBL)	B-cell precursors	Cutaneous masses and isolated lymph node masses		

*Reprinted with permission from P.A. Pizzo & D.G.Poplack: Principles and Practice of Pediatric Oncology, 5th edition 2006, Lippincott Williams & Wilkins, Philadelphia

76.2.2 Clinical Features

The various subgroups of childhood NHLs have different clinical behaviour and are also characterised by the occurrence in different parts of the body (Table 76.1).

Most frequent involved sites are mediastinum (mainly lymphoblastic precursor T-NHL), abdomen (mainly Burkitt and Burkitt-like lymphoma) (Fig. 76.1) and cervical lymph nodes (mainly lymphoblastic precursor B-NHL). Less frequent sites are Waldeyer's ring, skin or bone and rarely the CNS (Fig. 76.2). Even though patients may appear to have local disease, there is often submicroscopic dissemination in certain histologic subtypes to the bone marrow and the CNS and some patients, particularly with Burkitt's disease or mediastinal T-NHL may have a rapid and aggressive course

76.2.3 Diagnostic Work Up and Staging

To establish the diagnosis of suspected NHL in children, the least invasive procedure should be preferred so that the risk of general anesthesia may be avoided. Before surgery is considered examination of blood and bone marrow and in case of pleural effusion/ascites puncture (preferably under local anesthesia) with cytologic and immunophenotypic analysis should be done.

Only if the diagnosis cannot be established with these simple methods a diagnostic biopsy should be performed. Complete resection should be done only, if possible and without any risk or functional loss for the patient. These principles are particularly important in patients with high tumor burdens, resulting in significant respiratory distress, vena cava compression, pericardial tamponade and metabolic disturbances (Fig. 76.3). Particularly in certain patients with mediastinal NHL and significant airway narrowing all diagnostic and especially invasive diagnostic procedures should be postponed after a prediagnostic cytoreductive therapy with prednisone up to 48 h until clinical stabilisation. Under no circumstances should a critically large mediastinal tumor with clinical symptoms of respiratory distress be treated surgically. Caution should be also given to the tumor lysis syndrome in patients with high tumor burdens even before the start of cytoreductive treatment.

Further staging evaluation must be done quickly since most children with NHL have rapidly growing tumors that may cause life-threatening situations. It includes physical examination, complete blood count, bone marrow and spinal fluid aspiration, analysis of electrolytes, LDH, renal and liver function tests and imaging with X-ray, ultrasonography, magnetic resonance, computerized tomography and skeletal scintigraphy.

The most widely used clinical staging system was developed at the St. Jude Children's Research Hospital in Memphis, USA (Table 76.2).

For patients with Burkitt-NHL, the St. Jude staging system has been adapted by the French Society of Pediatric Oncology (SFOP) to a system which stratifies the patients to different treatment arms tailored to their risk and cumulative tumor burden (Table 76.3).

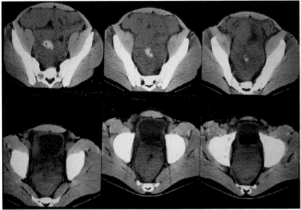
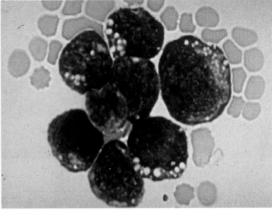
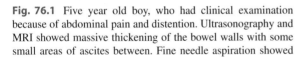

Fig. 76.1 Five year old boy, who had clinical examination because of abdominal pain and distention. Ultrasonography and MRI showed massive thickening of the bowel walls with some small areas of ascites between. Fine needle aspiration showed typical L-3 lymphoblasts with intensively basophilic cytoplasm and distinctive cytoplasmic vacuoles. Immunophenotyping and molecular studies confirmed the diagnosis of Burkitt lymphoma

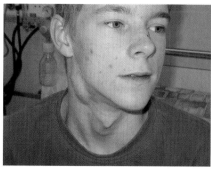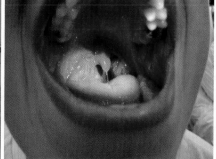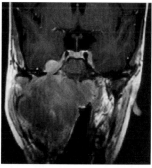

Fig. 76.2 Fifteen year old boy, complaining about difficulties in swallowing. Physical examination revealed right cervical lymphadenopathy with massive involvement of the Waldeyer's ring. MRI showed that the tumor mass infiltrated through the base of the skull with involvement of the CNS. Since CNS fluid and bone marrow aspiration were non-diagnostic, biopsy of the cervical lymph node under local anesthesia was done, demonstrating diffuse large B cell lymphoma

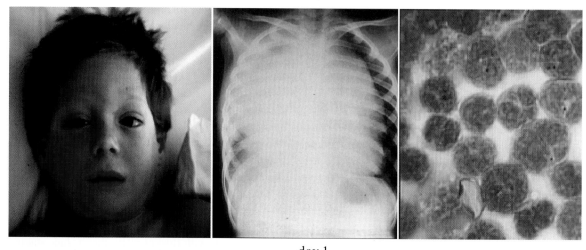

day 1

day 8

Fig. 76.3 Four year old boy with swelling and plethora of the face, cervical lymphadenopathy and respiratory distress in lying position. Chest X-ray showed a huge mediastinal tumor with pleural effusion on the right side. Pleural fluid aspiration in upright position with a thin needle using local anesthesia revealed convoluted lymphoblasts of T-cell type, positively stained with the acid phosphatase reaction and confirmed by immunophenotyping. After initiation of prednisolone there was a rapid tumor response with regression of the existing superior vena cava syndrome. Further treatment with a T-NHL/ALL-polychemotherapy protocol led to a complete and permanent remission

Table 76.2 St. Jude Children's Research Hospital staging system for non-Hodgkin lymphoma (Murphy et al. 1980)

Stage I

A single tumor (extranodal) or single anatomic area (nodal) with the exclusion of mediastinum or abdomen

Stage II

A single tumor (extranodal) with regional node involvement

Two or more nodal areas on the same side of the diaphragm

Two single (extranodal) tumors with or without regional node involvement on the same side of the diaphragm

A primary gastrointestinal tract tumor, usually in the ileocecal area, with or without involvement of associated mesenteric nodes only, grossly completely resected

Stage III

Two single tumors (extranodal) on opposite sides of the diaphragm

Two or more nodal areas above and below the diaphragm

All primary intrathoracic tumors (mediastina, pleural, thymic)

All extensive primary intraabdominal disease

All paraspinal or epidural tumors, regardless of other tumor site(s)

Stage IV

Any of the above with initial CNS and/or bone marrow involvement

---

Table 76.3 Risk stratification of B-cell non-Hodgkin lymphomas (SFOP) (Patte et al. 2001)

Group	Extent of Tumor
A	Resected stage I and abdominal stage II
B	Unresected stage I, non abdominal stage II, any stage III or IV, B-ALL-CNS negative (with < 70% blasts in BM)
C	CNS involvement or B-ALL with at least 70% blasts in the bone marrow

SFOP, French Society of Pediatric Oncology.

The stratification system utilizes the clinical stage assigned according to the St. Jude staging system.

Table 76.4 Staging system according to different risk groups in B-cell non- Hodgkin lymphomas used by the BFM- group (Seidemann et al. 2001)

Risk group 1:	Initial complete resection of the lymphoma manifestation
Risk group 2:	No or incomplete resection of lymphoma manifestation and one of the following criteria: only extraabdominal sites or abdominal sites and LDH less than 500 U/L
Risk group 3:	No or incomplete resection of abdominal lymphoma and LDH > 500 U/L, all patients with bone marrow involvement or/and CNS disease, or/and multifocal bone involvement

A similar staging system according to the different risk groups in Burkitt-NHL patients is being used by the BFM group (Table 76.4).

76.2.4 Treatment and Results

Nowadays clinical trials are available for all childhood NHL-types and participation in these studies is strongly recommended which guarantees treatment by an experienced multidisciplinary team of specialists. Chemotherapy is the mainstay of treatment. It is the same in lymphoblastic NHL of precursor B- and T-lineage as in precursor B- and T-ALL as the distinction between lymphoblastic NHL and ALL is largely arbitrary and simply based on the percentage of blasts in the bone marrow aspirate. CNS therapy is included in these regimes particularly for children with lymphoblastic and Burkitt-NHL, whereas the addition of radiotherapy does not have any benefit on survival except in rare cases (e.g. oncologic emergency).

Patients with diffuse large B-cell lymphomas (DLBCL), mediastinal large B-cell lymphomas and anaplastic large cell lymphomas (ALCL) are mainly treated on protocols either designed for Burkitt lymphoma or similar protocols with similarly good results. Overall more than 75% of children with NHL can be now cured with modern intensive polychemotherapy protocols and due to advances in supportive care to reduce the life-threatening complications of NHL and of therapy.

76.3 Hodgkin Lymphoma (HL)

76.3.1 Classification and Pathology

Two major subtypes of HL are differentiated according to the WHO classification:

Nodular lymphocyte predominant Hodgkin lymphoma (NLP HL) and classical Hodgkin lymphoma (cHL) subdivided in four histologic categories:

Lymphocyte-rich
Nodular sclerosis
Mixed cellularity
Lymphocyte depleted

In the cHL subtypes multinucleated Reed-Sternberg cells and their mononucleated variant Hodgkin cells are characteristic findings, expressing CD 30 antigen. Molecular studies have shown HL to be of B-cell origin. Only 0, 1–10% of the total cell population in HL are malignant cells, whereas the majority of the tumor consists of inflammatory cells (histiocytes, plasma cells, eosinophils, lymphocytes, neutrophils etc.) and fibrosis. This peculiar histologic pattern has been attributed to the secretion of different cytokines by the tumor.

76.3.2 Clinical Features

Most patients present with painless cervical or supra-clavicular enlarged lymph nodes which feel rubbery and firm at palpation. Differential diagnosis should include inflammatory conditions, especially with indolent course like atypical mycobacteriosis and toxoplasmosis, but also NHL, metastatic solid tumors (e.g. soft tissue sarcoma, neuroblastoma, nasopharyngeal carcinoma), histiocytoses and benign malformations. More than 60% of the patients with HL have also mediastinal involvement, sometimes causing symptoms of bronchial

compression or superior vena cava syndrome (Fig. 76.4). Axillary or inguinal lymphadenopathy is less frequent at initial presentation. Unexplained fever, weight loss of more than 10% within last 6 months and night sweats are considered as "B"-symptoms. Pruritus is another systemic symptom, sometimes leading to enormous scratching (Fig. 76.4).

76.3.3 Diagnostic Work Up and Staging

After diagnosis has been established by excisional biopsy, careful assessment of all lymph node regions by clinical examination and ultrasonography is essential. In addition complete blood count, analysis of electrolytes, LDH, renal and hepatic function tests should be done. The erythrocyte sedimentation rate, serum

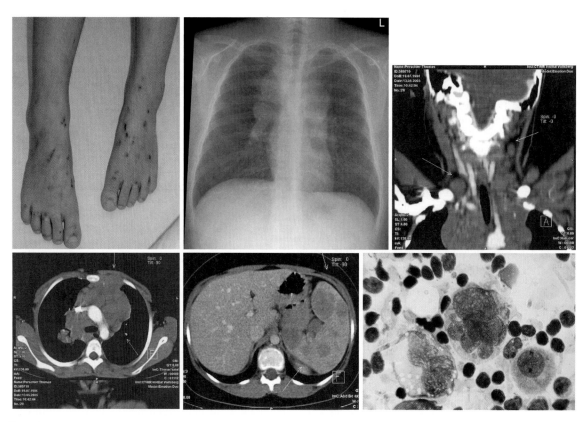

Fig. 76.4 The 12 year old boy had extensive dermatologic work-up because of itching and scratching. Chest X-ray revealed polycyclic bilateral enlargement of hilar lymph nodes. CT showed left cervical and right supraclavicular lymph node enlargement, a bulky mediastinal mass with anterior chest wall infiltration and a single left lung nodule as well as splenic involvement. Touch preparation smear of the excised supra-clavicular lymph node showed typical Reed-Sternberg and Hodgkin cells

copper and ferritin may be elevated as well as C-reactive protein, which can be used in follow-up evaluation. CT of the chest provides further information about the mediastinal lymph nodes as well as lungs, chest wall and pericardium. To evaluate the abdominal and pelvic lymph nodes and for diagnosis of splenic and hepatic involvement MRI may provide better information in children with the advantage of no radiation side effects. Positron emission tomography (PET) is being used as a promising new diagnostic tool for staging HL in adults; however prospective trials evaluating PET in pediatric HL are still awaiting. Since HL spreads along contiguous lymph nodes staging is based on the natural course of the disease (Table 76.5). Substage classification A means "asymptomatic" disease, substage B fever, night sweats and weight loss of more than 10% over the last 6 months and substage E extralymphatic disease. Bone marrow aspiration with biopsy should be reserved for patients with clinical stage III or IV or patients with B-symptoms, technetium-99 bone scan for patients with suspected skeletal metastases.

In the era when HL patients were only treated and cured with mainly radiotherapy, it was important to detect also minimal disease, so that exploratory laparatomy and splenectomy was the recommended staging procedure. Today, the success of diverse non-cross-resistant chemotherapy cycles in conjunction with the refinement in diagnostic imaging led to the abandonment of surgical staging. Laparotomy or better laparoscopic surgery is now reserved for females, who need transposition of the ovaries outside the irradiation field in case of pelvic irradiation.

76.3.4 Treatment and Results

Radiotherapy still is a fundamental part of current treatment protocols, however due to improvement of non-cross-resistant multiagent chemotherapy now can be reduced in dose and field. Chemotherapy mostly are derivates from the MOPP combination designed by Devita and ABVD regimen developed by Bonadonna given in alternating cycles according to the stage of disease. In some patients with favourable clinical presentation in early stage it is now investigated if the administration of risk-adapted multiagent chemotherapy alone can completely avoid involved – field radiation with the intention of sparing their late effects without impairing the results. Most current multicenter trials include central reviewing of all imaging studies by the study center in order to give a tailored risk-adapted treatment plan with precisely prescribed radiation fields and dosages in conjunction with the stage adapted chemotherapy. This has allowed not only for a more homogenous treatment stratification as well as comparison between the groups but also for further improvement of the already excellent treatment results in all treatment groups possibly also decreasing the acute and late side effects of treatment.

Further Reading

Carbone PP, Kaplan HS, Musshoff K et al (1971) Report of the Committee on Hodgkin's disease Staging Classification. Cancer Res 31:1860–1861

Dörffel W, Lüders H, Rühl E et al (2003) Preliminary results of the multicenter trial GPOH-HD 95 for the treatment of Hodgkin's disease in children and adolescents: Analysis and outlook. Klin Pädiatr 215:139–145

Jaffe ES, Harris NL, Stein H, Vardiman JW (2001) Pathology and Genetics of Tumours of Haematopoietic and Lymphoid Tissues. IARC Press, Lyon, France

Jerusalem G, Beguin Y, Fassotte MF et al (1999) Whole-body positron emission tomography using 18F-fluorodeoxyglucose for posttreatment evaluation in Hodgkin's disease and non-Hodgkin's lymphoma has higher diagnostic and prognostic value than classical computed tomography scan imaging. Blood 94:429–433

Mann G, Attarbaschi A, Steiner M et al (2006) Early and reliable diagnosis of non-Hodgkin lymphoma in childhood and adolescence: Contribution of cytomorphology and flow cytometric immunophenotyping. Pediat Hematol Oncol 23:167–176

Murphy SB (1980) Classification, staging and end results of treatment of childhood non Hodgkin's lymphomas: Dissimilarities from lymphomas in adults. Semin Oncol 7:332–339

Table 76.5 Staging classification for Hodgkin lymphoma (Carbone et al. 1971)

Stage	
Stage I	Involvement of a single lymph node (I) or of a single extralymphatic organ or site (I_E)
Stage II	Involvement of two or more lymph node regions on the same side of the diaphragm (II) or localized involvement of an extralymphatic organ or site and one or more lymph node regions on the same side of the diaphragm (II_E)
Stage III	Involvement of lymph node regions on both sides of the diaphragm (III), which may be accompanied by involvement of the spleen (III_S) or by localized involvement of an extralymphatic organ or site (III_E) or both (III_{SE})
Stage IV	Diffuse or disseminated involvement of one or more extralymphatic organs or tissues with or without associated lymph node involvement

Patte C, Auperin A, Michon J et al (2001) The Societe Francaise d'Oncologie Pediatrique LMB 89 protocol: Highly effective multiagent chemotherapy tailored to the tumor burden and initial response in 561 unselected children with B-cell lymphomas and L3 leukemia. Blood 97:3370–3379

Puri P, Höllwarth M (2006) Pediatric Surgery. Springer, Berlin, Heidelberg

Seidemann K, Tiemann M, Schrappe M et al (2001) Short-pulse B-non-Hodgkin lymphoma-type chemotherapy is efficacious treatment for pediatric anaplastic large cell lymphoma: A report of the Berlin-Frankfurt-Münster group trial NHL-BFM 90. Blood 97:3699–3706

Ovarian Tumors

77

Mary E. Fallat and Romeo C. Ignacio, Jr.

Contents

77.1 Incidence and Epidemiology

Ovarian tumors comprise a heterogenous group of benign and malignant lesions. Their clinical presentation can vary based on age of the patient, size of the tumor, hormonal activity, histology and local spread or metastasis. Although ovarian malignancies are the fifth most common cause of cancer among adult females, they are considered rare in children and adolescents. A significant proportion of ovarian tumors are potentially malignant. Therefore, a thorough understanding of the characteristics that distinguish malignant from benign ovarian tumors is necessary to optimize prompt evaluation, appropriate treatment and to consider the options for ovarian preservation in the event of a benign condition.

The annual incidence of ovarian masses in children is approximately 2.6 cases/100,000 girls per year. The majority of masses are benign, although various studies have estimated the occurrence of malignancy between 10–64%. This wide discrepancy in malignancy rate in case series is due to the biases in patient referrals, variable inclusion of benign lesions, and differences in data collection based both on the age groups and types of tumors included in these studies. As newer diagnostic imaging techniques have increased the detection of previously occult masses and cysts, the incidence of malignancy has declined. More recent series of patients have estimated malignancy rates at approximately 20%.

The majority of ovarian lesions have no specific etiology with regards to environmental exposure, genetic background or drugs. However, there are certain diseases, genes or hormonal factors that might increase the risk for certain ovarian tumors. Nulliparity, use of

P. Puri and M. Höllwarth (eds.), *Pediatric Surgery: Diagnosis and Management*,
DOI: 10.1007/978-3-540-69560-8_77, © Springer-Verlag Berlin Heidelberg 2009

Table 77.1　Syndromes and diseases associated with an increased risk of ovarian tumors

Syndrome/Disease	Description	Associated Ovarian Pathology
Basal cell nevus (Gorlin) syndrome	Rare autosomal disorder associated with two or more basal cell carcinomas, cysts of the jaw, characteristic facies, rib abnormalities and increased risk of medulloblastoma and cardiac fibromas	Ovarian fibromas
Chediak-Higashi syndrome	Oculocutaneous albinism, pyogenic infections and abnormalities of leukocyte granules resulting in defective phagocytosis	Sclerosing stromal tumors
Maffucci's syndrome	Multiple enchondromas, hemangiomas and bony deformities	Juvenile granulosa cell tumors
Muir-Torre Syndrome	Variant of HNPCC,[a] associated with multiple cutaneous neoplasms and visceral malignancies	Granulosa cell tumors
McCune-Albright syndrome	Café au lait spots, autonomic endocrine hyperactivity, polyostotic fibrous dysplasia	Recurrent ovarian follicles causing sexual precocity
Ollier's disease	Multiple enchondromas of the tubular bones of the hand and feet, increased risk for chondrosarcomas	Juvenile granulosa cell tumors
Peutz-Jeghers syndrome	Autosomal dominant disorder associated with melanocytic macules of the mouth, hamartomatous or adenomatous polyps of the gastrointestinal tract	Predominantly sex stromal tumors

[a]HNPCC—Hereditary non-polyposis colorectal cancer

ovulatory-inducing drugs, lack of oral contraceptive use, and high-fat diets are risk factors associated with later development of adult epithelial neoplasms. There are also numerous syndromes associated with various ovarian tumors (Table 77.1).

The most significant risk factor for ovarian cancer is genetic predisposition. The tumor suppressor genes BRCA1 and BRCA2 are responsible for 70–90% of familial cases of ovarian malignancy. The role for genetic testing in children and adolescents for such mutations is controversial since there are no medical benefits including preventive measures and therapy that have been studied in this population.

77.2 Pathology

Ovarian tumors can be classified as non-neoplastic or neoplastic (Tables 77.2 and 77.3). Approximately two thirds of these lesions are neoplastic, but only a small percentage (20%) have malignant changes. The most common clinical and pathologic staging methods of ovarian cancer are the International Federation of Gynecology and Obstetrics (FIGO) (Table 77.4) and the Children's Oncology Group (COG) staging systems (Table 77.5).

Table 77.2　World Health Organization histological classification of non-neoplastic ovarian lesions[a]

Solitary follicle cyst

Multiple follicle cysts (polycystic ovarian disease, sclerocystic ovaries)

Large solitary luteinized follicle cyst of pregnancy and puerperium

Hyperreactio luteinalis (multiple luteinized follicle cysts)

Corpus luteum cyst

Pregnancy luteoma

Ectopic pregnancy

Stromal hyperplasia

Stromal hyperthecosis

Massive edema

Fibromatosis

Endometriosis

Cyst, unclassified (simple cyst)

Inflammatory lesions

[a]Scully RE, Young RH, Clement PB: Atlas of tumor pathology, tumors of the ovary, maldeveloped

Gonads, Fallopian Tube and Broad Ligaments, 3rd ser, fascicle 23. Washington DC, American Registry of Pathology, Armed Forces Institute of Pathology, 1998

Table 77.3 World Health Organization[a] histological classification of tumors of the ovary

1. Surface epithelial-stromal tumors
   Serous tumors
   Mucinous tumors
   Endometrioid tumors including variants with squamous differentiation
   Clear cell tumors
   Transitional cell tumors
   Squamous cell tumors
   Mixed epithelial tumors
   Undifferentiated and unclassified tumors
2. Sex cord-stromal tumors
   Granulosa-stromal cell tumors
      Granulosa cell tumor group
      Thecoma-fibroma group
   Sertoli-stromal cell tumors
   Sex cord-stromal tumors of mixed or unclassified cell types
   Steroid tumors
3. Germ cell tumors
   Primitive germ cell tumors
      Dysgerminoma
      Yolk sac tumor (endodermal sinus tumor)
      Embryonal carcinoma
      Polyembryoma
      Non-gestational choriocarcinoma
      Mixed germ cell tumors (specify components)
   Biphasic or triphasic teratomas
      Immature
      Mature
   Monodermal teratoma and somatic-type tumors associated with dermoid cysts
      Thyroid tumor group
      Carcinoid group
      Neuroectodermal tumor group
      Carcinoma group
      Melanocytic group
      Sarcoma group (specify type)
      Sebaceous tumor group
      Pituitary-type tumor type
      Retinal anlage tumor group
      Others
4. Germ cell sex cord-stromal tumors
   Gonadoblastoma
   Mixed germ cell-sex cord-stromal tumor
5. Tumors of the rete ovarii
   Adenocarcinoma
   Adenoma
   Cystadenoma
   Cystadenofibroma
6. Miscellaneous tumors
   Small cell carcinomas, hypercalcemic type
   Small cell carcinomas, pulmonary type
   Large cell neuroendocrine carcinoma
   Hepatoid carcinoma

Primary ovarian mesothelioma
Wilms tumor
Gestational choriocarcinoma
Hydatidiform mole
Adenoid cystic carcinoma
Basal cell tumor
Ovarian wolffian tumor
Paraganglioma
Myxoma
Soft tissue tumors not specific to the ovary
Others
7. Tumor-like conditions
   Luteoma of pregnancy
   Stromal hyperthecosis
   Stromal hyperplasia
   Fibromatosis
   Massive ovarian edema
8. Lymphoid and hematopoietic tumors
   Malignant lymphoma (specific type)
   Leukemia (specific type)
   Plasmacytoma
9. Secondary tumors

[a] Jaffe ES, Harris NL, Stein H, Vardiman JW: WHO Classification of tumors: Pathology and genetics of tumours of the breast and female genital organs. IARC Press: Lyon, 2001.

Table 77.4 Staging of primary carcinoma of the ovary: International Federation of Gynecology and Obstetrics (FIGO)

Stage	Extent of disease
0	No evidence of primary tumor
I	Tumor confined to the ovaries
IA	Tumor limited to one ovary, capsule intact
	No tumor on ovarian surface
	No malignant cells in ascites or peritoneal washings
IB	Tumor limited to both ovaries, capsule intact
	No tumor on ovarian surface
	No malignant cells in ascites or peritoneal washings
IC	Tumor limited to one or both ovaries, with one of the following:
	Capsule ruptured, tumor on ovarian surface, malignant cells in ascites or peritoneal washings
II	Tumor involves one or both ovaries with pelvic extension
IIA	Extension to or implants on uterus or tubes or both
	No malignant cells in ascites or peritoneal washings
IIB	Extension to other pelvic organs
	No malignant cells in ascites or peritoneal washings

(continued)

Table 77.4 (continued)

Stage	Extent of disease
IIC	IIA or IIB with positive malignant cells in ascites or peritoneal washings
III	Tumor involves one or both ovaries with microscopically confined peritoneal metastasis outside the pelvis and/or regional lymph nodes metastasis
IIIA	Microscopic peritoneal metastasis beyond the pelvis
IIIB	Macroscopic peritoneal metastasis beyond the pelvis 2 cm or less in greatest dimension
IIIC	Peritoneal metastasis beyond the pelvis more than 2 cm in greatest dimension and/or regional lymph node metastasis
IV	Distant metastasis beyond the peritoneal cavity

Staging Classification and Clinical Practice Guidelines for Gynaecologic Cancers. FIGO Committee on Gynaecologic Oncology. Intl J Gynaecol Obstetr 2000; 70: 207–312.

Table 77.5 Clinical and pathologic staging of ovarian germ cell tumors: Children's Oncology Group (COG)[a]

Stage	Extent of disease
I	Limited to ovary (ovaries) peritoneal washings negative; Tumors markers are normal after appropriate half-life decline (AFP, 5 days; β-HCG, 16 h)
II	Microscopic residual or disease in lymph nodes < 2 cm; peritoneal washings normal; markers positive or negative
III	Gross residual disease or biopsy only; lymph nodes > 2 cm; contiguous spread to other organs (omentum, intestine, bladder); peritoneal washings positive for malignant cells; markers negative or positive
IV	Distant metastasis including liver

[a]von Allmen D. Malignant lesions of the ovary in childhood. Sem Pedr Surg 2005; 14:100–5

77.3 Diagnosis and Evaluation

77.3.1 Clinical Presentation

The clinical signs and symptoms associated with ovarian tumors are nonspecific. The most common complaint is abdominal enlargement or vague abdominal pain. Acute abdominal or pelvic pain can occur due to tumor torsion, hemorrhage or rupture. The occurrence of chronic pain varies depending on the type of ovarian tumor, its size and extent of disease. Large tumors can cause compression of adjacent organs causing cramping pain, constipation, or urinary symptoms. Abdominal distention can also be due to ascites, although rare in the pediatric population. Vaginal bleeding is an uncommon symptom. Recent studies have shown that genitourinary complaints may be associated with ovarian cancer. Regardless, there are no specific findings that indicate if the ovarian mass is malignant or benign.

The physical exam is usually revealing for an abdominal mass in children or pelvic mass in adolescents. Associated tenderness may occur with torsion, rupture or hemorrhage. A fluid shift may be detected in the presence of ascites. Pelvic examination is usually reserved for sexually active patients. Bimanual examination can aid in palpation of smaller adnexal masses. Bimanual rectal examination may be helpful in prepubertal children and infants.

Ovarian lesions that are hormonally active can cause precocious puberty or virilization. Features of isosexual or ambiguous development of the genitalia and breasts can be suggestive clues of a sex stromal tumor. The presence of hirsute or masculine features can be due to a Sertoli-Leydig tumor.

77.3.2 Laboratory Tests

The evaluation of suspected ovarian masses may include laboratory tests such as tumor markers, hormone levels and cytogenetic studies. All patients should have a quantitative human chorionic gonadotropin (β-HCG), since some ovarian tumors secrete β-HCG. In postmenarchal patients, this is also used to exclude an intrauterine or ectopic pregnancy. Ultrasound will help differentiate between these diagnoses.

Certain ovarian malignancies secrete specific tumor markers (Table 77.6). The main specific tumor markers for ovarian neoplasms are β-HCG, alpha-fetoprotein (AFP), lactic dehydrogenase (LDH) and CA-125. These tumor markers can aid in the diagnosis of certain ovarian pathologies, although they can also be elevated with other nongynecological tumors or medical conditions.

β-HCG is a glycoprotein with a similar structure to luteinizing hormone (LH). The two hormones only differ by the last 30 amino acids of the Beta subunit. β-HCG is secreted by syncytiotrophoblastic cells and functions to support the corpus luteum. β-HCG is positive in

Table 77.6 Tumor markers in relation to ovarian neoplasms and nongynecological conditions

Tumor marker	Associated ovarian neoplasms	Associated conditions
β-HCG	Mixed germ cell tumors[a]	Pregnancy
	Dysgerminomas	Seminomas
	Choriocarcinomas	
	Endodermal sinus tumors	
	Embryonal carcinomas	
	Hydatidiform moles	
AFP	Malignant teratomas	Hepatoma
	Endodermal sinus tumors	Neonatal hepatitis
	Embryonal carcinomas	Fetal neural tube defects
	Endodermal carcinoma	Omphalocele
	Sertoli-Leydig tumors	Gastroschisis
		Congenital nephrosis
		Fetal hemorrhage
		Hereditary tyrosinemia
LDH	Dysgerminomas (LDH-1)	Numerous causes depending on isoenzyme
CA-125	Endometrioma	Lung carcinomas
	Epithelial ovarian carcinomas	Liver carcinomas
	Carcinoma of the fallopian tubes, endometrium or endocervix	Pancreatic carcinomas
		Colon carcinomas
		Breast carcinomas
		Pregnancy
		Cirrhosis

[a]Mixed Germ Cell Tumors may secrete several markers depending on the components of the tumor.
B-HCG—human chorionic gonadotropin, AFP—alpha fetoprotein, LDH—lactate dehydrogenase

intrauterine or ectopic pregnancies and hydatiform moles. Neoplastic causes of a positive result include almost all cases of choriocarcinoma, 10–30% of seminomas and 5–35% of cases of dysgerminomas.

Alpha-fetoprotein is a product of fetal yolk sac, liver and gastrointestinal tissue and can remain elevated during the first 8 months of life. Maternal serum levels of AFP serve as an indicator of neural tube defects (spina bifida or anencephaly), ventral wall defects (gastroschisis or omphalocele), congenital nephrosis and fetal hemorrhage. As a tumor marker, it is a valuable test for primary malignancies of the liver, hepatic metastases for certain cancers (i.e. stomach or pancreas) and germ cell tumors of the testis and ovary. It is elevated in yolk sac tumors, embryonal carcinomas, malignant teratomas and Sertoli-Leydig carcinomas. Levels of AFP should return to normal after surgery and chemotherapy treatment. Recurrent elevations after treatment usually indicate relapse of cancer, often preceding clinical or radiographic evidence.

Serum CA-125 is a glycoprotein derived from coelomic epithelium. This tumor marker is associated with numerous malignancies in the liver, pancreas, breast, colon and lung. It is also associated with nonmucinous epithelial ovarian carcinoma, carcinoma of the fallopian tubes and endometrial cancers. CA-125 is useful in monitoring residual or recurrent disease after surgery. An elevated or rising level during chemotherapy is associated with poor response and progression of disease.

There are other nonspecific tumor markers that have some prognostic value. Carcinoembryonic antigen (CEA) is more commonly associated with colon cancer, but it is also present in 50–70% of cases of serous carcinoma of the ovary. Serum level of lactic dehydrogenase (LDH) may correlate with ovarian tumor activity due to high cell turnover. However, an elevated LDH is also associated with other malignancies such as neuroblastoma and lymphoma.

Approximately 10% of ovarian masses can produce hormones resulting in abnormal menses, early thelarche, precocious puberty or virilization. Elevated estrogen levels from ovarian cysts or sex stromal tumors can cause precocious puberty. Sertoli-Leydig tumors, yolk sac tumors and polycystic ovaries can produce high levels of androgens leading to virilization. These hormone tests should be selectively obtained based on the clinical history and physical examination of the patient.

77.3.3 Radiologic Studies

77.3.3.1 Ultrasonography

Ultrasound is the initial imaging study used to evaluate ovarian masses and can be done pre- or postnatally as an abdominal or pelvic exam. Prenatal ultrasounds commonly identify fetal abdominal cysts, and are helpful in distinguishing ovarian cysts from intestinal, uterine or genitourinary abnormalities. During infancy and early childhood, ovarian masses are typically intraabdominal due to the narrow and small pelvis. As the child grows, the use of transpelvic ultrasound is required. In age appropriate adolescents, transvaginal ultrasound can be done. Ultrasonography is used to distinguish cystic versus solid ovarian masses, and there are imaging clues that aid in determining whether a mass is benign or malignant (Table 77.7).

77.3.3.2 Computed Tomography

Computed tomography (CT) has the disadvantage of radiation exposure, a factor of particular importance in children. The average abdominal and pelvic CT is equivalent to 180–200 chest radiographs. Nevertheless, CT of the abdomen and pelvis is a valuable imaging study and useful in determining the anatomic location and origin of an ovarian mass, extent of local involvement and possibility of metastases. Suggestive findings

Table 77.7 Radiologic findings for the most common benign and malignant ovarian lesions

	Ultrasound	Computed Tomogram	Magnetic Resonance Imaging
Benign Lesions			
Ovarian Cysts	Thin walled Anechoic or hypoechoic mass	Thin walled fluid filled structure	Cysts which are fluid-filled have low signal intensity on T1-weighted images, high on T2-weighted images Hemorrhagic cysts will have high signal on T1 and T2 weighted images
Teratomas	Complex, hypoechoic mass (due to sebum or fluid) Peripheral mural nodules may appear as acoustic shadowing (due to hair, fat and sometimes calcifications) Central echogenic masses with "dot dash" pattern (due to sebaceous material and hair within the cystic lumen)	Fluid-filled mass with hair, fat and calcifications	Varied signal due to tissue composition. Fat will have high signal on T1 and T2-weighted images Serous fluid will have low signal on T1-weighted images, high signal on T2-weighted images
Malignant lesions			
Germ cell tumors (dysgerminoma, endodermal sinus tumor, embryonal carcinoma and choriocarcinoma)	Large tumors (>10–15 cm in size)	Direct extension to adjacent pelvic structures Stippled calcifications for dysgerminomas	Direct extension to adjacent pelvic structures. Useful in detecting tissue components and peritoneal implants
Sertoli-Leydig cell, Granulosa-theca cell, Undifferentiated tumors and Epithelial tumors	Variable appearance Solid or complex masses Irregular borders Thick septations Papillary projections	Presence of ascites, lymphadenopathy and hepatic metastases Similar findings to ultrasound	Presence of ascites, lymphadenopathy, peritoneal implants and hepatic metastases Similar findings to ultrasound

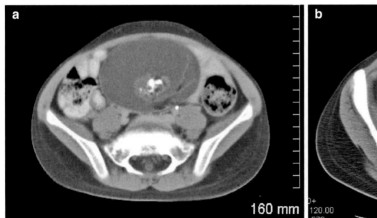 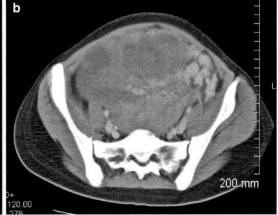

Fig. 77.1 CT scan of benign versus malignant ovarian tumor: (**a**) Demonstrates a benign ovarian tumor with no evidence of direct extension into the surrounding soft tissue structures. The teratoma was composed of adipose tissue, teeth and hair. (**b**) Demonstrates a large malignant tumor with irregular borders, thick septations, adenopathy and invasion into the adjacent pelvic organs. The final pathology was a mixed germ cell tumor

of malignancy include large mass size, solid nature of the tumor, peritoneal implants, ascites or suspicious calcifications (Fig. 77.1). Computed tomography is more accurate for disease staging than ultrasonography. This modality is also commonly used in detecting recurrent or metastatic ovarian cancer after treatment.

77.3.3.3 Magnetic Resonance Imaging

Magnetic resonance imaging (MRI) avoids radiation exposure to soft tissues. It is a useful adjunct in differentiating uterine tumors from ovarian masses. Based on signal intensity, MRI can further identify specific ovarian pathology such as dermoid cysts, endometriomas and ovarian torsion. However, similar characteristics seen on CT can aid in distinguishing benign versus malignant conditions, and a major disadvantage of MRI is the prolonged imaging time, which may contribute to motion artifact and mandate the use of sedation.

77.4 Treatment of Ovarian Tumors

The majority of ovarian masses are benign, making gonadal preservation an option. The treatment for malignant lesions is generally oophorectomy, depending on the specific tumor. Even with bilateral oophorectomy,

the option for uterine sparing should be considered for potential in-vitro fertilization. Each treatment option should be individualized based on the pathology, extent of the disease and patient and parental desire to preserve fertility. Most benign tumors can be approached laparoscopically, while it is generally agreed that laparotomy is preferred for malignant tumors.

77.4.1 Benign Tumors

77.4.1.1 Ovarian Cysts

Neonatal ovarian cysts have been described in detail in the literature. Most of these cysts are benign and tend to spontaneously regress. Incidental finding of a simple cyst on ultrasound requires only close follow-up at 6–12 week intervals. Intraoperative discovery of ovarian cysts in infants less than 12 months of age can be managed with aspiration or fenestration. Surgical management is recommended for cystic masses that are symptomatic, complex in character, increasing in size over time, or suggestive of malignancy.

Ovarian cysts are not uncommon in children and adolescents. The majority of these cysts arises from mature follicles and are benign. These cysts tend to be thin-walled, unilocular and unilateral, and can be discovered incidentally, during operations for other disease processes, or during evaluation for adnexal masses. The treatment for these lesions is based on symptomatology, endocrine activity and size. As ovarian cysts enlarge beyond 5 cm, they have an increased risk for torsion, rupture or hemorrhage. Some cysts have endocrine activity that can cause early isosexual development or premature thelarche. These latter groups of lesions should be excised with preservation of adjacent ovarian tissue. Operative approach can be through a midline laparotomy, Pfannenstiel incision or via laparoscopy. Other indications for cyst excision include persistence or size increase over 2–3 months of surveillance or concern for malignancy.

77.4.1.2 Mature Cystic Teratomas

The risk for malignancy in mature cystic teratomas (MCTs) is only 2%, and ovarian preservation with cyst removal via laparoscopy or laparotomy and postoperative surveillance is the preferred treatment. The postoperative follow-up consists of annual pelvic ultrasound in prepubertal children to evaluate any disease in the contralateral ovary or early signs of recurrent lesions, and annual pelvic exam or pelvic ultrasound in post menarchal adolescents.

77.4.2 Malignant Tumors

77.4.2.1 Malignant Germ Cell Tumors

Approximately two thirds of pediatric ovarian malignancies are germ cell tumors. These tumors vary in their presentation and malignant potential and can also arise in other areas of the body. Germ cell tumors originate from one or more embryonic cell layers (endoderm, mesoderm and ectoderm). Because of their variability in tissue origin and cellular behavior, they can be benign or malignant. Figure 77.2 is a schematic showing the various malignant germ cell tumors based on their embryologic differentiation.

Proper staging for malignant GCTs depends on intraoperative findings including extent of tumor involvement, peritoneal washings and results of tumor markers (Table 77.5). The surgical therapy for germ cell tumors is similar regardless of the tumor type. Operative management includes (1) surgical resection (i.e. unilateral oophorectomy or salpingo-oophorectomy) for optimal cure, (2) intraoperative evaluation of potential tumor involvement in the contralateral ovary, adjacent structures, regional and retroperitoneal lymph nodes, all peritoneal surfaces, diaphragm, and liver, (3) collection of peritoneal washings for cytology, and (4) omentectomy. Any suspicious lesions on the contralateral ovary are biopsied. Preservation of fertility options is considered and is dependent on extent of disease.

Chemotherapy regimens for germ cell tumors are predominantly platinum based. The most common regimen for advanced stages of dysgerminoma or endodermal sinus tumor consists of bleomycin, etoposide and platinol. The advantages of this regimen include less risk of future infertility and improved survival for children with endodermal sinus carcinoma. Embryonal carcinoma can be treated with the previously mentioned regimen or a cyclophosphamide-methotrexate-dactinomycin combination. Immature stage I or II teratomas can be treated with surgery only whereas higher stage tumors will require adjuvant chemotherapy such as vincristine, actinomycin D, cyclophosphamide with or without cisplatin.

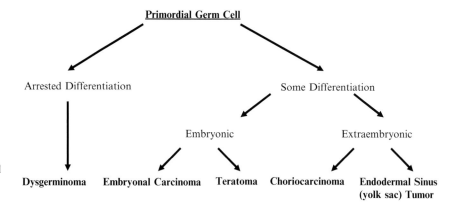

Fig. 77.2 Malignant germ cell tumors based on embryologic differentiation

77.4.2.2 Sex Stromal Tumors

The majority of the remaining one third of pediatric ovarian tumors are sex-stromal and epithelial tumors. Sex stromal tumors originate from stromal components of the ovary such as granulosa-theca cells or Sertoli-Leydig cells. These tumors are common in younger patients and account for 5–8% of ovarian malignancies. Occasionally, these tumors can produce hormones leading to androgenization or isosexual precocious puberty.

Juvenile granulosa-theca cell tumors are the most common sex stromal tumors and account for up to 10% of pediatric ovarian malignancies. These tumors are commonly functional and associated with pseudo-precocious puberty in 80% of patients. Other symptoms that have been described with these neoplasms are galactorrhea, menstrual abnormalities, vaginal bleeding, labial swelling, early development of axillary or pubic hair, and increase in overall growth. Due to high associated estrogen levels, a consequent increase in vascularity of these tumors can lead to significant hemoperitoneum and peritonitis if rupture occurs. These tumors tend to be more aggressive than their adult counterpart. The degree of malignancy is related to the proportion of granulosa cells present. Pure granulosa cell tumors are frequently malignant. Tumors composed of mixed granulosa and theca cells are less frequently malignant and pure thecoma cell tumors are usually benign. Most patients diagnosed with juvenile granulosa-theca cell tumors present with Stage I malignancies and have a favorable prognosis. These patients are adequately treated with a unilateral oophorectomy or salpingo-oophorectomy with survival rates close to 100%. However, those with more advanced disease (stage III) require hysterectomy with bilateral salpingo-oophorectomy, radiotherapy and multi-drug chemotherapy (i.e. carboplatin and etoposide).

Sertoli-Leydig cell tumors, also known as arrheno-blastomas, account for up to 30% of sex stromal neoplasms, but less than 0.5% of all malignant ovarian masses. Most of these tumors present with masculinizing changes such as amenorrhea, loss of female habitus, breast atrophy, hirsutism, thinning of hair, acne, clitoral enlargement and accelerated growth. The physiologic effects are due to the accumulation of testosterone, which can also be used as a biological marker for the tumors. These neoplasms tend to have elevated levels of AFP and CA-125. Treatment consists of surgery and chemotherapy. Unilateral oophorectomy or adnexal resection is adequate therapy and preserves potential child bearing options in the future. Advanced stages, bilateral disease, ruptured and/or poorly differentiated tumors require more aggressive surgical resection (similar to granulosa cell tumors) and chemotherapy. Gonadotropin-releasing hormone agonists and oral contraceptives can aid in treatment during and after chemotherapy.

77.4.2.3 Epithelial Tumors

Epithelial tumors derive from the germinal epithelium and are considered well-differentiated neoplasms. These ovarian tumors account for less than 20% of childhood ovarian malignancies. They are commonly serous or mucinous tumors and have an indolent course. CA-125 is a useful marker in malignant epithelial tumors and detecting recurrent disease after chemotherapy. Treatment of epithelial tumors is based on the FIGO staging system. Stage 1A disease is amenable to ovarian preservation with unilateral salpingo-oophorectomy. Stage IB tumors require bilateral salpingo-oophorectomy, with preservation of the uterus for potential in-vitro fertilization. Since serous tumors can be bilateral in 20% of cases, evaluation of the contralateral ovary is essential. More advanced disease requires surgical cytoreduction, total abdominal hysterectomy, bilateral salpingo-oophorectomy and omentectomy. Adjuvant chemotherapy has proved to have a 60–70% response rate, but the overall 5-year survival is only 20%. Radiation therapy for advanced epithelial tumors currently remains controversial.

Further Reading

Canis M, Rabischong B, Houlle C et al (2002) Laparoscopic management of adnexal masses: A gold standard? Curr Opin Obstet Gynecol 14:423–428

Dolgin S (2000) Ovarian masses in newborn. Sem Pediatr Surg 9:121–127

Fallat M, Brandt M (eds) (2005) Ovarian and tubal disorders. Sem Pediatr Surg 14:1–110

Lazar E, Stolar C (1998) Evaluation and management of pediatric solid ovarian tumors. Sem Pediatr Surg 7:29–34

Puri P, Höllwarth M (2006) Pediatric Surgery. Springer, Berlin, Heidelberg

Templeman CL, Fallat ME (2006) Ovarian tumors. In JL Grosfeld, JA O'Neill, EW Fonkalsrud, AG Coran (eds) Pediatric Surgery, 6th edn. Vol. 1 Mosby, Philadelphia, PA, pp 593–621, Chap 36

Templeman CL, Hertweck SP, Scheetz JP, Perlman SE, Fallat ME (2000) The management of mature cystic teratomas in children and adolescents. Human Reprod 15(12):2669–2672

Tozzi R, Köhler C, Ferrara A, Schneider A (2004) Laparoscopic treatment of early ovarian cancer: Surgical and survival outcomes. Gynecol Oncol 93(1):199–203

Vaisbuch E, Dgani R, Ben-Arie A, Hagay Z (2005) The role of laparoscopy in ovarian tumors of low malignant potential and early-stage ovarian cancer. Obstet Gynecol Surv 60(5): 326–330

Testis Tumors

78

Jonathan H. Ross

Contents

78.1 Introduction

There is a bimodal age distribution for testis tumors with one peak occurring in the first 2 years of life, and a second, much larger peak occurring in young adulthood. Therefore pediatric testis tumors occur in two distinct groups—prepubertal patients and adolescents. Testicular tumors in adolescents and children do have some similarities. Both usually present with a testicular mass and are treated initially with excision of the primary tumor. In both children and adolescents, malignant testis tumors are particularly sensitive to platinum-based chemotherapy, which has revolutionized the management of testicular cancer throughout the age spectrum. However, there are important differences between testis tumors occurring in children and adolescents. These differences occur in the tumor histopathology, malignant potential, and pattern of metastatic spread. The patients themselves are also dissimilar with different concerns regarding surgical morbidity and preservation of testicular function. These differences have resulted in a significantly different approach to testicular tumors in the two age groups.

78.2 Epidemiology

The incidence of pediatric testis tumors is 0.5–2.0 per 100,000 children accounting for 1–2% of all pediatric tumors. Testis tumors are categorized based on the presumed cell of origin into stromal tumors and germ cell tumors. The frequency and behavior of the various tumor types in prepubertal patients and adolescents is summarized in Table 78.1. Teratoma is the most common prepubertal tumor, followed by yolk sac whereas mixed germ cell tumors, which are malignant, account

Table 78.1   Tumor types and behavior in prepubertal patients and adolescents

Tumor type		Frequency of occurrence in prepubertal children	Frequency of occurrence in adolescents	Malignant potential
Germ Cell	Pure yolk sac	+++	0	Malignant
	Mixed germ cell tumor	0	+++	Malignant
	Pure seminoma	0	+	Malignant
	Teratoma	+++	++	Benign in children/Potentially malignant in adolescents
	Epidermoid cyst	++	++	Benign
Stromal	Leydig cell	+	+	Benign
	Sertoli cell	+	+	Occasionally malignant in patient over 5 years old
	Juvenile granulosa cell	+	0	Benign
	Undifferentiated stromal	+	0	Occasionally malignant
Gonadoblastoma		+	+	Benign (but can give rise to seminoma)

0 – virtually never, + – rare, ++ – uncommon, +++ – common

for the large majority of tumors in adolescents. Because teratomas (and most stromal tumors) are benign in children, the percentage of prepubertal testis tumors that have malignant potential is much lower than the 90% of tumors in adolescents.

78.3   Evaluation

The majority of patients with a testicular tumor will present with a testicular mass noted by the patient, a parent, or a health care provider. These masses are usually hard and painless. Occasionally patients may present with a hydrocele or pain due to torsion or bleeding into the tumor. Physical examination can usually distinguish testicular tumors from other scrotal masses such as hydroceles, hernias or epididymal cysts. When the physical exam is equivocal, an ultrasound of the testicles can resolve the issue. An ultrasound should always be obtained in a patient with a large or tense hydrocele that precludes palpation of the testis. Ultrasound can also assist in characterizing the lesion. While ultrasound cannot reliably distinguish malignant from benign testicular tumors, cystic tumors are more likely to be benign.

Tumor markers typically utilized in the evaluation and management of adolescent testis tumors include human chorionic gonadotropin (HCG) and alphafetoprotein (AFP). While HCG is elaborated in a significant number of mixed germ cell tumors, this tumor type is vanishingly rare in prepubertal patients. It is therefore not a helpful marker for the prepubertal population. On the other hand, AFP is elevated in 90% of patients with yolk sac tumor and can be very helpful in the preoperative distinction between yolk sac and other tumors (almost all of which are benign in children). One caveat is that AFP is quite high in normal infants. Though AFP levels are highly variable in infants; typical levels range from approximately 50,000 ng/ml in newborns, to 10,000 ng/ml by 2 weeks of age, 300 ng/ml by 2 months, and 12 ng/ml by 6 months of age. Therefore AFP levels among patients with yolk sac tumor and benign tumors overlap in the first 6 months of life making AFP less helpful in distinguishing tumor types in young infants.

The timing of a metastatic evaluation depends on the likelihood that a testis tumor is malignant. Delaying radiographic studies until pathology is available on the primary tumor avoids the unnecessary expense and radiation exposure for patients with benign tumors. However, changes related to orchiectomy, such as reactive lymphadenopathy or retroperitoneal bleeding, may confuse interpretation of post-operative radiographic studies. Since many, if not most prepubertal patients will have a benign tumor, the metastatic evaluation may be deferred until a histological diagnosis of the primary tumor is obtained for these patients. A preoperative metastatic evaluation may be undertaken in patients over 6 months of age with an elevated AFP level, who likely harbor a yolk sac tumor. A pre-operative evaluation is also appropriate in adolescents, particularly if tumor markers are elevated. Metastases from malignant testis tumors occur primarily in the retroperitoneal lymph nodes and lungs. A chest x-ray or chest computerized tomography scan (CT) and abdominal CT are obtained. For patients with very high tumor markers following chemotherapy or wide-spread pulmonary metastases, MRI of the brain should also be considered. Tumor markers are also followed post-operatively. The half-lives of AFP and beta-HCG are approximately 5 days and 48 h respectively. Failure of tumor markers to decline as expected after removal of the primary tumor is evidence of persistent metastatic disease.

78.4 Surgical Management

The standard initial treatment for a malignant testicular tumor in an adult or adolescent is an inguinal orchiectomy with early control of the vessels. In prepubertal patients, this approach should be applied only to patients greater than 6 months of age with an elevated AFP. In all other prepubertal patients a benign tumor is likely to be present, and the initial surgical management should be an excisional biopsy with frozen section analysis (Fig. 78.1). The exploration

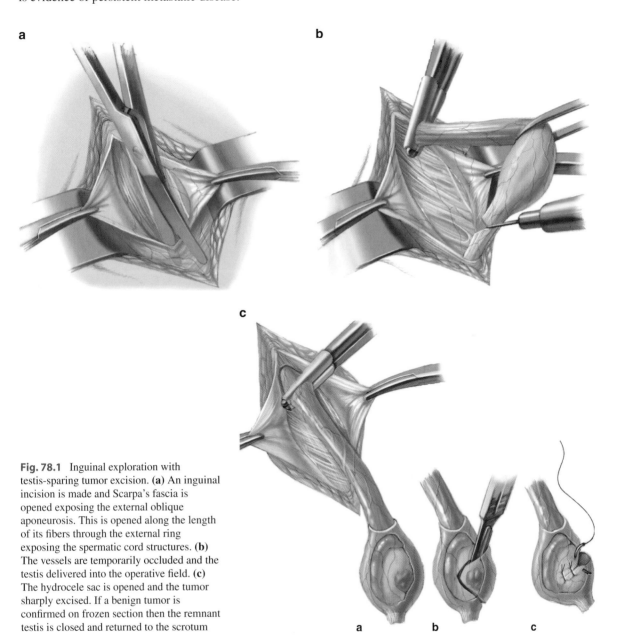

Fig. 78.1 Inguinal exploration with testis-sparing tumor excision. (**a**) An inguinal incision is made and Scarpa's fascia is opened exposing the external oblique aponeurosis. This is opened along the length of its fibers through the external ring exposing the spermatic cord structures. (**b**) The vessels are temporarily occluded and the testis delivered into the operative field. (**c**) The hydrocele sac is opened and the tumor sharply excised. If a benign tumor is confirmed on frozen section then the remnant testis is closed and returned to the scrotum

is accomplished through an inguinal incision with occlusion of the testicular vessels. Failure to follow these guidelines, particularly scrotal violations, may increase the recurrence rate if the tumor proves to be a yolk sac tumor. If the frozen section reveals a likely malignancy, then the entire testis is removed. If a benign histology is confirmed (usually teratoma), the remaining testis is closed with chromic suture and returned to the scrotum. Even large tumors can be enucleated with preservation of significant testicular tissue (Fig. 78.2).

One concern with this approach is the malignant potential of the remnant testicular tissue. In adults, 88% of testicles with teratoma harbor carcinoma in situ (CIS) elsewhere in the testis, and so orchiectomy is still an appropriate management in postpubertal patients. However, CIS is extremely rare in testicles of prepubertal patients harboring a teratoma. Testis-sparing surgery in this population appears to be safe and effective in preserving testicular tissue.

For some patients a retroperitoneal lymph node dissection is undertaken (see later discussion). Historically, this involved removing all lymphatic tissue from a template defined by the renal hila superiorly, the ureters laterally and the iliac bifurcations inferiorly. The classic complication of a standard RPLND is anejaculation due to disruption of the lumbar sympathetic nerves and hypogastric plexus. It was recognized that testis tumors tend to metastasize initially ipsilaterally in the retroperitoneum and so modified templates for right and left-sided tumors were developed which preserved the hypogastric complex and ejaculation (see Fig. 78.3). These modified templates became the standard approach for staging RPLND in stage 1 disease. Patients with positive nodes detected at the time of modified RPLND then underwent conversion to a full bilateral dissection. Recent advances have lead to intraoperative identification and preservation of the lumbar nerve roots. This allows preservation of ejaculation even when a full bilateral dissection is undertaken. Some centers have moved to a full bilateral nerve-sparing approach for all patients, while many still perform a modified template for staging RPLND's in low-risk patients.

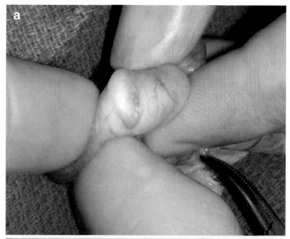
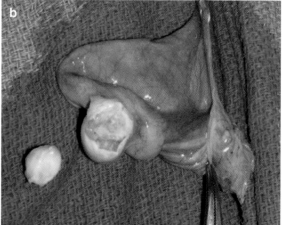
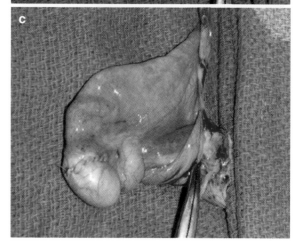

Fig. 78.2 Enucleation of a benign tumor (epidermoid cyst). **a** Through an inguinal approach, with the vessels occluded an incision is made in the testicular tunix exposing the tumor. **b** The tumor is enucleated from the testis. **c** The testis is closed with interrupted chromic suture

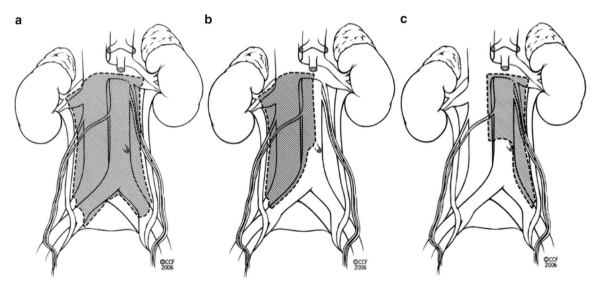

Fig. 78.3 Templates for a retroperitoneal lymph node dissection—**a** Standard bilateral template. **b** Modified template for a right-sided tumor. **c** Modified template for a left-sided tumor

78.5 Adjuvant Therapy for Malignant Adolescent Testicular Tumors

The typical mixed germ cell tumors (MGCT) seen in adults occur only after puberty. There is little data regarding the behavior of mixed germ cell tumors in adolescents, though they appear to exhibit behavior similar to that seen in adults. It is therefore assumed that they should be managed as adults with observation, retroperitoneal lymph node dissection, radiotherapy and/or chemotherapy depending on the specific histology and stage of the disease. This seems a reasonable approach until further studies in adolescents with testicular malignancies are undertaken.

Patients with MGCT limited to the testis and normalization of markers post-operatively may be managed with observation, retroperitoneal lymph node dissection (RPLND) or chemotherapy. The recurrence rate on observation is 25–30%. Recurrence may be prevented with a modified nerve-sparing RPLND or two cycles of platinum-based chemotherapy, but this "over-treats" the 70–75% of patients who do not have occult metastatic disease. On the other hand, when recurrence occurs on observation a longer course of chemotherapy is required and so patients may prefer an RPLND or short course of chemotherapy up front. Generally this dilemma is resolved by stratifying patients based on the local stage and histology of the primary tumor. Patients with low risk disease are usually observed with frequent chest x-rays, tumor marker measurements and abdominal CT scans. Nearly all recurrences occur within 2 years of orchiectomy and are treated with chemotherapy. Patients at higher risk for recurrence (such as those with vascular invasion, largely embryonal cell histology, or those who are poorly compliant with therapy) generally undergo a modified nerve-sparing RPLND. In Europe, some centers offer two courses of chemotherapy as an alternative. If microscopically positive nodes are found at the time of RPLND patients may elect a brief course of chemotherapy, although many with microscopic disease will be cured by the RPLND.

Patients with radiographic evidence of metastatic disease or persistently elevated tumor markers are treated with 3–4 cycles of BEP chemotherapy (bleomycin, etoposide and cis-platinum). RPLND may be considered for patients with very limited retroperitoneal lymph node disease and normalization of tumor markers as 70–80% of these patients are cured with RPLND alone. The relapse rate following chemotherapy for metastatic disease is approximately 15%.

Roughly one third of patients treated with chemotherapy for metastatic disease will have a residual retroperitoneal mass following therapy. These residual masses should be resected. 40–50% will contain only necrotic tissue and fibrosis, but 10–20% will have persistent malignancy and 40–45% will have mature teratoma in the mass.

78.6 Adjuvant Therapy for Prepubertal Malignant Germ Cell Tumors

Virtually all malignant germ cell tumors in children are yolk sac tumors. As with most malignancies, adjuvant therapy for yolk sac tumor is based on tumor stage. 85% of patients present with localized (Stage 1) disease. Recent studies suggest that these patients can be safely managed with observation. Observation should include frequent chest and abdominal imaging and measurement of AFP levels. The recurrence rate on observation is 17% and virtually all patients with recurrence can be salvaged with four courses of platinum-based chemotherapy. The overall survival of all patients receiving chemotherapy for recurrent or metastatic disease is 98%. The potential toxicities of the chemotherapy regimens employed include myelosuppression, ototoxicity and renal toxicity from platinum-based agents and pulmonary toxicity from bleomycin. High-grade ototoxicity is rare when carboplatinum is employed instead of cis-platinum. However, carboplatin is more myelotoxic.

RPLND plays very little role in the management of prepubertal testis tumors. The rationale for this dissection in select adolescent patients is the likelihood of retroperitoneal disease and the ability to avoid the morbidity of chemotherapy in some patients. Several characteristics of prepubertal tumors argue against its use in children. Most prepubertal patients have clinical stage 1 disease and the recurrence rate for these patients with observation alone is only 17%. Nearly all the recurrences can be salvaged with chemotherapy. For those with metastatic disease, it appears that only a minority of prepubertal patients have disease limited to the retroperitoneum. The majority have disease in the chest (with or without retroperitoneal disease). Finally, the morbidity of abdominal surgery is greater for children than for adults. Children have a particularly high rate of post-operative bowel obstruction. It is also unclear that a nerve-sparing approach is technically feasible in small children. For prepubertal testis tumors, RPLND is limited to patients with persistent retroperitoneal masses following chemotherapy—an extremely rare occurrence.

78.7 Teratoma and Epidermoid Cyst

Teratoma is the most common benign tumor in prepubertal patients. The median age of presentation is 13 months, with several patients presenting in the neonatal period. Histologically, teratomas consist of tissues representing the three germinal layers—endoderm, mesoderm and ectoderm. Epidermoid cysts are benign tumors composed entirely of keratin producing epithelium. They are distinguished from dermoid cysts, which contain skin and skin appendages, and from teratomas, which contain derivatives of other germ cell layers. Teratomas and epidermoid cysts are universally benign in prepubertal children. However, a small minority of teratomas in adolescents will behave in a malignant fashion.

For adolescents an inguinal orchiectomy is still the standard management for teratoma. However, in prepubertal patients a more conservative approach is undertaken. At the time of inguinal exploration, an excisional biopsy with frozen section is performed to confirm the diagnosis. In older children with teratoma, surrounding testicular parenchyma must be carefully evaluated. If there is histological evidence of pubertal changes then an orchiectomy should be performed. Biopsies of surrounding testicular parenchyma are probably unnecessary in prepubertal patients.

For all patients with epidermoid cyst and prepubertal patients with teratoma, no radiographic studies or follow-up for the development of metastatic disease are required. Because of the potential for malignancy, post-pubertal patients with teratoma should be evaluated and followed on the same protocol as adults with potentially malignant germ cell tumors.

78.8 Gonadal Stromal Tumors

Stromal tumors include Leydig cell, Sertoli cell, juvenile granulosa and mixed or undifferentiated tumors. Stromal testis tumors are rare in children, and there are no large series to guide their management. However, anecdotal reports and small series in the literature offer some experience on which to base therapy.

Leydig cell tumors are universally benign in children. They usually present between 5 and 10 years of age with precocious puberty. Congenital adrenal hyperplasia (CAH) can also lead to precocious puberty and testicular masses. Patients with Leydig cell tumors typically have elevated testosterone levels with low or normal gonadotropin levels, whereas patients with CAH will usually have elevated levels of 17-hydroxyprogesterone. Leydig cell tumors may be treated by testis-sparing excision. Persistence of androgenic effects may be due to a contralateral tumor, but this is rare in children. Because Leydig cell tumors are sometimes difficult to detect on physical exam, an ultrasound may be necessary to rule out a contralateral tumor. However, even after successful removal of a solitary tumor, androgenic changes are not completely reversible, and some children may proceed through premature puberty due to activation of the hypothalamic-pituitary-gonadal axis.

Sertoli-cell tumors are rare in children. Sertoli cell tumors are usually hormonally inactive in children, although they may occasionally cause gynecomastia or isosexual precocious puberty. While all reported cases to date have been benign in children under 5 years of age, there have been a few cases of malignant Sertoli cell tumors in older children and adults. Orchiectomy is usually sufficient treatment in infants and young children. A metastatic evaluation should be considered in older children and in patients with worrisome histological findings. When metastatic disease is present, aggressive combination treatment including RPLND, chemotherapy, and radiation therapy should be considered.

The large-cell calcifying Sertoli cell tumor is a clinically and histologically distinct entity with a higher incidence of multifocality and hormonal activity. These tumors are composed of large cells with abundant cytoplasm and varying degrees of calcification ranging from minimal amounts to massive deposits. While standard Sertoli cell tumors are more common in adults, large-cell calcifying Sertoli cell tumors are found predominantly in children and adolescents. Most present with a testicular mass. Approximately 1/4 of patients have bilateral and multifocal tumors. The presence of calcifications results in a characteristic ultrasound appearance including multiple hyperechoic areas.

Approximately one third of patients with large-cell calcifying Sertoli cell tumor have an associated genetic syndrome and/or endocrine abnormality. The two most common associated syndromes are Peutz-Jegher's syndrome and Carney's syndrome. Screening for these syndromes in patients with large cell calcifying Sertoli cell tumors is important since the patients and their first-degree relatives are at risk for the potentially lethal associated anomalies. While occasionally malignant in adults, large-cell calcifying Sertoli cell tumors have been universally benign in patients under 25 years of age and inguinal orchiectomy is sufficient treatment for children.

Juvenile granulosa cell tumor is a stromal tumor bearing a light microscopic resemblance to ovarian juvenile granulosa cell tumor. Granulosa-cell tumors occur almost exclusively in the 1st year of life, most in the first 6 months. Structural abnormalities of the Y chromosome and mosaicism are common in boys with juvenile granulosa cell tumor. Several cases have been described in association with ambiguous genitalia. These tumors are hormonally inactive and benign. Although these children should undergo chromosomal analysis, no treatment or metastatic evaluation is required beyond testis-sparing excision.

78.9 Gonadoblastoma

Gonadoblastomas are benign tumors that typically arise in dysgenetic gonads. They contain both germ cell and stromal elements. Gonadoblastoma arises almost exclusively in the dysgenetic gonads of patients with a Y chromosome or evidence of some Y chromatin in their karyotype. Dysgenetic gonads in patients without Y chromatin, such as patients with Turner's syndrome or XX gonadal dysgenesis, seem to be at little risk. Gonadoblastomas have been reported in 3% of true hermaphrodites, and 10–30% of patients with mixed gonadal dysgenesis or pure gonadal dysgenesis in the presence of Y chromatin. While gonadoblastomas are benign, they are prone to the development of malignant degeneration and overt malignant behavior is seen in 10% of cases. While most cases of malignancy occur after puberty, there have been cases reported in children as well. Therefore, early prophylactic removal of dysgenetic gonads should be performed. If malignant elements are present, a metastatic evaluation should be undertaken. Dysgerminoma (or seminoma) is the most common malignancy to occur in association with gonadoblastoma. Like their counterpart in normal testicles, these tumors are very radiosensitive, and the outlook for these patients is generally favorable.

Rare patients with persistent or recurrent testicular enlargement following chemotherapy should undergo testicular biopsy to confirm the presence of ALL. In most cases the patient will have relapsed at other sites and further systemic treatment will be required. Typically the testicles are also treated with radiation.

78.10 Leukemia

The role of testis biopsy for patients with acute lymphoblastic leukemia (ALL) has decreased markedly with modern chemotherapy. Approximately 20% of ALL patients have microscopic involvement at the time of diagnosis. However, with current chemotherapy, most patients with microscopic testicular involvement achieve a complete remission. Conversely, some patients without histological evidence of testicular involvement at diagnosis will ultimately relapse in the testicles. Therefore, pre-treatment testicular biopsy is not recommended since it does not predict those at risk for persistent or relapsing disease. Modern treatment has reduced the post-treatment relapse rate to less than 1%. Therefore, post-treatment biopsy in the absence of clinical evidence of persistent disease is also unnecessary.

Further Reading

Horwich A, Shipley J, Huddart R (2006) Testicular germ-cell cancer. Lancet 367:754–765

Klein E (2006) Nerve-sparing retroperitoneal lymphadenectomy. In AC Novick, JS Jones (eds) Operative Urology at the Cleveland Clinic. Humana Press, Totowas, NJ, pp 139–148

Ross J (2006) Testicular tumours. In P Puri, ME Höllwarth (eds) Pediatric Surgery, Springer Surgery Atlas Series. Springer-Verlag, Berlin, Heidelberg, New York, pp 477–482

Ross JH, Rybicki L, Kay R (2002) Clinical behavior and a contemporary management algorithm for prepubertal testis tumors: A summary of the Prepubertal Testis Tumor Registry. J Urol 168:1675–1679

Schlatter M, Rescorla F, Giller R et al (2003) Excellent outcome in patients with stage I germ cell tumors of the testes: A study of the Children's Cancer Group/Pediatric Oncology Group. J Pediatr Surg 38:319–324

Thomas JC, Ross JH, Kay R (2001) Stromal testis tumors in children: A report from the prepubertal testis tumor registry. J Urol 166:2338–2340

Part **X**

Spina Bifida and Hydrocephalus

Spina Bifida and Encephalocoele

79

Martin T. Corbally

Contents

79.1 Introduction

Neural tube defects (NTD: spina bifida (SB), encephalocele) are potentially serious congenital deformities of the spine and spinal cord that can have a major impact on the quality of life not only of the child but on the entire family. The precise aetiology is uncertain. Although the incidence appears to be decreasing there remain a significant number of newborns with this condition each year. In the past 10 years an awareness of the benefits of peri-conceptual folic acid and improved nutrition has significantly decreased the incidence of NTD. The impact of antenatal screening and therapeutic abortion in some jurisdictions has clearly further reduced the incidence. Surviving children face a varied future directly related to the severity of their NTD and to the quality of early interventional services and long term support structures. The patient with NTD is likely to require the expertise of many services and specialists over their lifetime including, the paediatric surgeon/neurosurgeon/urologist/orthopaedic/ophthalmic surgeon/paediatric radiologist/social workers/continence nurses and many other varied disciplines. Children with SB face the prospect of multiple surgical, urological and orthopaedic interventions for the duration of their lives and must cope with the effects of poor or zero ambulation, bladder and renal failure, hydrocephalus and the complexity of multiple shunt/bladder or bowel and shunt procedures.

The management objective for these children aims to provide as normal a life as possible, to minimise the effect of their disability in areas such as mobility, continence and education. In addition, urinary system monitoring is essential to safeguard against the complications of a neuropathic bladder and renal failure.

P. Puri and M. Höllwarth (eds.), *Pediatric Surgery: Diagnosis and Management*,
DOI: 10.1007/978-3-540-69560-8_79, © Springer-Verlag Berlin Heidelberg 2009

79.2 Embryology

A NTD is a congenital defect of the spine and neural tube with failure of fusion of the vertebral arches, and to a varying degree the development of the covering muscles and skin. In some cases the neural tube will protrude externally as a neural plaque without any covering of skin or muscle, as in a myelomeningocoele, but in others the neural tube is closed but there is a defect of the vertebral arch and muscles through which the dura and arachnoid protrude (meningocele) or it is entirely covered by skin (spina bifida occulta).

Essentially the defect arises as an abnormality of fusion of the neural tube. At the start of the 4th week of foetal life the neural plate (precursor of the neural tube) is a broad flat plate in its cranial portion that will become the brain and a narrow caudal portion that will become the spinal cord. At about 22 days the embryo undergoes ventral flexion and that portion of the neural tube cranial to the point of flexure (the mesencephalic flexure) is recognisable as the future forebrain, the point at the flexure is the midbrain and the point caudal to this point is the hindbrain. Rapid elongation over the next 7 days occurs with the narrow caudal portion (future spinal cord) occupying up to 60% of the neural tube. One of the most important events of the 4th week is conversion of the neural plate into a neural tube by a series of infolding of the plate called neurulation of the tube. This process begins along the future occipitocervical region of the plate and progresses caudally. During the process the lateral edges of the plate meet and fuse in the midline while detaching from the surface ectoderm, which then fuse and so cover the neural tube completely. The tube remains open at both ends during this process through small openings called the cranial and caudal neuropores. The cranial neuropore closes completely at day 24 and the caudal neuropore at day 26. The neural folds have essentially closed by 4 weeks. Subsequently the mesodermal somites form around the closed cord and the meninges, vertebral column and muscles result.

Failure of part of the neural tube to close disrupts both the process of differentiation of the central nervous system and the induction of the vertebral arches and can result in a variety of anomalies. This most commonly affects the caudal end of the spinal cord, which affects the lumbar and sacral regions of the central nervous system. Involvement of the cranial end of the tube can result at its most extreme end in anencephaly and in less severe cases form an encephalocoele.

Less severe anomalies of fusion are failure of the arch to fuse with or without meningocele protrusion (spina bifida occulta v meningocele respectively). More severe defects result in failure of the neuro-ectoderm with protrusion of the neural tube itself (myelomeningocoele). A similar process in the brain results in an encephalocoele. The process of lack of fusion can occur anywhere along the length of the spinal canal with varying levels of severity.

79.3 Classification

79.3.1 Anencephaly

Failure of the cranial end of the neural tube to close can result in disruption of differentiation of the CNS and is represented by an exposed mass of undifferentiated neural tissue (Table.79.1). These embryos often survive to late pregnancy but usually do not survive much after birth.

79.3.2 Encephalocoele

Although it is controversial whether this is truly a NTD defect it is probably best considered as such for the purposes of this discussion (Fig. 79.1). It results from bony defects in the cranial vault, which leads to a herniation of the meninges with or without differentiated brain tissue. The condition is more rightly called a meningoencephalocoele if dura and brain tissue herniate and a meningohydroencephalocoele if a part of the ventricular system also herniates.

79.3.3 Spina Bifida Occulta

At its mildest extreme the vertebral arches of a single vertebra fail to fuse but there is no underlying abnormality of the neural tube. The defect may occur anywhere along the spine but is most commonly found in the sacral region and its presence may only be signalled

Table 79.1   Types of Neural tube Defects

Anencephaly	Brain and skull poorly developed	Death inevitable
Myelomeningocoele	Failure of closure of neural tube	Significant lesion
	Failure of muscle and skin formation	Variable outcome
		Urgent closure
	Exposed neural tissue	90% need VP shunt
	Distal limb innervation affected	
	Neuropathic bladder	
Meningocoele	Failure of spinal fusion	Usually no neural
	Dural sac protrudes	consequences
		Rarely bladder function
		affected
	Skin covered defect	
Encephalocoele	Usually Occipital	Variable outcome
	Defect in cranial bone	
	Herniation of meninges and	Sometimes shunt needed
	Brain to varying degree	
Spina Bifida	Occulta Hamartoma at site	Excellent outcome
	Sinus occasionally	
	Skin intact	
	Bony vertebral arch deficient	

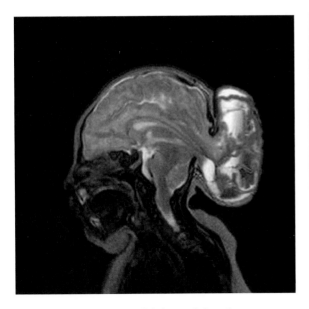

Fig. 79.1   MRI showing occipital encephalocoele

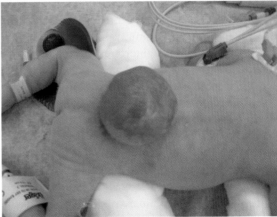

Fig. 79.2   Lumbosacral Myelomeningocele

gocoele. This cystic swelling is lined by dura and arachnoid.

79.3.4 Meningocoele

Abnormalities of the neural arch without underlying neural tube defects with the formation of a cystic swelling at the site of the lesion are called a menin-

by the presence of a small tuft of hair, small dimple, pigmented skin or vascular lesion overlying the lesion.

79.3.5 Myelomeningocoele

In this, the severest form of spina bifida, the tissues overlying one or more vertebra are deficient so that the neural tube tissue itself protrudes as a neural plaque to the surface (Fig. 79.2). This plaque may be completely or partially covered by arachnoid or exposed. It most typically involves the lumbar region but any portion of the spine can be affected.

79.4 Aetiology

The aetiology of NTD is clearly multifactorial and no single agent either genetic or teratogenic has been identified. However there is evidence of a genetic influence in some cases e.g. Spina bifida is more common in some parts of India and Ireland (1.1%) and is relatively rare in African Americans (0.035%). In addition, the presence on NTD in one sibling increases the risk among subsequent siblings to 1 in 20. In families with two siblings with NTD the risk increases to 1 in 8. In certain syndromes e.g. Meckel Syndrome, an autosomal recessive disorder, cranio-rachischisis may be seen. NTD may also be seen in the Waardenburg syndrome, which may result from Pax-3 gene abnormalities.

It also seems likely that environmental factors are important in the development of NTD. There has been a significant decline over the past 4 decades in the incidence of NTDS. Factors noted have been the association of maternal diabetes, the anti-epileptic drug sodium valproate and hyper-thermia. Valproate may interfere with folate metab-olism and there is also evidence that a significant number of infants with NTDS may have gene muta-tions that are involved in folate and vitamin B metabolism especially mutations of 5,10-methyltet-rahydrofolate reductase and methionine synthase reductase. The administration of periconceptual folic acid has probably been the single most impor-tant factor in the acknowledged decline in the inci-dence of NTD. Despite increased awareness of the benefit of periconceptual folic acid and its wide-spread use there remains a significant incidence of the problem. However, in women with a history of folic acid intake and a spina bifida child, it appears that the severity of the lesion is much reduced.

79.4.1 Incidence

The worldwide incidence of NTD is reported to be as high as 400,000 per annum. However the use of peri-conceptual folic acid has reduced the incidence by 70% in the past 20 years and also has reduced the severity of the lesion also. In Ireland the rate fell from 32 in 1979, to 22 per 10,000 in 1982 and con-tinues to fall.

79.5 Diagnosis

79.5.1 Antenatal

It is more preferable to make the diagnosis antenatally which allows for counselling and facilitates transfer to a paediatric surgical centre for appropriate management. Antenatal diagnosis may be made by careful ultrasound examination, chorionic villous sampling, maternal alpha fetoprotein (AFP) or amniocentesis. Varying sensitivi-ties have been reported but in experienced hands ultra-sound is a sensitive technique to detect a NTD. If antenatal ultrasound is suspicious of a NTD then mater-nal AFP combined with amniocentesis for AFP and ace-tylcholinesterase assay is confirmatory.

With improved prenatal care NTD are commonly detected before birth and arrangements can then be made for counselling and for the delivery and care of the infant. Delivery should be scheduled close to a surgical centre and consideration given to delivery by Caesarean section, which may confer a significant functional benefit to the child. Rarely hydrocephalus may need antenatal drainage to facilitate delivery.

79.6 Clinical Features

The diagnosis of a NTD is usually straightforward at birth if the lesion is a myelomeningocoele, meningo-coele or encephalocoele. Lesser lesions may not be clini-cally obvious and require more detailed investigations.

79.6.1 Myelomeningocoele

A myelomeningocoele presents as a large open lesion anywhere along the spinal column, although the lum-bar and sacral areas are the more frequently involved. It is unfortunately the commonest form of NTD. Typically there is a thin membrane covering the exposed neural plaque, which may be intact and appear cystic. Usually however the neural plaque is open to the environment and CSF leaks constantly. If there is little or no CSF leak the lesion will be raised. There may be occasional hamartomatous lesions associated with it is such as a haemangioma, lipoma or a naevus (Fig. 79.3). There may be associated deformities of the

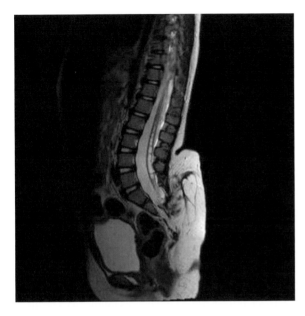

Fig. 79.3 MRI showing lipomyelomeningocele

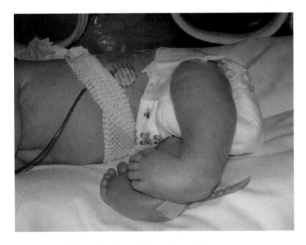

Fig. 79.4 Bilateral talipes deformities of feet

lower limbs with hip dislocation or subluxation, hypoplastic lower limbs, genu recurvatum, and talipes (Fig. 79.4). In addition there may be obvious hydrocephalus although this is uncommon at birth. The vertebral anomalies can be significant with severe kyphosis evident at birth. Neurological deficits include motor and sensory loss to the lower limbs. The effects of neural involvement include paralysis of lower limb muscle groups often with preservation of nerve supply to antagonistic groups, which results in more severe deformity. Occasionally there will be complete loss of innervation as in a flaccid paralysis while often there

will be an upper motor neurone lesion and a resultant spastic paresis.

While the internal anal sphincter is preserved due to its autonomic nerve supply the innervation to the external sphincter (puborectalis and pelvic floor muscles) are likely to be lost which results in a patulous anus. This may result in rectal prolapse but will not have any immediate impact on bowel emptying but clearly may affect faecal continence later.

At least 90% of patients with myelomeningocoele have a neuropathic bladder with disturbances of detrusor and sphincter muscle activity. This is manifest at birth by constant dribbling of urine but some do have an intermittent urinary stream. The management of the child with a NTD and a neuropathic bladder is quite complex and should involve the surgeon and paediatric continence nurse specialist. Frequent monitoring by renal ultrasound should be performed to allow early detection and intervention in the presence of upper tract dilatation, which occurs as a result of poor bladder compliance. Early introduction of clean intermittent catheterisation (CIC) may be required in some infants.

79.6.2 Meningocoele

A meningocoele is uncommon and presents as a sac and skin covered defect in the lower spinal column with no abnormality of the underlying neural tube. There is usually no neurological defect and the cord is normal. In addition the lower limbs are normal. Rarely some neural fibres may be adherent or contained within the sac and these require careful dissection from the sac during closure. This may be apparent on ultrasonic exam or MRI pre-operatively.

79.6.3 Spina Bifida Occulta

May be difficult to detect on clinical grounds and may only become apparent at a later stage during incidental spinal imaging. However the presence of a tuft of hair, pigmented naevus or vascular malformation in the midline along the spinal column may indicate the underlying vertebral anomaly of occulta. While the spinal cord is normal and there may be no overt evidence of neurological impairment it is important to be aware that functional disorders of the urinary tract may be related to an underlying occulta and would warrant a search for an underlying lesion. Occasionally there may be a sinus like tract connecting to the meninges and lying over the spine itself. This is an occasional cause of spinal sepsis and meningitis. It should not be confused with the quite common sacral or posterior anal dimple, which is a skin dimple attached to a normal coccyx and not related to NTD. It should be remembered that the defect usually includes a vertebral arch abnormality and normal cord and meninges but rarely the cord may be tethered and may be the cause of gait abnormalities or subsequent bladder abnormalities.

79.6.4 Encephalocoele

Is a midline defect in the bones of the skull, which allows protrusion of meninges only or gross herniation of brain tissue. In the latter condition there may also be an associated microcephaly or other macro-structural cerebral anomalies. Often these include Dandy-Walker cyst formation, hydrocephalus, and dysplasia of cerebellum and optic pathways. The usual bony site is the occipit but frontal encephalocoeles are more commonly seen in Asia.

There may be other congenital lesions such as NTD at other sites, cleft palate, cardiac, lung and renal anomalies.

79.7 Management

79.7.1 Myelomeningocoele

Surgical closure of the defect was not regularly attempted until the early twentieth century where survival of 23% was reported. The advent of asepsis and antibiotics improved survival and surgical closure became more widely practiced. Patients with extensive paralysis and hydrocephalus were not offered closure but the back lesion was allowed to slowly granulate and epithelialize. However death from infection and uncontrolled hydrocephalus was common. Improved surgical and anaesthetic techniques and antibiotics and the development of reliable valve regulated shunts led to more aggressive management of patients even with severe lesions. However many survivors were noted to have a poor quality of life with mental impairment, shunt and renal

problems that made their management difficult and tended to overwhelm existing medical resources. A review of the selection process generated a return to a conservative approach in patients with extensive paralysis, severe hydrocephalus, kyphosis, and major associated anomalies in the firm belief that the severity of the lesion was not compatible with an acceptable quality of life. Reports of unselected treatment for all patients with myelomeningocoele suggested that early mortality, the frequency of mental impairment, poor mobility, pressure sores, incontinence and other issues dictated a selected approach for all patients. However continued and increased survival of patients initially regarded as being of poor potential outcome indicated that survival could not always be based on the clinical appearance of the lesion or extent of associated problems alone. Moreover children surviving this initial conservative approach often suffered greater disabilities as a result of a non-operative attitude. A decision to withhold treatment cannot therefore be supported on clinical or ethical grounds alone. It must be noted however that this approach is not universally accepted and that parental wishes must also be considered. Nevertheless, the current standard of practice for children with myelomeningocoele is that the defect should be closed within the first 24–48 h of life, to place a ventriculo-peritoneal (VP) shunt if hydrocephalus is present and to monitor and treat aggressively their problems for the rest of their life.

Patients with myelomeningocoele should be transferred to a paediatric surgical centre and be prepared for early closure of the defect. It is important to protect the defect from contamination with faecal matter so chlorhexidine soaked gauze is applied to the lesion and this should be changed frequently. Broad spectrum antibiotics are usually given and the baby allowed feed on demand. Upon arrival at the surgical centre the baby undergoes a variety of investigations such as a cranial ultrasound, spinal x-ray (include back, pelvis and skull), muscle charting, thorough examination to rule out other problems, orthopaedic assessment, and a social work consult. An MRI scan may also be performed at this stage to document the presence or absence of other spinal lesions, although this can be performed at a later date and a spinal ultrasound is probably as sensitive. The surgeon should meet with both parents and discuss in detail the management plan and in particular the likely problems that may occur in the future. These include the possible need to treat hydrocephalus with a VP shunt, the possibility of shunt malfunction and its consequences, the likelihood of a neuropathic bladder and its significance, the possibility of orthopaedic treatment for talipes, dislocated hip, etc. and the issues of continence and intellect. The procedure is then scheduled for the next available time but generally within 24–48 h.

Although most patients with myelomeningocoele undergo surgical closure after birth considerable effort has been focused on in-utero repair in selected patients. This presents an alternative in their management and may carry significant advantages to the infant in terms of neurological outcome. The proposed mechanism of improved outcome with fetal intervention is to lessen the hindbrain herniation associated with Arnold-Chiari malformation and so reduce the frequency of significant hydrocephalus and shunt procedures. The results of randomized trials are awaited to determine if this approach will influence outcome.

79.7.2 Operative Approach

The procedure is carried out under general anaesthesia with the patient prone and in a warm ambient temperature (Fig. 79.5). A small roll may be placed beneath the hips and the lesion and surrounding skin prepped with an aqueous solution. It may be useful to cover the natal cleft with a non-porous tape to exclude the area from the sterile field.

Operating loupes are useful during all parts of the procedure. It is wise to plan the orientation of the incision before commencing the procedure as this may impact on the ease of the closure especially with large lesions.

The skin edge is incised just at its junction with the lesion and the membranes close to the plaque carefully dissected from the plaque. The plaque should be separated

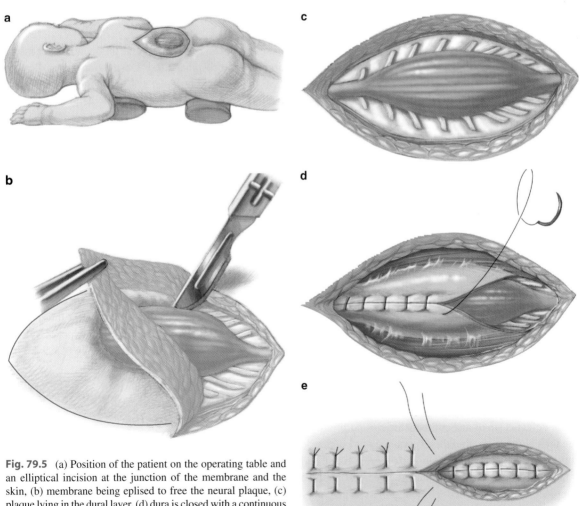

Fig. 79.5 (a) Position of the patient on the operating table and an elliptical incision at the junction of the membrane and the skin, (b) membrane being eplised to free the neural plaque, (c) plaque lying in the dural layer, (d) dura is closed with a continuous suture, (e) skin is closed with interrupted sutures

from all epithelial elements so as to prevent a theoretical epitheliod inclusion at a later date. When the plaque has been freed from all local attachments the dura is incised on its lateral surface in an elliptical manner around the neural plaque. This involves incising down to the underlying fascia and subsequently mobilising the dura so as to allow closure of the dura over the plaque. Closure is effected by a running 6/0 or 7/0 suture throughout the length of the dural sac. If possible the lumbar fascia can be mobilised to cover the dural repair although this is not essential. A small redi-vac drain is left in situ and the skin closed over the repaired defect. The skin is closed using a series of interrupted nylon sutures with alternating steri-strips. If the skin closure seems a problem the skin may be undermined or very rarely Z flaps used. It is normal practice to cover the repair with a semi-permeable dressing. Post operatively the patient is nursed prone or in a lateral position, the drainage is monitored and antibiotics continued until drain removal. If there is excessive CSF leakage it is generally not due to a problem with dural closure but to increasing hydrocephalus and a ventriculo-peritoneal shunt is indicated.

79.7.3 Meningocoele

Unlike myelomeningocoele there is usually no urgency to close a meningocoele. The surgical procedure can be scheduled electively after appropriate investigations. There is little risk of hydrocephalus although there may be neural elements adherent within the sac and an ultrasound and or MRI scan should be obtained pre-operatively. The skin edge is incised in an elliptical fashion around the defect and the protruding dura exposed. The dural sac is opened vertically on its lateral aspect taking care to avoid any adherent neural tissue (rare) and the sac then repaired removing the herniating portion. The skin is closed over a drain.

79.7.4 Encephalocoele

If the defect is small and contains little or no brain tissue then closure is within the experience of a paediatric surgeon, however if there is significant brain tissue and if there is associated microcephaly then a non-operative approach maybe indicated. Although there is generally

little urgency about closure of an encephalocoele there is the potential risk of further herniation which may compromise the child and make closure more difficult. In general these should be closed as soon as possible after appropriate imaging (MRI) is performed.

Surgery is performed with the child prone and intubated. In the case of occipital lesions a transverse incision is made over the apex of the lesion. The dural sac is exposed and opened away from the bone edges. Brain tissue should be preserved unless necrotic or grossly dysmorphic or likely to interfere with dural closure. The dura is closed with a continuous suture and a small drain left in situ. An acute rise in intra-cranial pressure may require an urgent VP shunt following repair.

Anterior encephalocoeles and meningocoeles are complex and may require the input of other specialist services such as neurosurgery and or otolaryngology.

79.7.5 Hydrocephalus

Results from an imbalance in the production and absorption of cerebrospinal fluid. Obstruction to the flow of CSF out of the ventricular system by the Arnold-Chiari malformation, tumour, aqueductal stenosis, haemorrhage, or obstruction of the fourth ventricle (Dandy Walker Cyst) causes a non-communicating hydrocephalus and is the most common type seen. Free flow of CSF due to lesions of the choroid plexus or following inflammatory conditions cause communicating hydrocephalus. In the newborn increasing pressure within the ventricles and cranial vault is somewhat compensated by the open fontanelles. Most patients with myelomeningocoele have hydrocephalus and approximately 90% of these will ultimately require insertion of a VP shunt to control it. Hydrocephalus in this group is associated with the Arnold-Chiari malformation which includes caudal displacement of the cerebellum and medulla through the foramen magnum, elongation of the aqueduct of Sylvius making it liable to blockage, various bony defects of the upper cervical vertebra and occiput.

79.7.6 Clinical Features

The most obvious is that of a symmetrically enlarged head either at birth or developing over the next few weeks. An ultrasound examination will easily show dilated ventricles and serial measurement of the head circumference will show increasing deviation over the standard measurements. The anterior fontanelle is wide and bulging and the sutures will appear separated. Consideration should be given to ventriculo peritoneal shunt insertion when there is a rapid increase in head circumference or when there is clear evidence of significant hydrocephalus on ultra-sound, CT or MRI. Newborn infants with a NTD and hydrocephalus tend not to have many symptoms of increased intracranial pressure as the open fontanelles and sutures can accommodate to some extent. However internal strabismus, setting sun sign due to pressure on soft orbital plates are seen with significant and untreated hydrocephalus. In addition optic nerve damage or occipital lobe damage may result in visual deficits if the hydrocephalus is not treated.

A description of the technique of VP shunt insertion is beyond the scope of this chapter. However shunt valves are selected on their opening pressure which is the pressure that the valve will open to allow CSF leave the ventricular system and enter the peritoneal cavity. Since it is possible to overdrain and cause a slit ventricle syndrome it is probably best not to use low pressure systems except in the very pre-term, small infant. The author's preference is to use a unitised single medium pressure system in the majority of cases.

Shunts are mechanical devices and are subject to problems such as blockage, breakage, malfunction and infection. Many or all of these problems can be found in the life of a single shunt.

79.8 Long Term Management

Most patients survive the trauma of back closure and surgical treatment of hydrocephalus. However as many as 23% may have died within 1 year of birth. Surviving patients face ongoing problems in relation to mobility, shunt issues, problems with faecal and urinary continence, problems specific to their neuropathic bladder, educational, intellectual and social issues. As many as 75% have normal intelligence but a significant number require special educational support. Many of these problems can and perhaps should be addressed at a special clinic to cope with the needs of this particular group. Individual care plans can be readily worked out for each patient and this can be modified on a fluid basis at the spina bifida clinic. It

can often be difficult to have all involved specialists attend such a clinic but the benefit to the parents and child are significant. Increasingly local agencies provide comprehensive care to NTD patients and their families such as Enable Ireland and the impact of a variety of voluntary agencies such as "The Association for Spina Bifida and Hydrocephalus" can not be overstated. Of particular importance is the ongoing surveillance of the urinary tract especially the results of 6 monthly renal ultrasound exams. This is chiefly to detect the early development of upper urinary tract dilatation due to a non-compliant neuropathic bladder. When this occurs the parents are instructed in the technique of clean intermittent catheterisation (CIC) which is performed every 4 h on average and serves to empty the bladder of urine and prevent reflux of static urine from high vesical pressures. Approximately 10–15% of patients will not have their high pressure bladder controlled by CIC and a vesicostomy may be necessary. Older children and children with small volume high pressure bladders will need the expertise of a paediatric urologist to assess the need for bladder augmentation. The input of paediatric continence nurses is invaluable especially in the performance of urodynamic studies and also in instructing older children in the often difficult task of overcoming manipulative skills to facilitate self CIC.

Bowel problems are generally treated using medications such as stool softeners and or regular stimulant enemas; however social "continence" can be achieved in up to 85–90% of children using a regular washout enema containing 200–300 ml of water and a stimulant like toilax. This generally gives clean results lasting up to 24 h. When this fails consideration should be given to performing an antegrade colonic enema (ACE) procedure using the appendix as a catheterisable conduit.

Ongoing issues of mobility and joint deformities need the continued input of orthopaedic surgeons and occupational physiotherapists. In addition social workers play a significant role in helping the family adapt the home environment to cope with mobility and toileting issues and to secure proper state funding for their needs.

The incidence of NTD continues to decline but for those born with this condition it can impose severe restrictions on the quality of their lives. The current standard of practice is that all patients with myelomeningocoele should be offered surgical repair within the first 24–48 h of life. Improvements in valve regulated ventriculo-peritoneal shunts have contributed greatly to quality of life. Long term review in special multi-disciplinary clinics facilitates review of renal function, status of urinary tracts, status of their valve-shunt and management of continence and education and social issues.

Further Reading

Corbally MT. In Puri P (ed) Newborn Surgery Operative repair of Myelomeningocoele, Arnold, London, pp 761–774

Corbally MT (2006) Spina bifida. In P Puri, ME Höllwarth (eds) Pediatric Surgery. Springer Surgery Atlas Series, Springer-Verlag Berlin Heidelberg, New York, pp 419–426

Dias MS (2005) Neurosurgical management of myelomeningocoele. Pediatric Rev 26(2):50–60

Finnell RH, Gould A, Spiegelstein O (2003) Pathobiology and genetics of neural tube defect. Epilepsia 44 Suppl 3:14–23

Hunt GM (1990) Open spina bifida: Outcome for a complete cohort treated unselectively and followed into adulthood. Dev Med Child Neurol 32:108–118

Lorber J (1971) Results of treatment of myelomeningocoele: An analysis of 524 unselected cases, with special reference to possible selection for treatment. Dev Med Child Neurol 13:279–303

Mitchell LE, Azdick NS (2004) Spina bifida. Lancet 364:1885–1895

Walsh DS, Adzick NS (2003) Foetal surgery for spina bifida. Semin Neonatol 8:197–205

Larsen WJ (2001) Human Embryology, 3rd edn. edited by Sherman LS, Potter SS, Scott WJ. Churchill Livingstone, New York

Hydrocephalus

80

Jerard Ross and Conor Mallucci

Contents

80.1 Introduction: Definition and Incidence

Hydrocephalus occurs in approximately 1 in 2000 births and is associated with a significant proportion of congenital malformation of the brain and spinal cord. While it is frequently diagnosed in infancy and early childhood, the complications and ramifications of the condition and its treatment continue through into adulthood.

Defining hydrocephalus is problematic, but in essence hydrocephalus can be said to be present when there is a relatively excess intracranial cerebrospinal fluid (CSF) in the closed compartment, that is, the cranium, resulting in raised intracranial pressure and brain dysfunction. There are variations of this but the important question to ask is 'is the intracranial pressure raised?' Ultimately ventricular volume is a secondary issue; small ventricles do not mean that a child does not have hydrocephalus and critically raised intracranial pressure. Therefore radiological definitions of hydrocephalus, although useful acutely, are doomed to failure.

The aim of this chapter is not to provide an exhaustive guide to hydrocephalus in all its guises, but rather to provide the non-specialist with a practical approach to the management of patients with hydrocephalus, both treated and untreated, as well as a rationale and set of algorithms to avoid serious complications.

80.2 Physiology of CSF Production

Understanding the pathophysiology of hydrocephalus requires some understanding of the physiology of CSF production and circulation. CSF is a result of active

P. Puri and M. Höllwarth (eds.), *Pediatric Surgery: Diagnosis and Management*,
DOI: 10.1007/978-3-540-69560-8_80, © Springer-Verlag Berlin Heidelberg 2009

secretion by the choroid plexus of the ventricular system and of water production in brain metabolism. CSF is produced at around 0.33 ml min^{-1} resulting in a total of 20 ml hour^{-1} and about 500 ml day^{-1} in an adult. At any point of time there is about 150 ml of CSF in the neuraxis of which around half is in the intracranial compartment; volumes are less in infants but adult values are reached by about 5 years of age. CSF circulates from the lateral ventricles through the foramina of Monroe into the third ventricle, through the aqueduct of sylvius and into the fourth ventricle in the posterior fossa. From the fourth ventricle, the CSF exits into the spinal subarachnoid space via the midline foramen of Magendie and the lateral foramina of Luschka, from where it circulates into the cerebral subarachnoid space and is reabsorbed by the arachnoid granulations (AG) abutting the dural venous sinuses. Reabsorption by the AG is not active but is pressure dependent and a pressure differential of 3–6 cm CSF^{-1} must be reached for reabsorption to occur.

80.3 Pathology

Hydrocephalus is most frequently due to the failure of absorption of CSF and only very rarely due to its overproduction. This failure occurs because of a blockage in the pathway to the AG or failure of the absorptive mechanism in the AG. In both the situations the CSF accumulates and pressure rises. The normal CSF pressure is 10–15 cm CSF^{-1} (as measured in the lumbar theca in the lateral position) and lower in neonates, this is approximately equal to 7–12 mm Hg^{-1}.

The historical classification into communicating or non-communicating (obstructive) has been superseded by understanding the obstructive nature of all hydrocephalus with block to circulation and hence reabsorption, either occurring in the ventricles or their outflow or thereafter in the subarachnoid spaces or arachnoid granulations. The pathoanatomical basis of a patient's hydrocephalus is vitally important in making rational management decisions.

The most common causes of hydrocephalus vary in different age groups and are detailed in Tables 80.1 and 80.2. This division into different age groups is also important to show how affected children in various age groups present themselves and these differences are explained by whether the sutures between the skull

Table 80.1 Etiology of hydrocephalus

Etiology	Congenital	Acquired
	Chiari malformation	Infectious (meningitis/TB)
	Aqueductal stenosis	Post-haemorrhagic (perinatal/trauma)
	Dandy Walker Complex	
	Venous outflow obstruction	Secondary to mass lesions (neoplasm/vascular)

Table 80.2 Etiology of hydrocephalus by age

Age group	Neonate/Infant	Child
Common Causes	Intraventricular haemorrhage	Aqueductal stenosis
	Meningitis Spina Bifida (Chiari 2 malformation)	Tumour

Table 80.3 Symptoms and signs of raised ICP

In the infant and young child

Irritability, impaired level of consciousness, vomiting, failure to thrive, poor feeding, developmental delay,

Head circumference crossing centiles, poor head control, tense anterior fontanelle, dilated scalp veins, 'setting sun' sign (the combination of upper eye-lid retraction and failure of up-gaze), bradycardia, apnoeic spells, seizures.

In the older child and adult

Headache, vomiting, drowsiness, diplopia, worsened seizure control

Impaired consciousness and coma, impaired upgaze, papilloedema

bones are fused (in a child the sutures fuse by the end of the second year). The symptoms and signs of hydrocephalus are detailed in Table 80.3.

The site of obstruction of CSF flow or absorption varies in the different conditions outlined in Table 80.1 and hence the approach to management may vary. Secondarily the treatment options may vary in different age groups.

80.4 Diagnosis of Hydrocephalus by Imaging

To reiterate, radiological investigations will diagnose the majority of cases of hydrocephalus but this will be based on ventriculomegaly, and normal sized ventricles do not always mean there is no problem with CSF flow and/or raised pressure.

80.4.1 Plain Radiography

Plain radiographs of the skull may show signs of raised pressure although they are not used as part of the standard diagnostic work-up of an infant or child with suspected hydrocephalus. Signs of raised pressure include 'copper beating' of the calvarium and erosion of the posterior clinoids at the dorsum sella. In addition the aetiology of the raised pressure may be noted, e.g., traumatic fractures or abnormal calcification associated with a pineal region mass obstructing the aqueduct.

80.4.2 Ultrasonography

Ultrasonography is a useful screening tool in children with an open anterior fontanelle. It allows the diagnosis of ventriculomegaly at the bedside but seldom allows a diagnosis of the aetiology of the hydrocephalus unless there is obvious intraventricular pathology.

80.4.3 Computed Tomography

Computed tomography (CT) is a widespread, rapid and easy-to-interpret tool in the diagnosis of hydrocephalus; it is unfortunately less good at defining the pathoanatomical substrate of the condition than is magnetic resonance imaging (MRI). In addition it exposes the child to radiation, the cumulative doses of which can be significant through a lifetime of treatment.

CT diagnosis of hydrocephalus is based on ventriculomegaly. Features suggestive of ventriculomegaly include ballooning of the frontal horns of the lateral ventricles, and periventricular low density suggesting trans-ependymal absorption of CSF secondary to raised pressure. There are radiological criteria that are quoted in the literature and these have been used diagnostically; however day-to-day cross-sectional imaging must be interpreted in the clinical context (history and examination) and with reference to previous imaging.

CT is frequently used to assess patients after insertion of ventricular catheters for CSF diversion, e.g., ventriculoperitoneal shunt catheters. The scan can indicate appropriate positioning as well as the state of the ventricles.

80.4.4 Magnetic Resonance Imaging (MRI)

MRI is the investigation of choice for delineating the ventricular size and the pathoanatomical substrate of the hydrocephalus. In addition to the axial assessment of ventricular size, the multiplanar imaging allows assessment of the third ventricle; the floor of which tends to be bowed down and backwards into the prepontine space and towards the dorsum sella respectively, whilst the roof and the corpus callosum are bowed back. One of the major advantages of MRI over CT is the ability to delineate small lesions adjacent to the CSF pathways particularly in the midbrain and to capture a better image the posterior fossa. MRI scans for assessment of *de novo* hydrocephalus should therefore be with and without gadolinium contrast as the enhancement characteristics of it is useful in diagnosis of mass lesions. (Figs. 80.1 and 80.2).

Like CT, MRI has a role in the post-operative imaging of patients with hydrocephalus; it is particularly useful in the assessment of internal CSF diversionary procedures, such as endoscopic third ventriculostomy, where particular imaging paradigms can be applied directly to image CSF flow (e.g., phase contrast MR). MR is less good at imaging implanted catheters than CT.

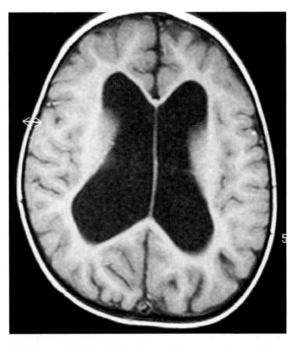

Fig. 80.1 Axial T1 weighted magnetic resonance image of ventriculomegaly in hydrocephalus

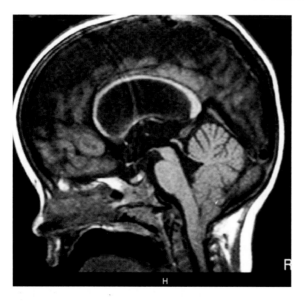

Fig. 80.2 Sagittal T1 weighted MRI demonstrating the thinned out corpus callosum bowed upwards and the downwardly displaced floor of the third ventricle. There is an associated Chiari malformation (type 1)

80.5 Treatment Options in Hydrocephalus

The indications for surgical intervention in hydrocephalus are straightforward. When there are signs or symptoms of raised intracranial pressure (Table 80.3) then hydrocephalus should be treated. There are caveats to hydrocephalus infection; CSF constituents, body weight and pathology. However, as a rule of thumb it stands up to scrutiny.

Lesional hydrocephalus is usually best treated by the removal of the causative lesion, i.e., a tumour in the anterior third ventricle causing obstruction of both foramina of Monroe, such as a colloid cyst, is best treated by operative removal. Similarly a posterior fossa tumour obstructing egress of CSF from the fourth ventricle is best resected.

In the cases of acute symptomatic hydrocephalus, secondary to an operable or potentially operable lesion, a short term CSF diversion may be employed to gain control of the immediate situation allowing time for further assessment of the situation. Insertion of an external ventricular drain (EVD) into the frontal horn of the lateral ventricle (usually the right side) allows control of raised ICP and more detailed investigations.

Hydrocephalus remains a surgically remediable condition. The treatment involves CSF diversion from the intraventricular compartment of the brain to another compartment either intra or extracranial. These *shunts* may be physically implanted or internally formed by creating an *ostomy* between cavities.

80.5.1 Implantable Shunts

Implantation of a shunt is one of the most commonly performed procedure in neurosurgical centres and often treated with disdain by trainees and surgeons alike. However the sequelae of a poorly positioned shunt, i.e., revision, and of a poor shunt insertion technique, e.g., infection and haemorrhage, can be so deleterious to future function that it is not an operation to be taken lightly.

CSF flow is most frequently diverted into the peritoneal cavity (a ventriculo-peritoneal or VP shunt) and the alternatives include the internal jugular vein (a ventriculo-atrial or VA shunt) and much less frequently the pleural cavity.

Shunts consist of a proximal (ventricular catheter), one-way valve and a distal catheter. They are usually made from synthetic silicone rubber, and the major differences between shunts usually lie in the characteristics ascribed to the valve.

The most frequent valves encountered are differential pressure valves; these can be fixed by opening pressure or, less commonly by variable (programmable) opening pressure. Most manufacturers provide differential valves with low (1–4 cm CSF^{-1}), medium (4–8 cm CSF^{-1}) or high (> 8 cm CSF^{-1}) opening pressures. It is important to realise that although valves may be of equivalent opening pressures they may have different internal resistances and behave quite differently in vivo.

Selection of valves and shunt types is a matter of preference without high quality evidence favouring one type over another. A randomised trial did not show any significant difference between standard valves and flow-limited valves designed to reduce over-drainage in the upright position.

For general surgeons who may come across intraperitoneal catheters it is similarly important to be aware that a very significant proportion of resistance to CSF flow comes not only from the valve but also from the distal catheter. Hence shortening a catheter in the peritoneum may have a marked impact on the function of shunt system.

80.5.2 Insertion of VP Shunt—the Technique

After induction of general anaesthesia and endotracheal intubation, a child receives prophylactic intravenous antibiotics and is positioned on the operating table. The position should allow access to the insertion sight on the cranium (usually occipito-parietal or frontal). Various reference points have been utilised for shunt insertion, however the truth of the matter is that insertion points vary depending on the child. The ideal insertion point traverses the least amount of brain and leaves the catheter in the biggest CSF space ideally not against the ventricular wall. However, even less than ideally placed shunts can work and the true impact of these sorts of insertions on longer term function is not known. The commonly used reference points include Keen's point, two finger's breadths above and behind the pinna and Frazier's point, 6 cm cephalad from the inion and 3 cm from the midline. Frontally burr holes are placed in the midpupillary line around the coronal suture. Shunt insertion is best done by two surgeons, with the opening of the cranium and the peritoneal cavity done simultaneously to shorten operative time. Cranial opening should be done with a small burr hole and a minimal dural opening, just wide enough for the catheter to minimise CSF bypass around the catheter. In babies a drill is often not required to open the soft calvarium. The catheter may be tunnelled from either wound, but tunnelling from the peritoneal wound to the head may allow easier avoidance of inadvertent intrathoracic passage. Wounds are closed in layers with absorbable sutures.

Postoperative radiological evaluation of a shunt's placement and efficacy in terms of resolution of ventriculomegaly is another area of controversy. Some surgeons like to see the shunt in the right place before discharge, even though early imaging does not usually demonstrate much change in ventricular dimensions. It is reasonable to image on

clinical grounds a child who is unwell post insertion or in whom there are some doubts about the operative placement (Figs. 80.3 and 80.4).

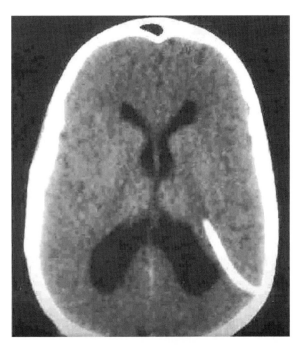

Fig. 80.3 Axial CT scan demonstrating a poorly positioned ventricular catheter

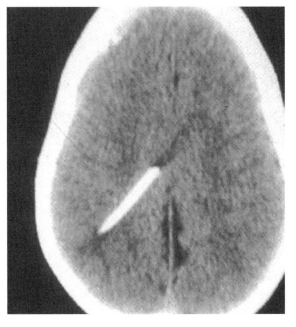

Fig. 80.4 Axial CT demonstrating a ventricular catheter *in situ* in slit like ventricles secondary to overdrainage of CSF

80.5.3 Complications of Implantable Shunts

There are a number of complications related to insertion of CSF shunts; these can be broken down into general complications related to surgery which are not covered here, complications related to shunts in general and complications to the particular route of drainage chosen.

Any shunt may become **obstructed** and this is the most common type of shunt malfunction. It usually occurs in the ventricle often due to the ingress of choroid plexus, less frequently in the valve or the peritoneum. It tends to present as symptoms of raised ICP in appropriate to the age of the patient and tends to be stereotypical for that patient, i.e., if the family of the patient think the shunt is blocked they are often right.

Infection is a common complication of shunt insertion and it becomes apparent in half of the cases within 2 weeks of the index operation. It is usually secondary to infection by skin commensals (particularly *Staphylococcus epidermidis*). On examining the patients with pyrexia, nausea and vomiting, anorexia and abdominal pain, there may be tenderness over the shunt, meningism and confusion. Infection is treated by conversion of the shunt to an externalised ventricular drain and systemic and/or intrathecal antibiotics before reimplantation (Fig. 80.5).

Overdrainage of the ventricular system can occur when an inappropriately low pressure valve is inserted into a shunt system, such that the cerebral mantle is allowed to collapse away from the overlying dura. This can result in tearing of delicate draining veins and the formation of subdural haematomas. Similarly overdrainage can be a positional phenomenon due to the

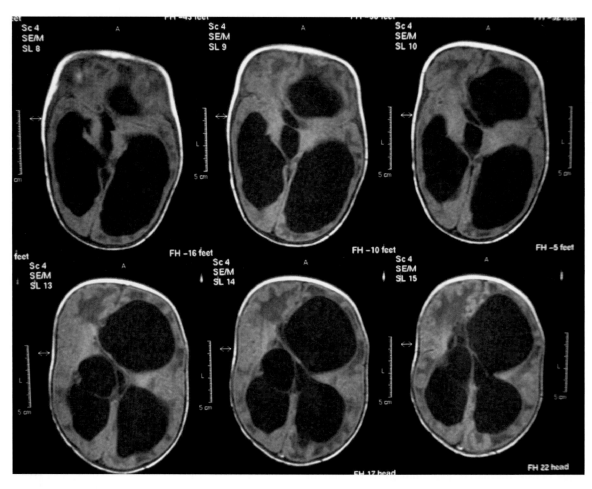

Fig. 80.5 Axial MRI sequence demonstrating a complicated loculated hydrocephalus secondary to intraventricular haemorrhage and infection

siphoning of fluid into the peritoneal cavity when upright. This can be limited by utilising shunt designs with incorporated antisiphon systems or gravitational valves which drain less in the upright position.

Chronic overdrainage of the ventricular system, especially in the context of previous infection can result in small ventricles that do not expand when the shunt is blocked, even when the pressure is very high. This is a particularly difficult problem termed the 'slit ventricle syndrome' and is one reason that ventricular volume *per se* is not a reliable index of shunt function.

VA shunts are indicated in patients with concomitant intraabdominal pathologies precluding the use of the peritoneum as a drainage site. Common coexistent pathologies include necrotising enterocolitis, peritonitis and extensive abdominal surgery. Complications specific to VA shunts include the need for repeated lengthening of the short distal catheter, higher risk of bacteraemia and sepsis as well as the risks of specific vascular complications such as thrombosis, microemboli with resultant pulmonary hypertension, macroemboli with pulmonary embolism and vascular perforation.

80.5.4 VP Shunts and Abdominal Surgery

Pediatric general surgeons will at times have to assess patients with VP shunts and potential abdominal pathology both in the acute and elective settings.

If, during an elective procedure without infection or contamination of the peritoneum, a peritoneal catheter is encountered then it should merely be pushed aside gently and excluded from the field. Significant contamination of the field mandates exteriorisation of the shunt.

Laparoscopic techniques are being utilised more frequently and these require induction of a pneumoperitoneum. This results in an alteration of the shunt dynamics and has been demonstrated in some reports to increase intracranial pressures. Others have reported no complications from induction of a moderate pneumoperitoneum. Laparoscopy should probably be done only after consultation with a neurosurgeon and due consideration to externalisation of the distal catheter or proximal drainage from the shunt reservoir. However at the pressures used frequently in paediatric laparoscopy (around 12 mm Hg^{-1}) harm is probably unlikely if only sustained for short periods.

Assessment of the acute abdomen with a shunt *in situ* is a difficult task and requires a holistic approach to the whole patient. Children may present with abdominal symptoms secondary to shunt malfunction and it is important to define early if there are clinical or radiological signs of shunt dysfunction and not concentrate solely on the abdomen; similarly it is vital that neurosurgeons seek an experienced opinion early in cases where the shunt seems to be functioning but the patient is symptomatic.

If there are abdominal symptoms and signs of peritonitis mandating laparotomy then the shunt should, at laparotomy be externalised into a specialised collection system, the CSF cultured and antibiotics started by the intravenous route. If the shunt is obviously infected in addition, i.e., signs of raised ICP, meningism, tracking along shunt, then the neurosurgical team should consider complete removal and insertion of a new EVD system.

There is some evidence that appendicitis is more frequent in the shunted population than in the general population. In an emergent appendectomy, if the appendix is inflamed but not perforated it is reasonable to leave the shunt *in situ*; if however there is any peritoneal soiling then the shunt must be externalised.

Other common, but usually non-emergent, complications of peritoneal catheters include peritoneal pseudocysts and ascites. Pseudocysts are wall-less fluid collections accumulating between matted bowel loops; they may be complicated by infection. If there are no features of infection then simple repositioning of the catheter in another portion of the peritoneum is all that is required. In the presence of infection, however, a whole new shunt system will be required after appropriate antibiotic therapy and externalisation. Ascites is now uncommon with the predominance of endoscopic techniques in the management of tumoural hydrocephalus, but again it is important to differentiate infection from peritoneal incompetence and this is done by paracentesis and aseptic shunt tap.

80.5.4.1 Endoscopic Third Ventriculostomy (ETV)

Traditionally hydrocephalus management has been a one-dimensional approach consisting of: to shunt or not to shunt!

The re-introduction of neuroendoscopy (with the advance in fibre-optics) in the late 1980s and early 1990s added a new dimension to the management of CSF disorders and importantly changed the way we think, investigate and manage hydrocephalus.

If there is an intraventricular blockage preventing the egress of CSF into the subarachnoid space then hydrocephalus will result. Common causes include tumours, aqueductal stenosis and problems around the foramen magnum such as the Chiari malformation (hernia of the cerebellar tonsils through the foramen magnum causing obstruction of CSF flow out of fourth ventricle).

The aim of ETV is to redirect the CSF through a 'shortcut' from the third ventricle into the subarachnoid space so that it can circulate and be absorbed naturally. It thus avoids the obstruction creating the hydrocephalus and offers a new route for the CSF to travel. The fundamental difference between ETV and a shunt is that this constitutes a natural internal pathway for CSF to re-route so that it can be absorbed physiologically. A conventional VP shunt on the other hand constitutes an external re-routing of CSF via an implant to another part of the body most frequently peritoneum or the venous system. This 'unnatural' pathway with its reliance on pressure differentials is perhaps why there have been so many long-term problems with the insertion of shunts.

80.5.4.2 ETV —the Technique

The technique of endoscopic third ventriculostomy is demonstrated in Figure 80.6 below. In short, a rigid endoscope (disposable or reusable) is navigated into the frontal horn of the lateral ventricle through a frontal pericoronal burr hole placed in the midpupillary line. After ventricular cannulation the endoscope is introduced and navigated through the foramen of Monroe into the third ventricle. On the third ventricle floor the landmarks usually visible, which include the mammillary bodies and the pituitary red spot. A hole is fashioned through the thinned floor of the ventricle usually by the passage of a small balloon, which is then inflated to create the ventriculostomy (Figs. 80.7 and 80.8).

ETV function is most simply seen on a sagittal T2 weighted image such as this one where CSF appears white when static but is demonstrated as a black flow void when moving (Fig. 80.9).

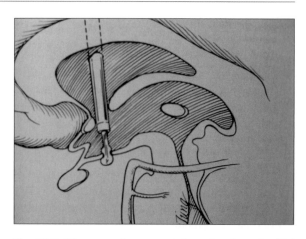

Fig. 80.6 Diagrammatic representation of endoscopic third ventriculostomy in the sagittal plane. It demonstrates the introduction of the endoscope into the lateral ventricle and through the foramen of Monroe. The balloon has been deployed through the floor of the third ventricle into the prepontine space adjacent to the basilar artery

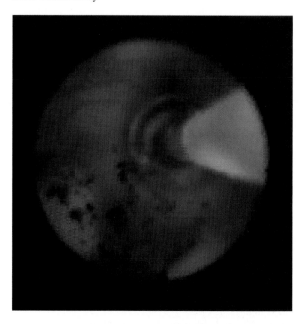

Fig. 80.7 Intraoperative picture of the balloon through the floor of the third ventricle. The mamillary bodies can be seen in the lower portions of the picture

80.5.4.3 Indications for ETV

ETV is indicated in all cases of intraventricular obstructive hydrocephalus including obstructions in the caudal portion of the third ventricle (pineal region), aqueduct, fourth ventricle and foramen magnum. Unfortunately these causes of hydrocephalus are rare in neonates and

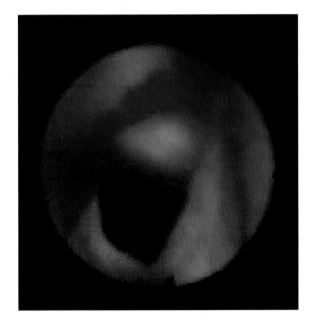

Fig. 80.8 The resulting hole in the floor of the third ventricle, the 'ostomy'

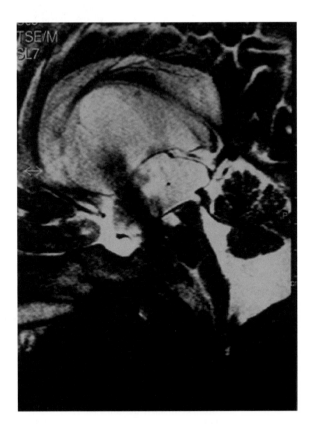

Fig. 80.9 A post-operative T2 weighted sagittal flow study which shows a very large flow void in front of the pons up into the third ventricle resulting from a successful third ventriculostomy

are more common in older children. The commonest causes we see in the developed world remain IVH and meningitis in neonates. ETV in these cases seldom works mainly due to the fact that the functional aetiology of the hydrocephalus is due to a problem in the subarachnoid space – – a blockage both to flow around the surface of the brain due to scarring and inflammation and a probable failure to absorb the CSF. Creating a communication between third ventricle and subarachnoid space is not adequate in these cases and the need for an 'external' shunt is usually inevitable.

ETV enjoys a success rate of 60–90% in children over the age of one when chosen as the primary treatment for true obstructive intraventricular hydrocephalus such as idiopathic aqueduct stenosis. Its success rate declines when used in very young children and when the aetiology of the hydrocephalus includes infection or haemorrhage.

In practice indications for a primary shunt are:

- Undisputed

    - IVH and prematurity
    - Neonatal meningitis

- Probables:

    - Newborn myelomeningocoele
    - Hydrocephalus after removal of post fossa tumours in the under 2's—indications for a primary ETV are:

- Undisputed

    - Over 2's with triventricular obstructive hydrocephalus

- E.g., Tumours – (pineal, tectal, posterior fossa), idiopathic or 'pure' aqueduct stenosis, arachnoid cysts

- For discussion:

    - Primary Aqueduct stenosis, all ages?
    - Chiari's and myelomeningocoele – fourth ventricle obstruction
    - Obstruction secondary to infection/ haemorrhage
    - ETV for shunt malfunction:

In a patient previously shunted who presents with a blocked or malfunctioning shunt, if scan or previous history indicates an originating obstructive hydrocephalus, then we consider ETV and removal of shunt as an alternative to shunt revision.

80.5.4.4 Complications of ETV

The main potential complication of ETV is the risk of damage to the basilar artery which lies very close where the hole is fashioned in the floor of the third ventricle. Such a perforation may be fatal and for this reason, ETV should be performed by experienced hands and is rarely left to trainees to perform unsupervised. Fortunately, perforation of the basilar artery is rare and is reported in less than 1% of cases. In our series of 350 ETVs this complication has thus far been avoided.

Other complications include damage to structures in the basal ganglia from inappropriate passage of the introducer for the endoscope. CSF leaks are potential to damage cranial nerves. These complications, however, may also be encountered when placing a shunt.

The main advantage of ETV over shunt remains in the short-term, a very low infection rate (1–2% in most series) versus a reported rate of shunt infection in most units of 5–15%. This is probably attributable to the fact that no foreign body is placed in the ventricle.

The other main advantage of ETV over shunts is the long term avoidance of functional drainage problems of over or under drainage as the ETV inevitably adjusts itself naturally to the physiological requirements, whereas with a valve one is constrained by the properties of the valve.

The prospect of obtaining an identical result without the insertion of a foreign body is surely one of the reasons for the success of ETV, both from the surgeon's and the patient's point of view.

Finally, long term follow up of ETV patients should be along the same lines as that of a shunted patient. One should always seek to exclude raised intracranial pressure as the cause of a patient presenting with acute or chronic symptoms in any one with a diagnosis of previously treated hydrocephalus, whichever the method or the technique was used.

80.5.4.5 Common Clinical Presentation

Three common presentations will now be discussed to give the non-specialist some insight into their management

80.5.4.5.1 Managing Posthaemorrhagic Hydrocephalus of Prematurity (PHHP)

Premature neonates are particularly at the risk of hydrocephalus because of their predisposition to intraventricular haemorrhage. They are prone to haemorrhage from the sub-ependymal region adjacent to the caudate nucleus where lies the **germinal matrix**, from which develop both the neural and glial elements at different stages of embryological and foetal development.

The lower the birth weight, the higher the incidence of intraventricular haemorrhage (IVH), with infants under 1,500 g being particularly at risk. Neonates tend to present with cardiorespiratory instability and new onset seizures. The open fontanelle makes US a good screening tool. IVH is graded accordingly on a scale of I–IV (Table 80.4) which correlates well with prognosis.

PHHP is defined by the combination of haemorrhage and clinical features of hydrocephalus. Once recognised, treatment varies depending on the neonate, some of whom are too unstable or small to undergo immediate VP shunting. Non-surgical options include administration of diuretics, lumbar puncture and percutaneous ventricular tapping all of which can be carried out at the bedside. Surgical options include insertion of a ventricular access device (a frontal subcutaneous reservoir with a catheter entering the ventricle) allowing repeated aspiration of CSF when the neonate is symptomatic. On average around 10 ml kg^{-1} is removed at any aspiration.

When to insert a VP shunt in a neonate with PHHP is controversial with different practices in different centres. Most authors prefer the infant to be at least 1,500 g and to be clear of other ongoing systemic medical problems, in addition many prefer the CSF protein to be less the 5 g l^{-1} although this is controversial.

Other causes of neonatal hydrocephalus are similarly likely to be treated by a VP shunt rather than endoscopic means; management in older age groups differs however.

Table 80.4 Grading of PHHP (Papile et al. 1978)

Grade	Description
I	Bleed confined to germinal matrix
II	IVH
III	IVH and ventriculomegaly
IV	IVH, ventriculomegaly and ICH

80.5.4.5.2   Approach to Newly Diagnosed Hydrocephalus in Childhood

Hydrocephalus in childhood has a different spectrum of causes than that in the neonatal period. Congenital causes of hydrocephalus, particularly aqueductal stenosis and tumoural obstruction of the CSF pathways are the prime causes of symptomatic hydrocephalus in this age group. The approach is outlined in algorithm 1.

Management is aimed first at making the clinical diagnosis of potential hydrocephalus, appropriate airway management if required and then radiological assessment. First line radiological assessment is CT scanning both with and without intravenous contrast. This alone may indicate a structural lesion resulting in hydrocephalus. In the event of a child who is anything less than fully conscious then consideration should be given to emergency insertion of an EVD to control the raised ICP associated with the hydrocephalus.

The vast majority of patients presenting with new onset hydrocephalus in childhood will be fully conscious but symptomatic often with features indicative of the underlying cause, i.e., truncal ataxia from cerebellar vermis tumours, limb ataxia and nystagmus from cerebellar lobar tumours, eye-movement disorders from midbrain/pineal region tumours and visual failure from tumours near the optic apparatus. Hydrocephalus may also present secondary to infections such as meningitis or bacterial abscess although with these latter pathologies there is usually a much more marked systemic illness (Fig. 80.10).

The main investigation for tumoural obstruction is MRI to assess the CSF pathways and plan operative intervention either to directly relieve the obstruction or to bypass the obstruction.

80.5.4.5.3   Approach to a Child with a Potentially Blocked Shunt

Children presenting with acute symptoms of shunt block, or presenting *in extremis* with no history available can be difficult to diagnose. Children still die from unrecognised shunt failure and a high index of suspicion is vital to save lives.

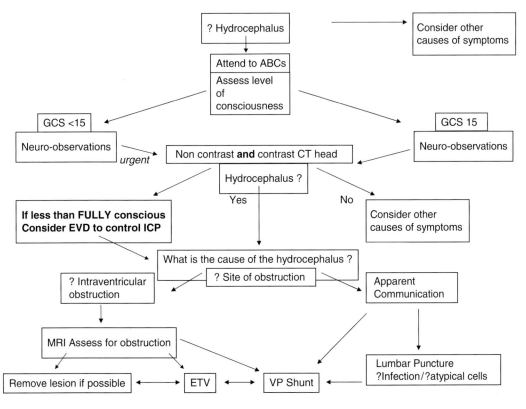

ALGORITHM 1

Fig. 80.10 An infant with chronic untreated hydrocephalus. Note the pressure sore on the parietal area

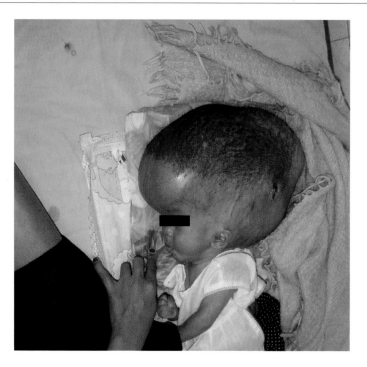

Symptoms of shunt failure are essentially those of raised intracranial pressure, but the presenting symptoms can be variable, with headache predominant in some, and vomiting in others. Children, however, tend to present stereotypically, i.e., on repeated episodes of block they tend to present the same way. Another crucial insight is that of the parents, if they say that the child is 'not right' then they are usually correct.

The approach is outlined in algorithm 2 and it relies upon attendance to the ABCs followed by urgent imaging and if possible comparison to the preceding imaging. The role of shunt series is to assess the integrity of the shunt in children who have no prior imaging or unchanged imaging. The shunt series does not have a role in a child who has clinicoradiological evidence of raised intracranial pressure.

80.5.4.6   Follow-Up of the Patient with Treated Hydrocephalus

Patients with treated hydrocephalus are followed up variably. Some clinicians rely on the fact that if the patient has a problem with their shunt they tend to come to the hospital and can then be assessed. Others will follow up patients as outpatients seeking signs of shunt dysfunction and imaging regularly. The best follow-up paradigm is not defined, however, base-line imaging after insertion of a VP shunt is necessary although its timing is controversial. Imaging too early will demonstrate large ventricles and the true shunted 'normal' will not be seen confusing assessment of the true shunt block.

80.5.4.7   Outcome of Treated Pediatric Hydrocephalus

Outcome in treated hydrocephalus has been evaluated in several long-term cohort studies. A study from The Paris group has demonstrated the severe morbidity of hydrocephalus. In 129 consecutive children with nontumorous hydrocephalus who underwent a first shunt insertion before the age of 2, neurological examination revealed a motor deficit in 60%, visual or auditory deficits in 25% and epilepsy in 30%. The final IQs were below 90 in 68% of the children with integration into the normal school system possible for 60% of

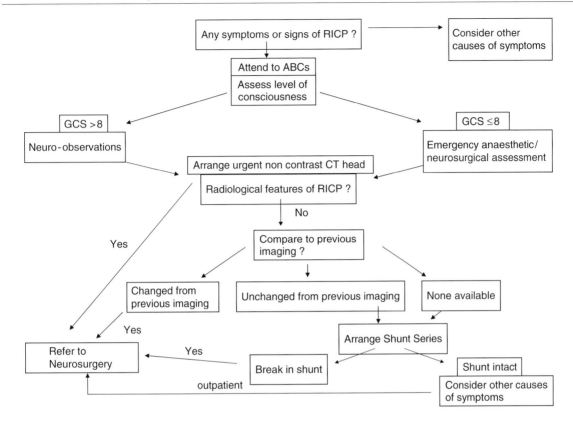

ALGORITHM 2

the children, but half of them were 1–2 years behind their age group or had some difficulties.

80.6 Summary

Hydrocephalus is a feature of many different pathological processes and it is apparent that understanding the underlying process is the key to appropriate therapy. Therapies are surgical but the choice, timing and intervention chosen is a matter of on-going debate. The condition is the source of a great deal of ongoing morbidity in the community and high quality early management influences the long-term outcome.

Further Reading

Arnell K, Olsen L, Wester T (2006) Hydrocephalus. In P Puri, ME Höllwarth (eds) Pediatric Surgery, Springer Surgery Atlas Series. Springer-Verlag, Berlin, Heidelberg, New York, pp 419–426

Cinalli G, Maixner WJ, Sainte-Rose C (2004) Pediatric Hydrocephalus. Springer, Milan

Drake JM, Sainte-Rose C (1995) The Shunt Book. Blackwell, UK

Drake JM, Kestle JR, Milner R et al (1998) Randomised trial of cerebrospinal fluid shunt valve design in paediatric hydrocephalus. Neurosurgery 43(2):294–303

Hoppe-Hirsch E, Laroussinie F, Brunet L et al (1998) Late outcome of the surgical treatment of hydrocephalus. Child Nerv Syst 14(3):97–99

Dermal Sinus and Tethered Cord

81

Andrew B. Pinter and László Bognár

Contents

81.1 Introduction

Dermal sinus and tethered cord are two significant lesions which are the result of an interference with the normal neurulation process which occurs in early pregnancy. Before dealing with these controversial anomalies, it is worth mentioning briefly the commoner defect seen on the lower back—the post anal dimple—which comes into the differential diagnosis of dermal sinus.

81.1.1 Post Anal Dimple or Pit

This anomaly has various alternative names including the post anal sinus and the coccygeal dimple or sinus. This lesion is a midline depression between the buttocks of the individual and may be sufficiently deep that there can be difficulty in clearing faecal material from it, but more often the pit is shallow and can easily be opened to see that the skin is simply tagged down to the lower end of the spine. It has been estimated to occur in 4% of individuals and is over 100 times more common than the dermal sinus.

This anomaly is not related to the neural tube and does not carry any long term sequelae related to the nervous system. Treatment of the deeper ones is advised as some of the individuals with this anomaly develop, during adulthood, pilonidal abscesses or sinuses. These cause significant morbidity and hence the advice for removal of the deeper dimples or pits.

P. Puri and M. Höllwarth (eds.), *Pediatric Surgery: Diagnosis and Management,*
DOI: 10.1007/978-3-540-69560-8_81, © Springer-Verlag Berlin Heidelberg 2009

81.2 Dermal Sinus

The dermal sinus is an abnormal epithelium-lined sinus from the skin, which may extend to communicate with the neuroectoderm. This indentation from the skin may communicate with the intravertebral or intracranial structures. It is the result of a defected primary neurulation process. It is a remnant of incomplete neural tube closure which occurs in the first month of pregnancy. Although dermal sinus can occur from the upper cervical region to the midsacrum, it is most commonly found in the lumbar or lumbosacral area.

Some dermal sinuses end blindly within the soft tissues, however most penetrate the vertebral canal and enter the dura. The connection between the subarachnoid space and the surface predisposes the patients to meningeal infections. The subcutaneous tract generally extends cephalad to a variable degree. The tract leading to the vertebral column or the skull may have a cystic termination (dermoid, epidermoid) or may be associated with tethered spinal cord. The cystic expansion may act as any other mass lesion and affect the neurological function by local compression. It may obstruct the normal circulation of the cerebrospinal fluid as well as impair the vascular supply. The epidemiology is unknown.

81.2.1 Clinical Features

A small sinus aperture may be overlooked on physical examination, and frequently a diagnosis is not considered until a child or an adult has suffered unexplained or recurrent meningitis or has developed signs of spinal cord compression. Therefore, the entire midline area of the skin from the skull to the sacrococcygeal region should be examined carefully for evidence of a dermal sinus. Cutaneous anomalies are frequently present along the midline (Table 81.1 and Fig. 81.1).

Table 81.1 Cutaneous findings associated with dermal sinus

Sinus aperture with a cephalically oriented tract
Angioma
Hypertrichosis
Skin tags
Abnormal pigmentation
Subcutaneous lipoma
Symptoms of infection such as erythema or induration

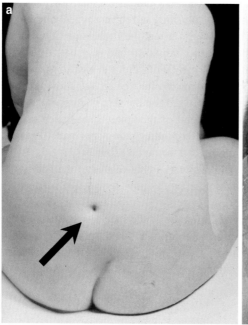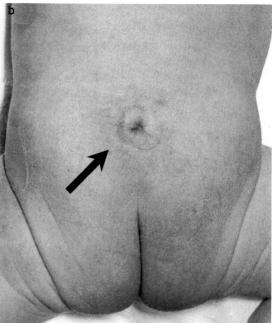

Fig. 81.1 Typical appearance of dermal sinus (*arrows*): (**a**) The asymmetric gluteal fold is a further indication of neural defect; (**b**) well visible sinus aperture probably with a cephalically oriented tract

These should initiate neuro-radiological evaluation as the development of investigative tools allows visualization of the pathology. Bacterial infection can occur through the fistulous tract that may communicate with the subarachnoid space.

Démodé cysts at the inner end of the tract can also cause episodes of aseptic meningitis due to cholesterol leakage into the subarachnoid space. Symptoms of spinal cord compression may develop due to the enlargement of the inclusion tumour.

81.2.2 Radiological Diagnosis

MRI is the choice of investigation to visualize the extraspinal tract, the spinal cord, and any inclusion tumour in axial, sagittal (Fig. 81.2.), and coronal views. Computed tomography and plain X-ray can only demonstrate the associated bony anomalies, i.e., spina bifida or dysraphic lesions, including vertebral anomalies or diastematomyelia. The usefulness of plain radiographs is limited in younger patients because of the delay in calcification in children, particularly those who are less than 18 months old. Ultrasonography can reveal the subcutaneous tract, sometimes the intraspinal inclusion tumours, and diminished cord pulsations, but the specificity and sensitivity are low. Invasive contrast studies are contraindicated.

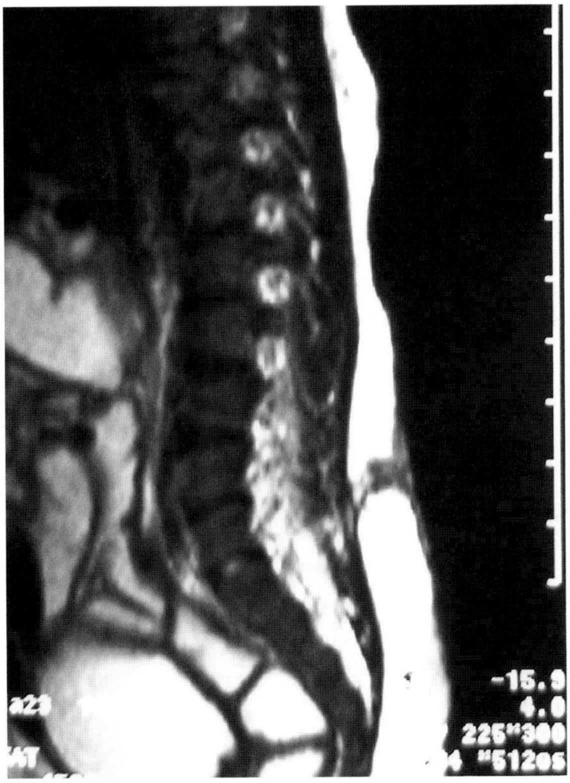

81.2.3 Differential Diagnosis

Coccygeal pits and dermal sinuses are distinctly different clinical entities. Dermal sinuses are located above the gluteal cleft which on occasions may be deviated as shown in Fig. 81.1a. This is further indication of significant hidden pathology and should add to the stimulus for investigation. The sinus usually has a cephalad oriented tract and is often associated with intradural pathology. In contrast, coccygeal pits located within the gluteal cleft, are oriented caudally and not associated with intradural pathology.

81.2.4 Management

Conservative management of dermal sinuses is not justified. These lesions should be selectively resected soon after diagnosis, before severe infection or progressive neurological deterioration occurs.

If preoperative MRI demonstrates intradural pathology, exploration and resection of the tumour is mandatory. If there is no visible intraspinal pathology then the excision is limited to the cutaneous mass and the tract to its deepest projection. Patients should be followed through puberty, with regularly scheduled detailed neurological examinations.

If the lesion is discovered during an episode of meningitis, laminoplasty and intradural exploration should follow after the infection has been controlled by antibiotics. Emergency surgery is required with rapid neurological deterioration, recurrent infection during antibiotic therapy, or when the infection cannot be controlled. The prognosis is good and chances of preserving the neurological function are high. In patients who already have some neurological deterioration, the prognosis mainly depends on the severity and duration of symptoms.

Fig. 81.2   MR image of dermal sinus: T2 weighted sagittal image of lumbar spine presenting dermal sinus tract

81.2.5 Complications

Postoperative infection is the most common complication. Meticulous closure of the dura prevents cerebrospinal fluid leakage. In the latter cases, repeated exploration, spinal drainage, and keeping the patient in prone position are mandatory. In cases of incomplete tumour resection, yearly follow-up MRI is recommended, and repeated surgery is advocated when there is any increase in size of the residuum.

81.3 Tethered Spinal Cord Syndrome

During normal foetal development, the spinal cord initially extends down to the lower end of the sacrum. After 16 weeks of gestation, the vertebral column lengthens more rapidly than the spinal cord. Therefore, the conus will migrate upwards reaching its final level at L1 or L2 by the 2nd month of life. The spinal cord is normally fixed by the cranial base, dentate ligaments and the filum terminale.

Tethered spinal cord (TSC) syndrome refers to an abnormal fixation of the spinal cord when the conus medullaris is below its normal vertebral level. Tethering is due to an inelastic structure anchoring the caudal end of the spinal cord. This abnormal fixation leads to stretching of the spinal cord, resulting in compromise of its blood supply and subsequent ischemia of the neural tissue. A spectrum of clinical presentations that are neurological, orthopaedic, dermatological, and urological may arise due to the tethering of the spinal cord and the consequent interference with the cauda equina function.

A variety of pathological conditions have been identified in the development of TSC syndrome, including adhesions that form after myelomeningocele repair, intraspinal lipoma, tumors, diastomyelia, and dermal sinus tract. However, TSC syndrome can occur also in patients who have a conus with a thickened filum in the normal position.

81.3.1 Clinical Features

The majority of patients with tethering lesions of the spinal cord come to clinical attention through detection of cutaneous, musculoskeletal or vertebral abnormalities encountered during routine childhood examinations (Table 81.2) that raise suspicion of spinal dysraphism. The presenting features of tethered spinal cord syndrome are in Table 81.3. Serial neurological, urological, orthopaedic examinations, and repeated spinal MRI scans are imperative in patients with TSC, to detect signs of gradual deterioration of spinal cord function.

Table 81.2 Anomalies associated with occult spinal dysraphism suggesting tethered cord syndrome

Cutaneous
  Subcutaneous lipoma
  Capillary hemangioma
  Hypertrichosis
  Dermal sinus
  Caudal appendage
Vertebral
  Hemivertebrae
  Sagittal cleft
  Block vertebrae
  Reduced number of bodies
Musculosceletal
  Scoliosis
  Club foot
Sacrum
  Complete or partial agenesis
  Splitting or deviation

Table 81.3 Symptoms of tethered cord syndrome

Genitourinary
  Neurogenic bladder
  Recurrent urinary tract infections
  Urinary incontinence
  Alterations of urinary frequency or urgency
  Sexual dysfunction
Gastrointestinal
  Bowel incontinence
  Constipation
Motor
  Delayed development or worsening of gait
  Asymmetrical strength or movement
  Lower limb muscular atrophy and spacticity
Sensory
  Back, leg or perineal pain
  Leg or perineal anaesthesia
  Painless skin ulceration
Musculoskeletal
  Club foot deformities
  Hip luxation
  Scoliosis

Midline and often multiple abnormalities of the overlying skin are seen in 70% of the patients with occult spinal dysraphism. The most common finding is subcutaneous lipoma and capillary haemangioma. They can vary in size and complexity. A meningocele that undergoes subsequent atrophy and fibrosis prior to birth, may present with epidermal atrophy, a midline patch of thin and tender skin.

Disrupted innervations of the urinary and anal sphincters cause changes in the function that may lead to urinary urgency, frequency, retention and incontinence, recurring urinary tract infections, constipation and faecal incontinence. Urodynamic investigations are essential for the diagnosis and follow-up of urological complications. Urodynamic abnormalities are found in up to two-thirds of patients under 1 year of age, with the most common urodynamic findings such as flaccid bladder, detrusor sphincter dyssynergia and detrusor hyperreflexia.

Neurological deficits are known to occur in patients with anorectal malformations, and these deficits are traditionally believed to be caused by developmental dysgenesis of the neural elements. However, it is important to recognize the association of anorectal malformations with occult dysraphic malformations which are commonly found.

81.3.2 TSC Following Repair of Myelomeningocele

All children in whom a myelomeningocele has been repaired will have a low-lying spinal cord that has at least some adhesions to the surrounding dura. It is caused by the inherent difficulty of closing the dura around the neural plate. Only approximately 10–30% of children with repaired myelomeningocele will develop neurological deterioration related to the tethered spinal cord. Thus the presence of a low-lying tethered spinal cord demonstrated on MR imaging does not indicate intervention. Exploration in that situation has not often resulted in significant improvement in the neurological status.

Bladder dysfunction is present in nearly 100% of the children and adults who have myelomenigocele. The urological presentation of TSC in these patients can be a significant change in voiding pattern.

81.3.3 Radiological Diagnosis

MRI is widely regarded as the definitive method for delineating intraspinal pathology. The visualization of the tethering and its relation to the cutaneous anomaly, mainly to the lipoma is a necessary part of presurgical evaluation (Fig. 81.3a and b.). In cases of myelomeningoceles (Fig. 81.4.), the MRI of the whole spine and the brain is mandatory to disclose other associated developmental anomalies such as Chiari malformation and hydrocephalus. Ultrasound remains only a screening tool for identifying occult spinal dysraphism in infants presenting with suggestive cutaneous abnormalities. Plain radiographs of the spine will show vertebral anomalies with a widened spinal canal in the majority of the patients, although the interpretation of such studies in infants with incomplete ossification of the skeleton may be difficult.

81.3.4 Differential Diagnosis

These include other congenital malformations, acquired infections, and traumatic and neoplastic diseases. Inherited degenerative diseases of the spine and neural and musculopathies must also be taken into account.

81.3.5 Management

Tethered cord syndrome is considered as a progressive disease. In infants with evident tethering caused by extra- and intra-spinal lipoma, the operation is advocated in around 4–6 months. In others, conservative expectant approach in the management of asymptomatic tethered cord appears to be safe. Later indication for surgery depends on the severity of clinical features, the degree of anatomical changes. Surgery should be undertaken before serious neurological dysfunction occurs.

Surgery consists of complete detethering of spinal cord, i.e., removal of tethering and reduction of intraspinal lipomas. A midline or perpendicular incision is used. After exposure to the tethering process and cranial laminectomy, a dural opening begins at this level. At all times the dissection should remain above the

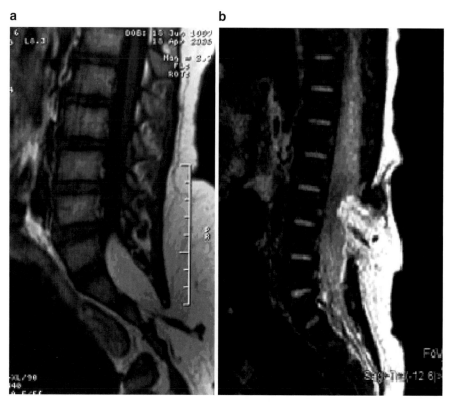

Fig. 81.3 MR image of tethered cord: (**a**) T1 weighted sagittal image of lumbar spine. Extra-intradural lipoma causes the spinal cord tethering; (**b**) T2 weighted image, extra-intradural lipoma with tethering

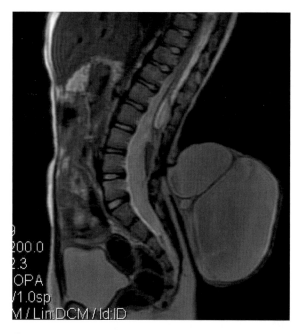

Fig. 81.4 T2 weighted sagittal image of lumbar spine. Meningocystocele and secondary tethering

dorsal nerve roots, within the sheet of lipoma to avoid injury to the neural tissues. The dural opening proceeds cranially until the spinal cord is free of adherent fatty tissue. Then reduction of the lipomatous tissue is performed. Complete removal is impossible because of anatomical reasons, thus can never be forced. If the filum terminale is identifiable, transection can be performed. The dura is closed to provide capacious space for cerebrospinal fluid circumferentially the newly released neural tissue and to provide a watertight seal to prevent cerebrospinal fluid leakage. Following closure of the dura, the repair should involve multiple layers of tissue including muscle, fascia, subcutaneous tissue, and skin. It may be necessary to make relaxing incisions in the fascia to facilitate closure. Drainage is not advocated. Postoperatively, the child is kept in a prone, flat position for 48 h.

In myelomeningocele patients, the primary goal of surgical correction is the release of the spinal cord from the adhering scar. The most common location for the spinal cord to be tethered is the area of the previous closure. The usual operative finding is a dense scar tissue between the posterior aspect of the spinal cord and the overlying dura. Complete untethering is often not achieved because of the high risk of injury to the functional neuronal elements. When surgery for scoliosis is required, previous detethering is mandatory.

A review of the literature on the effectiveness of spinal cord untethering in children revealed 25–50% and 36–66% improvement in clinical and urodynamic status, respectively.

81.3.6 Complications

The most common postoperative complication directly related to the surgical procedure is the cerebrospinal fluid leakage. The complete closure of the dura or sometimes patch insertion is necessary. In some cases reoperation or temporary lumbar drainage may solve the problem. New neurological and urological deficits may be present following surgery. Postoperative scar can cause retethering. Intraoperative electrophysiology can help to determine neural elements, identify the filum terminale, and avoid damage to nerves during operation.

Further Reading

Ackerman LL, Menezes AH (2003) Spinal congenital dermal sinuses: A 30-year experience. Pediatrics 112:641–647

Albright AL (ed) (2007) Principles and Practice of Pediatric Neurosurgery. Thieme, New York

Albright AL, Pollack IF, Adelson PD (eds) (2001) Operative Techniques in Pediatric Neurosurgery. Thieme, New York

Choux M, DiRocco C, Hockley AD (eds) (1999) Pediatric Neurosurgery. Churchill Livingstone, London

Greenberg MS (ed) Handbook of Neurosurgery. Thieme

Michelson DJ, Ashwal S (2004) Tethered cord syndrome in childhood: Diagnostic features and relationship to congenital anomalies. Neurological Research 26:746–753

Pinter AB (2006) Dermal Sinus. In P Puri, ME Höllwarth (eds) Pediatric Surgery, Springer Surgery Atlas Series. Springer-Verlag Berlin Heidelberg, New York, pp 427–432

Urinary Tract Infection

82

Jeremy B. Myers and Martin A. Koyle

Contents

Urinary tract infection (UTI) is a common infectious process in the pediatric age group. Unlike the typical and relatively benign course of UTI in the adult, there may be long-term sequelae of serious UTI in children, especially if there are coincidental urological anatomic abnormalities; potential hypertension and chronic renal insufficiency may be related to childhood renal involvement secondary to UTI. For this reason, it is important for clinicians to be cognizant of the risk factors, pathogenesis, and management of UTI in children. In addition, the pediatric urologist or surgeon needs to recognize how UTI may be a marker of serious urologic congenital and functional anomalies, which may be amendable by operative correction and cure.

82.1 Introduction

Urinary tract infections arise from a multitude of pathogens and can occur anywhere along the urinary tract including the kidney (pyelonephritis), bladder (cystitis), and urethra (urethritis).Anatomically, pyelonephritis is considered to be an upper urinary tract infection while cystitis and urethritis are considered to be the lower urinary tract infections. Pyelonephritis is most commonly accompanied by high fever and especially in infants and neonates, it can lead to renal scarring and permanent renal damage. Up to 40% of infants with a bout of pyelonephritis will show evidence of renal scarring upon subsequent nuclear imaging of the kidneys. This damage becomes more likely with every bout of recurrent upper tract infection. For this reason, the differentiation between upper and lower tract infections is critical.

Urinary tract infections are also classified in several other ways, other than the anatomic location of the infection.

P. Puri and M. Höllwarth (eds.), *Pediatric Surgery: Diagnosis and Management,*
DOI: 10.1007/978-3-540-69560-8_82, © Springer-Verlag Berlin Heidelberg 2009

A UTI can be categorized as complicated or uncomplicated, and also as the first infection or a recurrent episode. Several factors make UTI a complicated infection. One of the most important factors is known anatomic or functional abnormalities of the genitourinary system such as vesico-ureteral reflux (VUR). In addition, recent instrumentation or a retained foreign body,—such as a catheter, also makes a UTI complicated. UTIs that are accompanied by fever, and particularly those occurring in the neonatal and infant stages are also considered complicated infections. Uncomplicated UTIs are infections that arise in the absence of any of these factors.

Another important consideration that affects the management and clinical evaluation of a child is whether the UTI is the first or a recurrent infection. Recurrent infections fall into 3 categories. These are unresolved infections, infections with bacterial persistence and those that are true reinfections. In patients with unresolved bacturia, initial urinary cultures as well as all subsequent cultures will show persistence of the same bacteria. In these cases, the original bacterial infection has never been cleared from the urinary tract. In contrast, in bacterial persistence, the initial infection shows resolution, proven by sterile urine culture, and then infection recurs with the same organism. Similarly, in reinfection, the initial infection is resolved and then the patient documents recurrent UTI, however, unlike bacterial persistence, the recurrent infection is with a different pathogen or a separate serologic strain of the same pathogen (Table 82.1).

Table 82.1 Classification of UTI

Anatomic location:
  Upper – kidney (pyelonephritis)
  Lower – bladder (cystitis), urethra (urethritis)
Complicating factors:
  Complicated infection – infant or neonate, fever, foreign body or stone, anatomic or functional abnormalities
  Uncomplicated infection – simple lower tract infection without fever
Initial or recurrent infection:
  First infection – evaluate if complicated or uncomplicated
  Recurrent infection
  Unresolved – urine cultures are always + with the same pathogen
  Bacterial persistence – urine cultures become sterile after initial infection, recurrent infection occurs with the same bacteria
  Re-infection – the original infection is eradicated and then a different bacteria is isolated with recurrent infection

The first category of recurrent infection, unresolved bacturia, is often the result of inadequate treatment either because of poor compliance or antibiotic resistance. In recent years, uropathogens have developed increased resistance to commonly prescribed antibiotics for UTI. Notable examples of this increasing resistance are *Escherichia coli's* resistance to ampicillin and vancomycin resistant enterococcal infections. The urine culture, at the time of infection, will reveal not only the type of bacteria but also the resistance and sensitivity patterns to various antibiotics. A follow up of the results of a urine culture by the clinician can help prevent inadequate and inappropriate antibiotic treatments of the infection.

Bacterial persistence can indicate an occult nidus or reservoir for the infective process. The nidus for persisting infection can be a retained foreign body such as a piece of a catheter or ureteral stent, or a chronically infected stone. In addition to an actual physical nidus for recurrent infection, an anatomic or functional obstruction can also act as a reservoir for these infections. Obstruction of urinary flow eliminates the normal antegrade flow of urine and promotes urinary stasis and chronic infection. Anatomic obstruction of the urinary system may arise from bladder outlet obstruction from posterior valves or proximal (supravesicle) urinary obstruction from anomalies such as obstructed mega-ureter or uretero-pelvic junction obstruction. Functional obstruction can include conditions such as a neurogenic bladder, in which bladder emptying can be poor and the filling pressures of the bladder may be very high, causing hydronephrosis and a reservoir for infection either in the upper or lower urinary tract. Both, functional and anatomic obstructions promote recurrent infections by eliminating the normal antegrade flow of urine, an import physiologic host defense factor.

Reinfection of the urinary system with entirely different pathogens or different serologic strains of uro-pathogens may be a recurrent problem in patients who are genetically susceptible to UTI. In addition, those patients who have anatomic or functional anomalies of the urinary tract may also be prone to bacterial persistence as well as recurrent reinfections. Usually, the treatment with appropriate antibiotics, surgery to address anatomic anomalies if present, and prophylaxis with daily antibiotics if the reinfections are common or accompanied by complicating factors are successful treatment strategies.

82.2 Epidemiology

In a recent analysis of the incidence and cost of pediatric UTI, by the Urologic Diseases of North America Project, the yearly average risk in children under the age of 18 was 2.4–2.8%. There were 1.1 million visits to doctors' offices per year for UTI, which comprised 0.7% of all visits made by children. The economic burden of UTI was measured for acute hospitalizations and found to be US$180 million per year. This figure did not take into account the expenses occurred during follow up visits, outpatient doctors' visits, radiography, and subsequent surgical management. Of patients evaluated with UTI, infants were much more likely to require hospitalization and the average hospital bill was $5,100 for an episode of hospitalization, secondary to pyelonephritis.

After the 1st year of life, the incidence of UTI is much higher overall in girls than boys. During the 1st year of life, boys have an incidence of UTI of 2.7%, as opposed to girls of 0.7%. In adulthood, girls have a higher incidence. In children aged 1–5 years, the incidence of UTI per year in boys is 0.1–0.2% and in girls, it is 0.9–1.4%. From the age of 6–16, the reported incidence of UTI is stable. In boys, it is up to 0.4% per year and in girls, it approaches 2.3% per year (Table 82.2). With the onset of sexual activity, this incidence climbs to 11% in women, but is not very prevalent in men. Overall, about two-thirds of women will have a urinary tract infection throughout their life.

82.3 Pathogenesis

Some hypothesize that in the first several months of life, UTIs may be caused by hematogenous spread of pathogens from transient bacteremia. After this time period, however, most accept that UTIs arise from fecal pathogens more frequently. In these infections, ascending bacturia from contamination and colonization of the perineum and urethral meatus is thought to be the main factor in the development of UTI. This explains why females are at such higher risk than males. The peri-urethral folds and the moist environment of the vagina promote bacterial colonization around the urethral meatus. In addition, the shorter length of the urethra allows ascending infection to spread more easily to the bladder than in the male.

Once bacteria have gained access to the bladder, they colonize the bladder by adhesion to the bladder mucosa. This process of colonization and subsequent proliferation is a complex balance between the host's immune factors and the virulence factors expressed by the bacteria. Further, there is a proximal involvement of the kidneys, and the ascending bacterial cystitis causes pyelonephritis, which occurs by vesico-ureteral reflux or by another not yet understood phenomenon in non-refluxing patients.

82.3.1 Uro-Pathogens

Numerous organisms including viruses, yeast and bacteria can cause UTI. However, by far, the most common cause of UTI in an otherwise healthy child with a normal immune system is bacteria. Of the uro-pathogenic bacteria, in both adult and pediatric patients, *Escherchia coli* is the most common cause of UTI. *Escherichia coli* accounts for 77–93% of bacterial UTIs. Other common bacteria that cause urinary tract infections are *Enterococcus, Klebsiella, Enterobacter cloacae, Serratia, Staphylococcus aureus, Psuedomonus aeruginosa, Streptococcus* and *Proteus* species (Table 82.3).

Table 82.2 Yearly incidence of UTI in pediatric patients

Age	Boys %	Girls %
0–1 year	2.7	0.7
1–5 years	0.1–0.2	0.9–1.4
6–16 years	0.04–0.2	0.7–2.3

Table 82.3 Common uropathogens

Bacteria	Incidence
Escherichia coli	77–93%
Klebsiella	0–11%
Enterococcus	2–9%
Serratia	~1%
Staphylococcus aureus	~1%
Psuedomonas aeruginosa	~1%
Enterobacter cloacae	~1%
Streptococcus	~1%
Proteus	~1%
Enterobacter cloacae	~1%

82.3.2 Bacterial Factors (Virulence Factors)

Most pathogenic bacteria that cause UTI arise from a reservoir in the intestinal tract. *Escherichia coli* is by far the predominant bacteria to cause UTI and certain serotypes have the unique ability to adhere to the urothelium. One way of differentiating strains of *Escherichia coli* is based upon differences in the antigens elaborated on the polysaccharides capsule that surrounds the bacteria. These antigens are known as K antigens and it has been demonstrated that certain K antigenic *Escherichia coli* have a much higher propensity for causing UTI than other strains.

Perhaps the most significant predictor of a bacteria's uropathic potential is its ability to adhere to the epithelial membrane where they cause infection – in the urinary tract, the urothelium. Pili or fimbriae are long filamentous appendages, composed of protein, that project from the bacterial surface and allow this adhesion to take place. In *Escherichia coli,* type 1 pili is highly associated with bacteria that cause UTI. Type 1 pili bind uroplakin, a protein cap that is elaborated by the umbrella cell or urothelial cell. Another form of pili, P pili, named for its ability to bind the P antigen of blood group antigens, is highly associated with strains of *Escherichia coli* that cause pyelonephritis. Bacterial adherence, colonization and subsequent UTI is a complex process that involves a balance between bacterial virulence factors and the host's immune response to invasive bacterial infection and colonization. However, there are specific strains of enteric bacteria that cause UTI with a much higher virulence than many of the bacteria harbored in the gut. In addition, there are also individuals who are much more prone to UTI due to the complexity of the relationship between host and bacterial factors that allow adherence in the first place.

82.4 Risk Factors

82.4.1 Race and Gender

In infants, studies have suggested that Caucasian children are much more prone to UTI than African American children. This has been found particularly true in Caucasian girls, in whom the incidence of UTI during a febrile illness in the first 2 years of life was 16%. In African American counterparts the incidence was only 2.7%. Caucasian boys also had a higher incidence than African American boys, 2.6% versus 1.7%, however, this was not statistically significant. The authors observing this racial disparity hypothesize that the difference may be secondary to differences in blood group antigens expressed on the surface of uroepithelial cells and the ability of *Escherichia coli* to adhere to these urothelial cells.

As mentioned previously, gender plays a large role in susceptibility to UTI. During the 1st year of life, especially within the first 6 months after birth, uncircumcised boys have a higher incidence of UTI than girls. Thus, the foreskin appears, at least for a short period of a man's life, to be a harbinger of UTI. Thereafter and into adulthood, girls have a higher incidence of UTI, outnumbering males at least 4:1.

82.4.2 Previous Infection

One of the most significant risk factors for UTI is a previous episode of infection. This has been well recognized in adult women and it is also true in children. Of children who have a UTI in the 1st year of life, 26% of girls and 18% of boys are fated to have a further UTI in the several months following their initial infection. Of children who have an infection after their 1st year of life, 32% of boys and 25% of girls will have an additional infection in the future. The number of previous infections also increases the likelihood of a recurrent infection. After a girl has had three UTIs in her past, she has over a 75% likelihood of a return infection in the future. This risk may be reflective of changes that occur physiologically in the urinary tract after a UTI which predispose patients to recurrent infections or may also be secondary to selection of patients who are at high risk for UTI due to genetic or anatomic factors.

82.4.3 Circumcised Versus Uncircumcised

Circumcision is the most common surgical procedure performed and in the United States, the rate of circumcision of male infants born in the year 2000 has climbed to 62%. Circumcision is controversial for a variety of cultural, psychosocial and ethical reasons. However, very few refute the argument that circumcision decreases the risks of sexually transmitted diseases, HIV infection, development of penile carcinoma and also UTI. In boys who have not been circumcised, the risk of UTI has been consistently found to be approximately 10 times more likely in the 1st year of life. The physiologic reason for this increased incidence of UTI in uncircumcised males has been well elucidated. During the 1st year of life, there is increased colonization of the peri-urethral tissue of the inner prepuce allowing the retrograde ascent of infection more readily into the bladder. This peri-urethral colonization decreases after the 1st year of life and by the age of 5 years, little difference exists between an uncircumcised and a circumcised boy.

Twenty-nine percent of uncircumcised boys, less than 1 year of age, with UTI required hospital admission, compared to 18% of circumcised boys and 8% of female infants with UTI. Another important consideration is that the 1st year of life is also the time period when infants are most prone to renal scarring and permanent sequelae from UTI. The American Academy of Pediatrics circumcision policy, however, concludes:

> *Existing scientific evidence demonstrates potential medical benefits of newborn male circumcision; however, these data are not sufficient to recommend routine neonatal circumcision.*

In many pediatricians' opinion, the psychosocial aspects of circumcision may outweigh any potential medical benefits from the procedure. Circumcision is a hotly debated topic and it remains to be determined if the potential medical benefits outweigh the cost and other cultural factors.

82.5 Diagnosis

Diagnosis of UTI in an infant and a neonate may be quite difficult as the signs and symptoms of a UTI are nonspecific. Signs and symptoms of UTI in a febrile infant can include abdominal, suprapubic or flank pain, poor appearance, jaundice, foul smelling urine, and lack of other identifiable etiology for an unexplained fever. Among febrile infants in the first 2 years of life, without identifiable etiology for fever and a temperature greater than 38.5°C, it was found that the overall incidence of UTI was 3.3%. UTI is one of the more common serious causes of infant and neonatal sepsis and in the first 8 weeks of life, the incidence of UTI in a child with an unexplained febrile illness is as high as 13%. In any unexplained febrile illness in a child who is not capable of verbalizing the symptoms, a high suspicion of UTI must be maintained.

A urine analysis (UA) will provide information about the urine, which can suggest the presence of UTI. Nitrite, when present, suggests bacteria in the urine as it is a byproduct of bacterial metabolism of nitrates, however, finding nitrite in the urine is not sensitive and depends upon the time of collection – the first voided samples of the morning are best as it takes several hours for bacteria to elaborate nitrite. In addition, enterococci, the second or third leading cause of UTI in pediatric patients, does not produce nitrite. A UA in a patient with a UTI will often also show the presence of leukocyte esterase. Leukocyte esterase is an enzyme released when white blood cells are lysed in urine and indicates a significant degree of leukouria. An additional important part of the UA is a microscopic exam of the urine. In active infection, there will be many leukocytes and bacteria. Usually, the urine is centrifuged at 2,000 revolutions per minute for 10 min and the resultant pellet is examined under the microscope. When there are greater than five white blood cells (WBC) per high power microscopic field (hpf), significant leukouria exists. As the number of WBC/hpf increases, the positive predictive value of the microscopic exam for UTI also becomes higher. Additional sensitivity can be achieved with the use of a hemocytometer, which measures the number of WBCs in an uncentrifuged specimen of urine. The sensitivity of predicting UTI accurately by finding greater than ten WBC/- using the hemocytometer is 23% higher as compared to finding greater than five WBC/hpf on microscopic exam. Overall, the positive predictive value for a UTI when there is nitrite, leukocyte esterase, bacteria, and leukocytes in a sample of urine is virtually 100%. Similarly, the negative predictive value for UTI when these factors are not present also approaches 100%.

When a UTI is suspected based upon clinical suspicion and a UA showing nitrite or leukocyte esterase, accompanied by microscopic exam revealing leukocytes and bacteria, treatment should be initiated. However, bacterial culture of the urine remains the gold standard for establishing the diagnosis of UTI and for this reason, the patient's urine should be sent for bacterial culture before the initiation of antibiotic therapy. Traditionally, growth of greater than 10^5 colony forming units (CFU) of bacteria within a urine culture indicates significant infection. This limit has been challenged in adults and many symptomatic women, who are found to have fewer bacteria than 10^5 CFU and often develop a significant UTI if they are not treated. Similarly in febrile children, significant UTI can be present when fewer than 10^5 CFU, and up to 21% of febrile infants presenting with UTI only grow 10^4–10^5 CFUs upon urinary culture. For this reason, many pediatricians advocate that 10^4 CFUs should be the threshold for the diagnosis of UTI in children. Gram negative organisms are less likely to be contaminants particularly if found in a urine sample obtained by suprapubic aspiration, and treatment of 10^3 colony counts of gram negative rods, when found on a sample of urine obtained by suprapubic aspiration, has also been recommended by some. The urine culture will reveal the bacteria responsible for the UTI and also the antibiotic sensitivity and resistance pattern of the bacteria; this allows for focused antibiotic treatment strategies.

82.5.1 Urine Collection

The simplest collection method for a sample of urine for analysis and bacterial culture is a bag taped to the perineum. This method is helpful if the urine analysis is negative and therefore, infection is unlikely. However, it does not help if the urine suggests infection, since genital, perineal, and fecal contamination can easily give a false positive urine analysis. Two other methods have been commonly employed to obtain a sterile sample of urine when the correct diagnosis is critical, such as in an infant or neonate with unexplained febrile illness. These methods are suprapubic aspiration of the bladder and sterile urethral catheterization. To obtain a urine sample by suprapubic aspiration, a fine needle (23 or 25 gauge) is passed into the bladder by puncture directly above the symphis pubis. The needle is directed perpendicularly or with a slight caudal angle and aspirated as it is advanced until urine is obtained. Urethral catheterization is best accomplished with a five French feeding tube or specifically designed urethral catheter, which is usually a more compliant material. The technique should be performed with as strict adherence to sterile conditions as possible to prevent contamination of the sample.

Both suprapubic aspiration and urethral catheterization yield acceptable sensitivity for UTI, but in a recent analysis of pain perceived by caregivers and parents, urethral catheterization appeared to be better tolerated by infants and neonates than suprapubic aspiration, however, other studies have refuted this advantage. Urethral catheterization is a simple method, which may be better tolerated by patients and is possibly also perceived as less invasive by parents. Urethral catheterization may not be feasible when it is complicated by anatomic problems such as a tortuous or dilated urethra. In some instances, urethral catheterization may be aided by perineal pressure or gentle flushing of the catheter with sterile saline as it is advanced. When urethral catheterization is not achievable, a urine sample can usually be easily obtained by suprapubic aspiration.

82.6 Treatment

There are several controversies surrounding the treatment of pediatric UTI. These controversies include the timing of treatment initiation, the time course of adequate treatment, treatment with oral versus parenteral antibiotics, and the need and timing of radiologic imaging.

When an uncomplicated UTI, in the absence of fever, has been identified based upon symptoms or a UA suggesting infection or a positive urine culture, oral antibiotic therapy should be initiated. This therapy commonly consists of either amoxicillin or a sulfonamide-based antibiotic, such as sulfisoxazole or trimethoprim-sulfamethoxazole (TMP-SMX). The duration of oral antibiotic therapy has been an area of controversy in the treatment of children with UTI. Treatment in adults with as little as 3 days of TMP-SMX or flouroquinolone antibiotics has been found to be as effective as longer treatment regimens. A recent review of short-term therapy (2–4 days) versus long-term therapy (7–10 days), by the Cochrane collaboration, showed no evidence that long-term therapy was advantageous. The recurrence rate and reinfection rate remained the same up to 15 months after treatment with either short- or long-term therapy. Isolation of resistant organism showed a trend towards favoring short-term therapy, however, the authors concluded that there was not adequate evidence to recommend short- versus long-term therapy. It is important to emphasize that this was in the treatment of uncomplicated UTI and children without fever, toxemia, or suspected accompanying pyelonephritis. These children are more likely to be under the care of a primary care provider; the surgical consultant is usually involved with a child with a febrile UTI and a known or suspected genito-urinary surgical issue.

A common scenario presented to the consulting surgeon will be an unexplained high fever in a neonate or infant (Fig. 82.1). In this scenario, the clinician should make a clinical judgment about the need for admission to the hospital. If the child shows evidence of dehydration and toxemia and if admission to the hospital is warranted, usually parenteral antibiotics are administered. If there is no clear underlying etiology of the child's illness, a urine culture obtained by suprapubic aspiration or urethral catheterization should be performed. The unacceptably high false positive rate of a bagged collection of urine for UA excludes it as a practical method for a critically ill child. Broad-spectrum antibiotics are initiated and if the child improves in 24–48 h, these can be switched to oral antibiotics to complete a full course of treatment spanning 7–14 days. If the urine culture proves to be positive, antibiotic therapy can be tailored to the sensitivities of the bacteria responsible for the episode. Many antibiotic regimens have been utilized for the treatment of pyelonephritis. The Cochrane collaboration reviewed trials that compared regimens and outcomes of pyelonephritis and found no difference in the various treatment regimens published in randomized clinical trial for the treatment of

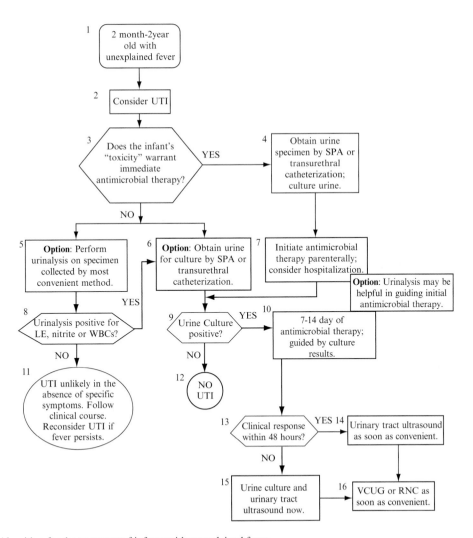

Fig. 82.1 Algorithm for the treatment of infants with unexplained fever

pyelonephritis. Most clinicians utilize a third or fourth generation cephalosporin, possibly in conjunction with an aminoglycoside during the acute phase of treatment and then transition the patient to an equivalent oral medication once fevers have abated, usually after approximately 48 h. Oral antibiotic agents that concentrate in the urine but obtain only poor tissue and blood levels should be avoided in patients who have had a febrile component to their UTI. Nitrofurantoin is one of these antibiotics, which remains a good choice for uncomplicated UTI and UTI prophylaxis but not for treatment of a febrile episode of UTI.

Not all patients with pyelonephritis will defervesce once treated with antibiotics and if fevers are persistent or the patient's condition worsens after the initiation of therapy, further steps should be taken in these patients' evaluation. In the first 24 h, 68% of patients less than 2 years of age with clinical signs of pyelonephritis will resolve their fevers when they are treated with parenteral antibiotic therapy. By 48 h, a total of 89% of these patients' fevers would have resolved. Some have refuted the need for further work up of infants who continue to have fevers after being on parenteral antibiotics, pointing to evidence that there is no difference in bacteremia rates or diagnosis of conditions such as vesico-ureteral reflux between patients who respond and patients who do not respond to antibiotics. However, the American Academy of Pediatrics still recommends that children with persistent fever after 48 h have another urine culture obtained and be evaluated with a renal-bladder ultrasound. The American Academy of Pediatrics in 1999 outlined a treatment algorithm for unidentified fever in a child and subsequent management of pyelonephritis (Fig. 82.1). The algorithm addresses the timing and urgency of imaging. If a child responds well to antibiotics, imaging can be postponed until after the infection has passed. The full spectrum of imaging to identify urologic pathology is beyond the scope of this chapter and will be addressed later in the text, however, the initial work up of a patient with fever and a UTI is a renal-bladder ultrasound and a voiding cystourethrogram.

After the bout of pyelonephritis has resolved, prophylactic antibiotic therapy should be initiated until a surgical consideration has been ruled out with imaging tests (Table 82.4). In several randomized trials, the use of prophylactic antibiotic therapy has been shown to decrease the incidence of recurrent UTI. The populations within these studies are heterogeneous. However,

Table 82.4 Surgical conditions leading to febrile UTI

Anatomic:
  Vesico-ureteral reflux
  Ureterocele
  Uretero-pelvic junction obstruction
  Posterior urethral valves
  Ureteral or renal calculi
  Obstructed megaureter/megacalicosis
Functional:
  Neurogenic bladder – Myelomenigocele
  Dysfunctional voiding – Hinman's syndrome

Table 82.5 Prophylactic antibiotic regimens for prevention of UTI

Trimethoprim – 2 mg/kg daily
Trimethoprim-sulfamethoxazole (TMP-SMX) – 2 mg/kg TMP, 10 mg/kg SMX daily
Nitrofurantoin – 1–2 mg/kg daily
Amoxicillin
Cefexime

most clinicians agree that beginning antibiotic prophylaxis is warranted after an episode of pyelonephritis until imaging studies have been completed. The basis of this practice is the well-recognized correlation between renal scarring and the number of episodes of pyelonephritis, especially in young infants. Many different antibiotics have been utilized to prevent recurrent UTI. The ideal antibiotic would have little effect upon the flora of the gut and be easy to administer for the child and the parent, since compliance is a major difficulty with these regimens. In randomized trials, nitrofurantoin has been compared to trimethoprim and to cefixime. Cefexime was found to be superior to nitrofurantoin, which was also found to be superior to trimethoprim, however, both cefexime and nitrofurantoin were associated with a high patient drop out mainly secondary to gastrointestinal side effects. At our institution, we utilize trimethoprim alone as daily prophylactic therapy and have not noted any adverse events associated with its administration. Several adequate prophylactic antibiotic regimens have been summarized in Table 82.5.

82.7 Conclusions

Urinary tract infection in pediatric patients can arise from a variety of causes, encompassing simple cystitis to life threatening urosepsis secondary to surgical anomalies of the urogenital tract. There are a number of complex host and bacterial virulence factors that also make children susceptible to UTI. It is important that the clinician be familiar with the spectrum of UTI and children at risk of UTI, so that infants and children who need to be evaluated for anatomic or functional abnormalities of the urinary tract are correctly identified. The hallmark sign of one of these children is an infant in the first few years of life with evidence of a UTI and a high fever. This child must be considered to have pyelonephritis and an anatomic abnormality until proven otherwise. These children should be begun on prophylactic antibiotics until proper imaging has been obtained to establish their diagnosis.

Further Reading

Chang SL, Shortliffe LD (2006) Pediatric urinary tract infections. Pediatr Clin N Am 53:379–400

Freedman AL (2005) Urologic diseases in North America Project: Trends in resource utilization for urinary tract infections in children. J Urol 173:949–954

The American Academy of Pediatrics (1999) Circumcision policy statement. Pediatrics 103:686–693

The American Academy of Pediatrics. Committee on Quality Improvement, Subcommittee on Urinary Tract Infection. (1999) Practice parameter: The diagnosis, treatment and evaluation of the initial urinary tract infection in febrile infants and children. Pediatrics 103:843–852

Puri P, Höllwarth ME (eds) (2006) Pediatric Surgery. Springer, Berlin, Heidelberg

Imaging of the Paediatric Urogenital Tract

83

Michael Riccabona

Contents

83.1 Introduction

When discussing imaging of the paediatric urogenital (UG) system, the basic rational of any imaging should be reconsidered and remembered: imaging should only be used if it has an impact on diagnosis, treatment, further management and/or patient outcome. Particularly, in paediatrics the imaging modality should be selected considering the specific paediatric needs and diseases: imaging should try to avoid ionising radiation whenever possible, the least invasive procedure applicable for the individual query should be selected (e.g., try to avoid catheterism if possible, reduce examinations that need sedation, etc.), and any imaging that does not impact management should be avoided. Furthermore, the recommended imaging method should be easily accessible and available. Another basic comment on imaging in children: children are not small adults, therefore state-of-the-art imaging of infants and children requires dedicated techniques (equipment, transducer, filtering…) as well as age-adapted investigation protocols (ultrasound, CT, MR, etc.). This means that everyone who deals with children needs to have not only the adequate equipment available, but also has undergone dedicated training in paediatric imaging.

83.2 Imaging Methods

There are a number of imaging methods that can be used and are applied for imaging the paediatric UG-tract (UGT): ultrasound (US), abdominal plain film, intravenous urography (IVU) (modified and adapted), voiding cysto-ureterography (VCUG) as well as other forms of urethra-or uretero- pyelography (antegrade or retrograde), including the therapeutic percutaneous nephrostomy (PCN), scintigraphy, computed tomography (CT) or magnetic resonance tomography (MRT). The details of specific imaging such as scintigraphy, CT or MRT in children are not discussed here, but the chapter briefly outlines the basic requirements for more commonly performed procedures such as US, IVU or VCUG which, in some centres, are in the hands of paediatric surgeons or paediatric urologists. Interventional radiology in the paediatric UGT is discussed in the respective chapters. Note that the role and potential of various imaging modalities is constantly evolving, as well as the patient treatment concepts and management strategies; this naturally has implications on imaging algorithms. And whoever performs paediatric uroradiologic studies, should have undergone dedicated training in paediatric imaging techniques to grant the optimal diagnosis at the lowest achievable invasiveness by high quality imaging and child adapted procedures.

Ultrasound has emerged from an initially orienting imaging tool to a dedicated high-end examination and a range of age adapted sector-, vector-, curved array-, and linear transducers are necessary to reliably perform the task. Today, modern techniques are included routinely such as amplitude-coded colour Doppler sonography (aCDS), motion mode, harmonic and high resolution imaging as well as image compounding, high frequency transducers, echo-enhanced (ee) US or three-dimensional US. These applications may help to reliably establish a final diagnosis in many conditions, reducing the need for other imaging in many conditions. However, to properly explore this quickly growing, vast potential of US, some prerequisites need to be considered:

- Investigations should always be performed in physiologically hydrated patients with a sufficiently filled bladder.
- Every US investigation includes the entire urinary tract (UT) and genital tract (GT).
- For a thorough evaluation, a detailed study of the renal parenchyma using linear transducers from a lateral, ventral or dorsal approach is mandatory as well as pre- and post-void assessment of the bladder, the retrovesical space, and the kidneys/the upper collecting system.
- An aCDS is mandatory in various conditions such as urinary tract infection (UTI).
- Kidney volume must always be calculated and assessed in relation to growth charts.

- In hydronephrosis (HN), standardised measurements of caliceal dilatation and of the width of the ureter and the renal pelvis are mandatory; grading of HN should be performed using standardised classifications such as the suggestion adapted from the Society of Fetal Urology (Table 83.1).
- Assessment of vesico-ureteral reflux (VUR) based on changing dilatation of the uretero-pelvic system is unreliable, only the use of US contrast-material (CM) instilled into the bladder (called ce-voiding urosonography = ce-VUS) enables a reliable and adequate sonographic assessment of VUR.

Note that particularly, initial studies should always include surrounding body compartments, i.e., an orienting overview ("sonoscope") of the other pelvic structures as well as of the liver, the pancreas, the spleen, the adrenal glands and adjacent intestinal parts, in order not to miss the potential disease that is clinically mimicking UT pathology or that is part of an underlying systemic or syndromal condition (e.g., US of the neonatal spine in patients with neurogenic bladder). Furthermore, it is recommended to thoroughly evaluate the inner GT in female neonates with severe UT malformations or single kidneys, as there is a relatively high incidence of embryologically determined associated genital malformations. The diagnosis of these conditions will be difficult after the first months of life due to the regression of the uterus und ovaries, whereas a reliable diagnosis can easily be achieved by sonographic genitography in the neonatal period (potentially supplemented by fluoroscopy using the same catheters). Furthermore, in certain conditions such as syndromal disease, adequate additional assessment of other body areas (heart, brain, spinal canal…) must be initiated, with many of these queries being sufficiently answered by US.

In spite of all US advances, *VCUG* still remains the most important investigation for VUR, particularly in countries where US CM is not approved for paediatric use. Furthermore, VCUG enables a detailed anatomic assessment of the urethra and is superior to US in depicting intermittently posing diverticula, in demonstrating intrarenal reflux and by offering a panoramic overview of the entire (refluxing) UT. However, VCUG poses a significant radiation burden, particularly to girls—thus indications must be very strict (and constantly reassessed), and a proper fluoroscopy technique is essential:

- The radiopaque CM should always be instilled into a (nearly) empty bladder, with CM instillation under physiologic pressure to avoid overextension and

Table 83.1 Hydronephrosis grading by US (Adapted suggestion, based on Fernbach SK et al. Ultrasound grading system of hydronephrosis: introduction to the system used by the Society for Fetal Urology. Pediatr Radiol 1993, 478–480, Riccabona et al., Pediatr Radiol 2008, 38: 138–145)

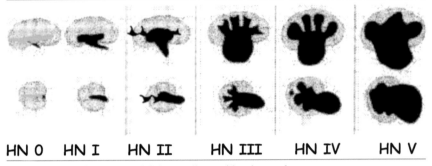

HN 0   HN I   HN II   HN III   HN IV   HN V

HN 0 = no collecting system visible, usually considered normal

HN I = just the renal pelvis visible with an axial diameter less than 5–7 mm, usually considered normal

HN II = axial renal pelvis diameter less than 5/7–10 mm, some calyces with normal forniceal shape visible

HN III = marked dilatation of the renal calyces and pelvis larger than 10 mm with reduced forniceal and papillar differentiation without parenchymal narrowing, often seen in dilating VUR and obstructive uropathy

HN IV = gross dilatation of the collecting system with narrowing of the parenchyma, in VUR and obstructive uropathy

HN V = in some places it is used additionally to communicate an extreme HN with only a thin, membrane-like residual renal parenchyma. Differentiation from MCDK is achievable, as in MCDK the residual dysplastic parenchyma is usually positioned centrally, with surrounding and exophytic cysts of varying size

non-physiological conditions. The way varies depending on the various centres, both transurethral as well as suprapubic puncture are used and the latter is particularly for psychological and socio-cultural reasons.

- Cyclic studies are recommended in neonates and infants to increase VUR detection rate.
- Adequate fluoroscopy units adapted for paediatric needs are mandatory—performing VCUG with blind spot films or using a C-arm device is inadequate.
- A VCUG should always include a fluoroscopic assessment during early filling phase in an anterior-posterior projection, an oblique view of the distal ureteral region, a lateral or oblique view of the urethra during voiding, an assessment of the upper collecting system during and after voiding, as well as a post-void assessment for residual urine and of potentially refluxed CM drainage dynamics.

Detailed guidelines on how to properly perform VCUG can be found in the paediatric radiology literature Riccabona et al. (2008); VCUG-based VUR grading has been standardised.

Plain film still has a roll in assessment of UT calculi as well as in assessment of various drains, catheters and devices; it, furthermore, is helpful for the assessment of associated skeletal changes such as spina bifida. It should be focussed at the kidney, the ureter and the bladder ("*KUB*") by using shutters; an age adapted technique (dose, grids, …) is essential.

Intravenous urography (IVU) allows for a reliable assessment of the collecting system anatomy and reveals information on renal function and urinary drainage. However, today it has lost most of its importance in the paediatric setting, as US, scintigraphy and MR-Urography (MRU) enable a superior assessment with less radiation in most paediatric queries. Still, in areas with restricted access to these modalities, for a focused pre- or post-operative assessment, in some conditions where maximal spatial resolution is indispensable for early diagnosis (e.g., for medullary sponge kidney), and in suspected urolithiasis that cannot be sufficiently assessed using the other means respectively, a modified and adapted IVU may still be a good option. If IVU is performed, the number of films should be restricted, and targeting (shutters, gonad protectors) as well as timing should be individually adapted to the diagnostically relevant moments and areas. X-ray dose, film-foil combination, grids and CM dose need to be adapted according to the patient's age. With this approach, a significant reduction of the film number (usually 2–4 films are sufficient for diagnosis) and of the delivered radiation dose can be achieved.

Scintigraphy is usually performed by paediatric nuclear medicine specialists according to the standardised protocols issued by the paediatric nuclear medicine groups. It uses tracers labelled with radioactive material (usually Technetium 99^m) that are specifically handled by the renal parenchyma and or secreted into the urine. The change in radioactivity over time is measured by a gamma camera, for functional assessment.

Static renal scintigraphy uses DMSA (dimercaptosuccinic acid). This tracer is specifically taken up by the tubuli, and it allows for an exquisite assessment of the functioning renal parenchyma. It is used for split renal size assessment and assessment of focal lesions such as acute pyelonephritis (aPN) or scars. Spatial resolution is restricted and can be improved using SPECT; however, due to an increased radiation burden this technique is rather reluctantly used in children.

Dynamic (diuretic) renography uses the glomerularly and tubularly handled MAG3 (Mercapto-acetyltriglycine) allowing for differentiation of an arterial phase, a parenchymal phase, an excretion phase and a drainage phase. Standardised hydration is essential as well as diuresis provocation using Furosemid to produce reliable results; a bladder catheter should be inserted in infants and in patients with VUR to avoid misdiagnosis by bladder filling induced "pseudo-obstruction". It is mainly used for assessment of obstructive uropathy such as pelvi-ureteral junction obstruction (PUJO) or megaureter (MU).

Radionuclide cystography (RNC) uses either the late phase of a dynamic renogram with the bladder filled by the renally excreted MAG3 (only applicable in toilet trained and cooperative patients), or the isotope (generally, Tc^99m colloid) is installed directly into the bladder via suprapubic puncture or transurethral catheter. Any activity increase in the upper collecting system proofs the VUR. Some grading and functional assessment are achievable but anatomic resolution is restricted; RNC, therefore, is used for screening purposes and for follow-up examinations.

CT and ***MRT*** are usually performed by paediatric radiologists and will not be covered in detail.

CT has a significant radiation burden and, therefore, is very reluctantly used in children. If UT-CT is considered in neonates, infants or children, age adapted low-dose protocols with adapted parameters, recon-

struction algorithms, as well as CM amount and timing are mandatory; normal protocols used in adults are not acceptable for routine paediatric use. The generally accepted indications for CT in children's UGT are: severe abdominal trauma, tumour assessment, assessment of renal abscesses (particularly if MR is not available), complex malformations that involve the pelvic skeleton (if this information is relevant for planning surgery, e.g. bladder exstrophy,…), and assessment of complicated urolithiasis and infections such as renal tuberculosis (Tbc) or xanthogranulomatous pyelonephritis (XPN). Note that increasingly, these queries are investigated by MRT if available.

MRT is becoming the ideal one-stop-shop imaging modality for particularly congenital UGT anomalies, as MRU constitutes a comprehensive investigation without radiation burden that allows for both anatomic and functional assessment. Its setbacks are the restricted availability, the sedation needs particularly in infants and young children, some spatial and temporal resolution issues, as well as artefacts derived from patient motion.

83.3 Typical Imaging Findings in Common Paediatric Urological Conditions

One of the most common queries is pre- or neonatally detected ***hydronephrosis*** (HN). The task of early imaging is to depict those neonates and infants who benefit from early treatment and appropriate management with consequent monitoring to prevent future harm to the kidney. Basically, a neonatal US study in the well hydrated patient at the end of the 1st week of life enables differentiation of the patients who do not need any further imaging, patients who need follow-up or additional studies, and patients who need urgent treatment, such as for severe bilateral obstruction or posterior urethral valve. The latter might need an earlier study if indicated by prenatal US findings. The most common diagnosis in this patient group is a "physiological" dilatation without any need for further studies or follow-up (Fig. 83.1). The other relevant group is those with (dilating) VUR and obstructive uropathy. The most important sonographic signs (constituting most of the "extended US criteria" that improve US diagnosis and differentiation, Table 83.2) that allow differentiation of obstructive versus non-obstructive dilatation are: thickening of the renal pelvic wall and the configuration of the calices which remain normally shaped in low pressure

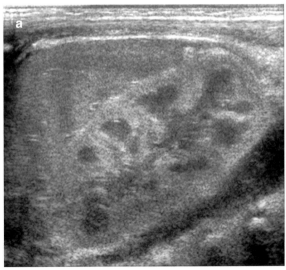 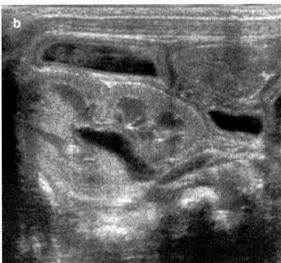

Fig. 83.1 US of a normal neonatal kidney. Longitudinal (**a**, no pelvo-caliceal distension) and axial (**b**, slight physiologic distension of the renal pelvis) section with a 14 MHz linear transducer: Note some echogenic papillae, with a physiologically pronounced cortico-medullary differentiation and echogenic cortex

Table 83.2 List of extended ultrasound criteria

These sonographic features may indicate UT pathology and should prompt further investigation:

Urethra: valve-like shape of open bladder neck

Bladder: atypical shape and size, bladder wall thickening and trabeculation, diverticula, ostium pathology, significant residual urine, persistent urachus

Ureter: dilatation, tortuousity, ureteral wall thickening, ectopic orifice, duplex ureter

Kidney: caliceal dilatation (HN III or higher, or obvious variation of dilatation during investigation), pelvic wall thickening, abnormal kidney size, parenchymal abnormalities (echogenicity, narrowing, cysts …)

pelviectasia, whereas they become distorted or rounded with more or less parenchymal narrowing in patients with increased intra-pelvic pressure. Additionally, the bladder wall changes or dilatation of the ureter—even if intermittent—may hint towards urine transport and drainage problems, particularly VUR. Note that already neonatally renoparenchymal changes due to hypodysplasia such as increased echogenicity, reduced corticomedullary differentiation or renal cysts may be present. These findings usually indicate a relatively restricted prognosis with high probability of renal insufficiency that sometimes manifests in infancy. Creative new sonographic approaches such as perineal US or ee-US can help in further specification of the condition by either directly showing an urethral valve or enabling a reliable assessment of VUR.

In high grade neonatal HN, early US may underestimate its severity as the physiologically reduced renal function during the 1st days of life will prevent the collecting system from reaching its maximum dilatation. Therefore, a repeated investigation after 2–4 weeks is necessary. The amount of dilatation does not necessarily equal the degree of obstruction or renal function; kidneys with significantly reduced function may exhibit less dilatation than systems that function well. Therefore, US is not sufficient for assessment and grading of obstruction. Earlier, IVU was generally used for assessment of urine drainage dynamics; today, this has been replaced by diuretic renography and MRU. Note that these functional studies (i.e., IVU, scintigraphy and MRU) should only be performed after kidney maturation, which is after the 6th week of life.

Particularly in patients with a dilated ureter, differentiation of obstructive uropathy from **VUR** is mandatory. In these cases—particularly in neonates and boys—VCUG is recommended as the modality of choice for comprehensive assessment of VUR including the bladder and the urethra. If VUR is detected, a base assessment of renal function by DMSA scintigraphy should be performed, usually at approximately 3–6 months of age. VCUG is also mandatory before surgery, whereas VUR follow-up can be performed by RNC or ee-US.

In *obstructive uropathy,* differentiation of the level of obstruction is important. Besides the rare but serious obstruction secondary to a tumour or a posterior urethral valve, the obstruction can be either at the level of the *uretero-vesical (UVJ)* or *pelvi-ureteric junction (PUJ).* In UVJ-obstruction (UVJO), an MU is present that can be usually and finely visualised by US, as well as a potential ureterocele and the often associated duplex system (Fig. 83.2a). Ultrasound can additionally assess and document (by motion-mode or using cine loop clips) ureteral peristalsis, particularly useful for follow-up (Fig. 83.2b). PUJO is sonographically characterised by significant dilatation of the renal pelvis (HN III–V) with more or less parenchymal narrowing without a visible ureter (Fig. 83.3a, b), unless a combined stenosis or a combination with dilating VUR is present. US examinations should always measure the maximum axial distension of the renal pelvis and the calices as well as the maximal narrowing of the parenchyma, and assess renal vascularity and perfusion. Colour Doppler sonography (CDS) may depict additional renal arteries compromising the PUJ, and Doppler trace analysis may exhibit asymmetrically elevated resistance indexes in severe acute obstruction, particularly under diuretic stimulation with Furosemid (= diuretic sonography). Furthermore, echoes and sedimentations may be present within a dilated system and may hint towards intraluminal infection. This condition is relatively frequent in MU patients under antibiotic prophylaxis and may be clinically silent; urine samples may produce equivocal results, as greater

amount of urine will be from the normal functioning non-affected contra-lateral healthy system.

Once the initial diagnosis is established, management varies: patients with non-obstructive dilatation or megacalycosis will usually be followed by repeated US examinations. Patients with obstructive uropathy or deterioration of mild ("non-obstructive") dilatation need additional imaging, particularly for deciding on surgery and for pre-operative anatomic assessment. US offers a non-invasive method for frequent follow-ups, but remains restricted in terms of functional assessment – therefore diuretic scintigraphy, at present, remains the standard investigation for grading and follow-up of obstruction; usually the decision for surgery is based on these findings (Fig. 83.3c). Increasingly, functional diuretic dynamic MRU is used for a combined approach to assess anatomy and function (Fig. 83.3d–h).

Another common paediatric condition is *urinary tract infection (UTI)*. Today, imaging increasingly focuses on differentiation of upper versus lower UTI, which clinically—particularly in infants—can be difficult. Potentially associated UT malformations need to be evaluated, but often these conditions have already been diagnosed by various screening programs.

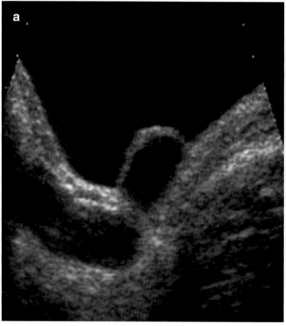
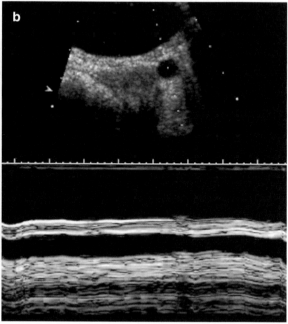

Fig. 83.2 US in megaureter. (**a**) US image of an ureterocele (using an 8 MHz curved linear array and harmonic imaging) protruding into the bladder at the ostium, with its corresponding distal megaureter (parasagittal section, slightly oblique).

(**b**) Cross section of a dilated distal left ureter behind the bladder in an infant using an 8 MHz curved linear array and harmonic imaging, with a motion-mode trace documenting lack of ureteral peristalsis

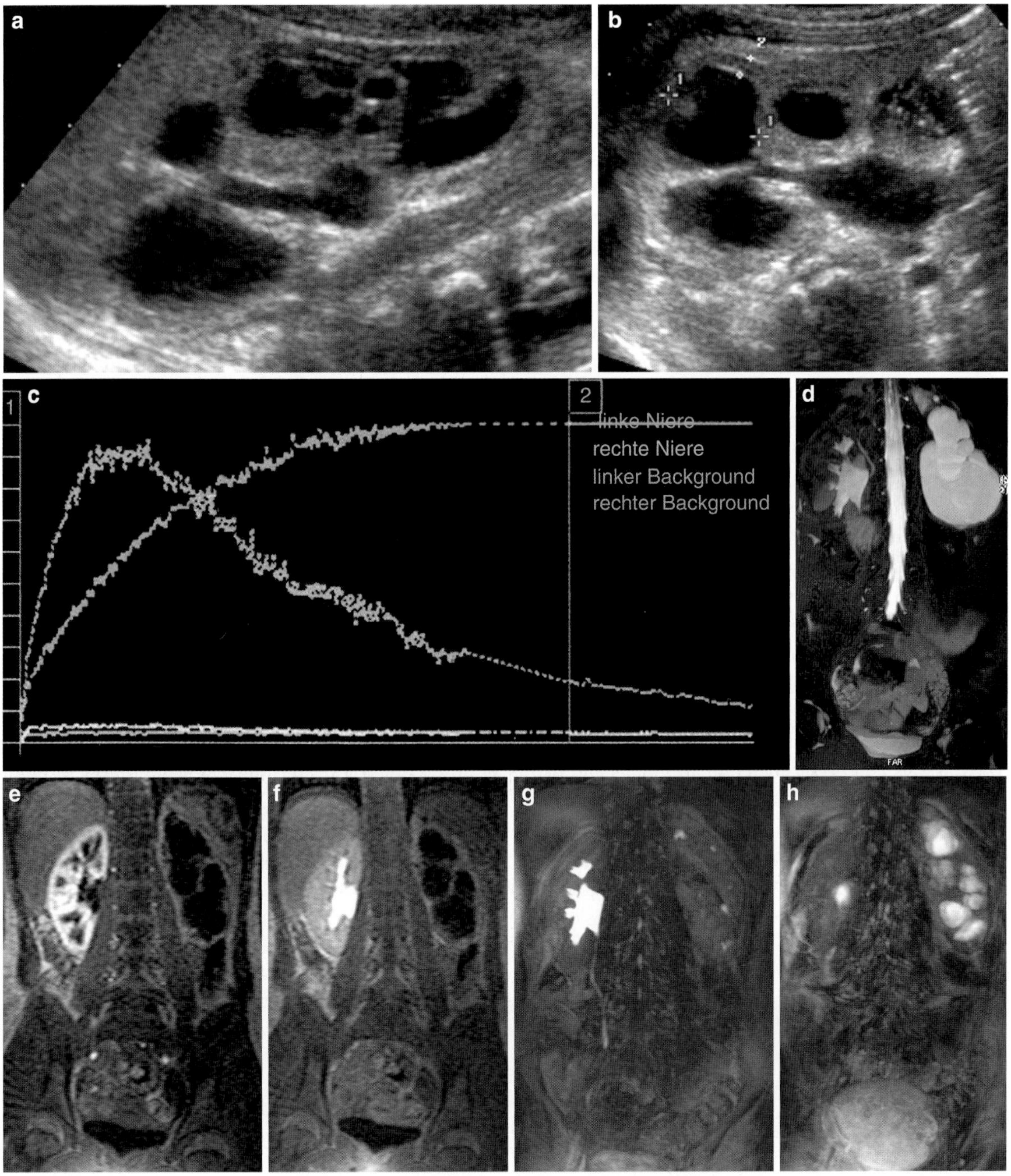

Fig. 83.3 Imaging in obstructive uropathy. (**a**, **b**) Typical US image of a pelvi-ureteric junction obstruction, with gross hydronephrosis, dilated calices (+ + 1) and parenchymal narrowing (+ + 2), in longitudinal (**a**) and axial (**b**) section using an 8 MHz curved linear array with harmonic imaging in an infant. (**c**) MAG3 dynamic diuretic renography showing the asymmetrically deteriorated drainage of the affected kidney (red line) in a decompensated pelvi-ureteric junction obstruction. (**d–h**) MRU in pelvi-ureteric junction obstruction: the T2-weighted "water image" shows the gross hydronephrosis with malrotated pelvocaliceal system on the left side (**d**). The serial T1 weighted gadolinium enhanced images show asymmetric uptake (**e**), asymmetric excretion (**f**), asymmetric diuretic response (**f**, 3d reconstructed image), and delayed excretion of contrast urine into the dilated left collecting system without sufficient urinary drainage (**h**, 3d-reconstruction)

The importance of bladder function disturbances is increasingly recognised; therefore—particularly in older girls—bladder function assessment constitutes an essential part of the work-up after UTI.

Again, US forms the mainstay of initial imaging allowing for assessment of UT anomalies, and using a supplementing aCDS enables a reliable assessment of renal involvement in UTI. Typical US criteria for (acute) pyelonephritis (aPN) are: enlarged kidney, focal or diffuse parenchymal changes, increased echogenicity of the perirenal sinus and thickening of the pelvic-, ureteral- and bladder wall (Fig. 83.4a). There may be echoes within the urine. Furthermore, focal or diffuse, particularly asymmetric perfusion or vascularity disturbances caused by inflammatory oedema, vascular compression or necrosis or scars can be reliably visualised by an aCDS (Fig. 83.4b). In patients with ambiguous, equivocal or inconsistent findings as well as in situations where aCDS is not available or of suboptimal quality, static DMSA scintigraphy is considered the gold standard for assessment of suspected aPN (Fig. 83.4c). CT and increasingly, MRT are used for evaluation of complications such as abscess formation, XPN, renal tuberculosis, as well as for differential diagnosis in sonographically unclear lesions such as complicated, infected cysts or tumours. VUR assessment is considered in all infants and in all patients with renal involvement or renal scarring.

Haematuria is a relatively rare event in childhood. There are a number of causes, most of them constituting a nephrologic problem such as glomerulonephritis or UTI including haemorrhagic cystitis. However, other severe UT conditions may also manifest with macroscopic haematuria such as haemolytic uraemic syndrome, renal vein thrombosis, or bladder and kidney tumours. Furthermore, conditions such as stress haematuria, retro-aortal left renal vein with nutcracker syndrome, idiopathic familiar microscopic haematuria, and haematuria associated with refluxing or even obstructing uropathy may also cause (microscopic) haematuria; renal infarction is an extremely rare event in children. In all these conditions, a comprehensive abdominal US including aCDS is indicated as the first imaging study to supplement urine (erythrocyte) microscopy and laboratory findings and often helps in the differential diagnosis.

If (macroscopic) haematuria is associated with flank pain or dysuria or even abdominal colics, ***urolithiasis*** must be considered. Ultrasound is the first imaging study allowing assessment of the collecting system and the renal parenchyma that may exhibit signs of nephrocalcinosis and other underlying nephropathies, or show different entities that need to be considered for differential diagnosis, for example, bleeding renal or bladder tumours such as large angiomyolipoma or rhabdomyosarcoma. Particularly, for detection of distal ureteral calculi a sufficiently filled bladder and a detailed study of the distal ureters are mandatory. CDS may be helpful by demonstrating the ureteric bladder inflow, enabling a differentiation of asymmetric urine inflow or complete obstruction (Fig. 83.5a, b). Furthermore, the "twinkling sign" may improve detection of even small calculi in poorly distended distal ureters (Fig. 83.5c). In the acutely obstructed kidney, US usually exhibits only little dilatation; the parenchyma is echogenic, and the kidney itself appears enlarged and swollen. Doppler

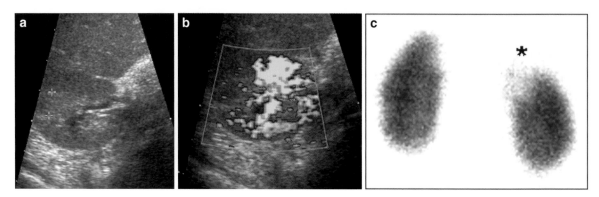

Fig. 83.4 Imaging in acute UTI. (**a**) Cross section with a 8 MHz curved array transducer in a child with febrile UTI demonstrating an area of increased parenchymal echogenicity and reduced corticomedullary differentiation (+ +), consistent with focal renal involvement. (**b**) Amplitude coded colour Doppler sonography (= power Doppler) in the same child depicts a focal perfusion defect at the site of the parenchymal abnormality, confirming renal segmental involvement in acute pyelonephritis. (**c**) Static renal DMSA scintigraphy in UTI, posterior acquisition, showing a photopenic defect in the upper pole (*) in a different child with acute pyelonephritis

flow profiles may demonstrate an asymmetrically elevated resistance index. The calculi themselves are echogenic, though blood clots and mixed concrements with low calcium content may also appear less echogenic and produce less shadowing, whereas intraluminal fungus may appear similar to a calculus (i.e., very echogenic, with some dorsal shadowing). In cases with ureteral obstruction, the PUJ often is wide open, the proximal ureter is dilated and thus can be followed to the level of the obstruction (Fig. 83.6a–c). Sometimes differentiation of papillary or wall calcifications from intraluminal concrements may be difficult—in these cases positioning manoeuvres that demonstrate floating of concrements may be helpful. Note that other sedimentations in the papillae or the distal tubules may also cause similar appearances and twinkling artefacts such as in nephrocalcinosis or the physiologic hyperechoic medullae and papillae of neonates.

In many cases, US supplemented by a KUB-film is sufficient for diagnosis (Fig. 83.6d). In some instances, particularly for planning lithotripsy, an adapted IVU may become necessary, for example for differentiation of a duplex system or assessment of multiple ureteral calculi (Fig. 83.6e, f). CT has become the major imaging method in adults with urolithiasis, but, at present, is still used reluctantly in children due to its radiation burden. Only some rare conditions such as prolonged complicated stone disease with infection, XPN or renal tumours with calcifications, as well as gross or complicated nephrolithiasis in an underlying problem as well as acute or traumatic haemorrhage, contrast-enhanced spiral CT may become indicated (Fig. 83.7a–c).

Kidney and bladder tumours are rare but important entities that only in part, manifest clinically. They often are detected incidentally when doing an US for various unspecific symptoms such as abdominal pain, haematuria, increased blood pressure or follow-up in various syndromes that are associated with a higher risk for renal tumours. The task of imaging is to detect and confirm the tumour, to try to give some information on the tumour entity, to properly stage the tumour and search for metastasis, to give the preoperatively necessary anatomic-topographic information and eventually, to monitor the patients for follow-up during and after treatment. US usually is the initial investigation, and it detects or confirms the tumour. MRT, at present, is basically propagated for assessment of bladder and kidney tumours. CT may become necessary for a thorough work-up, particularly concerning lung metastases or suspected calcifications (differential diagnoses versus e.g., neuroblastoma …), as well as in situations where (paediatric) MRT is not available.

In children, every *renal cyst* or *renal polycystic disease* should prompt a thorough family assessment and at least one follow-up examination. Basically, US is the primary investigation of choice in renal cysts which are usually diagnosed and followed by US. For a complete diagnostic work-up, a range of modalities may become necessary, including plain film, CT or MRT and scintigraphy, depending on the underlying setting, the clinical suspicion and method availability. Note that microcysts may remain invisible to imaging, just altering the (US) appearance of the renal parenchyma. Every complicated cyst or every undefined cystic

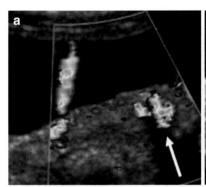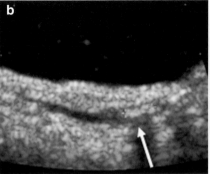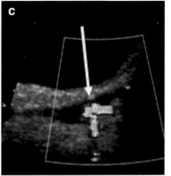

Fig. 83.5 Imaging in haematuria. (**a**) Colour Doppler sonography demonstrates the asymmetric urine inflow into the urinary bladder from the right ostium, and the twinkling colour signals at the area of the left ostium/left transmural ureter deriving from an ostial calculus (=>). (**b**) Longitudinal section of the distal ureter (curved array, harmonic imaging, 8 MHZ) in an infant with haematuria and hypercalcuria demonstrates a distal ureteral calculus (++), with dorsal shadowing (=>). (**c**) Same child, at maximum of peristaltic wave, with better dilated ureter, where the calculus exhibits twinkling signals on CDS (= "twinkling sign")

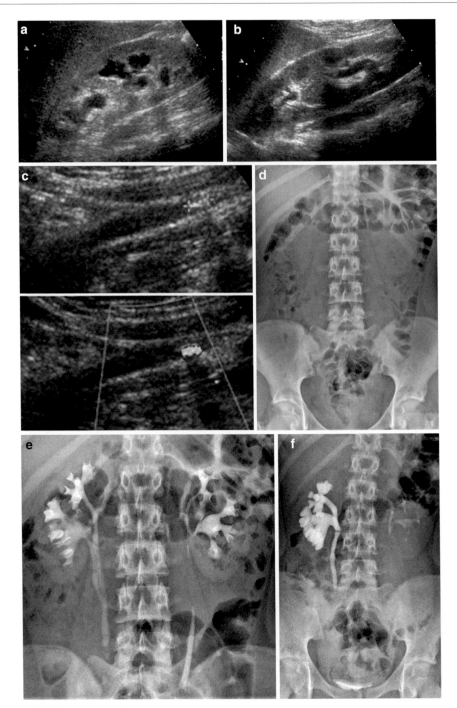

Fig. 83.6 Imaging in infants and children with urolithiasis. (a–c) US images pelvo-caliceal dilatation (a), an echogenic pelvic wall with indirect signs for a duplex system such as a central "parenchymal bridge" (b), and a calculus in the mid ureter (+ +) that exhibits the twinkling sign on CDS. (c) (d–f) KUB film (d) and adapted IVU using just two films for assessment of anatomy and drainage in the same girl as Fig 83.6 a–c with ureteral urolithiasis and suspected duplex system for planning shock wave lithotripsy (e = 15 min after contrast, f = 60 min after i.v. contrast)

disease (particularly if cyst size or number increases) must be investigated by additional sectional imaging such as CM-enhanced spiral CT or MRU.

Abdominal and urogenital trauma is relatively rare in children. Depending on the severity of trauma as well as the trauma mechanism and impact, different imaging

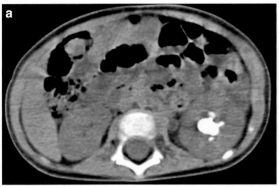
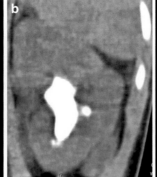
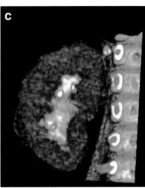

Fig. 83.7 Low dose unenhanced spiral multi-slice CT (adapted paediatric protocol). (**a–c**) Multi-slice CT (**a**) with sagittal reconstruction (**b**) and volume rendering (**c**) in an infant with a large concrement that filled the entire collecting system, performed for therapy planning (i.e., additional parenchymal calcifications that would obviate lithotripsy)

approaches are advocated. In mild trauma as well as after renal biopsy, a comprehensive US study may suffice with a mandatory follow-up after 12–24 h (Fig. 83.8a). In severe or multiple traumas, the role of US is restricted to the "one minute examination" in the emergency room used to check for free fluid; all other imaging is then achieved by contrast-enhanced multi-detector spiral CT. This approach grants a quick and reliable imaging of all necessary aspects (not only the kidney and ureter, but also other abdominal parenchymal organs, the spine, the major vessels and thorax, etc.) as necessary for proper patient management and decision making, particularly as a conservative approach is increasingly advocated. It also allows for detailed grading of the injury. In cases with suspected bladder injuries or ureteral as well as urethral tears, dedicated additional imaging should be performed such as fluoroscopic- or CT-cystography (complete filling of bladder essential) and retrograde or antegrade urethra- and ureterography.

Pre-operative imaging is outlined by the diagnostic imaging work-up of the various conditions discussed above. In order to enable an efficient use of imaging, a profound communication should be established between all physicians and specialties involved. For example, a PUJO has been diagnosed by US. Diuretic scintigraphy has shown decompensated obstruction with asymmetrically reduced renal function of the affected kidney. If any additional imaging is needed, the important questions to answer are: *Is there a duplex system? Is there VUR? Is there any vascular anomaly that may be associated with the UPJO or might pose a peri-operative risk?* In this situation, pre-operative imaging consists of VCUG, MRU with an included MR-Angiography sequence for the delineation of the exact anatomy of the collecting system, assessment of a potential duplex system and of renal vascular supply; IVU is not suitable to answer all these questions, and ee-US may miss short lasting VUR into a non-dilated ureter.

Usually, US is sufficient for post-operative and post-interventional monitoring (Fig. 83.8a–d). However, more intense *post-operative imaging* may become necessary in cases with a complicated post-operative course, as US may be restricted in reliably answering all management relevant function-related questions. Therefore, antegade pyelography (e.g., after pyeloplasty, using the peri-operatively placed drain) may be helpful; some centres even regularly perform an antegrade pyelogram as part of the assessment before drain removal. If no drain is in place (such as in patients after anti-reflux procedures), an adapted IVU (potentially only consisting of two delayed films) or scintigraphy may answer the question (Fig. 83.8e–g). Seldom may other imaging such as MRT or VCUG become necessary in the post-operative setting, except for rare cases after tumour- or trauma surgery.

83.4 Imaging Algorithms

In order to standardise the imaging procedures, to allow for comparison during follow-up, enable a reliable work-up even after working hours and grant some basic quality at reasonable costs as imaging algorithms are increasingly becoming important. They try to enable an effective use of the various modalities without increasing the risk of missing important conditions that would need urgent treatment. The European Society of Uroradiology as well as The European Society of Paediatric Radiology are engaged

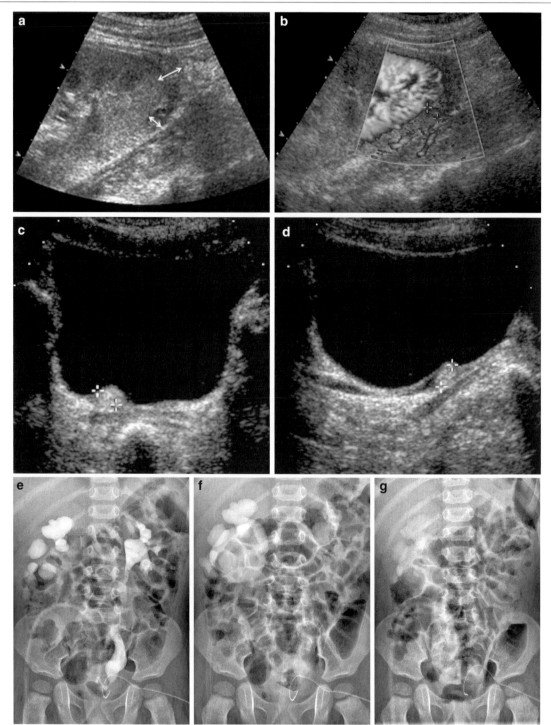

Fig. 83.8 Postoperative imaging. (**a**, **b**) Longitudinal US image of a perirenal/subcapsular haematoma at the lower pole of the left kidney in a patient after renal biopsy, much clearer visible using aCDS (+ +) than just on plain grey scale US (↔) (**c**, **d**) US after macroblast® injection for cystoscopic VUR treatment: note the echogenic deposit (+ +) at the left transmural distal ureter/ostium (**c**), with slight ureteral dilatation (**d**). (**e–g**) Adapted IVU after ureteral re-implantation and closure of a cutaneous ureterostoma in an infant with obstructive megaureter who sonographically exhibited gross dilatation with asymmetrically elevated resistance indices postoperatively. A series of three films demonstrates the partial obstruction after 20 min (**e**) and after Furosemide application (**f**), but sufficient clearance as response to gravitation after upright positioning (**g**) obviating intervention

in developing specific paediatric imaging recommendations for common queries related to neonatal HN, obstructive uropathy in childhood or imaging in UTI. They furthermore are issuing procedural guidelines that define a basic minimum standard for the various modalities used in paediatric uroradiology. These recommendations try to take specific paediatric considerations and growth variations into account (as the probability of various diseases as well as management approaches may differ depending on sex and age), and address radiation protection issues, as children are far more sensitive to ionising radiation than adults and need utmost radiation protection.

For example, the *imaging algorithm in UTI in childhood* shows slight differences for girls and boys (VCUG versus ce-VUS) and for infants versus older patients, where bladder function studies become very important while the need for VUR assessment constantly decreases (Table 83.3). The *imaging algorithm for neonatal HN* is strategised according to the amount of dilatation on prenatal US as well as the findings on the first post-natal examination (Table 83.4).

Note that all imaging recommendations and algorithms constitute a basic general minimum consensus; individual adaptation to the specific patient's condition as well as adjustment of the algorithms according to local facilities and availability and expertise remain essential. Furthermore, these recommendations need constant updating because,

Table 83.3 Flowchart "Imaging algorithm in UTI in infants and children" (Adapted from Riccabona et al., Pediatr Radiol 2008, 38: 138–145)

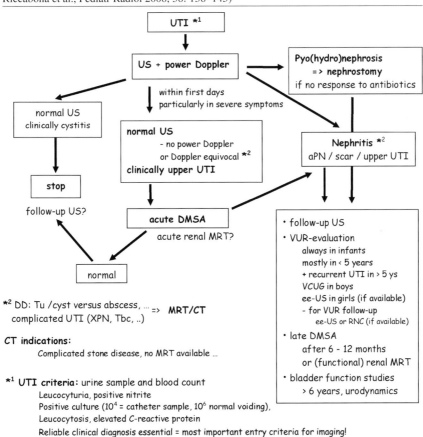

Suggested imaging algorithm in children with UTI

aPN = acute pyelonephritis, DMSA = static renal scintigraphy, ee-US = echo-enhanced urosonography, RNC = radionuclide cystography, Tbc = tuberculosis, Tu = tumour, US = ultrasound, UTI = urinary tract infection, VCUG = voiding cystourethrography, VUR = vesico-ureteral reflux, XPN = xanthogranulomatuous pyelonephritis

Table 83.4 Flowchart "Imaging in neonates with antenatal diagnosis of mild to moderate HN" (Adapted from Riccabona M, Fotter R, 2004, Reorientation and future trends in paediatric uroradiology: Minutes of a symposium. Pediatr Radiol 34, 295–301)

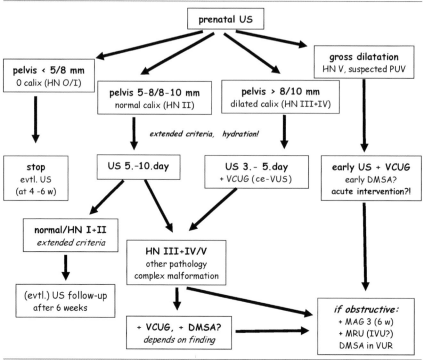

Suggested imaging algorithm in neonates with prenatally diagnosed mild to moderate HN: DMSA = static renal scintigraphy, HN = hydronephrosis, IVU = intravenous urography, MAG3 = dynamic renography, MRU = MR-Urography, PUV = posterior urethral valve, US = ultrasound, UT = urinary tract, VCUG = voiding cystourethrography, VUR = vesico-ureteral reflux

impact on management strategies are brought about not only by imaging techniques and potential changes, but also by new insights into pathophysiology and natural history of certain conditions, thereby inducing altered imaging requirement.

Abbreviations

(a)CDS	(amplitude coded) Colour Doppler sonography
(a)PN	(acute) Pyelonephritis
CM	Contrast media
CT	Computed tomography
DMSA	Dimercaptosuccinic acid
ee	Echo-enhanced
ee-US	Echo-enhanced ultrasound
ce-VUS	Contrast enhanced voiding urosonography
HN	Hydronephrosis
IVU	Intravenous urography
KUB	Kidney – ureter – bladder abdominal film
MAG3	Dynamic renal scintigraphy
MRT	Magnetic resonance tomography
MRU	Magnetic resonance urography
MU	Megaureter
PCN	Percutaneous nephrostomy
PUJ(O)	Pelvi-ureteral junction (obstruction)
PUV	Posterior urethral valve
RNC	Radionuclide cystography
Tbc	Tuberculosis
Tu	Tumour
UG(T)	Urogenital (tract)
US	Ultrasound
UT	Urinary tract
UTI	Urinary tract infection
UVJ(O)	Uretero-vesical junction (obstruction)
VCUG	Voiding cystourethrography
VUR	Vesico-ureteral reflux
XPN	Xanthogranulomatous pyelonephritis

Further Reading

Fotter R (2001) Pediatric uroradiology. Springer, Berlin, Heidelberg, New York

Gordon I, Riccabona M (2003) Investigating the newborn kidney update on imaging techniques. Semin Neonatol 8:269–278

Kao SC (2005) The urinary tract. In H Carty, F Brunelle, D Stringer, SC Kao (eds) Imaging Children, 2nd edn. Elsevier Science, New York, pp 537–882

Puri P, Höllwarth M (2006) Pediatric Surgery. Springer, Berlin, Heidelberg

Riccabona M (ed.) Paediatric Uroradiology. Elsevier, (2002)

Riccabona M, Fotter R (2006) Radiographic studies in children with kidney disorders: What to do and when. In R Hogg (ed) Kidney Disorders in Children and Adolescents. Taylor & Francis, Birmingham, pp 15–34

Riccabona M, Avni FE, Blickman JG et al (2008) Imaging recommendations in paediatric uroradiology: Minutes of the ESPR workgroup session on urinary tract infection, fetal hydronephrosis, urinary tract ultrasonography and voiding cystourethrography ESPR-meeting, Barcelona/Spain, June 2007. ESUR Paediatric guideline subcommittee and ESPR paediatric uroradiology work group. Pediatr Radiol 38:138–145

Management of Prenatal Hydronephrosis

84

Jack S. Elder

Contents

84.1 Introduction

An abnormality involving the genitourinary tract is detected in 1 in 50 to 1 in 100 pregnancies, depending on the sonographic criteria. The goal of management is to recognize and treat congenital anomalies that may adversely affect renal function or cause urinary infection or sepsis. Most structural abnormalities of the urinary tract are characterized by hydronephrosis, which generally is assumed to be obstructive. However, hydronephrosis is not often caused by obstruction; examples include vesicoureteral reflux, multicystic kidney, and certain abnormalities of the ureteropelvic and ureterovesical junction.

84.2 Development of the Kidney and Renal Function

The kidney is derived from the ureteral bud and the metanephric blastema. During the 5th week of gestation, the ureteral bud arises from the mesonephric (Wolffian) duct and penetrates the metanephric blastema, which is an area of undifferentiated mesenchyme on the nephrogenic ridge. The ureteral bud undergoes a series of approximately 15 generations of divisions, and by 20 weeks' gestation forms the entire collecting system, that is, the ureter, renal pelvis, calyces, papillary ducts, and collecting tubules. Under the inductive influence of the ureteral bud, nephron differentiation begins during the 7th week of gestation. By 20 weeks of gestation, when the collecting system is completely developed, approximately one third of the nephrons are present. Nephrogenesis continues at a nearly exponential rate and is completed by 36 weeks' gestation.

P. Puri and M. Höllwarth (eds.), *Pediatric Surgery: Diagnosis and Management*,
DOI: 10.1007/978-3-540-69560-8_84, © Springer-Verlag Berlin Heidelberg 2009

Throughout gestation, the placenta functions as the fetal hemodialyzer, and the fetal kidneys play a minor role in the maintenance of fetal salt and water homeostasis. Formation of urine begins between the 5th and 9th weeks of gestation. The rate of urine production increases throughout gestation, and at term, volumes have been reported to be 51 mL/h. The glomerular filtration rate (GFR) has been measured at 6 mL/min/1.73 at the 28th week of gestation, increasing to 25 mL/min/1.73 at term, and thereafter triples by the age of 3 months. The main factors responsible for this increase in GFR include an increase in the capillary surface area available for filtration, changes in intrarenal vascular resistance, and redistribution of renal blood flow to the cortical nephrons, in which most nephrons are located. A congenital obstructive lesion of the urinary tract may have a deleterious effect on renal function. Severe obstructive uropathy results in renal dysplasia.

84.3 Management of the Fetus with Antenatal Hydronephrosis

When a fetus is identified with a suspected urinary tract abnormality, the goals of management include determining the differential diagnosis, assessment of associated anomalies, and determining the fetal and postnatal risk of the anomaly.

Hydronephrosis is recognized by demonstrating a dilated renal pelvis and calyces. The ureter and bladder may also be dilated. The likelihood of having a significant urinary tract abnormality is directly proportional to the severity of hydronephrosis. In one of the series in which the renal pelvic diameter was more than 2 cm, 94% had a significant abnormality of the urinary tract requiring surgery or long-term urologic follow-up. Of patients whose maximal renal pelvic size was between 1.0 cm and 1.5 cm, 50% had an abnormality, and of patients whose dilated renal pelvis was less than 1 cm, only 3% had a significant abnormality. More recent studies have confirmed the 3% risk of having a significant obstructive uropathy if the fetus has minimal renal pelvic dilation. Currently a renal pelvic diameter of at least 4 mm before 33 weeks of gestation and at least 7 mm after 33 weeks of gestation is considered significant. The later the sonogram is performed, the more likely an existing abnormality will be detected, because the obstructed

renal pelvis gradually enlarges throughout gestation. Moreover, in utero, the fetus is usually upside-down and urine drains uphill. For example, Fugelseth and colleagues reported that only one third of a series of women carrying babies with a urologic anomaly had an abnormal ultrasound study at 15–21 weeks' gestation.

The differential diagnosis of antenatal hydronephrosis is provided in Table 84.1. Virtually all these conditions can cause bilateral hydronephrosis. A distended bladder is suggestive of bladder outlet obstruction, such as posterior urethral valves or a large ectopic ureterocele, but fetuses with high-grade vesicoureteral reflux or prune belly syndrome may also have bilateral hydronephrosis with a distended bladder.

In fetuses with a urologic anomaly, associated abnormalities are common. For example, in one series of fetuses with bilateral hydronephrosis and oligohydramnios, 16 of 31 (55%) had an associated structural or chromosomal abnormality. Congenital heart disease and neurologic deformities can often be detected, if they are present. In contrast, large bowel abnormalities, such as imperforate anus, are more difficult to detect by prenatal sonography, but recognition of small bowel anomalies, such as atresia, is usually straightforward.

The main considerations in determining fetal management include overall fetal well-being, gestational age, whether the hydronephrosis is unilateral or bilateral, and the volume of amniotic fluid. There are no guidelines for determining how frequently to image the fetus or whether specific intervention is necessary. If the hydronephrosis is unilateral, usually no specific fetal therapy is necessary.

Table 84.1 Causes of antenatal hydronephrosis

Anomalous UPJ/UPJ obstruction[a]
Multicystic kidney[a]
Retrocaval ureter
Primary obstructive megaureter[a]
Nonrefluxing nonobstructed megaureter[a]
Vesicoureteral reflux[a,b]
Midureteral stricture[a]
Ectopic ureterocele[a,b]
Ectopic ureter[a]
Posterior urethral valves[a,b]
Prune belly syndrome[a,b]
Urethral atresia[b]
Hydrocolpos[a,b]
Pelvic tumor[a,b]
Cloacal abnormality[a,b]

[a]May be unilateral or bilateral

[b]Bladder may be distended

For example, if the hydronephrosis is secondary to an ureteropelvic junction (UPJ) obstruction, even if the function is poor, the kidney has a significant capacity for improvement in function following neonatal pyeloplasty. Even with bilateral UPJ obstruction (characterized by bilateral hydronephrosis and a normal bladder), the amniotic fluid volume and pulmonary development are typically normal. Consequently, specific intervention, such as percutaneous drainage of the fetal kidney or early delivery to allow immediate urologic surgery, is unwarranted. These same principles apply to primary obstructive megaureter.

The primary life-threatening congenital urologic anomalies include posterior urethral valves, urethral atresia, and prune belly syndrome, which are usually characterized by bilateral hydroureteronephrosis and a distended bladder that does not empty in a male fetus. Approximately one third of infants with urethral valves eventually develop renal insufficiency or end-stage renal disease. Although prune belly syndrome is considered nonobstructive, neonates with this condition frequently have renal insufficiency. Urethral atresia is nearly always fatal, because the kidneys usually are dysplastic. A severe adverse prognostic factor is oligohydramnios, which prevents normal pulmonary development. In fetuses with severe obstructive uropathy and renal dysplasia, neonatal demise usually results from pulmonary hypoplasia rather than chronic renal failure.

Intuitively, it would seem that treatment of the obstructed fetal urinary tract by diverting the urine into the empty amniotic space might allow normal renal development to occur and restore amniotic fluid dynamics, stimulating lung development. Indeed, experimental procedures have been performed, including percutaneous placement of a vesicoamniotic shunt, creation of a fetal vesicostomy or pyelostomy, and even percutaneous urethral valve ablation through a miniscope. Unfortunately, the complication rate is high, including shunt migration, urinary ascites, stimulation of preterm labor, and chorioamnionitis. Furthermore, in most cases, irreversible renal dysplasia has already occurred, and although the procedure may be successful technically, often the baby is stillborn, dies of pulmonary hypoplasia, or is alive with end-stage renal disease. Nevertheless, some fetuses may benefit from aggressive intervention if the kidneys do not have irreversible dysplasia. Unfavorable prognostic factors include:

1. Prolonged oligohydramnios
2. Renal cortical cysts

3. Urinary Na > 100 mEq/L; Cl > 90 mEq/L; and osmolarity > 210 mOsm/L
4. B2-microglobulin > 6 mg/l
5. Reduced lung area and thoracic or abdominal circumference

Unfavorable urinary electrolytes may reflect stale urine in the fetal urinary tract. Obtaining one or two more samples every 2–3 days will yield fetal urine that is more reflective of true fetal renal function.

84.4 Management of the Newborn with Antenatal Hydronephrosis

84.4.1 Management in the Nursery

At birth, the abdomen is inspected to detect the presence of a mass, which most often is secondary to a multicystic dysplastic kidney or UPJ obstruction. In male newborn infants with posterior urethral valves, often a walnut-shaped mass, representing the bladder, is palpable just superior to the pubic symphysis. Newborn infants should also be evaluated for anomalies involving other organ systems. Renal function should be monitored with serial serum creatinine levels, particularly in infants with bilateral hydronephrosis. At birth, the serum creatinine level is identical to that of the mother's, but by the age of 1 week, the creatinine should decrease to 0.4 mg/dL. The exception is premature infants, in whom the creatinine may not decrease until these children reach 34–35 weeks of conceptional age because of the immaturity of renal function before that age.

Neonates with hydronephrosis are at risk of urinary tract infections (UTIs) and should be placed on antibiotic prophylaxis with either amoxicillin 50 mg per day or cephalexin 50 mg per day. At 2 months, the prophylaxis usually is changed to trimethoprim-sulfamethoxazole. In addition, circumcision should be considered in male neonates to minimize the likelihood of urinary tract infection.

84.4.2 Initial Radiologic Evaluation

Radiologic evaluation should be performed before infants are discharged to delineate the abnormality responsible for changes on prenatal sonography. Serial renal sonograms, a voiding cystourethrogram (VCUG), and a diuretic renogram, or excretory urogram (IVP) usually provide the diagnostic information necessary to guide management.

84.4.2.1 Renal Ultrasound

A renal and bladder sonogram should be obtained first. Typically this study is obtained shortly after delivery or the following day; however, because neonates normally have transient oliguria, a dilated or obstructed collecting system may appear normal for the first 24–48 h of life (Fig. 84.1). Ideally, if unilateral hydronephrosis

was present prenatally, the renal sonogram should not be obtained until 72 h to maximize its sensitivity; but with mothers being discharged within 24–48 h of delivery, it seems impractical to have the baby brought back to the hospital after discharge for sonography.

Renal length, degree of caliectasis and parenchymal thickness, and presence or absence of ureteral dilation should be assessed. The severity of hydronephrosis should be graded from 1 to 4 using the Society for Fetal Urology (SFU) grading scale (Table 84.2). Most significant urologic anomalies are associated with higher grades of hydronephrosis. In one report of 464 infants with 582 prenatally detected hydronephrotic kidneys, 80% of the patients who underwent surgical correction of a structural abnormality of the upper urinary tract had grade 3 or 4 hydronephrosis. More sophisticated analyses, such as the ultrasound renal resistive index, as well as urinary studies have been assessed, but efforts to demonstrate obstruction have been inconsistent.

The degree of pelvocaliectasis correlates closely with the likelihood that a significant urological condition is present. Lee et al. performed a meta-analysis of reports of antenatal hydronephrosis and determined that the risk of finding postnatal pathology was 11.9% with mild antenatal hydronephrosis, 45.1% for moderate, and 88.3% for severe antenatal hydronephrosis.

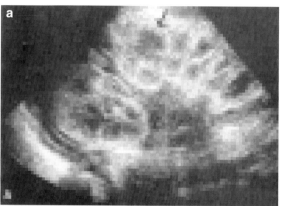

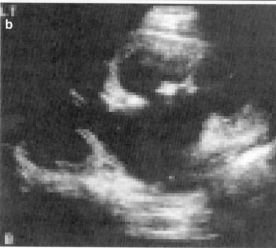

Fig. 84.1 (a) Ultrasound of left kidney taken shortly after birth. Normal study. Echolucent areas (*arrow*) in renal cortex are pyramids (normal finding). (b) Same patient. Ultrasound of left kidney at 6 weeks shows grade 4 hydronephrosis

Table 84.2 Grading of hydronephrosis

Grade of Hydrone-phrosis	Renal Image	
	Central renal complex	Renal parenchymal thickness
0	Intact	Normal
1	Slight splitting	Normal
2	Evident splitting, complex confined within renal border	Normal
3	Wide splitting pelvis dilated outside renal border; calyces uniformly dilated	Normal
4	Further dilatation of pelvis and calyces (calyces may appear convex)	Thin

Their definitions of mild, moderate, and severe hydronephrosis depended on gestational age at the time of diagnosis. Similarly, Sidhu et al. performed a meta-analysis and found that when postnatal hydronephrosis was SFU grade 1 or 2, there was stabilization or resolution of pelviectasis in 98% cases, whereas when there was SFU grade 3 or 4, there was stabilization or resolution in 51% cases.

The bladder should be imaged to detect a dilated posterior urethra (urethral valves), bladder wall thickening, ureteral dilation, inadequate bladder emptying, or a ureterocele. Perineal sonography may demonstrate a dilated prostatic urethra, which is consistent with posterior urethral valves.

84.4.2.2 Voiding Cystourethrogram (VCUG)

Next, a VCUG should be performed. This study may demonstrate vesicoureteral reflux, posterior urethral valves, or a bladder diverticulum. A radiographic cystogram is preferred over a radionuclide cystogram because the latter does not provide sufficient delineation of bladder and urethral anatomy and because reflux, if present, cannot be graded.

84.4.2.3 What if the Initial Sonogram Is Normal?

A common dilemma is whether a full evaluation is necessary if the initial renal sonogram is normal. Assuming that a significant degree of fetal renal pelvic dilatation (i.e., 4 mm anteroposterior pelvic diameter <33 w, 7 mm diameter after 33 w) was present, the child may have vesicoureteral reflux. For example, in one series, 17 of 42 (40%) infants with prenatally diagnosed reflux had mild antenatal renal pelvic dilation as the only sign of a urinary tract abnormality. Out of 982 children referred for treatment of antenatal hydronephrosis, among 255 renal units with reflux, the postnatal sonogram was normal in 177 (70%). Furthermore, in children with dilating grades of reflux, renal sonography is often normal. For example, Blane and colleagues reported that 12% of children with grade V, 31% with grade IV, and 80% with grade III reflux had a normal renal sonogram. Because reflux may cause intermittent renal pelvic dilation, theoretically these babies may have reflux; and early diagnosis and medical treatment of reflux may reduce the likelihood of developing reflux nephropathy. On the other hand, others have advocated performing a VCUG only if the postnatal sonogram was abnormal; however, in these reports neonates with a normal postnatal renal sonogram were not systematically evaluated to determine the real incidence of reflux in this group. This author generally does not recommend performing a VCUG unless the postnatal renal sonogram is abnormal.

84.4.3 Follow-Up Evaluation and Treatment

If bilateral hydronephrosis or unilateral hydronephrosis is present in one kidney, then close monitoring of the serum creatinine and electrolytes is necessary. If the hydronephrosis is caused by posterior urethral valves, then valve ablation should be performed before discharge. If the hydronephrosis is secondary to vesicoureteral reflux, the infant should be placed on prophylaxis and managed as described later in this article. If the hydronephrosis is grade 3–4 and bilateral UPJ or ureterovesical junction obstruction is suspected, prompt evaluation with diuretic renography is indicated.

If unilateral hydronephrosis and a normal contralateral kidney are present, abnormalities in serum creatinine or electrolytes are uncommon. Nevertheless, these serum studies should be drawn to document that renal function is normal. Usually follow-up functional radiographic studies can be delayed until the age of 4–6 weeks, when renal function is more mature and studies of renal function and obstruction are more likely to be accurate.

Only when the sonogram and VCUG are normal, a follow-up sonogram in 6–8 weeks is necessary. In general, if hydronephrosis is discovered on the initial postnatal sonogram, pediatric urologic or nephrologic consultation is advisable to direct subsequent radiologic evaluation and plan therapy.

84.4.4 Diuretic Renogram

The diuretic renogram is used to determine whether upper urinary tract obstruction is present. In general, it is used to assess renal function and efficiency of drainage in kidneys with grade 3 and 4, and occasionally grade 2, hydronephrosis. In newborn infants or young infants, mercaptoacetyl triglycine (MAG-3) is generally used, as the images and computer analysis seem more accurate than with diethyenetriamine pentaacetic acid (DTPA). MAG-3 is primarily secreted by the renal tubules.

In a diuretic renogram, a small dose of a radiopharmaceutical is injected intravenously. During the first 2–3 min, renal parenchymal uptake is analyzed and compared, allowing computation of differential renal function. Subsequently, excretion is evaluated. After 20–30 min, furosemide is injected intravenously, and the rapidity and pattern of drainage from the kidneys to the bladder are analyzed. If no upper urinary tract obstruction is present, then normally half of the radionuclide is cleared from the renal pelvis within 10–15 min, termed the *T 1/2*. In the presence of significant upper tract obstruction, the T 1/2 is greater than 20 min. A T 1/2 between 15 and 20 min is indeterminate. The images generated usually provide an accurate assessment of the site of obstruction.

The renal scan is considered superior to the IVP in infants and children with hydronephrosis. Because of the relative immaturity of renal function in newborn infants, visualization of the collecting system on an IVP is often suboptimal. In addition, bowel gas further obscures the renal cortical outline and detail of the collecting system. Finally, the diuretic renogram is a better functional study by providing an objective assessment of the relative function of each kidney. The diuretic renogram may be unreliable, however, if certain important variables are not controlled.

Numerous variables affect the outcome of the diuretic renogram. For example, newborns's kidneys are functionally immature, and in some cases even normal kidneys may not demonstrate normal drainage following diuretic administration. Dehydration prolongs parenchymal transit and can blunt the diuretic response. Giving an insufficient dose of furosemide may result in inadequate drainage. If vesicoureteral reflux is present, continuous catheter drainage is mandatory to prevent radionuclide from refluxing from the bladder into the dilated upper tract, prolonging the washout phase.

Because of the limitations of the diuretic renogram in newborns with hydronephrosis, and because the methodology for performing diuretic renography varies substantially, the SFU and the Pediatric Nuclear Medicine Club jointly developed a standardized methodology for performing diuretic renograms in infants, termed a *well-tempered renogram*. Few institutions use this term at present, but the principles of the standardized protocol are used by most children's hospitals in the United States, although some disagreement remains regarding a few details of the study such as whether a urethral catheter is absolutely necessary.

84.4.5 Ancillary Studies

In most cases renal sonography, the VCUG and diuretic renogram provide sufficient information to establish a diagnosis and plan management. Particularly in complicated cases, however, cystoscopy with retrograde pyelography, computed tomography (CT) scan, antegrade pyelography, or a Whitaker antegrade perfusion test is necessary.

84.4.6 Congenital Anomalies Causing Antenatal Hydronephrosis

84.4.6.1 UPJ Obstruction or Anomalous UPJ

The most common cause of severe hydronephrosis without a dilated ureter or bladder in newborn infants is UPJ obstruction, which results from an intrinsic fibrotic narrowing at the junction between the ureter and renal pelvis (Fig. 84.2). At times an accessory artery to the lower pole of the kidney also causes extrinsic obstruction, but this finding is rare in newborns with hydronephrosis. In kidneys with a UPJ obstruction, renal function may be significantly impaired from pressure atrophy. The anomaly is corrected by performing a pyeloplasty, in which the stenotic segment is excised and the normal ureter and renal pelvis are reattached. Success rates are 91–98%.

Lesser degrees of UPJ narrowing may cause mild hydronephrosis, which is usually nonobstructive, and typically these kidneys function normally. The spectrum of UPJ abnormalities has been referred to as *anomalous UPJ*. Another cause of mild hydronephrosis is fetal folds of the upper ureter (Fig. 84.3), which are also nonobstructive.

Hydronephrosis in many newborns gradually diminishes or resolves over months or years. The goal of early evaluation is to determine whether a true anatomic obstruction, that should be corrected, is present or whether it is safe to follow the infant nonoperatively. Definition what constitutes obstructive and nonobstructive hydronephrosis is a constant source of debate in pediatric urology.

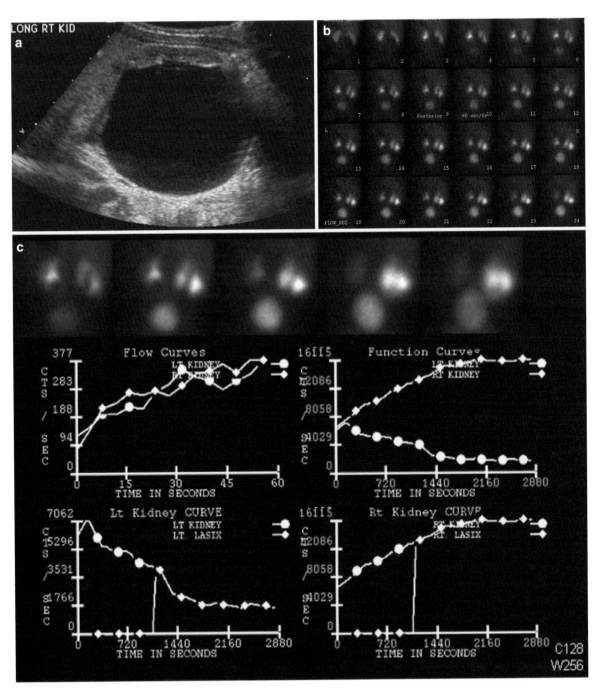

Fig. 84.2 (**a**) Ultrasound shows grade 4 hydronephrosis. (**b**) A 2-min image, diuretic renogram. The right kidney is on the right side of the image. Differential function left 67%, right 33% (normal, 50% each side). (**c**) Drainage curve following administration of furosemide shows obstructive pattern

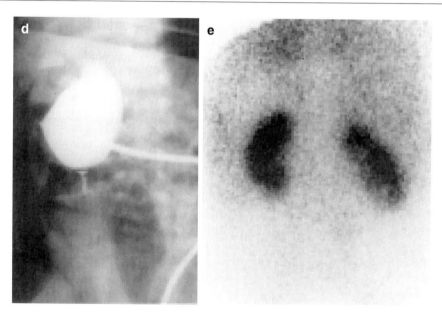

Fig. 84.2 (continued) (d), Patient underwent pyeloplasty at 2 months of age. Intraoperative antegrade pyelogram demonstrates ureteropelvic junction obstruction. (e and f) Diuretic renogram performed 7 months postoperatively shows 50% differential function in right kidney and normal drainage pattern

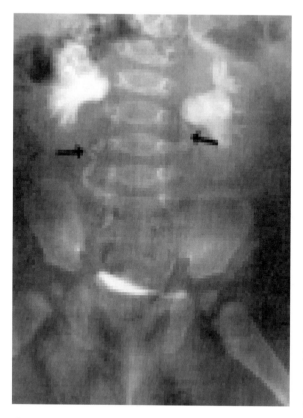

Fig. 84.3 Excretory urogram in infant with bilateral grade 2 hydronephrosis shows bilateral fetal folds of upper ureters (arrows). Note sharp calyces (normal)

Cartwright and colleagues studied 80 neonates with suspected UPJ obstruction. Of 39 with unilateral hydronephrosis and at least 35% differential renal function who were managed nonoperatively, only six (15%) later underwent pyeloplasty, primarily because of deteriorating differential renal function on renal scintigraphy. Following pyeloplasty, the differential renal function returned to its initial level in these patients. One might question whether early pyeloplasty in these patients would have allowed renal function to improve to 50% (normal). The remaining patients managed nonoperatively maintained differential function greater than 40%.

Koff and Campbell reported 104 consecutive neonates with unilateral hydronephrosis managed nonoperatively, with follow-up as long as 5 years. In follow-up, only seven (7%) underwent pyeloplasty because of reduction in differential renal function of more than 10% or progression of hydronephrosis. Pyeloplasty returned differential renal function to prepyeloplasty levels in all cases. Of 16 patients with significantly reduced renal function on initial scan and grade 4 hydronephrosis, rapid improvement was noted on follow-up diuretic renography in 15 and the washout curve became nonobstructive in six. In addition, hydronephrosis disappeared in six, improved in six, remained stable in three, and deteriorated in one. The physiology of the resolution or reduction in hydro-nephrosis and the improvement in differential renal function in these babies is unknown. In another more recent report from the same institution, of 19 newborns with bilateral grade 3 or 4 hydronephrosis, a total of 13 kidneys were subjected to pyeloplasty. Of those managed nonoperatively, 21 kidneys were grade 0–2 in 21 and grade 3 in 2 kidneys. The mean follow-up time to achieve maximum improvement in hydronephrosis was 10 months.

Although these studies suggest that it is safe or appropriate to manage neonates with a suspected UPJ obstruction nonoperatively, an infant's kidney has much greater capacity for improvement in differential renal function than an older child's. In addition, all of these studies base "differential renal function" on the uptake during the first 2–3 minutes of the study, and there is substantial variability in the way this percentage is calculated. Finally, these studies have not reported the pattern of washout on diuretic renography.

In a review of renal biopsies obtained at pyeloplasty at the author's institution, 63% showed minimal or no obstructive histologic changes; however, of those with differential function greater than 40%, 21% showed significant histopathologic changes, including reduced glomerular number, glomerular hyalinization, interstitial inflammation, and dysplastic glomeruli. Of the kidneys with a low differential function (less than 40%), 33% showed minimal or no histologic changes. Overall, in 25% of the patients the findings on renal biopsy did not correlate with the computed differential renal function and reflect the need for more sensitive markers of obstruction.

The approach of most pediatric urologists to neonates with a suspected UPJ obstruction is as follows. The hydronephrosis is graded from 1 to 4 using the SFU grading scale and a VCUG is obtained. Nearly all infants requiring pyeloplasty have grade 3 or 4 hydronephrosis. If a neonate has an abdominal mass from a hydronephrotic kidney, bilateral hydronephrosis, or a solitary kidney, a prompt "well-tempered" diuretic renogram is obtained. If signs of obstruction are apparent, prompt pyeloplasty is performed. Otherwise, the newborn is placed on amoxicillin 50 mg per day for prophylaxis, and the diuretic renogram is obtained at the age of 6 weeks. The study is not obtained right away in these cases because renal function in the newborn is immature. The GFR triples by 6 weeks, however, secondary to redistribution of intrarenal blood flow to the more populous cortical nephrons. If diuretic renography shows at least 35–40% differential renal function, and there is some drainage on the diuretic renogram, the child is managed nonoperatively, regardless of the drainage pattern (Fig. 84.4). At 2 months, prophylaxis is changed to trimethoprim-sulfamethoxazole suspension 1.25 mL per day. A follow-up well-tempered renogram is performed 3 months later. If there is deterioration in differential renal function or worsening of the diuretic washout curve, pyeloplasty is recommended; however, if these parameters remain stable or improved and the child does not develop a urinary tract infection, follow-up 3–6 months later with another diuretic renogram or an IVP is performed, and management is individualized. It is incumbent on clinicians caring for these infants to have a good understanding of the vagaries of the diuretic renogram and to monitor infants with a suspected UPJ obstruction

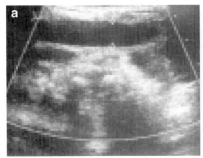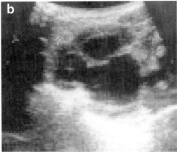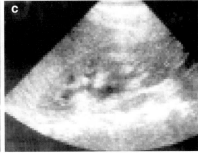

Fig. 84.4 Female newborn with nonrefluxing left megaureter discovered by prenatal ultrasound. (**a** and **b**) Newborn ultrasound shows grade 4 hydronephrosis and dilated ureter. Diuretic renogram, 8 weeks of age, showed 50% differential renal function in left kidney. Obstructive drainage pattern was noted following administration of furosemide. Patient managed nonoperatively. (**c**) Ultrasound 6 months later shows grade 1 hydronephrosis. Diuretic renogram later showed normal drainage pattern

closely. In addition, review of the radiologic studies (not just the radiology report) by the pediatric urologist is strongly encouraged.

There has been significant progress in the development of minimally invasive techniques in pediatric pyeloplasty, even in infants. Although infant pyeloplasty is performed through a small incision (lumbotomy or flank muscle-splitting) in most centers, an increasing number of pediatric urologists are performing the procedure with traditional laparoscopic techniques, and a few centers have utilized the daVinci robot for assistance. Success rates have been identical to series of open surgical repair, and hospital stay and narcotic use are less with the minimally invasive approach. Generally a transperitoneal approach has been used, with mobilization of the colon. However, on the left side the pyeloplasty can be performed with a transmesenteric approach.

84.4.6.2 Multicystic Dysplastic Kidney

A multicystic dysplastic kidney is composed of multiple non-communicating cysts of varying sizes with a stromal component that is composed of dysplastic elements. These kidneys do not function. Although multicystic kidney is the most common cause of abdominal masses in neonates, the vast majority of multicystic kidneys are detected by prenatal sonography. Some clinicians incorrectly assume that multicystic kidney and polycystic kidney are synonymous terms. Polycystic kidney disease is an inherited disorder and has an "adult form" (autosomal dominant) and an "infantile form" (autosomal recessive) and affects both kidneys. In contrast, a multicystic kidney is almost always unilateral and is not an inherited disorder.

Sonography of multicystic kidneys usually is diagnostic, demonstrating multiple echolucent cysts of varying sizes with no discernible cortex. Occasionally the cysts may resemble a severe UPJ obstruction with minimal parenchyma, termed the *hydronephrotic variant*. The contralateral kidney is abnormal in 5–10% of cases. A renal scan shows nonfunction and always should be performed to confirm the diagnosis. On occasion there is a segmental multicystic kidney affecting only the upper pole that is not apparent on sonography. A VCUG also is recommended because as many as 15% have contralateral vesicoureteral reflux.

The management of a multicystic kidney is becoming less controversial. If an abdominal mass that is symptomatic is present, early nephrectomy is indicated; however, left untreated, most multicystic kidneys become smaller relative to total body size, and some regress completely. Potential complications include malignancy and nodular renal blastema, which is a precursor to Wilms' tumor, and hypertension. In a review of 26 clinical series, no cases of Wilms' tumor were reported among 1,041 children, and the maximum estimated risk was 3.5 per 1,000 affected children. Tumors arise from the stromal, not the cystic, component of multicystic kidneys. Consequently, even if the cysts regress completely, the likelihood that the kidney could develop a neoplasm is not altered. With regard to hypertension, in a review of 29 studies, six cases were reported among 1,115 eligible children, and the mean probability was 5.4 per 1,000 affected children (95% CI 1.9 to 11.7 per 1,000).

Generally a follow-up sonogram is recommended at the age of 6 months. If any cysts enlarge, the stromal core increases in size, or hypertension develops, laparoscopic (or possibly open) simple nephrectomy is recommended. However, further follow-up sonography is unnecessary unless there is concern regarding the contralateral kidney, because finding a Wilms' tumor incidentally would be extremely rare. Because of the occult nature of hypertension, annual blood pressure measurement is recommended, and if hypertension occurs, nephrectomy should be considered.

84.4.6.3 Primary Obstructive Megaureter (Nonrefluxing)

Megaureter refers to a wide ureter and is associated with many significant urological conditions. Nonrefluxing megaureter results from an aperistaltic segment of the distal ureter that does not allow normal propulsion of urine. In this condition, sonography shows a dilated ureter and renal pelvis with variable renal parenchymal atrophy. VCUG shows no reflux in most cases. Before the sonography era, most patients with this condition presented with flank pain, flank mass, pyelonephritis, hematuria, or stone disease. Surgical correction consists of excision of the aperistaltic segment, tailoring (also known as tapering) of the ureter, and reimplantation of the ureter into the bladder.

Although severe hydronephrosis may be present, the natural history of this condition is that there is a tendency to gradual reduction in hydronephrosis over a period of several years. For example, in one series of 40 neonates with 57 nonrefluxing megaureters treated between 1986 and 1999, only four underwent early repair because of diminished renal function. With a mean follow-up of 6.8 years, none of the remainder showed deterioration in differential renal function or exhibited signs of obstruction. Similarly, Liu and colleagues found that 11 of 67 (17%) neonatal megaureters managed nonoperatively ultimately needed repair because of deteriorating renal function in eight and breakthrough UTIs in three. Consequently, most of these patients may be followed nonoperatively on antibiotic prophylaxis and serial monitoring of renal function and drainage.

In these neonates, a renal sonogram and VCUG should be obtained before discharge. Early management is identical to that of neonates with suspected UPJ obstruction. If an abdominal mass, solitary kidney, or bilateral hydroureteronephrosis is present, then a well-tempered diuretic renogram should be obtained promptly. Otherwise, the study is deferred until the age of 6–8 weeks. If the differential renal function is at least 40%, the child is managed nonoperatively and follow-up diuretic renograms are obtained every 3–6 months. In equivocal cases an IVP is recommended because even if marked ureteral dilatation is present, the calyces may not be dilated or blunted, indicating absence of obstruction.

Early repair of megaureter has a higher complication rate than in older children. For example, Peters and colleagues reported on megaureter repair in 42 infants operated on at a mean age of 1.8 months. In that series, early complications occurred only in those less than the age of 6 weeks and included transient apnea in three, UTI in one, hyponatremia in one, and meningitis in one. Reflux occurred postoperatively in six infants, and none developed postoperative obstruction. The reflux resolved spontaneously between 18 and 36 months in three patients, and the remainder underwent secondary ureteroneocystostomy. Greenfield and colleagues reported on repair of 11 megaureters in infants less than 6 months old. Of these children, two had transient ureteral obstruction immediately after stent removal and persistent grades 1 and 2 reflux in two children. In a series of older children

who underwent tapered ureteral reimplantation, the success rate was 90% for obstructive megaureter. The results were slightly better for intravesical compared with extravesical reimplantation.

There are two other reasonable treatment options if surgical repair seems necessary in the neonate or young infant. The first is to perform a temporary cutaneous ureterostomy, allowing the ureter to decompress over a period of 12–18 months. Subsequently, the ureterostomy can be taken down and ureteral reimplantation with or without tapering performed. In a series of children who underwent this procedure, when undiversion and ureteral reimplantation was performed, only 5 of 23 ureters required tapering. The other option is to insert a double J ureteral stent through the ureterovesical junction and leave it interposed between the bladder and the kidney. Castagnetti et al. reported ten infants, of whom five required open surgery for stent insertion. A total of seven had stent-related complications, including UTI in five and early stent removal was performed in two patients. Of the five who underwent subsequent surgical repair, none required ureteral tapering.

In summary, if differential renal function remains normal and the child is asymptomatic, it seems safe to follow these patients with diuretic renography to monitor renal function and drainage; however, if renal functional deterioration, slowing of upper urinary tract drainage, or UTI occurs, ureteral reimplantation is recommended. These infants should receive prophylactic antibiotics while stasis is present in the upper ureter and kidney.

84.4.6.4 Ureterocele and Ectopic Ureter

A ureterocele is a cystic dilatation of the distal end of the ureter and is obstructive. In children they usually extend through the bladder neck, termed *ectopic*, but may remain entirely within the bladder, termed intravesical or orthotopic. Ectopic ureteroceles and ectopic ureters occur more commonly in girls than in boys and usually are associated with the upper pole of a completely duplicated collecting system. In boys with a ureterocele, however, 40% drain a single collecting system. Prenatal sonography typically shows either hydroureteronephrosis or upper pole hydronephrosis with a dilated ureter. These conditions are bilateral in 10–15% of patients.

Early evaluation consists of:

- Sonography—shows a hydronephrotic upper pole connected to a dilated ureter; the ureterocele typically is visualized in the bladder.
- VCUG—shows whether reflux is present either into the lower pole moiety or whether the ectopic ureter refluxes, which usually occurs if the ureter inserts into the bladder neck.
- DMSA renal scan shows whether the moiety drained by the ectopic system functions; this study may be done at the age of 1–2 weeks because the result does not change with functional maturity. A DMSA renal scan is recommended rather than a diuretic renal scan, because there is generally not a question regarding "obstruction" and the DMSA provides excellent cortical imaging.

The management of neonates with a ureterocele is highly individualized. The least invasive initial form of therapy is transurethral incision (TUI), which can be performed either with a 3F Bugbee electrode or the holmium:YAG laser. The ureterocele is punctured several times at its junction with the bladder mucosa. If the ureterocele is ectopic, it must be punctured both in the bladder as well as in the urethra. TUI provides satisfactory upper tract decompression with a single procedure in > 90% of cases. However, there is a significant risk of post-operative reflux through the ureterocele into the upper pole moiety, which may require subsequent definitive treatment. If the ureterocele is orthotopic, approximately 30% reflux follow TUI, whereas if it is ectopic, 75% reflux follow TUI. Often TUI is the only procedure necessary.

TUI of a ureterocele draining a nonfunctioning moiety is unlikely to result in the development of any appreciable degree of function. Although the risk for subsequent reflux into the ureterocele is significant, TUI is a good minimally invasive alternative to an open partial nephrectomy. However, in recent years many centers have been performed minimally invasive (laparoscopic) upper pole heminephrectomy. Consequently, if the hydronephrotic upper pole does not function, the infant is put on antibiotic prophylaxis, and laparoscopic upper pole heminephrectomy (or nephrectomy, if the entire kidney does not function) is performed electively at the age of 6 months. If the DMSA scan shows significant upper pole function however, transurethral puncture of the ureterocele is recommended and should be performed during the first few weeks of life. An alternative is ureteropyelostomy, in which the upper pole ureter is anastomosed to the lower pole renal pelvis or ureter. Total urinary tract reconstruction in neonates and infants is not recommended because of the high complication rate caused by the small size of the infant bladder.

The upper pole moiety drained by an ectopic ureter is more likely to function than a moiety associated with a ureterocele, and ureteropyelostomy or ureteroneocystostomy or laparoscopic upper pole nephrectomy (if the moiety is nonfunctioning) is recommended.

84.4.6.5 Posterior Urethral Valves

The most common cause of severe obstructive uropathy in children is posterior urethral valves (PUV), which are tissue leaflets fanning distally from the prostatic urethra to the external urinary sphincter. Typically the leaflets are separated by a slit-like opening. Approxi-mately one third ultimately develop chronic renal failure or severe renal insufficiency. Prognosis is signifi-cantly better if a prenatal sonography study before 24 weeks' gestation was normal. In one study, 9 of 17 patients with PUV whose hydronephrosis was discovered before 24 weeks' gestation developed renal failure, whereas only 1 of 14 recognized after 24 weeks' gestation developed end-stage renal disease. Favorable prognostic factors include a serum creatinine level of less than 0.8–1.0 mg% after bladder decompression, unilateral reflux into a nonfunctioning kidney ("VURD syndrome"), ascites, and identification of the corticomedullary junction on renal sonography.

Early delivery of infants with a prenatal diagnosis of suspected PUV occasionally has resulted in premature neonates who require treatment of PUV. If severe bilateral renal dysplasia is present, pulmonary hypoplasia is often present as well, and problems with ventilation may result. Initially, a small feeding tube should be passed into the bladder for urinary drainage until electrolyte imbalances can be corrected. A Foley catheter is not recommended because the balloon may cause significant bladder spasm and impede upper tract drainage. A VCUG should be obtained to confirm the diagnosis, and a renal scan should be performed to evaluate the upper tracts.

In newborn infants, potential treatments include transurethral endoscopic ablation of PUV, cutaneous vesicostomy, and high diversion (cutaneous pyelostomy). The ideal initial treatment is valve ablation. In small neonates, the 8 or 9 French resectoscope may be too large for the urethra. An alternative is to use a small Bugbee electrode, as is used with TUI, or the holmium:YAG laser. Vesicostomy is reserved for those with a serum creatinine level that remains significantly elevated after bladder decompression. Cutaneous pyelostomy rarely affords better drainage compared with cutaneous vesicostomy and diverts urine away from the bladder, which may prevent normal bladder growth. However, in selected cases the Sober-en-T cutaneous ureterostomy is useful. In this procedure the upper ureter is brought out to the abdomen and transected, and the distal segment is anastomosed to the renal pelvis; this option allows urine to drain both through the ureterostomy as well as to the bladder.

84.4.7 Vesicoureteral Reflux

Some neonates with medium- and high-grade vesicoureteral reflux are detected by the finding of hydronephrosis on prenatal sonography. Approximately 80% of such patients are boys. The male predominance is thought to be secondary to transient urethral valve-like urethral obstruction in utero that resolves before birth. The high intravesical pressures generated seem to destabilize the ureterovesical junction. In the most severe cases of massive reflux, the bladder also may become distended from aberrant micturition into the upper tracts, termed the megacystis-megaureter syndrome. Neonates with reflux should undergo a baseline renal scan to determine whether scarring is present, which is detected in as many as 40%.

Initially neonates with prenatally diagnosed reflux are managed medically. Most are placed on amoxicillin prophylaxis for 2 months, followed by nitrofurantoin or trimethoprim-sulfamethoxazole prophylaxis, and circumcision is recommended for male neonates to decrease the risk for UTIs.

Neonates with reflux are more likely to show spontaneous resolution than older children. Indeed, 20–35% of ureters with grade 4 or 5 reflux have reflux resolution within 2 years; however, a significant proportion develop breakthrough UTIs, and antireflux surgery is recommended in these cases. The success rate for open surgical correction of reflux in infants can be as high as in older children. Another option is subureteral injection of the ureterovesical junction with dextranomer microspheres, in which the success rate is 69% with a single injection.

Summary

One per cent of newborn infants have a prenatal diagnosis of hydronephrosis or significant renal pelvic dilation. Hydronephrosis is often caused by nonobstructive conditions. The likelihood of significant urologic pathology is directly related to the size of the fetal renal pelvis, and 90% with an anteroposterior diameter more than 2 cm need surgery or long-term urologic medical care. Following delivery, antibiotic prophylaxis should be administered and a renal sonogram and VCUG should be obtained. If there is grade 3 or 4 hydronephrosis, usually a diuretic renogram is also recommended. Pediatric urologic or pediatric nephrologic consultation is helpful in planning evaluation and treatment. Prenatal recognition of hydronephrosis allows neonatal diagnosis and treatment of urologic pathology, preventing complications of pyelonephritis and obstruction. In the past decade significant progress has been made in the development of minimally invasive treatment options.

Further Reading

Castagnetti M, Cimador M, Sergio M, De Grazia E (2006) Double-J stent insertion across vesicoureteral junction—Is it a valuable initial approach in neonates and infants with severe primary nonrefluxing megaureter? Urology 68:870–875

Cendron M, Elder JS (2002) Perinatal urology. In JY Gillenwater, JT Grayhack, SS Howards, M Mitchell (eds) Adult and Pediatric Urology, 4th edn. Lippincott Williams & Wilkins, Philadelphia pp 2041–2127

Fefer S, Ellsworth P (2006) Prenatal hydronephrosis. Pediatr Clin N Am 53:429–447

Herndon CD (2006) Antenatal hydronephrosis: Differential diagnosis, evaluation, and treatment options. Scientific World J 6:2345–2365

Lee RS, Cendron M, Kinnamon DD, Nguyen HT (2006) Antenatal hydronephrosis as a predictor of postnatal outcome: A metaanalysis. Pediatrics 118:586–593

Maizels M, Mitchell B, Kass E et al (1994) Outcome of nonspecific hydronephrosis in the infant: A report from the registry of the Society for Fetal Urology. J Urol 152:2324

Onen A, Jayanthi VR, Koff SA (2002) Long-term followup of prenatally detected severe bilateral newborn hydronephrosis initially managed nonoperatively. J Urol 168: 1118–1120

P Puri, ME Hollwarth (eds) (2006) Pediatric Surgery, Springer-Verlag, Berlin, Heidelberg.

Shukla AR, Cooper J, Patel RP et al (2005) Prenatally detected primary megaureter: A role for extended followup. J Urol 173:1353–1356

Sidhu G, Beyene J, Rosenblum ND (2006) Outcome of isolated antenatal hydronephrosis: A systematic review and meta-analysis. Pediatr Nephrol 21:218–224

Walsh TJ, Hsieh S, Grady R, Mueiler BA (2007) Antenatal hydronephrosis and the risk of pyelonephritis hospitalization during the first year of life. Urology 69:970–974

Upper Urinary Tract Obstructions

85

Boris Chertin

Contents

85.1 Introduction

The advent of prenatal ultrasound (US) has enabled the physician to diagnose urinary tract abnormalities with far greater frequency than previously. Pelvi-ureteric junction (PUJ) and uretero-vesical junction (UVJ) obstruction are the most common causes of hydronephrosis detected antenatally. Management of these patients after birth remains controversial. In spite of the increased incidence of diagnosed urinary tract abnormalities the distinction between urinary tract obstruction and urinary tract dilatation still remains a challenging problem. The recognition and relief of significant obstruction is important to prevent irreversible damage to the kidneys.

85.2 Pelvi-Ureteric Junction Obstruction

The overall incidence of neonatal hydronephrosis which leads to the diagnosis of PUJ obstruction approximates 1 in 500 births. The ratio of males to females is 2:1 in the neonatal period, with left sided lesions occurring in 60%. In the newborn period, a unilateral process is most common, but bilateral PUJ obstruction was found in 10–49% of neonates in some reported series. PUJ obstruction is classified as intrinsic, extrinsic, or secondary.

Intrinsic obstruction results from failure of transmission of the peristaltic waves across the pelvi-ureteric junction with failure of urine to be propulsed from the renal pelvis into the ureter which results in multiple ineffective peristaltic waves that eventually causes hydronephrosis by incompletely emptying the pelvic contents. Extrinsic mechanical factors include aberrant renal vessels, bands, adventitial tissues and adhesions that cause angulation, kinking or compression of the pelvi-ureteric junction. Extrinsic obstruction may occur alone but usually coexists with intrinsic ureteropelvic junction pathology. Secondary PUJ obstruction may develop as a consequence of concomitant severe vesico-ureteric reflux (VUR) which occurs in 15–30% of children who have ipsilateral PUJ obstruction which a tortuous ureter may kink proximately.

Prenatal Diagnosis: The bladder is visualised by 14 weeks of gestation. The ureters are usually not seen in the absence of distal obstruction or reflux. The fetal kidney may be visualised at the same time as bladder. If not, they are always visualised by 16th week of gestation. However, it is not until 20–24 weeks of gestation, when the fetal kidney is surrounded by fat, that the internal renal structures appear distinct. Renal growth can then be assessed easily. Beyond 20 weeks, fetal urine production is the main source of amniotic fluid. Therefore, major abnormalities of the urinary tract may result in oligohydramnios.

Because of the distinct urine tissue interface, hydronephrosis can be detected as early as 16 weeks of gestation. An obstructive anomaly is recognised by demonstrating dilated renal calyces and pelvis. A multitude of measurement and different gestational age cut-off points have been recommended in the assessment of fetal obstructive uropathy.

Routine estimation of anteroposterior (AP) diameter of renal pelvis in fetus with hydronephrosis is considered as a useful marker for classification of renal dilatation and possible obstruction. AP renal pelvis threshold values ranged between 2.3 and 10 mm. Positive predictive values for pathological dilatation confirmed in the neonate ranged between 2.3% and >40% for AP renal measurements of 2–3 mm and 10 mm, respectively. Recently study which included more than 46,000 screening patients published the standards regarding renal pelvic measurement. This study clearly demonstrated that only fetuses exhibiting third- trimester AP renal pelvis dilatations >10 mm would merit postnatal assessment. In order to standardise postnatal evolution of prenatal hydronephrosis a grading system of postnatal hydronephrosis was implemented in 1993 by the Society for Fetal Urology (SFU). In SFU system, the status of calices is paramount while the size of the pelvis is less important. In SFU grading of hydronephrosis, there is no hydronephrosis in Grade 0. At Grade 1, the renal pelvis is only visualised. Grade 2 of hydronephrosis is diagnosed when a few (but not all) renal calices are identified in addition to the renal pelvis. Grade 3 hydronephrosis requires that virtually all cal-

ices are depicted. Grade 4 hydronephrotic kidneys will exhibit similar caliceal status with the involved kidney exhibiting parenchymal thinning. Often this classification is applied also on prenatal hydronephrosis. We have recently published our data regarding prenatal findings with the special emphasis on the natural history of hydronephrosis during postnatal period. Our data show that SFU grade of prenatal hydronephrosis is not a significant predictive factor for surgery in unilateral hydronephrosis. However SFU Grades 3–4 prenatal bilateral hydronephrosis indicates that the majority of the children will require surgical correction during postnatal period.

In case of severe prenatal bilateral hydronephrosis, severe hydroureteronephrosis or severe impairment of the solitary kidney fetal bladder aspiration for urinary proteins and electrolytes is recommended in order to predict the renal injury secondary to obstructive uropathy. Fetal urinary sodium level less than 100 mmol/L, chloride level of less than 90 mmol/L and an osmolality of less than 210 mOsm/kg are considered as prognostic features for good renal function.

Clinical Presentation: With the advent of prenatal ultrasonographic screening only sporadic cases present with clinical symptoms. Before the routine fetal ultrasonography, the commonest presentation was with abdominal flank mass. Fifty percent abdominal masses in newborns are of renal origin with 40% being secondary to pelviureteric junction obstruction. Some patients present with urinary tract infection. Other clinical presentations include irritability, vomiting and failure to thrive. Ten percent to 35% of pelviureteric junction obstructions are bilateral and associated abnormalities of urinary tract are seen in about 30%. PUJ problems are often associated with other congenital anomalies, including imperforated anus, contralateral dysplastic kidney, congenital heart disease, VATER syndrome, and oesophageal atresia. In patients with such an established diagnosis, a renal ultrasound examination should be performed.

Diagnosis: With the increasing number of antenatally diagnosed hydronephrosis it is difficult to interpret the underlying pathology and its significance. Severe obstructive uropathies are detrimental to renal function. However, on the other hand hydronephrosis without ureteral or lower tract anomaly is common. The important aspect of post-natal investigations is to identify the group of patients who will benefit from early intervention and those who need to be carefully followed up.

Ultrasound: Follow-up ultrasound examination is necessary in postnatal period in antenatally detected hydronephrosis. If the bilateral hydronephrosis is diagnosed in utero in a male infant, postnatal evaluation should be carried out within 24 h primarily because of the possibility of posterior urethral valves. If the ultrasound scan is negative in the first 24–48 h in any patient with unilateral or bilateral hydronephrosis, a repeat scan should be performed after 5–10 days, recognising that neonatal oliguria may mask a moderately obstructive lesion.

If hydronephrosis is confirmed on the postnatal scan, further careful scan of the kidney, ureter, bladder and in boys the posterior urethra is essential.

Ultrasonography depicts the dilated calyces as multiple intercommunicating cystic spaces of fairly uniform size that lead into a larger cystic structure at the hilum, representing the dilated renal pelvis (Fig. 85.1a). Peripheral to the dilated calyces, the renal parenchyma is usually thinned with the normal or increased echogenecity.

Typically the ureter is of normal calibre and not seen. But if it is dilated the size of ureter is also assessed ultrasonographically and graded 1–3 according to ureteral width <7, 7–10, >10 mm, respectively.

Radionucleide Scans: Diuretic renograms using 99 mTc DTPA augmented with furosemide were useful in the diagnosis of urinary tract obstructions for a long time.

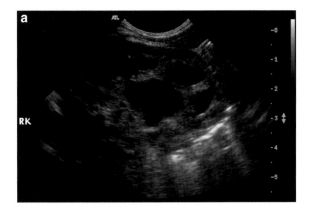

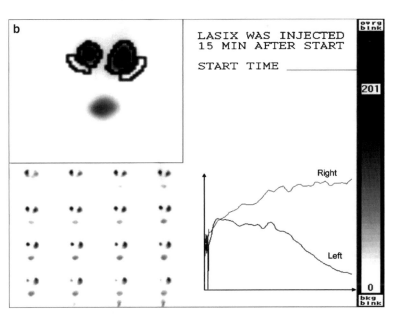

Fig. 85.1 (**a**) A sagittal plane scan through the obstructed right kidney confirms obstruction at the level of the pelvi-ureteric junction. (**b**) 99Tc MAG3 scan in the above patient. Clearance curve for right kidney confirming the high-grade obstruction on this side

DTPA is completely filtered by the kidneys a maximum concentration of 5% being reached in 5 min, falling to 2% at 15 min. Recently, it has been reported that use of tracers that rely on tubular extraction such as 123 I-Hippuran and 99Tc MAG3 (Fig. 85.1b) may improve diagnostic accuracy. The kidney of the young infant is immature; renal clearance, even when corrected for body surface, progressively increases until approximately 2 years of age. Therefore, the renal uptake of tracer is particularly low in infants, and there is a high background activity. Thus the traces such as 123 I-Hippuran and 99Tc MAG3 with a high extraction rate provide reasonable images enabling estimation of the differential kidney function during the first few weeks of life. It is also helpful in assessing the size, shape, location and function of the kidney. Diuretic augmented renogram is a provocative test and is intended to demonstrate or exclude obstructive hydronephrosis by stressing an upper urinary tract with a high urine flow. Obstruction usually is defined as a failure of tracer washout after diuretic stimulation. If unequivocal, it eliminates the need for further investigations. In equivocal cases, F15 in which furosemide is given 15 min before the test provides a better assessment of the drainage of upper urinary tract. Forced hydration prior to scan increases predictive value of non-obstructed pattern up to 94%. Since glomerular filtration and glomerular blood flow are still low in the newborn, the handling of isotype is unpredictable and can be misleading.

Diagnosis of pelviureteric junction obstruction can be made by intravenous urography. This investigation, although shows a dilated renal pelvis with clubbed calyces is often not helpful as concentration of contrast is unreliable therefore its routine use is abounded in paediatric urology.

85.2.1 Pressure-Flow Study

In the equivocal cases and in the presence of impaired function, the pressure flow study (Whitaker Test) and antegrade pyelography may be necessary to confirm or exclude obstruction. Whitaker test is based on the hypothesis that if the dilated upper urinary tract can transport 10 ml/min without an inordinate increase in pressure, the hydrostatic pressure under physiological conditions should not cause impairment of renal function and the degree of obstruction if present is insignificant. However, it is an invasive test and is

seldom required. Antegrade pyelography may be performed with ultrasound guidance in patients where diagnosis is difficult. Retrograde pyelography is seldom required to determine the status of ureters. The disadvantages include difficulty in ureteral catheterisation in neonates, trauma and oedema may change partial obstruction to the complete one. In patients where diagnosis is equivocal, serial examinations may be necessary.

A routine use of micturating cystourethrogram (MCUG) in patients with antenatal unilateral hydronephrosis is controversial. Some authors advocate a routine use of MCUG as a part of postnatal evaluation citing 15–30% of incidence of concomitant vesicoureteric reflux (VUR) either uni- or contra-lateral. Others recommend performing MCUG only in patients with SFU Gr III and IV hydronephrosis. We have abounded to perform MCUG routinely in children with unilateral antenatal hydronephrosis based on the fact that even if the reflux exists usually it is of low grade and does not require any treatment. We reserve MCUG only for patients with bilateral hydronephrosis or for those whose ureter was seen at any stage of antenatal or postnatal follow up.

Recently the role of dynamic contrast enhanced MR urography in the evaluation of antenatal hydronephrosis has become appreciated. This method allows precise understanding of the kidney anatomy while providing information regarding renal functioning without radiation exposure obviating need in the use of contrast media.

Treatment: A considerable controversy exists regarding the management of newborn urinary tract obstructions. Some authors advocate early surgical intervention to prevent damage to maturing nephrons, while others feel that early surgery carries no specific benefit. During late prenatal and early postnatal life, there is progressive increase in glomerular filtration rate. Additionally, this transition is associated with an abrupt decline in urine output from what appears to be a quite high in utero output to a rather low early neonatal level of urine production. These physiological observations may explain the common observation of hydronephrosis detected antenatally, which on postnatal follow-up reverts to an unobstructed pattern. Surgery is usually undertaken in infants whose renal function deteriorates during observation period. We have recently analysed our database of 343 children (260 males and 83 females) with antenatal diagnosis of hydronephrosis, which led to the postnatal diagnosis of PUJ obstruction, were deliberately followed up conservatively at our department over a 16 year period in order to define which factors lead to surgery. One hundred and seventy nine children (52.2%) required surgical correction in the course of conservative management. Average age at surgery was 10.6 months (range 1 month–7 years). Of these, 50% underwent surgery during the first 2 years of life and majority of the remaining patients underwent surgery between the 2nd and the 4th years of age, only two patients required surgery later on. Univariate analysis revealed that child sex, side of hydronephrosis are not significant predictive factors for surgery. However, SFU Grades 3–4 of postnatal hydronephrosis ($p < 0.0001$, Odds ratio 0.06281), RRF <40% ($p < 0.0001$, Odds ratio 0.1022) were significant independent risk factors for surgery.

A number of different operations have been described for surgical correction of PUJ obstruction. Dismembered Anderson-Hynes pyeloplasty is considered as a gold standard in the surgical treatment of PUJ obstruction. This operation may be performed through extraperitoneal approach via lateral flank incision or utilizing posterior lumbotomy incision. Recently a number of investigators have advocated a laparoscopic approach to the dismembered pyeloplasty showing good results in the different ages including infants. The basic principles of these operations is an excision of pelvi-ureteric junction with a subsequent oval shaped anastomosis between ureter and lower part of pelvis. Different types of stent are place for drainage usually for 6 weeks. The most popular are Double J Paediatric Stents or Pipi-Salle Stent nephrostomy (Cook, USA).

Although antegrade and retrograde endopyelotomy has been shown to be effective in children, this approach has not been recommended in neonates, infants, or young children. However, it should be considered in older children or in those with failed primary dismembered pyeloplasty.

Bilateral Pelvi-Ureteric Obstruction: Surgical correction of the symptomatic side or side with better function should take precedence. If a nephrectomy is considered on one side, the pyeloplasty should precede this.

Postoperative Complications: include infection, adhesive obstruction (transperitoneal approach), temporary obstruction at the anastomosis resulting in excessive urine leakage and failures due to postoperative stricture at anastomotic sites. An overall reoperation rate of 8.2% was reported in the early series. However, in the latest series, when temporally double-J stents were utilized, the reoperation rate was negligible.

Follow-up and Results: Follow up ultrasound may be performed 3–6 months after operation when maximum improvement can be seen. Follow up radionuclide scan should be done 6–8 months following pyeloplasty, in order to evaluate an improvement in the renal function and drainage. Pyeloplasty in the neonatal period when indicated gives excellent results.

85.3 Megaureter

Megaureter is a ureter, which is dilated out of proportion to the rest of the urinary tract and above the norms. Cussen and later Hellstrom et al., have established the normal measurement of the ureteral diameter in infants and children from 30 weeks of gestation to 12 years of age. Normal ureteral diameter in children is rarely greater than 5 mm, and ureters larger than 7 mm can be considered megaureters.

Classification: The Paediatric Urology Society in 1976 adopted a standard nomenclature for categorising megaureters, which is a useful guide for management. There are three types described.

1. Refluxing ureter which may be primary or secondary to distal obstruction or pathology
2. Obstructive: which may be primary and include intrinsic obstruction, or secondary due to distal obstruction or extrinsic causes
3. Non-refluxing, non-obstructed which may be primary-idiopathic type or secondary to diabetes insipidus or infection.

In 1980 King subsequently modified this classification by adding a fourth group consisting of the refluxing, obstructed megaureters.

85.3.1 Uretero-Vesical Junction Obstruction

The presence of an adynamic distal ureteral segment is the most common cause of primary obstructive megaureter. The presence of narrowed terminal portion of ureter will not convey the peristaltic wave or dilate enough to permit free passage of urine. This results in excess boluses of urine which coalesce and cause ureteral dilatation. The contraction waves become smaller and are unable to coapt the walls of dilated ureters. This along with infection could damage the renal parenchyma. The most common etiologic causes of obstructive megeureters are: (i) alteration in muscular orientation, (ii) muscular hypoplasia with fibrosis or excessive collagen deposition resulting in a discontinuity of muscular co-ordination, and finally (iii) disturbance in the electric syncytium along with the nexus injury causing pathological innervation.

Prenatal Diagnosis: Currently the vast majority of obstructive megaureters are discovered on prenatal ultrasound. Usually ureter is not seen in fetal scans. Visualisation of dilated ureter to the level of vesicoureteric junction without abnormal bladder may suggest obstruction or reflux. However this may be a transient phenomenon. Fetal urine flow is 4–6 times greater before birth than after and is due to differences in renal vascular resistance, glomerular filtration and concentrating ability. This high outflow contributes to ureteral dilatation. Other contributing factor is increased compliance of the fetal ureter. The most intriguing question on prenatal evaluation is which children will require follow up only and who will need surgery in order to rescue the renal function. We have recently analysed at our database of 79 children with antenatal diagnosis of obstructive megaureter. Antenatal SFU grade of hydronephrosis had no predictive value for the surgery in postnatal follow up. However, those children who had ureteric diameter more than 1.4 cm are more likely to require surgery postnatally.

Clinical Features: Although the commonest mode of presentation of obstructive megaureter is on antenatal US, some children present with urinary tract infection, microscopic hematuria due to disruption of mucosal vessels of the ureter secondary to ureteric distension. Primary obstructive megaureter is more common in males than females, and the left ureter is more likely to be involved than the right. Seventeen to 34% patients have bilateral megaureters.

Postnatal Diagnosis: Antenatally diagnosed ureteral dilatation needs further evaluation to confirm or exclude obstruction, reflux or both. The clinician should confront the common clinical dilemma in paediatric

antenatal hydronephrosis. And to distinguish between those patients who will have deterioration in renal function while on surveillance protocol and therefore will benefit from early surgery and those who have non obstructive hydronephrosis. In antenatally detected cases, ultrasonography should be performed between 3 and 5 days after birth to confirm antenatal findings. If no dilatation is seen, repeat ultrasound should be performed after a few weeks as neonatal oliguria can mask dilatation. If dilatation persists on a repeat ultrasound, radionuclide scan is performed at the age of 4–6 weeks. In males infants with bilateral ureterohydronephrosis, MCUG should be performed during 72 h since birth to role out posterior urethral valve.

Ultrasonography classically shows hydroureter and variable hydronephrosis, with hyperperistalsis of a lower ureter that terminates shortly above the bladder in a narrow, adynamic segment. (Fig. 85.2a) However, the narrow segment may not always be visualised and therefore MCUG is necessary to exclude vesicoureteric reflux. Intravenous Urography (IVP): may be necessary in equivocal cases to establish the diagnosis (Fig. 85.2b). It delineates the anatomy showing dilated, obstructed ureter. However, it is better to wait for a few weeks for renal maturation to allow concentration of contrast reliability. Occasionally, Whitaker test and antegrade pyelography may be required to establish the diagnosis.

Recently Fung et al. explored ureteral opening pressure as a novel parameter for evaluating paediatric ureterohydronephrosis. Renal pelvic pressure is assessed while simultaneously documenting the passage of contrast material from the distal ureter into the bladder. A pressure increase of 14 cm H_2O within renal pelvis is consistent with distal ureter obstruction.

Management: It is being increasingly recognised that many antenatal and neonatal ureteral dilatations improve with time. Surgery is indicated in patients with progressive ureteral dilatation and deterioration in renal function. In our series of the 79 children with antenatal diagnosis of hydronephrosis who led to postnatal confirmation of UJL obstruction, only 25 (31%) children required surgical correction during over 16 year conservative follow up. Univariant analysis did not reveal statistical significance in those children who required surgical correction and in those who followed conservatively neither from the side of obstruction nor sex of the patient. However those children who required surgery had ureteric diameter more than 1.4 cm., renal

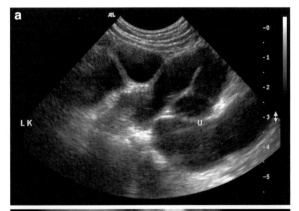

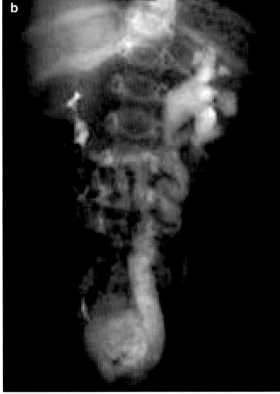

Fig. 85.2 (**a**) Longitudinal renal scan demonstrates severe left ureterohydronephrosis. (**b**) Intravenous urogram shows severe left ureterohydronephrosis

function less than 30% and SFU Grades 3 and 4 of hydronephrosis.

Operation: There are various techniques of reimplanting the ureter in a non-refluxing manner after excision of adynamic, narrow segment. The initial approach to the ureter can be either intravesical, extravesical or combined. The most commonly used techniques for intravesical approach are Cohen's transtrigonal reimplantation and Politano Leadbetter operation. The basic principle of these operations is an excision of adynamic, obstructive terminal narrow portion of the ureter and reimplantation of the remaining ureter into the bladder in antirefluxing fashion. In those cases a significant dilated tapering of the ureter is required. Non-excisional techniques such as Folding (Kalikinski) or Plication (Star) of ureteral wall are also available. Although these techniques have the advantage of avoiding a suture line with potential urinary leakage, they are inappropriate for very dilated ureter as it reduces diameter by only 50% and in neonates it can become too bulky for the tunnel. In these cases excisional tapering technique utilizing Hendren clamps where part of the ureteral wall is excised by using knife and scissors is recommended.

Recent progress in endoscopic tools (such as mini-scopes, balloons and guide wires) has led to widespread use of endoscopy for ureteral repair mainly in adult population. The technique consists of incision of the obstructive segment of ureter through all of the layers in order to expose the periureteral areolar tissue via an ureteroscope inserted into ureteral orifice. The role of endoureterotomy in the treatment of megaureters in children population has not yet been established.

85.3.2 Postoperative Course

Patients are fasted for 24 h in case of development of ileus. In the cases of intravesical approach drain is removed after 24–48 h. Stents are removed after 7–10 days followed by suprapubic catheter. Ureteral reimplantation using extravesical approach can be performed without stenting. Indwelling urethral catheter is placed usually for 3–5 days to avoid urinary retention.

Complications: wound infection, vesicoureteral reflux due to short tunnel with no effective flap valve mechanism, or obstruction due to a fibrotic distal end secondary to ischemia especially in children who underwent excisional type of ureteric remodelling.

Follow-up and Results: US is performed 3 months following surgery with radiologic studies at 6 months after repair in order to assess renal function and drainage. MCUG is performed at the time of radionuclide scan to role out denovo reflux into reimplanted previously obstructed ureter.

Further Reading

Chertin B, Fridmans A, Knizhnik M, Hadas-Halpern I, Hain D, Farkas A (1999) Does early detection of ureteroplevic junction obstruction improve surgical outcome in terms of renal function? J Urol 162:1037–1041

Chertin B, Pollack A, Koulikov D et al (2006) Conservative treatment of uretero-pelvic junction obstruction in children with antenatal diagnosis of hydronephrosis: Lessons learned after 16 years of follow up. Eur Urol 49(4):734–739

Chertin B, Pollack A, Koulikov D et al (2008) Long-term follow up of antenatal diagnosed megaureters. J Ped Urol 4:188–191

Chertin B, Rolle U, Farkas A, Puri P (2002) Does delaying pyeloplasty affect renal function in children with a prenatal diagnosis of pelvi-ureteric junction obstruction? BJU Int 90:72–75

Churchill BM, Feng WC (2001) Ureteropelvic junction anomalies: Congenital UPJ problems in children. In JP Gearhart, RC Rink, PDE Mouriquand (eds) Pediatric Urology. W.B. Saunders, Philadelphia, pp 318–346

Fretz PC, Austin JC, Cooper CS, Hawtrey CE (2004) Long-term outcome analysis of Starr plication for primary obstructive megaureters. J Urol 172(2):703–705

Koff SA, Campbell K (1992) Non-operative management of unilateral neonatal hydronephrosis. J Urol 148:525–531

Koo HP, Bloom DA (1999) Lower ureteral reconstruction. Urol Clin N Am 26(1):167–173

Kutikov A, Resnick M, Casale P (2006) Laparoscopic pyeloplasty in the infant younger than 6 months—Is it technically possible? J Urol 175(4):1477–1479

Onen A, Jayanthi VR, Koff SA (2002) Long-term followup of prenatally detected severe bilateral newborn hydronephrosis initially managed nonoperatively. J Urol 168(3):1118–1120

O'Reilly PH, Brooman PJ, Mak S et al (2001) The long-term results of Anderson-Hynes pyeloplasty. BJU Int 87(4):287–291

Puri P, Höllwarth M (2006) Pediatric Surgery. Springer, Berlin, Heidelberg

Shukla AR, Cooper J, Patel RP et al (2005) Prenatally detected primary megaureter: A role for extended followup. J Urol 173(4):1353–1356

Ureteric Duplication Anomalies

86

Thambipillai Sri Paran and Prem Puri

Contents

86.1 Introduction

Incomplete and complete duplication anomalies of the upper urinary tract are estimated to be present in up to 0.8% of the normal population. Majority of these anomalies have normally developed renal moieties and cause no functional problems. When detected during the antenatal scans, it is of paramount importance that the clinician keeps in mind that the vast majority of these anomalies are benign, incidental findings.

Ureteric duplications overall are more common in females than in males. In 15% of patients the ureteric duplication is bilateral. There is an increased incidence of up to 12% within some families, suggestive of an autosomal dominant inheritance.

However, a percentage of ureteric duplications are associated with ureterocoele, ectopic ureter, vesicoureteric reflux, and pelviureteric junction obstruction. One or more of these abnormalities are frequently found in the presence of complicated complete duplication, where two separate ureters are seen to insert separately into the bladder or into an ectopic opening. In incomplete duplication, the two bifid ureters may join at any level from the ureteropelvic junction to the bladder and open as a single entity into the bladder.

86.2 Incomplete Duplication

The ureteric bud appears at 5 weeks of gestation from the Wolffian duct. Premature division of a single ureteral bud before it reaches the metanephric blastema is thought to result in incomplete duplication of the ureter. The premature division may occur at variable distance from the kidney, but there is only one ureteric orifice present on

P. Puri and M. Höllwarth (eds.), *Pediatric Surgery: Diagnosis and Management,*
DOI: 10.1007/978-3-540-69560-8_86, © Springer-Verlag Berlin Heidelberg 2009

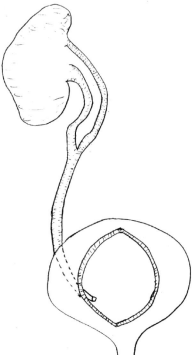

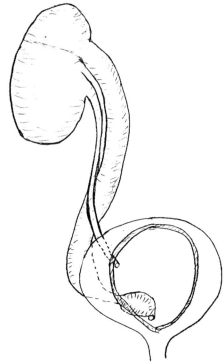

Fig. 86.1 Incomplete duplication. The two ureters unite well above the bladder and open into the bladder with a single opening

Fig. 86.2 Complete duplication with intravesical ureterocoele associated with the upper pole ureter. Lower pole normal ureter inserts superiorly and laterally with a short intramural tunnel

the affected side. Incomplete duplication is three times more common than complete duplication. The commonest complications seen with this type of anomaly are vesicoureteric reflux and pelviureteric junction obstruction. The management of these complications will be discussed later in this chapter (Fig. 86.1).

86.3 Complete Duplication

This anomaly is thought to result when two ureteral buds arise from the Wolffian duct instead of one. The ureteral bud that gives rise to the upper pole ureter is more closely associated with the Wolffian duct and is carried medially and caudally along with the Wolffian duct. This is thought to result in the upper pole ureter opening more medially and inferiorly than the lower pole ureter into the bladder (Weigert-Mayer law). Sometimes this upper pole ureter has an abnormally prolonged or close attachment to the Wolffian duct, which may result in it opening at an ectopic location

such as the urethra, seminal vesicles, vas deferens, or even epididymis (Fig. 86.2).

The upper pole ureters are associated with ureterocoeles and ectopic insertions while the lower pole ureters are associated with vesicoureteric reflux and pelviureteric junction obstruction. These pathologies and their clinical manifestations together with their management are discussed below.

86.4 Investigations

86.4.1 Renal Ultrasound

Following on from either antenatal scan or clinical history suggestive of renal pathology, renal ultrasound is the first line of investigation. It may identify ureteric duplication and associated renal pelvic or ureteric dilatation clearly. Usually the kidney in ureteric duplication is larger in size than a normal kidney, and the upper pole has fewer numbers of calyces (usually one third of the total). When VUR is present, lower pole hydronephrosis and ureteric dilatation will be seen. When the renal parenchyma is hypoechoic, then renal dysplasia should be suspected. Ultrasound can also identify a ureterocoele well. Ectopic dilated ureters may mimic a ureterocoele during ultrasound study.

86.4.2 Voiding Cystourethrogram (VCUG)

This study is best performed with a feeding tube rather than with a foley catheter, which has a balloon that may confuse the diagnosis of an ureterocoele. The bladder should not be overfilled, as it may compress the ureterocoele. It is also important to take an oblique view to demonstrate the ureterocoele, which is posteriorly placed.

This is the study of choice to demonstrate VUR and its severity. It is important to appreciate that an ectopic ureter, opening at the bladder neck, can show reflux and have features suggestive of obstruction as well. It may be necessary to repeat the study to demonstrate this complex phenomenon (Fig. 86.3).

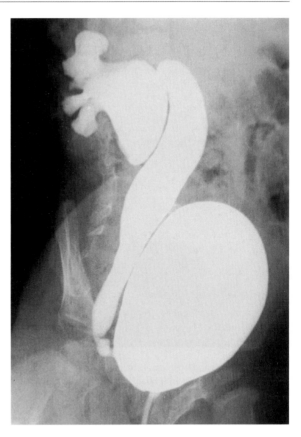

Fig. 86.3 Voiding cystourethrogram showing gross reflux into the lower pole ureter

86.4.3 Intravenous Pyelogram (IVP)

Though the use of this investigation has become infrequent in pediatric urology, when confronted with a dilemma of demonstrating an ectopic ureter, IVP still has a role to play. When the bladder is filled with contrast, an ureterocoele could also be clearly demonstrated. A "drooping lily sign," which is the inferior and lateral displacement of lower renal moiety by the nonfunctioning upper renal moiety, is a good sign of occult duplex kidney with an ectopic ureter (Figs. 86.4 and 86.5).

86.4.4 DMSA (^{99m}Tc Dimercpatosuccinic Acid) Scan

Unlike the MAG3 scans, DMSA scans result in renal tubular labelling and are unaffected by obstruction to drainage. Therefore, they provide more accurate assessment of function and also highlight any scarring within the parenchyma. Since the newborn kidneys

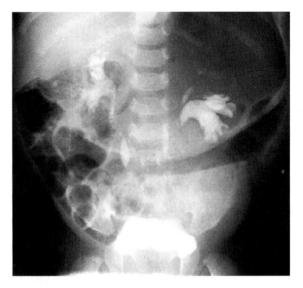

Fig. 86.4 Intravenous pyelogram demonstrating PUJ obstruction in the lower pole ureter

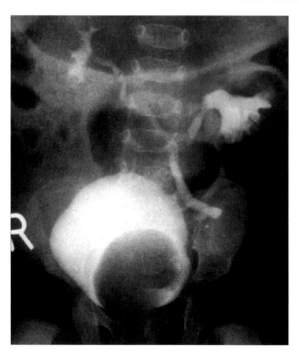

Fig. 86.5 Intravenous pyelogram demonstrating a large ureterocoele on the left side with no uptake of contrast seen within the upper renal moiety (dysplastic moiety)

may not uptake the radionuclides properly, all such studies should be deferred until 6 weeks after delivery to allow for maturation of renal function.

86.4.5 MAG3 (Mercaptoacetyltriglycine) Scan

This study combines information regarding the relative renal function with that of any degree of obstruction to drainage. As mentioned above, in the presence of obstruction, the relative function values may be somewhat inaccurate. As with DMSA scans, MAG3 should also be postponed to allow maturation of neonatal kidneys.

86.4.6 Computed Tomography (CT) and Magnetic Resonance Imaging (MRI) Scans

These should be reserved when the anatomy, especially that of a possible ectopic ureter, cannot be clearly demonstrated with the above studies. MRI is becoming

increasingly useful in cases where occult dysplastic renal moieties, ectopic ureters, and ureterocoeles are suspected and not clearly defined by all other modalities of investigation.

86.4.7 Vesicoureteric Reflux (VUR)

VUR is the commonest problem associated with both complete and incomplete ureteric duplications. It is more common in girls than in boys. In complete duplications, it is mostly seen in the lower pole ureter, which inserts superiorly and laterally, resulting in a short intramural tunnel. However, following ureterocoele puncture, or excision and reimplantation, VUR may also be seen in the upper pole ureter.

The management of VUR in ureteric duplication is the same as in normal nonduplicated systems. Studies have shown that the rate of resolution of minor grades of reflux is similar to that seen in nonduplicated systems. In the newborn period, it is essential to start chemoprophylaxis, until all the problems associated with ureteric duplication are identified. High grades of reflux, associated breakthrough infections in spite of adequate chemoprophylaxis, and progressive renal scarring are all indications for an antireflux surgical intervention.

Surgical options include reimplantation of the ureter(s), endoscopic subureteric Deflux injection, ureteroureterostomy, or heminephrectomy when the function within the associated renal moiety is poor. Reimplantation of the refluxing ureter could only be undertaken in isolation, if it can be safely isolated from the normal ureter without causing ischemic injury. If this is not possible or when there is documented reflux into both ureters on the same side, then common sheath reimplantation (where both ureters are reimplanted without being separated) could be done (Fig. 86.7). Recurrence of reflux is well reported within these reimplanted ureters, and may necessitate further surgery.

Endoscopic correction of VUR (with submucosal injection of Deflux) has been shown to be highly effective for high-grade reflux in single nonduplicated systems by several authors. Puri et al. have shown that this technique could be safely and effectively adopted in ureteric duplication as well. The injection is made under the bladder mucosa, 2–3 mm below the refluxing ureteric opening (which is usually the one belonging to the lower renal moiety that opens superiorly and laterally in the bladder) at the 6 o'clock position. The needle needs to be advanced fully and enough material is injected until a "volcanic" bulge of the mucosa is seen around both ureteric orifices, resulting in a slit-like appearance of both orifices.

Ureteroureterostomy, where the markedly dilated ureter is anastamosed to the side of the normal ureter, was initially used to overcome obstructed ureters secondary to ureterocoeles. However, this approach has been successfully used in dilated ureters secondary to severe VUR as well. But, de novo ipsilateral VUR of the normal ureter has been noted following ureteroureterostomy. The advantages of this approach are that it could be performed laparoscopically with minimal morbidity, shorter hospital stay, and better cosmetic results.

When the refluxing ureter is associated with a poorly functioning or nonfunctioning dysplastic renal moiety, then heminephrectomy would be the best option (Fig. 86.9). At times, both upper and lower renal moieties may have very poor function and nephroureterectomy will become the option of choice. Most reports show that a second incision to remove the residual ureteric stump is not necessary in most children and could be safely undertaken in the minority of children who develop problems related to residual ureteric stump. However, when heminephrectomy or nephrectomy is undertaken laparoscopically, complete removal of the ureter(s) could safely be carried out at the same time.

86.5 Ureterocoele

Ureterocoele is a cystic dilatation of the terminal intramural segment of the distal ureter. It is usually associated with the dilatation of the ureter and calyces with a dysplastic poorly functioning renal moiety. Uretero-coeles can be classified into intravesical and extravesical based on the position of their opening. In the intravesical ureterocoele, the opening of the ureterocoele is located between the normal position of the ureteric orifice and the bladder neck. The extravesical ureterocoele opens ectopically at the bladder neck or urethra, and the opening is usually proximal to the external sphincter. These ectopic ureterocoeles are associated with significant obstruction and dysplastic upper renal moieties. A large ureterocoele could be seen prolapsing through the vestibule (Fig. 86.6).

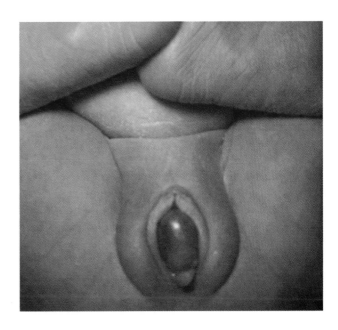

Fig. 86.6 Large ureterocoele seen to prolapse through the vestibule

Ureterocoeles have been reported to be 4–8 times more common in females than in males. In females, 95% of the ureterocoeles are associated with complete duplication of ureters, while in males only two thirds are associated with complete duplication; the remainder is associated with single system normal kidneys.

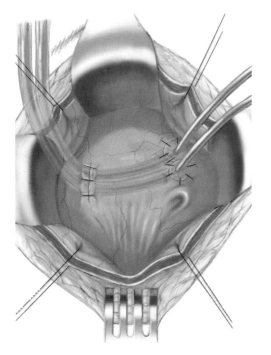

Fig. 86.7 The two ureters, which are bound closely, are dissected out together and reimplanted en bloc to avoid ischemic injury to the lower segments of the ureters

The cystic swelling of the ureterocoele and the dilated ureters associated with them are easily identified in the antenatal scans, after 20 weeks of gestation. In neonates with an uninfected ureterocoele discovered by antenatal scans, endoscopic puncture of the ureterocoele alone may be sufficient. If a dysplastic renal moiety is identified in these asymptomatic children following the deroofing, on functional imaging studies, one could adopt a wait-and-see policy or elect to carry out heminephrectomy at a convenient time. Of late, the consensus has shifted to minimal intervention in these antenatally diagnosed asymptomatic children during the 1st year of life and subsequent evaluation as to what surgical reconstruction, if any, is required.

In those infants with infected ureterocoele, early endoscopic puncture of the ureterocoele must be undertaken. Imaging studies such as DMSA scans should be delayed until 6–8 weeks, following the endoscopic deroofing, to attain accurate values. The overall incidence of VUR following endoscopic puncturing of the ureterocoele is much less than with open surgical procedures. Studies have shown that almost 90% of intravesical and 50% of extravesical ureterocoele renal moieties show useful function, if drained in early life. Therefore, full anatomic and functional assessment should be delayed till 1 year of age, and appropriate reconstructive surgery must then be undertaken.

In almost 50% of extravesical and 15% of intravesical ureterocoeles, further reconstructive surgery will be required. A dysplastic nonfunctioning upper moiety, prone to recurrent infection is better removed. When the upper moieties have reasonable function, then ureteroureterostomy or excision of ureterocoele followed by ureteric reimplantation can be carried out. The final management must be tailored according to the functional and anatomical findings in each child, and demands a flexible approach.

Studies have shown that in up to 50% of those who were treated with heminephrectomy and extended ureterectomy, a second bladder surgery is necessary to deal with VUR of the lower pole ureter or rarely for bladder outlet obstruction. However, the management of VUR that only occurs following heminephrectomy could be guided by the same principles as discussed above.

86.6 Ectopic Ureters

Ectopic ureters are nearly three times more common in females than in males. As with the ureterocoeles, the vast majority of the ureters are associated with duplication in females. In males, the majority of ectopic ureters are associated with single system kidneys. The commonest sites of ectopic ureteral openings in males are posterior urethra and prostatic urethra; a small percentage is seen to be associated with seminal vesicles and epididymis. In females, the commonest sites of ectopic ureteric openings are the urethra, vestibule, and vagina.

When ureteric duplication is detected in the antenatal scans, then a thorough evaluation must include a search for ectopic openings. However, when present later in life, the females tend to present with a history of normal voiding pattern, with damp underwear day and night. In males, the symptoms may be one of urgency and frequency or epididymo-orchitis. The most important factor in diagnosing ectopic ureters is high index of clinical suspicion.

The ectopic ureters are usually associated with the upper renal moiety, and may be seen easily with the initial ultrasound scanning. However, at times, demonstrating an ectopic ureteric opening with imaging studies can be highly challenging. Intravenous pyelography, contrast-enhanced delayed CT scan, and MRI scan have all proven useful in the diagnosis of an ectopic ureteric opening and the associated nonfunctioning, nondilated renal moiety.

When diagnosed later in life, there has already been a period of infection and dysplasia in the associated renal moiety, and heminephrectomy is the treatment of choice in these children. Of late, due to early detection following antenatal diagnosis, the upper moieties could be saved by ureteropyelostomy, ureteroureterostomy, or ureteric reimplantation, when good relative function is confirmed with imaging studies.

At times, when continued vaginal discharge or local infection is noted, a second surgery may be necessary to deal with the residual distal segment of ureter following the initial surgery.

86.7 Pelviureteric Junction Obstruction (PUJO)

Though PUJO in ureteric duplication is relatively rare, when present it is mostly seen in association with the lower renal moiety (Fig. 86.4). On renal ultrasound, a dilated lower pole renal pelvis, with no dilatation of the ureter is seen. MAG3 scintigraphy is necessary to confirm the degree of obstruction and the relative function of the affected renal moiety.

Depending on the exact anatomy, a standard pyeloplasty or a pyeloureterostomy (anastomosing the lower pole pelvis to the upper pole ureter) could be carried out (Fig. 86.8). During pyeloureterostomy, the remainder of the distal ureter should be removed to avoid VUR into this remnant ureteric stump and associated infections in future. However, if the function in the associated renal moiety is poor, then heminephrectomy will become the treatment of choice.

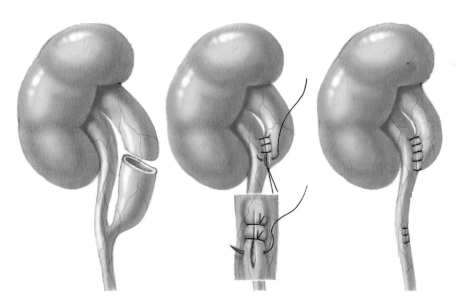

Fig. 86.8 The dilated upper pole ureter should be cut at its insertion with the lower pole ureter. Following repair of the lower pole ureteric defect, the upper pole ureter is anastamosed end to side to lower pole renal pelvis

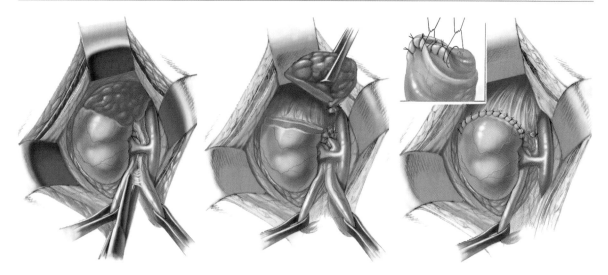

Fig. 86.9 Through a subcostal loin incision and retroperitoneal approach the duplex kidney is exposed. The entire hilar vessels, including that of the lower pole should be clearly identified, before the upper pole vessels could be tied off. The upper pole is usually dysplastic with a clear demarcation from the healthy lower pole. The defect following the heminephrectomy is closed to achieve hemostasis

Further Reading

Fernbach SK et al (1997) Ureteral Duplication and its Complications. Radiographics 17(1):109–127

Keating MA (2007) Ureteral duplication anomalies: ectopic ureters and ureteroceles. In SG Docimo (eds) Clinical Pediatric Urology. Informa Healthcare, Oxon, pp 593–647

Puri P, Miyakita H (2003) Duplication anomalies. In P Puri (eds) Newborn Surgery. Arnold, London, pp 831–836

Puri P, Höllwarth M (2006) Pediatric Surgery. Springer, Berlin, Heidelberg

Schulman CC (2006), Ureteric duplication. In P Puri, M Hollwarth (eds) Pediatric Surgery, Springer Surgery Atlas Series. Springer-Verlag Berlin, Heidelberg, New York, pp 515–522

Vesicoureteral Reflux

87

Prem Puri

Contents

87.1 Introduction

Primary vesicoureteral reflux is the most common urological anomaly in children. It occurs in 1–2% of the paediatric population and in 30–50% of children who present with urinary tract infection. The association of vesicoureteral reflux, urinary tract infection and renal damage is well known. Parenchymal injury in vesicoureteral reflux occurs early, in most patients before age 3 years. Most renal scars are present when reflux is discovered at initial evaluation for urinary tract infection.

The hereditary and familial nature of vesicoureteral reflux is now well recognized and several studies have shown that siblings of children with vesicoureteral reflux have a much higher incidence of reflux than the general pediatric population. Prevalence rates of 27–51% in siblings of children with VUR and a 66% rate of VUR in offspring of parents with previously diagnosed reflux have been reported.

87.2 Aetiology

The ureterovesical junction (UV) acts as a valve and closes during micturation or when the bladder contracts. The UV is structurally and functionally adapted to allow the intermittent passage of urine and prevent the reflux of urine in the bladder. The main defect in patients with vesicoureteral reflux (VUR) is believed to involve the malformation of the UVJ, in part due to shortening of the submucosal ureteric segment due to congenital lateral ectopia of the ureteric orifice. Since VUR primarily involves abnormalities of the ureter and ureteric orifice, it has been suggested that the timing and positioning

P. Puri and M. Höllwarth (eds.), *Pediatric Surgery: Diagnosis and Management*,
DOI: 10.1007/978-3-540-69560-8_87, © Springer-Verlag Berlin Heidelberg 2009

of branching of the ureteric bud from the Wolffian duct may be related to VUR. The underlying abnormality could be due to mutations in one or more developmental genes that control these processes.

87.2.1 Mechanism of Renal Scarring

The association between VUR and renal scarring is now widely recognized. Scarring is directly related to the severity of reflux. Belman and Skoog assessed renal scarring in 804 refluxing units and found renal scars in 5% of those with grade I reflux, 6% of those with grade II reflux, 17% of those with grade III Reflux, 25% of those with grade IV reflux, and 50% of those with grade V reflux.

The mechanism by which reflux produces renal scars is still not clear. It is essential to distinguish between the commonly acquired segmental scarring associated with VUR and infection, and the primary scarring seen congenitally, in which the etiology is very different and linked to abnormal metanephric development. There is no doubt that bacterial pyelonephritis produces renal scars experimentally and clinically. Dimercaptosuccinic acid (DMSA) scans have allowed us to follow sequentially the evolution of a scar from an area of decreased blood flow during the acute inflammatory phase to a parenchymal defect indicative of a mature scar. Yet only half of patients with acute pyelonephritic will have such a scar. What converts an acute inflammatory process into a scar in some patients and not in others is not clearly understood. Factors implicated in the formation of a mature scar include magnitude of the pressure driving the organisms into the tissues, the intrinsic virulence of the organism itself, and the host defence mechanisms. Furthermore, some of the worst examples of renal injury associated with VUR are those that are present at birth. As renal damage at that time cannot be the consequence of infection, such injury is assumed to be developmental in origin, but the pathophysiology of this is not entirely clear.

The three mechanism considered potential etiologies for renal scar formation are (1) reflux of infected urine with interstitial inflammation and damage, (2) sterile, usually high grade reflux, which may damage the kidney through a mechanical or immunological mechanism and (3) abnormal embryological development with subsequent renal dysplasia. Patients in the latter group may also have urinary tract infection in the postnatal period, resulting in extensive parenchymal damage. It is well recognized that in the first 2 groups of renal parenchymal damage it is essential to discover reflux early before damage can be initiated. In the third group, it is clear that congenital damage currently cannot be prevented. However, in these patients it is mandatory to discover reflux at the early stages to prevent exposure to urinary tract infection and avoid the possible progression of renal parenchymal damage.

87.3 Clinical Presentation

It is obviously important to diagnose VUR at the earliest possible age, preferably in infancy. There are a number of clinical presentations, which should raise the suspicion of VUR in an infant. As antenatal ultrasound becomes increasingly routine, many cases will be suspected before birth and should be investigated within the first month of life. Infants with antenatally detected VUR show a male preponderance. Infants with a poor urinary stream as in posterior urethral valves or infants with spina bifida have a high incidence of VUR, while early investigations are indicated in the first-degree of patients with high-grade VUR.

In most cases, VUR is discovered clinically after investigation of urinary tract infection (UTI). The incidence of VUR in children with UTI is 30–50%, with even higher incidence in infants. Infants and children with VUR may also present with symptoms of voiding dysfunction such as frequency, urgency and incontinence.

87.4 Radiological Investigations

87.4.1 Ultrasound

Sonography should be performed in any infant with suspicion of VUR. The kidneys and upper ureters should be examined both in B-mode and real time. The bladder and lower ureters are assessed by real-time examination at each uretero-vesical junction for dilatation, configuration, peristalsis, and continuity with the bladder base. VUR is suspected in the pres-

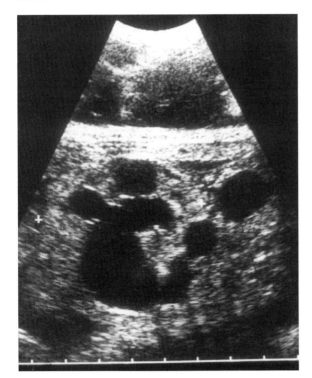

Fig. 87.1 Ultrasound in an infant with grade V VUR, showing hydronephrosis and hydroureter

ence of a dilated pelvicaliceal system, upper or lower ureter, unequal renal size, or cortical loss and increased echogenicity (Fig. 87.1). Sonography is not sufficiently sensitive or specific for diagnosing VUR. The intermittent and dynamic nature of VUR probably contributes to the insensitivity of routine renal sonography in the detection of even higher grades of reflux.

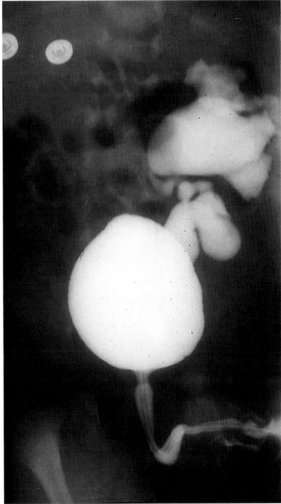

Fig. 87.2 Voiding Cystourethrogram in a male infant showing grade V left VUR

87.4.2 *Micturating Cystography*

VUR is a dynamic process. Bladder filling and voiding are necessary for its elucidation which requires catheterization for adequate documentation.

Micturating cystogram remains the gold standard for detecting VUR (Fig. 87.2).

Despite the high radiation dose and unpleasant nature of the procedure, it has a low false-negative rate and provides accurate anatomical detail, allowing grading of the VUR. It is commonly performed as first-line investigation, together with ultrasound.

Some investigators employ nuclear cystography for diagnosing VUR. This can be either direct or indirect using technetium-labelled diaminotetra-ethyl-pentaacetic acid (DTPA). In direct nuclear cystography, DTPA is instilled into the bladder by urethral catheter or suprapubic injection and the ureters and kidneys are observed on camera during bladder filling and voiding. In indirect nuclear cystography, DTPA is injected intravenously. After the bladder is filled, the patient is instructed to void and the counts taken over the ureters and kidneys are used to assess the presence of VUR. Indirect nuclear cystography requires a co-operative patient and therefore is of no value in infants. The main disadvantage of nuclear cystography is that it does not give anatomical detail and VUR cannot be graded according to international classification.

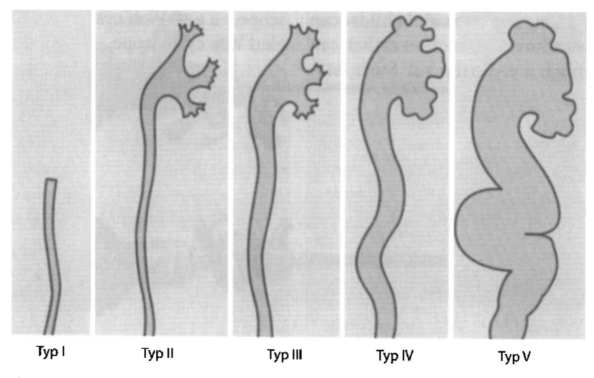

Fig. 87.3 International Classifications of VUR (grades I–V)

According to the international classification of reflux, there are five grades of reflux:

– Grade I, reflux into ureter only
– Grade II, ureter, pelvis, and calices - no dilatation, normal caliceal fornices
– Grade III, mild dilatation and/or tortuosity of the ureter and mild dilation of the renal pelvis - minor blunting of the fornices.
– Grade IV, moderate, dilatation and/or tortuosity of the ureter and moderate dilatation of the renal pelvis and calices-complete obliteration of the sharp angle of fornices but maintenance of the papillary impressions in the majority of calices.
– Grade V, gross dilatation of the renal pelvis and calices (Fig. 87.3)

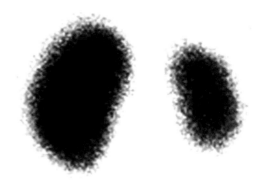

Fig. 87.4 DMSA scan in an infant with VUR shows small scarred L Kidney

87.4.3 DMSA Scan

DMSA is the most sensitive technique for detecting renal scarring. When performed in the course of acute urinary tract infection, the DMSA scan is currently the most reliable test for diagnosis of acute pyelonephritis. The scan, when performed within 4 weeks of the UTI, detects transient areas of abnormality that may not develop into scars on long-term follow-up. To avoid misleading results of the DMSA scan, it is mandatory to establish under what clinical condition the test was undertaken (Fig. 87.4).

87.5 Management

Management of VUR has been controversial. The two main options available for the treatment of VUR are medical or surgical.

87.5.1 Medical Management

This strategy is based on three important assumptions:

1. Sterile low grade VUR in most cases is not harmful to the kidneys and has no relevant effect on kidney function.
2. Children can outgrow VUR, at least the lower grades.
3. Continuous low-dose antibiotic prophylaxis can prevent infection for many years while VUR is still present.

The patient is required to take low dose daily antibiotics with or without bladder training and anticholinergics and annual ultrasound and VCUG are performed to assess if the reflux has resolved. However, the International Reflux Study Group in children showed that 84% of the children with grade III and IV reflux randomly allocated to medical treatment still have reflux after 5 years. In those with bilateral reflux, 91% had persistence of reflux after 5 years.

87.6 Surgical Treatment

87.6.1 Antireflux Procedures

The majority of the open antireflux procedures entail opening the bladder and performing a variety of procedures on the ureters such as transvesical reimplantation (Politano-Leadbetter technique) and transtrigonal advancement of the ureters (Cohen technique). These procedures although effective, involve open surgery, prolonged in-hospital stay and are not free of complications, even in the best hands. Although open surgery achieves a success rate of 92–98% in grade II-IV VUR, the American Urological Association report on VUR, reported persistence of VUR in 19.3% of ureters after reimplantation of ureters for grade V reflux. The rate of obstruction after ureteral reimplantation needing reoperation reported by the American Urological Association in 33 studies was 0.3–9.1%

87.6.2 Endoscopic Treatment of VUR

Endoscopic treatment has several advantages over the other two options. In contrast to long-term antibiotic prophylaxis, it offers immediate cure of reflux with a high success rate, its success does not rely on patient or parent compliance and the procedure is virtually free of adverse side effects. Long-term administration of antibiotics implies the danger of bacterial resistance with promotion of breakthrough UTIs and antibiotics are usually needed for years. In 2001, Deflux® was approved by the Food and Drug Administration (FDA) as an acceptable tissue augmenting substance for subureteral injection therapy for VUR. Since then, endoscopic treatment has become increasingly popular worldwide for managing VUR and Deflux® is the most widely used tissue augmenting substance.

87.6.3 Indications

- High Grade primary VUR (Grade III-V)
- VUR in duplex renal systems
- VUR secondary to neuropathic bladder and posterior urethral valves
- VUR in failed reimplanted ureters

87.6.4 Technical Notes

- All cystoscopes available for infants and children can be used for this procedure.
- The disposable Puri flexible catheter (STORZ) or a rigid metallic can be used for injection.
- A 1 ml syringe filled with Deflux® is attached to the injection catheter.
- Under direct vision through the cystoscope, the needle is introduced under the bladder mucosa 2–3 mm below the affected ureteral orifice at 6 o'clock position.
- In children with Grade IV and V reflux with wide ureteral orifices, the needle should be inserted not below but directly into the affected ureteral orifice (Figs. 87.5–87.8).

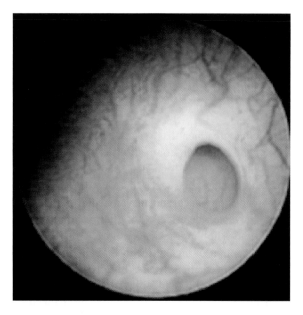

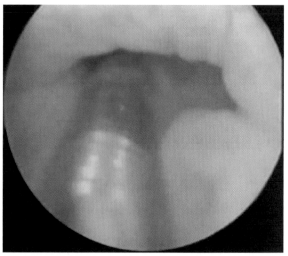

Fig. 87.7 In grade reflux the needle for injection is inserted under the mucosa directly inside the affected ureteral orifice

Fig. 87.5 Endoscopic appearane of a grade V refluxing ureteral orifice prior to injection

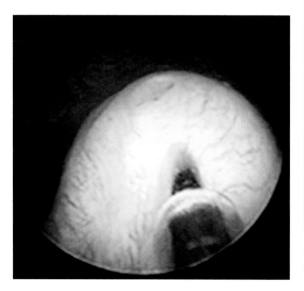

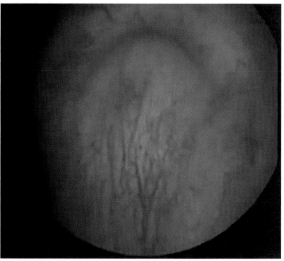

Fig. 87.8 At the end of the injection the ureteral orifice has a slit-like appearance

Fig. 87.6 During the injection the needle is slowly withdrawn until a "volcanic" bulge of paste is seen

- Patients are treated as day cases and a voiding cystourethrogram and ultrasound are performed 6–12 weeks after discharge (Figs. 87.9 and 87.10).

- The needle is advanced about 4–5 mm under the mucosa and the injection started slowly.
- As the Deflux® is injected a bulge appears in the floor of the submucosal ureter.
- A correctly placed injection creates the appearance of a nipple on the top which is a slit-like or inverted crescent orifice.

Endoscopic subureteral injection of Deflux® is excellent first line treatment in children with 87% success in high grade Vesicoureteral Reflux after one injection. This 15-min outpatient procedure is safe and simple to perform, and it can be easily repeated in failed cases.

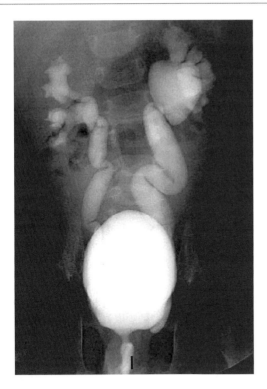

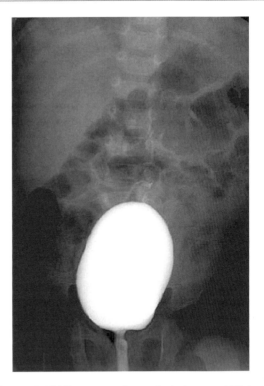

Fig. 87.9 Voiding cystourethrogram showing bilateral grade V reflux

Fig. 87.10 Voiding cystourethrography in the same child showing no evidence of reflux 3 months after the STING procedure

Further Reading

Menezes M, Puri P (2007) The role of endoscopic treatment in the management of Grade 5 primary Vesicoureteral Reflux. Eur Urol 52:1505–1510

Puri P (2006) Endoscopic Treatment of Vesicoureteral Reflux. In P Puri, ME Höllwarth (eds) Pediatric Surgery. Springer Surgery Atlas Series, Springer-Verlag Berlin Heidelberg, New York, pp 493–498

Puri P, Pirker M, Mohanan M et al (2006) Subureteral dexranomer/hyaluronic acid injection as first line treatment in the management of high grade vesicoureteral reflux. J Urol 176:1856–1860

Posterior Urethral Valves

88

Paolo Caione and Simona Nappo

Contents

88.1 Definition and Incidence

Posterior urethral valves (PUV) are the main cause of bladder outflow obstruction in male infants, and the most common obstructive uropathy leading to chronic renal failure in childhood. Their incidence is estimated at 1/5,000 to 1/8,000 male births, but these figures are probably underestimated due to fetal and perinatal demise. Despite occasional reports of PUV occurring in twins and in siblings, PUV are generally sporadic. Chromosomal anomalies are uncommon and associated anomalies are also very rare. Cryptorchidism only occurs more frequently in VUP patients (12%) compared to the 0.8% expected incidence in common children.

88.2 History and Classification

Morgagni was the first to report PUV in 1717. Subsequent descriptions were made by Lagenbeck (1802) on an autopsy finding, and by Tolmatschew (1870) who first recognized PUV as a pathological entity. Finally a systematic classification of PUV was

P. Puri and M. Höllwarth (eds.), *Pediatric Surgery: Diagnosis and Management*,
DOI: 10.1007/978-3-540-69560-8_88, © Springer-Verlag Berlin Heidelberg 2009

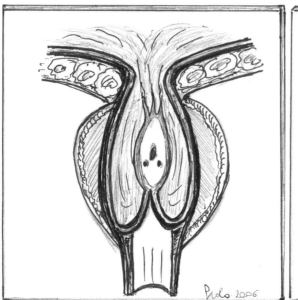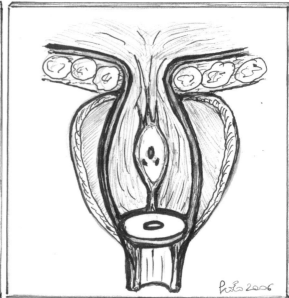

Fig. 88.1 Type 1 and Type 3 PUV according to Young's Classification

created by H. Young. He recognized three types of PUV: type I are a pair of leaflets originating from the lower border of the veru montanum extend laterally and distally on the lateral wall of the membranous urethra, to fuse anteriorly at 12 o'clock; type II valves are folds that arise from the veru montanum but proceeds proximally towards the bladder neck to divide into membranes; type III valves are a congenital urethral diaphragm with a central perforation, not related to the veru montanum but located either above or below it (Fig. 88.1).

Over the years several criticisms have been moved to Young's classification. Type II folds are now regarded as not obstructing. Most PUV encountered in the clinical practice are classified as type I while type III is less common.

In the early 1990s Dewan et al. proposed a different classification: in their series they noted that if endoscopy was performed before passing any urethral catheter, a diaphragm could always be detected. The diaphragm (type III valves) would therefore be disrupted by the urethral catheter, transforming it in type I valves. The authors proposed a new name for PUV, which they termed COPUM (Congenital Obstructing Posterior Urethral Membrane). According to recent anatomical findings in a fetus with PUV, Dewan's classification

could reflect the real embryogenesis of PUV. Nonetheless, Young's classification is the one commonly in use.

88.3 Embryology

The precise embryology regarding PUV remains unclear.

At the 6th week of gestation the mesonephric duct opens in the cloaca at the Muller's tubercle, at midpoint between the cranial and caudal portion of the primitive urogenital sinus. During the 7th week the urorectal septum divides longitudinally the cloaca in the urogenital sinus, anteriorly, and the anorectal canal posteriorly. The cranial portion of the urogenital sinus will give rise to the bladder and the prostatic urethra, while the caudal portion will become the definitive urogenital sinus. In the male the definitive urogenital sinus will become the lower part of the prostatic urethral, just below Muller's tubercle, and the membranous urethra; the anterior urethra will form from tubulization of the urethral plate, a phenomenon which is dependent on the peripheral transformation of testosterone by the 5-alpha reductase.

Tolmatchew considered PUV as the abnormal overgrowth of the normally present anatomical folds and ridges of the posterior urethra. Bazy (1903) thought they were the remnants of the urogenital membrane. Lowsley (1914) was the first to offer a theory of PUV based on microscopic examination: noting that valves were primarily composed of dense connective tissue fibers and sparse smooth muscle fibers, with a stratified squamous epithelium, he considered PUV of mesodermal origin, as the result of anomaly of the mullerian and Wolfian duct origin. Stephens (1955) in a similar theory suggested that PUV would result from an abnormal anterior insertion of the mesonephric duct in the cloaca: the development of the rectourethral septum would impend the migration of the mesonephric duct cranially and posteriorly, giving rise to anterolateral folds. The study of Roberts and Hayes (1969) further supported the hypothesis of an extraurethral or wolffian origin of PUV.

88.4 Pathophysiology

The urethral obstruction due to PUV appears early in the fetal life. As a consequence, all the urinary apparatus above the membranous urethra develop in the presence of a significant distal obstruction and therefore of high pressures. The posterior urethra, the bladder, ureters and kidneys will show different degree of damage according to the degree of the urethral obstruction. Futhermore, fetal urine is one of the main components of amniotic fluid, which is essential for lung development: in the more severe cases of PUV oligohydramnios may develop, with subsequent risks of pulmonary hypoplasia.

88.4.1 Urethra

The prostatic urethra above the PUV dilates and elongates.

88.4.2 Bladder

Bladder outlet obstruction during fetal life determines hyperplasia and hypertrophy of the detrusor muscle, which appears significantly thickened. At prenatal ultrasound a huge dilated bladder with a thickened wall, so–called "megacystis", can be detected. At birth the bladder can be visible and palpated as a hard suprapubic mass. At cystoscopy it will have a typical appearance with pseudodiverticula and severe trabeculation, with the ureteral orifice hardly visible. Histology of the bladder wall shows infiltration of the smooth muscle with collagen type III and elastin. Alterations in local neurotransmitter have also been described, leading to bladder overactivity. The result is at birth a low-compliant, small capacity, high pressure bladder.

88.4.3 Vesico-Ureteral Reflux and The "Vurd" Syndrome

About 50% of patients with PUV show vesicoureteral reflux (VUR) at the time of diagnosis. VUR can be due either to the high bladder pressure that induces the development of diverticula and the anatomical incompetence of the uretero-vesical junction, or to the congenital embryological lateral placement of the ureteral bud, according to Stephens' theory.

Once obstruction is relieved, at long term follow-up between 30% and 50% of VUR will show significant improvement or will disappear, and 30% more will be adequately managed with antibiotic prophylaxis, without the need of surgery.

Between 15% and 20% per cent of patients with PUV have unilateral VUR associated with unilateral significant renal damage or dysplasia. Duckett termed this condition "VURD syndrome" (posterior urethral Valves, Unilateral Reflux, Dysplasia) (Fig. 88.2). Greenfield (1983) subsequently reported that the contralateral kidney in boys with VURD syndrome was normal, concluding for a protective role of the condition: the unilateral VUR with associated dysplasia would act as a "pop-off" mechanism, relieving the pressure in the urinary system and therefore protecting the contralateral kidney. Three other possible pop-off mechanisms were proposed by Rittenberg et al. (1988), and namely a giant bladder diverticulum, a perirenal urinoma and urinary ascites.

Recently Cuckow (1997) found that patients with VURD present a dramatic increase of serum creatinine along with age, suggesting that adequate follow-up is warranted before drawing any conclusion.

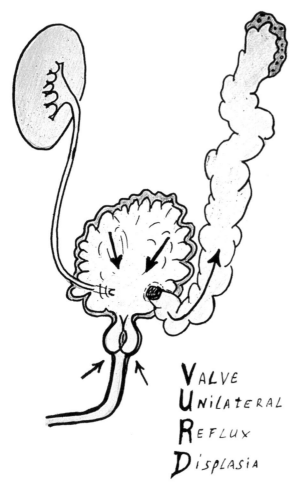

Fig. 88.2 The "VURD syndrome": Unilateral vesicoureteral reflux and renal Dysplasia in PUV patients

88.4.4 Urinary Ascites and Urinoma

The increased pressure in the urinary tract may lead to rupture of the caliceal fornix with subsequent perirenal urinoma. Urinary ascites can also develop, whose mechanism is yet unclear. These entities can be detected at prenatal ultrasound (Fig. 88.3). During the following gestational weeks the site of the rupture may heal spontaneously and no lesion be visible at birth. Just like a unilateral reflux in the VURD syndrome or giant bladder diverticula, both urinary ascites and a urinoma may act as a pop-off mechanism.

88.4.5 Renal Dysplasia

Renal dysplasia is the result of congenital anomaly of tissue development. At histology it is characterized by the presence of primitive ducts, modest disorganization and foci of cartilage; microcysts are present in the renal cortex. At prenatal or postnatal ultrasound, dysplastic kidneys appear small and hyperechoic, with small cortical cysts (Fig. 88.4).

According to Stephens, dysplasia results from the congenital lateral displacement of the ureteral bud that meets the metanephric blastema. This is confirmed by the frequent report of dysplasia associated with lateral displacement of the ureteral orifice at cystoscopy in

Fig. 88.3 Prenatal ultrasound showing urinary ascites in a male fetus with bilateral hydroureteronephrosis

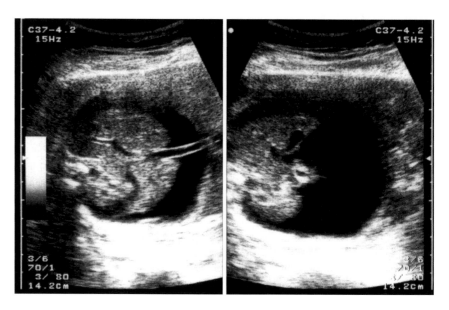

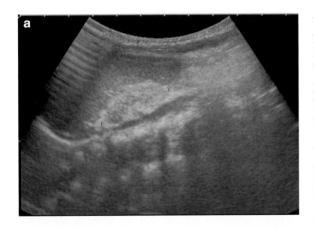

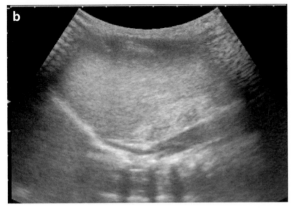

Fig. 88.4 Postnatal ultrasound of renal dysplasia (small hyperhecoic kidneys) in a baby with prenatal bilateral hydronephosis and last term oligohydramnios

PUV patients. However Beck demonstrated that dysplasia may also result from maturation of the renal blastema in the presence of high pressure. Whether dysplasia is caused mostly by a developmental defect or by high pressure is impossible to determine. Dysplasia must be regarded as a negative prognostic factor since it is not reversible, determines reduced renal functional reserve and leads to chronic renal failure.

88.4.6 Renal Failure

In PUV patient's renal damage involves either the tubular or the glomerular function.

Tubular damage may indeed precede glomerular injury. It manifests with impaired ability to acidify urine, and therefore acid-base imbalance and metabolic acidosis, and impaired ability to concentrate urine and therefore polyuria. Acidosis and polyuria are particularly dangerous in newborns and infants with PUV, where continuous monitoring of hydric and salt balance is warranted. At long term polyuria may induce persistence of upper urinary tract dilatation, despite the relief of the obstruction, and worsen bladder function (see "the valve bladder syndrome").

Glomerular damage with chronic renal failure may be due to different mechanisms. First congenital dysplasia, which strongly reduces the amount of functioning renal parenchyma. Secondly urinary infections, which in the presence of urinary dilatation and bladder dysfunction, can lead to further renal scarring. Third, somatic growth at puberty, which determines an increased requirement for renal function and may face with a situation of reduced functional renal reserve. Glomerular hyperfiltration of residual glomeruli, with proteinuria, glomerulosclerosis and progressive glomerular damage can also play a role in the progression towards end stage renal disease.

88.4.7 Lung Development

For normal pulmonary development, both mechanical and chemical factors produced by the kidney are necessary. Before the 16th week of gestation the contribution of fetal urine to the amniotic fluid is scarce; later in gestation up to 90% of amniotic fluid is made of fetal urine. In the most severe cases of PUV, the decreased urinary output due to renal dysplasia or severe hydronephrosis results in oligohydramnios. This in turn interferes with alveolar development and leads to lung hypoplasia and perinatal death. Patients show at birth the typical facial features, lung hypoplasia and lower limb deformities of Potter's syndrome.

88.5 Diagnosis: Symptoms and Signs

88.5.1 Prenatal Diagnosis

Prenatal ultrasound has dramatically changed the diagnosis of PUV, with the majority of patients nowadays diagnosed in the prenatal age.

Screening obstetric ultrasound series have determined that the incidence of hydronephrosis varies from 0.48%

to 1.4% of fetuses. The diagnosis of PUV must be suspected in a male fetus in the presence of hydronephrosis (unilateral or bilateral), and a thick walled bladder that does not empty. Additional sonographic finding can be the dilatation of the posterior urethra (the "keyhole" sign as described 1994) (Fig. 88.5), and occasionally the appearance of a urinoma or urinary ascites (Fig. 88.3). The development of oligohydramnios during pregnancy is the main factor with a negative prognostic significance in fetus with suspicion of bladder outlet obstruction. The sonographic report of increased parenchymal echogenicity and/or cortical cysts, suggestive of renal dysplasia, is also a poor prognostic factor, but the report of "normal" fetal echogenicity does not exclude the finding of dysplasia after birth. The skill level of the ultrasonographer, the ability to delineate the normal from the abnormal and the time of gestation have a profound impact on the correct diagnosis (Table 88.1).

It is not clear yet whether a prenatal diagnosis is per se related to a worse prognosis compared with a postnatal diagnosis. Several reports nonetheless agree that an early prenatal diagnosis (<24 week gestational age) is followed by a worse prognosis in terms of pulmonary hypoplasia or renal failure than a later prenatal diagnosis (>24 week)).

In summary, sonographic criteria have been defined which allow identifying with considerable accuracy the fetuses with suspected PUV: male fetus dilated bladder, hydroureteronephrosis and dilated posterior urethra (Table 88.1). Predictors of poor prognosis include: dilatation present <24 week, moderate/severe hydro-ureteronephrosis, thick-walled bladder, oligohydramnios, sonographic evidence of renal dysplasia (hyperechoic cortex, cortical microcysts).

88.5.2 Neonatal Diagnosis

In the absence of a prenatal diagnosis the newborn with PUV may present with an abdominal mass, failure to thrive, urosepsis or urinary ascites. Respiratory distress can also be the presenting sign soon after birth. Abdominal distention can be due to urinary ascites. In most cases the bladder can be palpated as a firm mass in the suprapubic region. In a third of cases the presentation is dramatic with vomiting, dehydration, renal failure with increased creatinine, acidosis, hyperkalemia, and risk of life. Urinary stream is often weak, or urine comes out in drops, but the presence of a normal stream does not exclude PUV (Table 88.2).

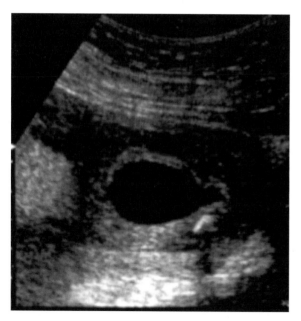

Fig. 88.5 Prenatal ultrasound showing dilated thickened-walled bladder and dilated posterior urethra ("keyhole sign") typical of PUV

88.5.3 Diagnosis in Childhood and Later

PUV presenting in older children are generally minor forms at the end of the spectrum. It may still happen though to see young boys complaining only of voiding

Table 88.1 Prenatal ultrasonographic signs suggestive of PUV (in a male fetus)

Hydronephrosis (unilateral/bilateral)
Ureteral dilatation
Distended thickened walled bladder ("Megacysts")
Distended bladder + Dilated urethra ("Keyhole sign")
Oligohydramnios
Hyperechoic kidneys (renal dysplasia)

Table 88.2 Presenting symptoms and signs of PUV in newborns

Respiratory distress
Abdominal suprapubic mass (urinary retention)
Abdominal distention (urinary ascites)
Urinary sepsis (failure to thrive, vomiting, dehydration, hypotonia, fever)
Metabolic acidosis
Electrolyte imbalance (Hyponatremia, hyperkalemia)

symptoms, with misdiagnosed renal failure. School-age children may present with urinary incontinence, enuresis, and urinary tract infections. Late acquisition of urinary control is often reported. Hematuria can occur after minor trauma. A careful micturition chart will reveal symptoms of urgency and frequency but also hesitancy, weak stream, abdominal straining to void. An urgency/frequency syndrome not responding to anticholinergics and associated with increased bladder thickness and postvoid residual at the ultrasound should demand careful further investigations.

88.5.4 Differential Diagnosis

In the prenatal age, differential diagnosis between upper urinary tract dilatation due to PUV and hydronephrosis due to primitive UPJ obstruction or obstructive or refluxing megaureter is not always possible. The presence of other signs of infravesical obstruction (megacysts, dilated urethra, oligohydramnios, renal dysplasia) improve diagnostic accuracy.

The differential diagnosis between PUV and other causes of infravesical obstruction is even harder. Among the other causes: urethral atresia, prune-belly syndrome, neurogenic bladder, and megacystis-microcolon-hypoperistalis syndrome (the latter occurring in female fetuses) (Table 88.3).

In school age children presenting with voiding dysfunction, other causes of bladder outlet obstruction must be ruled out, from meatal stenosis to urethral stenosis due to previous urethral trauma (Table 88.4). Careful inspection of the genitalia, personal history of

Table 88.3 Differential diagnosis of PUV in the newborn

Hydronephrosis from uretero-pielic junction (UPJ) obstruction
Vesicoureteral reflux
Obstructive megaureter
Ureterocele (obstructing bladder neck)
Prune-belly syndrome
Neurogenic bladder
Microcolon, megacystis, hypoperistalis syndrome

Table 88.4 Differential diagnosis of PUV in school age children (minor forms of PUV)

Meatal stenosis
Urethral stenosis (post traumatic)
Anterior urethral valves
Overactive bladder

previous urethral trauma, uroflowmetry, urinary ultrasound and mostly VCUG will lead to diagnosis.

88.6 Diagnosis: Imaging

88.6.1 Ultrasounds

Both in the prenatal and postnatal period ultrasound is fundamental to evaluate the effects of PUV on the urinary tract. PUV will be suspected in the presence of unilateral or bilateral hydronephrosis with ureteral dilatation, associated with increased thickness of the bladder wall; eventually hyperechoic renal parenchyma, dilatation of the posterior urethra, a urinoma or urinary ascites can be associated signs (Figs. 88.3, 88.4, 88.5, 88.6).

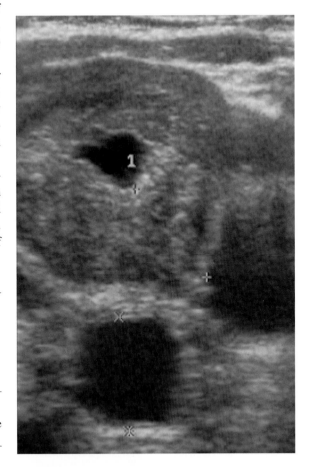

Fig. 88.6 Postnatal ultrasound in a newborn with PUV, showing a significantly thickened walled bladder and bilateral ureteral dilatation

In older children complaining of voiding symptoms, the sonographic report of increased bladder thickness and significant post void urine residual will require further diagnostic investigations (VCUG, uroflowmetry + EMG, cystoscopy).

88.6.2 Voiding Cystourethrogram (VCUG)

VCUG is the gold standard for the diagnosis of PUV. Adequate antibiotic therapy and absence of urinary tract infection are mandatory to perform VCUG.

In the newborn, transurethral catheterization can be performed with a 6 or 8 Ch Nelaton catheter or feeding tube. With the introduction of the contrast medium, the bladder will be evaluated: bladder capacity and if present pseudodiverticula, giant diverticula and vesicoureteral reflux will be recorded.

At bladder capacity, the transurethral catheter will be removed and the urethra evaluated during micturition. In PUV patients the posterior urethra will typically appear dilated and elongated, ending with a U shape at the membranous urethra. Distal to the obstruction, the urethra will be of reduced diameter (Figs. 88.7 and 88.8). Reflux of contrast medium in the seminal vesicles may occur. Overdistention of the bladder with bladder rupture during VCUG has been occasionally described and must be carefully looked into.

At VCUG differential diagnosis of PUV is easily made from urethral atresia, neurogenic bladder and prune-belly syndrome. In prune-belly syndrome the urethra is dilated and scoliotic and may narrow at the membranous urethra, but no obstacle to the outflow is present, the bladder neck is wide open and the bladder is large and with smooth walls.

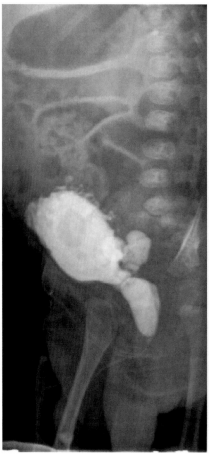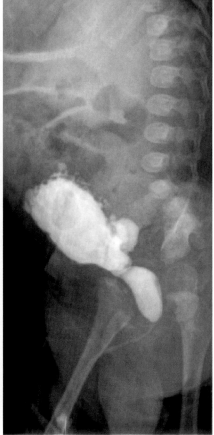

Fig. 88.7 In the same patients VCUG shows a trabeculated bladder with multiple small pseudodiverticula, dilated posterior urethra, absence of VUR

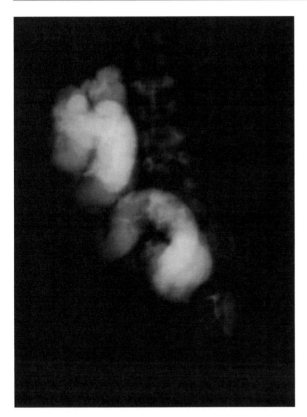

Fig. 88.8 VCUG showing a small trabeculated bladder and a high grade VUR with dilated pielocalicel system in baby with VURD syndrome

88.6.3 Urodynamics

Both non invasive urodynamics (voiding chart, uroflowmetry + EMG, residual urine) and invasive urodynamics (cystometry, pressure/flow study, videourodynamics) are particularly useful in the follow-up of patients with PUV, especially after the age of acquisition of urinary control. (See "incontinence and voiding dysfunction".)

88.6.4 Radioisotopic Scan

Both DMSA renal scan and MAG3 renal scan are routinely performed in PUV patients. The first is mostly accurate in assessing split renal function and the presence of renal scarring. MAG3 renal scan is more useful in assessing the degree of urinary tract obstacle in cases of persisting upper tract dilatation.

Table 88.5 Fetal urine value indicative of good renal function

Total protein < 20 mg/dl
β2-Microglobulin < 4.0 mg/dl
Sodium < 100 mg/dl
Calcium < 100 mg/dl
Chloride < 90 mg/dl
Osmolality < 200 mosm/l

From Thomas DFM. Fetal urology and prenatal diagnosis. In Belman B et al. Clinical Pediatric Urology. Dunitz Ed. 2002, pp. 65–81

88.7 Management

88.7.1 Prenatal

Antenatal treatment of bladder outlet obstruction still remains controversial. Bladder drainage by serial vesicocentesis, continuous drainage by vesico-amniotic shunt or open bladder surgery were adopted enthusiastically in the Eighties. The metanalysis of the published studies shows that although bladder drainage improves survival relative to no drainage due to ameliorate postnatal pulmonary function, results of prenatal treatment have been generally disappointing as far as renal function is concerned (Table 88.5).

The futility of treating severely affected fetuses with irreversible renal dysplasia has been recognized. Similarly, antenatal intervention is not recommended in cases with normal amniotic fluid. Efforts are therefore directed towards selecting those fetuses with deteriorating but potentially recoverable function, which would potentially benefit from intervention. Criteria for patient selection are considered: oligohydramnios, presence of a normal male karyotype, absence of other life-threatening malformations, and absence of sonographic findings renal dysplasia, electrolyte and protein contents on fetal urinary samples considered of good prognosis (Table 88.6).

Open fetal surgery as first reported by Harrison in the Eighties, still has to be considered experimental. Minimally invasive surgery with laparoendoscopic technology as suggested by Quinter et al. is now being developed in some centers. The aim is to create a vesicostomy under direct vision or directly treat the urethral obstruction in utero using a semirigid fetal cystoscope.

The generally accepted modality of antenatal treatment is the creation of a vesico-amiotic shunt. Under sonographic guidance the bladder is punctured with a

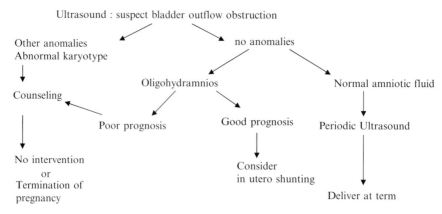

Table 88.6 Flow-chart of management of the fetus with supect bladder outflow obstruction

trocar and a cannula introduced through the maternal abdominal wall, the uterus and the fetal abdominal wall, and a JJ or a pigtail catheter inserted into the fetal bladder. Complications occur in up to 40% of cases, including shunt malfunctioning and dislodgement, chorioamnionitis, damage to adjacent anatomical structures or prenatal labour. Modifications in catheter design and in anaesthesiology, with more accurate shunt placement, will hopefully reduce the complication rate.

In cases of late occurrence of olygohydramnios, there is insufficient evidence to justify elective preterm delivery, which should indeed be performed as close as possible to term. But when premature labour occurs spontaneously after 34 weeks, it seems reasonable to allow it proceed once adequate lung maturity is established. A planned C section in a hospital with neonatal intensive care staff is warranted in order to adequately manage a respiratory distress if present.

In summary, prenatal intervention with vesico-amniotic shunting is still object of debate because (1) Differential diagnosis may be not accurate; (2.) we are not able yet to identify those patients which benefit from a shunt; (3) prenatal intervention is possible at a fetal age when renal dysplasia has already occurred and is not reversible; (4) complications of prenatal intervention are not negligible.

88.7.2 Neonatal

In newborn with suspicion of PUV aggressive treatment of electrolyte and fluid imbalance, sepsis and acidosis is mandatory. Adequate bladder drainage must be provided even before the diagnosis is confirmed at the VCUG, for the high risk of sepsis till the urethral obstruction is not relieved. Bladder drainage can be achieved trans urethram or through a suprapubic catheter. A 6 Fr or 8 Fr Nelaton Catheter or a 5 Fr feeding tube inserted per urethram gives generally adequate drainage. These catheters, with a straight tip, may actually bump on the hypertrophic bladder neck or curl in the posterior dilated urethra: should this happen, a little finger inserted in the rectum may help in elevating and straighten the prostatic urethra, thus facilitating the catheter placement into the bladder. As an alternative a Tieman 6 Fr or 8 Fr catheters with a bent tip will be easily inserted. We prefer the insertion of a 6 Fr or 8 Fr Foley catheter with a balloon as fixing device; in PUV patients however the balloon can be incorrectly inflated in the dilated posterior urethra, therefore the correct position of the catheter must always be checked.

Once bladder drainage is obtained, transient polyuria with increased water and sodium urinary loss is generally observed. Careful monitoring of fluid balance with records of in and out fluids, daily body weight and electrolytes check are of utmost importance in PUV newborns and infants (Table 88.7).

Table 88.7 Management of a newborn with suspicion of PUV

Drain the urinary tract (transurethral catheter, suprapubic)
Provide venous access
Correct metabolic acidosis
Correct electrolyte and water imbalance
Provide antibiotic coverage
Check in/out fluids, body weight, blood pressure, serum analysis

88.7.3 Valve Ablation

Historically valve ablation was attempted both with a non operative approach and with open surgery. The first consisted of introducing an indwelling catheter that was left in place for prolonged time, with the hope it would erode the valves: the risks of sepsis and failure in valve ablation were particularly high. Open surgical valve ablation was performed either through a perineal approach or through an anterior retropubic or transpubic approach. Others proposed the rupture of the valves by retrograde passage of urethral sounds through a vesicostomy or by a percutaneous sheath, or by forceful withdrawal of an inflated Fogarty catheter introduced per urethram, but major urethral trauma can be associated with these procedures. Whitaker designed a specific hook electrode for valve ablation: the procedure was performed under fluoroscopic control under general anesthesia. These procedures are now abandoned or reserved for particular cases (such as babies too small to allow the introduction of a cystoscope) or logistic situation, in favour of and endoscopic approach where the valves are resected under visual control. Hugh Young first described (1919) a rudimental urethroscope and a miniature punch able to resect PUV transurethrally. Since the advent of fiberoptic lighting and Hopkins rod lenses, endoscopic valve ablation has today to be considered the first choice treatment for PUV.

Cystoscopy is first performed with a neonatal cystoscope: the urethra is evaluated, and the valves visualized: gentle pressure on the bladder can create an antegrade flow thus inflating the leaflets valves. The protruding bladder neck, bladder wall trabeculation and morphology of the ureteral orifices are evaluated at this first cystoscopic inspection. Then the cystoscope is withdrawn and a 10 Ch resectoscope is introduced (A more recent 6 Ch neonatal resectoscope is also available). The narrowest site along the urethra is generally the meatus: progressive dilatation with 8–12 Nelaton catheter can be required before the introduction of the resectoscope. The introduction must be gentle and smooth, and the urethra straightened in order to avoid false passage and urethral bleeding. The electroresection (with short burst of cutting current) of the valves at 5 and 7 o'

clock position is then performed under visual control with a right-angle "hook" electrode. When a third leaflet is present, resection at 12 o'clock position is also warranted (Fig. 88.9). As an alternative a "Bugbee" electrode is used by some urologists for resection, but the hook allows better engaging the leaflets and evaluating the complete valve resection. Bladder overdistention during the procedure must be carefully avoided. We prefer to position a Foley catheter soon after the procedure and keep it in place for 48 h, in order to avoid dysuria and better monitor the diuresis in the post-obstructive period. However, when the procedure is correctly performed and urethral bleeding is negligible, the placement of a Foley catheter is not strictly necessary. VCUG is generally repeated after 2–3 months (Fig. 88.10). An endoscopic "second look" is often required in order to complete PUV resection.

Despite the hypertrophy of the bladder neck, bladder neck resection at the time of the endoscopic valve ablation must never be performed. Such treatment in the past has led to persistent urinary incontinence and must therefore be avoided.

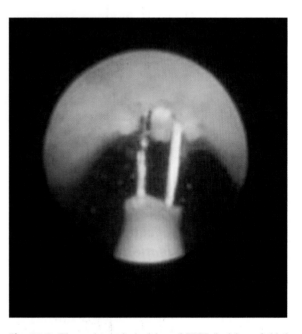

Fig. 88.9 The endoscopic incision of PUV (incision of third leaflet at 12 o'clock position)

Fig. 88.10 VCUG after the
endoscopic incision of PUV,
showing good resolution of the
obstruction with a non dilated
posterior urethra but persistent
VUR

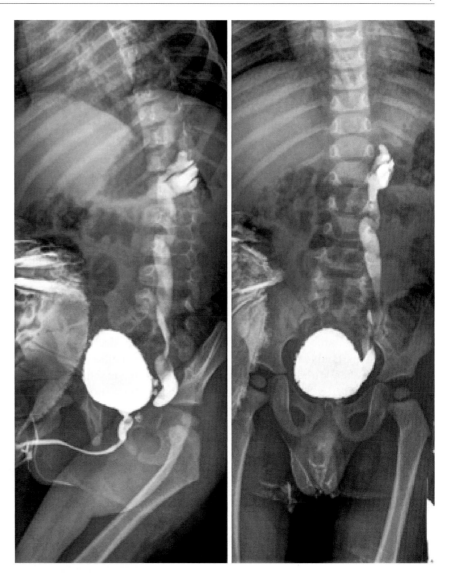

88.7.4 Early Complications of Valve Ablation

If the endoscopic technique of valve ablation is correct, bleeding is generally negligible or very poor. Should this occur, a transurethral Foley catheter should be kept in place until its resolution. The additional placement of a percutaneous suprapubic catheter can be required if blood clotting obstructs the transurethral catheter.

Urethral stenosis nowadays occurs in less than 10% of cases after PUV resection. Stenosis can be imputed to direct urethral trauma by the instrumentation, to longstanding urethral catheter or to the use of the electrode. Most urethral stenosis occurs in the bulbar or membranous urethra, are thin and can be easily resected endoscopically. In rare cases the stenosis is long and fibrotic, requiring repeated transurethral procedures and eventually open surgery. Of particular concern are those babies undergoing valve ablation and concurrent or subsequent urinary diversion: the "dry" urethra after valve ablation seems particularly at risk of stenosis.

88.7.5 Urinary Diversions

Urinary diversion is still regarded by some authors as a valid alternative to valve ablation.

In our opinion endoscopic valve resection has to be considered the gold standard in the treatment of PUV. Urinary diversion should be reserved to particular situations, such as very small babies, patients with renal failure not improving after resolution of urethral obstruction and patients with persistent very dilated upper tract and/or recurrent urinary sepsis.

88.8 Vesicostomy

Vesicostomy is generally performed according to Blocksom technique: through a 2 cm transverse incision, performed half-way between the umbilicus and the pubis, and an extraperitoneal approach, a small stoma is performed on the posterior bladder wall. The great advantage of vesicostomy, as stated by Duckett, is that it allows decrease of bladder pressure and satisfactory upper urinary tract drainage while at the same time guarantees bladder cycling, which is necessary to maintain bladder elasticity.

88.9 Upper Tract Diversion

Upper tract diversion in the form of percutaneous nephrostomies or different forms of ureterostomies has been advocated by some as routine procedures in PUV patients.

In our opinion these procedures should be reserved to very selected cases such as patients with renal failure and absence of creatinine improvement after PUV ablation or vesicostomy, and in patients with a single, very dilated, functioning kidney. In such cases a high diversion can be justified as salvage procedures. Since the preservation of bladder cycling is important in PUV patients in order to maintain or improve bladder compliance, we prefer surgical techniques of

diversion that preserve bladder cycling. Bilateral Sober "Y" ureterostomy can assure upper tract decompression and at the same time partial urinary flow to the bladder. As an alternative, in cases of bilateral high grade VUR, a unilateral ureterostomy can be performed on the less damaged kidney, leaving the contralateral side undiverted: the unilateral ureterostomy will allow adequate drainage and bladder cycling will be preserved.

88.10 Long Term Outcomes

88.10.1 Vesico-Ureteral Reflux

From 20% to 70% of PUV patients show some degree of VUR at the time of diagnosis, bilateral in 50% cases. In the past, early reconstruction of the upper urinary tract with tailoring of the dilated ureters and ureteroneocystostomy was advocated by some authors. The reimplantation of dilatated ureters in a thickened small capacity bladder carries a high risk of complication, up to 30% of cases, and does not prevent the evolution towards end stage renal disease.

Long term follow-up of PUV patients has indeed shown that there is no rationale for early repair of VUR in these patients.

Mild VUR often disappear spontaneously after valve ablation, without requiring further treatment.

VUR in VURD syndrome on the contrary generally shows little or no improvement after relief of obstruction, and in these cases early nephroureterectomy around 1 year of age was advocated by Duckett. More recently the dilated upper tract of VURD syndrome has been successfully used for bladder augmentation, avoiding the need of an intestinal segment. Ureteral bladder augmentation seems to have less complication than intestinal augmentation. Preserving the refluxing dilated unit of VURD syndrome till older age is therefore recommended: it will be beneficial as pop-off mechanisms for the high bladder pressures in the 1st year of life, and could be used for bladder augmentation in older age, should the augmentation be necessary.

Persisting bilateral high grade VUR may finally require surgical repair. Before any attempt at VUR correction, however, bladder function must be accurately investigated and corrected when needed, fear a high risk of complications after surgery (obstruction, persisting VUR). In selected cases of VUR and good compliance bladder, the endoscopic treatment of VUR with bulking agents can be performed successfully.

88.10.2 The "Valve Bladder" Syndrome

"Valve bladder syndrome" was defined by Mitchell (1980) as a condition with progressive upper tract dilatation despite adequate PUV ablation, a markedly reduced sensation of bladder fullness and elevated intravesical pressure at low filling volumes. Older PUV patients present with incontinence, persistent upper tract dilatation secondary to a non-compliant thick walled bladder, and large urinary output. In these patients with persistent upper tract dilatation three different patterns of Whitaker test are recognised, unobstructed during bladder filling and after voiding; obstructed both during bladder filling and after voiding; obstructed during filling and unobstructed after voiding.

This condition does not appear to be congenital, since many patients show a significant improvement in the upper tract dilatation soon after the relief of the obstruction. The valve bladder syndrome seems indeed an acquired condition, due to a combination of postnatal factors such as a reduced bladder compliance, a reduced bladder sensitivity, an increased post void residual and polyuria.

Reduced bladder compliance is strictly related to the hypertrophy and hyperplasia of the detrusor muscle induced during fetal life by the urethral obstruction. These are initially a rather protective phenomenon and provide for better contractions in the effort of improving voiding. With prolonged obstruction, bladder contractility and compliance are reduced due to increased fibrosis of the bladder wall.

Whether temporary upper tract diversion worsens or ameliorates bladder compliance is still object of debate. Tanagho first noticed that prolonged bladder defunctionalization could result in a small non compliant bladder, and Duckett stated that valve bladder was an acquired phenomenon due to supravesical diversion: he recommended vesicostomy for urinary diversion in order to preserve bladder cycling. Other authors nonetheless (Jayanthi, Koury) do not agree on the negative impact of diversion on bladder function, and assess that poor bladder compliance is inherent in the detrusor and not acquired from the period of temporary defunctionalization.

The increased post void residual can be due to several mechanisms: inefficient bladder emptying with true residual; reflux of urine in a refluxing ureter during voiding with subsequent bladder refilling (so called "pseudo-residual"); functional obstruction of the uretero-vesical junction during bladder filling, with drainage of the dilated upper urinary tract soon after voiding.

The other main factor in valve bladder syndrome is polyuria. Polyuria is described in as many as 75% of boys with PUV. The reduced tubular ability to concentrate the urine determines an increase in the urinary output which leads to progressive and/or persistent upper tract dilatation.

The "valve bladder" is indeed an evolving condition; an initially low capacity, hyperactive, low compliant bladder can progressively decompensate and become overdistended and overcompliant, with supervening hypocontractility. Insensitivity to bladder filling and failure to recognize a full bladder worsen the risk of overdistention and incomplete voiding.

88.10.3 The Defunctionalized Bladder

Much as been written about the ultimate outcome on bladder function of upper urinary tract diversion versus primary valve ablation. A normal bladder, after supravesical diversion, shows significant reduction of capacity and compliance. Once the urinary tract is restored, however, bladder capacity will increase to normal values. What happens to PUV bladder is still object of debate. Tanagho felt that PUV bladder diverted for long time had a great risk of failing to expand after undiversion, and cautioned against prolonged diversion. Lome et al. attributed the reduced bladder compliance not to the length of defunctionalization, but to the chronic infection which would lead to bladder wall fibrosis. Khoury et al. recognized the potential detrimental effect of infections but underlined that reduced bladder compliance was not related to defunctionalization; probably diversion was performed in the worst bladder, which would be non compliant anyhow, regardless the initial form of management. Duckett on the contrary was strongly against supravesical diversion, underlining the importance of bladder cycling in order to maintain and improve bladder compliance and proposed vesicostomy as superior to supravesical diversion. Furthermore he suggested that valve bladder does not occur after primary valve ablation. More recently Jareguizar et al. compared long term bladder function in patients treated by either primary valve ablation or supravesical diversion. They found no significant difference in bladder function between the two different groups; they conclude that temporary urinary diversion has no adverse effect on ultimate bladder function and that low compliance is probably the result of fetal detrusor muscle damage.

The subject is still object of debate. It is not clear yet how often, if ever, a supravesical diversion causes reduced bladder compliance and to what extent the initial bladder status determines the final bladder function, irrespective of the initial urological management.

88.10.4 Incontinence and Bladder Dysfunction

Incontinence is described in 19–81% of 5 year old boys with a history of PUV. In the newborn with PUV, chronic obstruction typically produces a small capacity, scarcely compliant bladder, often associated with upper tract dilatation. After successful valve ablation, progressive reduction of upper dilatation and improvement in bladder capacity and compliance are expected. However, not all bladders become "normal". Up to 75% of boys with PUV show abnormal bladder dynamic.

Urodynamic studies have to identify four different patterns of bladder dysfunction in boys with PUV: bladder instability (overactivity); low compliance; high voiding pressure and myogenic failure.

Bladder overactivity and low compliance are considered the direct consequence of detrusor hypertrophy and hyperplasia during the fetal age. The risk of high tract deterioration in the presence of high bladder pressures has prompted some authors to recommend early aggressive anticholinergic therapy even in small children.

High voiding pressures after valve ablation can be secondary to residual valve leaflets, urethral stenosis or bladder neck obstruction. Historically, during the 1950s and 1960s the bladder neck was perceived as an important cause of bladder outlet obstruction in PUV patients. This led several authors to perform bladder neck endoscopic incision; at long term incontinence resulted in some cases. Recently the use of alpha blockers in PUV patients with outflow functional obstruction has been revisited and encouraging results have been reported.

Safer drugs are also available, despite none of them approved for the use in children so far.

"Myogenic failure" is not easy to diagnose. The diagnosis is based upon a urodynamic study showing the inability to sustain a voiding contraction, rather than on the sole basis of a large post void residual. Post void residual in fact is also found in patients with high grade reflux, due to urine refluxing in the upper tract during voiding and in those with megaureter and functional ureteral obstruction during filling. Patients with myogenic failure can generate only weak bladder contractions; they void with abdominal straining and have large post void residual. Several authors have reported that capacity and compliance increase with age, and in some patients reach or even overcome normal values. Myogenic failure is considered the end point of a progressive increase in capacity and compliance of a valve bladder that eventually decompensates (Holmdahl, De Gennaro). Several factors are thought to increase the risk of evolution towards myogenic failure: persistent bladder outlet obstruction due to residual valves, urethral stenosis or hypertrophic bladder neck; polyuria which induces progressive bladder overdistention and worsen bladder emptying. Glassberg does not accept detrusor hypocontractility as the normal evolution of the valve bladder and consider the "myogenic failure" as the result of secondary bladder neck obstruction, persistent detrusor overactivity and aggressive anticholinergic therapy. Bladder overactivity would induce tightening of the pelvic floor, in the attempt to counteract detrusor contraction, with subsequent worsening of outlet obstruction.

Given the complexity of bladder dysfunction in PUV patients, the evaluation of boys complaining of incontinence is not an easy one. Accurate micturition chart, urinary tract ultrasound and flowmetry with measurement of post void residual represents the first line non invasive urodynamic tools. A normal flowmetry does not exclude the presence of a urethral obstruction, since the bladder may exert particularly high pressure in order to overcome the obstruction. Standard urodynamics, pressure-flow study or videourodynamic are required in many patients in order to accurately rule out the bladder dysfunction. Should a high voiding pressure be detected, any anatomical obstruction must first be ruled out at cystoscopy.

Overactive bladder will be treated with antimuscarinics. Oxybutinine has been widely used so far, but newer drugs such as Tolterodine have the advantage of fewer side effects.

An hypocompliant bladder could improve with anticholinergics, but in case of failure a bladder augmentation could be required.

High voiding pressure is now successfully managed with alpha blockers, while more complex is the approach to myogenic failure which may require scheduled double voiding, alpha blockers, nocturnal bladder drainage and intermittent clean catheterization.

88.10.5 Bladder Augmentation

The indications to bladder augmentation have progressively decreased in the past years in boys with PUV. First, the improved knowledge in valve bladder pathophysiology has shown that PUV bladder is in continuous evolution with spontaneous progressive increase in capacity and compliance over the years. Secondly, the greater attention paid to bladder rehabilitation and urotherapy and the more "aggressive" conservative treatment (anticholinergics, rehabilitation, alphablockers, clean intermittent catheterization, and overnight bladder drainage) have progressively reduced the indications to bladder augmentation in PUV patients.

When necessary, augmentation with a dilated ureter in patients with VURD syndrome can provide adequate improvement in bladder capacity with significant reduction of complications if compared with augmentation with an intestinal segment.

In a small percentage of PUV patients, an intestinal bladder augmentation with an ileal or colonic segment, with or without a Mitrofanoff appendicocutaneovesicostomy, will eventually be required.

88.10.6 End Stage Renal Disease (ESRD)

The incidence of end stage renal disease varies in the different series from 25% to 44%. In one third of cases ESRD develops in the newborn age, mostly due to renal dysplasia. The other two thirds reach ESRD in the late puberty or adulthood. In these latter patients renal function was satisfactory at birth; during the years a combination of urinary infections, bladder dysfunction, hyperfiltration and increased metabolic demand at puberty may lead to decompensation. The longer the follow up of these patients into adulthood, the higher the incidence of end stage renal disease.

Several studies have tried to identify prognostic indicators for evolution to ESRD, including age at presentation in utero and after birth, presence of voiding dysfunction, nadir serum creatinin, presence or absence of pop-off mechanisms. Nadir creatinine seems one of the main prognostic factors: a nadir serum creatinine of 0.8 mg/dl or less during the 1st year of life is significantly correlated with a good prognosis.

Incontinence is a poor prognostic factor. It is reported that incontinence at 5 years to be associated with a 46% incidence of renal failure, versus an incidence of 5% in continent children. It is further reported that bladder dysfunction, and particularly reduced bladder compliance and myogenic failure, are significantly related to ESRD, while bladder overactivity was associated with the lowest incidence of renal failure. Ultrasound evidence of renal dysplasia (hyperechoic cortex and absence of definable medullary pyramids) as well as proteinuria has a poor prognostic significance. It is yet debated whether presence or absence of VUR, and laterality (unilateral versus bilateral) has any prognostic significance for ESRD development (Table 88.8).

88.10.7 Renal Transplantation

A significant reduction in renal graft survival in PUV patients was first reported by Churchill in 1988. Others noted a similar graft survival but reduced graft function with higher serum creatinine levels and increased urological complications.

Table 88.8 Prognostic factors for ESRD

Favorable prognostic signs
- Prenatal detection >24 week (provided a normal ultrasound <24 week)
- Sonographic hypoechoic pyramids (at least in 1 kidney)
- Nadir serum Creatinine <0.8 mg/dl in the 1st year
- No VUR
- Continence at the age of 5 years
- Presence of pop-off mechanisms
- Unilateral VUR

Unfavourable prognostic signs
- Prenatal detection <24 weeks
- Hyperechoic kidneys, no evidence of pyramids
- Nadir serum Creatinine >0.8 mg/dl in the 1st year
- Bilateral VUR
- Incontinence
- Absence of pop-off mechanisms

It is possible that inadequate assessment of bladder function or long term bladder defunctionalization (anuric patients) may have led in the past to renal transplantation on dysfunctional bladders which could increase the risk of graft failure.

With the better knowledge of valve bladder pathophysiology, accurate urodynamic assessment of PUV patients before admission to the waiting list and adequate management of bladder dysfunction, graft survival rate comparable to other patients are expected. Even after bladder augmentation, transplantation can be as successful as in other groups of patients.

ment of ESRD, still represent a heavy burden for these patients. Even prenatal intervention has not significantly improved the prognosis of renal function in boys with PUV. Urodynamic studies have helped us to understand the pathophysiology of valve bladder, and its effect on the urinary tract at long term follow-up. Hopefully an earlier correction of abnormalities of bladder storage and emptying will improve the drainage of the upper urinary tract and will delay or impend the occurrence of ESRD in these patients.

88.10.8 Sexual Function and Fertility

Impaired fertility and sexual function are both reported in PUV patients. Scarring of the posterior urethra secondary to valve ablation, reflux into the seminal vesicles and the ejaculatory duct and cryptorchidism, which occur in 12% of PUV patients, are all factors that could account for a reduced fertility rate. Woodhouse et al. reported a high incidence of slow ejaculation, which they imputed to the persistence of a dilated posterior urethra, but did not find evidence of retrograde ejaculation. More recently hyperprolactinemia was found in 62% of adults with PUV, which can be responsible of slow ejaculation and have an impact of fertility status. Impaired sexual function is on the contrary mostly to be imputed to ESRD.

88.11 Conclusions

Mortality rate in PUV patients has significantly decreased in the last 30 years, from 50% to less than 10% of patients, due to prenatal diagnosis, improvements of respiratory support and resuscitation at birth, and adequate management of ESRD. Nonetheless, morbidity related to PUV, and particularly the develop-

Further Reading

Glassberg KI (2001) The valve bladder syndrome: 20 years later. J Urol 166:1406–1414

Glassberg KI, Horowitz M (2002) Urethral valve and other anomalies of the male urethra. In Belman B, King LR, Kramer SA (eds) Clinical Pediatric Urology, Dunitz, London, pp 899–945

Kaplan GW, Scherz HC (1992) Infravesical obstruction. In PP Kelalis, LR King, B Belman (eds) Clinical Pediatric Urology. W.B. Saunders, Philadephia, pp 821–864

Koff SA, Mutabagani KH, Jayanthi VR (2002) The valve bladder syndrome: Pathophysiology and treatment with nocturnal bladder emptying. J Urol 167:291

Koh CJ, Diamond DA (2006) Posterior urethral valves. In P Puri, ME Höllwarth (eds) Pediatric Surgery. Springer Surgery Atlas Series, Springer-Verlag Berlin Heidelberg, New York, pp. 523–528

Krishnan A, De Souza A, Konijeti R, Baskin LS (2006) The anatomy and embryology of posterior urethral valves. J Urol 175:1214–1220

Lopez Pereira P, Martinez Urrutia MJ, Jaureguizar E (2004) Initial and long term management of posterior urethral valves. World J Urol 22(6):418–424

Puri P, Höllwarth M (2006) Pediatric Surgery. Springer, Berlin, Heidelberg

Thomas DFM (2002) Fetal Urology and prenatal diagnosis. In B Belman, LR King, SA Kramer (eds) Clinical Pediatric Urology, Dunitz, London, pp 65–81

Smith GHH, Duckett JW (1996) Urethral lesions in infants and children. In Gillenwater JY, Grayhac JT, Howards SS, Duckett JW, (eds), 3rd edn. Adult and Pediatric Urology, Mosby, St. Louis, Mo, pp 2411–2443

Neurogenic Bladder

89

Yves Aigrain and Alaa El Ghoneimi

Contents

89.1 Introduction

The prevalence of children with a neurogenic bladder dysfunction secondary to spina bifida has been decreased in the last decades after the wide prenatal ultrasonographic screening and the prophylactic use of folic acid during pregnancy. Nevertheless, there are still many children presenting with signs of neurogenic bladder for other causes than spina bifida. In this chapter we will deal only with neurogenic bladder secondary to neurological lesions, we have not considered the important variant of non neurogenic bladder dysfunction.

Although the management of these children has been significantly modified during the last decades, the main goals of the treatment did not change: preventing urinary tract deterioration and obtaining continence at the expected social age to improve the social insertion of these children.

The first step in investigating a child with a suspected bladder dysfunction is a thorough clinical examination (Table 89.1). This routine examination is very important, especially in occult spinal lesions, not to miss any underlying neurological pathology in children with voiding dysfunction. Once the clinical examination is done, and the voiding diary is established, we usually start with non invasive investigations: renal and bladder ultrasound, urine flowmetry associated with EMG and post void residual estimation. More invasive investigations are done according to these results and on the underlying neurological pathology.

There are many classifications describing neurogenic bladder dysfunction. Most of these classifications are depending on the site of the neurological lesions, well adapted to adult pathology but not to congenital spinal lesions. In fact, in children there is poor correlation between the spinal level of the lesion and

P. Puri and M. Höllwarth (eds.), *Pediatric Surgery: Diagnosis and Management,*
DOI: 10.1007/978-3-540-69560-8_89, © Springer-Verlag Berlin Heidelberg 2009

Table 89.1 Clinical history and exams done when suspecting neurogenic bladder dysfunction. Investigations are required according to the clinical findings and the medical history

History
- Prenatal diagnosis
- Perinatal complications
- Socio-familial conditions
- School activities
- Bladder and bowel habits
- Pattern of incontinence

Physical Examination
- Spine
- Lower extremities reflexes
- Muscles testing
- Sensations
- Gait
- Thorough perineal examination
- Central nervous system, Manual dexterity, Motor coordination

Laboratory
- Urine analysis and culture
- Urine osmolarity
- Serum creatinine level

Imaging
- Renal and bladder ultrasonography
- Voiding cystourethrogram
- Spine plain radiography
- Spinal cord ultrasound (less than 3 months)
- MRI spine and cerebral (more than 3 months)
  UroDynamics
- Non invasive simplified urodynamic studies:
  Flow rate, residual urine, EMG external urethral sphincter electromyography.
- Full urodynamic study:
  Cystomanometry, urethral pressure profiles. (Static, filling, and voiding)

the clinical impact. For this reason, classification based on clinical disorders and urodynamic findings are more practical to be used in children. Main dysfunction is due to either detrusor or urethral sphincter dysfunction. The four main anomalies are defined as: overactive detrusor, under active detrusor, overactive sphincter, or under active sphincter. Many patterns can be the results of combinations of these four anomalies. The most common is the DSD (Detrusor Sphincter Dyssynergia), which is usually secondary to overactive detrusor with overactive sphincter.

Because urodynamic investigation has become such an integrated part of any discussion of the management of neurogenic bladder, it is mandatory to know the definition and specificity correlated to children. The standardisation of the terminology to be used in chil-

dren's bladder dysfunction has been established by the International Children's Continence Society.

The first difficulty to perform urodynamic study in a child is to give the optimal conditions and to do it in a cooperating child. It is important to explain the full procedure to the child and his family assisted by a booklet with simplified explanations. A detailed past and present history is taken. Voiding diary is filled out by the parents before coming to the urodynamic study. Any constipation should be treated efficiently by a bowel program to empty the rectum on the day of the study. Premedication is sometime needed in sensitive children, in our current practice we use routinely the Meopa® to introduce the catheter, and then the child is under no medication during the study to be able to detect his first voiding desires and also to be able to void when needed during the study.

There are many methods of urodynamic studies, but the common basic principles specific to children are the following: smaller catheter, rectal pressure measurement, urethral profile is measured, the rate of bladder filling should be adapted to the expected bladder capacity (usually divided by 10 min), EMG of external sphincter measured either by needles under local anaesthesia or by surface patches. The study is usually completed by measuring the voiding pressures, if the child is able to void by himself.

Video urodynamic has gained popularity in the last decades. Visualisation of the bladder and bladder neck during filling and the urethra during voiding has added more accuracy in the determination of voiding dysfunction, confirming the location of the external sphincter during measurement, or measuring the bladder pressure when reflux is associated.

The most common cause for neuropathic bladder dysfunction in children is the congenital spinal anomaly. The main lesions are summarised in Table 89.2. We are going to describe the expected findings and the modalities of follow up of the most common of these pathologies.

89.2 Myelodysplasia Patient

In cases of MyeloMeningoCele (MMC) the workup is done in the neonatal period, usually after the surgical closure of the defect. This initial workup will serve later as baseline information for the follow up of the child. The workup will include renal and bladder ultrasound, urodynamic study, voiding cystourethrogram.

Table 89.2 Aetiology of neurogenic bladder dysfunction

- Myelomeningocele
- Occult dysraphism
  - Tethered spinal cord
  - Spinal lipomas
  - Filum terminale anomalies
  - Other occult anomalies (Sacral agenesis, Diastematomylia)
- Intraspinal lesions (tumours and cysts)
- Spinal cord injuries
- CNS infections
  - Encephalitis
  - Myelitis
  - Meningitis
- Surgical trauma
  - Pelvic and perineal tumours
  - Anorectal malformations

This baseline information can be compared with subsequent studies to be able to identify children at risk for urinary tract deterioration: poor compliant or overactive detrusor or outflow obstruction as a part of DSD. The identification of such risk factors will justify initiating the prophylactic measures before deterioration of the upper urinary tract.

It is not enough to look at just the radiological appearance of the upper urinary tract, detailed functional screening of the lower urinary tract is necessary to allow an early preventive therapy before the late appearance of upper tract deterioration.

The neurological lesion produced by MMC can be variable. The vertebral level provides little or no clue to the exact neurologic level or lesion produced. The neurologic lesion produced by MMC influences lower urinary tract function in a variety of ways and cannot be predicted by looking at the spinal anomalies or the neurogenic function of the lower extremities. The neurologic lesion in myelodysplasia is a dynamic disease process in which changes take place throughout childhood.

Three categories of lower urinary tract dynamics may be detected: synergic (26%), dyssynergic with and without poor detrusor compliance (37%) and complete denervation (36%). Fifteen percent of newborn have abnormal urinary tract that developed in utero.

Dyssynergy: when the external sphincter fails to decrease or actually increases in its activities during a detrusor contraction or a sustained increase in intravesical pressure as the bladder is filled to capacity. In general, a poorly compliant bladder with high pressure occurs in conjunction with dyssynergic sphincter, resulting in a bladder that empties only at high pressures.

Synergy is characterized by complete silencing of the sphincter during a detrusor contraction, so voiding pressures are usually within normal range. Complete denervation: is noted when no bioelectric potentials are detectable in the region of the external sphincter at any time during micturition cycle or in response to sacral stimulation or Credé manoeuvre.

Within the first 3 years of life 71% of newborn with DSD had urinary tract deterioration on initial assessment or subsequent studies whereas 17% of synergic children and 23% of completely denervated developed similar changes. It appears that outlet obstruction is a major contributor to the development of urinary tract deterioration in these children. It is not only the leak point pressure but also the detrusor filling pressure, which is a significant marker to predict upper tract deterioration. Detrusor filling pressures should be maintained lower than 30 cm H_2O.

When detrusor filling pressures exceed 30 cm H_2O and voiding pressure exceeds 100 cm H_2O, clean intermittent catheterisation (CIC) is necessary.

Sequential urodynamic studies, on a yearly base during the first 5 years of life, provide a safe monitoring of these children.

Anal incontinence is unpredictable and is not correlated to urinary incontinence. The mechanism of anal continence is different from that of urinary sphincter. The external anal sphincter is innervated by the same nerves as the external urethral sphincter, but the internal anal sphincter is influenced by more proximal centres and moreover the internal anal muscle relaxes in response to anal distension.

When the child reaches teenage years the topic of sexuality should be approached and managed according to the diagnosed dysfunction. Men with neurological lesions at S1 or lower are likely to have normal or adequate reproductive sexual function, but only 50% of those with lesions above that level have adequate function.

89.3 Other Spinal Dysraphisms

This group of congenital defects affects the formation of the spinal column but does not result in an open vertebral canal. In children younger than 3 months the vertebral bones have not ossified, thus a window of opportunity exists for ultrasound to screen spinal cord lesions. In children with voiding dysfunction, it is necessary to do a meticulous clinical examination of the sacral area. 90% of children with various occult dysraphic status have cutaneous lesions. This varies from small dimple or skin tag to a tuft of hair, a dermal vascular malformation, subcutaneous lipoma, or a asymmetrically curving gluteal cleft.

On careful inspection of the lower extremities, we can detect a high arched foot, alteration of configuration of toes, or pressure zones on the feet with atrophic lesions on the skin. Some other symptoms like back pain, absent perineal sensation are common in elder children.

Lower urinary tract function is abnormal in 40–90% of affected elder children.

Lipomeningocele, intradural lipoma, and other rare anomalies of filum terminale may be present.

The majority of these children have a normal neurological examination. Urodynamic evaluation reveals abnormalities in one third of infants younger than 18 months of age. These congenital anomalies produce different neurologic findings. Lipomas invariably cause upper motor neuron lesion alone or in combination with lower motor neuron lesion. The reason to consult a specialist may be difficulty in toilet training, urinary incontinence after an initial period of successful dryness (especially during the period of pubertal growth) recurrent UTI, and fecal soiling.

When such lesions are suspected by the urinary symptoms and the cutaneous signs, MRI studies are needed and a full urodynamic evaluation with EMG should be done. The therapeutic measures should be discussed with a neurosurgeon during a multidisciplinary outpatient clinic.

89.4 Sacral Agenesis

Sacral agenesis is defined as the absence of part or all of two or more lower vertebral bodies. The aetiology of this anomaly is uncertain. In familial cases associated with Curarino syndrome (presacral mass, sacral agenesis, and anorectal malformation) deletions in chromosome 7 resulting in HLXB9 mutation have been found. The presentation is variable. More than three fourth of the disorders are detected in early infancy and the remainder detected later in childhood.

When not detected prenatally or at birth, the diagnosis is delayed until failed toilet training brings the child to consult his paediatrician. The main difficulty to detect these children is that they have normal skin sensation and the lower extremities are often normal without any orthopaedic anomalies. The diagnosis

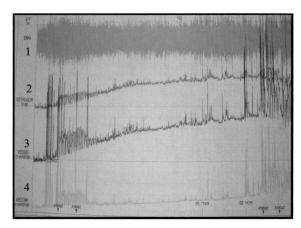

Fig. 89.1 Urodynamic study in a child with sacral agensis showing typical findings of upper motor lesions; overactive detrusor (3), overactive sphincter on the EMG (1), resulting in detrusor sphincteric dyssynergia. This combination has resulted in low compliant bladder and deterioration of the upper urinary tract

may be clinical with the palpation of flat buttocks, and even absent vertebrae in palpating the coccyx. The diagnosis can be confirmed by a simple lateral plain x-ray of the sacral area. MRI will either confirm or exclude sacral anomalies in case of doubt, and it will define associate spinal cord anomalies (sharp cut-off of the conus at T12.

Urodynamic findings: these may show either upper motor neuron lesion (35%) or lower (45%) and 25% have no sign of denervation. Upper motor lesions are characterized by an overactive detrusor, exaggerated sacral reflex and DSD and no evidence on EMG of denervation of the sphincter (Fig. 89.1). The VCUG shows thick trabeculated bladder with closed bladder neck. On the other hand, the lower motor lesions show an acontractile detrusor with open bladder neck on the VCUG, small thin walled bladder.

The neurological lesions are stable and rarely progress with time. The management will depend mainly on the urodynamic findings and the morphological aspect on the VCUG.

89.5 Neurologic Bladder Associated to Anorectal Malformations (ARM)

Spinal cord anomalies (tethered cord, filum terminale anomalies, and a lipoma) may be found in up to 50% of cases of ARM, specially in high type ARM.

Intraspinal imaging is mandatory as not all patients with spinal cord anomalies have a bony defect. Neurogenic bladder dysfunction is a frequent finding, specially when spinal cord anomalies are found. The aetiology of bladder dysfunction can be unclear either due to the congenital spinal anomalies or secondary to the surgical trauma during the surgery. The most common finding on urodynamic studies is an upper motor lesion with DSD. Some authors advise the routine pre-operative urodynamic studies as a baseline information, and others advise doing urodynamic studies when spinal anomalies are detected or urinary symptoms are apparent later in childhood. In our current practice we reserve urodynamic studies to children who have symptoms or abnormalities on the simplified urodynamic studies (flowmetry, EMG, postvoid residual).

89.6 Cerebral Palsy

Cerebral palsy is a non progressive injury of the brain occurring in the perinatal period. Most children with cerebral palsy develop total urinary control. Incontinence is a feature in some, but the exact incidence has never been determined. The most recent publications of Karaman et al. have found urodynamic abnormalities in all children explored. Overactive detrusor with DSD is the most common finding.

89.7 Traumatic Injuries of the Spine

Most common injuries are of the cervical and high thoracic regions; the high spinal lesions will produce an upper motor neuron lesion with overactive detrusor and DSD, thus a high risk for urinary tract deterioration. Urodynamic studies are done after stabilisation of the spinal trauma, usually 2 months after the injury and to be repeated 6–9 months after. It is mandatory to distinguish the type of motor neuron lesions on urodynamic study, the low ones (associated with sacral spinal injuries) are less common and the findings are acontractile detrusor with inactive external sphincter, so low risk for the urinary tract but needs specific measures for incontinence (Fig. 89.2).

89.8 Management of Neurogenic Bladder

The principle of management of a child with a neurogenic bladder has the main objective to preserve a normal upper urinary tract. The second main objective is to improve the social life and the quality of life of these children, giving them urinary and fecal continence. These goals need a reservoir (the bladder) with adequate

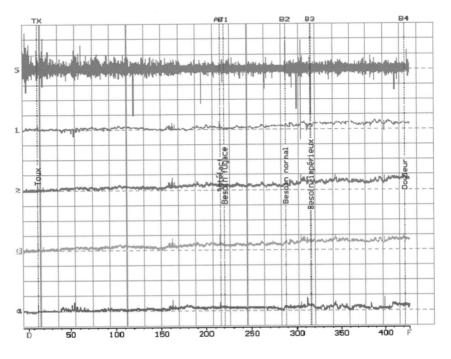

Fig. 89.2 Urodynamic study in child, done 3 years after spinal trauma. The pattern is a typical lower motor neuron lesion: underactive detrusor with underactive sphincter. The main complaint is the urinary incontinence, but the upper tract is protected by the low detrusor pressure and the denervated sphincter

capacity and low storage pressure, able to empty itself with a normal micturation pressure. In a child with a neurogenic bladder none of these characteristics are present. The management will have to be tailored to each individual case in function of his urodynamic results and of his motor and intellectual capacities.

The treatment has to achieve a complete emptying of the bladder, maintain or restore an adequate bladder capacity and compliance and reinforce the sphincter outlet resistance when needed.

89.9   Clean Intermittent Catheterization (CIC)

CIC was introduced by Lapides in 1971 and remains the most important tool in the management of a child with a neurogenic bladder. Intermittent catheterization is a clean but not sterile procedure. It allows a complete emptying of the bladder, lowering the risk of urinary tract infection (UTI) and protecting both the upper urinary tract against high bladder pressure and a degradation of the bladder wall. It may be sufficient to induce dryness of the child if the bladder capacity and the sphincter pressure are sufficient. CIC is enhanced by the availability of single use lubricated catheters but it may be realized with classical Nelaton catheter kept in an antiseptic solution.

CIC should be started as soon as possible to avoid UTI and deterioration of the bladder in case of congenital neurogenic bladder, and there is no more role for Crédé or Valsalva maneuvers. These authors report a favorable outcome in 19 children with upper tract dilatation and or reflux and UTI. When CIC is impossible we rather consider a tubeless cystostomy when the cystometry shows a low compliant bladder and a leak point pressure above 40 cm of water. CIC may be realized through the urethra or through a continent cystostomy (the Mitrofanoff principle). This is another revolution in the management of these children allowing the introduction of CIC when the child or his parents have difficulties in catheterizing the urethra. It may also reduce the risk of prostatitis in post-pubertal boys.

In selected cases where despite adequate CIC urinary tract deterioration occurs, the overnight catheter drainage of the bladder may be successfully tried. Overnight drainage may increase bladder compliance and capacity, avoiding augmentation in some children.

89.10   Pharmacologic Treatment of Neurogenic Bladder Overactivity

As discussed above the maintenance of a normal bladder compliance and capacity rely first on adequate drainage by CIC and sometimes overnight drainage. However this is not always sufficient and the preservation of the reservoir may need either pharmacological manipulation or surgery.

Oxybutinin remains the gold standard of treatment of bladder overactivity. It is acting as an anticholinergic agent. Even if it has not been approved for use in children younger than 5 years, in most cases, oxybutinin is well tolerated and may be introduced early in life after the initiation of CIC. Oxybutinin has the side effects of most anticholinergic agents including mouth dryness, constipation, headaches. These side effects may be reduced or suppressed by direct instillation of the oxybutinin in the bladder during CIC, but the sterile solution is not available everywhere. Other anticholinergic agents have been tested and share the same efficacy: tolderodin, and more recently propiverine. These agents are claimed to reduce the side effects.

Alpha receptor blocking agents have a very limited place in the management of neurogenic bladder.

Botulinum toxin A has been shown to be very effective to reduce bladder overactivity, enhance bladder capacity and compliance. Botulinum toxin A is injected in the detrusor muscle under cystoscopic guidance at 5 IU/kg body weight with a maximum dose of 300 IU. The sites of injection are spread through the bladder except the trigone not to induce reflux. The effect lasts between 6 to 9 months. The procedure, which is minimally invasive, may be repeated after ruling out any allergic reaction.

Sacral modulation has been shown to be effective on bladder overactivity and is currently under investigation in a prospective study.

89.11   Bladder Augmentation

The goal of bladder augmentation is to protect the upper urinary tract when the less invasive procedures are ineffective, and to induce dryness in children where the incontinence is related to low compliance and capacity. There is no ideal tissue for bladder augmentation and each digestive segment has been used has its own side effects.

Bladder auto-augmentation by opening of the sero-muscular layers of the bladder was considered at the beginning as alternative to intestinal augmentation to avoid all the side effects of the use of intestinal segments. The case selection is based on bladders which do not have a major reduction in capacity. The results can be improved by the insertion of a balloon within the bladder to distend the opening of the sero-muscular layers during the initial post-operative period. The auto-augmentation may at least in these cases help to postpone a classical intestinal augmentation.

The stomach, ileum and sigmoid colon have been used for bladder augmentation. The sigmoid has the main advantage to be just behind the bladder lowering the risk of post-operative adhesions. However we are reluctant to its regular use because it may modify the consistence of the feces and compromise fecal continence. Even when it is used as a detubularized patch, it seems that it conserves a significant contractility leading in some cases to urinary incontinence.

The stomach has the advantage of little mucus formation and to lower the metabolic consequences of bladder augmentations avoiding the acidosis that may be induced by ileal or sigmoid augmentation. These advantages are counterbalanced by the haematuria induced by the acid secretion and most authors have abandoned the use of stomach for bladder augmentation.

Ileum is our material of choice for bladder augmentation. The length of the graft is about 30 cm and the last 20 cm of ileum should be preserved to keep to their specific absorptive capacities. The ileum is used as a detubularized patch (clam cystoplasty) after opening the bladder from the bladder neck on its anterior face to the trigone.

When reflux is present at the time of bladder augmentation of a neurogenic bladder, it is secondary to the high bladder pressure and bladder augmentation is usually sufficient to resolve without the need for reimplantation.

Bladder augmentation should only be realized in a patient emptying their bladder by CIC and a neurogenic bladder if the CIC is impossible by the urethra, sensitive or technically impossible because of disability. It is often associated with the construction of a catheterizable channel (Mitrofanoff principle) either through the appendix or through a Monti-tube constructed from an additional 2 cm ileal segment.

89.11.1 Complications of Bladder Augmentation

The augmentation induces per se many complications, some being preventable, others having to be looked for during the life-long follow-up. These complications are mainly infections, stone formation, metabolic complications, perforation and cancer.

It is important to distinguish the presence of a bacteruria which is nearly always found in a child with an augmented bladder under CIC and true clinically significant UTI. Most authors agree not to treat the asymptomatic bacteruria, reserving the use of antibiotics to symptomatic UTI in order to reduce the selection of multi resistant germs. However, the presence of bacteruria may be associated with an increase in the incidence of stone formation. The indications of probiotics and/or of medications reducing the adhesion of E. coli (cranberry juice) are currently under evaluation.

There are many etiologies of stone formation after bladder augmentation: infection, mucus and metabolic are the main factors. Stones are infective in origin in 86% of the cases but additional metabolic factor maybe found in 80%: among these raised urinary pH and hypocitraturia are the most frequent. Mucus is another well known factor of stone formation in these patients. Bladder irrigation with saline once a day during the 1st months following augmentation has been shown to reduce the risk of stone formation.

The reservoir perforation is a rare but life threatening complication which may occur in 2 different situations: fall on a full bladder, but more frequently poor compliance with catheterization. The diagnosis is not easy and should be suspected in case of abdominal or shoulder pain. US is the most useful exam for the diagnosis showing free fluid in the abdomen when the contrast cystography does not show the leak in every case. The treatment of the perforation is surgical in most cases.

The risk of a cancer on an augmented bladder is now well established. This risk is enhanced by the association with tobacco use, exstrophy and immunosuppression (PUV patients with kidney transplantation and bladder augmentation). There is a 12% incidence of adenocarcinoma after a mean follow-up of 18 years in this last case. This implies an adequate patient's (and his/her family) information and a close follow-up after 10 years with US and cystoscopy.

The failure rate of bladder augmentation is low but in rare occasions, the bladder capacity or compliance remains low even after an augmentation and a redo procedure is necessary. The main cause of failure is the ischemia of the intestinal segment due to poor vascular supply. This may be worsened by poor compliance to the CIC regimen and over distension of the bladder.

89.12 Outlet Resistance

In the vast majority of patients with a neurogenic bladder, augmentation and CIC are efficient in obtaining dryness interval compatible with a normal social life. However in some patients where the outlet resistances are broken down, their reinforcement is necessary.

This may be obtained by the peri-urethral or peri-cervical injection of bulking agents, an open cervico-plasty, a sling suspension of the bladder neck, an artificial urinary sphincter or the bladder neck closure.

The injection of bulking agents around the urethra or the bladder neck has the advantage of being a non invasive technique. Various agents have been tested including dextranomer (Deflux®) or silastic particules. We have recently published our experience with dextranomer injections in 61 patients. The incidence of dryness or improvement at 6 months was 51% and this result was maintained during long-term follow-up.

Many techniques of cervicoplasty for patients with a neurogenic bladder have been published suggesting that no one gives perfect results. Urethral lengthening following Kropp tube or its modification by Pippi Salle seems to give better results than the classical Young Dees procedure. The cervicoplasty is usually associated with the bladder augmentation and the construction of a catheterizable channel to avoid difficulties in catheterizing the native urethra in the post-operative period.

Bladder neck sling is considered by many authors as the procedure of choice in females and it has also been advocated in male patients by some. The sling is made of autologous material in most cases (rectus fascia). In selected patients where an augmentation is not needed, the sling may be realized through a vaginal approach using synthetic materials such as small intestinal submucosa (SIS®). Castellan et al. report 88% of good continence with a mean follow-up of 4 years in 58 patients.

The Artificial Urinary Sphincter (AUS) is considered by many authors as the procedure of choice in boys when a reinforcement of outlet resistance is needed to gain adequate continence. Its ideal indication is when one may hope for spontaneous voiding of the child when the pericervical component of the AUS is deflated. This is rarely the case in children with a neuropathic bladder, most of them being under CIC. Continence rates between 80% and 90% are reported among children where the AUS has not been removed due to erosion, sepsis or dysfunction. Children with AUS undergo many procedures due to device technical problems: hence 63/107 children of the French multi-institutional study had to be reoperated on and 42 of them more than once. Most authors do not recommend implantation of an AUS device before puberty.

Bladder neck closure was initially proposed by Mitrofanoff in the management of children with a neuropathic bladder. It has the obvious advantage to theoretically prevent any leakage through the urethra but it exposes the bladder and upper urinary tract to a high risk of deterioration in case of bad compliance to CIC. The surgical procedure to close the bladder neck is not an easy one and fistula between the bladder and urethra are not exceptional. We reserve bladder neck closure as a secondary procedure in case of failure of a sling suspension or a cervicoplasty in girls. After puberty, the bladder neck closure may be realized through a vaginal approach.

89.13 Complications of Surgical Procedures Increasing the Outlet Resistance

Any of these procedures imply the risk of bladder and upper urinary tract deterioration with renal insufficiency. It is difficult to predict with the cystomanometry the post-operative evolution of an apparently compliant and non overactive bladder after outlet procedures. A close follow-up is mandatory to detect any change in the urodynamic profile and any dilation of the upper urinary tract.

89.14 Urinary Diversion

Despite the widespread acceptance of CIC, there are some patients unable or unwilling to perform self-catheterization. Quadriplegia, limited dexterity, devastating cognitive impairment or lack of ancillary support are the main factors leading to the decision of urinary diversion to prevent either upper urinary tract deterioration or refractory perineal problems. The urinary diversion is most often realized by an ileal conduit (Bricker's procedure). A report on a cohort of 33 adult patients who underwent an ileal conduit with or without concomitant cystectomy to prevent the occurrence of a pyocystitis had a good post-operative evolution. Four of these patients experienced one episode of acute pyelonephritis but kept a normal upper tract on IVP. Hence, urinary diversion through an ileal conduit, even if rarely indicated, remains one option in the treatment of children with a neurogenic bladder.

89.15 Bowel Management

The quality of life of a child with a neurogenic bladder is as much altered by the feces incontinence as by the urine leaks. It is then important to consider bowel management. Some of these children may be continent with the use of retrograde enemas but they then need the help of one of their parents. The use of the antegrade colonic enemas as described by Malone (MACE) offers an alternative. The colonic access may be either through a continent caecostomy (though the appendix or through a Monti tube) or by the percutaneous insertion of a cecal tube. The left colonic access has been also suggested in order to reduce the evacuation time but seems to induce an increased morbidity. The time needed for the antegrade enema is the major draw-back of the procedures, since the evacuation lasts between 30 to 45 min. Some patients will suffer from abdominal pain during the infusion. Most will be able to stay continent when they have one enema every 2nd day. The most frequent complication of the procedure is the occurrence of a stenosis of the continent stoma which is best prevented by a regular twice a day cannulation.

89.16 Conclusion

The management of a child with a neurogenic bladder needs a multidisciplinary team and has to be tailored to each peculiar child in function of his familial environment, and his orthopedic and or mental limitations. CIC is the most important part of the treatment and should be started as early as possible after birth and repair of the spinal defect. It will not always be sufficient to gain continence but it is mandatory to protect the upper urinary tract which is the main goal of the treatment.

Further Reading

Bauer SA (2007) Neuropathic dysfunction of the lower urinary tract. In AJ Wein, LR Kavoussi, AC Novick, AW Partin, CA Peters (eds) Campbell-Walsh Urology, 9th edn. W.B. Saunders Elsevier, Philadelphia, PA, pp 3625–3655

Castellan M, Gosalbez R, Labbie A, Ibrahim E, Disandro M (2005) Bladder neck sling for treatment of neurogenic incontinence in children with augmentation cystoplasty: Long-term follow-up. J Urol 173(6):2128–2131

Dik P, Klijn AJ, van Gool JD, de Jong-de Vos van Steenwijk CC, de Jong TP (2006) Early start to therapy preserves kidney function in spina bifida patients. Eur Urol 49(5):908–913

Guys JM, Haddad M, Planche D, Torre M, Borrione C, Breaud J (2004) Sacral neuromodulation for neurogenic bladder dysfunction in children. J Urol 172:1673–1676

Karaman MI, Kaya C, Caskurlu T et al (2005) Urodynamic findings in children with cerebral palsy. Int J Urol 12:717–720

Kiddoo DA, Canning DA, Snyder HM 3rd, Carr MC (2006) Urethral dilation as treatment for neurogenic bladder. J Urol 176(4 Pt 2):1831–1833

Lopes Pereira P, Somoza Ariba I, Martinez Urrutia MJ, Lobato Romero R, Jaureguizar Monroe E (2006) Artificial urinary sphincter: 11-year experience in adolescents with congenital neuropathic bladder. Eur Urol 50(5):1096–1101

Lottmann H, Margaryan M, Aigrain Y, Läckgren G (2006b) Long-term effects of peri cervical injection with dextranomer in 61 patients. J Urol 176(4 Pt 2):1762–1766

Lottmann H, Margaryan M, Lortat-Jacob S, Bernuy M, Läckgren G (2006a) Long-term results of bladder autoaugmentation in 31 children. J Urol 175(4):1485–1489

Nguyen MT, Pavlock CL, Zderic SA, Carr MC, Canning DA (2005) Overnight catheter drainage in children with poorly compliant bladders improves post-obstructive diuresis and urinary incontinence. J Urol 174(4 Pt 2):1633–1636

Nørgaard JP, van Gool JD, Hjalmas K, et al (1998) Standardization and definitions in lower urinary tract dysfunction in children. International Children's Continence Society. Br J Urol 81(Suppl 3):1–16

Puri P, Höllwarth M (2006) Pediatric Surgery. Springer, Berlin, Heidelberg

Sarica K, Erbagci A, Yagci F, Yurtseven C (2003) Multidisciplinary evaluation of occult spinal dysraphism in 47 children. Scand J Urol Nephrol 37:329–334

Woodhouse CRJ (2005) Myelomeningocele in young adults. Br J Urol 95(2):223–230

End Stage Renal Disease and Renal Transplantation

90

Atif Awan

Contents

P. Puri and M. Höllwarth (eds.), *Pediatric Surgery: Diagnosis and Management,*
DOI: 10.1007/978-3-540-69560-8_90, © Springer-Verlag Berlin Heidelberg 2009

90.1 Introduction

End stage renal disease (ESRD) is defined as a glomerular filtration rate (GFR) of $10\,ml/min/1.73\,m^2$ (SA) or less. This represents a residual renal function mass of less than 5%. Renal replacement therapy (RRT) in the form of dialysis and/or transplantation therefore becomes necessary at this stage. The incidence of end stage renal disease in paediatrics remains low. The incidence ranges from 7.4 per million age adjusted population in the UK to 6.4 per million of children less than 16 years old from Sweden. The prevalence of children receiving RRT has been reported 53.4 per million age adjusted population in the UK. There is increased prevalence of ESRD in Asian children, as compared to Caucasians in the U.K. (40 vs 15 per million children).

90.2 Etiology

The vast majority of children who require RRT are born with renal dysplasia/hypoplasia with or without urological malformations. It is however uncommon for RRT to be commenced soon after birth, as the progression to ESRD is often slow.

In the underdeveloped countries glomerular diseases are reported more frequently as leading cause of ESRD than renal dysplasia/hypoplasia and may be related to under reporting or under diagnosis of these conditions.

Various conditions which lead to ESRD are outlined in Table 90.1.

90.3 Presentation and Diagnosis

Presentation of children who progress to ESRD and require RRT is variable.

Signs and symptoms may be related to their primary renal disease and/or complications of ESRD.

Advances in technology and expertise in antenatal screening have led to increased awareness and diagnosis of potential renal and/or urological abnormalities in the *newborn*. Antenatal scan may reveal reduced liquor, severe hydronephrosis, cysts or increased echogenicity of the renal parenchyma with or without associated bladder anomalies. These point towards serious

Table 90.1 Conditions causing ESRD

Congenital abnormalities (largest group accounting for ≥ 40–50 %)
1. Dysplasia/aplasia(rare) /hypoplasia.
2. Obstructive uropathy
3. Reflux nephropathy
4. Prune belly syndrome

Hereditary conditions (second largest group accounting for 13–25 %)
1. Juvenile nephronophthisis/medullary cystic disease
2. Hereditary nephritis with or without nerve deafness (e.g. Alport's)
3. Polycystic kidney disease (autosomal recessive)
4. Congenital nephrotic syndrome
5. Cystinosis
6. Primary oxalosis

Glomerulonephritis (less common 10–20 %)
1. Focal segmental glomerulosclerosis
2. Other glomerulonephritides

Multisystem disease (uncommon up to 7 %)
1. Systemic Lupus erythematosus
2. Haemolytic uraemic syndrome (typical and atypical)
3. Henoch-Schönlein purpura/IgA nephropathy
4. Other multisystem diseases

Miscellaneous (rare)
1. Renal vascular disease
2. Denys-Drash syndrome
3. Kidney tumour

Chronic renal failure
Cause unknown

underlying renal/urological abnormalities. These findings should be confirmed postnatally. Some conditions which are suspected prenatally and lead to renal impairment and progression to ESRD include infantile polycystic kidney disease, severe renal dysplasia with or without posterior urethral valves and/or vesicoureteric reflux.

Infants/young children may present with urinary tract infection and subsequent investigations reveal serious underlying conditions such as severe reflux nephropathy (Figs. 90.1 and 90.2). Children presenting with failure to thrive, pallor, fatigue or polydipsia and polyuria, with or without enuresis should have further evaluation for potential underlying renal problem.

Urinary tract infection is the most common cause of macroscopic haematuria, but in the absence of UTI, urgent investigations should be performed to rule out serious underlying renal disease. If associated with proteinuria, impaired renal function and/or hypertension, then an urgent referral to paediatric nephrologist

3 yr old UTI 6 months ago

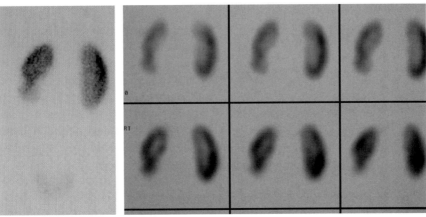

Planar images   SPECT (single photon emission computed tomography)

Fig. 90.1 Bilateral renal scarring

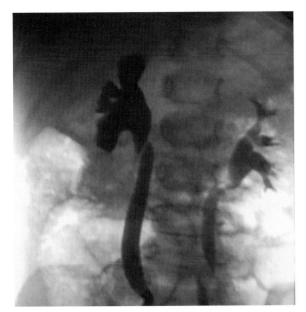

Fig. 90.2 Bilateral vesicoureteric reflux. Grade 4 on the right, grade 3 on the left

Table 90.2 Investigations to diagnose causes of ESRD

1. Urinalysis (protein, creatinine ratio, cast, etc.)
2. Urine microscopy and culture
3. Renal tract ultrasound (hydronephrosis, echogenicity, size, cysts etc.)
4. Radio-isotope scans,: DMSA, MAG3, (renal scarring, dysplasia, obstruction)
5. Micturating cystourethrogram (vesicoureteric reflux, posterior urethral valves)
6. Intravenous urogram (where radio isotopes not available or conclusive, rarely used)
7. C3, C4, antinuclear antibody, anti-DNA antibodies, anti-GBM antibodies, ANCA (glomerulonephritides)
8. Renal biopsy
9. White cell cystine level
10. Oxalate excretion

90.4 Assessment and Investigation of End Stage Renal Disease

Some of the common investigations which are helpful to point towards specific diagnosis leading to ESRD are outlined in Table 90.2.

90.5 Complications and Management

As ESRD approaches, glomerular filtration, tubular secretion/re-absorption and ability to concentrate urine are seriously impaired. In addition, production, metabolism

should be sought for further investigations, including serology, renal biopsy etc.

Some children may fail to recover from acute renal failure, and are left with significant renal impairment, requiring subsequent RRT, for example in some cases of Haemolytic Uremic Syndrome or rapidly progressive glomerulonephritis, etc.

and/or excretion of hormones are deranged. Similarly drug excretion is altered and the dosage should be reduced according to the GFR.

Some of the changes in metabolism which occur as a consequence and their management are described below:

90.5.1 Fluid Requirements

Children with ESRD may be polyuric or oligoanuric. Fluid requirement therefore depends on how much urine a child produces.

Children with conditions like dysplasia are polyuric and any attempt to restrict fluid intake will lead to severe dehydration and further deterioration in renal function.

In patients with none or low urinary output states, $400\,\mathrm{mls/m^2}$ (insensible losses) plus replacement of any urinary output achieves adequate homeostasis.

90.5.2 Sodium

Conditions like renal dysplasia and obstructive uropathy lead to salt losing state. Continued sodium depletion leads to contraction of extra cellular fluid volume and impairs growth and renal function. It is therefore imperative to replace adequate sodium to maintain normal sodium homeostasis. Patients are monitored clinically (for example oedema or hypertension) and biochemically by estimating urine and blood electrolytes to ensure a balanced sodium intake is achieved. Daily requirements of salt supplements may be in the range of 1–6 mmol/kg/day.

Some children on the other hand require salt and fluid restriction to control hypertension and fluid overload (such as in patients with advanced stages of glomerulopathy).

90.5.3 Potassium

Hyperkalemia primarily occurs due to reduced fractional excretion of potassium. Metabolic acidosis and insensitivity to aldosterone may further enhance hyperkalemia.

Bicarbonate supplements, diuretics, dietary modification and change in dialysis prescription (for children on dialysis) are essential to control hyperkalemia.

90.5.4 Calcium and Phosphate

Calcium phosphate metabolism is deranged leading to stimulation of PTH (parathyroid hormone). Reduced intestinal calcium absorption and phosphate excretion in combination with low levels of vitamin D3 lead to strong stimulation of PTH. This results in diffuse parathyroid hyperplasia and secondary hyperparathyroidism. If untreated this may lead to nodular parathyroid hyperplasia with tertiary hyperparathyroidism.

This results in rickets of renal disease, called renal osteodystrophy (Fig. 90.3).

Vitamin D supplementation in the form of 1α-hydroxycholecalciferol should be used in all patients. It is also essential to reduce the phosphate intake and to use phosphate binders when necessary (non aluminium based).

PTH levels should be closely monitored, particularly in children who are experiencing growth spurt.

90.5.5 Anaemia

Anaemia is typically normochromic and normocytic, and is primarily due to severe reduction in the production of erythropoietin.

Recombinant human erythropoietin (rEPO) is routinely used to maintain a target haemoglobin (Hb) level of between 10–12 g/dl. This is injected subcutaneously

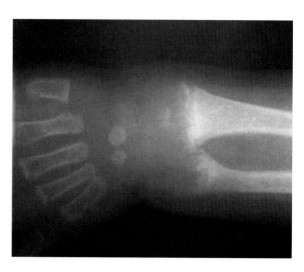

Fig. 90.3 Rickets of renal disease (renal osteodystophy)

2–3 times per week. Response is monitored by measuring Hb, ferritin levels, percentage (%) hypochromia and reticulocyte count (for instance a high % hypochromia and normal/high reticulocyte count points towards iron deficiency rather than deficient rEPO and vice versa).

Patients on haemodialysis are routinely given intravenous iron supplementation and erythropoietin to maintain the target haemoglobin.

90.5.6 Growth and Nutrition

Growth is severely effected in up to 50% of children with chronic renal disease. This is much more pronounced in children requiring RRT in the first 2 years of life. It is a result of poor nutrition, as growth at this stage is primarily dependent on provision of adequate nutrition. Nasogastric or gastrostomy route should be used to feed these children. It is advised to fashion gastrostomy early in the course of disease, particularly when peritoneal catheter insertion is envisaged within a few weeks to months. Feeds should be well balanced with adequate mixture of all of the essential nutrients and provide calories of at least 100% of the recommended daily allowance.

Children who remain growth retarded, despite adequate supportive therapy for renal failure or after early withdrawal of steroids post transplantation, require growth hormone treatment.

90.5.7 Hypertension

Hypertension leads to significant morbidity and hastens the progression of renal failure. Various mechanisms may be responsible for hypertension, such as salt and water retention leading to fluid overload, vascular wall rigidity due to excessive lipid and/or calcium phosphate complex deposition and finally hyperreninemia. Conditions like autosomal recessive polycystic kidney disease and reflux nephropathy may cause significant hypertension.

Hypertensive encephalopathy and/or congestive cardiac failure due to hypertension should be treated with intravenous anti-hypertensive agents with proper monitoring in paediatric intensive care unit. It is critical

Table 90.3   Common antihypertensive drugs

Calcium channel blockers—Nifedipine, Amlodipine
Diuretics—Furosemide Metalozone
Cardio selective beta blockers—such as Atenolol
ACE inhibitors—Captopril, Enalapril
Peripheral vasodilators—Prazosin, Minoxidil (rarely)

to reduce the blood pressure gradually and not to use sublingual Nifedipine which can lead to severe neurological damage.

A persistent blood pressure of more than 95th centile for the child should be treated and the drug therapy would depend on the underlying condition leading to renal failure and clinical evaluation of an individual child. (e.g. oedema, low or high urinary output conditions etc)

Angiotensive converting enzyme inhibitors (ACE) should be used with caution in chronic kidney disease as they may lead to hyperkalemia and/or further deterioration in renal function. Some of the common anti-hypertensives used in paediatric ESRD are outlined in Table 90.3.

90.6   Renal Replacement Therapy (RRT)

Renal transplant is the only treatment for children with end stage renal disease. Dialysis is regarded as a temporary means of keeping the child well, so that ultimately a successful renal transplant is achieved. Supportive therapy whilst on dialysis is essential to prevent the complications of ESRD.

90.7   Dialysis

Over the past 2 decades there has been immense improvement in the way the dialysis is delivered to children, leading to favourable outcomes. Decision to embark on dialysis/type of dialysis not only depends on biochemical numbers but also clinical status of patient and underlying disease.

The usual indications include fluid overload, uncontrolled hyperkalemia, severe acidosis and hyperphosphatemia. Once GFR has fallen to or below 10 ml/min/m^2 dialysis is usually commenced.

90.8 Peritoneal Dialysis (PD)

This remains the preferred choice amongst paediatric nephrologists and majority of families. It is technically easy and is delivered at home. It is suitable for very young and small patients and does not require intense fluid restriction.

Peritoneum acts as a semi permeable membrane for bi-directional passage of water and solutes. Diffusion and convection help to clear small and large solute molecules/water respectively.

90.8.1 Types of PD

1. CAPD (continued ambulatory peritoneal dialysis). The dialysis solution is constantly present in the peritoneal cavity. This is manually changed four times a day with drainage of the dialysate and inflow of fresh solution. The twin bag system with Y-line is used in paediatric PD programmes. This carries less risk of peritonitis as the dialysate is emptied into the empty bag, thus flushing any bacteria which may have contaminated the connection.
2. Automated peritoneal dialysis (APD). A small machine (Fig. 90.4) which regulates dialysate volume (cycle volume), dwell and drain times, number and duration of exchanges required (usually 7–12 cycles over 10–12 h). This is done at night time. Some children may require small amounts of dialysis fluid left in the peritoneal cavity once the cycling

therapy is finished and is called last bag fill. This is particularly important in children with reduced or no urinary output as it improves fluid removal and acts as an extra exchange during the day.

90.8.2 Types of PD Catheters and Solution

There are various types of PD catheters available but most commonly used are double cuff Tenckhoff. These are inserted surgically under general anaesthesia. The first cuff is sutured at the peritoneum with the purse string suture and the second cuff is approximately 1 cm from the exit site. The exit site should be fashioned, directed downwards and ideally should be above the "jeans line". The exit site should be swan-necked to reduce the chances of tunnel infection.

Partial omentectomy helps to prevent catheter blockage. It is routine to prescribe IV antibiotics prior to surgical procedure which are continued for 48 h afterwards.

Three different types of peritoneal dialysis solutions are routinely used in isolation or combination of each other. Glucose concentration of each dialysate, 1.36%, 2.25%, and 3.86% represents the increasing strength of each type of fluid. Children requiring large amounts of fluid removal need stronger strength dialysis solution.

90.8.3 PD Prescription

Where possible the dialysis catheter should be rested for 4–6 weeks to reduce the risk of leakage, although in certain circumstances particularly in infants it may not be possible. It is usual to commence dialysis with an exchange volume of 300 ml/m^2 for the first 48 h. This is then gradually increased to a maximum of 1,300 ml/m^2 after a week. The dialysis prescription is individualised to the patient's need. A child who maintains good urinary output may only require 5–6 nights of dialysis as opposed to someone with none or low urinary output who needs dialysis every night of the week.

It is essential for the parents to have proper training in order to prevent complications of peritoneal dialysis. This is undertaken by senior renal nurse specialist and may take up to 3 weeks.

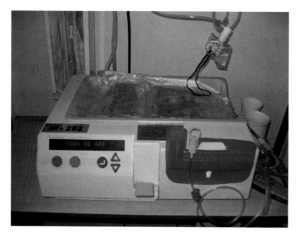

Fig. 90.4 Automated Peritoneal Dialysis machine

90.8.4 Complications of PD

Peritonitis

Peritonitis remains the most important and serious side effect of peritoneal dialysis and can lead to removal of dialysis catheters and switch over to haemodialysis treatment.

The diagnosis of peritonitis is made if the dialysate is cloudy, cell count is more than 100/mm^3 with predominance of neutrophils. Abdominal pain, fever, rigors, nausea and vomiting are other clinical features pointing towards peritonitis.

The most common isolated organism is coagulase negative staphylococci but the most serious are staph aureus, pseudomonas and fungal organisms often leading to catheter loss.

If the child is haemodynamically stable then therapy with intra peritoneal (IP) antibiotics is started. Vancomycin and ciprofloxacin combination provides a good initial therapeutic regimen for peritonitis. Duration and choice of antibiotics therapy depends on the cultured organisms. However, if the child is unwell, intravenous and I.P. antibiotics are used for first 24–48 h. Heparin at a dose of 500 units lu/l should be used while the dialysate remains cloudy.

Exit Site Infection

In presence of swelling, tenderness and/or pus discharge at the exit site, antibiotics should be used to prevent tunnel infection and peritonitis.

Hernia/Hydrocele

Inguinal hernias are not uncommon in infants initiating peritoneal dialysis and should be corrected surgically when they occur.

Catheter Malposition/Blockage

If there is problem in drainage of catheter then a simple abdominal X-ray will outline the position of catheters as it may have moved and cause poor drainage of dialysate. We perform partial omentectomy in our center to prevent possibility of catheter blockage.

90.9 Haemodialysis (HD)

Significant improvements have been made in delivering safe and effective haemodialysis, even to the children weighing below 10 kg. This is due to new types and sizes of dialysis filters, extra corporeal lines and the dialysis machines.

Haemodialysis is provided by a highly skilled and experienced staff and should be equipped with personnel to give supportive therapy to children whilst on dialysis. These include dietician, teacher, play therapist, in addition to social worker and psychologist.

90.9.1 Physiology of HD

The clearance is achieved by diffusion and convection. Haemodialysis entails clearance (solute removal) and ultra filtration (fluid removal) through blood perfusion of an extra corporeal filter membrane, across which, runs a counter current electrolyte solution.

A good vascular access is essential for effective haemodialysis. Central venous line catheters are commonly used and are particularly useful in small children. Other ways of creating vascular access is by the formation of arterio venous fistula (AVF). The creation of AVF is dependent on the local expertise and can be achieved even in small children, though it is unusual in children less then 20 kg. Preferred choices of insertion of central line are internal jugular or where possible external jugular veins.

90.9.2 HD Prescription

Acute HD

To prevent disequilibrium syndrome, first session should be short with low urea clearance. Gradually blood flow, duration of the sessions are increased as adaptation to haemodialysis occurs.

Chronic HD

Most children will require up to three times per week of 3–4 h haemodialysis sessions. This achieves optimal clearance and dry weight by the end of each session. Children weighing less then 10 kg may require more sessions every week to achieve adequate dialysis. The weight gain between the dialysis session should not be more then 8% and preferably no more than 5% of the dry weight. Weight gain over 10% of dry body weight in between haemodialysis session is often due to non compliance and can be potentially life threatening due to pulmonary oedema.

Complications of HD

1. **Catheter Blockage**
   Fibrin deposits around the catheter causing obstruction.

   In the absence of fibrin sheath, to unblock the line, therapeutic agents such as urokinase/alteplase locks are used. However, in the presence of fibrin sheath, urokinase infusion and/or Tinzaparin (subcutaneously) are used (monitor factor anti X a)

2. **Infection**
   With strict aseptic techniques, the infection rate should be low and when suspected blood cultures, CRP and other routine bloods should be performed and IV antibiotics administered. Vancomycin, Teicoplanin, Ceftriaxone are the common drugs used.

3. **Catheter slippage**

4. **Hypotension**
   Generally due to excess removal of fluid and requires correction of intravascular volume.

5. **Disequilibrium syndrome**
   This is due to swift removal of urea in the early dialysis session. It manifests as nausea, vomiting, headaches, disorientation, seizures, coma and can lead to death. Mannitol should be used to treat.

90.10 Renal Transplantation

90.10.1 Transplant Evaluation for Recipient

It is unusual for children weighing less then 10 kg and be younger than 18 months to be considered for a renal transplant.

Since most of the children requiring transplants have dysplasia/hypoplasia with or without severe urological abnormalities, a proper urological evaluation by a paediatric urologist should be undertaken. Bladder capacity, pressure and/ or evidence of obstruction are assessed. Any abnormality found should be dealt with prior to being considered for a transplant. This is particularly true of children with a history of neurogenic bladder, posterior urethral valves, Prune Belly syndrome, vesicoureteric reflux etc. In addition to urological evaluation a full medical evaluation should be done, including status of immunisation, virology, wrist x-ray, echo and dental examination.

90.10.2 Donor Characteristics

It is unusual to accept cadaveric kidney from a patient less then 5 years or more than 50 years old for transplantation.

90.10.3 Indications of Bilateral Nephrectomies Prior to Transplantation

1. Congenital nephrotic syndrome. It is essential for these children to have bilateral nephrectomies and a period of dialysis to correct their hyper-coagable state and provide optimum time for vaccination.
2. Resistant hypertension. If a child is on three or more antihypertensive medications nephrectomies should be considered.
3. Patient with bilateral Wilm's tumour, Denys-Drash syndrome.
4. Patients with recurrent and chronic kidney infections, in association with severe reflux and/or stones.
5. Patients with FSGS as an underlying condition of their renal failure.

90.10.4 Pre-Emptive Transplantation (PET)

Once the GFR falls to or below 15 ml/min/1.73 m² children should be considered for pre-emptive renal transplantation. This means transplant without dialysis. Most of the children with renal dysplasia/hypoplasia will have low clearance renal failure and maintain growth and normal activities until puberty. These patients will benefit from PET. PET should be encouraged and account for up to 24% of kidney transplants reported by North

American Paediatric Renal Transplantation Corporative Study(NAPRTSC) in 2001.

90.10.5 Risk of Recurrence of Primary Disease

Though recurrence of primary disease in a renal transplant leads to less than 5% graft failure, there is increased morbidity associated. For instance in patients with FSGS, there is a risk of 30% recurrence post transplant. This risk increases to 80–100% in the second transplant.

Other conditions like membranoproliferative glomerulonephritis type II have 80% risk of recurrence in the transplant and leads to 20% of graft loss in these patients. Atypical Haemolytic Uremic Syndrome patients who require renal transplants have a recurrence risk of 10% but have increased risk of graft loss of approximately 50%.

90.10.6 Surgical Technique

The technique of renal transplant in children more than 15 kg is similar to that in adults. These children have kidney placed in the right or left iliac fossa, where renal vein is anastomosed to one of the iliac veins, the renal artery to common or external iliac artery.

Children less then 15 kg have their kidneys put intra-abdominally and renal vessels anastomosed to aorta and inferior vena cava.

At the time of unclamping careful attention should be paid to recipient's haemodynamic status and it is advisable to maintain central venous pressure of more than 15cm of H_2O and blood pressure near the adult range before unclamping.

The ureteric anastomosis is performed either by leadbetter-politano re-implant procedure or non-refluxing extra vesicoureteric neo-cystostomy (preferred). The short length of ureter in latter technique ensures adequate distal ureteric blood supply.

90.10.7 Surgical Complications

1. Graft thrombosis may result due to hypotension or pro-coagulant status of the nephrotic child. The transplant kidney may not be salvageable.
2. Vascular anastomosis Haemorrhage (unusual, would require urgent surgical intervention).
3. Urinary leakage: Urinary leakage from vesico ureteric junction may occur but improved technique and placement of Stent or use of suprapubic catheter may prevent this happening.
4. Ureteric necrosis: This may occur as a result of damage to the vascular supply to the ureter or acute rejection.
5. Ureteric stenosis: This may occur as late complication and is prevented by ureteric stenting.
6. Renal artery stenosis is uncommon and may require angioplasty.

90.11 Transplant Immunobiology

Human leucocytes antigens (HLA) differ in individuals in their expression of cell surface antigens. T lymphocyte recognise antigen as peptides bound to these molecules. The two important types of HLA in humans, in relation to transplant are class I and II. HLA class I's subdivided into HLAA, and HLAB and HLAC. The HLA class II are further sub divided into three sub groups, HLADR, HLADP and HLADQ. HLA class II molecules present antigen to helper T cell, resulting in proliferation and amplification of immune response.

Alloresponse is a process where lymphocytes from an individual interact with cells from an unrelated individual, these lymphocytes recognise antigens on the unrelated tissue as non self and are activated. These cells then proliferate in numbers and differentiate to activate other important factors of the immune system like interleukins, interferon, natural killer cells and transforming growth factors.

Rejection can be hyper acute, (associated with pre formed antibodies), acute or sub acute with cellular infiltrates, as a result of increased activity of the immune system or chronic rejection which is associated with vascular and interstitial changes.

90.11.1 Immunosuppressive Treatment

1. The intensity of immunosuppression prescribed is directly related to degree of HLA miss-matching.

2. Most centres use induction therapy to avoid early acute rejection.

3. Multiple drugs are used simultaneously to maintain immunosuppression. They act on different molecular targets, and have added beneficial effect, thus preventing toxicity of individual drug.

4. Each event of graft dysfunction should be investigated urgently. It is imperative to assess underlying cause which may be due to rejection, infection, drug toxicity, obstruction or combination of any of these.

5. The ideal combination of drug regime is one which provides effective immunosuppression with minimal side effects.

6. Immunosuppressive therapy is a life long therapy.

The optimal induction immunosuppressive therapy to prevent acute renal transplant rejection remains controversial. Some of the agents used are briefly mentioned below.

90.11.2 Monoclonal Antibodies

1. Anti-thymocyte globulin (ATG) and OKT 3 have been shown to reduce acute rejection episodes, though there was no improvement in the long-term outcome of transplant.

2. IL-2 receptor antibodies have become a popular choice as induction immunosuppression therapy. These are partially human monoclonal antibodies, such as Dacluzimab and Basiliximab. The former is 90% and latter is 70% human. These antibodies are directed against IL-2 receptor thus inhibiting IL-2 induced activation of T Cells and interrupt the immune response towards the allograft.

90.11.3 Maintenance Immunosuppressive Therapy

Calcineurin Inhibitors

The most effective immunosuppressive drugs used as maintenance therapy are the calcineurin inhibitors (Cyclosporin A, Tacrolimus). Though the general mechanism of action of the two drugs are similar, they are structurally unrelated and bind to different but related molecular targets in the cells.

The Calcineurin Inhibitors act by targeting intracellular signal pathways like translocation and transcription, therefore preventing production of IL-2 and other early activation genes. This leads to markedly reduced T-cell activation and helper T-cell function.

Tacrolimus is preferred over Cyclosporin in most of the paediatric transplant programmes. Both drugs require careful monitoring of drug levels to avoid nephro-toxicity and other serious side effects. Some of the children under the age of 5 may require three times dosage rather than the usual twice a day regime due to difference in rate of drug metabolism.

Azathioprine and Mycophenolate Mofetil

Mycophenolate Mofetil is a far superior drug then Azathioprine and is particularly used in the transplant protocols where steroids are either avoided or tapered soon after transplant. These drugs inhibit nucleotide biosynthesis and hence inhibit lymphocyte proliferation, antibody formation and cell adhesion.

The major side effect of Mycophenolate therapy is gastrointestinal intolerance. Other side effects include anaemia, leucopoenia, and thrombocytopenia.

Steroids

Steroids exert multiple effects on immune system. They acutely reduce peripheral lymphocytes count. They also down regulate pro-inflammatory cytokines like IL1, IL6 but have little or no effect on humoral immune system.

The major side effects include glucose intolerance, hypertension, poor wound healing, vascular necrosis of the bone and osteopenia.

90.12 Other Drugs Used at the Time of Transplant

1. Antibiotics: Broad spectrum antibiotics like co-Amoxiclav is used for 48 h at the time of transplantation pending the results of transport medium culture.

2. H2 receptor blockers, should be used until the child is on daily steroids and then stopped.

3. Cotrimoxazole: Most of the transplant programmes would use Cotrimoxazole prophylaxis for up to

6 months. This prevents urinary tract infection and protects against pneumocystis carinii infection.

90.13 Medical Complications of a Renal Transplant

Despite immense improvement in the immunosuppressive therapy in the past 2 decades medical complications like hypertension, drug toxicity and infections pose major challenge to the transplant team.

90.13.1 Post Transplant Hypertension

This may be due to immunosuppressive therapy (steroid, calcineurin inhibitors), allograft dysfunction, (acute rejection, calcineurin inhibitor), renal artery stenosis (rare), or persistent hypertension due to underlying renal disease prior to renal transplant.

Angiotensin converting enzyme inhibitors should be avoided in post transplant recipients particularly in the first 3 months after surgery.

90.13.2 Infectious Complications

Infectious complications lead to significant morbidity and mortality after transplantation.

1. Bacterial infection: Most common post transplant bacterial infections are due to urinary tract infections. Use of cotrimoxazole for the first 6 months post transplant reduces the risk of urinary tract infections.

90.13.3 Viral Infection

CMV Infection

CMV can be transmitted via the donated organ and unusually through the blood transfusion. Transplanted children should only receive CMV negative blood. Children who receive CMV donor kidney and are non-immune receive IV Ganciclovir for 10 days post transplantation. Oral Ganciclovir or Valaciclovir is then used for 3 months post transplant to prevent the occurrence of CMV disease.

Epstein Bar Virus (EBV)

Most of the children do not have immunity against EBV and thus acquire primary infection post transplant. Careful monitoring of the EBV viral load with quantification PCRs and serology in combination with tailored immunosuppression is undertaken to prevent the occurrence of post transplant lymphoproliferative disorder (PTLD). An acute rejection rate of up to 30% has been reported in patients with tailored immunosupresion. This entails stoppage of Azathioprine or Mycophenolate and reducing the dose of Calcineurin inhibitor to minimal acceptable level.

90.13.4 Malignancy after Transplant

Skin cancers have been reported in approximately 3% of paediatric transplant population. PTLD remains the most serious malignancy post transplant in paediatrics. Most of these are non Hodgkin's lymphomas, are of the lymphocytes origin and triggered by EBV infection. Close collaboration with paediatric oncologist is imperative to treat these malignancies.

90.14 Long term Graft Survival

Data supports superiority of living donor(LD) outcomes compared with cadaveric donation (CD) at 1% in 5 years. The European Dialysis and Transplant Association Data from 1984–1993 shows 1 year graft survival for LD of 91% and 5 years of 74%. The outcomes for cadaveric grafts at 1 year was 80%, falling to 60% at 5 years. Near similar outcomes have been supported by NAPRTCS, improved survival of LD of 10% at 1 year and 14.5% at 5 years over cadaveric graft.

Several factors, independently or in combination can adversely influence the graft survival. Some of these factors which lead to negative outcome include recipient age less than 2 years, high degree of miss matching between the donor and the recipient, acute rejection episodes, particularly in the first 6 months post transplant. This is supported by the data from NAPRTCS, that a single episode of acute rejection increases the relative risk for development of chronic rejection, threefold. Chronic rejection is the commonest cost of long term graft failure.

Delayed graft function (need for dialysis during the 1st week post transplantation) occurs in up to 5% recipient of live donation (LD) and 19% for cadaveric donation (CD). Children who had DGF had inferior graft outcome as compared to those with no delayed function. This difference is 41.6% versus 89.6% for LD and 49.5% versus 80.2% for cadaveric kidneys.

The recurrence of primary disease in the graft (as outlined before in this chapter) results in subsequent graft loss in majority of these patients.

Further Reading

Avner ED, Harmon WE, Niaudet P (2004) Paediatric Nephrology. Lippincott Williams & Wilkins, Philadelphia

Ellis EN, Yiu V, Harley F et al (2001) The impact of supplemental feeding in young children on dialysis: A report of the North American Pediatric Renal Transplant Cooperative Study. Pediatr Nephrol 16:404–408

European Society for Paediatric Nephrology Handbook (2002)

Webb N, Postlethwaite R (2003) Clinical Paediatric Nephrology. Oxford, New York

Puri P, Höllwarth ME (eds) (2006) Pediatric Surgery. Springer, Berlin, Heidelberg

White CT, Gowrishankar M, Feber J, Yiu V and Canadian Association of Pediatric Nephrologists (CAPN) and Peritoneal Dialysis Working Group (2006). Clinical practice guidelines for pediatric peritoneal dialysis. Pediatric Nephrol 21:1059–1066

Intersex Disorders

91

Maria Marcela Bailez

Contents

91.1 Introduction Including Definition and Incidence

Patients with ambiguous genitalia mostly present in the newborn period requiring a multidisciplinary team which includes a pediatric surgeon/urologist to assign the sex of rearing as soon as possible after a thorough genetic, anatomic, functional and socioeconomic workup.

The diagnosis of "ambiguous genitalia" is based on a meticulous perineal exam and gonadal palpation. External genitalia exam includes the visualization of both faces of the phallus, looking for the urethral orifice, defining its localization and aspect. Inguinal and perineal palpation looking for gonads is the other diagnostic key.

Feminine phenotype presents a normal looking clitoris and no palpable gonads.

Masculine phenotype presents a normal looking penis and two scrotal testicles

Although exceptions to this pattern occur e.g.: a female with an inguinal hernia or a male with a mild hypospadias or an undescended testicle; if a combined abnormal gonadal palpation and external genitalia appearance are detected, sexual ambiguity should be studied (Figs. 91.1a and 91.2). Isolated severe defects like a perineal hypospadias or bilateral nonpalpable gonads in a patient with a normal looking phallus should also be investigated (Fig. 91.1b).

Occasionally, patients with previously unrecognized disorders of sex development present later in infancy or puberty.

P. Puri and M. Höllwarth (eds.), *Pediatric Surgery: Diagnosis and Management*,
DOI: 10.1007/978-3-540-69560-8_91, © Springer-Verlag Berlin Heidelberg 2009

Fig. 91.1 (**a**) A newborn with bilateral nonpalpable gonads, hypospadias, and hyperpigmentation of labioscrotal folds. Further studies confirmed the diagnosis of CAH. She was female sex assigned, (**b**) An older patient with a non salt losing CAH male sex assigned when newborn. She had a normal looking phallus but bilateral nonpalpable gonads and should have been studied before sex assignment

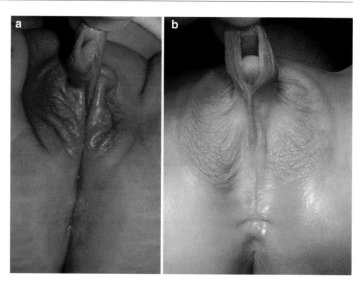

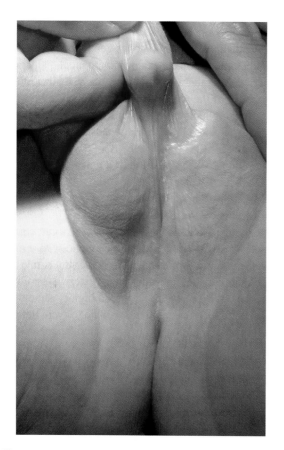

Fig. 91.2 A 3 month old patient with asymmetric ambiguous genitalia. Final diagnosis was Mixed gonadal dysgenesis and was female sex assigned

91.1.1 Classification

Advances in identification of molecular genetic causes of abnormal sex with heightened awareness of ethical issues and patient advocacy concerns necessitate a reexamination of nomenclature. Terms such as "intersex, "pseudohermaphroditism," "hermaphroditism," "sex reversal," and gender-based diagnostic labels are particularly controversial. These terms are perceived as potentially pejorative by patients and can be confusing to practitioners and parents alike. The consensus statement on management of intersex disorders propose the term "disorders of sex development" (DSD), as defined by congenital conditions in which development of chromosomal, gonadal, or anatomic sex is atypic.

Traditionally DSD patients were classified in three groups based on gonadal structure.

1. Presence of two well defined ovaries with ambiguous or male external genitalia (female pseudohermaphroditism; now called overvirilized XX female).

    These patients have a 46 XX karyotype and virilization of the external genitalia results from exposure to high level of androgens in utero while they have female internal genitalia. Congenital adrenal hyperplasia (CAH) is the most common disease in this group and accounts for 50–80% of all the cases of ambiguity, depending on the population analyzed. The most common enzymatic defect is 21-hydroxylase deficiency. The incidence of 21-hydroxylase deficiency is 1 in 15,000–40,000 newborns. Other defects are 11-hydroxylase (hypertension) and 3 b-ol dehydrogenase or aromatasa.

2. Presence of two well defined testicles with ambiguous or female external genitalia (male pseudohermaphroditism; now called undervirilized XY male). These patients have a 46 XY karyotype and ambiguity of the external genitalia results from a failure of the masculinization of the male fetus. This can be due to a failure in androgenic synthesis or in the biological response. This group includes rare defects of the biosynthesis of testosterone, defect of the 5 alpha-reductase (enzyme that converts testosterone in dihydrotestosterone) and partial androgen insensitivity syndrome (partial defect of androgenic receptors).

   It is important to recognize that patients with a 46 XY karyotype and dysgenetic testicles are sometimes included in this group in the literature.

3. Presence of incomplete differentiated gonads or coexisting ovarian and testicular tissue with ambiguous or female external genitalia. This is a heterogeneous group with one common factor which is a structural defect in gonadal differentiation with or without a chromosome alteration. Patients with mixed gonadal dysgenesis, testicular dysgenesis and true hermaphroditism (now called ovotesticular disorder of sexual development) are included in this group.

For the purpose of investigation they are divided in:

1. Disorders of chromosomes (chromosomal DSD)
2. Disorders of gonad development (gonadal DSD, sex determination)
3. Disorders of sex steroid synthesis and action (phenotypic/anatomic DSD, sex differentiation)

91.2 Etiology

Sex differentiation refers to the anatomic development of the internal and external genitalia as male or female dependent on the presence or absence of functioning androgens.

Genital development is constitutively female and non-dependent on oestrogens prenatally. In contrast, male sex differentiation is mandatory androgen-dependant and requiring optimal ligand activation of the androgen receptor.

91.2.1 Gonad Development

Fifteen years have passed since the discovery of SRY as the primary "testis-determining gene" in Koopman et al's classic experiment showing that transgenic expression of SRY in xx mice results in testis development and male phenotype. Studies in mice are continuing to provide exciting information about differential structural changes and gene expression in normal gonad development (testis versus ovary) as well as the effect of targeted deletion of key genes involved in this process.

WT1, SF1, SOX9, DHH, DMRT, SIDDT and ARX are some of the genetic determinants of normal gonad development and gonadal dysgenesis.

91.2.2 Androgens

The production of androgens by fetal Leydig cells is initially gonadotropin independent. Placental hCG is the one that ensures high concentrations of androgens during the first half of gestation to stabilise Wolffian duct development and differentiation of the external genital anlage. Wolffian duct stabilization is dependent on high local concentrations of testosterone diffusing in a gradient along the duct from the adjacent ipsilateral gonad. This accounts for the asymmetric development of Wolffian ducts in some DSD.

The androgen receptor (AR) is a transcription factor that mediates male sexual differentiation in utero and is responsible for the development and maintenance of male sexual characteristics. The AR gene is located on the X-chromosome. Mutations in the AR gene may lead to diseases like androgen insensitivity syndrome (AIS). In AIS gonadal males had a spectrum of abnormalities ranging from individuals with a female phenotype (complete AIS CAIS) through genital ambiguities in the partial form (PAIS) to men with fertility disturbances in minimal AIS (MAIS). More than 500 mutations have now been documented in AIS.

In summary, circulating testosterone is responsible for virilization and is dependent upon 5-alpha reductase (transforms testosterone in dihydrotestosterone) and the presence of appropriate receptors.

91.2.3 Anti Mullerian Hormone

The pre Sertoli cells secrete a glycoprotein hormone the Anti Mullerian Hormone (AMH). It causes involution of the Mullerian ducts and stimulates the Leydig cells to produce testosterone. It is also responsible for the first stage of testicular descent.

The AMH receptor is different from the AR. Persistent Mullerian structures in 46 xy DSD patients may be due to failure of the production of the hormone from the testes (50%) or to receptor deficiency.

91.2.4 Steroids

Problems in the early stages of steroidogenesis can result in abnormalities of adrenal steroid synthesis which may result in external virilization of a gonadal female like adrenal hyperplasia (CAH) or underandrogenization of the 46 xy fetus.

The 21-hydroxylase is encoded by a gene on chromosome 6. Its deficiency is inherited in an autosomal recessive fashion.

Tremendous progress has been made in the past 15 years in understanding the role of mutation of factors involved in the steroidogenesis process (e.g. STAR, CYP11A, HSD3B2, and CYP17).

Considerably more research is needed to be able to translate this new knowledge into effective patient care and to understand the long term outcome in specific conditions.

91.3 Diagnosis Investigation and Management of DSD

According to the Consensus Statement on Management of Intersex Disorders, optimal clinical management of individuals with DSD should comprise the following:

1. Gender assignment must be avoided before expert evaluation in newborns

2. Evaluation and long-term management must be performed at a center with an experienced multidisciplinary team
3. All individuals should receive a gender assignment
4. Open communication with patients and family is essential, and participation in decision-making is encouraged
5. Patient and family concerns should be respected and addressed in strict confidence

The initial contact with the parents of a child with a DSD is important, because first impressions from these encounters often persist. A key point to emphasize is that the child with a DSD has the potential to become a well-adjusted, functional member of society. Although privacy needs to be respected, a DSD is not shameful. It should be explained to the parents that the best course of action may not be clear initially, but the health care team will work with the family to reach the best possible set of decisions in the circumstances. The health care team should discuss with the parents what information to share in the early stages with family members and friends. Parents need to be informed about sexual development.

A detailed personal and familiar anamnesis can give important information. Some of these pathologies recognize a sex linked transmission (x link) and the mother will be able to transmit the defect to 50% of the sons/males (complete or partial androgen insensibility). Many have an autosomal recessive transmission (CAH, deficit of the testosterone synthesis, deficit of 5-alpha reductase, deficit of the LH receptor.)

The finding of a neonatal death in the 1st days of life of male babies may be due to an unecognized CAH.

As previously mentioned gonadal palpation and perineal exam are the key to choose the sequence of diagnostic procedures to reach an etiologic diagnosis.

Each patient needs to be considered on an individual basis.

Still diagnostic algorithms are useful as a guideline to simplify the study of these complex patients. Table 91.1 resumes the sequence of investigations used in a newborn with a suspected DSD, according to gonadal palpation. A karyotype is mandatory but this always requires some days. In the absence of palpable gonads, the first blood test are those to exclude problems that can put in risk of life (blood electrolytes) commonly found in the event of salt losing CAH. The blood sexual steroids must be determined and among them the level

Table 91.1 Diagnostic algorithm

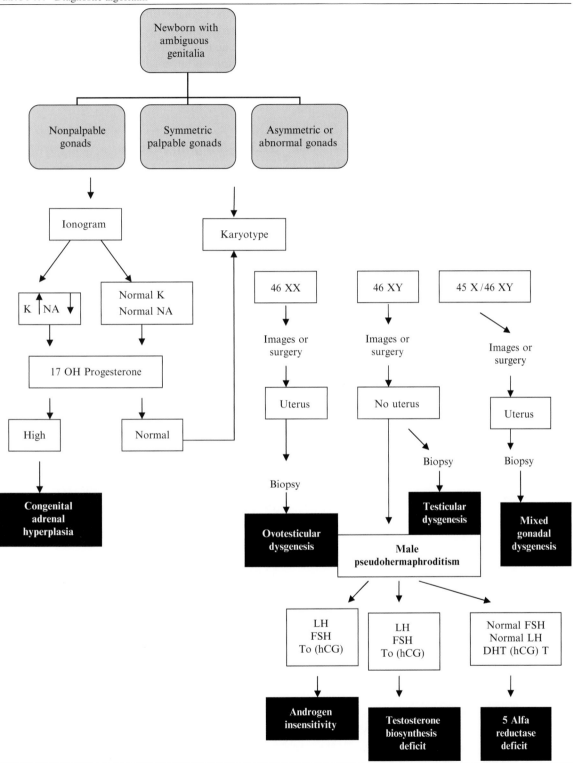

of 17·OH progesterone that, if elevated will help diagnose the most common cause of DSD.

The estimation of other steroids (testosterone, dihidrotestosterone, delta4 ·androstenedione, DHEA, 17 OH pregnenolone); ACTH, cortisol and renin will allow to get a precise picture of the gonadal and adrenal steroidogenesis.For example, the relation T/DHT with a value larger than 10 is suspicious of deficit 5-alpha eductase enzyme.

The most valuable stimulation tests for evaluating steroidogenesis are:

hCG test for the study of testicular functionality.
ACTH test for the study of adrenal steroidogenesis.
Low values of testosterone can be the sign of testicular dysgenesis if associated with low levels of all the other testicular steroids or of an enzyme defect of the steroidogenesis path if they are associated to high levels of their precursors.
Normal or elevated levels of T and DHT may be suggestive for a receptor resistance to androgens.

The possibility of the ambiguous genitalia to virilize can be estimated after an hCG test or an appropriate stimulation trial with testosterone or topical DHT. This can be estimated by demonstrating the increment of the penile dimensions or indirectly by the dosage of androgen sensitive circulating substances (SHBG). Its

values are reduced if the patient tissues present sensitivity for the virilizing effect of androgens.

Molecular biology techniques are more sensitive and specific tests for assessment of the tissue sensibility to androgens but not always available.

Histology is only required for diagnosis in patients with abnormal gonads (group 3).

91.3.1 Imaging Tests

The primary objective of this test is the study of the internal genitalia anatomy. The pelvic ultrasound for the demonstration of the presence of Mullerian structures is an important diagnostic element. Genitography is very useful for the study of vaginal morphology, dimension and relation to the urethra (Fig. 91.3). We look for the onset of the vaginal outlet in the urogenital ginus with special attention to the proximal urethra to plan the urogenital reconstruction (See surgical treatment).

91.3.2 Sex of Rearing

Factors that influence gender assignment include diagnosis, genital appearance, surgical options, need for

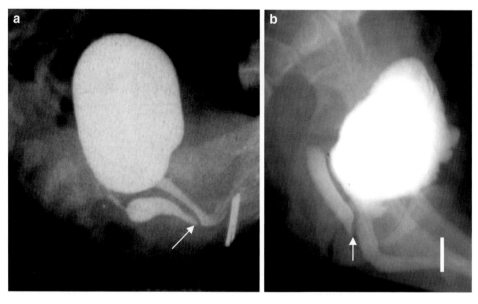

Fig. 91.3 Genitography showing vaginal morphology, dimension and relation to the urethra. The white arrows show the onset of the vaginal outlet in the UGS in a low variant (**a**) and in an intermediate, high one (**b**)

lifelong replacement therapy, potential for fertility, views of the family, and, sometimes, circumstances relating to cultural practices.

More than 90% of patients with 46,XX CAH and all patients with 46,XY CAIS assigned female in infancy identify as females. Evidence supports the current recommendation to raise markedly virilized 46,XX infants with CAH as female.

A consistent penile development constitutes a basic element for the male choice of rearing even if today the criteria that must guide this choice are objects of debate.

A good response in testosterone levels after hCG test and an increase in penile length after administration of testosterone in neonatal age will be useful to decide the choice in male sense.

In some patients the possibility of future virilization at puberty has to be taken into account (deficit of 5-alpha reductase and the defect of synthesis of testosterone from 17 bHSD deficit.). Nowadays diagnosis is easier due to the possibility of molecular genetic investigations.

Approximately 60% of 5-alpha reductase (5α RD2)-deficient patient's assigned female in infancy and virilizing at puberty (and all assigned male) live as males. In 5-alpha reductase and possibly 17 hydroxysteroid dehydrogenase deficiencies, for which the diagnosis is made in infancy, the combination of a male gender identity in the majority and the potential for fertility (documented in 5α RD but unknown in 17 hydroxysteroid dehydrogenase deficiencies) should be discussed when providing evidence for gender assignment.

Among patients with partial androgen insensitivity syndrome (PAIS), androgen biosynthetic defects, and incomplete gonadal dysgenesis, there is dissatisfaction with the sex of rearing in 25% of individuals whether raised male or female.

Available data support male rearing in all patients with micropenis, taking into account equal satisfaction with assigned gender in those raised male or female but no need for surgery and the potential for fertility in patients reared male.

Those making the decision on sex of rearing for those with ovotesticular DSD should consider the potential for fertility on the basis of gonadal differentiation and genital development and assuming that the genitalia are, or can be made, consistent with the chosen sex.

In the case of mixed gonadal dysgenesis (MGD), factors to consider include prenatal androgen exposure, testicular function at and after puberty, phallic development, and gonadal location.

91.4 Surgical Management

The role of surgery consists in:

1. Gonadal treatment
2. Feminizing genitoplasty
3. Urethral/penile reconstruction in the undervirilized child

91.4.1 Gonadal Treatment

Gonadal histology is required for diagnosis in intersex patients with abnormal gonadal development like mixed gonadal dysgenesis (MGD) and true hermaphroditism (TH), recently called ovotesticular DSD. Although sex may be assigned before the biopsy is taken, histology in these patients is required for definitive diagnosis.

Gonadal biopsies must be taken along the longitudinal axis of the gonad as both ovarian and testicular tissue may be found at the polar ends of the gonad (Fig. 91.4). Depending on the result of the frozen section biopsy and the previous studies, the gonad is removed. Patients with TH may have an ovary (O) and testicle (T); bilateral ovotestes (OT) and an O and OT.

Surgical management in DSD should also consider options that will facilitate the chances of fertility. Ovarian component of an ovotestes may be separated and the testicular tissue removed, using zoom lens, although it must be kept in mind that these gonads need to be followed closely.

If a streak gonad is recognized like in most patients with MGD, it is removed without prior biopsy together with the surrounding peritoneum and the ipsilateral gonaduct (Fig. 91.5). This gonad has to be removed, avoiding previous biopsy, as it has a 25–50% chances to develop a gonadoblastoma and or dysgerminoma and as there is the possibility of an in situ tumor at the time of the procedure. It is usually associated with an intrabdominal or inguinal dysgenetic testicle, which is removed at the same time in patients with female sex assignment. Although there is the same risk of malignancy in the contralateral gonad (dysgenetic testicle) it may be biopsied and preserved in the scrotum of patients with male sex assignment because this gonad is functional.

The highest tumor risk is found in TSPY (testis specific protein Y encoded) positive gonadal dysgenesis and

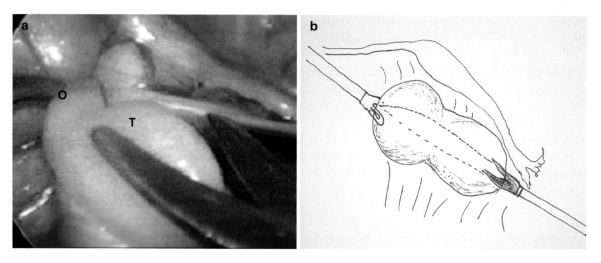

Fig. 91.4 (**a**) A laparoscopic view of an ovotestes. O: Ovarian portion T: Testicular component, (**b**) Illustration of the technique for gonadal biopsies along the longitudinal axis of the gonad

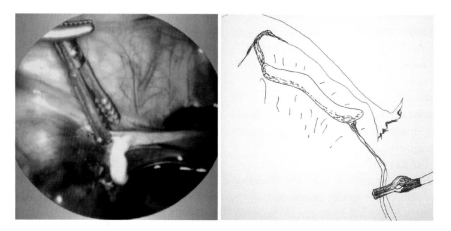

Fig. 91.5 (**a**) A laparoscopic view and (**b**) illustration of a streak gonad

partial androgen insensitivity (PAIS) with intraabdominal gonads, whereas the lowest risk (5%) is found in ovotestis and complete androgen insensitivity (CAIS).

Laparoscopy gives better visualization and quicker access to intraperitoneal gonads and has encouraged us to schedule simultaneous gonadal and genitalia procedures with good results. Nowadays, following a preoperative workup by an experienced multidisciplinary group, we do laparoscopic biopsies followed by gonadal resection if required at the same time of feminizing genitoplasty in female sex reassignment patients in a single stage initial approach.

Sex may be assigned prior to laparoscopy in patients with 45 XO/46,XY gonadal dysgenesis. This is based on a functional and psychosocial basis in combination with the results of the karyotyping, hCG testing and interview of the parents.

We have never found functional ovarian tissue in these patients but we always wait for the result of frozen section biopsy before removing any other gonad than a classical streak.

TH patients do not have such a classical pattern and definitive histology is often necessary for sex assignment. Although the most common karyotype is 46,XX and the most common gonadal combination ovary/ovotestes, each case is unique and should be treated on an individual basis. Sometimes the macroscopic aspect of the gonad and gonaduct as well as the result of a

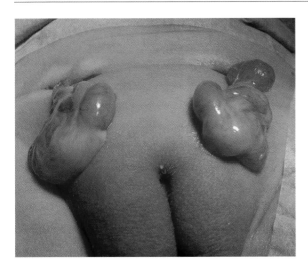

Fig. 91.6 An inguinal approach for gonadectomy in a CAIS patient with two palpable gonads

frozen section biopsy strongly favors gonadectomy in patients with previous sex assignment. There is an advantage of a laparoscopic approach in these patients requiring secondary pelvic exploration, especially because many of them are potentially fertile.

An additional role of laparoscopy is excision of mullerian structures, prostatic utricle and orchidopexy in patients raised as males. In patients with a symptomatic utriculus, removal is best performed laparoscopically to increase the chance of preserving continuity of the vas deferens.

An inguinal approach may be indicated in patients with palpable gonads (Fig. 91.6). We still prefer a laparoscopic approach in most of them as it enables not only better visualization of potential Mullerian structures but also allows for treatment of a patent peritoneal sac, when removing the gonads, with better cosmetic results. In addition, most of these patients have asymmetric gonads with one of them being intra-abdominal. We reserve the inguinal approach for xy patients with symmetric palpable gonads introducing the telescope through the associated hernial sac in order to rule out the presence of Mullerian structures.

91.4.2 Feminizing Genitoplasty

Fortunately there have been many advances in ambiguous genitalia reconstruction with many surgeons contributing. Cosmetically a near normal appearance can now be achieved, but long term functional results with newer techniques are still unknown.

Timing for this type of surgery is controversial. It is now our belief that one stage total reconstruction can be done in most patients in the early months of life.

Regardless of the timing or the procedure elected, the surgery must be done meticulously with a clear understanding of the anatomy and only be undertaken in centers with great experience and after all aspects of controversy have been explained in detail to the parents.

It consists in: (A) Management of clitoral enlargement; (B) Reconstruction of the urogenital sinus (UGS); and (C) Labioplasty

(A) Management of clitoral enlargement remains controversial because of the ablative nature of the structure so vital to psychological body, image and gender. Initial techniques consisted in total clitorectomy based on the belief that it was necessary to prevent gender dysphoria. However new understanding that an intact clitoris plays a crucial role in the development of female sexuality has stimulated more conservative surgical approach but recession of the clitoris, keeping the corpora may lead to painful erections during sexual arousal. The most used technique has been that based in Kogan's reduction clitoroplasty including removal of the corporal erectile tissue with preservation of the neurovascular bundle to the glans (Fig. 91.7). Glans reduction is accomplished by superficial excision on the epithelium of the glanular groove avoiding a scar in the glans tissue which is fixed to the pubis attachment.

Recently a non ablative and potentially reversible technique that dismembers the corporal bodies keeping them in the labia majora has been described in response to new understandings that an intact clitoris plays a crucial role in the development of female sexuality but no long term follow up is available.

(B) UGS abnormalities are a spectrum that goes from a labial fusion to an absent vagina depending on the location of the vaginal confluence in the UGS. Powell described four types: (I): labial fusion (II) distal confluence (III) proximal confluence (IV) absent vagina. In 1969 Hendren described different procedures required for reconstruction depending on the location of the vaginal confluence in the UGS

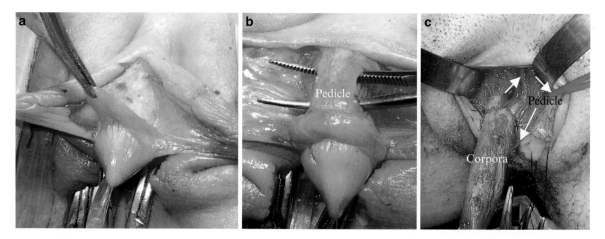

Fig. 91.7 Reduction clitoroplasty including removal of the corporal erectile tissue with preservation of the neurovascular bundle to the glans, (**a**) Dorsal incision of skin. (**b**) Isolated neurovascular bundles. (**c**) Corporal erectile tissue ready to resect. Arrows show the isolated preserved neurovascular bundle and glans

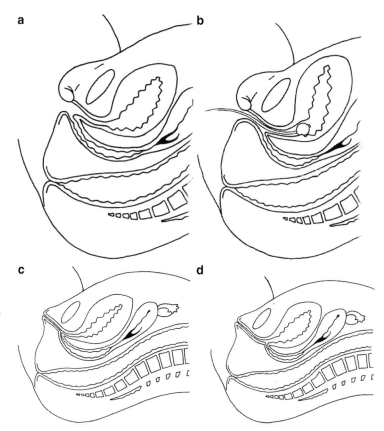

Fig. 91.8 Illustration of the spectrum of UGS abnormalities depending on the location of the vaginal confluence in the UGS and the presence of enough proximal urethra (between the bladder neck and the onset of vagina), (**a**): Lower variant. The vagina is very near the entrance of the UGS, (**b** and **c**) Intermediate variants. Spectrum between both, (**d**) Highest variant. The vagina is very near the bladder neck

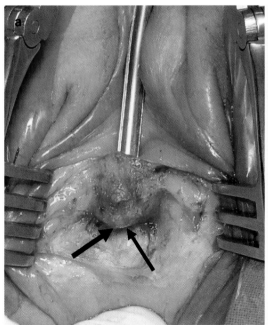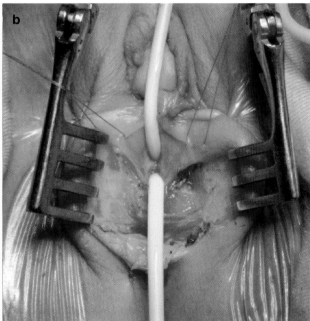

Fig. 91.9 (**a**) Dissection of the posterior vaginal wall, separating it from the rectal wall before sectioning the UGS, (**b**) A Foley catheter was introduced in the vaginal opening to help dissection to the perineum with traction. Even in low type UGS we advocate an aggressive dissection of the posterior vaginal wall before it's opening. We prefer to bring the vaginal wall to the perineum

related to the external sphincter (low when distal and high when proximal to the sphincter).This has been very helpful for reconstructive understanding but the vagina is not always high or low and the sphincter not well seen.We have found vaginas located from a normal position to an entrance in the bladder in a wide spectrum (Fig. 91.8).

The low confluence can be easily repaired by a "flap vaginoplasty" and the mid to high by a "pull through vaginoplasty".

Even in the low type, we advocate for a very aggressive dissection of the posterior vaginal wall, separating it from the rectal wall. The vagina is then cut in the midline well back into its normal caliber and at this point a wide cutaneous flap can be sewn using delicate sutures (Fig. 91.9).

Exteriorization of the high vagina in the severely masculinized female is a surgical challenge.The vagina must be detached from the UGS and then connected to the perineum. The pull through principle consists in placing a Fogarty balloon catheter into the vagina cystoscopically to locate it by palpation deep in the perineum later (Fig. 91.10). The UGS is approached like a bulbous urethra. Perineal anatomy in severe cases is like that of a normal male. The vagina is incised over the balloon,detached from its entry point in the UGS and the anterior wall carefully dissected off the overlying urinary tract. The vaginal walls to reach the perineum may be constructed using a combination of inverted U cutaneous flap (Fortunoff), prepucial flap (Gonzalez), redundant tissue from the UGS (Passerini flap).

In the middle of these two points we found what we called intermediate UGS.Although the vaginal opening is far from the UGS opening, there is enough proximal urethra to avoid urethra vaginal dissection and separation. After Alberto Peña's description of "total urogenital mobilization" (TUM) for the treatment of cloacas in 1997, we started using this maneuver to treat intermediate UGS abnormalities. The UGS is mobilized in block to the perineum.We use it in the lithotomy position, mobilize it without previous opening to prevent bleeding and never amputate the sinus tissue until the end as it may be used in the repair (Fig. 91.11). Each patient must be individualized and this technique can be combined with a pull

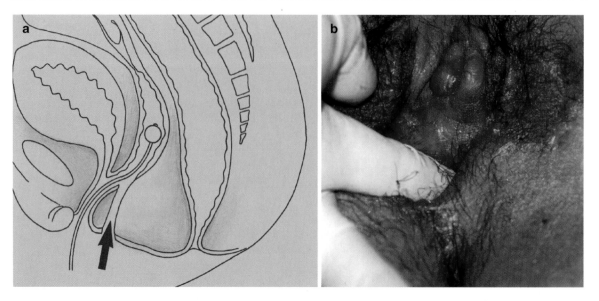

Fig. 91.10 (**a**) Illustration showing the pull through technique for the reconstruction of the high UGS. A balloon catheter has been introduced through the cystoscope and the vagina is reached through a perineal approach preserving the distal UGS sinus,

(**b**) Cosmetic appearance after a pull through technique with Ricardo Gonzalez modification (the phallus dorsal skin is used to reach the anterior vaginal wall after it has been detached from the UGS

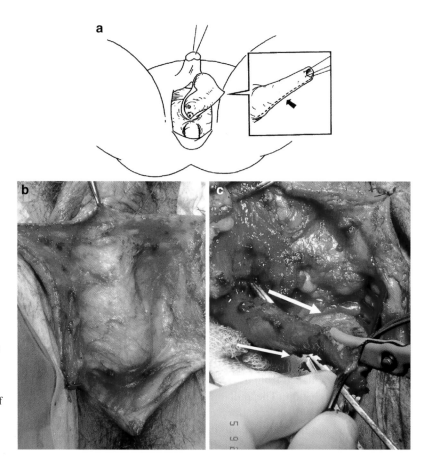

Fig. 91.11 Total UGS mobilization (TUM).The UGS is mobilized in block to the perineum. We do it in the lithotomy position, mobilize it without opening to prevent bleeding and never amputate the sinus tissue until the end. (**b**) The posterior wall of the UGS is the first to be dissected. It may be incised in the ventral wall of the UGS (**a**) or in the dorsal one (**c**)

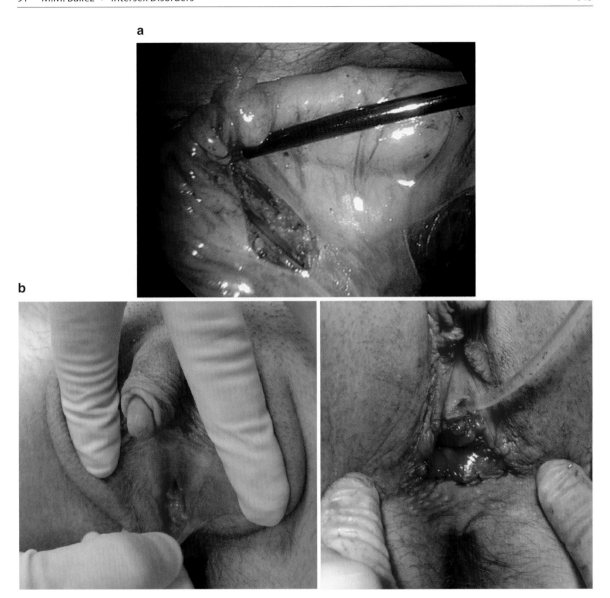

Fig. 91.12 Laparoscopic sigmoid vaginal replacement. (**a**) Laparoscopic aspect of an isolated piece of sigmoid colon. (**b**) Pre and postoperative perineal appearance of an XY patient who underwent this operation

through if required but it has simplified many of these repairs.

Richard Rink has recently described a variant that he calls partial urogenital mobilization (PUM), stopping dissection at the level of the pubourethral ligament. Currently regardless of the level of the confluence he starts with PUM, allowing a unified approach to all repairs.

A posterior sagital approach has been also by Peña described to correct intermediate and high UGS.

Those patients with absent vagina (type IV) should undergo vaginal replacement. Most of them are undervirilized males and a bowel vagina (colon if possible) is preferred. We have been doing it completely laparoscopically since 1999 (Fig. 91.12).

(C) Labioplasty is performed by dividing the clitoral hood skin in the midline (Byers) sewing the flaps around the clítoris and along the central mucosal strip down to the lateral vaginal walls (Fig. 91.13).

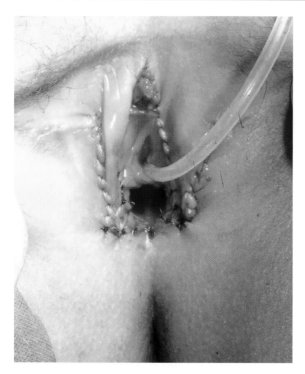

Fig. 91.13 Immediate postoperative perineal aspect of a 4 months old CAH patient who underwent feminizing genitoplasty

91.4.3 Urethral/Penile Reconstruction

This will be addressed in the hypospadias reconstruction chapter.

91.4.4 Timing of Surgery

The rationale for early reconstruction is based on guidelines on the timing of genital surgery from the American Academy of Pediatrics. The beneficial effects of estrogen on tissue in early infancy, and the avoidance of potential complications from the connection between the urinary tract and peritoneum via the Fallopian tubes.

The surgeon must be familiar with a number of operative techniques to reconstruct the spectrum of urogenital sinus disorders.

We have experienced reconstruction in both postpuberal and early months and we feel that the most important point is strategy and combination of different approaches if necessary. The goal is having a visible urethral and vaginal opening without functional damage. At this point if an introitoplasty may be necessary in the future for sexual function, it won't be a big deal. At any time it is important to have a stable patient which means well medicated and psychologically evaluated.

91.5 Outcome

The pattern of surgical practice in DSD is changing with respect to the timing of surgery and the techniques used. It is essential to evaluate the effects of early versus later surgery in a holistic manner, recognizing the difficulties posed by an ever-evolving clinical practice.

Some studies suggest satisfactory outcomes from early surgery (Fig. 91.14). Nevertheless, outcomes from clitoroplasty identify problems related to decreased sexual sensitivity, loss of clitoral tissue, and cosmetic issues.

Techniques for vaginoplasty carry the potential for scarring at the introitus necessitating repeated modification before sexual function.

The risks from vaginoplasty are different for high and low confluence of the urethra and vagina. Analysis of long-term outcomes is complicated by a mixture of surgical techniques.

The outcome in undermasculinized males with a phallus depends on the degree of hypospadias and the amount of erectile tissue. Feminizing genitoplasty as opposed to masculinizing genitoplasty requires less surgery to achieve an acceptable outcome and results in fewer urologic difficulties. Long-term data regarding sexual function and quality of life among those assigned female as well as male show great variability. There are no controlled clinical trials of the efficacy of early (12 months of age) versus late (in adolescence and adulthood) surgery or of the efficacy of different techniques.

Gender-role change occurs at different rates in different societies, suggesting that social factors may also be important modifiers of gender-role change.

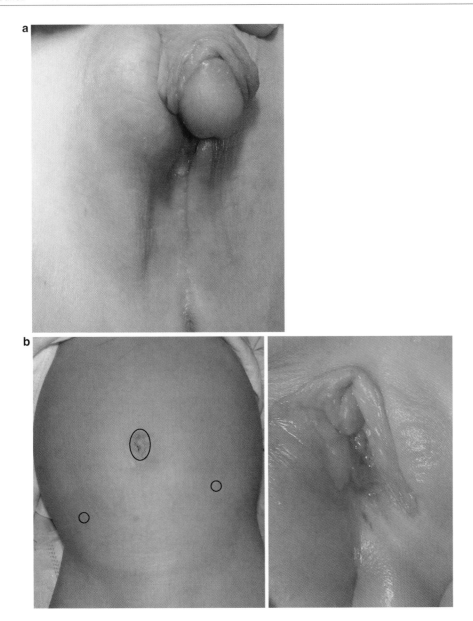

Fig. 91.14 (**a**) External genitalia of a patient with mixed gonadal dysgenesis; (**b**) cosmetic results after early simultaneous laparoscopic gonadectomy and feminizing genitoplasty

Further Reading

Bailez M, Fraire C (1998) Total mobilization of the urogenital sinus for the treatment of adrenal hyperplasia. BJU 81:76

Grumbach MM, Hughes IA, Conte FA (2003) Disorders of sex differentiation. In PR Larsen, HM Kronenberg, S Melmed, KS Polonsky (eds) Williams Textbook of Endocrinology, 10th edn. W.B. Saunders, Heidelberg, Germany, pp 842–1002

Lee PA, Houk CP, Ahmed SF, Hughes IA, in collaboration with the participants in the International Consensus Conference on Intersex organized by the Lawson Wilkins Pediatric Endocrine Society and the European Society for Paediatric Endocrinology Department of Pediatrics, Penn State College of Medicine, Hershey (2006) Consensus statement on management of intersex disorders. Pediatrics pp 118:488–500

Peña A (1997) Total urogenital mobilization—An easier way to repair cloacas. J Pediatr Surg 32:263–268

Puri P, Höllwarth M (2006) Pediatric Surgery. Springer, Berlin, Heidelberg

Cryptorchidism

John Hutson

Contents

92.1 Introduction

Congenital or cryptorchid testes are testes that are not located normally in the scrotum. At birth approximately 4–5% of boys have testes which are out of the scrotum, although during the first 3 months after birth about one half of these descend, leaving approximately 1–2% of boys with undescended testes at 3 months of age. The testicular position has significant implications for subsequent life with a decreased outcome for fertility and also risk of developing testicular tumour in young adult life. Because of these, as well as the obvious cosmetic abnormality, surgery for undescended testes is an extremely significant part of paediatric urology.

92.2 Embryology

The testes originally form in the aneomedial part of the urogenital ridge in the abdominal cavity of the embryo. Prior to 7–8 weeks of gestation gonadal position is identical in both sexes, but with the onset of sexual differentiation hormones produced by the early testis then trigger internal and external genital development and subsequent descent of the testis. A testis produces three known hormones in the early embryo; testosterone from the Leydig cells, as well as newly described hormone insulin-like hormone 3 (Insl3), as well as Müllerian Inhibiting Substance (anti-müllerian hormone) (MIS/AMH) from the Sertoli cells. With regression of the mesonephros in the urogenital ridge, and also regression of the paramesenephric duct or müllerian duct by MIS/AMH, the testis and adjacent mesonephric duct (Wolffian duct) are held to the posterior abdominal wall cranially by the cranial suspensory ligament, and caudally to the anterior

P. Puri and M. Höllwarth (eds.), *Pediatric Surgery: Diagnosis and Management,*
DOI: 10.1007/978-3-540-69560-8_92, © Springer-Verlag Berlin Heidelberg 2009

abdominal wall by the genitoinguinal ligament or gubernaculum. With regression of the mesonephros the testis acquires a mesentery or "mesogenitale" which enables it to be suspended in the abdominal cavity. The cranial suspensory ligament and the gubernaculum are in peritoneal folds attached to the testis.

During the first phase of descent the cranial suspensory ligament regresses under the action of androgens. This is quite a prominent ligament in animals, but is less prominent in humans. In the male fetus the caudal end of the gubernaculum that is embedded in the anterior abdominal wall becomes thickened, known as the swelling reaction. This is mediated primarily by Insl3 from the Leydig cells. In the female, by contrast, the gubernaculum remains thin and ultimately develops into the round ligament and ligament of the ovary. The swelling reaction in the male gubernaculum holds the testis very close to the inguinal abdominal wall as the abdominal cavity enlarges with growth of the fetus. This produces a relative descent of the testis compared with the ovary. The inguinal canal forms by the abdominal muscles differentiating around the gelatinous end of the gubernaculum. In addition, the peritoneum forms an annular diverticulum inside the gubernaculum to form the processes vaginalis. The first phase of descent is complete by about 15 weeks of gestation (Fig. 92.1).

At about 25 weeks of gestation the processus vaginalis elongates within the gubernaculum creating a peritoneal diverticulum within which the testis can descend. A central column of gubernacular mesenchyme remains attached to the epididymis and lower pole of the testis. The distal end of the gubernaculum then bulges out of the abdominal musculature and begins to elongate towards the scrotum, eventually arriving there between 30 and 35 weeks of gestation. The testis descends inside the processus vaginalis, which remains open until descent is complete, and then undergoes proximal obliteration. This second phase of descent is controlled by testosterone from the testis acting not only directly on the gubernaculum, but also indirectly via the sensory branches of the genitofemoral nerve, which in a rat release a neurotransmitter, calcitonin gene-related peptide (CGRP), that provides a chemotactic gradient for migration of the gubernaculum to the scrotum. Descent of the testis inside the processus vaginalis is aided by the intra-abdominal pressure. The cremaster muscle develops in the wall of the gubernacular mesenchyme outside the processus vaginalis, and does not appear to be derived from the internal oblique muscle as previously proposed.

92.3 Etiology

Congenital undescended testis can be caused by any anomaly of the hormonal control or anatomical processes required to produce normal testicular descent. Hormonal

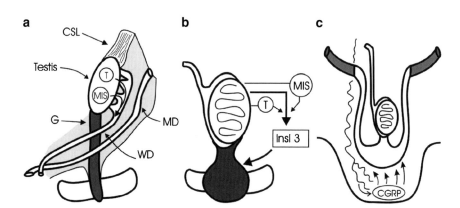

Fig. 92.1 Schema showing the different gonadal positions during the two stages of testicular descent (**a**) Initially the testis is in the urogenital ridge with the Wolffian duct (WD) and the Müllerian duct (MD) and the two main supporting ligaments, the cranial suspensory ligament (CSL) and the genitoinguinal ligament or "gubernaculum" (G). Testosterone (T) and Müllerian Inhibiting Substance (MIS) are secreted down the WD (**b**) During the transabdominal phase, the testis is held by the enlarged gubernaculum close to the inguinal region as the fetus enlarges. Insulin 3 stimulates gubernacular swelling, augmented by MIS, and T, which also causes regression of CSL (**c**) In the inguinoscrotal phase, the gubernaculum migrates out of the abdominal wall and elongates towards the scrotum (with the testis inside the peritoneal diverticulum, processus vaginalis) under androgenic control partly direct and partly indirect via the genitofemoral nerve and release of calcitonin gene-related peptide (CGRP) (Reproduced with permission from Elsevier)

defects in androgen, MIS/AMH or Insl3 are rare but well recognised causes of cryptorchidism. Abnormalities of the first or transabdominal phase of descent are also rare, probably because there is little mechanical movement with enlargement of the gubernaculum to hold the testis near the groin during enlargement of the fetal abdomen. Not surprisingly, therefore, intra-abdominal testes are relatively rare (less than 5–10% of cryptorchid testes). By contrast, inguinoscrotal migration during the second phase of descent is a complex, hormonally-regulated anatomical process, and anomalies are common. These are secondary to failure of gubernacular migration to the scrotum, leaving the testis palpable in the inguinal region. The exact cause of most of these remains unknown, but poor placental function producing inadequate fetal androgens or inadequate gonadotropin stimulation from the fetal pituitary are all likely possibilities. Compounds in the environment with oestrogenic properties may play a role in the apparent increase in cryptorchidism in the last 20–30 years. Rare ectopia of the testis during migration is most likely to be caused by anomalous location of the genitofemoral nerve causing migration to an abnormal site.

Some connective tissue and nervous system disorders are associated with cryptorchidism, such as arthrogryposis multiplex congenita, spina bifida and hypothalamic disorders. The role of abdominal pressure is observed in the increased frequency of undescended testis in abdominal wall defects such as exomphalos, gastroschisis, and bladder exstrophy. Prune belly syndrome is a special case where the enlargement of the bladder probably prevents the gubernaculum forming normally in the inguinal region, or even tearing of the gubernaculum from the inguinal abdominal wall because the bladder becomes so big. This then prevents the processus vaginalis forming a normal inguinal canal and hence the testes remain intra-abdominal on the back of the enlarged bladder.

Many undescended testes where there has been low hormone levels *in utero* are associated with deficient development of the epididymis, which may be partially separated from the testis.

92.4 Clinical Presentation

At birth 4–5% of boys show cryptorchidism, but this reduces to 1–2% by 12 weeks after term. Cryptorchidism is more common in premature infants, who are born before the normal process has been completed. Beyond 12 weeks of age spontaneous descent is rare. A cryptorchid or undescended testis is defined as a testis that cannot be manipulated to the bottom of the scrotum by 12 weeks of age (Fig. 92.2). In most cases, the testis is near the neck of the scrotum or just outside the external inguinal ring. It often is located a little bit lateral to the external inguinal ring in the subcutaneous space under Scarpa's fascia, described by Denis Browne as the "superficial inguinal pouch". This is not usually ectopic migration of the gubernaculum causing this position, but the testis displaced laterally by the fascial layers of the abdominal wall. The testis even when undescended is still on a mesentery inside the tunica vaginalis, which may or may not be still patent. The presence of the mesentery means that the undescended testis will be mobile within the tunica vaginalis on palpation. About 10% of undescended testes are impalpable because they are either intra-abdominal or have undergone perinatal torsion and atrophied ("the vanishing testis"). Truly ectopic testes are rare (Fig. 92.3).

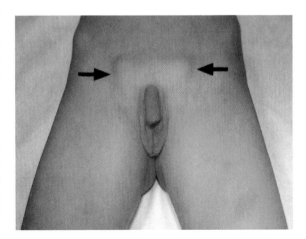

Fig. 92.2 Bilateral undescended testes in the inguinal region

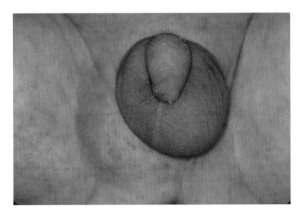

Fig. 92.3 Perineal ectopic testis

The length of the spermatic cord in babies is approximately 4–5 cm from the external inguinal ring to the top of the testes. By contrast, in 10–year-old children the spermatic cord is approximately 8–10 cm in length. This is because as the child grows the distance from the external inguinal ring to the scrotum enlarges with changes in the shape of the pelvis. This necessity for the spermatic cord to elongate postnatally is now recognised as the probable cause of the newly described acquired cryptorchidism. Acquired undescended testes are thought to be those testes that descended relatively normally to the scrotum at birth, but where the spermatic cord fails to elongate normally postnatally. The testis appears to be in the scrotum at birth but then ascends gradually out of the scrotum with age. However, what is actually happening is that the scrotum is getting further from the inguinal region with age and the testis is actually stationary in most cases (Fig. 92.4). In early stages the testis might be thought to be retractile, as it can be pulled into the scrotum. However, on release the testis retracts out of the scrotum. This usually implies that there is residual fibrous tissue from the processus vaginalis which is preventing normal elongation of the spermatic cord with age. In children with cerebral palsy and spastic diplegia, acquired undescended testes are caused by abnormal spasm of the cremaster muscle, but in most children the cause of acquired undescended testis appears to be failure of

obliteration of the processus vaginalis leaving a fibrous remnant which does not elongate with age.

There has been much controversy in the literature about the definition of retractile testes and ascending testes. Here retractile testes are defined as those testes which retract out of the scrotum on stimulation of the sensory branch of the genitofemoral nerve, but then return to the scrotum within 10–20 s. An ascending testis is a testis that was in the scrotum at 3 months of age but then reascends out of the scrotum with progressive increase in size of the boy. In the latter case there is commonly a history of delayed postnatal descent in the first 3 months after birth. As mentioned above, these are usually caused by a persistence of an obliterated fibrous remnant of the processus vaginalis, although occasionally it is actually even patent as a potential hernia.

92.5 Diagnosis

The clinical examination aims to locate the testis if palpable, and to determine the lowest position to which it can be manipulated without undue tension on the spermatic cord. This corresponds to the caudal limit of the tunica vaginalis in most cases. In babies the diagnosis is straightforward as the scrotum is thin and

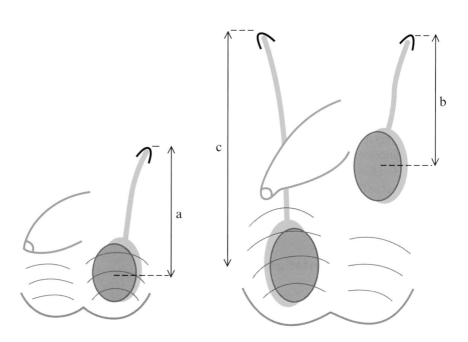

Fig. 92.4 Acquired maldescent is likely to be secondary to failure of spermatic cord elongation over the first 5–10 years, caused by a fibrous remnant of the processus vaginalis

pendulous. Indeed, in a newborn male the scrotum often reaches almost to the knee of the baby! Hypoplasia of the hemiscrotum suggests that it has not contained a testis. In older boys diagnosis can be more difficult particularly if the boy is obese. The squatting position is sometimes useful to cause automatic relaxation of the cremaster muscle and allow the testis to descend if it is merely retracted normally out of the scrotum. When the testis is located in the groin, it is important to remember that it is on a mesentery within the tunica vaginalis and will therefore be quite mobile. This mobility can be used to diagnose the malposition by attempts to milk to testis from lateral to medial and down into the scrotum (Fig. 92.5). Compression of the inguinal region from the anterior superior iliac spine medially to the pubic tubercle and then down into the scrotum will often deliver the testis into the scrotum and the waiting contralateral hand.

In a situation where the testis is impalpable, two physical signs should be sought: one is the presence of an open external inguinal ring or possible membranes of a processus vaginalis in the pubic region. If these are present this suggests that the testis is just inside the inguinal canal. Also, the size of the descended testis should be noted, as where the cryptorchid testis is absent the contralateral descended testis will often undergo compensatory hypertrophy. Should the palpable testis be larger than normal, it usually means that the cryptorchid testis is absent or atrophic.

92.6 Investigations

Investigations for cryptorchidism are rarely required, except when both testes are impalpable. In this case hormonal investigations such as hCG stimulation test, androgen serum levels, MIS/AMH levels, or even chromosome analysis may be appropriate. The aim of the tests is to confirm that a testis is present and is producing measurable hormones. Once a testis is known to be present (because of hormone levels) then the testis is best located by laparoscopy. Ultrasound examination is often unreliable, while magnetic resonance imaging and particularly magnetic resonance angiography might be required in very special cases. However, the current gold standard for a impalpable undescended testis is laparoscopy to identify the position and to potentially perform orchidopexy in one or two stages.

92.7 Rationale for Management

A testis located in the scrotum is 4°C cooler than the core temperature of the body, which provides the testis with optimal function. Cryptorchidism leads to an abnormal temperature of the testis which causes progressive derangement of the gonadal biochemistry and physiology. In the first year, the normal testis responds to a surge of gonadotropin secretion in the first few months, with a transient but significant production of testosterone between 2–6 months, as well as significant production of MIS/AMH between 6–12 months of age. This hormone production is likely to be intimately involved in regulating development of the neonatal germ cells. At birth the neonatal germ cell, known as a gonocyte, transforms into a Type A spermatogonium between 4–12 months of age. The neonatal gonocyte is in the middle of the seminiferous tubule, but the

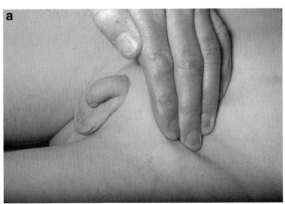

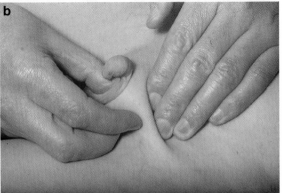

Fig. 92.5 Milking the mobile testis from the groin into the upper scrotum where it can be snared by the other hand

Type A spermatogonium is abutting the basement membrane of the tubule and surrounded by the Sertoli cells. This change in position with development of the germ cells is important in allowing them to mature into Type A and then subsequently Type B spermatogonia, and then finally into primary spermatocytes about 3–4 years of age. The primary spermatocyte is located in the centre of the seminiferous tubule similar to the neonatal gonocyte, but its physiology and biochemistry is now quite different. These cells then remain relatively dormant from 3–4 years of age until the onset of puberty.

In undescended testes transformation of the neonatal gonocytes into Type A spermatogonia is impaired (Fig. 92.6), and this is thought to lead to two significant consequences for the person. An inadequate pool of Type A spermatogonia will lead to infertility, as the

Type A spermatogonium is the stem cell for spermatogenesis. Furthermore, the neonatal gonocytes which fail to transform into Type A spermatogonia would normally undergo apoptosis. However, at the abnormal temperature of the undescended testis it is quite likely that apoptosis is impaired, leaving some neonatal gonocytes persisting in the cryptorchid testis. These may eventually mutate into carcinoma-in-situ and then invasive seminoma in early adult life. Although the exact cause of testicular cancer in men with previous cryptorchidism is not known conclusively, it would now appear that failure of the neonatal transformation of gonocytes into Type A spermatogonia is the key event leading to not only infertility but also malignancy risk. Hence, this information has had a major impact on determining the choice and timing of treatment for undescended testes. Despite this, however, the optimal

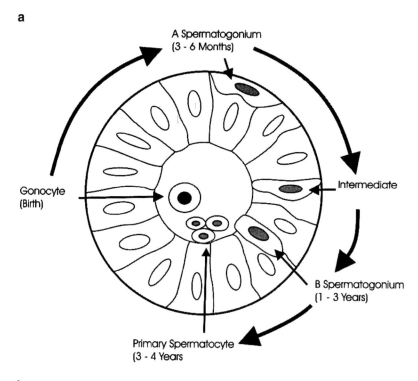

Fig. 92.6 Postnatal germ cell development from gonocyte to A spermatogonium, B spermatogonium and eventually to primary spermatocyte. Cryptorchidism inhibits the first step from gonocyte to A spermatogonium, which occurs at 3–6 months, and is the biological basis for recommending surgery at this time

time for surgical intervention with orchidopexy is still not known, as the long-term follow-up of children having surgery in the first year of life is not yet accomplished. It will be some years before we know whether orchidopexy in the first year can prevent infertility and malignancy. Furthermore, it is not known whether the risks of infertility and malignancy in children with acquired cryptorchidism are the same as for those with congenital cryptorchidism. Recent evidence suggests that the cancer risk in ascending testes may be very low. If this is the case then acquired cryptorchid patients are at risk of decreased fertility but not of a higher risk of cancer.

92.8 Treatment

Hormone treatment remains controversial, as both gonadotropin and LHRH have been shown to have success rates between 10% and 50%. In particular, higher success rates have only been found in those children that might be regarded as having pathologically retractile or acquired ascending testes. In children with congenital failure of migration of the gubernaculum to the scrotum, hormonal treatment appears to have a very low success rate. The reasons for this are unknown, but it may be that the anatomical processes following hormonal stimulation are too complex to respond to hormone treatment given postnatally.

The principle behind surgical management is to mobilise the testis and relocate it within the scrotum. For testes at the neck of the scrotum or in the inguinal region this is a relatively straightforward orchidopexy. The details will not be discussed at length here. For intra-abdominal testes laparoscopy is used in most places to identify the testicular position, and then a decision can be made about whether a one stage or a two-stage orchidopexy can be performed. The two stage, Fowler-Stephens operation, with initial division of the testicular vessels, is used now for those testes which cannot be brought to the scrotum in one operation. A simple test for determining this laparoscopically is whether the intra-abdominal testis can be pulled with graspers to the contralateral internal inguinal ring. If it reaches the contralateral ring then it should reach the scrotum without division of the vessels being necessary.

Based on the germ cell development, the optimal timing for orchidopexy should be somewhere between 3 and 12 months of age, with 6–12 months being a convenient time. There is no evidence that orchidopexy at this age carries any greater risk of complications than orchidopexy done in older children, as long as the surgeon has been adequately trained in paediatric surgical techniques.

92.9 Complications

The complications of orchidopexy include wound infection and haematoma, but the most serious complication is atrophy of the testis. This occurs in a small percentage of testes, that is probably in the range of 5–10% depending on the severity of the original abnormality. Certainly, the risk of atrophy with an impalpable testis is significantly greater than in a testis palpable in the groin. Also, the risk of atrophy is greater in children with a primary abnormality of testicular development where the testes are smaller than normal at the time of surgery. A final factor that increases the risk of atrophy is whether or not previous surgery has been performed.

92.10 Prognosis

The current predictions of fertility and malignancy remain very controversial, because of the dramatic changes in understanding and management of undescended testes in the last 25 years. Currently quoted figures in the literature suggest possible infertility in a quarter of adult males with previous unilateral undescended testes and maybe in three quarters of those with a history of bilateral undescended testes. The risk for malignancy is quoted to be about 5–10 times greater than normal for a man with known previous unilateral cryptorchidism. As mentioned previously, it is not known whether these prognostic factors will improve with the much younger age of surgery currently than was done in a previous generation. At present we can only hope that the risks for infertility and cancer will improve with surgery in infants, and improved discrimination between congenital and acquired undescended testes, where the prognosis appears to be different.

Further Reading

Docimo SG (1995) The results of surgical therapy for cryp-
    torchidism: A literature review and analysis. J Urol 154:
    1148–1152

Hutson JM, Clark MCC (2007) Current management of the
    undescended testicle. Semin Ped Surg 16:64–70

Hutson JM, Hasthorpe S (2005) Testicular descent and cryp-
    torchidism: The state of the art in 2004. J Pediatr Surg
    40:297–302

Hutson JM (2006) Orchidopexy. In P Puri, ME Höllwarth (eds)
    Pediatric Surgery. Springer Surgery Atlas Series, Springer -
    Verlag Berlin Heidelberg, New York, pp 555–568

Ong C, Hasthorpe S, Hutson JM (2005) Germ cell develop-
    ment in the descended and cryptorchid testis and
    the effects of hormonal manipulation. Pediatr Surg Int
    21:240–254

Patil KK, Green JS, Duffy PG (2005) Laparoscopy for impal-
    pable testes. BJU Int 95:704–708

Acute Scrotum

93

Amulya K. Saxena and Michael E. Höllwarth

Contents

Testicular torsion or spermatic cord torsion is the most common genitourinary tract emergency of childhood. This clinical entity is commonly referred to as "the acute scrotum" and is the most serious of the conditions in a pediatric patient with swelling, redness and tenderness in the area of the scrotum. Other differentials in this entity are torsion of the appendices and epididymis as well as epididymitis which are discussed in this chapter.

93.1 Testicular Torsion

93.1.1 Introduction

Testicular torsion refers to twisting of the spermatic cord structures, either in the inguinal canal or just below the inguinal canal. Torsion of the testis or of the spermatic cord is a surgical emergency as it causes strangulation of testicular blood supply with subsequent testicular necrosis and atrophy. The number of twists determines the amount of vascular impairment, but generally there is a 6–8 h window before significant ischemia damage occurs affecting long-term testicular morphology and sperm formation. Testicular torsion is a true surgical emergency and acute scrotal swelling in children indicates torsion of the testis until proven otherwise. In approximately 60% of patients, history and physical examination are sufficient to make the definitive diagnosis.

93.1.2 Etiology

There are two main types of testicular torsion: extravaginal and intravaginal torsion.

93.1.2.1 Extravaginal Torsion

Extravaginal torsion comprises approximately 5% of all torsions. Up to 20% of cases are synchronous, and 3% are asynchronous bilateral. This type is characterized by testes that may freely rotate via the tunica vaginalis prior to the development of testicular fixation within the scrotum. Since the tunica vaginalis likely becomes adherent to the surrounding tissues by 6 weeks of age, this type manifests in the perinatal period. Perinatal testicular torsion can be further divided into two subtypes: pre- and postnatal torsion. Prenatal torsion characteristically presents at birth as a hard, non-tender mass in the hemiscrotum with underlying dark skin discoloration and fixation of the skin to the mass. Postnatal torsion on the other hand presents with acute inflammation with erythema and tenderness. This difference is important in the planning of the clinical strategy, since the postnatal torsion requires emergency exploration. Testicular salvage is generally rare in perinatal torsion, however encouraging reports are emerging with varying degrees of success.

93.1.2.2 Intravaginal Torsion

Intravaginal torsion occurs beyond the perinatal period due to abnormal fixation of the testicle and epididymis within the tunica vaginalis. Normally, the tunica will invest the epididymis and posterior surface of the testi-

cle, which fixes it to the scrotum and prevents it from twisting. If the tunica vaginalis attaches in a more proximal position on the spermatic cord, the testicle and epididymis hang free in the scrotum and can twist around the longitudinal axis of the spermatic cord within the tunica vaginalis. This abnormal fixation is described as the "bell-clapper" deformity which predisposes to testicular torsion in older children (Fig. 93.1). Peak incidence occurs in adolescents aged 13 years, and the left testis is more frequently involved. Bilateral cases account for 2% of all torsions. Contraction of the spermatic muscles is presumed to apply the rotational force which is mainly responsible for the initiation of testicular torsion in these patients. Furthermore, rapid growth and increasing vascularity of the testicle during puberty may also be precursors to intravaginal torsion.

93.1.3 Pathophysiology

Torsion of the spermatic cord interrupts blood flow to the testis and epididymis. The degree of torsion is variable with a range from 180–720°. At the onset of torsion, an increased testicular and epididymal congestion is encountered which further promotes the progression of the torsion.

The extent and duration of torsion directly influence both the immediate salvage rate and late testicular atrophy. Testicular salvage can be expected if the duration

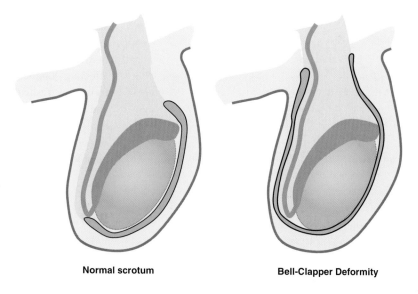

Fig. 93.1 In normal testis (*left*) the tunica invests the epididymis and posterior surface of the testicle, which fixes it to the scrotum. In "Bell-clapper deformity" (*right*) the tunica vaginalis attaches in a more proximal position on the spermatic cord leaving the testicle and epididymis to hang free in the scrotum and twist within the tunica vaginalis

Normal scrotum   **Bell-Clapper Deformity**

of torsion is less than 6–8 h. If however 24 h or more elapse, testicular necrosis develops, and the salvage of the affected testicle is not possible.

93.1.4 Diagnosis

In all cases in which the clinical presentation strongly points out to testicular torsion, surgical exploration for detorsion and fixation is mandated. The physical examination should include thorough investigation of the abdomen, inguinal region, and scrotum. Although precise preoperative diagnosis is the goal, excessive pre-surgical evaluation should be avoided that may further substantially delay surgery and add further risk to the affected testicle.

93.1.5 Clinical Features

Prenatal torsion manifests as a firm, hard, scrotal mass, which is discoloured, ecchymotic and edematous does not transilluminate in an otherwise asymptomatic newborn male. On the other hand, postnatal torsion is a unique phenomenon in that it is generally a subacute or chronic process by the time the infant is delivered. Postnatal torsion accounts for 10% or less of all cases of testicular infarction from torsion. Distinguishing neonatal torsion from incarcerated hernia may necessitate urgent operation, but a salvaged testis is rarely the outcome if torsion is confirmed. In such cases complete infarction is present and detorsion does not lead to the recovery of the testis. Surgery of neonatal testicular torsion is therefore mainly utilized to fix the contralateral testis to prevent its future loss due to torsion.

In older boys, the classic presentation of testicular torsion is the sudden onset of severe testicular pain followed by inguinal and/or scrotal swelling. However, reduced pain may be seen in patients who have a longstanding torsion. If a history of previous bouts of intermittent testicular pain is present it may suggest previous episodes of torsions and spontaneous detorsions. Approximately 33% of patients also have gastrointestinal upset with nausea and vomiting. In some patients, scrotal trauma or other scrotal disease (including torsion of appendix testis or epididymitis) precede the occurrence of subsequent testicular torsion. Depending on the duration of torsion, the physical examination may reveal various degrees of swelling, tenderness and indurations. In classical cases, a high riding testicle is found which has a transverse orientation or an anteriorly located epididymis. The absence of the cremasteric reflex in a patient with acute scrotal pain supports the diagnosis of torsion. In later stages of testicular torsion, a reactive hydrocele, scrotal wall erythema, and ecchymosis become more prominent and mask the above mentioned landmarks making examination more difficult. A low-grade fever may be present, but urine analysis is generally clear.

93.1.6 Differential Diagnosis

The differential diagnosis for unilateral acute pain, mass or swelling varies with the age of the patient. Trauma to the testis may produce a tender scrotal mass from testicular rupture, hematoma and hematocele. Testicular rupture requires urgent exploration to salvage the gonad, and severe testicular hematoma may even lead to infarction from the increased pressure within the intact tunica albuginea. Epididymal orchitis is more frequently the diagnosis in febrile patients with pyuria and among those who are sexually active, although it can occur in any age group. Torsion of the appendages presents initially with more focal pain and if the scrotum is examined before the onset of diffuse scrotal edema, a discrete nodule may be palpated along the superior pole of the testicle. A subcutaneous "blue dot" may also be apparent on transillumination and is pathognomic for torsion of the appendix testis. Idiopathic scrotal edema is an allergic condition producing painless swelling of the perineum and groin, most commonly in prepubertal children.

If the patient does not show clinical evidence of testicular torsion, a urinalysis and culture may exclude urinary tract infection and epididymitis as the etiology of the scrotal complaints. Leukocytosis indicates testicular torsion but is not specific.

93.2 Imaging Studies

93.2.1 Scrotal Doppler Sonogram

Color Doppler sonography is a sensitive tool in most of the age groups to diagnose testicular torsion, but it may be more difficult in neonates and prepubertal boys (Fig. 93.2). In the pediatric population it has a 90–100% sensitivity compared with nearly 100% by scintigraphic studies. Although scintigraphy and color Doppler sonography have comparable sensitivities in the evaluation of intratesticular flow, color Doppler sonography provides additional valuable information, is non-invasive, and can be obtained generally with less delay. In small gonads, the intratesticular blood vessels are of a smaller calibre, and blood flows at a lower average velocity. The sensitivity of the examination is dependent up to a large extent on the capabilities of the equipment and the experience of the examiner. In older patients, the examination is easier to perform and the contralateral asymptomatic testis is used as a control.

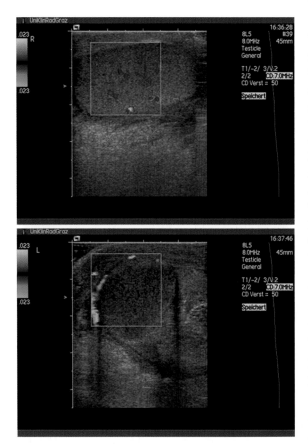

Fig. 93.2 Color Doppler ultrasonography showing blood flow in the unaffected testis (*above*) and lack of perfusion in the testicle affected by torsion (*below*). Note increased blood flow around the left superior margin of the testis which corresponds to the location of the epididymis/cord complex. These vessels represent hyperaemic collateral arteries from the arteries supplying the epididymis

93.2.2 Radionucleotide Scans

Radionucleotide scans were previously the gold standard for determining the presence of testicular perfusion, but in recent years, Doppler ultrasonography has become popular because it provides equally accurate assessment of flow along with valuable anatomic clues. Radionucleotide scans and color Doppler ultrasonography are both limited in the diagnosis of intermittent torsion, because perfusion studies reflect flow at only one particular moment in time. Detorted testicles have return of flow and may be associated with reactive hyperemia.

93.3 Management

There are many controversies surrounding the management of prenatal testicular torsions. These include (a) the timing of exploration of torsed gonad, (b) whether to remove or replace the grossly necrotic gonad, and (c) the indication of contralateral orchidopexy. Because prenatal torsion has progressed to chronic torsion by the time of delivery, the testicle can seldom be salvaged. Exploration need not be performed as an emergency but should be executed promptly depending on the overall condition of the newborn. In newborns, the main objective in the management should be prompt exploration for potential salvage of the contralateral gonad. Any delay in diagnosis and treatment may have an adverse effect on the endocrine function and fertility in the long term.

At the time of exploration, the testicle may be edematous or necrotic. Bleeding from an incision of the tunica albugenia is the best prognostic sign for potential viability (Fig. 93.3). The previous concept to replace the necrotic testis back in the scrotum and fix it in order to preserve any potential endocrine function is now redundant. Necrotic testicles that have been replaced have found to be atrophic on later examinations. Experimental studies in rodents have shown such testicles to liberate antigens that may have adverse immunological effects on the contralateral testicle. Early exploration and removal of the necrotic testicle is the most appropriate management. The only exception to this concept is the neonate with bilateral necrotic testicle from prenatal torsion, where salvage of one of the gonads is the only potential for preservation of endocrine or reproductive function.

93.3.1 Surgical Approach

In case of perinatal torsion, many surgeons prefer an inguinal approach to the affected side, which allow easier access and removal of the necrotic, fixed gonad. This approach is also more appropriate when an alternative pathology is suspected. Contralateral exploration is however performed through a scrotal transverse skin incision in these patients with the secure placement of the testis in the dartos pouch between the external spermatic fascia of the scrotum and the dartos layer.

Older patients are best explored trans-scrotally, unless there is an any evidence of a concomitant testicular tumor. Once the torsion is relieved during surgery, the testicle should be placed in warm moist gauzes while exploring the opposite hemiscrotum, since contralateral trans-scrotal orchidopexy should be performed at the same time. Orchiectomy of the testis should be performed only when necrosis is clearly evident. Otherwise, if signs of viability are evident, the affected testis should be returned to the scrotum and fixed in place. All orchidopexy procedures should consist of three-point fixation between the tunica albugenia and scrotal wall or septum. The lateral suclus between the testicle and epididymis is a helpful landmark for this purpose.

Patients with suspected intermittent torsion should also undergo bilateral trans-scrotal exploration and orchidopexy. It should be noted that testicular fixation is not an absolute guarantee against the possibility of future torsion, since cases of torsion after fixation have been reported. Patients presenting with acute scrotum after torsion and orchidopexy should therefore be treated and managed the similar way as prior to the fixation.

Patients requiring an orchiectomy because of a non-viable testis may benefit from the placement of a testicular prosthesis. The placement of a testicular prosthesis should be delayed for 6 months after orchiectomy surgery, until healing is complete and inflammatory changes resolve. There are three types of silicone elastomer implants currently available as testicular prosthesis: saline filled, soft solid and solid forms. Gel-filled prosthesis that were used in the last decade, are no longer available. The solid silicone prosthesis used in Europe are available in three sizes (31 × 23 mm; 37 × 28 mm; 42 × 32 mm). Testicular implants may be placed in a small child, however they have to be replaced by a larger implant as the child matures and grows, if the child or his parents wish to

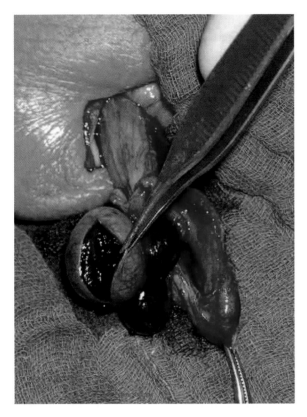

Fig. 93.3 Absence of bleeding from an incision of the tunica albugenia is not a good prognostic sign for potential viability of the testicle

In older children, depending on the tolerance of the patient, detorsion of the testicle should be attempted in a medial to lateral rotation. If this is successful, the testicle will drop lower in the scrotum and a sudden relief in pain will be reported by the patient. In approximately two-third of the patients this "open book" rotation may be helpful; however, if unsuccessful a rotation in the other direction may be attempted. Manual detorsion improves the symptoms of the patient and decreases the degree of ischemia, but it is not a substitute for surgical exploration.

Contralateral orchidopexy is recommended in all cases of unilateral torsion regardless of the age of the patient of the type of torsion intra- or extravaginal at the time of initial exploration. This minimal invasive procedure does not cause any harm to the contralateral gonad and can be extremely beneficial in the future for the patient who has already lost one testicle in torsion.

maintain a size that closely matches the child's other healthy testicle. Complications with testicular prosthesis include scrotal hematoma, keloid formation and scrotal edema. In addition, infection or extrusion (when the implant shifts and presses out through the skin) may also require additional surgery.

93.3.2 Complications

Delay of more than 6–8 h between onset of symptoms and the time of detorsion reduces the salvage rate to 55–85%. As mentioned above, a correlation exists between the duration of torsion and abnormal semen parameters, and some reports suggest that retention of an injured testis can induce pathologic changes to the contralateral testis.

Success in the management of spermatic cord torsion is measured by immediate testicular salvage and incidence of late testicular atrophy, which are, in turn, directly related to the duration and degree of testicular torsion. Delaying surgical intervention worsens the intraoperative testicular salvage and increases the incidence of subsequent testicular atrophy. The delay between the onset of symptoms and the time of surgical or manual detorsion is of utmost importance in achieving a viable testis.

93.3.2.1 Epididymitis

Acute epididymitis is the most common condition that causes acute scrotal pain. The exact incidence in children is unknown; however studies from larger pediatric centers report about 5–40 cases of acute epididymitis per year. Distinguishing between acute epididymitis and testicular torsion is important because their treatments differ significantly. Typically epididymitis has a slow onset, with scrotal pain and swelling worsening over a period of days rather than hours. There is generally no nausea or vomiting in the history. However, fever and pyuria may be present at the time of presentation. Physical examination reveals an enlarged and tender epididymis that can be separated from the scrotum. The pain is relieved by elevating the scrotum to the symphysis pubis (Prehn sign). Usually, the cremasteric reflex is present. Sonography, clinical history taking, and physical examination are the mainstays in diagnosing

acute epididymitis. Urinanalysis and urine culture should be performed in all children; and urethral swabs samples from patients who are sexually active. Acute epididymitis may be classified depending on the etiology as infectious, reactive or traumatic. However, it is important to note that recent reports have demonstrated no association to etiologic factors in majority of the patients.

Both specific and non-specific infections are reported to be causative. The bacterial infection is presumed to reach the epididymis in a retrograde fashion via the ejaculatory ducts, and can be associated with a urinary tract infection or urethritis. Usually, acute epididymitis in pubertal boys is caused by *Chlamydia trachomatis* or *Neisseria gonorrhoeae* who are sexually active. Other uncommon pathogens identified in this age group are *Escherichia coli, Proteus mirabilis, coagulase negative Staphylococci, Acinetobacter, Streptococci viridans* as well as *Psedumonas aeruginosa*. Common urinary pathogens including coliforms, and mycoplasma species have been found more probable in younger children. Despite the implication of the above pathogens, in a large number of clinical cases no bacteria can be identified. However, when bacterial infection is suspected, appropriate antibiotic treatment should be commenced.

Once the infection has resolved, radiographic studies which include ultrasound examination and voiding cystourethrograms should be obtained since acute epididymitis can be linked to anomalies of the urinary tract. In older children careful questioning regarding voiding symptoms is necessary and non-invasive urodynamics may confirm suspected dysfunctional voiding. Uropathies such as ectopic ureter, ejaculatory duct obstruction, posterior urethral valves, congenital stenosis of the urethra, utricular reflux, rectourethral fistulae, and seminal vesicle reflux should be ruled out with imaging studies. The association of urinary tract anomalies with acute epididymitis is again not confirmed in most of the patients.

Viral infections such as mumps are the most common cause of orchitis and usually require no intervention. Mumps orchitis affects approximately 33% of postpubertal boys affected by virus and is fortunately on the decline in the present era of immunization. Other viruses such as adenovirus, enterovirus, influenza and parainfluenza virus have also been reported in the etiology. Symptomatic therapy is warranted in the management and antibiotics are not indicated.

Rarely, acute epididymitis has been associated with systemic diseases such as tuberculosis (especially in patients with AIDS), sarcoidosis, Hennoch-Schönlein purpura, Kawasaki's disease, brucellosis and leprosy. Noninfectious causes such as trauma and drugs such as amiodarone have also been linked with acute epididymitis.

93.3.2.2 Torsion of the Testicular Appendage

In several retrospective reviews of pediatric patients who presented to the emergency department with acute scrotal pain, the incidence of torsed testicular appendages ranged from 46–71% and represented the most common cause of scrotal pain. Age ranges vary from infancy to adulthood with more than 80% of cases occurring in children aged 7–14 years. This condition rarely presents in adulthood probably due to local fibrosis of the appendages. The vestigial tissues forming the appendices are commonly pedunculated and are structurally predisposed to torsion. The most common affected appendages are the testicular appendage, a remnant of the paramesonephric (müllerian) duct, and the epididymal appendage, a remnant of the mesonephric (wolffian) duct. The testicular appendage is present in 92% of all testes and is usually located at the superior testicular pole in the groove between the testicle and the epididymis. The epididymal appendage is present in 23% of testes and usually projects from the head of the epididymis, but its location may vary.

Torsion of an appendage leads to ischemia and infarction. Necrosis of appendages causes pain and local inflammation of surrounding the tunica vaginalis and epididymis (acute hemiscrotum). Classically, in the acute stages this is associated with the "blue-dot sign" when the inflamed and ischemic appendages can be seen as a subtle blue-colored mass through the scrotal skin (Fig. 93.4). In later stages, this may be accompanied by presence of a thickened scrotal wall, a reactive hydrocele, and enlargement of the head of the epididymis. Torsion of the testicular appendages is virtually a benign condition, but again, must be distinguished from testicular torsion, which can have permanent consequences on testicular viability.

Physical findings reveal an afebrile patient with normal vital signs. An unreliable marker of pathology, the cremasteric reflex is usually present. Several studies indicate that the presence of a cremasteric reflex in the

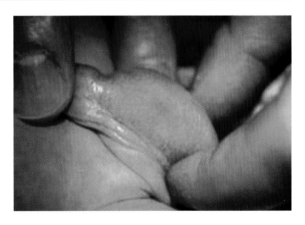

Fig. 93.4 The "blue-dot sign" is evident when ischemic appendages can be seen as a subtle blue-colored mass through the scrotal skin

acute scrotum is unlikely to be testicular torsion. The testis is nontender to palpation. If present, tenderness is localized to the upper pole of the testis. The combination of a blue-dot sign with clear palpation of underlying normal, nontender testis allows for the exclusion of testicular torsion on clinical grounds alone. However, as local inflammation progresses the epididymitis, testis, and superficial tissues become edematous, making the diagnosis more difficult. Urinary symptoms are absent. Dysuria and pyuria are not associated with torsion of the testicular appendages.

On ultrasound, testicular appendage torsion appears as a lesion of low echogenicity with a central hypoechogenic area. Early ultrasound can be diagnostic, but later examinations may only show increased blood flow on color Doppler ultrasound to the adjacent epididymis and testis and possibly a reactive hydrocele, resulting in the misdiagnosis of acute epididymitis or epididymoorchitis. However, the role of color Doppler ultrasound in prepubertal patients is somewhat controversial and less accurate due to low-velocity blood flow in the prepubertal testis. Radionucleotide scan is another alternative imaging study for the diagnosis of torsion of testicular appendages. A positive sign for testicular appendix torsion is the "hot-dot" sign, which is an area of increased tracer uptake. Radionuclide images do not show a positive result if symptoms have been present for fewer than 5 hours. The test is reported to be 68% sensitive and 79% accurate.

Necrotic tissue of the testicular appendices causes no damage other than damage to itself. Most cases, therefore, are treated conservatively. Pain usually resolves

Fig. 93.5 Schematic representation and localization of the five testicular appendages

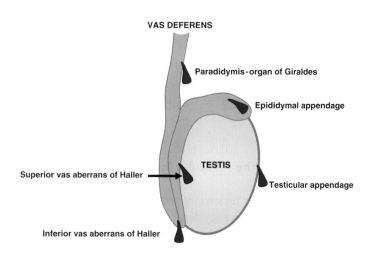

within 1 week but rarely persists for several weeks. Non-steroidal anti-inflammatory drugs (NSAID) and ice are the mainstays of therapy for inflammation. Reduced activity and scrotal support are indicated. As the torsed appendage infarcts and necroses, the pain resolves. Even after resolution of torsion, recurrent torsion of appendage can be observed in the same hemiscrotum, as there are potentially five appendages that may be prone to torsion (testicular appendage, epididymal appendage, paradidymis-organ of Giraldes, inferior and superior vas aberrans of Haller) and that more than one appendage may be present at a given site (Fig. 93.5).

Torsion of testicular appendices is a diagnosis of exclusion in patients presenting with acute hemiscrotum. Surgical intervention is indicated in cases where the diagnosis of testicular torsion cannot be ruled out with certainty or when the symptoms persist and spontaneous resolutions of the symptoms do not occur. Excision of the torsed appendage through a small scrotal incision is the best approach with excellent results in the relief of symptoms.

Further Reading

Brandt MT, Sheldon CA, Wacksman J, Matthews P (1992) Prenatal testicular torsion: Principles of management. J Urol 147(3):670–672

Lewis AG, Bukowski TP, Jarvis PD et al (1995) Evaluation of acute scrotum in the emergency department. J Pediatr Surg 30(2):277–281

Noske HD, Kraus SW, Altinkilic BM (1998) Historical milestones regarding torsion of the scrotal organs. J Urol 159(1):13–16

Puri P, Höllwarth M (2006) Pediatric Surgery. Springer, Heidelberg

Schalamon J, Ainoedhofer H, Schleef J, Singer G, Haxhija EQ, Hollwarth MR (2006) Management of acute scrotum in children—The impact of Doppler ultrasound. J Pediatr Surg 41(8):1377–1380

Hypospadia

94

Göran Läckgren and Agneta Nordenskjöld

Contents

94.1 Introduction

Hypospadia is a common congenital malformation in boys that implies an abnormal opening of the meatus urethrae on the ventral side of the penis. Hypospadia arises due to a premature arrest of the male urethra development during gestational week 8–16. Depending on when the arrest arises the malformation will have different severity with the meatus on the ventral side of the penis, in the scrotum or in severe cases in the perineum. The word is derived from the Greek words *hypos* meaning "under" and *spadon* "opening". The incidence is about 1:300 boys and varies between 0.4–8.2 per 1,000 newborn boys in different populations, due to genetic and environmental differences as well as different reporting to birth defect registries.

94.2 Etiology

In an embryo with a normal male karyotype, 46,XY, the undifferentiated gonads will develop into testes during gestational week 8. Human chorionic gonadotropin from placenta will stimulate hormone production in the Leydig cells. Testosterone is secreted from the testis and is converted by steroid 5-alpha reductase to dihydrotestosterone that will cause growth and development of the genital tubercle through binding to the androgen receptor in the target genital organs. The meatus is primarily located in the perineum but during male genital development the urethra will gradually elongate when the phallus grows and the urethra forms by fusion of the urethral folds until the opening will be located on the glans after 16 weeks of gestation (Fig. 94.1). The last event of male genital development

P. Puri and M. Höllwarth (eds.), *Pediatric Surgery: Diagnosis and Management,*
DOI: 10.1007/978-3-540-69560-8_94, © Springer-Verlag Berlin Heidelberg 2009

Fig. 94.1 Penile development during fetal life

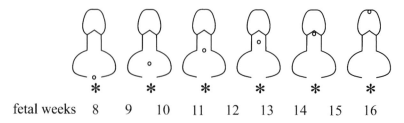

fetal weeks   8   9   10   11   12   13   14   15   16

is fusion of the prepuce. A premature arrest of urethral development will subsequently, depending on the timing of the arrest, causing varying degrees of hypospadias.

This malformation is a complex or multifactorial disorder meaning that both a genetic predisposition and environmental factors contribute to the developmental failure of the urethra. There are many families described with an autosomal dominant inheritance. The concordance in dizygotic twins is 9% as compared to monozygotic twins, that are concordant in 27%, supporting the notion of a strong genetic factor. The risk for a brother of a hypospadiac boy is reported to be around 12–14% and the risk for a son is around 7–9%. If there are two first degree relatives, the risk for the next sibling is as high as 26%. In about 10% of the cases there is an additional relative with hypospadias, however, most cases are sporadic.

There are several gestational factors that are associated with hypospadias and the most important is low birth weight, both adjusted for gestational age and twinning and correlated to severity of the phenotype. This growth restriction is an early event since it is also associated with low head circumference and low body length. Maternal risk factors are preeclampsia, diabetes mellitus, epilepsy and influenza during the first trimester. Hypospadias may also be associated with chromosomal aberrations and is part of many malformation syndromes, possibly due to lower birth weight in a majority of cases.

Environmental factors, like estrogenic chemicals, have rendered much attention during the last decades due to findings of increased incidences of hypospadia, as well as cryptorchidism and testicular cancer, in several countries, not readily explained by genetic factors.

94.3   Pathology and Classification

The abnormal positioning of the meatus is located along the ventral side of the penis, in the scrotum or in the perineum. Hypospadias have traditionally been described due to the position of the urethral meatus on the shaft of the penis and by the extent of ventral penile curvature and therefore have been classified as glandular, coronary, penile, penoscrotal, scrotal or perineal, with the mildest form being an isolated cleaved prepuce. In rare cases the malformation is covered by a normal prepuce and discovered later when retraction of the foreskin is possible or when circumsicion is performed.

Consequently, the surgical techniques were also based on the position of the meatus and the curvature of the penis. However, the location of the urethral opening may be misleading. For example, a boy with a subcoronal meatus may have a distal urethra without a surrounding corpus spongiosum and that consists only of a thin epithelial tube extending from the point where the corpus spongiosum divides. Consequently the preoperative assessment may often mistake the location of the normal urethral end-point and thus underestimate the severity of the hypospadia.

Nowadays, the division of corpus spongiosum is regarded as marking the distal part of a normal urethra and the position of the urethral meatus. In order to help the surgeon to make a correct classification of the hypospadia it is very important to distinguish the division of the ventral rafe of the penile skin, which is the point where the corpus spongiosum deviates.

Therefore a classification based on embryology and anatomy, proposed by Mouriquand and Mure, may better describe the different types of hypsopadia.

(A) Glanular hypospadias. The very distal hypospadias with a normal penile urethra.

(B) Hypospadia with a distal division of the corpus spongiosum associated with little or no chordee. The coronary, penile and some penoscrotal hypospadias belong to this group.

(C) Hypospadia with a proximal division of the corpus spongiosum associated with chordee. Included in this group are the proximal hypospadias with a hypoplastic non-elastic distal urethra and where distal urethral substitution may be necessary.

94.3.1 Ventral Curvature

The urethral plate distal to the hypospadic meatus lies as a plate on the corpus cavernosum. In most penile or distal hypospadias the corpus spongiosum and the urethral plate are well preserved and the current surgical techniques are based on the preservation of the urethral plate that can be reconstructed to a "normal urethra" with all its layers.

However, in the more proximal, penoscrotal or perineal hypospadias there is often chordee due to different mechanisms. The chordee is a consequence of the abnormal proximal division of corpus spongiosum and the hypoplasia of the ventral tissues. Chordee is related to tethering of ventral hypoplastic skin onto the underlying structures and a fusion of Buck's fascia, corpus spongiosum and tunica albuginea.

From 1960s to 1980s four different types of ventral curvature including chordee associated with hypospadias have been distinguished. In the first type, the spongiosum is absent in the distal urethra and a fibrous layer prevents the penis from being straight. This type occurs in the perineal and penoscrotal hypospadias with a hypoplastic urethral plate.

In the second type the urethra is completely developed with corpus spongiosum but Buck's fascia and the Dartos fascia are abnormal. This is common in the penile hypospadias were the dissection of the urethral plate often is sufficient to get a good correction of the curvature.

The third type has been described as skin chordee and is caused by an abnormality of the superficial Dartos fascia. Often a degloving and reconstruction of the penile skin is sufficient to correct the curvature.

In a few cases with ventral curvature a transection of the urethral plate and resection of chordae may not suffice to straighten the penis thus constituting the fourth type of ventral curvature due to corpora cavernosal disproportion resulting in a persistent bending after the penis has been degloved. Corporoplasty, without transection of the urethral plate, is therefore the only solution to achieve a straight penis in those cases.

94.4 Clinical Considerations

The diagnosis is usually obvious from birth due the typical appearance. Most important neonatally is to identify if there is an associated meatal stenosis that in pronounced cases will have to be treated urgently. Later during childhood, the boy may be unable to void in a standing position due to the ventral orientation of the urine. Chordee that is diagnosed during erection, can vary to a large extent and can be assessed by compressing the corpora cavernosa against the symphyseal bone or preferably during surgery with an artificial erection test. If untreated, chordee can unable normal intercourse. The fourth consideration is the cosmetic appearance of the penis with different degrees of chordee and the cleaved prepuce that is mainly located on the dorsal tip of the penis described as a "hood". Fertility might be affected in uncorrected hypospadias due to mechanical reasons or otherwise mainly due to the underlying cause of hypospadias, like steroid 5-alpha reductase deficiency that seldom is compatible with fertility due to the small prostate gland.

When the hypospadias is very severe the child is born with an uncertain sex. Usually, a team consisting of pediatric endocrinologist, pediatric surgeon, psychiatrist, clinical geneticist should gather urgently after birth to perform a proper investigation and inform and involve the parents during the process of assigning the child a sex as accurately as possible according to up-to-date knowledge of sex development. The investigation includes karyotyping, hormone analysis, like 17-OH-progesterone, especially in order to diagnose 46,XX with congenital adrenal hyperplasia that untreated can be life-threatening during even the first days of life. In order to clarify the anatomical conditions of the malformation, ultrasonography of the abdomen, urethroscopy, laparoscopy with biopsies of the gonads may be needed as well as hormone testing and mutation analysis, for example of the 5-alpha reductase or androgen receptor genes.

94.5 Associated Malformations

The most common associated malformation is cryptorchidism that is found in up to 10% of the hypospadiac boys. Milder forms of hypospadias are often isolated as an anomaly but in severe hypospadias renal malformations like hydronephrosis, vesicoureteric reflux, renal agenesis are found in a few percent of the cases. Other minor penile anomalies, that can be found in combination with hypospadia, are torsion of the penis, concealed penis or webbed penis. In the more severe cases a bifid scrotum is seen and sometimes partial or total penoscrotal transposition.

94.6 Management

The treatment is surgery and the goal is to restore the urethral meatus to its normal position on the glans and to correct the penile curvature if necessary and to reconstruct the glans and also the foreskin with or without circumcision. The goal is preferably achieved in as few surgical procedures as possible. In addition one should strongly advise against performing a circumcision prior to surgery since the prepuce may be essential for the urethroplasty or to cover the penile shaft. Surgery should be performed between 6–12 months of age, before the boy is aware of his body image, but also because the tissues are easier to handle during that period. The mildest form of hypospadias variant is cleaved prepuce and that can easily be corrected at any age by a prepuceplasty for the sake of psychological reasons if the parents or the child prefer that.

94.7 Preoperative Androgen Treatment

Severe hypospadias combined with micropenis can be treated preoperatively with testosterone injections or dihydrotestosterone locally. The same treatment as is sometimes used diagnostically in DSD (Disorder of Sexual Development) cases neonatally.

94.8 Surgical Techniques

The surgical technique differs depending on the position of the meatus and the eventual curvature of the penis. During the last century, a vast number of surgical techniques have been described in order to repair hypospadias. However, each hypospadias surgeon should familiarise with some techniques that are appropriate for different severity of hypospadias since there is no technique that can correct all malformations.

Twenty to 40 years ago, a two-stage procedure was the most common in penile or more proximal hypospadias repair. As the first stage a penile straightening with resection of chordee, including the urethral plate, was performed and as the second stage a complete urethroplasty using various skin flap techniques was used (most commonly according to Dennis –Brown and Crawford).

One-stage repairs were initially introduced in the sixties and have been used even in proximal hypospadias with different kind of vascularized flaps. During the last 15 years the preservation of the urethral plate has been advocated and has led to many modifications of the tubularized urethral plate according to Thiersch-Duplay. The urethral plate consists of the tissues distal to the hypospadia meatus that are unique structures with a mucosal layer on an underlying corpus spongiosum, in essence constituting all the layers of a normal urethra. The preservation of the urethral plate has probably been the most important advancement in the reconstruction of penile and even proximal hypospadias and has changed our surgical techniques significantly. The urethral plate can be primarily tubularized without additional skinflaps after a midline relaxation incision of the urethral mucosa is made. The incorporation of the urethral plate (including spongioplasty) into the neourethra may reduce surgical complications. In addition, the urethral plate is rarely the cause of penile bending. The technique has been popularised by Snodgrass and is named as the Snodgrass' procedure (Tubularized Incised Plate = TIP).

The most common surgical techniques that are used today are demonstrated in Fig. 94.2–94.9.

94.9 Correction of Chordee

The degloving of the penile skin sorts out the chordee related to the tethering of the ventral skin. If the angulation persists after freeing the skin, the dissection of the urethral plate from the ventral surface of the corpus cavernosum

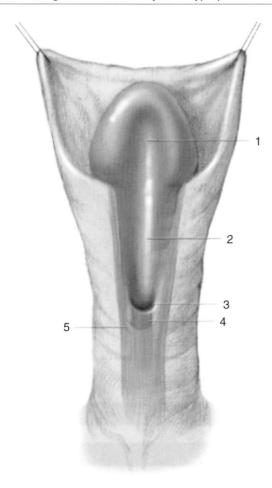

Fig. 94.2 Hypospadia from the tip to the base of the penis: the ventral aspect of the glans is wide opened (1). The urethral plate (2) and extends from the apex of the glans down to the hypospadic meatus (3). The point where the corpus spongiosum (4) deviates marks the proximal limit of the urethral malformation (5). This is also the point where the ventral raphe of the foreskin is separated

from the glans down to the normal urethra allows in most cases a straight penis. In a few cases when the bending still persists, and that is caused by a disproportion between the dorsal and the ventral parts of the corpus cavernosum, a dorsal plication may be needed. In the severe forms (scrotal or perineal) the urethra is dysplastic with associated chordee. Therefore these structures has to be resected to get a straight penis before urethroplasty.

94.9.1 Urethroplasty

Reconstruction of the missing urethra and the technique chosen depends on the size and quality of the urethral plate. In the very distal cases with a normal penile urethra the MAGPI-procedure may still have a place (Fig. 94.3). However, the Snodgrass procedure have replaced even the very distal reconstructions, with better cosmetic result.

In most cases the urethral plate is wide and healthy and can be tubularized either according to the Thiersch-Duplay technique (Fig. 94.4) or the Snodgrass' technique with incision of the urethral plate (Fig. 94.5). In some cases, where the urethral meatus is < 2 cm from the tip of the glans a complete mobilisation of the penile urethra (Koff) may be sufficient to get urethral meatus to the tip of the penis (Fig. 94.6). If the distal plate is too narrow there are optional techniques using a flap of the ventral penile skin according to Mathieu (Fig. 94.7) or either an inlay flap in the incision of the urethral plate or using a pedicularized preputial flap as an onlay urethroplasty (Fig. 94.8).

In rare cases in perineal or penoscrotal hypospadias the urethral plate may be hypoplastic and is not appropriate to use for the urethroplasty. The plate has to be divided in order to straighten the penis and to resect the chordee. A tube needs to be made to replace the missing urethra either using a pedicularized preputial flap (Asopa-Duckett technique) (Fig. 94.8) or a two-stage technique using buccal mucosal graft according to Bracka. When the urethra has been reconstructed it is very important to cover the sutureline with either a vascularised Dartos flap or a flap from the Buck's fascia or surrounding tissue, thus preventing fistula formation. Even if a proper spongioplasty can be performed, covering of the sutureline is necessary.

94.10 Glanuloplasty

The reconstruction of the glans is very important as it determines the final cosmetic outcome of the surgery. The tubularization of the urethra allows a slit-like urethral opening and necessitates a dissection of glandular wings to cover the glanular part of the urethra to get the best cosmetic result.

94.11 Foreskin Reconstruction

In distal hypospadias there is always a possibility to preserve the foreskin. Depending on the cultural or

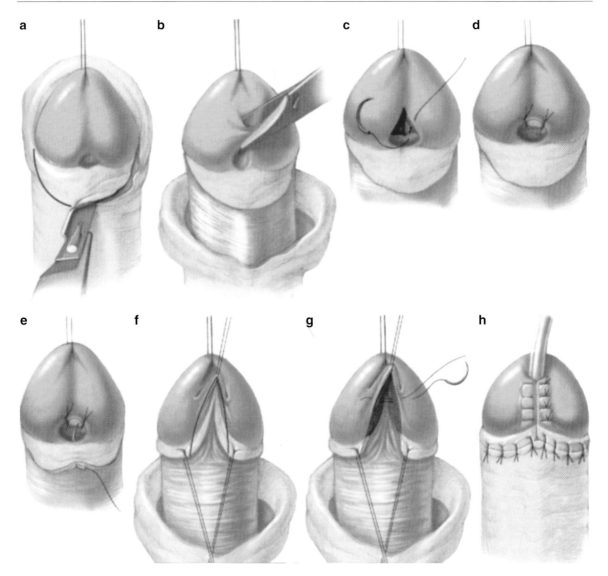

Fig. 94.3 (a–h) The MAGPI Procedure (Meatal Advancement and GlanuloPlasty(I).
The incision line is drawn 5 mm behind the meatus (**a**). The glanular groove is incised (**b**). The dorsal meatus opens up and a diamond-shaped defect is created. This is closed transversely with 2–3 sutures (**c**, **d**). The ventral lip of the urethra is fixed with a holding stitch and brought forward (**e**). This allows the lateral wings of the glans to rotate to the ventrum (**f**, **g**). A sleeve approximation of the penile skin is done, excising all redundant tissue and leaving a circumcised appearance (**h**). No stent or catheters are required and the procedure can be done on outpatient basis. Secondary retraction of the meatus is quite common and therefore this procedure has become less popular

religious traditions in each country either a circumcision is performed or the foreskin can be preserved and reconstructed (Fig. 94.9). This is a simple procedure that in most cases of distal hypospadias even saves operative time. The skin incision is performed between the inner and outer layer of the foreskin.

After the urethral and the glanular reconstruction have been performed, the inner layer is sutured with continuous 6-0 or 7-0 sutures till the tip of the foreskin, leaving an opening that allows the foreskin to be retracted without difficulty. The inner layer may be covered with a subcutaneous layer. Thereafter the

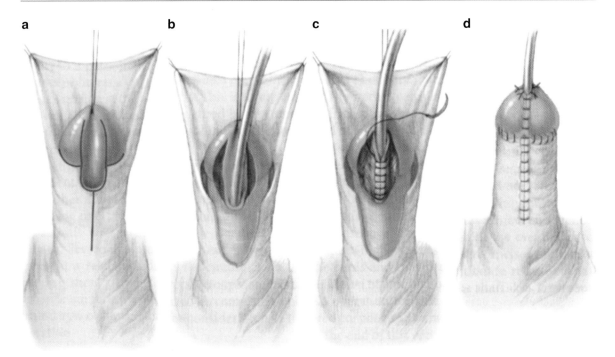

Fig. 94.4 (a–d) Thiersch-Duplay-procedure. Parallell incisions along the hypospadic urethral plate to the tip of the glans. The urethra is dissected proximal to the division of the corpus spongiosum (**a**, **b**). Deep glanular incisions are made and the urethral plate is tubularized around a 6–8 Fr Catheter (**c**). The sutured urethra is covered with a Dartos-flap before the glanular wings are sutured (**d**). This technique is applicable in distal hypospadias with a deep glanular groove and a wide urethral plate. The corpus spongiosum should be dissected and the surgeon should aim at doing a spongioplasty to further strengthen the urethra

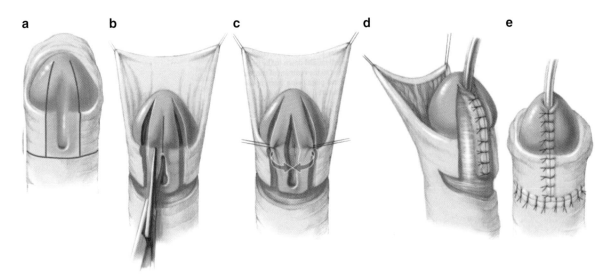

Fig. 94.5 (a–e) The TIP (Snodgrass)—procedure. The Snodgrass' procedure is a development of the Thiersch-Duplay technique, saving even a narrow urethral plate for tubularization. The incisions are the same (**a**) and the distal urethral plate including corpus spongiosum is dissected (**a**). Deep glanular wings are created. The urethral plate is incised longitudinally in the midline from meatus up to the tip of the glans (**b**). The urethral incision leaves a dorsal raw area in the urethra which will subsequently epithelialize (**c**). This allows the plate to be tubularized around a 6–8 Fr catheter (**d**). The dorsal foreskin is either resected (**e**) or saved and reconstructed This technique may also be used even in proximal hypospadias with a good urethral plate

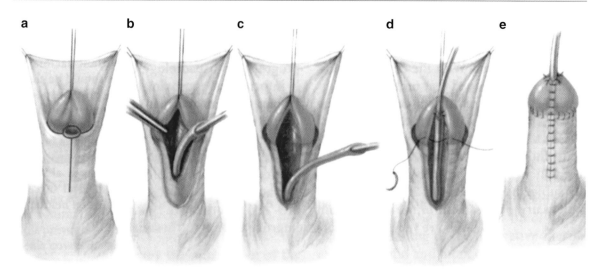

Fig. 94.6 (a–e) Urethral mobilisation technique (Koff). This technique is based on the elasticity of the urethra. When the distance from the tip of the glans to the ectopic meatus is <2 cm it is possible to mobilize the penile and even the bulbous urethra to get a good "extra length", which is enough to get the normal urethra to the tip of the glans without causing ventral bending. After dissection of the urethra from the ectopic meatus and proximally enough to get the desired length (**b, c**) a deep incision in midline of the glandular urethra is performed (**c**). The dissected urethra is sutured to the tip of the glans and the glans wings are sutured to cover the distal urethra (**d, e**). A 6–8 Fr catheter is often left in place, but can be removed shortly after the operation because the distal urethra is "normal". Thus, the great advantage with this technique is that there are no urethral sutures and less risk for fistulas and strictures

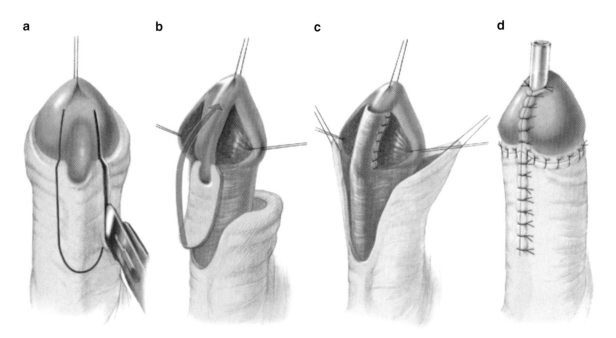

Fig. 94.7 (a–d) The Mathieu Procedure. The incisions are made on both sides along the distal urethra (**a**). A skin flap from the ventrum of the penile foreskin is prepared (**b**). This flap is based and attached to the distal urethra and is sutured to the dissected distal urethral plate. Deep glanular flaps are dissected (**c**) down to corpus cavernosum and enough to cover the distal urethra (**d**).There is also a possibility to reconstruct the foreskin if wanted. The Mathieu technique gives often a transverse meatus, which gives a less satisfactory cosmetic result

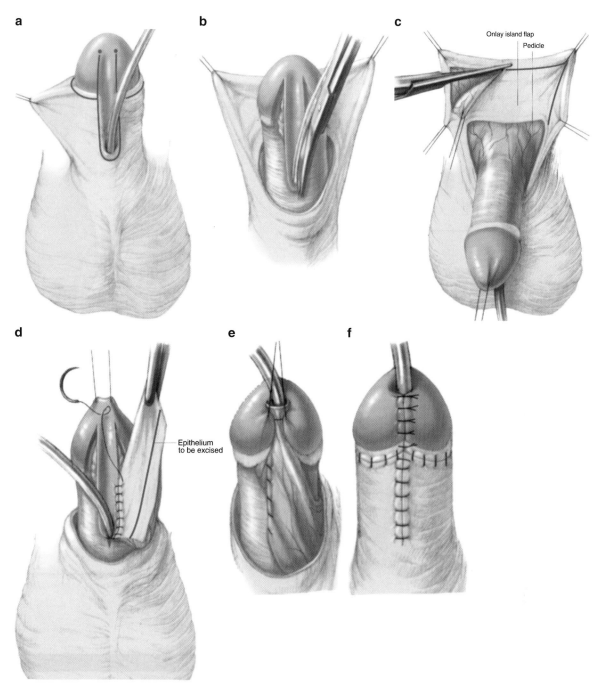

Fig. 94.8 (a–f) Onlay Plasty with the Transverse Island Flap Technique. In cases with a narrow urethral plate that do not allow tubularization even with a TIP, the plate may be preserved. Providing the penis is straight an onlay procedure may be the method of choice. The penis is degloved (**b**) and a rectangle flap of the inner preputial mucosa is pediculized (**c**) and transferred to the ventrum of the penis to be layed on the urethral plate using interrupted or a running 6/o or 7/o suture over an 8 Fr catheter (**d**). The sutureline is covered with a Dartos-flap (**e**) and deep glanular wings are dissected and sutured and the foreskin is reconstructed (**f**). In the severe hypospadias (scrotal or perineal), the urethral plate is often dysplastic and associated with severe chordee causing ventral bending of the penis. The plate is then too poor to be kept and a full-tube urethroplasty needs to be performed using either a pediculized flap from the inner preputial layer or a buccal mucosal graft. The main disadvantage of these techniques is the risk of proximal urethral anastomosis stricture and dilatation of the distal neourethra. There is a high complication rate associated with the tubularized flap-techniques and therefore these techniques have been less popular and more and more the two stage procedures using either preputial flaps or buccal mucosal graft as replacement of the urethral bed in a first stage and tubularization as the second stage procedure (Bracka)

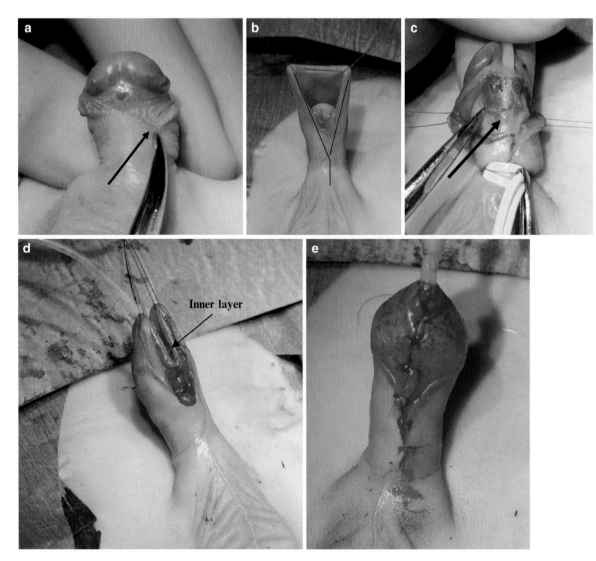

Fig. 94.9 Preservation of the foreskin in Hypospadia reconstruction (**a**) Point of the deviation of the ventral raphe (arrow). (**b**) Outline of the incision. (**c**) End point of the normal urethra. (**d**) Reconstruction of inner and outer preputial layer. (**e**) A well-preserved foreskin

outer foreskin is sutured with intracutaneous 6-0 sutures. Hypospadiac cases with an abundant dorsal foreskin (a big dorsal "hood") may have to be reconstructed in several stages.

94.12 Postoperative Care

The milder cases are treated as out-patients. In most cases even in distal hypospadias an urethral stent is left in place. We prefer the Cook double diaper catheter that is sutured to the glans. The catheter is kept for 1 week and used as a dripping urethral stent with a double diaper. The dressing is variable from one center to another and also the time of catheter drainage. One commonly used dressing is a Tegaderm dressing that will be removed together with the stent during which time an antibiotic is given prophylactically.

94.13 Postoperative Follow-Up

The first postoperative follow-up is due after 1–3–6 months followed by medical evaluations at 5, 10 and 15 years of age. These patients are important to follow because there is a risk of recurrent curvature and also there maybe a risk of urethral stricture that has to be controlled with fluometry and residual urine after the age of 5 years. The final postoperative result can be judged only at puberty and the boys should be motivated to come for a final examination.

94.14 Complications

Early and more common complications are bleeding, infections and urinary retention that can be treated appropriately in the postoperative period. Later complications are listed below and treated accordingly. Urethrocutaneous fistulas, that have to be reoperated, are reported in several percent in different degrees depending on the severity of the malformation. Meatus stenosis and urethra stricture are examined postopera-

tively by checking the urinary flow. The most common treatment is meatoplasty and urethral dilatation, respectively but sometimes internal urethrotomy is required. Diverticulum of the reconstructed distal urethra can arise especially after two-stage procedures and if the meatus is relatively stenotic. Residual curvature is examined at puberty since it will need further surgery. Balanitis xerotica obliterans (BXO) can arise after surgery and render residual strictures. Rupture of reconstructed foreskin can happen and will also need a reoperation. The cosmesis is important and should be recognised as of significant importance to the patient. Sometimes the initial result is not optimal and will require smaller skin corrections. Also the patient should be informed about a large potential for better cosmesis depending on the underlying condition and due to growth at puberty.

94.15 Conclusion

Important advances of the etiology and the management of hypospadia have been done over the last 20 years. The increased knowledge of the embryology and the genetic background can help us to better select the correct surgical treatment of boys born with hypospadia.

A distal meatus may be a penoscrotal hypospadia. It is very important that the surgeon recognises the diagnostic signs for the different types of hypospadia in order to give a correct information and treatment. We have to accept that there are no minor hypospadias.

We have gone from two-stage surgery, even in simple cases, to one-stage procedures in almost all. A step, that in the severe cases of hypospadia, may have been too big. Therefore we have to accept that a two-stage operation with grafts may be considered not only in the surgery of the hypsopadia cripples but also as a first treatment in some severe cases. It is, thus, very important that each surgeon familiarises with different techniques and judge each case individually. It is also very important to follow the patients long-term as there are many that will require further surgical reconstructions and the controls should continue until the boys have passed puberty.

Further Reading

Baskin LS (2006) Hypospadias. In MD Stringer, KT Oldham, PDE Mouriquand (eds) Pediatric Surgery and Urology: Longterm Outcomes. Cambridge University Press, New York, pp 611–620

Baskin LS, Ebbers MB (2006) Hypospadias: Anatomy, etiology and technique. J Pediatr Surg 41(10):1786

Bracka A (1996) Hypospadias repair: The two-stage alternative. Br J Urol 76 (Suppl 3):31–41

Hadidi AT, Azmy AF (eds) (2003) Hypospadias Surgery. Springer, Berlin, Heidelberg, New York

Mouriquand P (ed) (2007) Etiological aspects of hypospadias. Dialogues in Pediatric Urology, 28:4–7

Mouriquand P, Mure PY (2004) Current concepts in hypospadiology. BJU Int 93 (Suppl 3):26–34

Mouriquand P, Mure P-Y (2006) Hypospadias. In P Puri, ME Höllwarth (eds) Pediatric Surgery, Springer Surgery Atlas Series. Springer-Verlag, Berlin, Heidelberg, New York, pp 529–542

Snodgrass W (2006) The "learning curve" in hypospadias surgery. BJU Int 97(3):593–596

Circumcision and Buried Penis

95

Martin Kaefer

Contents

95.1 Introduction

Historically, several reasons have been cited to justify circumcision; at various times circumcision has been reported to cure or prevent over 100 diseases. The majority of newborn boys in countries where there are no religious reasons given for circumcision, retain their prepuce. However, with a validation based to a large degree in folklore, the majority of boys in the United States have been circumcised during the 20th century. Recent data suggests that circumcision may be beneficial in certain high risk populations as a part of a comprehensive effort to limit the transmission of HIV.

The term Buried Penis encompasses a spectrum of conditions in which the penis does not appear to adequately extend from the abdominal wall as an organ distinct from the scrotum. Since the term Buried Penis comprises such a wide spectrum of conditions with widely varying severity no specific incidence can be stated.

95.2 Definitions and Etiology

95.2.1 Prepucial Anatomy

During the third month of gestation the prepuce can be seen protruding from the level of the coronal sulcus. This tissue grows and eventually projects distally to gradually envelop the glans. The preputial and glanular surfaces then fuse with the process usually complete by the 5th month of gestation. Natural separation of the two structures, which is to some degree androgen-dependent, begins in utero and continues through childhood. In a newborn the foreskin is rarely retractile,

P. Puri and M. Höllwarth (eds.), *Pediatric Surgery: Diagnosis and Management,*
DOI: 10.1007/978-3-540-69560-8_95, © Springer-Verlag Berlin Heidelberg 2009

but by 1 year of age sufficient separation of the two structures has occurred to allow preputial retraction in 50% of infants. By age 4 years nearly 90% can be retracted without causing trauma. If a decision is made not to perform neonatal circumcision the foreskin should not be forcefully retracted. Forceful retraction at an early age replaces the natural preputial-glanular fusion with two opposing layers of traumatized tissues and risks iatrogenic scarring. The parents must then become committed to daily retractions of the prepuce to avoid abnormal healing, and the child experiences repeated unnecessary discomfort.

95.2.2 Buried Penis

Various forms of Buried Penis are recognized based on etiology. These include the concealed or hidden penis (due to poor penile skin attachments and/or prepubic obesity), webbed penis, and trapped penis. The concealed or hidden penis is most commonly caused by inadequate attachment of the penile skin to the shaft and inelasticity of the dartos fascia. Extension of the penis is restricted because the penile skin is not anchored to the deep fascia (Figs. 95.1 and 95.2). As a result the penis is concealed by the suprapubic fat pad (Fig. 95.3).

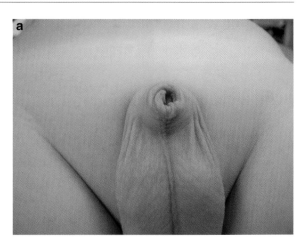

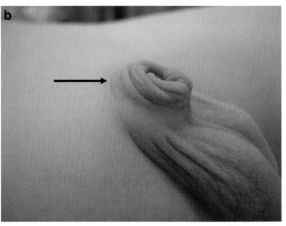

Fig. 95.2 A 1 year old boy with concealed penis following neonatal circumcision (**a**) Frontal view; (**b**) lateral view with arrow demonstrating poor attachments of skin at penopubic angle

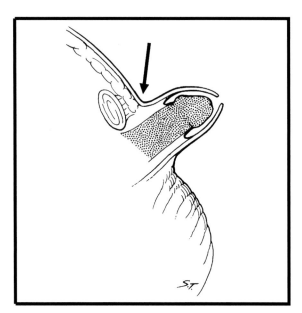

Fig. 95.1 Normal Penile-Prepucial Anatomy. Arrow demonstrates adequate penopubic angle definition due to adequate penile skin attachments

Further increase in weight as the child matures into an adult may accentuate this problem (Figs. 95.4 and 95.5). It is important to examine the patient in both the supine and the standing position. Full appreciation of the effect of the prepubic fat pad on the penis (as it relates to the buried penis phenotype) may only be appreciated with the patient in the later position.

The webbed penis represents an abnormality of the attachment between the penis and the scrotum (Fig. 95.6). In this condition the scrotal skin extends up the ventral aspect of the penile skin.

The trapped penis is an iatrogenic form of Buried Penis in which a dense post-circumcision cicatrix develops over the glans (Figs. 95.7 and 95.8). As a result the penis becomes embedded in the suprapubic fat pad. Performing a neonatal circumcision in a patient with poor definition of the boundary between shaft

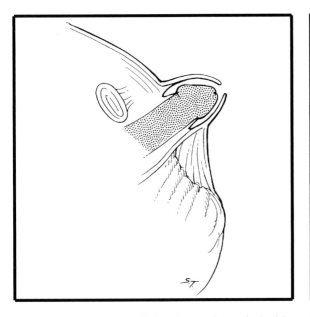

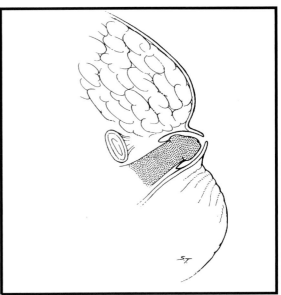

Fig. 95.3 Congenital concealed penis secondary to inelasticity of the dartos layer of the penis and poor attachment of penile skin to the base of the penis

Fig. 95.5 Acquired concealed penis, a result of marked suprapubic weight gain
@IUSM Visual Media

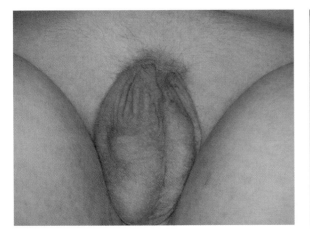

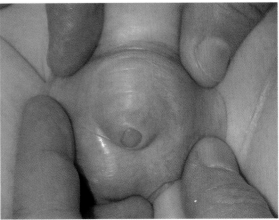

Fig. 95.4 A 14 year old boy with acquired concealed penis secondary to excessive abdominal weight gain

Fig. 95.6 A 3 week old boy with penoscrotal webbing. Note poor demarcation of penile skin from the scrotum

skin and neighboring skin of the scrotum and abdominal wall (e.g. large hydroceles or poor attachments at the penopubic angle) may lead to this deformity due to excess removal of shaft skin.

Buried penis can be associated with hypospadias, epispadias, chordee and can clearly result from repair of these conditions if great care is not taken to secure the shaft skin to the base of the penis after complete degloving of the penis.

95.3 Rational for Treatment

95.3.1 Circumcision

Parents often cite several indications for circumcision, including custom, beauty, and promotion of health. Current therapeutic indications for circumcision include trauma, phimosis, paraphimosis,

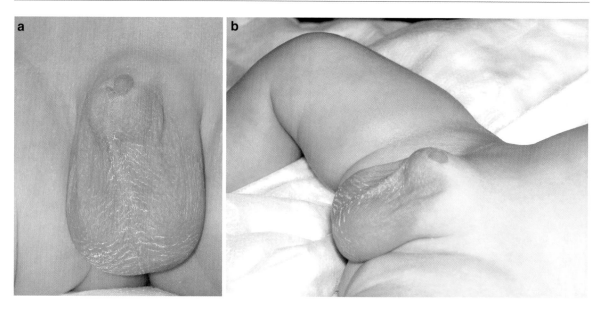

Fig. 95.7 A 1 month old boy with trapped penis secondary to severe cicatrix formation distal to the glans penis. (**a**) Frontal view; (**b**) lateral view. Nearly all shaft skin had been resected at the time of circumcision. Repair required scrotal skin flaps for ventral shaft coverage

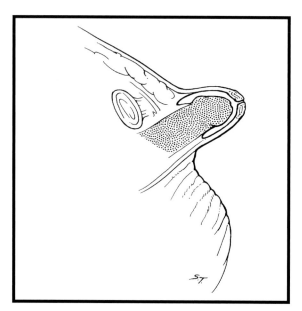

Fig. 95.8 Trapped penis. Distal cicatrix of shaft skin results in trapping of the glans penis below the skin surface. In more severe cases no residual shaft skin may remain

balanitis, decreased risk of penile or cervical cancer, decreased incidence of neonatal urinary tract infections, and decreased transmission rates of certain sexually transmitted diseases. These reported advantages should take into consideration the incidence of certain disease entities within the population and be weighed against the complications of circumcision, including infection, bleeding, adhesions, meatal stenosis, as well as other more rarely reported problems.

Urinary tract infection: Studies involving neonates have established a tenfold (1.12% vs 0.11%) increase in urinary tract infections in uncircumcised infants compared with their circumcised peers. Nevertheless, whether it is beneficial and cost-effective to circumcise approximately 100 babies to avoid problems in one remains open to debate. In contrast it is known that in boys with recurrent UTI or high grade vesicoureteral reflux, the risk of UTI recurrence is 10% and 30% respectively and many surgeons may therefore have a lower threshold for recommending circumcision in this high risk population.

Sexually Transmitted Diseases: Three randomized trials now provide firm evidence that the risk of acquiring HIV is halved by male circumcision in endemic areas of Sub-Saharan Africa. It has been predicted that circumcision of all men in Africa could prevent 2 million new cases of HIV/AIDS and avert 300,000 deaths in the next 10 years. The effect after 20 years would be even greater with predicted 3.7 million fewer infections and 2.7 million deaths averted. There is mounting evidence that there are certain cells within the prepuce (e.g. Superficial Langerhans' cells) having a large number of receptors for the HIV-1 virus which could help explain this phenomenon. A similar predisposition to preputial colonization with bacterial organisms responsible for sexually transmitted disease has been reported. The strongest associations exist for ulcerative STDs such as chancroid and syphilis. Evidence that circumcision leads to a lower incidence of herpes and condylomata accuminatum is less convincing.

Penile Cancer: The intact prepuce may also predispose to carcinogenesis. Neonatal circumcision has been established as a prophylactic measure that virtually eliminates the occurrence of penile carcinoma, because it eliminates the closed preputial environment where penile carcinoma develops. Studies show that penile cancer is rare among neonatally circumcised individuals but more frequent when circumcision is delayed until puberty. In contrast, adult circumcision appears to offer little or no protection from subsequent development of the disease. In one study, DNA sequencing implicated papilloma virus in the etiology of half the lesions in males with penile cancer. This carcinogenic threat to uncircumcised men raises additional concerns for their sexual partners since the same virus is thought to play an etiologic role in the development of cervical cancer.

95.3.2 Buried Penis

The buried penis can cause secondary phimosis, recurrent balanitis, difficulty in holding the penis resulting in inability to void while standing, or parental/patient concern for social embarrassment. Older patients may also complain of the inability to achieve adequate sexual intercourse. In addition, penoplasty may improve the psychological status of the patient.

95.4 Management

95.4.1 Presurgical Considerations

95.4.1.1 Circumcision

In children the most common medical indication for circumcision is uncomplicated phimosis. Steroid cream (betamethasone 0.05%) applied topically three times a day for 6 weeks is a highly effective form of treatment for this condition. Adhesiolysis for asymmetric or pronounced adhesions between foreskin and glans is a simple procedure that may be performed in the office setting following the application of topical anaesthetic.

Contraindications to circumcision include the presence of any penile anomalies, including hypospadias and chordee, where the prepuce might be necessary for reconstruction. Results of circumcision may be suboptimal in the low birth weight child with a small penis and in those individuals who have a buried penis phenotype. The procedure should also be deferred in infants who are compromised by other childhood illness (e.g. major congenital cardiac disorders). Although relatively minor in its technical challenge, the stress of circumcision and its potential for complications increase the risk in these infants considerably.

95.4.1.2 Buried Penis

Need for and timing of reconstruction for buried penis should take into consideration the fact that the size of the neonatal prepubic fat pad may change significantly as the child matures. As the child enters the 2nd year of life a redistribution of prepubic fat often occurs. As a result, the penis often appears less buried either resulting in the parents electing not to proceed with surgery or, if the surgical procedure is still desired, decreasing the number of steps needed to achieve the desired cosmetic and functional result. If the penis continues to maintain a buried appearance well into the 2nd year of life then surgery is undertaken prior to 2 years of age so that the child has minimal memory of a genital surgery being performed.

In the older patient with truncal obesity it can be beneficial to obtain consultation from a multidisciplinary weight-loss team prior to embarking on surgical intervention. It is important for the obese patient to understand that buried penis may to a great extent be a symptom of a much larger problem. Additionally they should be fully informed that additional weight gain following the procedure may serve to once again obscure the penis.

95.4.2 Surgical Technique

95.4.2.1 Circumcision

Contemporary variations of circumcision fall into one of four categories: dorsal slit, shield, clamp, and surgical excision. The dorsal slit offers a simple and effective release of the distal preputial cicatrix that leads to phimosis and paraphimosis. The prepuce remains, but when done correctly the slit should prevent further genital problems and provide permanent access to the glans to permit proper cleansing. The shield borrows from the principle of tools used in ritual circumcisions. A grooved shield is placed over the outstretched prepuce and redundant distal tissue is excised. Devices such as the Mogen clamp are typical examples. Clamps such as the Gomco and Plastibell are the modality most commonly used for neonates in the United States. With both techniques the prepuce is freed from the glans and the device placed between the two structures. The inner and outer layers of the prepuce are crushed by the device to achieve hemostasis, and the redundant tissue is excised.

In older infants and adults clamp techniques are far less effective and are associated with an increased incidence of bleeding. Larger prepucial vessel size resulting from postnatal testosterone stimulation of the foreskin is the presumed reason for this increased complication rate in the older population. Surgical excision, the most accurate modality, is used for most individuals over age 3 months of age. Two circumferential incisions are made—one at the distal aspect (approximately 5 mm proximal to the coronal margin) and one at the proximal aspect of the prepuce. The underlying soft-tissue layers are separated from Buck's fascia and the foreskin is removed. Exact reapproximation with fine sutures is done to ensure adequate alignment and to prevent iatrogenic torsion.

All circumcision techniques except surgical excision are performed with the patient awake. The cortical and subcortical centers responsible for sensing pain are present in the newborn and are usually fully developed by the third trimester. Cardiovascular, respiratory, and hormonal changes have been documented as indicators of pain during circumcision. Dorsal penile nerve blocks reduce these physiologic responses. Perioperative oral sucrose has also been suggested as a means of modifying the infant's response to pain.

95.4.2.2 Buried Penis

Various techniques for repair of the buried penis have been described. The complexity of the operation is dependent on many factors including age of the patient,

size of the penis, size of the suprapubic adipose tissue mass and amount of penile shaft skin.

The shared step in the correction of nearly all forms of buried penis is complete degloving of the penile shaft followed by proper fixation of penile skin so that it can no longer prolapse over the glans. In the young child the base of the penile skin can be sutured to Buck's fascia in one or multiple locations (most commonly at the 3 and 9 o'clock positions so as to avoid the neurovascular bundles) with permanent suture resulting in excellent cosmetic results. In the older, obese patient more sturdy fixation of the skin directly to the rectus fascia may be necessary. In severe cases additional suture placement to attach the subcutaneous tissue of the scrotum to the ventral aspect of the base of the penile shaft should be undertaken. In severe cases where there is a marked paucity of ventral shaft skin, penoscrotal z-plasty, rotational flaps or grafts may be needed for coverage. In the most severe cases, the suspensory ligament of the penis may be divided.

An additional step that may help in correction of the webbed penis may be incision of the penoscrotal web transversely, separating the penis from the scrotum, and closing the skin vertically. The scrotum should be secured to the base of the penis to prevent recurrence of the webbed appearance.

The buried penis in overweight children and adults who have had substantial weight gain may require additional surgical steps to provide an adequate functional and cosmetic result. Debulking the suprapubic adipose tissue is most commonly performed using suction lipectomy through two small incisions near the anterior superior iliac spine. Following suction lipectomy the patient wears an abdominal binder to minimize the potential for developing a subcutaneous seroma. Suction lipectomy alone may not completely correct the problem. The laxity of the prepubic skin (that is often seen in adults that have had massive weight gain and subsequently undergone liposuction) may continue to obscure the penis. These individuals may benefit from a formal abdominoplasty with anchoring of the pubic and penile skin directly to the rectus fascia. If formal abdominoplasty is indicated the suprapubic skin incision should be marked with the patient in the standing position.

When permanent sutures are placed for fixation of the penile skin many authors elect to place the patient on a short course of antibiotics to minimize the chance of complication.

95.5 Complications

95.5.1 *Circumcision*

Complications accompany every surgical procedure and circumcision is no exception. Numerous studies have found a complication rate of 5% or less, most of them minor. These include bleeding, inclusion cysts, persistent glanular-preputial adhesion, iatrogenic chordee and hypospadias (due to urethral incorporation into the clamp) and trapped penis. There are often concerns about skin separation, (especially when a clamp has been used) although even complete separation can be managed conservatively with antibiotic salve until healthy granulation and epithelialization resolve the problem. Meatitis and subsequent stenosis, a process that rarely occurs in uncircumcised boys, can develop after circumcision. The newly exposed meatus is probably injured from exposure to ammonia produced by the action of urea splitting organisms on urine in the diapers. Meatal stenosis is far less common in males who are circumcised later in life. Fortunately, more serious complications, such as injury to the glans or urethra and urinary retention are rare.

95.5.2 *Buried Penis*

Recurrence of the buried penis phenotype has been reported to be as high as 16%. Distraction of the fixation sutures and additional postoperative weight gain are two possible reasons for suboptimal results. On rare occasion acquired cryptorchidism may occur following suction lipectomy due to the highly mobile adolescent testicle migrating to the newly created plane in the suprapubic location. This complication should theoretically be completely avoidable if proper attention is paid to assuring that the testicles sit in the dependent scrotum following completion of the procedure.

With repair of the adolescent more often requiring liposuction and generally coming at a time when there is increased perception and anxiety regarding the genitalia, it should not be surprising that there overall satisfaction rate is lower than in younger non-obese patients in whom this surgery is undertaken.

Further Reading

Check E (2007) Trio of studies makes headway in HIV battle. Nature 446(7131):12

Cuckow P (2006) Phimosis and Buried Penis. In P Puri, ME Höllwarth (eds) Pediatric Surgery. Springer Surgery Atlas Series, Springer-Verlag Berlin Heidelberg, New York, pp 543–554

Gray RH, Kigozi G, Serwadda D et al (2007) Male circumcision for HIV prevention in men in Rakai, Uganda: A randomised trial. Lancet 369(9562):657–666

Maizels M, Zaontz M, Donovan J et al (1986) Surgical correction of the buried penis: Description of a classification system and a technique to correct the disorder. J Urol 136(1 Pt 2):268–271

Puri P, Höllwarth M (2006) Pediatric Surgery. Springer, Berlin, Heidelberg

Shenoy MU, Srinivasan J, Sully L et al (2000) Buried penis: Surgical correction using liposuction and realignment of skin. BJU Int 86(4):527–530

Wiswell TE, Smith FR, Bass JW (1985) Decreased incidence of urinary tract infections in circumcised male infants. Pediatrics 75:901

Hydrometrocolpos

96

Devendra K. Gupta and Shilpa Sharma

Contents

96.1 Introduction

Hydrometrocolpos is a condition in which the uterus and vagina are distended by retained fluid other than blood, in the presence of distal vaginal outflow obstruction. The incidence of hydrometrocolpos is 1 in 16,000 live births. The condition is now being increasingly diagnosed prenatally. The incidence is higher in communities having a high degree of consanguinity. The rarity of this anomaly quoted in the earlier literature was probably due to the difficulty in diagnosis and high mortality resulting from infections and associated anomalies, even before the diagnosis could be established.

96.2 Embryology

During the second month of fetal life, Mullerian ducts develop as tubular invaginations of the coelomic mesothelium parallel to mesonephric ducts. The caudal ends (which form the uterus and vagina) fuse in the midline and make contact with the urogenital sinus. The distal portion of the fused Mullerian ducts is temporarily completely occluded by a solid cord of cells, the Mullerian tubercle, the caudal end of which becomes the hymen. Failure of degeneration of the epithelial plate in the Mullerian tubercle results in imperforate hymen, and persistence of a portion of the solid cord of cells in the fused Mullerian ducts above the level of the hymen results in atresia of the vagina. Presumably, a transverse septum of the vagina would result from incomplete coalescence of the vacuoles that develop as the epithelial cord begins to degenerate.

P. Puri and M. Höllwarth (eds.), *Pediatric Surgery: Diagnosis and Management,*
DOI: 10.1007/978-3-540-69560-8_96 © Springer-Verlag Berlin Heidelberg 2009

96.3 Etiopathogenesis

For the development of hydrometrocolpos, there should be both, an accumulation of excessive fluid in the female genital tract due to estrogenic stimulation as well as vaginal obstruction. Thus, the condition occurs at the extremes of childhood—in infancy, when there is a high level of maternal hormones, and in early puberty, when the patient herself begins to elaborate estrogenic hormones. If there is a low level of maternal hormones in the presence of vaginal obstruction, the obstruction remains unnoticed until puberty and presents as hematocolpos at the time of menarche. The common causes of distal vaginal obstruction are imperforate hymen, transverse vaginal septum, and vaginal atresia with or without persistence of a urogenital sinus or cloaca. The distal vaginal outflow obstruction is usually because of an imperforate hymen (60–70%) that forms a thin translucent membrane bulging between the labia or atresia of the vagina. These anomalies may result either from a local error of development or as an inherited disorder, e.g. McKusick-Kaufman syndrome.

The newborn female infant under the effect of maternal hormones, in addition to having enlarged breasts, usually displays swollen vulva and a slight mucoid leukorrhea with a low pH and many Doederlein's bacilli. The vagina has thick stratified squamous epithelium consisting of an active basal layer and 20–30 layers of large vacuolated cells containing abundant glycogen. By the age of a month, the vaginal secretion becomes scanty and alkaline. The epithelium is thin, the individual cells small and devoid of glycogen, and the basal layer comparatively inactive. Rarely, hematocolpos will develop in the newborn infant with estrogen-withdrawal bleeding from the uterus. Secondary infection of the vaginal fluid, usually with colonic organisms, is not uncommon.

Types – depending upon the type of fluid

1. Secretory

This is the most common type, consisting of mucoid material secreted mainly by the cervical part of uterine glands in response to maternal estrogenic hormones, operating prenatally and to some extent,

postnatally. The fluid is viscid, pear gray in color and may accumulate up to one liter in volume. The retained fluid is usually acidic and serous or mucoid with a large number of desquamated epithelial cells and leukocytes.

2. Urinary

In urinary hydrometrocolpos, urine collects in the vagina as a backwash during micturition although there is no distal vaginal mechanical obstruction. This is usually in association with urogenital sinus or cloaca.

The terms hematometrocolpos and pyometrocolpos are used for the presence of blood and pus respectively in the uterus and vagina.

96.4 Classification

This is based on the type and level of obstruction. Hydrometrocolpos has thus been classified into five types (Fig. 96.1)

(I)   Low hymenal obstruction
(II)   Mid-plane transverse membrane or septum
(III) (a) High obstruction with distal vaginal atresia
       (b) High obstruction with distal vaginal atresia and gluteal swelling
(IV)   Vaginal atresia with persistence of the UGS
(V)   Vaginal atresia with cloacal anomaly

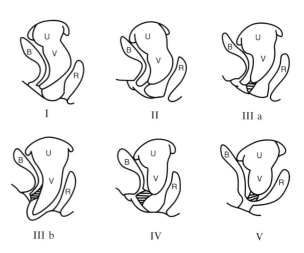

Fig. 96.1 Classification of Hydrometrocolpos

96.5 Associated Anomalies

Hydrometrocolpos may be associated with inherited disorders like McKusick-Kaufman syndrome (MKKS) and Bardet-Biedl syndrome (BBS).

McKusick-Kaufman syndrome is a rare, autosomal recessive disorder characterized by hydrometrocolpos, postaxial polydactyly, and congenital heart disease and less often, urinary and gastrointestinal anomalies. Less than 100 cases had been reported in the literature till 2005, mainly in the Amish population. Bardet-Biedl syndrome is a group of autosomal recessive disorders characterized by retinal dystrophy or retinitis pigmentosa (appearing usually between 10 and 20 years of age), postaxial polydactyly, obesity, nephropathy, and mental disturbances or occasionally, mental retardation. The phenotypic overlap of Bardet-Biedl syndrome and McKusick-Kaufman syndrome, both autosomal recessive syndromes, including hydrometrocolpos and postaxial polydactyly in the neonatal stage may cause diagnostic confusion initially.

Typically, MKKS is diagnosed in very young children whereas the diagnosis of BBS often is delayed to the teenage years. A series of nine patients diagnosed in infancy with MKKS because of the presence of vaginal atresia and postaxial polydactyly, who later developed obesity and retinal dystrophy, thus turning out to be instances of BBS has been reported. Thus, some authors recommend that all children seen in infancy with a diagnosis of MKKS be re-evaluated for other signs of BBS including mental retardation, obesity, and retinitis pigmentosa. MKKS may be considered as a variant of BBS. It has been postulated that mutations in MKKS cause Bardet-Biedl syndrome.

In the inherited type of hydrometrocolpos, obstruction is mainly due to transverse vaginal septum or vaginal atresia.

Rare variants may be seen with fused labia or ipsilateral hydrometrocolpos in patients with uterus didelphys and septate vagina. It may be associated with congenital heart disease, genitourinary and gastrointestinal anomalies.

Associated gastrointestinal anomalies include anorectal malformation, esophageal atresia, duodenal atresia, paraesophageal hiatus hernia, and congenital intestinal aganglionosis. Associated genitourinary anomalies include bicornate uterus and double vagina, duplication of the uterus and vagina, bifid clitoris, congenital urethral membrane, double ureter, ureteral stenosis, urethral atresia, absence of vulva, renal agenesis, and ambiguous genitalia. Rare associations include Mullerian dysgenesis syndrome, staphyloma of the left eye, and severe hydrops. Other additional findings include vertebral segmentation anomalies, lung hypoplasia, corpus callosum hypoplasia, and single umbilical artery. Patients with multiple congenital anomalies have a bad prognosis, thus, awareness about associated anomalies is necessary for proper diagnosis and treatment.

96.6 Antenatal Diagnosis

In recent years, prenatal diagnosis has been made possible by routine antenatal ultrasound scan. Antenatal hydrometrocolpos may be associated with oligohydramnios. It may be initially misdiagnosed as a large bladder, representing actually the dilated proximal vagina. Ultrasonographic findings include a large retrovesical septate hypoechogenic mass in the fetal abdomen. Fetal female urogenital anomalies are often difficult to evaluate by ultrasonography, especially in late gestation. However, when sonographic findings are inconclusive, magnetic resonance imaging is a useful complementary tool for assessing fetal urogenital anomalies. It has been useful to diagnose a hydrometrocolpos with septate vagina and uterus didelphys. In acutely distended patients, planned delivery by cesarian section may be considered.

96.7 Clinical Features

About 80% of the cases are less than three months of age. The typical presentation in a neonate is a lower midline mass associated with abdominal distension, calling for a surgical emergency. The female baby is usually sick due to the gross distension. The upper vagina becomes enormously distended, usually producing a palpable abdominal mass arising from the pelvis. The uterus, with its less distensible, thick muscular wall, is involved to a lesser degree but is always larger than normal. Examination of the abdomen reveals a tensely cystic, rounded mass arising from the pelvis and occasionally reaching as high as the costal margin. The tumor may seem lobulated because of the anteriorly distended bladder and the moderately enlarged uterus surmounting the vagina. The Fallopian tubes are usually normal, although occasionally, they may be distended, even allowing escape of fluid into the peritoneum rarely. Compression of adjacent structures may cause acute respiratory distress that becomes life threatening. The patient may also have respiratory infection, neonatal sepsis, and fever. Extensive squamous cell peritonitis has been described to result from vaginal atresia with hydrometrocolpos and squamous cell reflux through the genital system.

Associated features include urinary retention with obstructive uropathy causing scanty and infrequent urination. The upward pull of the enlarging vagina elongates and angulates the urethra, producing dysuria and acute urinary retention. Pressure of the vagina on the ureters at the pelvic brim results in hydronephrosis and hydroureter.

Besides abdominal distension, renal failure is also a common presentation in hydrometrocolpos. In addition, there may be presence of abdominal ascites.

Compression of the vena cava and iliac vessels will cause cyanosis, edema, and ecchymosis of the perineum, lower extremities, and abdominal wall. The rectum is less commonly involved, but constipation, ribbon stools, and actual intestinal obstruction may complicate hydrometrocolpos. Obstruction in the urinary tract alone may be seen in up to 33% cases, in the urinary tract and venous system in 10% cases, and in the urinary and intestinal tracts in 7% cases.

The perineal examination in lithotomy position under adequate illumination may help to identify a bulging hymenal membrane. Rectal examination reveals the pelvic component of the mass. The translucent bulge of an imperforate hymen will be seen to increase in size when the infant cries or when pressure is exerted on the abdominal mass. In vaginal atresia, the upward pull of the enlarging vagina rising out of the pelvis may retract the atretic lower portion of the vagina up into the pelvis and make examination difficult. If a major portion of the vagina is absent, the external genitalia may seem quite normal, and the diagnosis will be missed unless the vaginal orifice is deliberately sought.

In some cases, a transverse septum higher in the vagina will be seen to protrude through a normally perforated hymen, apparently representing a congenital diaphragm. Obstruction may be caused by atresia of the vagina usually in the lower portion but occasionally extensive, involving most or the entire vagina. In the absence of clearly demonstrable patency of the vagina, the mass should be considered to be vagina until proven otherwise.

In atresia of the vagina, the appearance of the external genitalia differs markedly from that seen with imperforate hymen. Instead of a bulging membrane protruding from the labia, with unusual prominence of the vulva and perineum, the area normally occupied by the vaginal orifice may be retracted upward into the pelvis as a result of the enlarging upper vagina escaping from the small pelvis into the more capacious abdominal cavity.

Rarely, abdominal mass may be associated with gluteal swelling or acute abdomen with paralytic ileus.

In McKusick-Kaufman syndrome, hydrometrocolpos is always associated with postaxial polydactyly and less often with congenital heart disease, urinary and gastrointestinal anomalies.

For obstruction at a higher level, identification and probing of perineal orifices, endoscopy and radiological studies are essential. When three perineal orifices are present, it is type II anomaly; with two orifices it is type III or IV; and with one orifice it is type V. Type IIIb will have cystic gluteal bulge. In type II anomaly, there is mild depression at the vaginal site with a small orifice, which can be dilated. Types III and IV can be differentiated by endoscopy and radiological studies.

96.8 Late Presentation

Rare cases presenting in the prepubertal group, from 12 to 15 years of age, may present with complications like leukorrhea through a pinpoint opening in the hymen. In asymptomatic hydrometrocolpos, the diagnosis is made only after accidental discovery of a bulging membrane. The early symptoms attributed to this condition are nonspecific indications of discomfort followed by urinary, venous, or intestinal obstruction, respiratory distress, or superimposed infection of the urinary tract or of the fluid retained in the vagina.

Adolescent patients may present with abdominal pain, voiding dysfunctions and backache. Adults may present with inability to consummate and infertility.

96.8.1 Differential Diagnosis

These include congenital, inflammatory, or neoplastic cyst. When the diagnosis is in doubt, exploratory laparotomy gives the definitive diagnosis.

96.9 Investigations

In addition to routine investigations, special preoperative investigations are necessary not only to differentiate hydrometrocolpos from other neonatal pelvic masses, e.g. presacral or ovarian teratoma and rectosigmoid duplications, but also to confirm the type of hydrometrocolpos and plan surgery.

These include:

1. Plain x-ray of the abdomen—anteroposterior view and lateral view to identify location of mass. The small intestinal loops will be displaced into the epigastrium by a rounded homogenous mass in the lower abdomen. Neonatal peritoneal calcifications along with the ascites have also been described in cases of hydrometrocolpos secondary to imperforate hymen, without the evidence of gastrointestinal tract obstruction.
2. Abdominal ultrasonography to identify dilated vagina and upper urinary tract anomalies, especially ipsilateral renal agenesis. Transperineal ultrasonography can help measure a caudally placed obstructive septum in vaginal atresia and thereby help in planning reconstructive surgery. Ultrasonography after drainage of the bladder with a catheter may help in the diagnosis of hydrometrocolpos
3. Retrograde genitourethrogram to identify the urogenital sinus and its communication with vagina (Fig. 96.2). This may be combined with a hysterovaginogram to delineate the site of vaginal obstruction. When a bulging membrane can be visualized clearly, aspiration of some of the contained fluid and injection of a water soluble radio-opaque material will outline the distended vagina and uterus.
4. Endoscopic evaluation of vaginal, urethral (Type III, IV) and rectal orifices (in Type V) in addition to

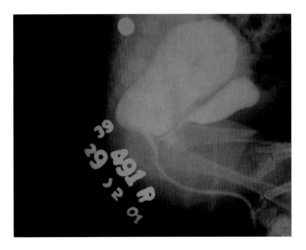

Fig. 96.2 A Retrograde genitourethrogram of a baby with hydrometrocolpos and anorectal malformation (pouch colon). The faint shadow of pouch colon can be seen that opens in the vaginal septum (bifid vagina). The outline of the Urinary bladder with urethra anteriorly and Hydrometrocolpos with bifid vagina posteriorly along with the urogenital sinus with 3 cm common channel can be appreciated

radiological procedures to give a composite and accurate picture. Endoscopic catheterization of vaginal and urethral orifices in urogenital sinus and vaginal, urethral, and rectal orifices in cloacal anomaly, in order to establish the internal anatomy by contrast studies. An invertogram may be of help to identify a rectovaginal fistula in cloacal anomaly.
5. Skeletal x-rays to assess vertebral anomalies and digital skiagrams in the presence of digital or syndromal anomalies.
6. Echocardiogram to rule out cardiac anomalies.
7. Chromosomal studies may be needed rarely in cases of ambiguous genitalia to establish the genotype.
8. Intravenous Urography or computed tomography helps to delineate the anatomical details to assess the anatomy while planning corrective surgery. The Urogram will demonstrate anterior and superior displacement of the bladder and, possibly, hydronephrosis and hydroureter.

96.10 Management

Early operation is indicated when grossly distended hydrometrocolpos is present with bulging hymen or is associated with complications. Laparotomy is indicated for high vaginal obstruction, treatment of abdominal obstruction, and abdominal complications or associated anomalies.

96.11 Preoperative Preparation

Patients presenting with complications should be given incubator care with head-end elevated, parenteral antibiotics, and intravenous fluid. In the case of respiratory distress, prompt decompression of gastrointestinal tract by nasogastric aspiration and administration of oxygen and humidity is indicated. If vomiting is present with or without constipation, in addition to nasogastric decompression, fluid and electrolytes imbalance should be assessed and corrected. When dribbling or retention of urine is present, a Foley catheter should be inserted into the bladder for better drainage of urine. When huge distended abdominal mass is present in the ill neonate, a preliminary drainage by puncturing the vagina under ultrasonographic guidance may be done 24–28 h prior to corrective surgery. Where experience is available, vaginal septum (type II anomaly) can be incised safely under ultrasonographic guidance and x-ray imaging in two planes, in a criss cross manner.

96.12 Surgical Management

A definite protocol, awareness, and appropriate investigations before surgery can avoid complications (Fig. 96.3). The management is simple with low anomalies (Type I and II). However, patients with Type III, IV, and V usually suffer from obstruction and infection. In complicated cases, the attempt should be to drain the infected material through the suprapubic vaginostomy and allow the dilated vagina to shrink, followed by a definitive procedure later (staged procedure). All previous attempts to drain and simultaneously reconstruct the vaginal tract in the newborn stage carried very high risk of mortality and are not recommended presently. In the presence of fused labia or adhesion, separation of adhesion followed by vaginal drainage is adequate. In others, it is a temporizing procedure and can be achieved by drainage into the perineum.

96.12.1 Drainage Procedure

The drainage procedure may be the definitive treatment in Type I and II, while it will be a temporizing procedure in the other types. The majority of Type I

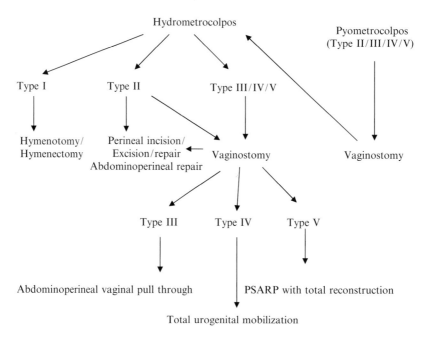

Fig. 96.3 Algorithm for treatment of Hydrometrocolpos

and II patients may be managed by vaginal drainage into the perineum. Sometimes, however, in Type II anomaly, a perineal procedure may be deferred either due to secondary infection or complex anomalies and these babies may need suprapubic drainage by catheter or a vaginostomy. The proximal diversion stoma not only helps in decompressing the vagina but also provides a portal for detailed radiographic studies to delineate the anatomy. If the atretic lower portion of the vagina has been retracted up into the pelvis, it may be desirable to open the vagina through a laparotomy incision to avoid damage to the urethra, bladder, and rectum.

96.12.2 Hymenotomy/Hymenectomy

A bulging membrane in an infant with imperforate hymen or transverse septum of the vagina may be incised without anesthesia, but if the hymen is thickened or the obstruction recurrent or the patient an adolescent, excision is probably preferable. Hymenotomy may resolve the laboratorial and clinical abnormalities of a patient with hydrometrocolpos due to imperforate hymen presenting as acute renal failure. In all cases, it is desirable to maintain patency of the opening by use of a drain and/or repeated dilatation.

In the lithotomy position, the bulging hymen becomes visible as a grayish membrane. If necessary, the abdomen may be compressed to make the hymen more prominent. A no. 8 Foley catheter is inserted into the bladder to decompress it and to identify the urethra during surgery. A stay suture is placed at the center of the hymen and, with a no. 18 needle, an amount of fluid is aspirated and sent for microscopic examination and culture. A circular hymenal segment is excised using a no. 11 blade (Fig. 96.4). The cut margin is oversewn with vertical mattress sutures and a soft silastic catheter is inserted into the vagina. A skiagram is taken while injecting contrast in order to delineate the internal anatomy. The catheter left in the vagina acts as a stent and helps drainage as well.

In the postoperative period, the vagina is irrigated three times a day for a week with normal saline and suitable parenteral antibiotics may be given for 1 week to 10 days.

96.12.3 Vaginostomy

A vaginostomy may serve as a temporizing drainage procedure for cases with infected Type II, Type III, Type IV and Type V. A tubed vaginostomy avoids the use of any indwelling catheter and at the same time provides excellent drainage and an easy access for performing dye studies to outline the pathological anatomy of the condition.

96.12.4 Abdominoperineal Repair

In Type II anomaly, the patients may have a minute opening at the site of the vaginal orifice in the septum (Fig. 96.5) and in case of a well formed septum, it may be prudent to drain the vagina by a laparotomy approach and then, under vision, the septum may be incised. If the septum is 1 cm thick, it is wiser to drain the vagina from above by laparotomy and then incise the septum under direct vision after defining the anatomy in order to prevent injury to the urethra and rectum during dissection. When a low transverse vaginal septum is present as a bulging membrane, excision and drainage may be done by the perineal route (Fig. 96.6). A Foley catheter is inserted into the bladder and the rectum is packed with Vaseline gauze. A transverse lower abdominal incision is made. The top of the dilated uterus and abdominal part of the distended vagina are visualized. In general, the mass occupies almost the whole of the abdominal cavity. The adhesions due to spillage from the Fallopian tube are gently separated and the abdomen is explored. The cystic uterovaginal mass is delivered into the wound (Fig. 96.7). In the case of hydrometrocolpos, the bladder is retracted forward until the lower cervical part of the uterus is exposed.

In Type III, following initial vaginostomy and drainage during the definitive procedure, the vagina is exteriorized onto the perineum by an abdominoperineal pullthrough.

96.12.5 Total Urogenital Mobilization

In Type IV, initial vaginostomy and drainage are done. During the definitive procedure, total urogenital mobi-

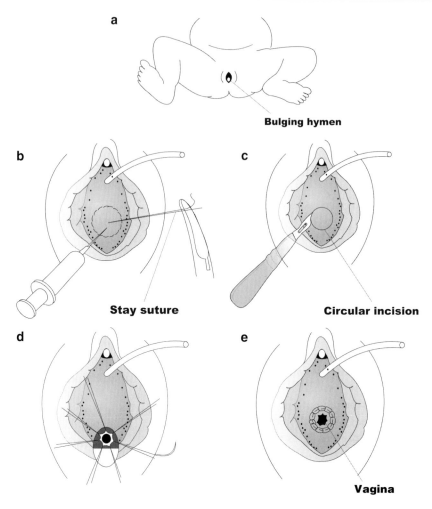

Fig. 96.4 Hymenectomy: (**a**) lithotomy position showing bulging hymen; (**b**) aspiration of vaginal fluid; (**c**) circular hymenal incision; (**d**) cut margin retracted by vertical mattress sutures; (**e**) sutures tied exposing the vaginal cavity

lization is done. The vagina is exteriorized onto the perineum and the urogenital sinus is left behind to function as the urethra. If the length of the common channel is less than 3 cm, then total urogenital mobilization would be the treatment of choice. However, if the length of the common channel is more than 3 cm, then vaginal replacement would be required. An Anterior Sagittal Transanorectal approach (ASTRA) in cases of neonatal urinary hydrometrocolpos associated with a persistent urogenital sinus has also been described, though not widely practiced.

96.12.6 Vaginal Pullthrough Along With the Posterior Sagittal Anorectoplasty

In the cloacal anomaly (Type V), the hydrometrocolpos may be secretory or urinary. In this condition, it is more acceptable to do a temporizing drainage procedure and then do the pullthrough via the posterior sagittal anorectoplasty route. This route is also preferable for all cases with associated anorectal malformation,

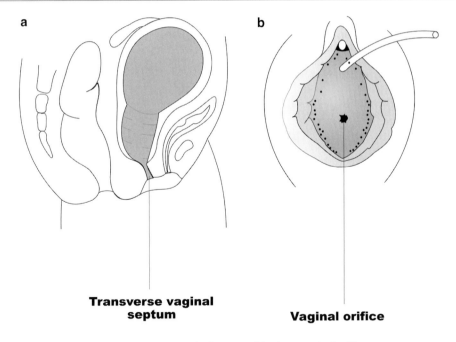

**Transverse vaginal
septum**

Vaginal orifice

Fig. 96.5 Type II Hydrometrocolpos: (**a**) Transverse vaginal septum; (**b**) minute vaginal orifice

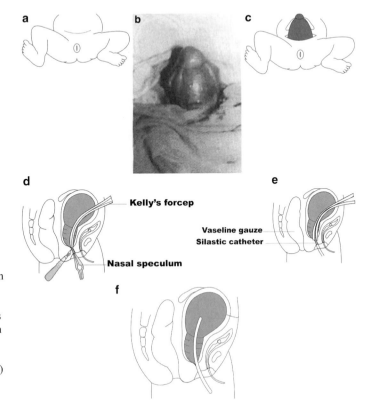

Fig. 96.6 Abdominoperineal repair of Type II
Hydrometrocolpos: (**a**) Low transverse abdominal
incision; (**b**) Hydrometrocolpos delivered from
abdominal wound; (**c**) purse-string suture on
vaginal wall; (**d**) Kelly's forcep introduced through
the hysterotomy and tip advanced to the most
depended part of the dilated vagina; (**e**) Vaginal
septum is being incised while the vaginal orifice is
spread open by the nasal speculum and the septum
is pushed downwards by Kelly's forcep—the
septum is incised and Kelly's forcep pushed down
and out, grasping the tip of the Silastic catheter; (**f**)
Vagina being drained by an indwelling perineal
catheter

Kelly's forcep

Nasal speculum

Vaseline gauze
Silastic catheter

Fig. 96.7 Operative photograph of the same patient with the Rectum (pouch colon) held with silk suture posteriorly, the vagina—reconstructed from hydrometrocolpos around the Foley catheter and the urogenital sinus with the urethral meatus high up that was used to reconstruct the urethra

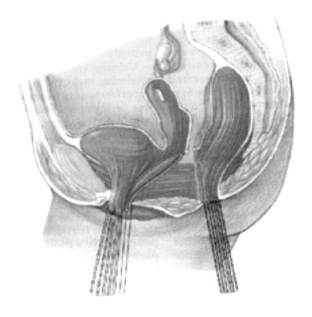

after the initial vaginostomy and colostomy (Fig. 96.7). The vagina may occasionally open to the bladder with a small orifice. Vaginal pull-through surgery and closure of the communication may be required for a vagina occasionally opening into the bladder.

96.13 Morbidity and Mortality

The causes of morbidity include recurrent infection due to inadequate drainage, discomfort due to tube vaginostomy, open vaginostomy that continuously drains secretions and urine in cases of Type IV and V. Colostomy done for Type V and for cases with associated anorectal malformation or Hirschsprung's disease has its own inherent complications and associated morbidity.

As hydrometrocolpos is associated with serious anomalies, many cases are still born.

Associated genitourinary anomalies in more than half the cases with hydrometrocolpos are responsible for high morbidity and mortality in this entity. Other causes of mortality include inadequate drainage, urinary infection, spontaneous rupture, and generalized peritonitis.

96.14 Follow-Up

On follow up (range 1–15 years; mean 7), more than 60% patients have menstrual irregularity, endometriosis, and infertility. A comprehensive management is imperative to preserve the reproductive potentials as significant proportion of patients may experience sexual difficulties following vaginal reconstruction.

Further Reading

El-Messidi A, Fleming NA (2006) Congenital imperforate hymen and its life-threatening consequences in the neonatal period. J Pediatr Adolesc Gynecol 19:99–103

Gupta DK, Sharma S (2009) Hydrometrocolpos. In DK Gupta (ed) Neonatal Surgery—Diagnosis and Management. Jaypee Brothers, Delhi (in press)

Hayashi S, Sago H, Kashima K et al (2005) Prenatal diagnosis of fetal hydrometrocolpos secondary to a cloacal anomaly by magnetic resonance imaging. Ultrasound Obst Gyn 26:577–579

Nazir Z, Rizvi RM, Qureshi RN, Khan ZS, Khan Z (2006) Congenital vaginal obstructions: Varied presentation and outcome. Pediatr Surg Int 22:749–753

Gynaecologic Conditions of Childhood

Lina Michala and Sarah M. Creighton

Contents

97.1 Introduction

Gynaecological problems are rare in childhood and adolescence but can cause significant distress to affected children and their families. These children may first visit paediatric surgeons and paediatricians who may not be familiar with gynaecological ailments. It is important that paediatric surgeons are aware of these problems to ensure correct management with appropriate referral if necessary. This chapter describes common gynaecological conditions occurring in children.

97.2 Prepubertal and Adolescent Anatomy

During childhood, the ovarian hormonal function is inactive and circulating oestrogens are low. External genitalia are infantile in appearance. Pubic hair is absent, the labia majora are flat and the vaginal mucosa is thin and fragile.

By the age of 9 years, the hypothalamic pituitary axis starts to mature. GnRH is secreted in pulsations and as a result of this, ovarian function is stimulated and oestrogen is produced. Breast budding is the first sign of puberty and is known as thelarche. The development of pubic hair is dependant on adrenal androgens and adrenarche usually follows thelarche in a few months. As the amount of oestrogen increases, the body of the uterus enlarges and the endometrium thickens, and around the age of 13, menstruation begins. In the first few cycles after menarche, ovulation does not necessarily occur and bleeding in the young adolescents can be irregular, heavy and prolonged. By the age of 16 years, breast and pubic hair have reached

P. Puri and M. Höllwarth (eds.), *Pediatric Surgery: Diagnosis and Management,*
DOI: 10.1007/978-3-540-69560-8_97, © Springer-Verlag Berlin Heidelberg 2009

adult levels of development and the menstrual cycles usually become more regular.

97.3 Gynaecological Conditions Occurring Prior to Puberty

97.3.1 *Vulvovaginitis*

Vulvovaginitis is the most common gynaecological disorder in prepubertal girls. A child is more susceptible to genital infection, as she lacks the protective features that depend on adequate oestrogenisation. The vaginal mucosa is thin, the vaginal pH is raised and the vulva lacks its protective hair and labial fat pads. To these are added the relative proximity of the anus to the vagina and the possible inadequate hygiene of the child after micturition and defecation.

In most cases, the presenting complaint is of vaginal discharge, soreness and pruritus, which may be associated with dysuria. The discharge may be yellow or green in colour and have an offensive odour. Vaginal bleeding is not a symptom of vulvovaginits, and needs careful evaluation. The symptoms of vulvovaginitis are usually present for weeks or months and can relapse and recur. Physical examination should include inspection of the vulva and the perianal area. Erythema, mild oedema and excoriations may be present along with evidence of poor perineal hygiene. If a discharge is noted, then a low vaginal swab should be taken. The diagnosis is usually made based on the history and the inspection of the perineum. A vaginal swab may be helpful but is commonly negative. An examination under anaesthetic is not usually required. However, when the symptoms are more severe and persistent, or when there is associated vaginal bleeding, then a more thorough vaginal examination is warranted, usually under general anaesthesia.

In the majority of cases, the cause is a non-specific bacterial infection. Swabs will show a mixed bacterial flora with anaerobes. Where a specific infective agent is detected, it is most commonly group A beta-haemolytic streptococcus. Candida is rarely found in the prepubertal child. Detection of sexually transmitted infections such as chlamydia and gonorrhoea should always trigger a referral to child protection services for further investigation.

Other causes of vulvovaginitis include chemical irritants such as soaps and bubble baths and this may be more common in children who already suffer from eczema or atopic dermatitis. Sand-box play can also cause vulval irritation. Some systemic infections such as varicella, rubella measles and shigella can be associated with concomitant vulvovaginitis, which usually resolves as the systemic symptoms improve.

Foreign bodies are a rare cause of vaginal discharge, but need to be considered if the discharge is bloody or foul smelling or if the child gives a history of inserting something into her vagina. In unusual cases, a persistent watery vaginal discharge may indicate the presence of an ectopic ureter. Nocturnal itching may indicate threadworm infestation, which can sometimes present as vaginal itch.

There are no specific treatments for vulvovaginitis. If a pathogen is isolated, antimicrobial therapy should be instituted. Instructions should be given on improving hygiene, avoiding irritants such as bubble bath or harsh soaps and preferring loose cotton to tight nylon underwear. Simple emollients and barrier creams are also useful. Nevertheless, the symptoms commonly relapse and resolution may not be complete until puberty approaches.

97.4 Labial Adhesions/Labial Fusion

Labial adhesions are reported to occur in 1.8% of girls. They are never present at birth and usually develop after the 1st year of life. The adhesions lead to fusion of the labia minora, obscuring the introitus and usually leaving a small opening anteriorly. The aetiology is unknown, but they are thought to result from a combination of vulvitis that leads to local inflammation and thinning of the mucosa, and lack of oestrogen stimulation.

The vast majority of cases of labial adhesions are asymptomatic. If symptoms are present, they are usually urinary, as urine can pool behind the adhesions and cause irritation, infections and post-micturition dribbling.

The diagnosis is easily made on examination of the child. Typically, there is a thin membranous line in the midline, at the junction of the labia. No other investigations are clinically required. However, in some cases, the possibility of an absent vagina and uterus has been suggested to the parents and an ultrasound will allay the fear.

If the condition is asymptomatic, no treatment is required as resolution usually occurs spontaneously at puberty. In symptomatic cases, therapy consists of local application of oestrogen cream. A pea-sized amount of oestrogen cream is applied daily over the midline of the labia for a maximum of 6 weeks. As oestrogen can be systematically absorbed through the mucosal membranes, treatment can cause transient side effects, such as breast enlargement and vaginal spotting, and parents need to be warned of this possibility.

Surgical treatment is rarely required, however, it is sometimes performed in refractory cases and where urinary symptoms are severe and persistent. Oestrogen cream should also be used postoperatively to avoid recurrence. Unfortunately, recurrence is common after both, hormonal and surgical treatment and parents need to be aware of this. It is important to reassure them that the condition is benign and self-limited and that it will have no implications for the future reproductive life of their daughter.

97.5 Congenital Uterovaginal Anomalies

Uterovaginal abnormalities result from the abnormal development of the Mullerian system. Simple anomalies are usually asymptomatic and are incidental findings during routine gynaecological or obstetric procedures in adult life. The more complex ones, however, can present in childhood or adolescence. Mullerian anomalies can be separated into two groups: those causing obstruction to menstrual flow and those conditions in which the uterus and vagina are absent. The latter group usually presents to the gynaecologist with primary amenorrhoea. However, conditions causing vaginal obstruction can frequently present to the paediatric surgeon for investigation of pain or a pelvic mass.

In addition, congenital gynaecological anomalies can occur in children with complex anomalies of other organs within the lower genital tract.

97.6 Imperforate Hymen

97.6.1 Neonatal Presentation

The hymen is a thin septum lying between the sinovaginal bulbs and urogenital sinus. Failure of this septum to perforate during foetal life can cause the vagina to fill with retained vaginal secretions and lead to a hydrocolpos. This can occasionally present during pregnancy when a pelvic collection is seen on antenatal ultrasound scan. Presentation can also be at birth with the findings of pelvic or abdominal mass or a bulging hymen seen on perineal inspection.

Treatment is by a simple incision and drainage, usually carried out by a paediatric surgeon or urologist, and is curative. There are no follow-up data available on whether this group of girls are more likely to present with vaginal stenosis during adolescence, but this would seem unlikely and routine follow-up into adolescence is not currently recommended.

97.6.2 Adolescent Presentation

This condition presents more commonly during adolescence with a haematocolpos. The typical presentation is with pelvic pain but no periods in an adolescent girl. The menstrual flow collects behind the hymen in the vagina and causes pain, which is initially cyclical but can become constant with time. Otherwise, pubertal development is normal. The resulting haematocolpos is often palpable as a pelvic mass. On inspection of the vaginal introitus, it is usually possible to see the imperforate hymen as a bulging blue membrane. Treatment is simple, with a cruciate incision on the hymen to allow drainage of the haematocolpos and excision of the redundant skin.

97.7 Other Obstructive Anomalies

97.7.1 Transverse Vaginal Septum

This is a rarer condition that presents with symptoms very similar to an imperforate hymen such as cyclical pain, amenorrhoea and a haematocolpos. In this case, however, the septum occurs due to failure of the Mullerian ducts and urogenital sinus to canalise in utero. The septum is most commonly located at the level of the middle third of the vagina and a significant length of the vagina may be involved in the septum. A pelvic mass is often palpable, but on inspection of the vagina, however, the introitus looks normal. An MRI scan is usually required to localise the septum and measure its thickness. If the septum is low and thin, the excision can be made vaginally. In cases where the septum is located higher in the vagina, more complex reconstructive surgery using a combined abdominal and perineal approach is usually required. Reanastomosis may be difficult in cases of large septa, where the vaginal defect left after the excision may need to be bridged by using a skin graft or bowel segment.

97.7.2 Obstructed Uterine Horn

The incidence of uterine anomalies has been estimated to be between 0.5–2%. Uterine anomalies may be asymptomatic but have been associated with infertility and pregnancy related complications. In adolescence, an obstructed uterine horn may present with severe pelvic pain and a pelvic mass. In this situation, there are two uteri. One is connected via a cervix to the vagina and the second horn is not connected to the vagina (Fig. 97.1). Both function normally and menstruate, but menstrual blood accumulates in the non-communicating horn leading to the formation of a palpable pelvic mass and causing pain that becomes increasingly severe. The diagnosis is commonly delayed as there is normal menstrual flow from the unobstructed side. Treatment is by removal of the obstructed uterine horn and this can be done laparoscopically.

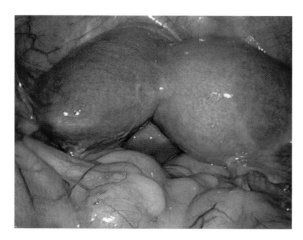

Fig. 97.1 Laparoscopic picture of double uterus. The left horn is non-communicating

97.8 Mullerian Agenesis (Mayer-Rokitansky-Kuster-Hauser Syndrome)

The syndrome is characterized by the congenital absence of the uterus and part of the vagina. It is estimated to affect one in 5,000 to 20,000 female births. The most common presentation is with primary amenorrhoea in a girl with otherwise normal secondary sexual characteristics. Further investigations reveal a normal karyotype, and imaging either in the form of ultrasound or MRI scans identify normal ovaries, but an absent or rudimentary uterus. It is also important to image the upper urinary tract as in 30–40% of affected individuals, there are associated renal anomalies. Treatment focuses mainly on psychological support and the creation of a vagina to enable penetrative intercourse. The method of choice for this is using dilators to stretch the existing vaginal area. When dilation therapy is not successful, surgical treatment can be offered.

97.9 Gynaecological Anomalies Associated with Complex Congenital Conditions

Gynaecological anomalies can occur in children with conditions affecting development of the lower genital tract. Many of these conditions are now successfully treated because of the advances in paediatric surgical and medical care. As these children reach adolescence, it is important that gynaecological difficulties are anticipated. For example, it is recognised that girls with anorectal and cloacal anomalies have a high incidence of mullerian anomalies; however, prediction of uterine potential is extremely difficult, especially in the neonate. This can lead to removal of a potentially useful uterus or conversely, presentation in adolescence with a haematometra in a girl in whom the uterus was deemed vestigial. In other conditions, surgery on the urinary tract or bowel may compromise the vagina leading to scarring and stenosis. Involvement of a gynaecologist in the care of these girls as they approach puberty should allow anticipation of problems and better planning of treatment if needed.

97.9.1 Congenital Adrenal Hyperplasia (CAH)

CAH is the commonest cause of ambiguous genitalia. Immediate management is medical with the introduction of steroid replacement therapy, which the child will need lifelong. Current surgical management is a feminising genitoplasty within the first year of life to reduce the size of the clitoris and open the lower vagina. Repeat surgery in adolescence is common and poor cosmetic, anatomical and sexual outcomes have been reported. The requirement for and timing of genital surgery is currently under debate. While the early surgical management is the remit of paediatric surgeons, it is important to have gynaecological involvement at puberty to ensure optimum outcome for sexual activity and fertility. This is best done within a multi-disciplinary team.

97.10 Ovarian Cysts

Ovarian cysts may present during childhood acutely with pain or more chronically with a pelvic mass. Most cysts are functional cysts, and develop as a result of gonadotropin stimulation of the ovary. They are therefore most commonly seen in the neonatal period and again in the prepubertal and pubertal years.

Cysts of smaller size are usually asymptomatic and require no treatment as they resolve spontaneously. In some cases, cysts can attain considerable size and become palpable abdominally or lead to an increase in the abdominal girth. They may also lead to severe pain if they become haemorrhagic, if they rupture or if ovarian torsion occurs. Surgical treatment becomes necessary in the latter cases and is usually amenable to a laparoscopic approach. Preferably, an ovarian cystectomy rather than an oophorectomy should be performed in order to preserve healthy ovarian tissue. It is thought that the ovary of a prepubertal and adolescent girl may be more at risk of torsion because of its higher anatomical location and the longer ovarian ligament. Contralateral ovariopexy is not part of routine gynaecological management unlike orchidopexy, however, it should be considered.

In addition to functional cysts, pathological cysts can also occur. The commonest of these is a benign cystic teratoma (dermoid cyst). Treatment is with surgical excision, which is usually laparoscopic, and reconstruction of the remaining ovarian tissue. Malignant cysts are unusual in children and adolescents but can occur. Malignant germ cell tumours (immature teratomas), endodermal sinus tumour and mixed germ cell tumours account for the majority. The diagnosis is usually suspected on ultrasound scan. Referral to a specialised oncology team is essential. With the use of combined surgery and chemotherapy, high cure rates have been reported and in most cases, fertility preservation is possible.

97.11 Pelvic Inflammatory Disease

In the UK, it is estimated that one in 4 teenage girls under the age of 16 is sexually active. Despite increasing efforts to improve sex education among youngsters, the proportion that does not use any form of contraception remains high, particularly among 13–15 year olds. Indeed, sexually active teenagers are more likely to acquire sexually transmitted diseases than adults. The most commonly implicated organism is *Chlamydia trachomatis*. Although many of those infections remain subclinical, a proportion of affected girls will present with symptoms of pelvic inflammatory disease (PID). Initial presentation is usually with abdominal pain, offensive vaginal discharge and fever. In some cases, *Chlamydia* can cause a peri-hepatitis (Fitz-Hughes-Curtis syndrome). Symptoms of right hypochondrial pain can be severe and can lead to a surgery in the first instance. Early and effective antibiotic therapy is necessary in order to reduce the risk of long-term gynaecological and reproductive complications. Chlamydia infections can lead to chronic PID causing persistent pelvic pain and tubal infertility (Fig. 97.2). If the girl is very young, a child protection referral must be considered.

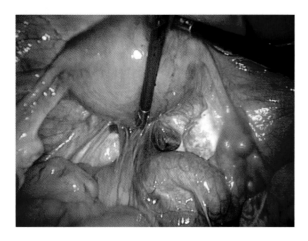

Fig. 97.2 Severe pelvic inflammatory disease following Chlamydia infection in a 14 year old girl admitted with pelvic pain. The right fallopian tube is swollen and infected. This child presented with a fever and right iliac fossa pain

97.12 Pregnancy Related Complications

Pregnancy related complications should also be kept in mind when assessing an adolescent girl presenting with abdominal pain. It is important to remember that in England, over 7,000 13- to 15-year olds become pregnant every year. Both, ectopic tubal pregnancy and miscarriage can occur. A high index of suspicion is necessary to make the diagnosis of an ectopic pregnancy as the clinical presentation can vary and unusual vaginal bleeding is not always present. The condition can rapidly deteriorate leading to internal haemorrhage, hypovolaemic shock and eventually, death. Extreme vigilance is required to make an accurate diagnosis. Urinary pregnancy tests are very accurate and are available in all Accident and Emergency departments. Treatment of an ectopic pregnancy is almost always possible by laparoscopy and removal of the pregnancy by salpingostomy or salpingectomy.

97.13 Conclusion

Gynaecological problems can occur at any age including infancy and adolescence. Conditions such as vulvovaginitis, labial adhesions and congenital anomalies may be typical of young age group. As adolescence approaches, girls may present with problems similar to those seen in adult life, such as ovarian cysts, pelvic infection and pregnancy related complications.

In most cases, the conditions are benign and self-limited. However, some may have important repercussions on the future sexual and reproductive life of the child. These conditions need to be treated with careful and accurate medical management as well as sensitive and gentle discussion with the child and her family.

Further Reading

Aittomaki K, Hille E, Kajanoja P (2001) A population-based study of the incidence of mullerian aplasia in Finland. Fertil Steril 73(3):624–625

Alizai NK, Thomas DFM, Lilford RJ, Batchelor GG, Johnson F (1999) Feminizing genitoplasty for adrenal hyperplasia: What happens at puberty. J Urol 161:1588–1591

Muram D (1999) Treatment of prepubertal girls with labial adhesions. J Pediatr Adolesc Gynecol 12:67–70

Puri P, Höllwarth ME (eds) (2006) Pediatric Surgery. Springer, Berlin, Heidelberg

Stricker T, Navratil F, Sennhauser FH (2003) Vulvovaginitis in prepubertal girls. Arch Dis Child 88:324–326

Warne SA, Wilcox DT, Creihton S. Ransley PG (2003) Long-term gynaecological outcomes of patients with persistent cloaca. J Urol 170:1493–1496

Wellings K, Nanchahal K, Macdowall W et al (2001) Sexual behaviour in Britain: Early heterosexual experience. Lancet 358:1843–1850

Index